ALLE · ZEIT · WACH · 1842

LÁSZLÓ BURIS

FORENSIC MEDICINE

DIAGNOSIS AND SIGNS OF DEATH / SPECIAL AUTOPSY TECHNIQUES / INJURIES AND ACCIDENTS / WOUNDS AND WOUND HEALING / SUDDEN, UNEXPECTED DEATH / SUFFOCATION, INFANTICIDE, SEXUAL OFFENCES, CRIMINAL ABORTION / PATERNITY / TOXICOLOGY / IDENTIFICATION OF VICTIMS.

Springer-Verlag
Budapest Berlin Heidelberg New York London
Paris Tokyo Hong Kong Barcelona 1993

Author:

László Buris M. D., D. Sc.
Medical University Debrecen
Institute for Forensic Medicine
Debrecen, Nagyerdei krt. 98.
Hungary

The publication of the book was sponsored by Hewlett-Packard Co.

ISBN 978-3-642-48886-3 ISBN 978-3-642-48884-9 (eBook)
DOI 10.1007/978-3-642-48884-9

Softcover reprint of the hardcover 1st edition 1993

BURIS, László: Forensic Medicine/László Buris. Budapest; Berlin; Heidelberg; New York; London; Paris; Tokyo; Hong Kong; Barcelona: Springer-Verlag, 1993.

ISBN 978-3-642-48886-3

Felelős kiadó:

Springer Hungarica
Prof. Dr. István Árky
Medical University Debrecen
Prof. Dr. László Buris

Printed on acid-free paper

CONTENTS

Foreword

Chapter 1.

SIGNS OF DEATH 11
Early signs of death 14
Cooling 16
Rigor mortis 17
Desiccation 18
LATE CHANGES OF DEATH 20
Putrefaction 20
Formation of grave wax 25
Mummification 27
Damage to the dead body caused by animals 27
MEDICOLEGAL AUTOPSY 31
SPECIAL AUTOPSY TECHNIQUES 38
THE SCENE OF THE CRIME 43
References 46

Chapter 2.

TYPES OF INJURIES 49
Incising injuries 50
Stab wounds 53
Hacking injuries 61
Alterations caused by blunt instruments ... 64
Traffic accidents 95
Electrical injuries 106
Gunshot wounds 120
Injuries caused by high and low temperature 140
References 149
VITAL INJURIES 155
References 159

Chapter 3.

THE EXTENT OF WOUND HEALING 161
The medicolegal certificate 161
The medical certification 166

Chapter 4.

EXAMINATION OF BIOLOGICAL TRACES 169
Procedures for testing blood stains 169
Examination of hair 177
Examination of seminal stains 180
Examination of bite marks 184
References 188

Chapter 5.

SUDDEN DEATH 191
Alterations in the circulatory system causing sudden death 192
Alterations of the respiratory system causing sudden death 206
Diseases of the abdominal organs causing sudden death 209
Diseases of the central nervous system causing sudden death 210
Sudden infant death syndrome (SIDS) 213
Sudden death in youth 214
References 216

Chapter 6.

DEATH BY SUFFOCATION 219
Hanging 223
Strangulation by ligature 227
Manual strangulation 227
Drowning 231
Thoracic restriction 234
External occlusion of air 234
References 235

Chapter 7.

INFANTICIDE 237
References 252

Chapter 8.
SEXUAL LIFE IN RELATION TO THE LAW 253
Rape 253
Sexual deviation 261
ABORTION 269
References 275

Chapter 9.
EXAMINATIONS FOR DETERMINING PATERNITY 277
Proof of paternity 286
References 291

Chapter 10.
DISABILITY 293
Common conditions resulting in disabilityoccurring in the practice of forensic medicine 300
Permanent injuries resulting from accidents 301
The role of the forensic medical specialist in compensation process 307
References 311

Chapter 11.
TOXICOLOGY 313
Metabolism of toxic substances 315
Metal poisoning 318
Carbon monoxide 325
Cyanide poisoning 327
Poisoning by corrosives 328
Pesticides 332
Insecticides 333
Herbicides 336
Rodenticides 338
Narcotic poisoning 338
Tranquilizers 343
Alcohol intoxication 345
Mushroom poisoning 353
Expectations and capabilities of toxicological tests 357
References 369

Chapter 12.
IDENTIFICATION 373
References 386

Chapter 13.
LEGAL ASPECTS OF MEDICAL PRACTICE 389
The right of the physician 390
The responsibilities of the practicing physician 391
Responsibilities of the physician 395
References 401

Preface

In recent years numerous excellent books have appeared on the subject of legal medicine in the field of forensic pathology. All of these deal in detail with the different subjects belonging to forensic medicine and the questions that arise in forensic medical practice with respect to the characteristics of the country from which they originate. The development of legal medicine in Europe goes back centuries and the countries of Central Europe have played a significant role. For this reason we considered, along with the publisher, to produce a book specifically published in Hungary in English translation to provide the reader with an appropriate image of Hungarian forensic medical practice.

The author has spent decades in the practice and teaching of pathology along with forensic medicine. This is particularly apparent in some chapters, especially that dealing with sudden death, or those sections on histopathological recognition. The short case stories illustrating the practical work lend insight into the results and provide useful information which may be of assistance not only to the practicing forensic medical specialist, but also to medical students, lawyers and policemen.

The choice of the individual chapters was made to reflect the practical, everyday necessities and those alterations which are encountered most frequently in practice. The more detailed content of the toxicological section with attention to the metabolization of damaging substances cannot be neglected in the forensic medical practice. Likewise the significance and methods of trace element examination in the daily practice of forensic medicine is indispensable.

Two chapters are included in the book which reflect the characteristics of Hungarian circumstances, one of which being the evaluation of disability and the other being the health regulations. These include health regulations which apply not only to Hungary but represent the regulations recognized by the European Economic Community as a whole.

The illustration of the book consists primarily of color prints which in a book dealing with morphology are, in the opinion of the author, essential since they convey far more information than black and white photos do.

Naturally, the translation cannot be perfect, although the translator not only possesses an excellent command of the Hungarian language, but experience in the specialty which made possible the accurate rendering of the text. For this I owe a special debt of thanks to

Dr. Lloyd Sparks and to Prof. A. Carmi, Prof. Y. Hiss and Dr. Stephen Görömbey for their excellent checking of the manuscript.

I thank them for their work and trust that with their help an easily understandable and useful text has been provided to the reader. May this book be a helpful companion in the everyday practice.

Debrecen, 1993.

Preface to the Hungarian edition

The most useful Hungarian practical forensic medicine handbook was published almost 80 years ago by Balazs Kenyeres under the title, "Legal Medicine". Some chapters of the three-volume work are useful even today in the practice of forensic medicine, as a classical example of a good readable textbook.

In 1964 Somogyi Endre compiled and published the book "Forensic Medicine", in which selected shapters were written by the current leaders in their fields. It has found use more as a handbook than as a text.

The textbook entitled "Fundamentals of Forensic Medicine" has survived several printings. It has served in the education of medical students, as the author recommends in the foreword to the first edition, but it is also used in preparation fot the board examination in absence of a detailed text in Hungarian. A handbook which could serve for the preparation of the forensic specialist has not apeeared in the last 20 years. This has been prepared as a detailed, up-to-date contribution to the literature.

This book exceeds the dimensions of a university text. It was not my intention to write a book destined only for the use of university students. I hoped to create a work that would be appropriate both for board examination preparation as well as for use by medical students in their study of forensic medicine. The bibliographies included in several chapters will be of help for further study in the course of preparation for the board exam. In several chapters more detailed discussions have been included to emphasize the more important practical elements of the profession, in that injuries, toxicological tests and the recognition of disability to work are areas which cannot be neglected.

The illustrations, which adds a very important dimension to any forensic medical text, has been collected over my 34 years of practice and I have endeavored to select such photographs that provide the greatest amount of information. In the few cases where I used photographs obtained from other institutions, their places of origin are annotated.

The opportunities I have come across while writing the book have been rather unique in that over the last three years I had the privilege of spending 14 months as visiting professor in Gainesville at the Florida State University Center for Drug Design and Delivery.

The powerful periodical and information processing system at the university library assured the conditions under which the survey of not only the forensic, but also the most current scientific research results could be included in the composition of several chapters. It allowed for the opportunity in several instances to include explanations from the pathological, pathophysiological and biochemical points of view. I am grateful to my friends Professor Nicholas Bodor, director of the Center for Drug Design and Delivery, who allowed me every opportunity to use the result of his latest reserarch in the elucidation of drug metabolism in my work. The help of the employees of the university library eased my labors enormously.

For the proof-reading of several chapters, and the clarifying of the occasional controversial parts I called upon the talents of such outstanding experts whose familiarity with certain areas and whose friendly advice hopefully made it possible to avoid many errors.

I thank L. Kalabay for the proof-reading and criticism of the chapter on reduced capacity for work, A. Zsindely for checking the chapter on toxicology, Gy. Bujdosó for the writing of the paternity tests section, and L. Szabó for his valuable advice.

I am greatly indebted to my coworkers who were of assistance in the writing of this book, especially N. Kapusz, assistant lecturer, for the preparation of the diagrams, and to Margit Szabó for her hard and tedious work with the preparation of the text.

I thank Professors Endre Somogyi and Péter Sótonyi for their attention and helpful advice, and the employees of the Alföldi Publishing Company for their excellent quality work.

Debrecen, 1993.

Dr. Buris László

Chapter 1
Signs of death

The determination of the time of death is an important question in forensic medicine. However while many methods have been developed establish the exact time of death, we can hardly speak of definitive results. In most cases of death, it is not relevant. However during many criminal and civil proceedings such questions may be presented which make the establishment of the time of death important. One of the most exact definitions given about the onset of death, is linked to the name of GENERSICH: "Death is the final and complete paralysis of the central nervous system, the consequence of which is the decline to the minimum of the physiological activities of the circulatory and respiratory functions, which, in a short time cease completely."

Three factors determine the function of a living organism: circulation, respiration and integrity of the central nervous system. Any damage to one of the three results in functional disturbance to the other two. In clinical practice, the cessation of breathing or circulation determines the onset of death. In a significant number of cases, heart function can be observed for a short time after respiration ceases. There fore cessation of breathing and heart function *mean clinical death.* In this state, a number of organs and tissues survive. This state is called intermediate life. The time of survival of the tissues is relevant from the standpoint of transplantation. Those tissues with a low oxygen demand can be used for transplantation hours after death, whereas the organs with a greater metabolism or oxygen demand suffer irreversible damage after a short period of time and *biological death* sets in. The widespread use of transplantation has made a demand for the precise diagnosis of the onset of death.

One is declared dead when:

a) circulatory and heart functions irreversibly cease

b) there is complete and irreversible cessation of cerebral function.

Signs indicating irreversible cessation of brain function:

a) unconsciousness, (coma)

b) absence of spontaneous breathing,

c) moderately or more frequently maximally dilated pupils, pupils which do not react to light,

d) absence of the oculocephalic reflex,

e) absence of corneal reflex,

f) absence of reaction to painful stimulus in the area of innervation by the trigeminal nerve,

g) absence of laryngeal and bronchial reflexes.

The ability to elicit the autonomic spinal reflexes does not exclude *the determination of brain death.* Extensive examinations have been developed for the determination of brain death, since medical technology makes possible the maintenance of respiratory and circulatory function – in the presence of irreversible brain damage. These tests are, at present, only of theoretical significance. PÁSZTOR described the existence of brain death in detail. *Brain death can be declared* with certainty if,

1. the capacity for reception of stimulation and reaction to stimulation are completely absent,
2. spontaneous breathing is completely absent,
3. reflexes are absent.

This is reflected by the flat EEG. In brain death circulation in the brain stops, and thus numerous supplementary tests are necessary.

The literature lists the *criteria for establishing brain death,* which are:

1. EEG silence; isoelectric curve, with examination of the brain with deep electrode, absence of spontaneous discharge,
2. caloric vestibular test; no eye movement,
3. electronystagmography; flat curve,
4. echo-encephalography; no echo pulsation,
5. the temperature of the brain lower than that of the body,
6. intracranial pressure measurement, very high pressure,
7. carotid and vertebral angiography, no contrast filling of the brain vessels, blood flow measurements; no circulation.
8. determination of brain oxygen consumption.
9. radioisotope scintigraphy, or gamma chamber examination; verifies cessation of cerebrospinal fluid circulation.

The MOLNÁR test for extremely high pyruvate and lactate concentrations in the cerebrospinal fluid may be of value as a sign of brain death. In certain instances the determination of brain death is not a simple task. Of the above mentioned diagnostic procedures each one has its own disadvantage which, when applied to different forms of death, does not provide sufficient information as to the time of death. For example, the flat, isoelectric EEG curve does not necessarily means brain death, and must be considered with caution in the cases of death due to drug overdose or hypothermia, as well as in cases of death due to metabolic and endocrine disturbances or following neuromuscular blockade.

The cessation of circulation, breathing or brain activity brings about individual *clinical or somatic death.* Despite the above assertion that the diagnosis of death is not a simple task, it may be simple if the last minutes of a person's life are spent under the supervision of a physician. The atony of the musculature, the cessation of thoracic expansion and pulse all indicate the onset of death. These changes indicate that circulation and breathing have stopped and within a few minutes irreversible brain damage will occur. Practically speaking, however, these signs merit careful consideration. The detection of cessation of heartbeat by auscultation is made significantly more difficult if the patient is obese, or the presence of severe emphysematic changes make the sounds of a weakened heart undetectable. As mentioned above, the diagnosis of the time of death is more difficult in certain manners of death, such as in the cases of electric shock, drowning, hypothermic death, and sleeping pill overdose. In these cases intense efforts must be directed toward resuscitation.

Somatic death is followed by, *molecular biological death.* Biological death of the central nervous system occurs within

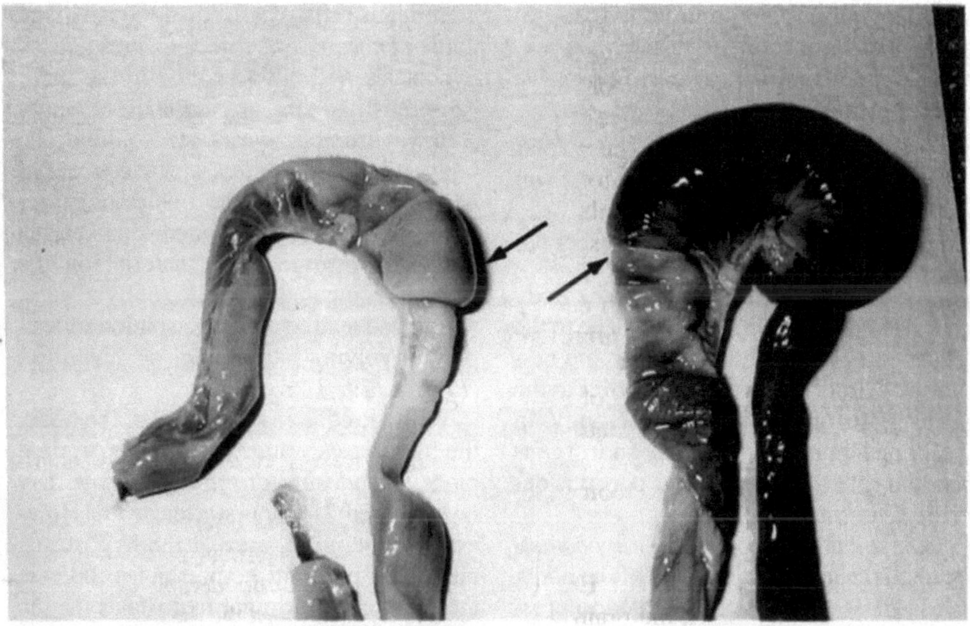

Fig. 1. Agonal and vital invagination from an infant.
With invagination occurring during life there is hemorrhagic necrosis; with postmortal invagination there are no vital signs.

five minutes after the cessation of blood flow to the brain, while the muscle tissue survives for a significantly longer time. This property is used in the postmortal electric excitability test. Likewise several tissue reactions are preserved after death, such as the pupil's ability to dilate in response to atropine for four hours after the onset of death.

The *agonal-life* and it's phenomena can only be explained by the survival of the organs. In the agonal phase, the heart may continue to function after respiration has ceased to function. This may be especially significant in premature or asphyxic newborns, where the continued heart function following cessation of respiration, helps to explain the different pathological findings. The heart may continue to function for minutes in the case of hanging as well.

The retained functional ability of both the smooth and the striated musculature is similar to that of the heart. Thus muscles of the intestines urinary bladder, seminal vesicles and pregnant uterus contract, which may result in defecation, urination, ejaculation or the delivery of a fetus, (so called coffin birth). Another sign of the agonal-life can be appreciated in the circular contractions and intussusception of the stomach, the "hour-glass stomach" formation or the postmortal invagination of the small bowel, especially noticeable in the body of infants. The absence of vital reactions unambiguously verifies that the phenomena are in fact those of the agonal-life *(Fig. 1)*. Similarly, agonal phenomena of the smooth muscle cause goose pimples on the dead body due to rigor mortis of the musculus arrectores pylorum.

Among the manifestations of agonal

life involving skeletal muscle is the idiomuscular contraction in response to external stimulus, which can occur up to five hours postmortally.

Early signs of death

The first noticeable alteration in the body after death is the *change in color* due to the cessation of the circulation. With the cessation of circulation the blood settles to the lowest parts of the organs of the body. In the higher portions, the skin and organs become pale, while the lower portions develop hypostasis.

The so-called *post-mortal hypostasis* forms at the lowest lying parts of the body, and in those tissues not subjected to pressure. In this case, sometimes they may reflect an imprint of an object pressing on the body or the surface on which the body was lying. The hypostases are particularly large, confluent indistinct dark red areas which blanch under pressure which forces the blood out of the vessels. The blood, however, returns to fill them after the pressure is released and the hypostases can again be seen. Cutting into the areas of hypostasis, blood flows from the vessels and can be removed from the neighboring tissue by use of a water jet. Hypostases appear within a short time after the cessation of circulation in the internal organs, especially in the low lying areas of the lungs (in the case of poor circulatory flow we can see similar bluish purple areas on the back of neck in a supine patient), and within 20–30 minutes after death on the skin, soonest on the back of the head and neck. In the beginning the hypostases form small, scattered areas which within 3/4 of an hour to 4 hours later will begin to be confluent. Intensive wide-spread hypostases form between 3 and 12 hours after death. (Hypostases do not form in the parts of the body subject to pressure so hypostasis will not be found in the mark caused by hanging, nor at the place where some instrument was used to hold the body up. In numerous instances errors have been made by the misleading presence of a tightly buttoned shirt or the pressure of some other material on the neck resulting in the absence of hypostasis which had lead to a false suspicion of foul play involving strangling or hanging.) *(Fig. 2, Fig. 3)*

With the change in position of the body, the hypostases wander from their original place. *Wandering of the hypostases* may be observed 2–6 hours after death. However, in the initial area of the hypostasis, numerous pinpoint hemorrhages indicate the area of the original hypostasis. In the bodies of the elderly the confluent hypostases covering large areas may resemble *per rhexim* hemorrhages, and in many cases, has mislead an examiner to conclude that foul play has taken place.

- At the coroner's inquest into the hanging of an elderly man foul play was suspected because hypostasis was found on the back of the body and the doctor conducting the inquest believed it improbable in that the hypostasis hadn't appeared in the lower extremities instead. A bleeding wound was also found on the head of the deceased, which raised the question of foul play. The later inquest and the subsequent autopsy verified the wandering of the hypostasis. Great many pinpoint hemorrhages were found on the lower extremities in the areas of the original hypostasis, showing that the hypostasis had wandered. The head wound was postmortal in origin having been caused by the falling of the body after the instrument of suspension had been cut.

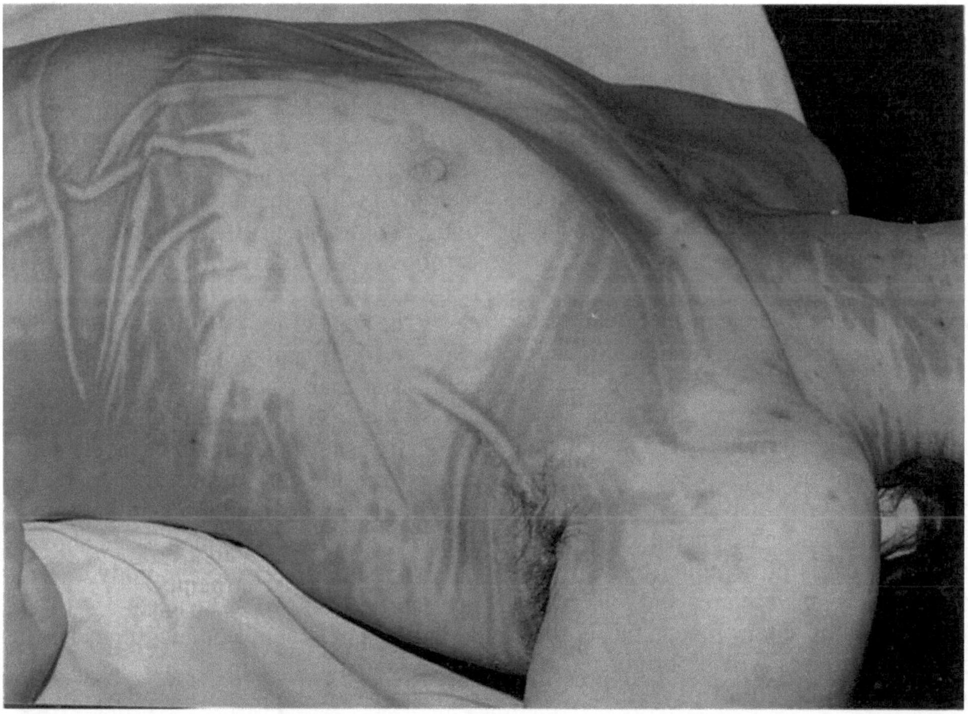

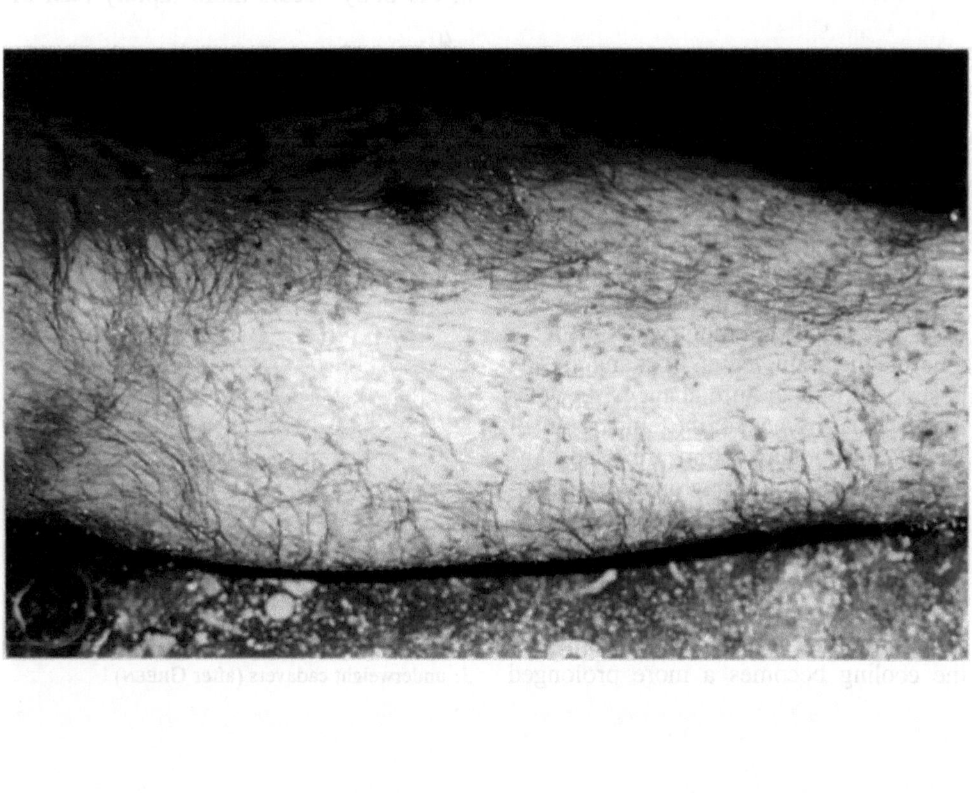

The blood in the vessels undergoes *hemolysis,* stains the internal membranes of the vessels, also penetrating the neighboring connective tissue. This process forms the *imbibition* which will not blanch under as hypostases does. The imbibition may occur or appear at earliest, eight hours after the onset of death and by 24 hours later extensive alterations can be found.

In many cases the hypostases may provide some clue to the cause of death. The *color of the hypostasis* is characteristic for certain types of poisoning. In carbon monoxide or cyanide poisoning the hypostasis is bright red ("cherry red"), or in methemoglobin-forming poisons the hyhypostasis is brownish-red, in suffocation the hypostasis is an extensive, dark bluish red, or in cases of bleeding to death the hypostasis is small in area and pink in color. In a damp environment the borders of the hypostases will be bright red due to postmortal uptake of oxygen.

Cooling

The cooling of the body was one of the earliest described signs of death. The decrease in body temperature is one of the signs of death which also provides the possibility to establish the time of death. Various methods for measuring temperature were tried: attempts were made to measure the brain, rectal, liver and muscle postmortal temperature changes. In practice the measurement of the temperature of the brain and the rectum are used. The *cooling* of the body may occur by *radiation* and *conduction* and there fore external temperature and the immediate surrounding of the body are very significant factors. The temperature of the dead body drops rapidly in the first hours, after which the cooling becomes a more prolonged process. According to experimental data the postmortal cooling of the body follows an exponential curve. *Over the first 3–4 hours* the decrease in temperature is *regular* at 1 °C per hour measured rectally. (In practice the rectal temperature is used, measured with a thermometer inserted into the rectum, about 10–15 cm deep). This is followed by an irregular cooling of the body and many factors influence the process. The state of the nutrition of the body plays a significant role. Thinner bodies cool faster than obese bodies. The thickness of the layers of clothing and its ability to retain heat also cannot be neglected. Due to the greater surface area to body weight ratio, the bodies of infants and children cool faster. As mentioned above, the external temperature and body covering exert a decisive influence.

The loss of heat by conduction makes it understandable that in a cold, wet environment for example in water, the cooling of the body occurs more rapidly than in

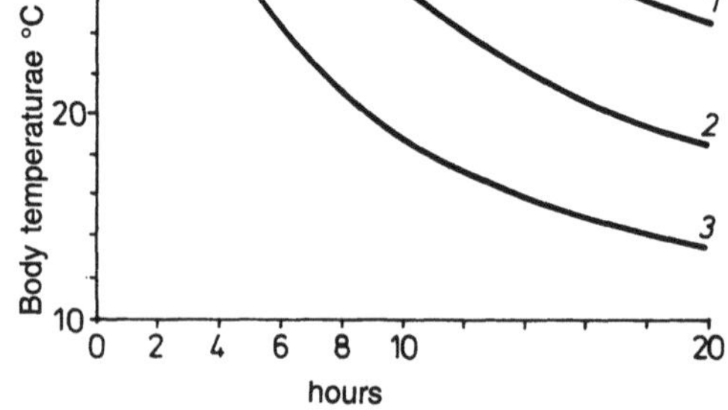

Fig. 4. Rectal temperature from a 10 °C environmental temperature.

1: overweight

2: normal

3: underweight cadavers (after GREEN)

warm, dry environments. There fore the measurement of the rectal temperature is of value in determining the time of death only in the first hours. Things are made more difficult, in thất the starting temperature is unknown.

In some cases we do encounter a decline in temperature, but rather a rise in *rectal temperature,* after death. In certain circumstances of suffocation the rectal temperature has been observed to go up *(Fig. 4).* Also, in tetanus, strychnine poisoning or septic processes we may observe a rise in postmortal. The postmortal temperature of the brain is one of the most well described methods in the literature in that, according to the authors, the tissue of the brain is not subjected to outside temperature changes and the placement of a thermometer in the cranial cavity ensures constant conditions. If the brain temperature is 25 °C, there is a great probability that death occurred approximately 2.5 hours before the measurement was taken. A temperature below 25 °C means that death occurred at least five hours previously.

Rigor mortis

Following death the musculature first goes limp and loses its tone. As a result, the temporomandibular joint relaxes and the wrinkles in the face smooth out due to atonic state of the facial muscles thus the body gives the impression of a younger person. Rigor mortis follows this muscular atonic state affecting both striated and smooth muscle. The biochemical explanation of rigor mortis even to this day is still incomplete. According to some theories, following death there is a rise in *lactic acid* in the muscle tissue which causes a cramp-like contracture. Another view holds that the amount of ATP, which in relaxed muscle is high, decreases following death. The drop in ATP level results in contracture of the muscles. The role of ATP in muscular contraction is known. Actinomyosin is contractile in vitro, if ATP and KCl are present. A rapid fall in ATP level occurs following death and the postmortal excitability of the muscles lasts only as long as there are sufficient stores of ATP in the system for the contraction of muscle tissue. If the ATP decomposition is complete, the rigor mortis is irreversible. After this point, relaxation is due to the decomposition, and decay of muscle tissue. Not only skeletal muscle, but smooth muscle is also affected. Rigor mortis of the musculus arrectores pylorum causes *goose pimples* on the skin of the corpse and gives the impression of postmortal growth of the hair. Later the muscles of facial expression undergo rigor mortis giving the face the expression known as *risus sardonicus* (the sardonic smile).

Rigor mortis does not take effect in all muscles at the same time. According to Nysten rigor mortis begins in the muscles of mastication and in the muscles in the nuchal region spreading to the face, the neck, the upper extremities, the trunk musculature, and the lower extremities. Rigor mortis starts first in the heart muscle 30 minutes after death. Visible external signs, however, may be observed between 2–4 hours after death. Six to 12 hours later the whole body is involved. Rigor mortis sets in within eight hours following the initial relaxation. Between 20–84 hours the body can be stiff enough to be stood up. The body may become completely limp again 24–140 hours. This relaxation is a result of the process of decomposition of the body which return the musculature to a limp state.

The development of rigor mortis is dependent upon many factors. It depends on the age, the musculature of the corpse, and in a significant degree the environmental temperature. In young, muscular persons rigor mortis occurs more quickly, more obviously and remains for a longer time than in the case of an elderly, emaciated patient. Certain diseases intensify and hasten the onset of rigor mortis such as cholera, tetanus, injuries (e.g. spinal injuries), burns, and certain poisonings (cyanide, strychnine). Other factors cause a delay in onset, such as death by asphyxia or carbon monoxide poisoning.

A special form of rigor mortis of which the existence is doubted by many must be discussed. This is the so-called *"cataleptic rigor mortis"* in which the musculature of the deceased assumes the state of rigor mortis at the moment of death and appears fixed in the position of his last act. Cataleptic rigor mortis can be seen in the case of cramps caused by poison or in tetanus. The sudden onset of rigor mortis has been described following spinal or brain stem injury.

The heat-induced muscular contraction, may resemble rigor mortis, in corpses subjected to high heat (burning, hot liquids) the muscle proteins denature and coagulate. In contrast to rigor mortis, the damaged muscle fiber bundles power fully shorten and cause a characteristic pose, for example the gladiator a position. This does not mean that a burn occurring during life causes similar heat induced coagulation as in the dead body.

The stiffening effect of cold on the soft tissues of the body must not be mistaken for rigor mortis. The effect of cold on the plasticity of the soft tissues varies, being most noticeable on the body of the infant at +4 °C.

The *electrical excitability* of the skeletal musculature is a long recognized supravital phenomenon. It has been employed in recent years in forensic medicine to assist in the establishment of the time of death. The simplest variation was demonstrated by Popvassilev and Prokop: with the use of needle electrodes inserted into the muscle, the stimulus, whether by current from flashlight batteries or car batteries, elicits contraction. This excitability remains for a variable time after death. Arranged in order of occurrence, the muscles around the eyes retain their excitability for the longest time (8 hours), followed by the perioral group and lastly the musculature of the extremities. From the experiments conducted by Nagy, we know that in the first 20–30 minutes following death some muscle groups show an expressed contraction with a gradually decreasing excitability over 1.5–2 hours. According to observations made on skeletal muscle, its excitability in the first hours following death appears to be independent of environmental temperature, age or state of nutrition.

Appearance of rigor mortis		
Onset	1/2	4 hours
Renewed onset after relaxation	2	8 hours
Fully developed	6	12 hours
Relaxation	24	140 hours

Muscular electric excitability		
Intensive movement of extremities	1/2	2 hours
Extremity muscle groups	1.5	2 hours
Facial muscles	2.5	8 hours

Desiccation

Desiccation is one of the signs of death. An the skin of the dead body, the areas covered with thinner epithelia, and in the

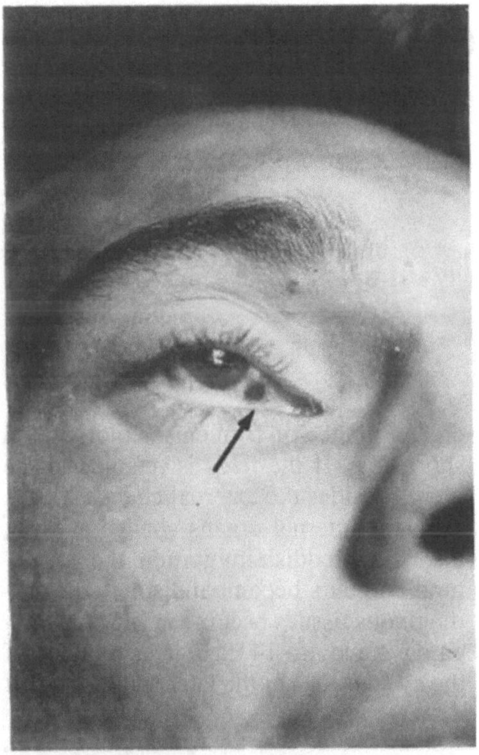

Fig. 5. Postmortal drying of the sclera, the Larcher spot

areas covered by mucous membranes develop sharply bordered, parchmentlike, dry yellowish-brown and in some places bacon rind patches which vary in shape and size. Desiccation may be observed the earliest on the cornea off the open eye. It forms an almost triangular area next on the sclera and appears as a dark grey area, and is called the *Larcher spot (Fig. 5)*. Desiccated areas may form in places where the skin is injured, whether by chaffing or by deeper wounds, or in those areas where the skin is soaked. Very often, in women the mucous membranes of the labia minora or majora dry out and in men the skin of the scrotum becomes discolored to a brownish, parchment-like appearance. Often on the skin of infants these characteristic desiccated areas are mistaken for previously inflicted injuries or are assumed to be the result of acid burns. The desiccation of the abrasions in the furrow occurring during hanging whether originating in life or postmortally, causes a brownish-yellow, bacon rind-like drying in the area. Similarly desiccation occurs in the area of abrasions in the area of wounds caused by the fingernails during manual strangulation. Desiccation in an area of an injury may occur either in life or postmortally. Judging whether the marks are in fact wounds received during life or damage occurring postmortally damage is therefore difficult. For this reason we must pay much more attention to the presence of vital reactions (see later chapter). Desiccation may occur not only in connection with wounds, but within the internal organs as well, a characteristic form is seen in an as in elderly body where the pericardium lies against the emphysematic lungs and assumes a hardened, parchment-like appearance.

Late changes of death

Putrefaction

Autolytic processes following death start early. One form is *maceration.* In the uterus, the skin of a dead fetus becomes bloated and loosens and large pieces flake off, and the subcutaneous tissue becomes imbibed with a dirty reddish discoloration, and later if the macerated fetus is delivered, will take on a greenish color, after a short time. If the fetus is retained in the uterus besides the external changes of the skin, the internal organs change as well, they show reddish imbibition, their structural contours become indistinct, the cartilaginous tissues become imbibed in seven days and 12–14 days later the lens of the eye as well. In the later stages the soft

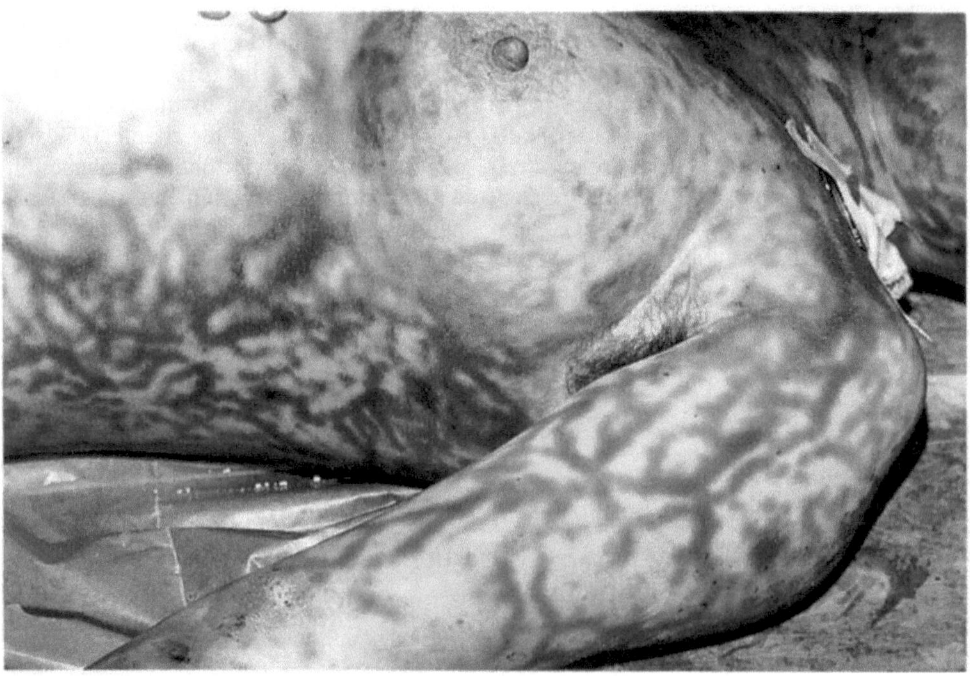

Fig. 6. Decomposition, imbibition, outlining of the superficial veins

tissues of the fetus liquify, and minerals may be deposited in the soft tissues and the *lithopaedion* (stone fetus) is formed.

The visible signs of deterioration in a dead body may be seen within 48–72 hours depending on the temperature and humidity of the external environment. The optimal environmental temperature for the processes of decay is 20–40 °C, at lower temperatures the intensity of putrefaction is slowed because of the slowed chemical processes, and at higher temperatures is slowed because of the denaturation of proteins.

Decay is a result of *bacterial and enzymatic action.* The bacteria, partly from the flora of the body and partly from the external environment, initiate the process. Of the bacteria in the body, those living in the intestines are the primary initiators of the putrefactive processes, and the first sign of this is a circumscribed discoloration of the skin of the abdomen beginning on the lower abdomen. The greenish-black discoloration of the skin is caused by the bacterial production of sulfhemoglobin which spreads, discoloring the whole abdominal wall, the skin of the thorax, the neck, the soft tissues of the face and finally the extremities. The superficial vessels of the skin are outlined in the discolored skin, this being due to the decay of blood in the veins *(Fig. 6).*

In a decomposed body areas of hemorrhage and bruising are also imbibed, there fore making it difficult to recognize hemorrhages due to injury, near to or in the imbedded areas. In the early stages of decomposition microscopic examination may provide valuable information in that we may see red blood cells in the area of an injury or the shadows of erythrocytes that have leached out.

In the process of decay, we see finger-

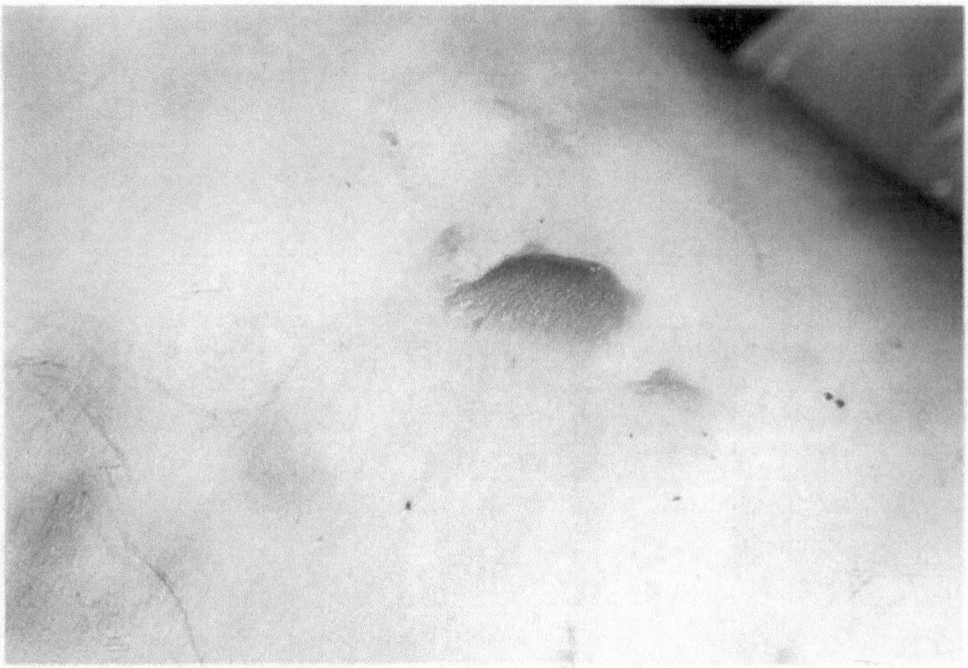

Fig. 7. Decomposition blister on the skin

tip-sized and later larger blisters which are formed by the detachment of the cornified layer of the skin *(Fig. 7)*. These fill with gases and fluids resulting from decay (these must be distinguished from second-degree burns, by demonstrating a significantly higher protein content and showing leukocytes as vital reaction). The loose surface epithelium detaches upon contact, and thus the external appearance of the body shows gas bubbles, displaced flakes of cornified epithelium and the skin appears dirty green. In the places where epithelium is stripped off – the skin dries, has a dirty green color and turns stiff, the further processes of decay are significantly slowed.

The process of decay significantly changes when the body is submerged in water with the saturation of the cornified layer, the scalp and body hair are simultaneously loosened, and the thicker skin of the hands and feet may be pulled off like gloves complete with the nails. In numerous instances this, has led to the possibility of misinterpretation *(Fig. 8, Fig. 9)*.

Gases from decomposition form in the cavities of the dead body so that the abdomen swells up or bloats and becomes tightly stretched. Similarly, gases form in the thoracic cavity and in the soft tissue areas and musculature so that crepitation similar to that caused by the gas gangrene-producing bacteria may be palpated in the muscle tissues. The significant pressure which builds up in the body cavities from the gas-producing decay brings its own characteristic signs such as deformation of the face, bulging or protruding of the eyes, the protruding of the tongue between the teeth and the prolapse of the uterus in women due to the pressure in the abdominal cavity, or the expulsion of a fetus if she was pregnant (the so-called *"coffin birth"*). With an average temperature in the range of 20–25 °C, this

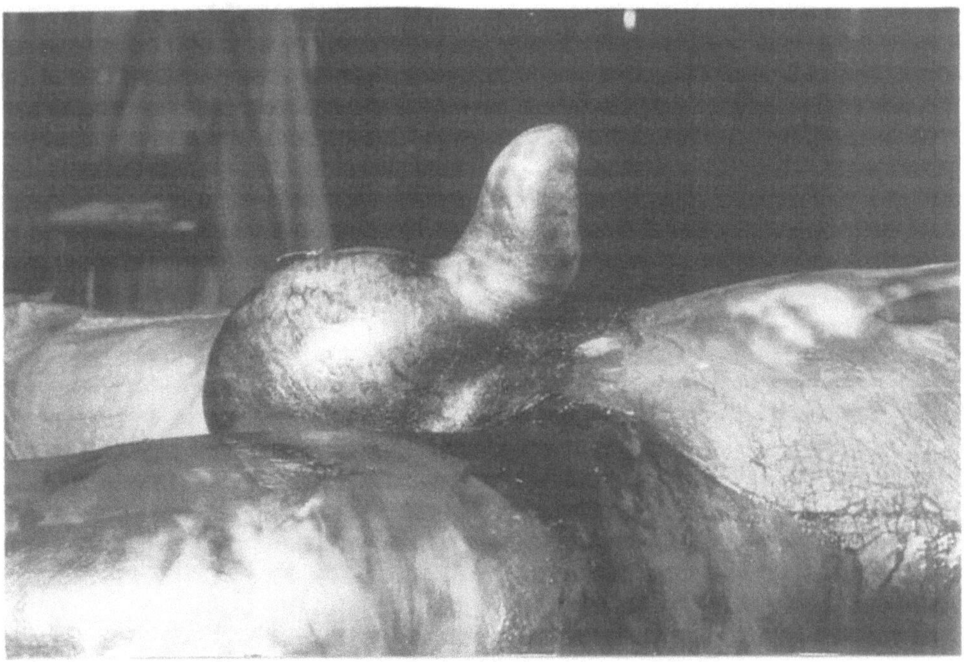

Fig. 8. Decomposition swelling of the scrotum and penis

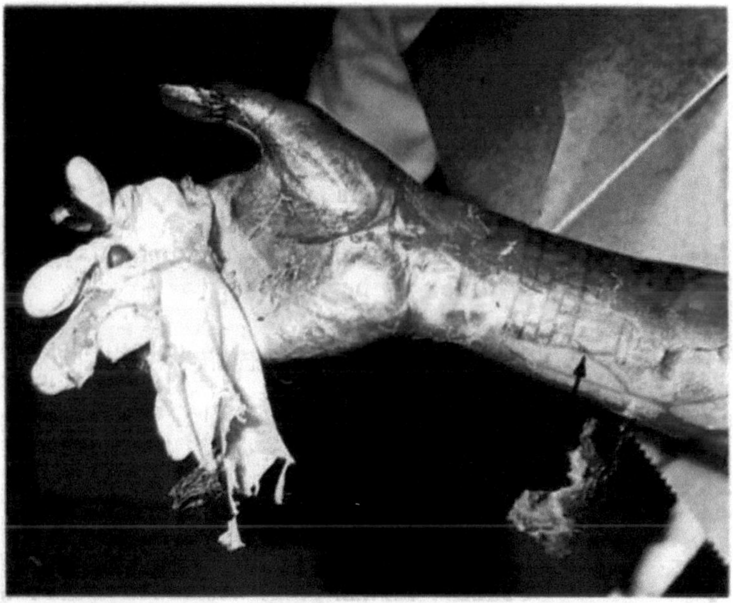

•*Fig. 9.* Loosening of the cornified layer of the skin on a body soaked in water, the skin removable from the hand like a glove (the tattoo prints still visible afterwards)

process can take place in the span of one to two weeks. The microorganisms involved in the process that originate in the body include *E. coli, B. proteus,* various streptococci, staphylococci and clostridia.

Sometimes fungi significantly damage the body surface. Depending on the environmental temperature and humidity, the fungi usually occupy those parts of the body where superficial wounds can be found. In the articles written by Woorde the time of death may be deduced on the basis of the presence and extent of fungal colonies and knowledge about the previous environmental temperatures by the study of mycelia grout in the culture medium and air, as well as the sporulation time. The article emphasizes that the determination the time of death on the basis of fungal growth is very complex and difficult *(Fig. 10).*

The postmortal autolytic processes result in *the self-digestion* of the gastric mucosa. Gastromalacia in the stomach changes the mucous membranes to a greyish-black with the vessels being outlined in a dark grey color and the mucosa in some places may become softened and friable resulting in the emptying of the contents into the abdominal cavity. Sometimes, due to moving the body, the contents of the stomach may get into the airway and lungs. The pneumomalacia produced in this way resembles gangrene of the lung, but as in every postmortal process, the vital reaction is lacking.

During the decomposition of the body the fatty tissues also decay. The tissue's fatty components break down, the triglycerides from the fat tissue undergoing hydrolysis to form glycerin and fatty acids – oleic, palmitic and oleinic acids – and are present in the form of a rancid smelling fluid in the body cavities, and is soaked into the soft tissues. The free fatty acids, combine with the environmental calcium and magnesium ions, from the soil undergo saponification to form a gray, lumpy, soft material.

Rarely, in cases of advanced decomposition on the endocardium we may find pinpoint to pinhead sized ball-like forma-

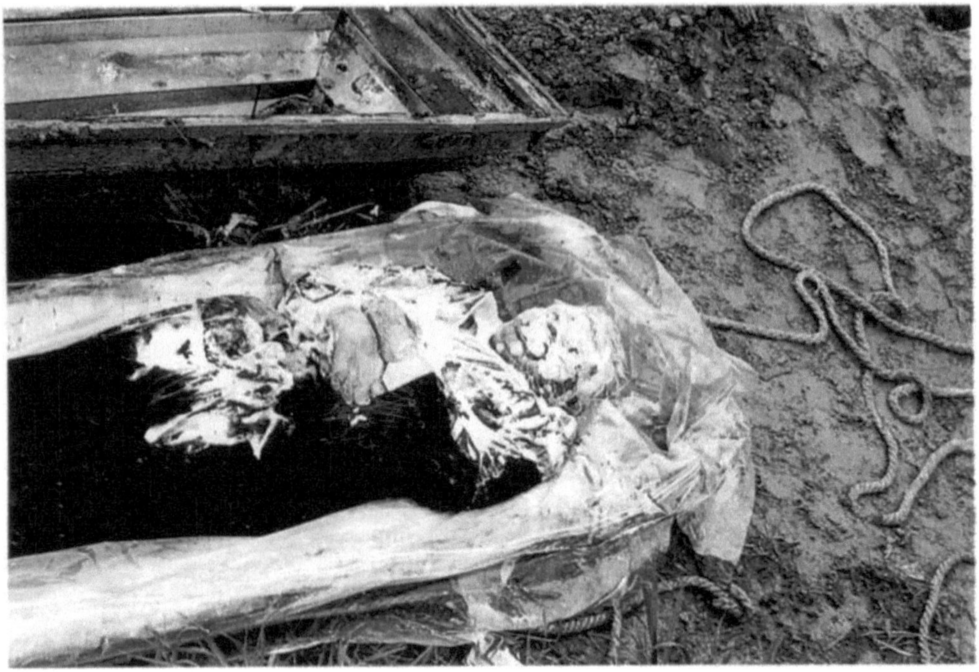

Fig. 10. In moist areas fungus appears on the body

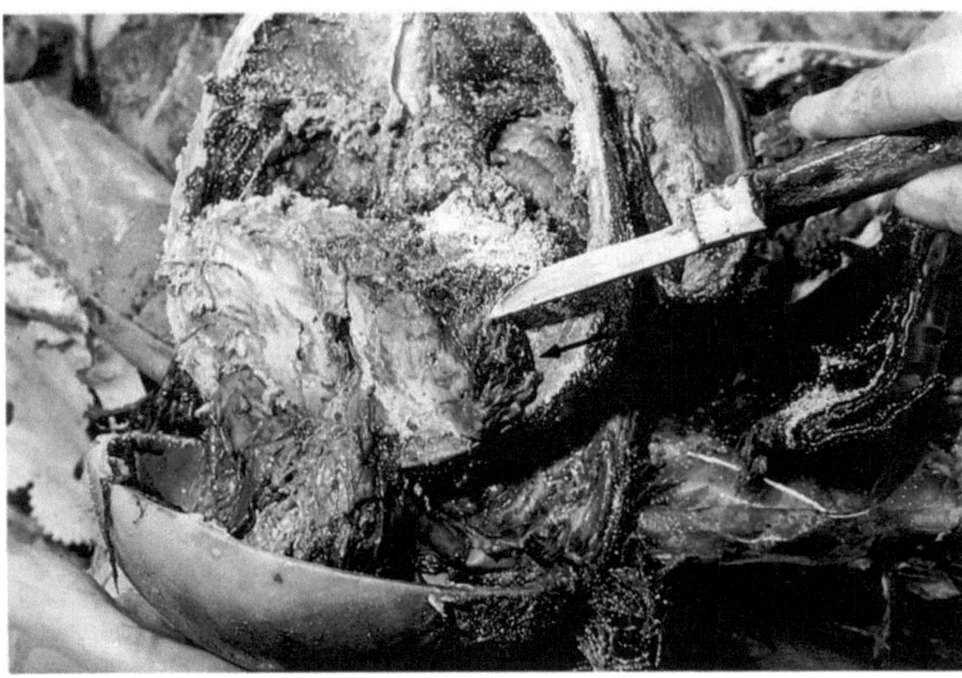

Fig. 11. Exhumation with autopsy months after burial showing subdural hemorrhage

tions, which are clumps of decaying proteins and bacterial masses.

The decay of the internal organs is completed with time. In the area of the gall bladder, yellowish imbibition of the liver, small intestines, large intestines is also a sign of putrefaction. The permeability of the gall bladder increases and when it does, the bile stains the surrounding organs. The gas-producing ability of the decomposition processes does not spare the internal organs. The alterations in the liver are most expressed which, due to the ongoing decay in its tissues and the gas production, resemble the spongy inside of a loaf of bread. The decomposition of the blood in the vessels also produces gas. This develops in a relatively short period of time after death and in several instances has been mistaken for air embolism.

Over the course of decomposition a significant amount of fluid is released. This appears partly in the body cavities and partly outside, leaking into the external environment. The practical significance is that a significant amount of water soluble toxins wash into the environment, or into the soil.

After death the microscopic arrangement of the tissues change with the course of decay. In many cases during exhumation we get a still well-identifiable histological picture of certain organs, and at others times, due to the progress of decay, all that may be seen of the erythrocytes in the area around of a wound are the shadows of their cells. On the other hand, the formation of hemosiderin, characteristic of the vital reaction, may be demonstrated for a long time *(Fig. 11)*.

The striations of the striated muscle disappear and only the sarcolemma may be recognized. Smooth muscle cells maintain their structure, particularly in the more massive organs. Thus the arrangement of the uterine tissues can be recognized for a long time after death and may be useful in identification. The integument resists decay for a long time. The body and head hair fades, losing its hue, a property which makes it impossible to tell the original color. The cartilage and fibers of the dense connective tissues retain their form for a relatively long time (3–5 years). The bones and teeth remain recognizable for the longest time.

The course of decay or putrefaction depends on the *environmental temperature*, (and in numerous instances, upon the consequences of certain forms of death). Decay is most pronounced in an environmental temperature of 25–30 °C. At higher temperatures decomposition caused by bacteria slows to a stop and the process of decay is significantly delayed, or will not occur at all. In bodies found in the cold the appearance of the signs of decay is prolonged. In the septic state, decomposition is more rapid and pronounced, while in certain poisonings, such as arsenic and mercury, the process is decreased or inhibited.

Formation of grave-wax

Adipocere, or grave-wax, is a greyish-white material of oatmeal-like consistency with a soft outer appearance which may form on the surface of the body over varying spans of time after death on certain organs. The cause is the putrefactive decomposition of the fatty tissues. Following death the decay of the adipose tissues occurs simultaneously with the other tissues, yielding fatty acids and glycerin. This decay may be caused by bacteria and fungi and during the hydrolysis glycerin, palmitic acid and stearic acid are produced in significant quantities. In life the adipose tissues contain only insignificant amounts of free fatty acids, but after death the pro-

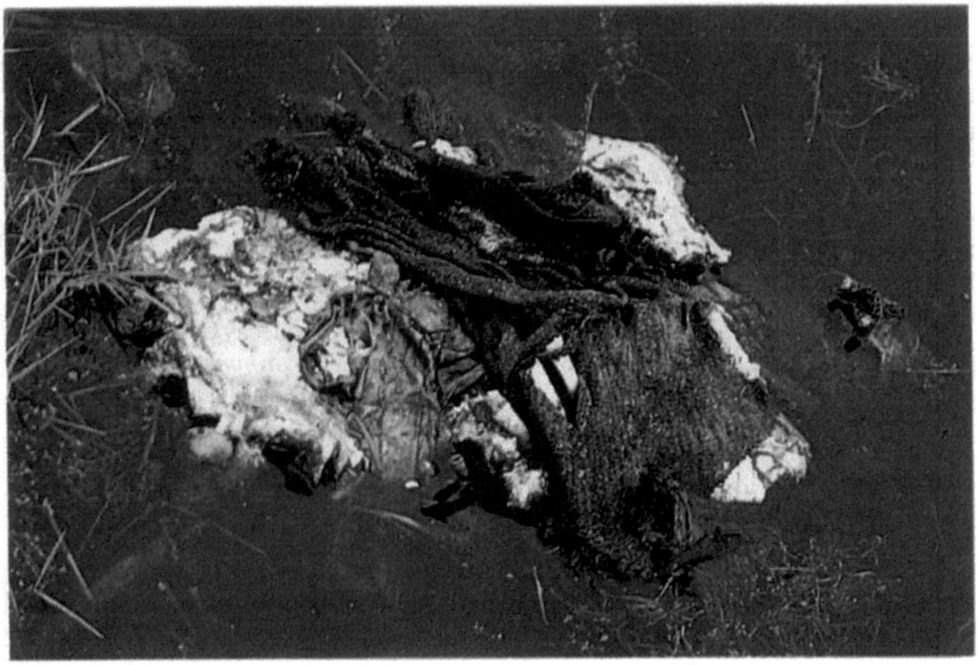

Fig. 12. Grave-wax formation in a body found in the water

cess of decay results in their increase in amount. Three months after death 70% of the triacylglycerols in the organs are decomposed to free fatty acids. The fatty acids combine with the calcium, magnesium and sodium ions in the environment to form soaps, the consistency of which is dependent upon the environmental calcium, magnesium and sodium content. Grave-wax formed from calcium soap is rock hard. During decay the fats are not only hydrolyzed, but also oxidized and decarboxylated by bacterial and fungal action, and the products of decay thus produced give the fatty tissues and therefore the grave-wax it's pungent rancid odor. The formation seems to be dependent on a damp, oxygen free environment – and takes a long time. The first indications of the formation of grave-wax may be seen on the skin and subcutaneous areas 1–2 months after death. For the transformation of the muscle tissues at least six months of decay is required. The complete transformation of the soft tissues (the grave-wax ensheathes bones, like a "coat of armor") occurs within two years. The formation of grave-wax occurs most commonly on bodies found in water, and the formation depends upon the surrounding temperature, the depth of the water and the presence of underwater currents *(Fig. 12)*.

If the body is kept submerged for a long time in deep water, grave-wax forms more rapidly and more extensively, and the consistency of the calcium and magnesium soaps is less plastic. The mass of the grave-wax formed from other than fat tissue, may be more dense, and contains untransformed muscle fibers and perhaps nerve bundles. The formation of grave-wax in the internal organs is not insignificant and preserves the form and sometimes the alterations left by such disease processes as tuberculous cavities or severe coronary sclerosis. The formation of grave-wax occurs under damp, oxygen-free conditions and may be seen quite often with bodies buried in mass graves. In examinations of mass graves the formation of grave-wax preserved injuries and external wounds for a longer period and the transformation of some organs in to grave-wax can sometimes be useful in identifying or determining the sex of a body.

Mummification

The course of changes in the body after death can deviate from the usual depending upon the effects of the environment. If the temperature is high, the air dry and the airflow or ventilation sufficient, the signs of decay in the wet tissues will be less and the soft tissues will dry out resulting in mummification of the body. The soft tissues of the body become dry, hard and brown, and the weight of the body is significantly decreased. Mummification, which depends primarily on the removal of the water may also occur in such cases where the temperature is not dominant, but rather between minus 20 °C and plus 40 °C. In these temperatures, a frozen corpse loses large amounts of water (although at a much slower rate) and under these conditions bacterial activity may be slowed or stop completely, and the body will become mummified over decades or centuries.

The dried tissues preserve their injuries relatively well and the alterations in the internal organs are well-visible, and the cause of death may occasionally be deduced. Successful histological tests can in many cases be applied to mummified tissues. Mummification of adult bodies is a rare occurrence in central European countries. Bodies of newborns and infants may also mummify, under suitable conditions.

Damage to the dead body caused by animals

The decisive role in the destruction soft tissues of the body is played by *flies.* Flies lay their eggs in the unprotected, moist areas covered by mucous membranes. This may occur in such large a number that the nose, mouth and, eyes have the appearance as if a fungus were growing out. Damage the corpses is caused primarily by the e housefly, the bluebottle fly and the blow-fly. Within 10–12 hours maggots hatch from the eggs, and grow rapidly, and three days later are 2–5 mm in length, growing to their full 7-8 mm length within a week. On the eighth day they enter the pupa state and on day 14 a new generation of flies takes wing. Thus if we find in a body maggots and empty pods, at least 14 days have elapsed since death. We use the SCHRANZ table of the development for the most commonly occurring flies *(Table 1).*

The *maggots* produce proteolytic enzymes which rapidly destroy the soft tissue areas. Circumscribed areas of missing flesh on the skin of a body dead a few days shows the damaging effect of the maggots. Later the internal organs also disappear and it may occur that following to total destruction of the soft tissues, only the dry honeycombed like skin covers the bones. These small circumscribed areas of missing flesh resemble shotgun pellet wounds, and a careless examination may result in a misdiagnosis *(Fig. 13).*

Chewing by *ants* appears as superficial, reddish, moist wounds, on the edge of

Table 1. Development of the most commonly occuring types of flies according to SCHRANZ

	Hatching of Housefly eggs 10–12 hours	Hatching of Bluebottle fly eggs 12–16 hours	Hatching of Greenbottle fly eggs 12–16 hours	Blowfly eggs move immediately (vivipara)
2. day	2 mm	3–4 mm	2 mm	3–4 mm
3. day	2–3 mm	5–6 mm	2–3 mm	5–6 mm
4. day	4–5 mm	7–8 mm	3–4 mm	7–9 mm
5. day	6–7 mm	10–12 mm	5–6 mm	10–12 mm
6. day	8–8 mm	13–14 mm	7–8 mm	13–14 mm
7. day	8 mm	pupation	8–9 mm	15–16 mm
8. day	pupation	pupa 9–10 mm	pupation	16–18 mm
9. day	pupa 5–6 mm	pupa	pupa 6–7 mm	19–20 mm
10. day	pupa	pupa	pupa	pupation
12. day	pupa	pupa	pupa	pupa 10–12 mm
14. day	fly away 7–8 mm	fly away 12–13 mm	fly away 7–9 mm	pupa
16. day				pupa
18. day				fly away 16–18 mm

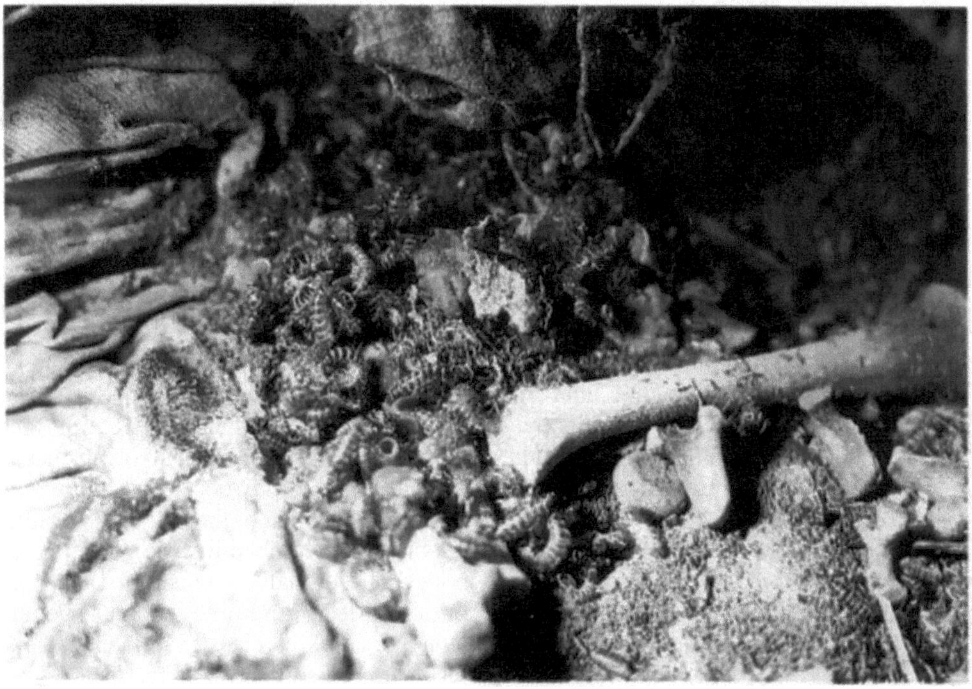

Fig. 13. Destroyed soft tissue, bony remains, empty fly pods (In the cadaver of a newborn discovered a year after death)

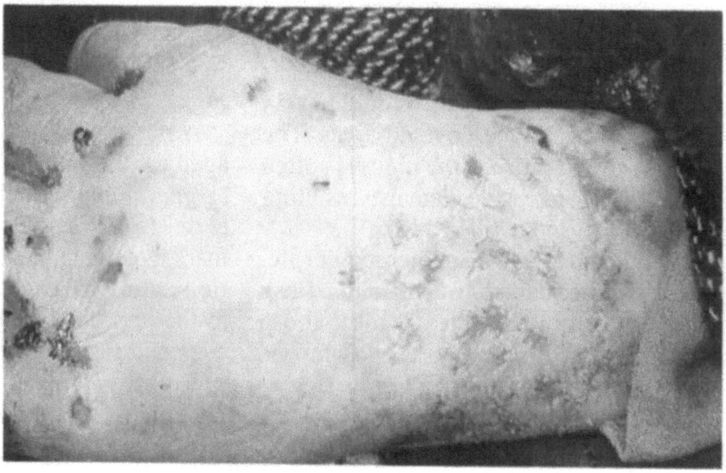

Fig. 14. Ant bites on the hand (from the collection of Prof. Ökrös)

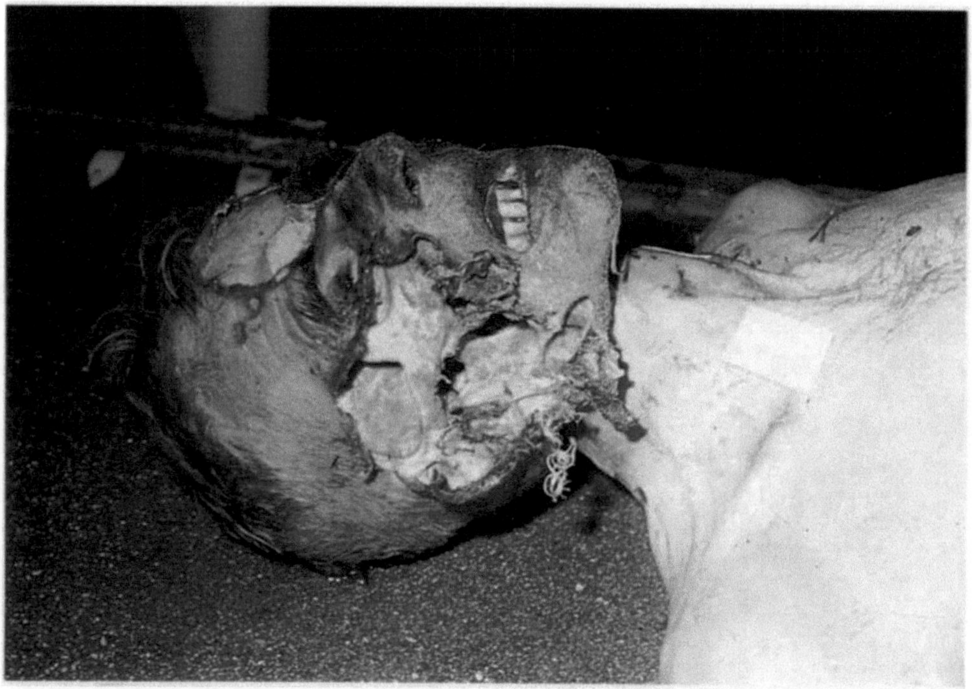

Fig. 15. Rat bites, extensive soft tissue destruction

which fine indentations may be seen. The formic acid introduced into the area of the wound increases its size, the corrosive effect being especially effective on thin skin or mucous membrane-covered areas. The chewing by ants around the mouth is often mistaken for corrosive damage resulting from acid poisoning *(Fig. 14)*.

Fish may damage a submerged corpse. Circumscribed areas of missing flesh may result from fish bites into the loose pieces of soft tissue, which was in one case were mistaken for gunshot wounds. The surface of a body that has been lying in water may be covered by a slimy green algae.

A body lying in the open may be damaged by the bites of *mice and rats, or of larger animals* such as foxes and dogs *(Fig. 15)*. We may easily recognize the marks of their teeth on the bones. Carrion-eating birds cause damage primarily to the unprotected soft areas, namely the eyes and face.

Medicolegal autopsy

"An autopsy is a detailed examination of a corpse carried out by one or more qualified medical practitioners in order to ascertain the primary cause of death and any other ancillary or contributory abnormalities and, in certain circumstances, to establish the identity of the deceased."

The dead body, which includes that of the still-born infant, may be removed from the place death occurred for autopsy, burial, or cremation only after medical examination to establish the fact of death has been performed. Medical examination to determine death must be accomplished within six hours after the notification of the incident. The physician performing the coroner's inquest is responsible for establishing:

– the fact of death

– the time and cause of death

– whether the death was caused by an infective disease

– whether the death was unusual

to arrange for the disposal of the body. The coroner's inquest has significance to the law, public health, death statistics and criminal statistics. When a death takes place, the cause and time of death must be determined, the death certificate issued, and the body disposed of. If the cause of death is unknown, after writing a short history of the case, an autopsy is to be performed. Determining correctly the death certification was reported by FERNANDO. Only 38% of the certificates contained the correct causes of death.

If it is suspected that the death was not from normal causes – *unnatural death* - the police must be notified. In these cases, a forensic autopsy is mandatory. The official autopsy is mandated by regulation. It is stated, in case of unnatural death, the forensic autopsy must be ordered. An unnatural death is that death which occurs under circumstances which make a natural death doubtful. These include:

a) circumstances that raise the suspicion of crime,

b) traffic or industrial accident, or suspicion thereof,

c) various accidents (e.g. household) in which the establishment of death demands investigation assignment of responsibility,

d) suicide or circumstances that lead to that suspicion,

e) result of medical treatment with the doctor or health practitioner suspected of malpractice (e.g. transfusion, anesthesia, operation, insufficient treatment),

f) unknown antecedents or circumstances and information cannot be obtained which makes it fundamentally possible to determine the cause of death, with regards to whether the death occurred in a natural manner (unexplained death).

In the case of unnatural death, investigative procedures must be instigated – until the identity is established – in those instances when the identity of the deceased is unknown.

In accordance with the laws, the exammining physician, if noticing circumstances indicating unnatural death, must inform the police and ensure that the body and the scene be preserved in their original condition until they arrive.

In a case of unnatural death occurring in a medical institution, the examining physician is also required to notify the head of the department, who also informs the local police. If an accident, suicide or crime against life happens in a medical institution, care must also be taken in this situation as well to ensure that the body and the surroundings remain untouched and unaltered.

In the case of unnatural death, the police hold a coroner's inquest in cooperation with a medical examiner. If possible the coroner's inquest must be performed by a qualified forensic medical specialist. In the absence of this, a police surgeon or, if the coroner's inquest can not be delayed, another physician must be requested. This physician, however, may not be one who has treated the deceased previously although, he must provide information about the deceased's treatment and diseases. The physician serves at the scene as an expert or advisor, and it is desirable later, for the same physician to be present at the autopsy. The physician may take photographs of the scene, the body and the surroundings as it may later aid in the expert's work.

After the examination of the body the *clothing* of the deceased must be examined and each item of clothing must be recorded. On the clothing tears, soiling, and in cases of traffic accidents traces of paint are searched for. The tears and injury to clothing must be meticulously examined and matched to any injury alteration found on the surface of the body. The examination of the clothing is of special significance in certain violent crimes, such as in the case of a stab wound where the location of the wound and the hole in the clothing must match. The examination of clothing may later provide information in the determination of the amount of force which could have caused the injury. In gunshot wounds, the examination of the clothing provides case winning evidence. It is likewise essential to look for traces from vehicles e.g. in the case of traffic accidents *(Fig. 16)*.

In the examination of clothing the soiling is more easily separated and recognized if we shake the clothes out over wrapping paper or a plastic sheet. Damp clothing, especially if there is a significant amount of blood on them must be treated appropriately after the examination and only then packaged. Appropriate treatment primarily means drying out the cloth. Damp clothing kept in plastic bags will be significantly damaged, the type of the decayed blood will be impossible to determine, and the signs of injury will also be destroyed. It is therefore a basic requirement that following appropriate drying, the clothing be packed in paper or material which allows a good free circulation of air and should not be packed in plastic wrap. In traffic accidents it is especially important to examine the shoes. On the shoes we especially look for skid marks on the soles and if we find them, must photograph them.

Following the basic clothing examination, we strip the corpse naked. The clothing may be taken away if necessary and directed by the physician participating in the coroner's inquest. The naked corpse is then examined in the prescribed manner and observations recorded. During the

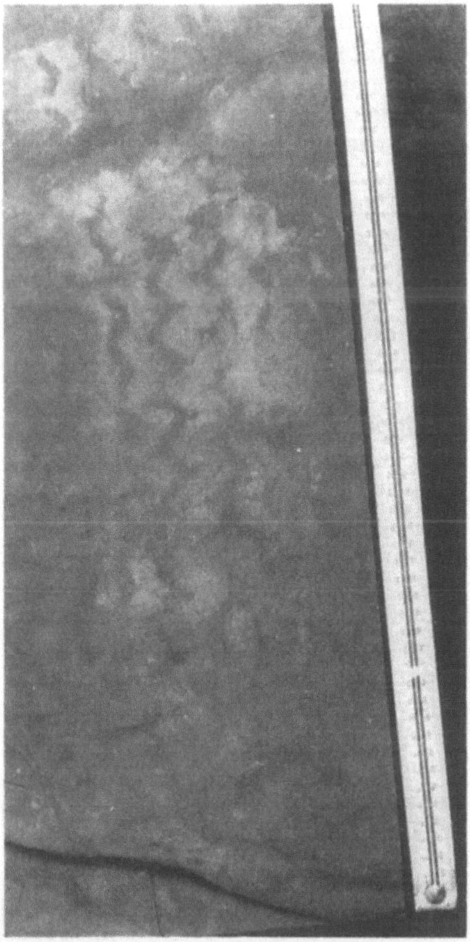

Fig. 16. Tire prints on the clothing of a traffic accident victim

course of the inquest we must take notice of any superficial marks, with special attention being drawn to the so-called hidden body areas, hair-covered skin of the scalp, body creases, the external genitalia and the anal opening. On the body patches of lividity can draw our attention to the cause of death: bright red patches suggest carbon monoxide or cyanide poisoning, brownish red patches to the effect of methemoglobin-type poisoning, and small and vague pale patches suggest significant bleeding. Pinpoint hemorrhages in the conjunctiva and conjunctival sacs point to death by suffocation, while bits of foreign matter in these places can originate from the area the corpse was found in. Alterations found in the area of the neck must be examined with special care: here may be reflected the evidence of a too-tight collar or strangulation by a scarf which can only be recognized by careful study. Likewise injuries appearing on the neck – nail marks, bruises – may point to manual strangulation. We must pay attention to foreign odors coming from the mouth, alcohol and certain poisons (parathion, nicotine) which have characteristic smells. Corrosions around the mouth are often caused by poisoning by caustics; and at other times by postmortal stomach acid and the resultant corrosion of the mucous membranes may give further guidance. In examining the extremities we must look for unnatural ranges of motion, and injuries which may suggest defense or struggle. These must be carefully recorded and studied. Especially relevant are the palms and soles of the feet in the case of electrocution in which the entry and exit points of electricity leave characteristic marks (sometimes circumscribed, hyperkeratotic changes can be mistaken for electric burns). With the examination of the corpse the attention of the examining physician must be turned to the contamination of the surroundings and the characteristic forms of blood traces. With an unknown body the special identifying signs must be described.

The time of death must be declared, and an opinion should be given as to whether the cause of death came about by natural means or by criminal means and whether any signs are present which suggest contagious disease. (In the latter case, the pathologist has to report it to the Health Service).

The law defines separately, those cases where autopsy must be performed to determine the cause of death. If during the course of the diagnostic autopsy signs are uncovered which raise the suspicion of an unnatural death, the autopsy must be interrupted, the head of the medical institution and the police notified. If in the case of other than unnatural death the examining physician may advise a judicial autopsy, only under extraordinary circumstances.

In the case of unnatural death samples must be taken from the body, in those instances where the suspicion arises of such a poisoning in which the material would change with the passing of time, or deteriorate so that later examination of the material would not produce useful results. The examining physician is required to both take and record the sample.

In cases of unnatural death the police arrange for the autopsy and disposal of the body while the examining physician issues the death certificate.

When the autopsy or judicial autopsy of a patient who died in a medical institution is to be performed, the department head or the chief resident of the department must be notified of the time. The attending physician may be present at the autopsy only if his presence would not jeopardize the investigation or contribute to the investigating authority's conduct of the autopsy. A copy of the record of the official autopsy must be given on request to the head of the medical institution by the permission of the office authorizing the autopsy.

Among the regulations regarding the corpse, there are rules governing the performance of the autopsy. The purpose of the autopsy is to certify a clinical diagnosis, and in the case of natural death, to determine the cause. The patient who dies in hospital usually undergoes diagnostic autopsy, in the pathological department of the hospital with the consent of the next of kin, under the cooperation of the leaders of the attending medical department and the department conducting the autopsy. "The autopsy must be carried out by a trained and experienced forensic pathologist who follows a protocol which is according to the protocol of profession".

Burial is conducted in accordance with regulation. The regulation also deals with cremation. An official permit is required for cremation issued by the appropriate health department office and the coroner must indicate on the death certificate, the fact if autopsy was performed or not. If the office of health deems necessary an autopsy before cremation, they must arrange for it. It must be pointed out that cremation is not allowed for a patient dying in hospital without prior autopsy. The physician conducting the autopsy must record on the examination certificate that the remains may be cremated. The remains must be kept in cold storage until cremation, which must be carried out after 72 hours but before 15 days. The body or amputated parts can be kept only in places where there is a proper morgue, and should be transported immediately after the examination, or at least within 16 hours, to appropriate cold storage facilities. The body must be transported to a funeral home or burial facility after 16 hours and at most in 4 days. The corpse must be buried no sooner than 48, or no later than 72 hours after death, with the exception that the examining physician issues a permit of exemption, or if there are proper cold storage facilities available. In that case the burial may be permitted between 48 hours and 8 days after death.

The coroner's investigation is followed by the autopsy, if necessary. In the case of unnatural death, a forensic medical exam is ordered and is assigned to either a police medical examiner, a forensic pathologist or to pathologist. If during the process of autopsy suspicion of criminal activity surfaces, the autopsy must be interrupted and the assigning authorities must be notified and all observations must be reded, including the suspicion of the nature of the crime. In the suspicion of criminal activity, a forensic autopsy is arranged which is performed by two forensic pathologists.

The law details the responsibilities of the medical specialist and guides as to which questions must be answered. For every injury on the corpse an assessment must be made as to, presumably how did it occur, how long did it occur before or after death and whether it was self-inflicted or inflected by others.

In the case of injuries found on the body, an opinion must be given as to whether the death

a) could have been caused by the injuries?

b) could have been related with the injuries together with previous alterations e.g. illness of the injured person.

c) could have been brought about by such a cause which originated from the injuries, and if not, what was the presumed healing time of the injuries

d) could have occurred at about at the same time without the injury, so that death would have resulted shortly after

e) could have been avoided had proper care been administered in time?

In the case of multiple injuries, an opinion must be given as to the origin of the multiple injuries, and which among them would have been capable of causing death, and further how much time would have been required for their healing.

The *autopsy record* must be written during the autopsy. A conspicuous reminder must be attached to the record that it should be clear, understandable and relevant. It is done along with the autopsy and every injury is recorded. The autopsy record consists of three main parts: the personal data, findings and opinion. In the first part we find the personal data of the deceased, the authority arranging the autopsy, the time and place of the autopsy, the conducting physician or specialist, and the name of the person writing the record, and the official taking part in the autopsy. The observation and findings section is divided into two subparts: the *external examination* and the internal examination. The external examination describes the general appearance of the corpse indicating the age, sex, height, state of nutrition, skin color, physique, location of the patches of lividity, their extent, form, color, compressibility, the appearance of rigor mortis or decay. The length of the hair, color, state of the pupils and conjunctiva, alterations of the ears, nose and mouth, the shape of the thorax, character of the external genitalia and anal region and state of the extremities must also be described. Injuries on the surface of the body are described separately. The description of the injuries are put down in the chapter about injuries. Here we want to record the injuries in a systematic fashion starting with the head, the trunk, the upper and then the lower extremities so that even the most insignificantly appearing injury is not left out. The injuries must be described precisely, giving their size in centimeters or millimeters and it is not allowed to describe them comparatively (plum-sized, peanut-sized, hand-breadth, etc). The location must be related to fixed anatomical points. Certain injuries are especially important, as in the true measurement to the plane of the sole of gunshot wounds, traffic accident injuries or stab wounds. In the event that no injuries can be found on the body, that also must be noted.

Following the external examination, the *internal examination* is performed.

In the recording of the internal organs, we also record the pathological particulars describe them from a pathologist's point of view. Otherwise, we note such alterations which are important from a forensic point of view.

We start with the displacement of the scalp to open the skull. Here we must note hemorrhages, their place, extent and form. Special attention must be given to the localization of the injuries because this provides information as to the mechanism. The bones of the calvaria and base of the skull must be studied with special care, looking for fractures, but they must not be mistaken for the impressions of vessels. In suspicion of a fracture, examination of the plane cut by the saw can clear up the difficulty in that impressions of vessels are only found on the internal surface and do not extend to the outer layer. The localization of intracranial bleedings are caused by different vessels. Epidural hemorrhages are caused most commonly by injury to the arteria meningea media while subdural hemorrhage usually comes from injury to the emissary vessels, or possibly the venous sinuses. Subarachnoid hemorrhage may be due to trauma or be spontaneous. In the region of the basilar artery network at the base of the brain a massive bleeding is suspicious for a ruptured aneurysm. In these cases the search for a ruptured dilation of a vessel can be decisive. After removal of the brain the venous sinuses must be carefully examined, along with the network of the basilar artery, and the presence of a thrombus either in the venous sinuses or basilar arteries sought. If the circumstances demand, we must examine the nasal and pharyngeal cavities, the facial sinuses and open the branch of the carotis interna in the base of the skull as well.

Upon opening the thoracic and abdominal cavities and removing the organs, we must pay attention to the position of the organs and to the character of the odor coming from them. When pneumothorax or air embolism is suspected, we employ a special opening procedure. In the case of *pneumothorax,* after stripping off the skin, first one side and then the other side we open the chest cavity under water and any escaping bubbles confirm the diagnosis. Care must be taken so that no fluid gets into the thorax which might cause misleading results later in the examination. In the case of suspected *air embolism* we fill the pericardium with water and open the right ventricle. Here as well, the escaping bubbles show evidence of air embolism. In some instances the thoracic organs merit a special dissection which is discussed in the chapter about special autopsy techniques.

Examination of the *gastric contents* in many instances provides the possibility to establish the *time of death.* If we know the time of the person last meal, the state of emptying of the stomach can help us. According to the literature, after the consumption of liquids, emptying starts within a few minutes and is complete within one or two hours. A meal of solid food usually takes four to six hours to leave the stomach, but this is influenced by many factors. In childhood the emptying of the stomach takes two to 2.5 hours, but if the meal was large, a child's stomach empties in 4.5 to 7.5 hours. Age slows stomach emptying, as does smoking either between or after meals, alcohol, fatty foods, gastritis, and stress. Large quantities of fluid or duodenal ulcer speeds the gastric emptying.

In the abdomen special attention must be paid to accumulations of fluids, which may be blood, transudate or exudate. In the case of bleeding we try to find the source while preserving the original abdominal situation. With the accumulation of exudate, we try to find the place from where the inflammation originated. The abdominal organs, the stomach, liver, spleen and kidneys are removed as a complex or individually. When rupture of esophageal varices and bleeding is suspected, we remove the thoracic and abdominal complexes together to find the place of bleeding. In every case our dissection technique must be guided by purpose. The usual dissection procedures cannot be dogmatically followed in the practical work of the forensic medical specialist. Many times we must deviate from standard procedures, for example in splenic injury we can count on adhesions around the spleen and must take extra care in dissecting out the spleen from under the ribs so that in looking for the injury we don't find one we caused ourselves. Likewise in other organs we must employ appropriate methods in preparation, removal and examination. (After gynecological operations the kidneys must purposely be removed with the ureters along with the pelvic organs as a unit so the territory of the operation can be examined for the position of the ureters and their cavities.)

Injury to the vertebrae may necessitate removal of the spinal cord. Injuries appearing in the area of the spinal cord may show bleeding under the meninges and perhaps a softening of the tissue of the spinal cord. It is practical to examine the spinal cord after formalin fixation when the softened areas become more apparent. In the case of hemopoetic diseases or in the case of administration of drugs, known to be toxic to bone marrow a marrow sample must be taken from the long bones for histological examination.

Tissue sections taken during the autopsy for histological examination must be fixed quickly, the excised material should be no thicker than 1–2 mm, because if the fixation is imperfect the organ's histological structure will be significantly damaged and practically useless. Fixation is done in 10% formalin, the appropriately fixed specimen also being prepared for electron microscopic examination upon occasion.

Removed and excised specimens must also be recorded in the autopsy record, just as for such organs and parts of organs which are removed for transplantation. The law does not prohibit the removal of organs, during an autopsy for the purpose of healing (e.g. organ transplantation) unless the person refused permission while alive.

Special autopsy techniques

In the practice of forensic medicine in certain cases we must perform the autopsy to meet appropriate requirements. The dissection technique called for in such instances must aid the specialist in the recognition of the injury, the causal mechanism, clarification of the injury's character, and formulation of a precise opinion about it. In some injuries – traffic accidents, gunshot wounds, stabbings – the location of the injury must be indicated by measuring from the plane of the sole, in that this may help to clarify the originating mechanism.

With every injury group we will mention the purpose for a specific dissection technique. The following is a summary of techniques used in specific cases.

In *infanticide* we may gain numerous points of evidence if the autopsy is performed in the appropriate order and prescribed protocol. The maturity of the newborn can be assessed from body measurements and besides the weight, we can observe the disappearance of the lanugo, the length of hair, the descent of the testes into the scrotum, the form of the external genitalia, and we measure the diameter of the ossification center at the distal end of the femur, which in the matured newborn measures about 5 mm in diameter *(Fig. 17)*. During the external examination we look for vernix caseosa on the body surfaces, which can be found in abundance in the axillae, and between the thighs and buttocks of the mature newborn. In the autopsy of the newborn after dividing down of the scalp we look for the presence of a serous swelling on the presenting part of the head *(caput succenadeum)*, or the formation of the so-called *cephalhematoma*, which is a collection of blood under the periosteum extending to the border of the bone. We open the skull by the BENEKE method (wicker basket method), thus exposing the sinuses and the emissary vessels. The incision is shown on the schematic diagram, as well as the exposure of

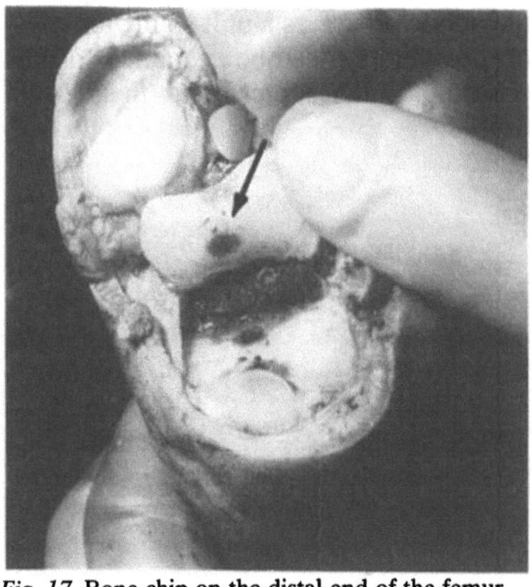

Fig. 17. **Bone chip on the distal end of the femur**

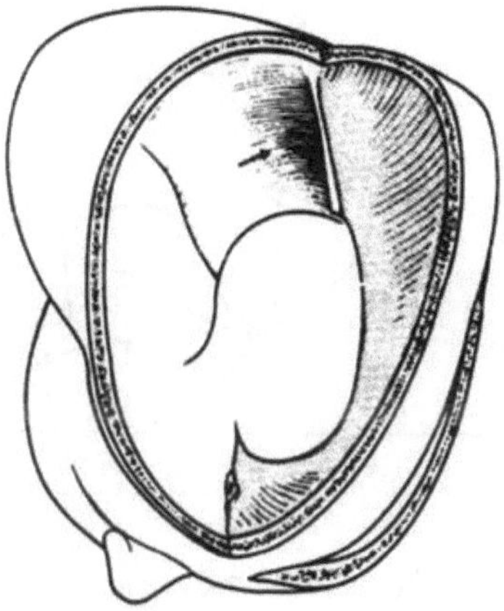

Fig. 18. Opening of the cranium of the newborn and the most common site of injury to the tentorium

the skull bones *(Fig. 18).* After folding back the two parietal bones of the skull, we look at the form of the sinuses and emissary vessels under the cerebral hemispheres by pushing them up, and examine the falx cerebri and the tentorium cerebelli. After a section through the corpus callosum and the cerebral peduncles the cerebral hemispheres can be removed. Again we examine the tentorium cerebelli and note any injuries to it. We open the chest and abdomen with a medial incision branching in a Y-shape at the umbilicus, thus exposing the umbilical vein and enabling us to examine the umbilical arteries as well. Of special significance in the autopsy of the newborn is the *lung* and *gastrointestinal tract air test.* The "lung float" test was first described by RAYGER in 1770 and later adopted into the practice of forensic medicine. The lungs are lifted individually out of the chest and small pieces are incised to see whether they float in water. Following the first breath the weight of the lung is significantly reduced due to the air in the lung tissue, and thus the inflated lung floats. Gas from decaying lung tissue can give a false positive result as can any condition when the density of the lung becomes less than that of water, such as inhalation of a large quantity of vernix caseosa. We obtain a positive float test if we fix the lung with alcohol first. A frozen lung also gives a false positive. In the examination of the thoracic organs of the newborn we must look for Botallo's duct (ductus arteriosus) and test for patency of the foramen ovale. The gastrointestinal air content test indicates the length of time the live-birth newborn survived, since the infant, while taking the first breath, will also swallow air, and this is the explanation of now air gets into the gastrointestinal tract. To the estimate the presence of the air in the stomach the organ must be tied off at the cardia and pylorus and then removed for the float test, after which the stomach contents are examined which in many cases provides evidence of prior breathing and swallowing movement (inhalation or swallowing of meconium). The air content of the small intestine can verify the amount of time the baby lived after birth, as air arrives in the small intestine of the newborn after six hours and into the large intestine by 12 hours *(Fig. 19).* (Naturally, the processes of decay render the results meaningless. These processes can be indicated if in the small intestine the air containing sections of the small intestine alternate with the airless ones.) The course of destruction of the fetal red blood cells can give information the question of how long the infant lived in the consequences of the so-called urate infarct appearing in the kidney tissue, in that for two weeks after birth in the medullary part of the kidney parallel golden yellow streaks appear.

In the autopsy of the victims of *traffic accidents,* the external examination must be conducted with care. We search for such marks in the hairy and bare areas of the body which were left by the colliding vehicle. The so-called primary effect im-

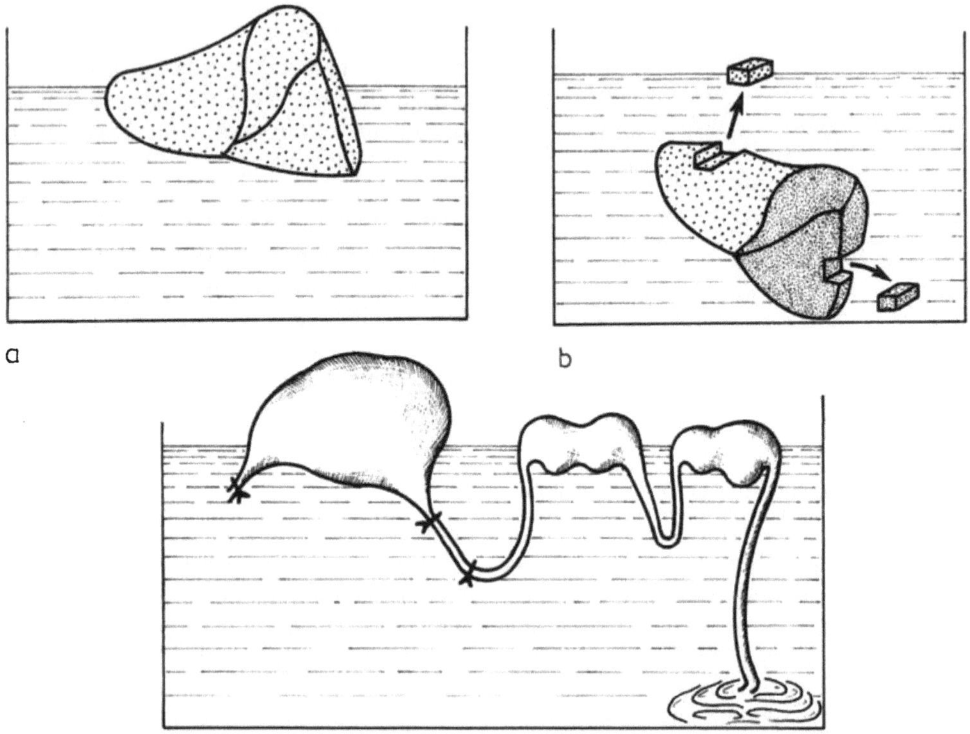

Fig. 19. Schematic drawing of the float test for the lungs and gastrointestinal tract

pression of the colliding vehicle leaves a sign of initial impact on the injured person and can provide relevant informations for the expert as to the type of vehicle. In *the place of the primary impact,* which is generally caused by the foremost protruding part of the vehicle, we can expect serious soft tissue injuries and fractures, and in the case of a fast, powerful hit the bones show a characteristic fracture, the so-called *wedge fracture,* which also indicates the direction of the impact. Following the primary impact, other alterations to the injured person come about which partially form bruises in the direction of the hit and abrasions are seen. These injuries occasionally form *characteristic impressions* (pattern of tyre), so that a rubber-covered object may leave no surface abrasions, but only damaged subcutaneous connective tissue and muscle tissue with hemorrhages at the site of the injury. For this reason in the case of traffic accidents it is necessary to search the soft tissues of the back for suffused hemorrhage during the autopsy. In traffic accident cases, it is also necessary to record the distance of the injury from the plane of the sole of the foot, whether it is the primary place of impact or other secondary forms of injury. Injuries due to traffic accidents consist largely of injuries to the extremities and facial protrusions.

Precise recording of the external injuries is the goal in *strangulation-type deaths* (hanging, garotting, manual choking). The description of the hanging mark left by the noose or the strangler's cord, its direction, and the signs of prolonged hypoxia in the case of manual strangulation are to be given. Such injuries leave internal hemorrhages in the area of the application of force, and we modify the dissection technique to better demonstrate the injuries. We look for hemorrhages in the soft tissues under the marks found on the neck, but as a precaution (during autopsy postmortal bleeding can infiltrate the soft tissue areas) we first remove the brain and heart so the vessels of the neck will drain and not cause postmortal hemorrhage. We dissect the cervical fascia, platysma of the neck in a layered fashion. This means that, after peeling back the skin of the neck, we examine the subperiosteal areas at the insertion of the sternocleidomastoid at the clavicle. In hanging we will find here an infiltration of blood. We prepare the superficial and deep muscle layer of the neck, and the carotid sheath, dissect out; the superior horn of the thyroid cartilage, the thyroid cartilage, removing from it the thyroid gland and the small muscles lying over it. We prepare the hyoid bone, seeking fractures which are identified by hemorrhages of the tissue surrounding it (sometimes the hyoid may be naturally moveable, and this should not be mistaken for an injury). Then we examine the processes of the thyroid cartilage for integrity, together with the joints of the larynx: the cricopharyngeal joint and the cricoarytenoid joint. In the case of an application of a strong force to the neck, we will find hemorrhages in these joints and their capsules. In the preparation of the soft tissues of the neck, we may find fine, parallel, transverse-lying ruptures in the intima of the common carotid artery perpendicular to the long axis of the vessel as it found in the case of hangings. This is the so-called *Amussat sign.* In cases where the nose and mouth are grasped, many times we find no external marks, but the loose connective tissue of the face and the periosteum of the facial bones may contain small or large hemorrhages. It is therefore necessary to peel back the skin of the face in the areas around the soft tissues of the face, namely the nose and the mouth to find hemorrhage in the muscle tissue and under the periosteum.

In *drowning,* fresh water gets into the pulmonary circulation and dilutes the blood feeding into the left side of the heart. One of the signs of drowning is a difference in the concentration of the blood between the right and left side of the hearts which we purposely check in these cases by measuring the dry weight content of the blood.

In the case of *gunshot wounds* the special autopsy technique begins the external examination. During the external examination we must determine, as much as possible, which is the *entry wound* and which is the *exit wound.* The distances of both the entry and exit wounds must be measured from the plane of the sole and from the midline, which will give us coordinates of the entry and exit wounds and, in the ideal case, provide the direction of the path of the projectile. In gunshot, as well as stab injuries, we uncover the wounds in layers while describing the characteristics of the *projectile path* (occasionally in the initial portion of the path, we discover relevant parts of the burned and unburned powder particles, gases or at other times the presence of material from the external environment helps to indicate the projectile's entrance). We describe the direction of the path of the projectile (in gunshot wounds the early straight part of the projectile's entry indicates the direction of the shot). In cases of wounds caused by a projectile remaining in the body, we must take care in searching for it. The entry point in a flat bone can reveal the diameter of the projectile, and we must preserve this mark before continuing our search.

The *age of the injuries* is relevant from the standpoint of determining a sequence of events. For this reason histological examinations are indispensable.

"Apart from total dissection of all three body cavities (head, chest and abdomen), it should comprise all additional forms of examination (X-ray, normal photography, special photography, microscopy, histology, histochemistry, odontology, hematology, serology, chemistry, toxicology etc.) which will bring the causes and circumstances of death to light and which may reconstitute a chain of events leading to death."

The scene of the crime

The scene of the crime is the locus where a significant illegal act has taken place. Procedures connected with the scene of the crime are fixed in Hungarian Law under Criminal Procedures "Examination of a scene of a crime warranted if to prove or to deduce facts it is necessary to inspect individuals, objects or places." The tools for gathering evidence at the scene of the crime occupy a relevant place, providing a means of systematically uncovering and discovering material proof. It follows that all the surroundings at the scene must be recorded in detail, if possible and necessary, photographed, or sketched, and material evidence must be searched for and collected. The purpose is to reconstruct the crime from the characteristics of the scene and examination of the related alterations. In connection with the scene of the crime PUSZTAI writes that unavoidable changes in the original state of the scene come about due to necessary investigations, and no matter how well the scene is reconstructed, it can never be restored to its original state, but occasionally from the undestroyed lasting signs, for example blood drops, the scene can be recognized.

The examination of the scene of a crime must be mentioned to medical students, since with events at a scene involving especially crimes against the life, it is a physician who is usually the first to arrive. In the work related to the scene of the crime, the actions of the physician can decisively influence the examinations.

The criminal proceedings in connection with the scene show that in the case when personal investigation may be necessary in the search for evidence of injuries, the scene must also be examined. A personal examination is performed if such injuries occur as a result of crime, which understanding of the originating mechanism by examination the severity of the injury can be given.

A personal examination occurs within the coroner's inquest at the scene as well, the recording of which doesn't differ from the coroner's inquest proceedings, and the coroner's inquest the scene of the crime includes its essential elements. In connection with this the opinion of VEDRES can be raised: "The examination of the body at the scene of a murder plays a special part."

The tasks of those taking part in the investigation of the scene of the crime are well-defined. Among the permanent *committee members* besides the investigators are criminal technicians and recording investigators, while among the occasional members forensic pathologists most commonly play a role. According to the opinion of some experts, the committee which investigates scenes of crimes against life should have medical specialists as permanent members, and this especially emphasizes the value of the forensic specialist, whose special knowledge can provide help from time to time in uncovering evidence. The involvement of the specialist is purposeful from the start of the investigation in that only such questions are taken up in this stage which are related to his special area of knowledge. In crimes against life it is very important whether a specialist with little practical experience takes part in the investigation at the scene of the crime. Later, technical blunders originating from inexperience are practically irreparable. From the above it is obvious that the work of those investigating the scene of the crime must be that of a team, where everyone knows his responsibilities and only with the harmonizing of assignments can satisfactory results be achieved.

Among the events at the scene we can differentiate single location crimes. These are where events begin and end at one place.

With multiple location crimes, the start, progress and finish of the act cover more than one locus and the investigation schedule can give valuable insight with each phase at the appropriate scene.

● (A body burned beyond recognition was found on the outskirts of Debrecen at the edge of a harvested wheat field. At autopsy an extensive injury caused by a blunt instrument was found in the area of the neck with lacerations of the entrance to the throat and injury of the thyroid cartilage. The injuries were characteristic of a karate blow. The corpse resembled the body of a man about 25 years old. The time of death, based on the contents of the stomach had occurred within an hour of his last meal. Later investigations verified that the victim had been attacked by two karate assailants Budapest, who had transported the corpse from the primary scene of the crime to Debrecen in the trunk of a car, and at the second locus of the crime had poured gasoline over the body to burn it. In identification of the victim, dental examination played an important role as the victims teeth were X-rayed and identification was made on the basis of comparison with previous dental records).

As previously mentioned, the practical work of the physician starts when he is notified of the occurrence of a crime against life, and in many cases is the first to arrive on the scene. The preservation of the scene and the preservation of the original state is not the responsibility of the practicing physician. This belongs to the law enforcement authorities. Nevertheless, it is a great help if he can prevent significant alterations of the scene of the crime until the police or the committee arrives.

(Following a rape case the doctor who had been summoned to the scene cleaned it up so well that he also destroyed so many traces that the eventual capture of the perpetrator of the crime was made almost impossible)

The performance of the duties of the physician after arrival at the scene should be limited to treating the injured, inasmuch as that is possible, and if it is necessary to alter things at the scene, it should be made known by the members of the committee. If death has occurred, only the most essential examinations are applied to the victim and in no case are they to exceed the scope of their practice.

The examination of a scene of the crime is divided into two parts. At first in the static phase it is the responsibility of the committee to get oriented to the scene without disturbing it, to record the data of the scene, including those signs and information that would help in the reconstruction of either the crime or the scene.

DERI in his Handbook of Criminology writes concerning the static phase: "By investigation of the scene of the crime in the appropriate manner information can be gathered concerning the conduct of the crime and its perpetrator.

Thus: This gathered information may given an idea as to:
whether the place was familiar to the perpetrator (the place of entry and exit and the line of approach),
whether the perpetrator knew the victim,
what was the perpetrator's physical condition,
what was his modus operandi,
what were the criminal motives, when did the crime take place,
what was the target of the attack,
who changed or set up the scene?"

The answer to these questions can provide information about the period the time took place, the means by which it was accomplished, and sometimes the identity of the perpetrator.

Answering these questions in some cases lies within the responsibility of the special forensic medical expert. From the information given by the location of the injuries, their number and character, we may deduce the physical characteristics of the perpetrator. The determination of the time of death lies squarely within the field of the medical specialist. It is inadequate, if it was not attempted to try to deduce the time of death at the scene, and to raise the question days later at the autopsy. When untangling the data of the signs of death, the longer we delay in dealing with them, the harder it becomes to establish an accurate time of death.

The character and location of the injuries in numerous instances can mislead even those experts in criminology who do not personally take part in the practical work, thus the evaluation of particularly seldom occurring cases of suicide occupy the greater part of the medical specialist's time and care. (The scene of a combination suicide with numerous injuries and wide-spread splattering of blood can mislead not only the examiner, but even the most experienced practicing specialist as well.)

● (The body of a 52-year-old woman was found in her apartment. She was lying in her room in a pool of blood around which were claw marks. At the edge of the pool was a hatchet. Numerous injuries – hacking wounds to the head, cuts to the legs and a stab to the left side of the thorax – led the police to consider murder. Hacking wounds to the head are rare in cases of suicide, and about 100 hacking injuries penetrating the scalp and reaching the lamina externa of the skull were found. Old scars were also found on the scalp. Such wounds are often inflicted by the sufferers of trigeminal neuralgia on themselves to relieve the excruciating headaches. According to the testimony of a brother, his sister had suffered attacks from childhood, and at these times used to hit her head with a hatchet. We found these marks. This so-called combination suicide can often leave the impression of a murder both to the investigators and the doctor).

The *dynamic phase* of the examination follows the static phase at the scene of the crime. This means that the objects found at the scene must be examined. In this phase the responsibility of the committee is to evaluate and put into logical order the evidence found. Here the entrance of the medical specialist into the committee takes on significance in that with crimes against life the examination of the corpse, the recording of the injuries, the examination of the clothing from the standpoint of information sheds essential light.

Likewise the responsibility of the medical specialist includes among other things the so-called search for biological signs and to confirm further examinations. We must search for blood at the scene. The place and form of the blood stains may indicate whether the victim suffered the injuries at the same place at which the body was found. The forensic pathologist may look for blood stains around the body, on the furniture and not rarely on the wall and ceiling as well. He must examine the quantity of blood and the form of blood stains. The forms may be drops, depending on distances others likened to exclamation marks and smears.

We must seek secretions. These include looking for remnants of saliva, semen and feces, examining them and ensuring future examination. Occasionally human remains and parts of tissues must be sought from under the fingernails which may result from a struggle, the examination of which modern equipment can serve to shed significant light. Especially in the pursuit of injury to the newborn, we must deal with the examination of the amnion, meconium and fetal membranes, placenta etc. It is important that hair found in the vicinity of the corpse be collected and packaged in the appropriate manner.

In certain crimes we may find it necessary to employ other specialists. In these instances, the collection of the team of experts may be drawn from several disciplines. Thus at the scene of traffic accidents, the auto mechanic may work side by side with the medical specialist, and a weapons expert is indispensable in gunshot wounds.

References

[1] Assemblée parlementaire. N de l'Europe (Report on the harmonization of autopsy rules – Morris) Doc. 6332

[2] Berg, S., G. Bode, L. Sekardi: Radiochemische Untersuchungen über den Verwendungsstoffwechsel von Leichenhaut in der Supravitalphase. Beitr. z. Gericht. Med. XXXII, (1974) 280–285

[3] Boglioli, L. R., M. L. Taff: Religious objection to autopsy. An ethical dilemma for medical examiners. Am. J. Forensic Med. Pathol. 11, (1990) 1–8

[4] Brown, A., T. K. Marshal: Body temperature as a means of estimating the time of death. Forensic Sci. 4, (1974) 125–133

[5] Davis, J. H.: Gastric emptying time. Am. J. Forensic Med. Pathol. 10, (1989) 271–272

[6] Déri, P.: A helyszíni szemle. Kriminalisztika BM, Bp. (1961) 329–411

[7] Fernando, R.: Medical certification of cause of death in the General Hospital, Colombo. Ceylon Med. J. 35, (1990) 71–74

[8] Földes, V., Harsányi, L.: Kihantolással bizonyított közlekedési baleset. Morph. és Ig. Orv. Szemle 7, (1967) 150–152

[9] Földes, V.: Orvosszakértők szerepe a helyszíni szemlén. BM kiadvány (1972)

[10] Gantner, G. E.: The autopsy and the law. Am. J. Clin. Path. 69, (1978) 235–237

[11] Green, M. A., J. C. Wright: Postmortem interval estimation from body temperature data only. Forensic Sci. Int. 28, (1985) 35–46

[12] Green, M. A., J. C. Wright: The theoretical aspects of the time dependent Z equation as e means of postmortem interval estimation using body temperature data only. Forensic Sci Int. 28, (1985) 53–62

[13] Hansen, J. P., J. Meldgaard, J. Nordquist: Mummies of Qilakitsoq. National Geographic 167, (1985) 191–207

[14] Hegarty, P. V. J., J. J. A. Heffron: Partial reversal by adenosine triphosphate of the rigorinduced decrease in the diameter of skeletal

muscle fibres. Comp. Biochem. Physiol., 50A, (1975) 675–680
[15] HENSSGE, C., B. BRINKMANN, K. PÜSCHEL: Todeszeitsbestimmung durch Messung der Rektaltemperatur bei Wassersuspension der Leiche. Z. Rechtsmed. 92, (1984) 255–276
[16] HENSSGE, C.: Death time estimation in case work I. The rectal temperature time of death nomogram. Forensic Sci. Int. 38, (1988) 209–236
[17] HENSSGE, C., R. FREKERS, R. BECKMANN, E. R. BECKMANN: Todeszeitbestimmung auf der Basis simultaner Messung von Hirn- und Rektaltemperatur. Z. Rechtsmed. 93, (1984) 123–133
[18] IWASA, Y., T. ONAYA: Postmortem changes in the level of calcium pumping adenosine triphosphatase in rat heart sarcoplasmic reticulum. Forensic Sci. Int. 39, (1988) 13–22
[19] JAFFE, F. A.: Stomach contents and the time of death reexamination of a persistent question. Am. J. Forensic Med. Pathol. 10, (1989) 37–41
[20] JASTREMSKI, M., D. POWNER, J. SNYDER, J. SMITH, A. Grenvik: Problems in brain death determination. Forensic Sci. 11, (1978) 201–212
[21] KATSUMATA, Y., K. SATO, S. YADA: Green pigment in epidermal blisters of decomposed cadavers. Forensic Sci. Int. 28, (1985) 167–174
[22] KNIGHT, B.: A comparative survey of the medico-legal aspects of death in Europe. Med. Law 2, (1983) 137–156
[23] KROMPECHER, T., O. FRYC: Experimentelle Untersuchungen an der Leichenstarre. Beitr. Gerichtl. Med., 36, (1978) 345–349
[24] KROMPECHER, T., O. FRYC: Experimental evaluation of rigor mortis III. Comparative study of the evolution of rigor mortis in different sized muscle groups in rats. Forensic Sci. Int. 12, (1978) 97–102
[25] KROMPECHER, T., O. FRYC: Experimental evaluation of rigor mortis IV. change in strength and evolution of rigor mortis in the case of physical exercise preceding death. Forensic Sci. Int. 12, (1978) 103–107
[26] MALAGELADA, J. R., G. F. LONGSTRETH, W. H. J. SUMMERSKILL, V. L. W. Go: Gastroenterology, 70, (1976) 203–210
[27] MARSHALL, T. K.: The use of the cooling formula in the study of postmortem body cooling. J. Forensic Sci. 7, (1962) 189–210
[28] MARSHALL, T. K., F. E. HOARE: Estimating the time of death The rectal cooling after death and its mathematical expression. J. Forensic Sci. 7, (1962) 58–81
[29] MARSHALL T. K.: The use of body temperature in estimating the time of death. J. Forensic Sci. 7, (1962) 211–221
[30] MINIMI, H., R. W. MCCALLUM: The physiology and pathophysiology of gastric emptying in Humans. Gastroenterology 86, (1984) 1592–1610
[31] MOLNÁR, L.: The death of the brain and the CSF. In: Meyer J. S., H. Lechner, M. Reivich, O. Eichhorn: Cerebral Vascular Disease. G. Thieme Publ. Stuttgart (1973) 192–196
[32] MOLNÁR, L., L. CSIBA: Changes in composition of cerebrospinal fluid and cytoplasmic NADH/NADU+ ratio of stroke patients during agony and after death. Luxury oxygenation of the brain. In: Meyer J. S., H. Lechner, M. Reivich, E. O. Ott, A. Aranibar: Cerebral Vascular Disease 3 Excerpta Med. Amsterdam, (1981) 187–192
[33] NOKES, L. D. M., B. HICKS, B. H. KNIGHT: The post-mortem temperature plateau-factor fiction? Med. Sci. Law 25, (1985) 263–264
[34] NOKES, L. D. M., B. HICKS, B. KNIGHT: The use of trachea temperature as a means of determining the post-mortem period. Med. Sci. Law 26, (1986) 199–202
[35] PÁSZTOR, E.: Az agy akut sérülései. Ideggyógyászati Szemle 29, (1976) 484–497
[36] ROSSI S., D. REALE, E. GRANDI: Correlation of clinical diagnosis with autopsy findings. IARC Sci. Publ. 112, (1991) 99–108
[37] SCHRANZ, D.: A legyek jelentősége törvényszéki orvosi szempontból. Orvosi Hetilap 78, (1934) 716–719)
[38] SEELYE, R. N., T. J. NEVALAINEN, J. B. GAVIN, V. J. WEBSTER: Physical and biochemical changes in rigor mortis of cardiac muscle. Biochem. Med. 21, (1979) 323–332
[39] SOMOGYI, E., SZUCHOVSZKY, Gy.: Fekvőbeteggyógyintézetben elhaltak hatósági boncolásáról. Orvosi Hetilap 107, (1966) 75–78
[40] SOMOGYI, E., SZUCHOVSZKY, Gy.: Az orvos halottkém eljárása rendkívüli halál esetén. Medicus Univ. II/6, (1969) 13–16
[41] SUGIYAMA T., T. FUJIMORI, S. MAEDA: Autopsy rates in medical schools and hospitals in Japan IARC Sci. Publ. 112, (1991) 245–252
[42] TAKATORI, T., A. YAMAOKA: The mechanism of adipocere formation. Forensic Sci. 9, (1977) 63–73
[43] TAKATORI, T., N. ISHIGURO, H. TARAO, H. MATSUMIYA: Microbiol production of hydroxy and oxo fatty acids by several microorganismus as a model of adipocere formation. Forensic Sci. Int. 32, (1986) 5–11
[44] VOORDE, H., P. J. VAN DIJK: Determination of the time of death by fungal growth. Z. Rechtsmed. 89, (1982) 75–80
[45] WEBB, P. A., H. J. TERRY, D. J. GEE: A method for time of death determination using ultrasound. J. Forensic Sci. Soc. 26, (1986) 393–399

Chapter 2
Types of injuries

Injuries to tissues can bring about such alterations which, from tissue to tissue, or with temporary or permanent damage to organ function can cause anatomically related changes. It can interrupt tissue continuity – at the sides of the wound – or deficit of material, in which a part is more or less destroyed (gunshot, explosion) or removed from the area (bite or tear wounds).

The largest group of injuries consist of those cases in which the practical occurrences in forensic and clinical medicine overlap. Their categorization and description can determine, or make possible the later identification of, the mode of origin, the amount of applied force and the detection of the instrument used. Indeed, expert medical knowledge can be applied in the examination to answer questions of any kind. It is not by accident that the description of the injury, the occasional identification of the instrument used, the determination of whether the injury was self-inflicted or by another, and the differentiation between injuries occurring in life or postmortally make up the greater part of every book on forensic medicine.

The complete knowledge of the characteristics of the various types of injuries is not only the obligation of the forensic medical specialist, but of every physician who deals with injuries. With injuries found on the living body, and much more so on the dead one, the preparation of scaled photographs lends great help in their analysis. This is not only a job for the

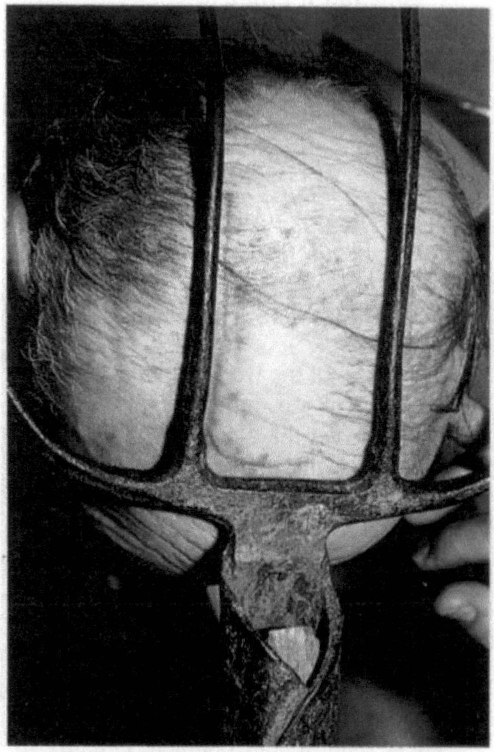

Fig. 20. Comparison of the injuries with the instrument. The course of the scar matches the imprint of the instrument

criminal technician, but for one who is familiar with the signs of injury, a well-trained forensic pathologist or at least an experienced photographer *(Fig. 20)*. (In numerous instances we have seen a criminal technician take insufficient picture with a wide-angle lens in which the injury could not be made out at all. The work of a good criminal photographer requires lots of practice, and even with this the description of the injuries requires certain special forensic medical experience).

The examination of the injuries must settle:

1. The type of injury – continuity-interruption or missing material.
2. What caused it, and with what force?
3. How did it originate?
4. Whether it is self-inflicted or by another?
5. Whether a lethal condition resulted?
6. To what extent had the wound healed?
7. Did the alteration occur in life?

In characterization of the injury, the components of the wound must be described (Fig. 21).

The *dimensions* of the wound: length, width

The *shape* of the wound: sharp, uneven, undercut, covered, indented

The *edges* of the wound: singular, multiple, sharp, dull, uneven (slipped crease)

The *side* of the wound: smooth, bulging, uneven, undercut, bridged by connective tissue

The *base* of the wound: the wound's deepest

The *area* surrounding the a, dirtied, swollen.

These data appear characteristically in certain injuries and if we describe the characteristics of the wound sufficiently.

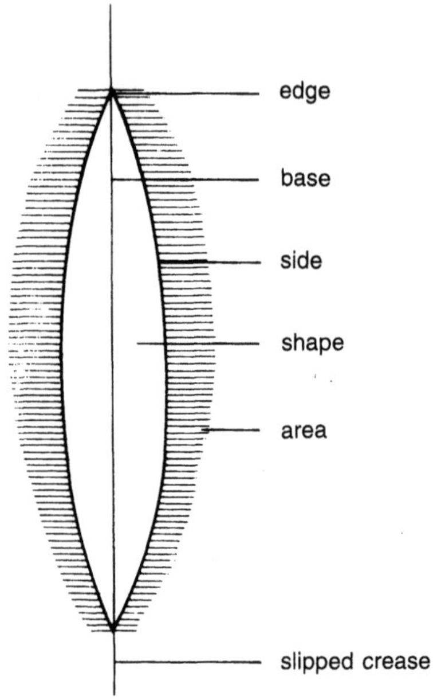

Fig. 21. Parts of the wound

We can conclude later correctly nature of the wounds but the insufficient data will make it impossible.

The categories into which an injury can be placed include:

1. incising injuries
2. stab wounds
3. hacking injuries
4. alterations caused by blunt instruments
5. traffic accidents
6. electric injuries
7. gunshot wounds
8. heat-induced injuries

Incising injuries

The effect of a sharp-edged instrument comes about by moving the edge over material along the direction of its axis.

Among the small cutting angled instruments, the knife, razor, and a piece of glass, or the characteristic form of toothed instruments, i.e. saw, may cause characteristic effects. (Under the *sharp edge* we usually find a fine angle of the sides, in that the finer the cutting angle of the instrument, the less it lacerates.)

In incising wounds the greatest expanse of the *injury* is its *length*, the alteration depending on the region of the body, and the extent of separation by the cutting line in relation to the cleavage plane of the skin, but this gap must not be mistaken for missing material, if the sides of the wound can be realigned together perfectly. The *edges* at the ends of the wound are sharp. From the ends of the wound, depending on how fast the instrument sank into the soft tissues and how fast it came out, laceration can result, resulting in the so-called *"skid mark"*, from which the start of the injury cannot be exactly discerned. The *shapes* of the wound are cut sharply. If the instrument was not dirty, the shape of the wound is usually raised, and if it was dirty we find bits of the material wiped off in the sides of the wound. The *base* of the wound is sharply cut, more or less in a V-shape. Whereas fatty tissue bulges in a little, muscle tissue retracts and pulls the sides away.

The single effect of force usually leaves one angle at each end of a wound (an attack on well-wrinkled skin or when the skin becomes folded under the instrument may leave several wound angles), and with multiple attacks, if not done in the place of the previous injury, or into the base of the wound, or at its end, the number of attacks can be easily seen. The area containing the most cut ends suggests the minimal application of force, or if we find on the base of the wound multiple injuries, that will also show the number of thrusts.

Among the characteristic forms of the incised wound, that is caused by an uneven edged instrument, for example a wound caused by a saw, where the wound angle and sides are finely indented and uneven, the teeth of the saw cause an abraded border which becomes dry and brownish over time and this can be characteristic of the instrument used. Likewise the form of the lobulated cut is unique, where the cutting instrument digs under the edge detaching the soft tissues from their base. The components of the cut correspond to those mentioned above, a small cutting angled instrument showing a characteristic finely elevated wound angle, sharp edges and a visible wall. These kind of cuts can always be seen with attacks to protruding parts of the body, like the ear or nose.

The results of the attack depend on the sharpness and cutting plane of the instrument used. Sharp, fine-angled instruments can cause a deep incision with little force, while the alterations caused by a cut on the bone is caused by a stronger effect.

Incising wounds can cause profuse bleeding, especially if the incised vessel is cut only partly and can not retract.

Incising wounds make up a significant percentage of cases examined. It must also be decided whether they are self-inflicted or by someone else. The appearance of wounds in the places that have a so-called predilection for self-inflicted wounds, that is, where such wounds commonly occur, such as the wrist, the crook of the elbow and the region of the neck, helps us to judge their origin. Around the wounds we find *tentative marks* extending from superficial scratches to the deeper injuries parallel to each other, which originate from trial of the instrument *(Fig. 22)*.

The unique form of the so-called *self-defense type* of alterations, in which the victim grabbed the stab-cutting instrument, appears as multiple, deep incis-

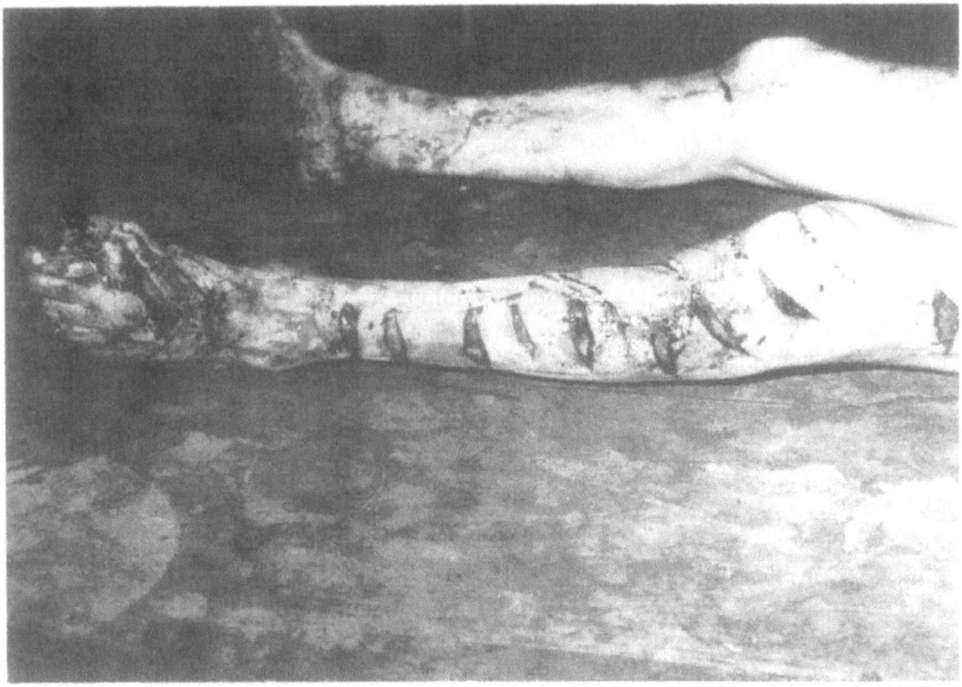

Fig. 22. Unusually placed self-inflicted incision injuries

ing wounds to the palms. Cuts to the palms can usually be accepted as self-defense type wounds.

Incising wounds cause only shallow damage to the surrounding tissue and tend to heal well. If a superficial incision is treated by primary intention, it heals within eight days. Injuries to nerves, tendons and ligaments or deeper injuries naturally take more time to heal, and in these cases the factors affecting the healing must be taken into account during the examination.

Differentiating between wounds to the neck that are self-inflicted or inflicted by others is not an easy task. We may also see multiple neck cuts resulting from attack, however, these are more likely to be deep, cutting the windpipe or the tracheal cartilages and often reaching the cervical vertebrae. In self-inflicted wounds we rarely find injuries that serious. The direction of lie of the incisions to the neck is not unambiguous. The idea that with self-inflicted wounds the right-handed assailant places the corner of the cut higher on the left side cannot be generally accepted. In a significant portion of cases, self-inflicted cuts to the neck do indeed start higher on one side and end lower on the other, but the existence of a horizontal cut doesn't argue against self-inflicted alterations. Air embolism is a common complication of incisions to the neck which open the veins. In other cases, in especially deep cuts as usually caused by an assailant, severe drainage of blood can result, which occurs in wrist or elbow cuts after a longer period of time. The injured person may keep activity and self defence capability for a longer period. The prognosis in a cut to the neck is always du-

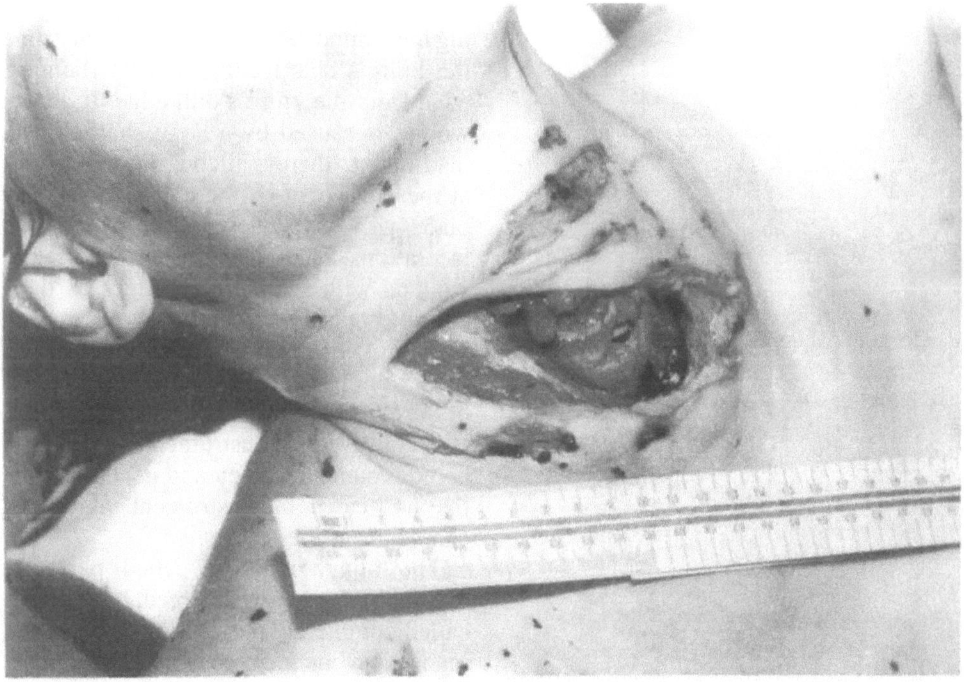

Fig. 23. Multiple homicidal incision injuries to the neck

bious. The practicing physician is not able to judge the seriousness of the wound, and therefore must send the victim to the hospital for the treatment of the severed deep neck vessels that may be there, or for other appropriate care *(Fig. 23).*

- A 25-year-old lady suffered a cut to the neck region. The general practitioner bandaged it and sent her home without further examination. The following morning the victim died. The cause of death was an incising injury to a vessel feeding the thyroid and the resultant bleeding to death.

In incising wounds, *the identification of the instrument* can only be carried out in the cases where some bits of dirt carried by the instrument are left in the wound, or when parts of the instrument break off and remain in it.

The *cause of death* may be haemorrhage on account of the injuries of arteries. In other cases the injuries of the neck may result air embolism, due to injuries of great veins.

Stab wounds

The stab wound is caused by an instrument with a pointed ends. The *impact force of the attack* follows the axis of the instrument. The character and form of the wound depends on the shape of the instrument used. Dull-pointed, round-bodied instruments – spikes – cause wounds with rounded sides, the wound being formed in part by the effect of withdrawal on the line

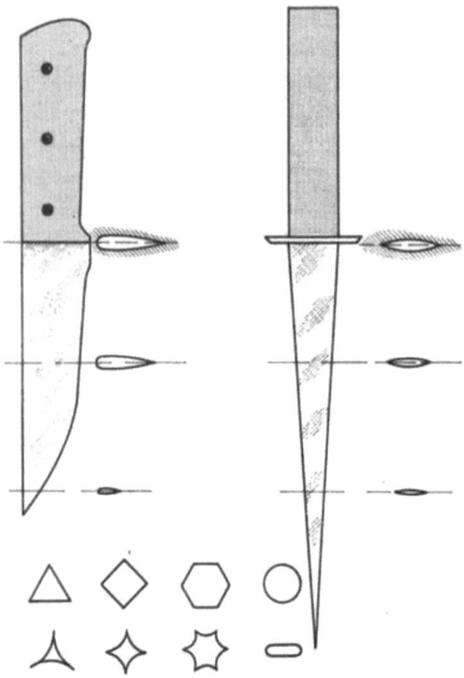

Fig. 24. Schematic drawing of stab injuries comparing the cross-section of the instruments with the visible injuries on the skin

of cleavage of the skin, leaving it gaping a little in a somewhat spindle shape. If the point of the instrument is dull, it first stretches the skin inward causing characteristic abrasion marks around the wound shapes. If the diameter of the instrument was less than 1 mm – hypodermic needle or awl – the wound will form a nearly round discontinuity in which the lines of cleavage of the skin play no role *(Fig. 24).* This must not be mistaken for missing tissue.

A single edged instrument such as a butcher's knife or a pocket knife cause characteristic marks. The unsharpened back of the blade slides against the one end of the cut while the instrument's sharp edge incises the tissue at the other end, cutting the fibers of the skin and giving the wound its single pointed edge from the knife's sharp edge, and its rounded edge from the knife's dull edge. If a stab wound is caused by a large sharp edged instrument, there will be fine abrasions at the edge of it or the extraction of the blade will have caused little superficial lacerations. Two-edged instruments cause wounds with two-pointed edges as they cut in both directions, both edges being sharp. In multiple edged instruments (for example, a sharpened file) the imprint of the edges of the instrument can be seen. With three-edged instruments, three-cornered wounds are seen and depending on the surface of the instrument, abrasions can occur at the shapes.

The injury may be called perforating if a body cavity is pierced, but may be called completely perforating or penetrating if the wounded area is pierced through and an exit wound is caused at the other side.

A characteristic form of the stab wound is the so-called *piercing incision injury.* The piercing incision injury is caused by the application of two separate forces, one due to the turning of the instrument or the victim, and the other due to the instrument being pulled out causing another wound, which is in general butterfly shaped *(Fig. 25, 26)* in which the back of the instrument forms the rounded wound wall and edges of both the entry wound and the extraction wound are sharp.

With stab wounds, the length of the break in continuity reveals the width of the blade. The length of the break in continuity is at least as long as the blade is wide, the length of the wound depending on its relationship to the skin's line of cleavage. If they are perpendicular, the wound may be a little shorter because of the resistance of the lines of cleavage, and if parallel to them, it may be longer than the width of

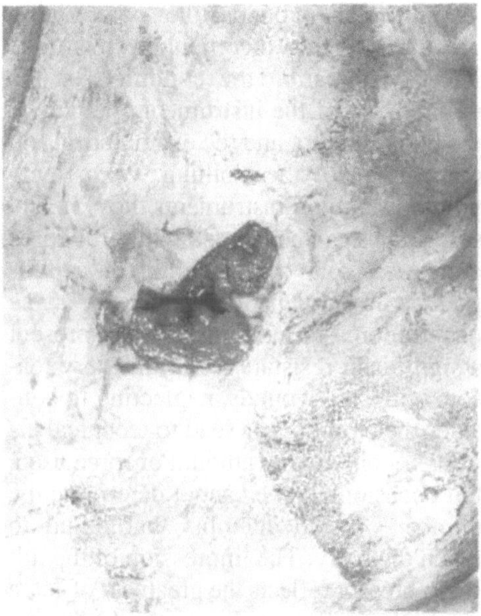

Fig. 25. Stabbing incision injury

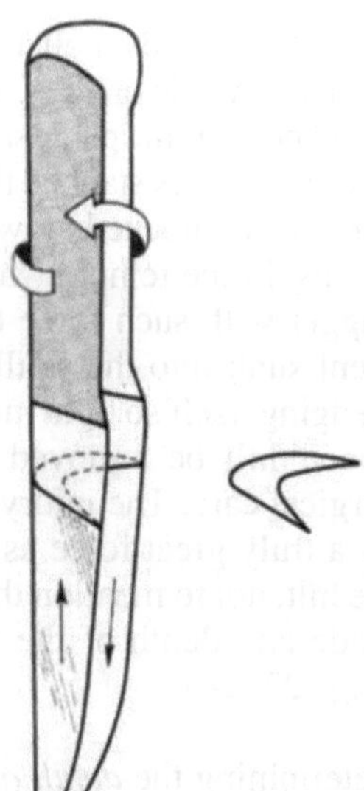

Fig. 26. Schematic drawing of a stabbing incision injury

the blade due to the tendency of the lines of cleavage to pull apart. Usually the stabbing instrument cleaves the soft tissues ahead of its edge and the blade of the instrument causes a wound longer than the blade's width. As already mentioned, the appearance of the walls of the wound depends on the shape of the instrument that caused the wound. Abrasions on the edges or shapes of the wound may appear depending on the surface of the instrument, its sharpness and quality of its point, but we can also count on finding abrasions at the edges or around the injuries if the instrument was applied to the body with great force so that scratch marks are caused on the surface and here the scratches form characteristic abrasions and contusions. With stab wounds into fatty tissues the sides of the wound bulge in and deep wounds are hard to follow.

The base of the wound can be hard to find and the length of the channel of the wound in a living victim may be impossible to determine in many cases.

The marks *caused by scissors* are of a character different from those mentioned so far in that beside the two rounded wound corners, depending on the degree that the blades were apart from each other, an open V-shaped discontinuity is formed with abrasions at the edges.

The stab wound can originate from a direct application of force where the stabbing instrument is plunged straight into the body. It can be caused by any pointed instrument.

● An inebriated 57-year-old man suffered a stab wound to the eye from a burning skewer while roasting bacon. The injury was treated at the ophthalmology department, but due to difficulties in healing, the injured eye became enucleated. The base of the wound for a long time showed signs of healing by second intention and a half a year after discharge from the hospital central nervous system complaints began. He became disturbed and the possibility of a brain tumor suggested itself with the result that he was sent to the department of neurosurgery. The ensuing examinations and tests revealed no tumor, and after a few days of treatment at the clinic, he died. At the autopsy we found a brain abscess on the left side caused by an 8 cm piece of the skewer which had been left inside. The skewer had entered the brain tissue through an injury of the orbital wall and the broken end could be easily felt sprouting on the base of the granulation wound during the autopsy.

Such injuries can be caused by thrown instruments, whether in sports or by other pointed instruments.

- The committee arriving on the scene for the coroner's examination of the body of a 29-year-old man established that the victim had been gathering wood the edge of a forest when he was attacked by an unknown assailant and struck on the forehead with an axe. The inquest revealed that in the right internal orbital wall and the bridge of the nose there was a typical stab wound caused by a two-edged instrument, with the two sharp edges. The wound penetrated into the brain tissue, injured the sinus cavernosus and the victim died of an air embolism. Examination of the vicinity of the scene to determine the origin of the injury then verified that the marks of a pointed instrument could be found on the door of the house, and later it was shown that the inebriated victim had been hit while standing at the target where someone was throwing knives.

With stab wounds the determining greatness of the force applied must take into consideration the condition of the pointed end of the instrument, the part of the body injured, and the examination and comparison of the clothing. With finely pointed stabbing instruments the skin and soft tissues can be pierced with little force compared with that required of a dull-pointed instrument to produce the same penetration. The clothing may also present a significant resistance. For this very reason, with stab wounds, neglecting to consider the clothing can lead to technical errors, not only in the amount of force used, but occasionally we cannot determine the number of stab attempts that failed to reach the body. The impression of the hilt when present reflects the greatness of force used. Wounds that pierce the bones require quite a lot of force, especially if the bone was thick or if the depth of penetration by the blade is conspicuous.

- A 23-year-old police officer was wounded while on duty. The victim was attacked by multiple assailants, and one of the attackers stabbed the victim, who had been knocked down and unconscious, in the temple with a two-edged dagger with such force that the instrument sunk into the skull up to the hilt wedging itself so tight into the sella that it couldn't be removed during neurosurgical care. The injury was produced by a truly great force as the imprint of the hilt, not to mention the length of the blade and depth of the wound, attests *(Fig. 27, 28)*.

Determining the *depth of the wound* in the examination of the corpse is usually an easy task. In the living person to whom surgical care of the wound isn't given in every case, the character, depth and exact description and examination is practically

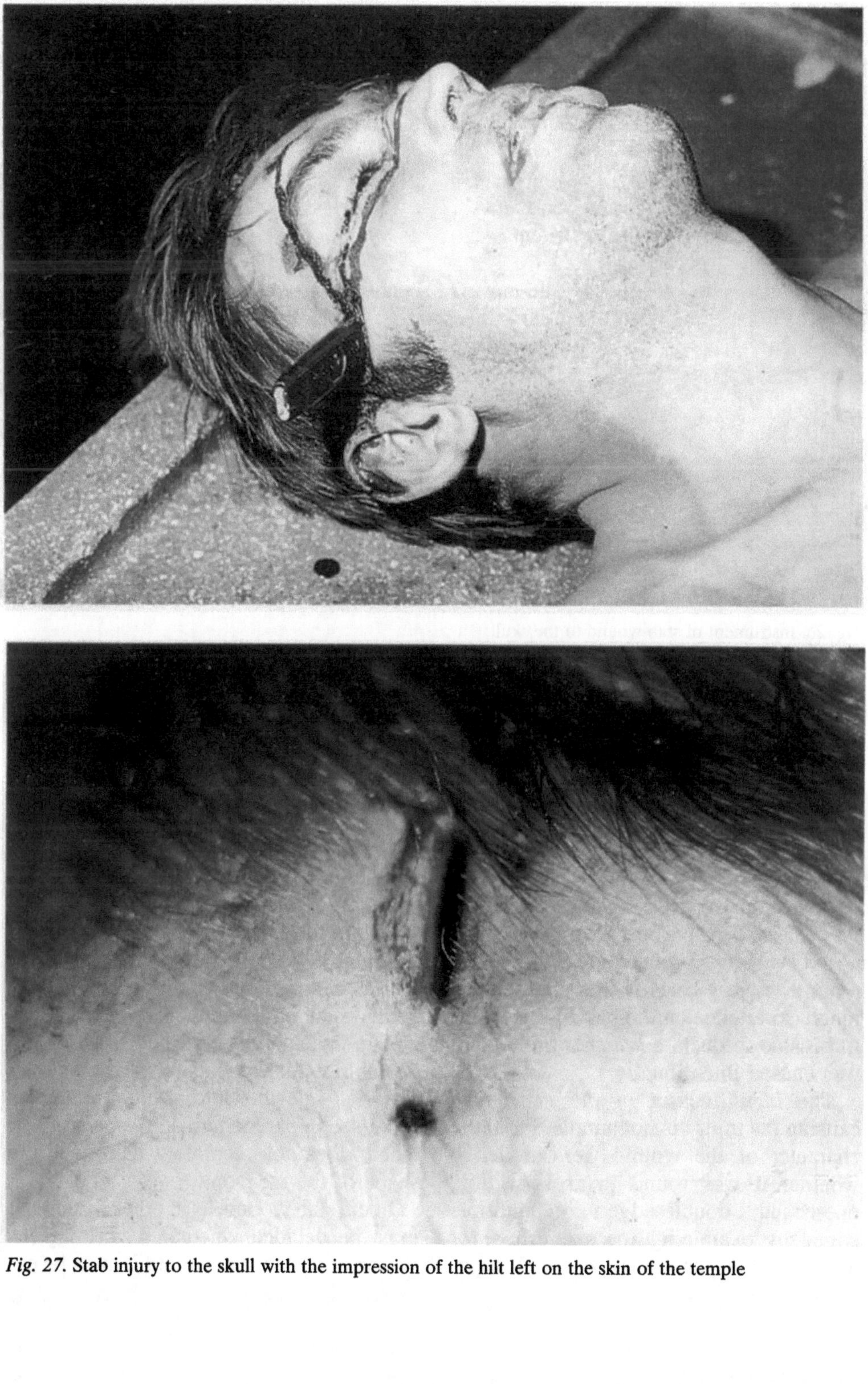

Fig. 27. Stab injury to the skull with the impression of the hilt left on the skin of the temple

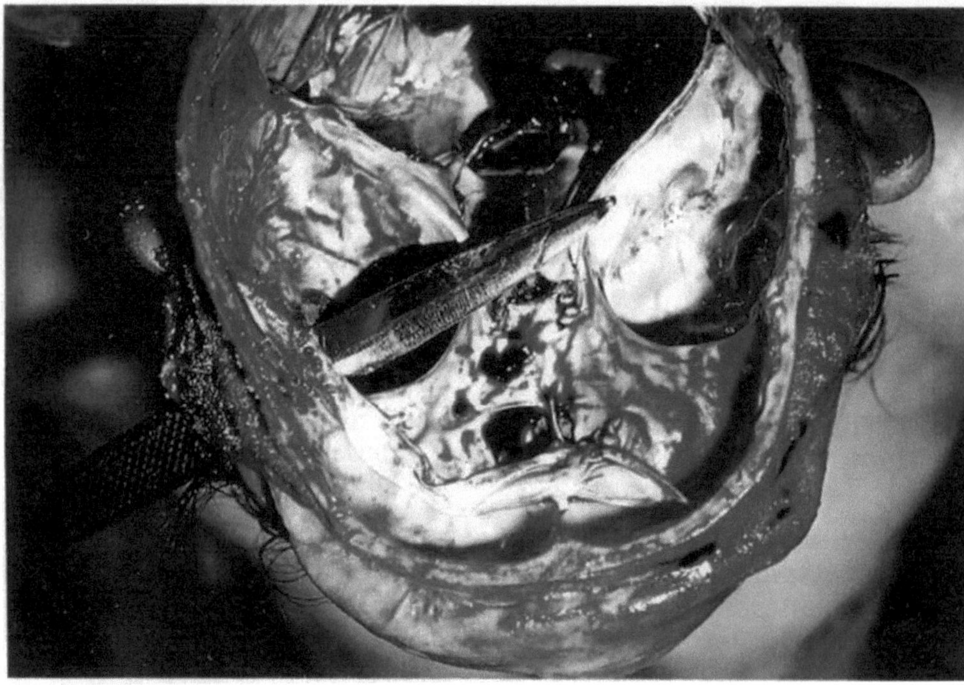

Fig. 28. Instrument of stab wound to the skull

impossible. Especially the stab wounds to the back present diagnostic problem. The missed occult injuries may cause elevated morbidity. With computer tomography increases the diagnostic possibility of the penetrating injury to the back. We have already touched upon the types of stab wounds previously. In numerous instances the question is raised whether the injury was caused by a purposeful movement or not. It is not an easy question to answer. It requires a very careful examination and much experience on the part of the expert to be able to declare whether the wound was caused intentionally.

The *identification of the instrument* causing the injury is not simple. From the character of the wound we can derive whether it was round in cross-section, one-edged, double-edged or multiple edged by examining the size, shape or length of the penetration channel, especially in wounds that pierce the body cavities, but these pieces of information give us little help in identification of the weapon itself. In stab wounds that penetrate bone the identification of the instrument is a little easier in that the width of the blade and perhaps even its edge can be seen and occasionally it can be used in the identification of the instrument. Instrument identification has been tried experimentally in artificially produced stab wounds filled with X-ray contrast material, and is now being used in criminal investigations as well. Our experience in the identification of stabbing instruments by use of contrast material injected into wound channels produced in parenchymal organs has been that it does not accurately reproduce the shape of the weapon.

In the stab wound, as in other wounds, it must be decided whether it was *self-inflicted* or with a stab wound it must be established whether it occurred during life. The self-inflicted injuries have places of predilection to which stabs tend to be directed, such as toward the heart and abdomen. We may find tentative marks, but it doesn't mean any thing in regards to self-infliction if we don't. In these instances we must find so-called "internal tentative marks" in the internal organs in which the instrument caused multiple injuries from being pulled back while an external force was applied. Establishing that a stab wound was self-inflicted may be a gradual revelation as the injured region is uncovered.

- A 24-year-old male while being reated at the dermatological clinic suffered a stab wound to the cardiac area and died in hospital. Because of the character of the wound – the stab wound being made on the cardiac region as a single injury – the possibility of homicide raised itself. The autopsy unequivocally established the wound as self-inflicted in that in the heart, pericardium, the left ventricle areas on the epicardium were found numerous tentative marks along with a stabbing slash which opened widely the right and left ventricles.

Similar cases were also published. Four isolated stab wounds of the heart were examined without other injuries. The differentiation between self inflicted or homicidal injuries was given by autopsy records.

In wounds caused by an assailant multiple injuries can also be found on various parts of the body, and here can be found the characteristic so-called *self defense marks* on the palms from the grabbing the stabbing-slashing instrument *(Fig. 29)*.

The time of healing of the stab wound depends on the location of the wound and its depth. Superficial stab wounds to the extremities, if the depth of the stab channel doesn't necessitate muscle suturing, heals in eight days without complications. The fate and time of healing of stab wounds that open body cavities vary. Most stab wounds are directed into the thoracic or abdominal cavities, and according to the literature, while the possibility of healing of thoracic wounds is considered good – with modern thoracic surgical care stab wounds to the heart have a 76% chance of healing – death from a wound to the abdomen without appropriate treatment was 88%. The opinions of medical specialists concerning the care of wounds opening the body cavities is not unified. In the view of some, the operative care of wounds opening the body cavities should only be performed in the case of unmistakable complications. An abdominal injury raises the concern for peritonitis, thoracic wounds for bleeding or injury to thoracic organs. In the view of others, only superficial abdominal injuries do not require laparotomy. Fullum at all published 100 consecutive cases of stab

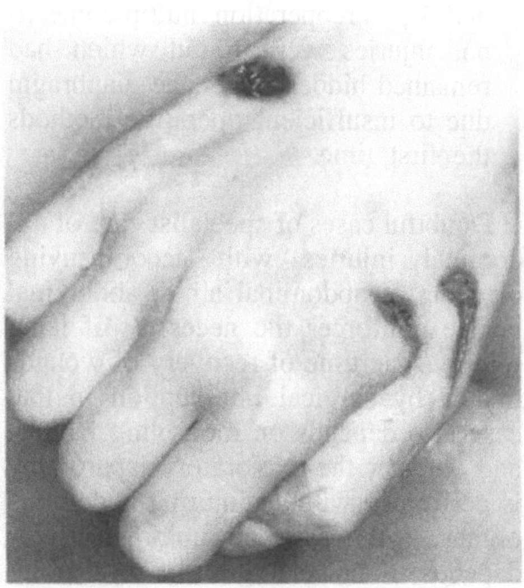

Fig. 29. **Self-defense stab and incision injuries to the hand**

wounds to the chest. 44 patients were treated successfully with tube thoracotomy, 14 required thoracotomy, 17 persons having minor ptx were only observed, and 25 patients were asymptomatic. The overall mortality was 4%, and the operation mortality 7,1%. The accepted position is that abdominal injuries that open the abdominal cavity are an indication for surgery to identify internal injuries.

- A 28-year-old male was admitted to general surgery for a stab wound to the chest and then to the pulmonary surgery clinic because of the presence of thoracic injuries, where upon opening the chest a stab wound piercing the diaphragm was discovered. Exploration of the abdominal injury through a little diaphragmatic incision they revealed that the wound penetrated a few centimeters into the neighboring abdominal structures causing no damage, so they treated the thoracic wound. Twelve hours later the patient developed peritoneal irritation and pronounced symptoms of peritonitis emerged. Upon reoperation multiple intestinal injuries were found which had remained hidden under the diaphragm due to insufficient operative methods the first time.

Doubtful cases of specialist care of abdominal injuries with accompanying bleeding or abdominal air or abdominal lavage reinforces the necessity of laparotomy. The time of recovery of wounds treated by surgical intervention in that case also depends on modifying factors, and whether the exploratory laparotomy is performed without injuring abdominal organs. In this case the time of recovery depends on the healing of the surgical intervention. In thoracoabdominal injuries if organ damage is discovered, it means a serious life-threatening situation. The diagnosis of injuries penetrating the thorax is especially difficult in that case where significant accumulation of thoracic bleeding or air are not found. In some cases an accumulation of as little as 15 ml of fluid in the pericardial sac can be detected by echocardiography. The formation of subcutaneous emphysema can verify a lung injury. Among the influential factors affecting the time of recovery we must not forget the effect adhesions from a healing thoracoabdominal injury have in producing later complaints, or in stab injuries to the cranium, the later complications of aneurysm or carotideo-cavernal fistula.

In the victim's autopsy of a stabing injury the precise location of the wound and its height, which is taken usually from the plane of the sole, and its distance from the midline, is measured. We dissect the stab channel in layers and establish the direction of the attack, and in the area of the channel describe the injuries to the organs we come across, measuring exactly the wound and when possible taking photos of the injuries. The depth of the stab channel can only be determined by dissection. With a stab wound to the abdomen, the depth of the stab channel does not yield the length of the blade in that compressible body parts can show a longer channel than the blade of the knife which caused it.

In the dissection of the stab wound we also surmise the number of thrusts, taking care that rarely one stab may produce two wounds, so a thrust that penetrates the arm may pass on through into the thorax as a continuation of one channel *(Fig. 30)*. From the standpoint of examination of the clothing, we have mentioned that not only the origin, but the greatness of the force, causing the injuries and the number of the thrusts are relevant matters.

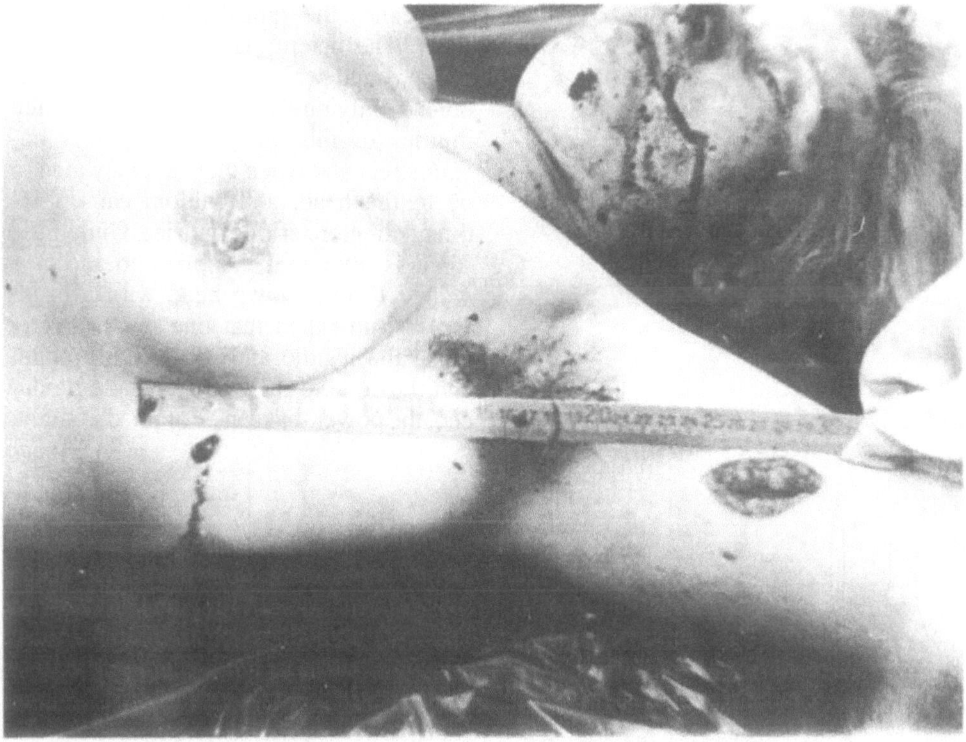

Fig. 30. Multiple injuries caused by one thrust

Hacking injuries

The hacking injury, like the incision injury, is caused by an instrument with a sharp edge. The instrument is a more massive, large-bladed object which may be a heavier knife, hatchet, axe, etc. The direction of motion is perpendicular to the length of the edge and the character of the wound reveals the size of the blade, the sharpness of the instrument, and the strength of force applied. A wound caused by a smaller, sharp-bladed hacking instrument looks almost exactly like an incision injury *(Fig. 31).* The edge of the wound, if the sharp part of the instrument penetrated, are pointed, the sides of the wound are sharp, the walls of the wound in fatty tissue bulge slightly, and the depth of the wound depends upon the force applied and the type of tissue met. If the blade of the hacking instrument is larger and the edge dull, we will find abrasions around the sides of the wound, which may be wider depending upon the sharpness of the hacking instrument, and may cause contusions. The state of the edges of the wound depends upon whether the end of the blade penetrated. A discontinuity with two pointed *edges* reflects the impression made by the hacking instrument. If the sharp edge of the instrument and one of its corners penetrate, only one wound edge will be sharp. In the peaked part an appropriately irregular, rounded, abraded injury can be found in the area of the wound edge, and occasionally fine superficial laceration wounds can be noticed on

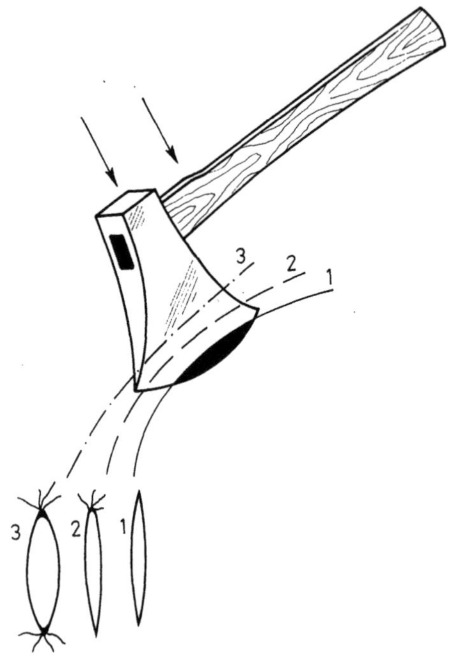

Fig. 31. Form of hacking injuries depending on the edge of the instrument

the skin. If the entire breadth of the hacking instrument penetrates the body, both wound corners will be similar. The depth of the injury, as mentioned, depends on the weight, sharpness and applied force.

A hacking instrument can produce *significant wounds to bony areas.* If it happens that the blade glances off the bone at an angle, it produces a smooth superficially cut injury. The wedge effect of a large-bladed instrument on the other side of a bone creates the outward break as a V-shaped loss of tissue on which one side is smooth, and the broken out side is rough *(Fig. 32).* This alteration caused by the hacking instrument is also known as a crush. The hack wound depends both upon the strength of force and the weight of the instrument, a heavy instrument being able to cause a serious injury with rather little applied force, and likewise, a light instrument can do the same if wielded with great force. The determination of whether the hack wound was self-inflicted or by another is only rarely in doubt. Self-inflicted injuries of this category are rarely encountered, and when they are, they tend to be to the head, and seldom cause life-threatening or serious injuries. Quite little force is able to be applied to inflict a wound to one's own head with a hacking instrument in that one must directly grasp the handle and the meeting point, and thus due to the limited torque produced, the power that can be applied is slight.

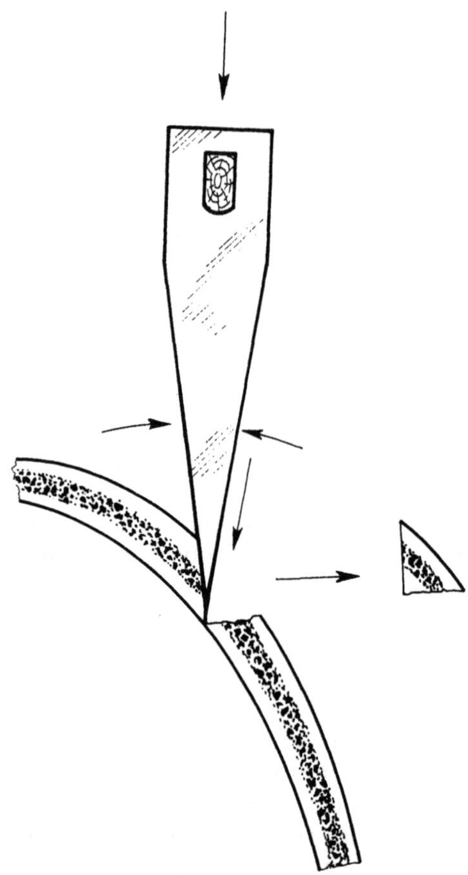

Fig. 32. Schematic drawing of the alterations due to the effect of the instrument, piece of the bone chipped out

For this reason, only superficial cuts are caused to the scalp leaving the characteristic superficial tissue loss over the skull *(Fig. 33).* Due to the scarcity of self-inflicted hacking injuries, every one encountered is suspected to be caused by an assailant, inasmuch as in these cases besides a high number of superficial injuries, there are usually other lethal alterations, occasionally stabs or hanging, and it is the task of the specialist to decide on the possibility of self-infliction for each injury. In hacking injuries produced by an assailant, the wounds are rough and serious, causing wide-spread lacerations, usually to the head *(Fig. 34).* In some instances self-defense injuries can be found on the palms and forearms. The healing ability of hacking injuries is worse than that of incision injuries. In the side of the injury, especially in injuries caused by dull-bla-

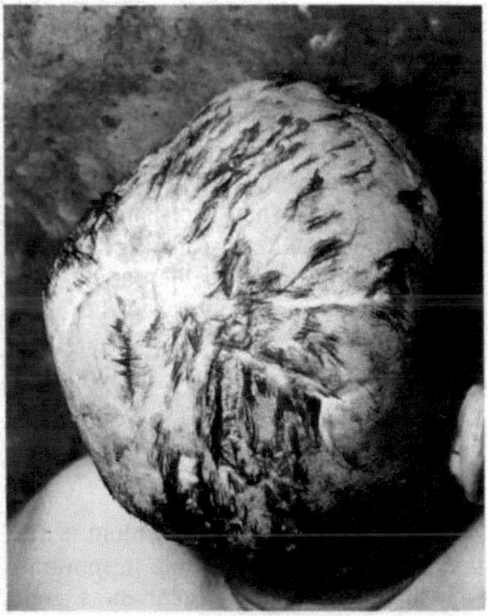

Fig. 33. Self-inflicted hacking injuries to the scalp and the scars of previous laceration injuries

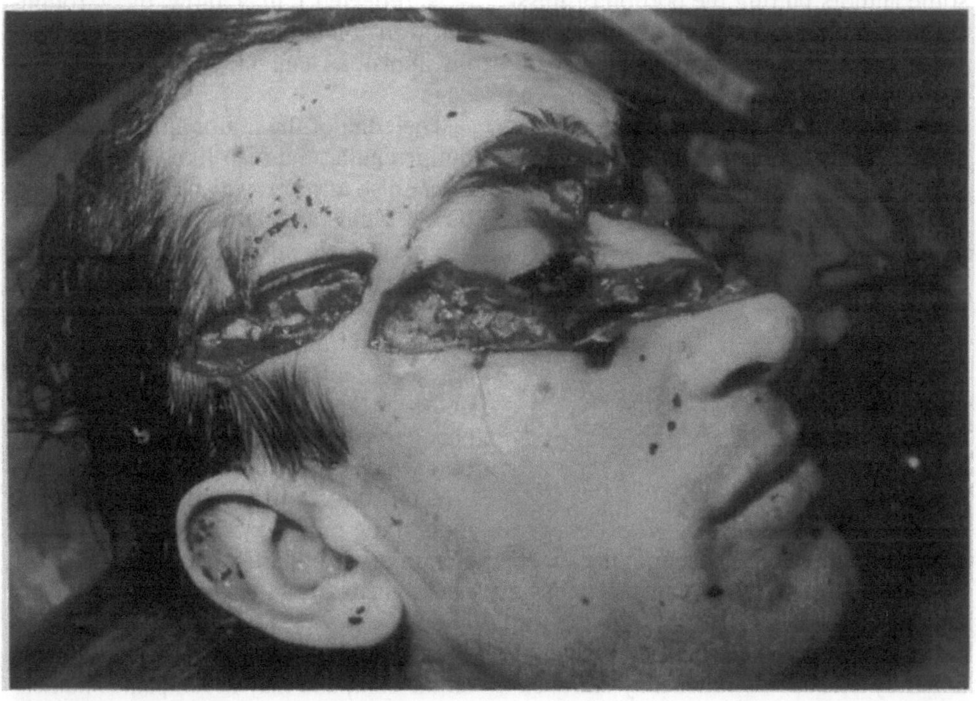

Fig. 34. Parallel hacking injuries on the face and skull (the sleeping victim was struck in the brain by his wife with an axe)

ded instruments, wide local tissue necrosis spreads, which does not occur in incisions of first intention, and they heal by second intention only rarely within eight days. Other factors come into play in the healing of bones that happen to get injured. An attack to the head that opens the cranial vault is a life-threatening situation. Clinical examination of the patient must involve exclusion of injury to the brain.

Alterations caused by blunt instruments

Wounds caused by attack by blunt instruments play a prominent role in mortality statistics. The injuries occur more commonly in men than in women. The number of wrong diagnoses is also significant, some authors putting the portion of missdiagnosed injuries by blunt instruments at 16%. The unrecognized cases are usually injuries to the chest and abdomen. The cause of death is usually multiple injuries and the leader among these is brain injury.

The categories of injuries from blunt instruments is as follows:

a) abrasion,
b) contusions,
c) laceration,
d) bone fractures,
e) injuries of the body parts.

Abrasion

The alterations usually occur in the superficial layers of the skin, but the damage may reach the dermis, too. While the former is generally a superficial injury which is hardly bleeds, the latter may show extensive hemorrhage. The injury occurs when a rough surface object applied moves the superficial layer of the skin, or the body moves over the blunt instrument. The origin in both cases is similar. The abraded part rolls up and that indicates the direction of attack as well. The wound may also show the effects of light force which brings about small *raised splinters* of chaffed skin *(Fig. 35).* The free sides of the splinters face the direction of the attack. In other cases where there is no movement during the injury, an irregular wound does not occur, but rather the impression of the object may be clearly reflected, which can be of use in identification of the instrument. (Especially characteristic of traffic accidents is the impression left by the protruding part of the vehicle, or the tire print left by a rubber bumper on the skin *(Fig. 36)*, or the mark left by the ligature in hanging, in which the instrument – twisted or rough-surfaced – is reflected.) In a blow by a rough-surfaced blunt instrument, characteristic abrasions can be found around the edges.

The edge of the injury appears washed out, irregular and map-like. A superficial injury also turns brownish due to the dried tissue fluid and dries parchment-like, whereas deeper injuries involve congealed blood which forms scabs later. If the injury does not reach the dermis, it heals within eight days without a scar, if there are no complications. The determination of the weapon can be made only if it leaves characteristic impressions, otherwise at best we can only follow the instrument's effects – direction, irregular surface – without more precise description. The abrasion injury is of particular relevance to forensic medicine in that:

1. indicate, some force has been applied on the skin, and may accompanies numerous other injuries,
2. it can show the direction of attack,

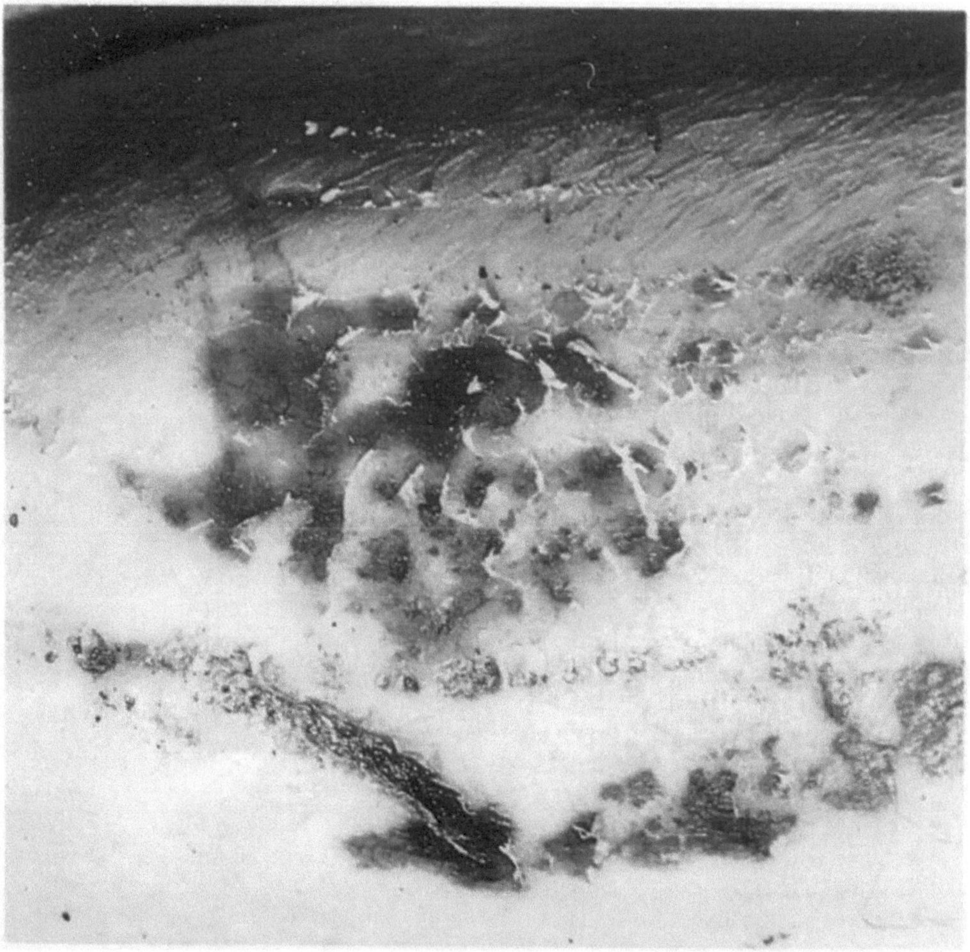

Fig. 35. Abrasion injury with skin flakes pointing in the direction from which the injury came

3. it can sometimes reveal the instrument used,
4. the age of the wound can be determined on the corpse.

Examination, especially of the corpse, must be performed carefully, so as not to destroy the splinters of abraded skin which show the direction of attack (for example, washing the corpse before examining it removes the blood stains and dried foreign material left by the attack). We must search for foreign material and tissue stuck in the abraded wound which can be of much help in identifying the origin of the injury and sometimes the degree of force applied as well (in the area of strong attacks we often see superficial abrasions which show up as parallel, fine, brownish, dried, superficial cracks on the epidermis) *(Fig. 37).* One form of the abrasion injury is the scratch mark, which is characterized by 0.5-2 mm wide, several cm long abrasion wounds which,

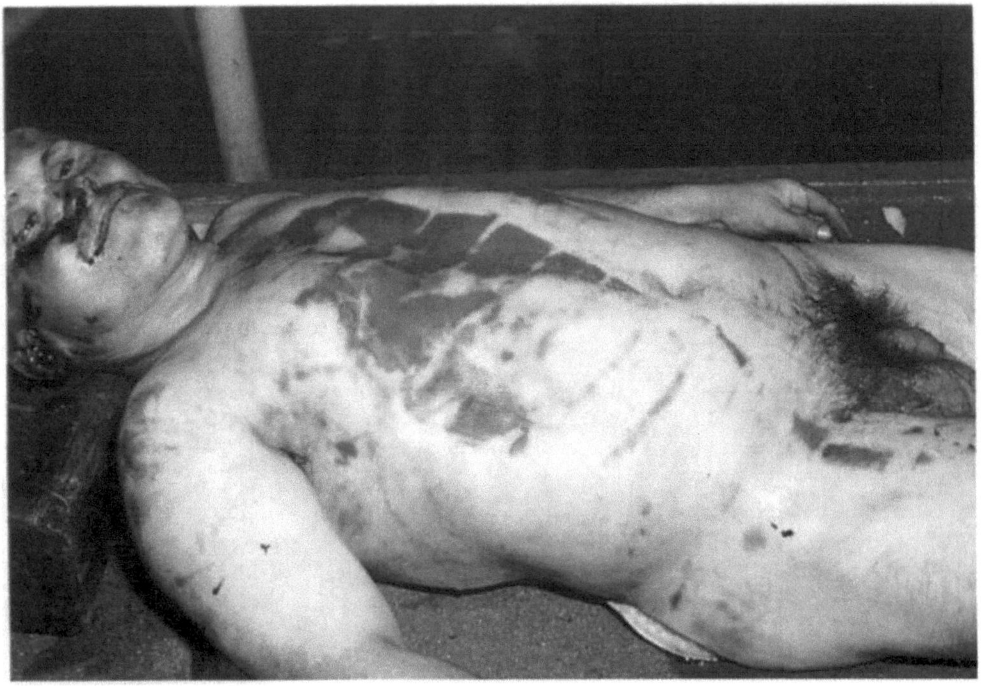

Fig. 36. Tire marks on the skin

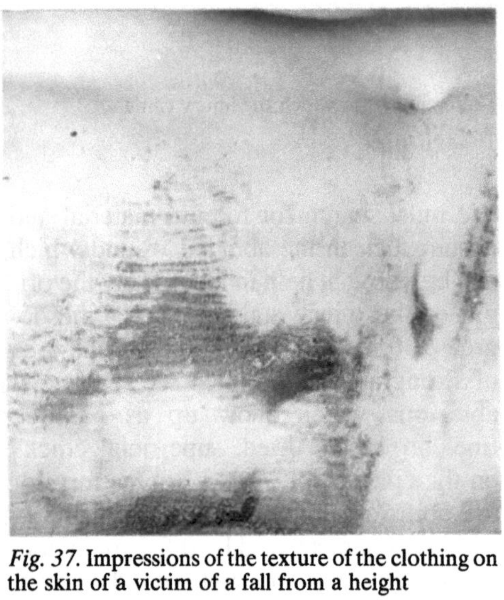

Fig. 37. Impressions of the texture of the clothing on the skin of a victim of a fall from a height

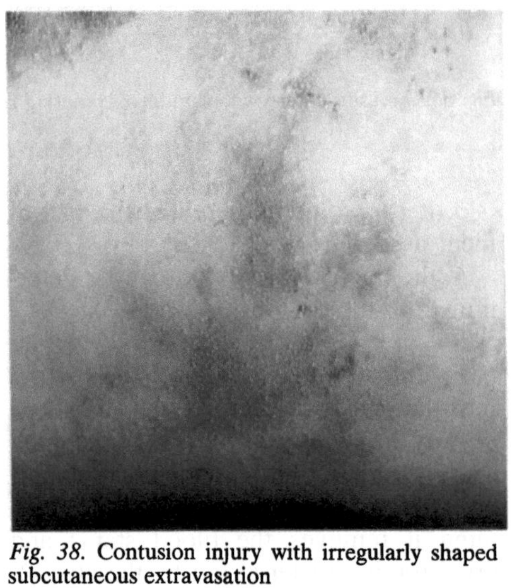

Fig. 38. Contusion injury with irregularly shaped subcutaneous extravasation

with accompanying skin splinters, are followed by drying to a brownish color. They are brought about by a circumscribed attack by pointed, blunt-surfaced instruments, for example, fingernails. The form of the injury can be characteristic, in that fingernails leave the imprint of crescent-shaped scratch abrasions in the area that was gripped.

Contusions

Attack by a large blunt instrument into a tissue area with rapid compression injures small blood vessels, lacerating the subcutaneous connective tissue, muscle tissue and perhaps organs such as lungs, liver heart and kidneys. The skin covering the injury is intact and the injured tissues turn it purple. Occasionally the area swells and local edema may accompany it. Abrasions are not found over bruises in every instance, and for that reason it isn't easy in every case to distinguish between bleeding caused by an injury and simple subcutaneous hemorrhage *(Fig. 38)*. Bleeding due to injury is very similar to that caused by non-injury bleeding from disorders of hemostasis or hyperfragility of vessel walls. This circumscribed form of pin-point hemorrhages, or petechia, can form confluent, larger bleedings and suffusions. Recognition of the underlying disease causing the bleeding can unambiguously solve the problem. In infants, children and the elderly and the above mentioned disorders, a slight amount of force can result large suffusions. In other cases the settling patches of lividity on the corpse can be mistaken for bruises. Distinguishing between a patch of hypostatic lividity and a bruise is done easily in the corpse. The suspicious area is incised and blood drains from the vessels in the area of the lividity. In the area of a bruise, the blood has infiltrated the fatty tissue, connective tissue and occasionally the muscle tissue. The character of a bruising injury is revealed when the fresh alteration on the skin in the form of a bluish-red discoloration appears, remaining in the indistinct edges. In highly pigmented skin the alteration is hardly noticeable. Its recognition can be difficult not only in life but in the fresh dead corpse. One or two days later the injury is easier to recognize not only in life, but postmortally as well, the latter case being due to the production of sulfhemoglobin by the processes of decay. In some cases the preliminary examination or the superficial coroner's inquest accepts what the practicing specialist knows well, that with the earlier processes of decay the identity of the deceased is hardly discernible, and the presence of contusion injuries remains hidden. In contrast to the abrasion injuries, the contusion injuries do not reveal the direction of attack, but can reveal the character and shape of the instrument used. We have already discussed in connection with determining the direction of attack by a long instruments that rough surfaced objects cause the formation of abrasions around the edges of abrasion injuries *(Fig. 39)*. Blows produced by smoother elongated instruments such as rubber batons and clubs, cause contusion injuries *(Fig. 40)*.

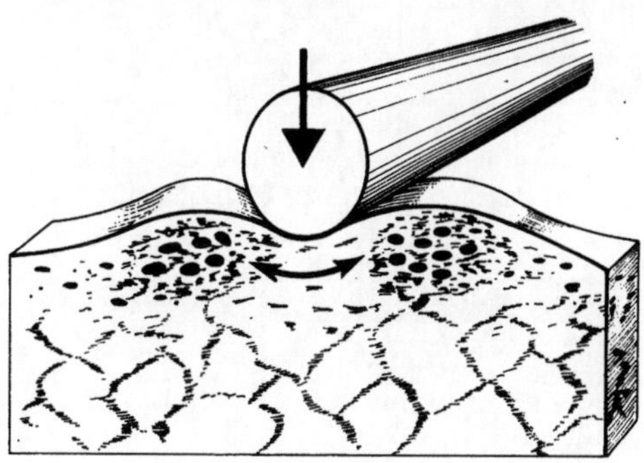

Fig. 39. Schematic drawing of the formation of a contusion caused by a long instrument

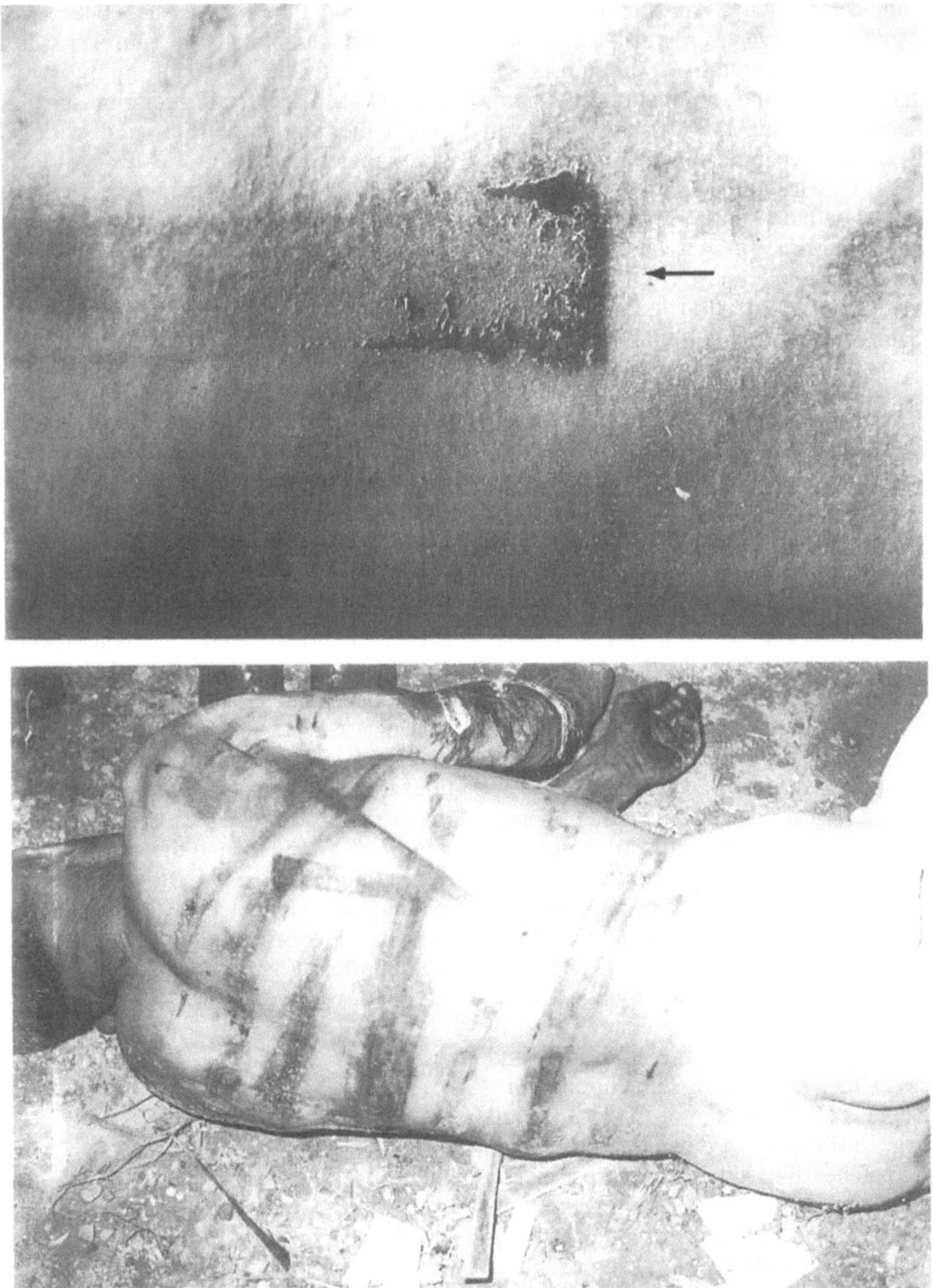

Fig. 40. Contusions caused by a long instrument, chaffing at the edges, punctate hemorrhages under the imprints of the instrument

The injury of blood vessels in a rapidly applied compression play a role in that at the center of the injury pin-point hemorrhages form, while at the periphery interconnected, parallel marks or abrasions revealing the shape of the instrument may be found. The extent of the injury not only reflects the amount of force applied in the attack, but the nature of the body area as well. In those areas where the subcutaneous connective tissue is loose, such as around the eyes, a smaller amount of force can cause bruising and such tissue is more susceptible to a wider spread local edema. If the covering tissue of another area, such as the back or the extremities, suffers a contusion, we cannot always count on finding a striking alteration, although tissue edema also develops, if only to a lesser degree than that which was previously mentioned. The color of the bruise reveals the age of the injury. A fresh injury is reddish-purple. The deterioration of the blood pigments causes a greenish discoloration at the edges of the bruise within 4-7 days, and 10-14 days later it is yellow. In the area of this injury the results of the vital reaction can be seen, which will be discussed in detail later. The localization and form of the alteration indicates its origin. Circumscribed, 1-2 cm diameter bruises on the upper arm are characteristic grip marks. Similar alterations found on the neck, with accompanying crescent-shaped abrasions or scratches indicate the injuries were caused by a grip to the neck, in cases of throttling, or strangle marks. In other cases the extent and seriousness of injuries to the lower extremities, the buttocks, or the back, especially if the injury involves a separation of the underlying loose connective tissue, so-called *blood blisters* form from the effect of great force and indicate a traffic accident

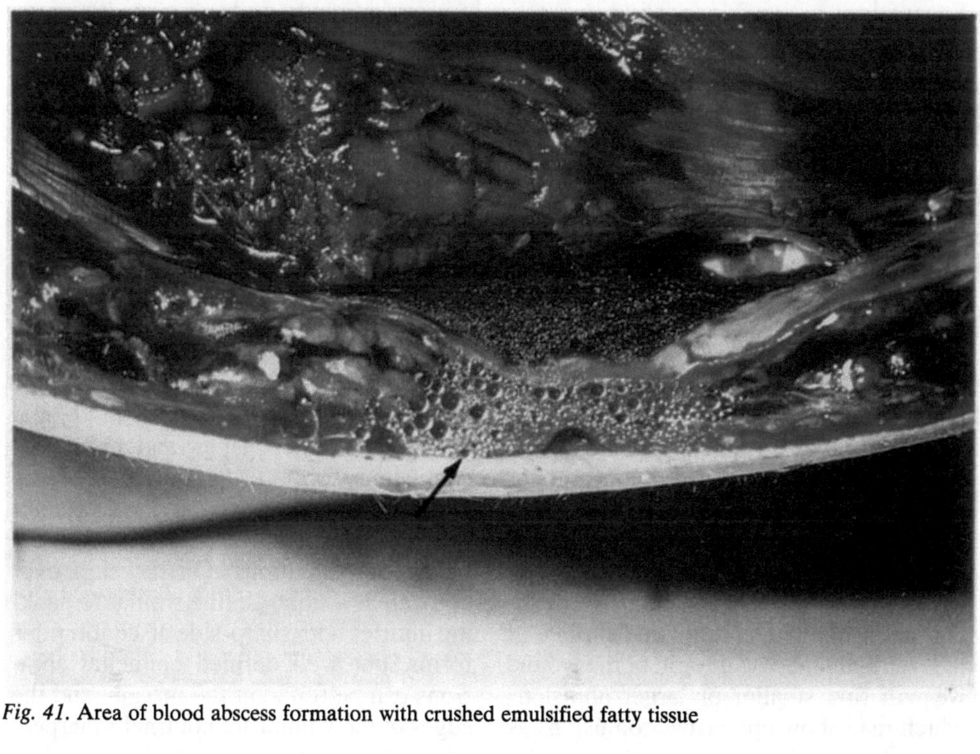

Fig. 41. Area of blood abscess formation with crushed emulsified fatty tissue

(Fig. 41). In these cases, the subcutaneous fatty tissue separates in layers forming blood-filled pockets in which suffusions of fluid blood containing bits of tissue and fatty tissue pieces can be found, and in many instances serious or even deadly fat embolism or tissue embolism can result *(Fig. 42).*

Contusions found on the forearms, especially on the ulnar surface, are typical for self-defense alterations. The amount and extent of bleeding into the tissues is a measure of the force applied which caused the injury *(Fig. 43).*

The speed of recovery depends upon the extent and seriousness of the bleeding into the tissues. Minor bruises heal within eight days, whereas larger contusions, especially those involving a joint contusion naturally take much longer.

Laceration

A blunt-surfaced instrument can cause lacerations, because the mechanism is similar to the contusions, the two types of injuries are often associated. For an instrument with a small surface area applied on a body part having massive soft tissue to cause such an injury, a great amount of force is required. The characteristic form is found in places where skin directly overlies bone. The configuration of the injury is varied being X or H shaped. The line of the injury is irregular with the *shape* discontinuous, roughly indented, with the *edges* of the injury irregular and sometimes covered. The *sides* of the wound are bridged by unbroken strands of connective tissue, which are thicker fibers and occasionally vessels and nerves. Depending on the applied strength and surface of the instrument, at the margin of the wound we will find smaller or larger abrasions which may show epidermal contusions as

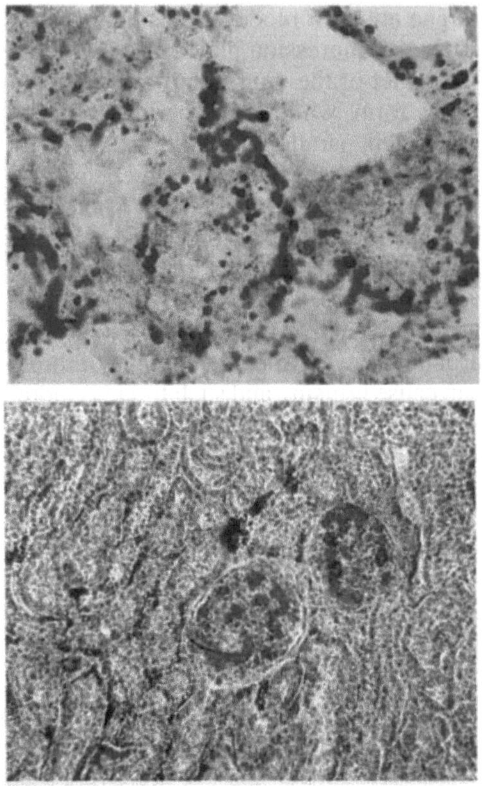

Fig. 42. Fat embolism in the pulmonary vessels, fat embolism in kidney glomerulus

well. In this case the margin of the injury not only dries brownish, but takes on a bluish lividity in which can be found pinpoint hemorrhages if great pressure has been applied.

On bony areas, if the applied instrument had a wide area of contact, we find in the middle a laceration injury with dermal abrasions at the shapes and epidermal contusions form. From the base of the wound the skin is removed, little pouches separate, and thus the injury is undercut from both directions. On the skin over bony areas – tibia – a line similar to hacking injuries with sharp-side discontinuities forms, but well defined epithelial abrasions can be found at the margin, and the edges of the wound are not finely sharped.

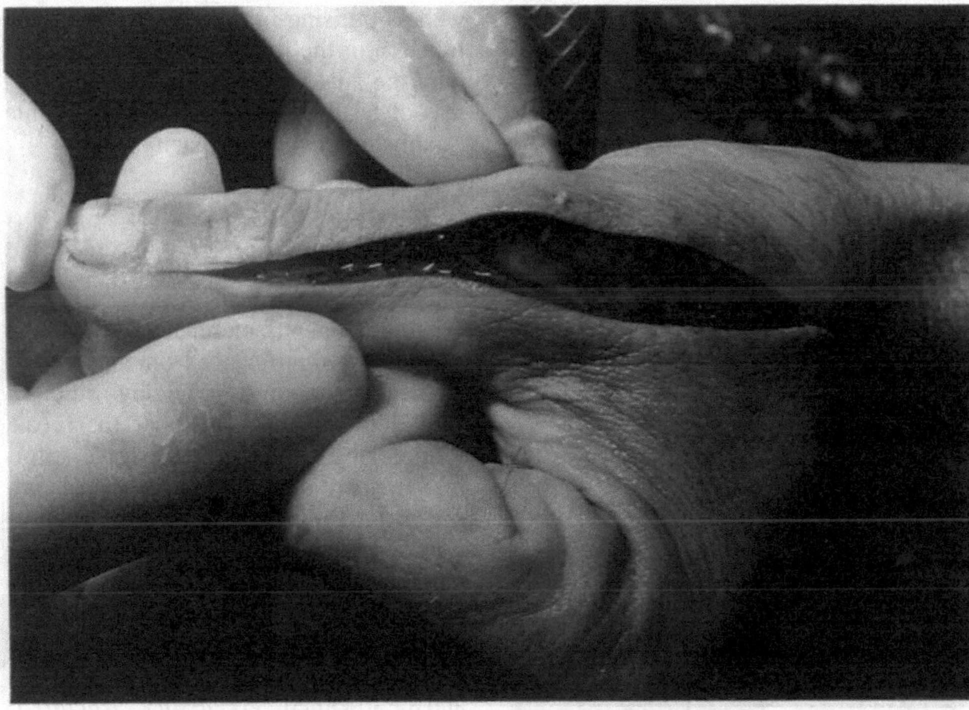

Fig. 43. Self-defense type contusion injury with subcutaneous tissue showing blood imbibition

If a blunt surfaced instrument is applied to the surface of the body at an angle, it will cause a *lobulated laceration injury,* in which the wall of the wound opposite the direction of attack is undercut, covering the other side which slopes down under it, and here also we can find connective tissue bridges. One form of the laceration injury is the *flaying injury,* in which the blunt instrument peels up the superficial skin separating it from the underlying tissue and the injury separates into a lobulated form, removed however with numerous connective tissue bridges. The above-mentioned epithelial contusions and bruises at the margins and outside pin-point hemorrhages indicate the severity of the force applied. Similarly means a great force the free hair bulbs in the side of head injuries or broken hairs are found stuck in the fractured bones itself. With laceration injuries special characteristics can clarify the manner of origin. Laceration injuries found in the area of the head *(Fig. 44)* justifiably raise the suspicion of foul play, since in numerous cases we find such lacerations on the scalp which originate from falls or blows. The character of these and the manner of origin in a significant percentage of cases can be clarified by recognition of conditions at the scene. We can suppose that injuries in the area of the temples, orbits, or occiput originated in a fall even though these injuries result in serious cranial fractures, concussions, and intracranial bleeding. Inebriated, unconscious or incapacitated individuals often suffer such alterations in falls. In other cases a laceration injury found in the area of the parietal bone raises suspicion of assault *(Fig. 45).* Laceration injury found on the arms, especially the ulnar surface, is

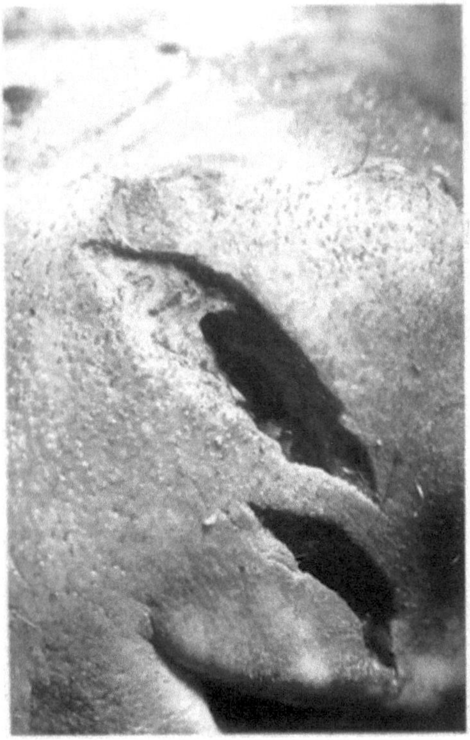

Fig. 44. Laceration injury to the face. Irregular lines and angles of the wounds, connective tissue bridges between the walls of the wounds

typical of self-defense injuries, or may be caused by a fall or blows. Laceration injuries to the head, if resulting in skull fractures, may cause injury to the dura mater, and open wounds carry with them the danger of infection and are therefore considered life-threatening.

The prospect of healing of laceration injuries is significantly worse due to the extensive tearing, as in the injuries previously discussed. Without proper attention, healing by second intention will occur in which the scar formation will require more than eight days. However, if it is properly surgically attended in a medical facility, healing by first intention will ensue within eight days.

Laceration injuries to joint areas, as well as bruising injuries, can damage the function of the joints and in this case not only the anatomical but functional progress of healing must be monitored while establishing healing capacity.

Fractures

The general surgical classification of fractures – open fracture, closed fracture – carries little significance from the forensic medical standpoint, providing little insight into the mechanism of the break. Radiological signs provide more information about the origin of the injury. *Spiral fractures* give evidence of the application of torque to the injured area, *bending fractures* are significant in the ribs, *separation fractures* appear at the attachments of muscles, shearing fractures are typical of the second cervical vertebra, and the so-called *"green-stick" fracture* is characteristic of subperiosteal fracture in children. The diagnosis of the alteration can be problematic even for experienced radiologists, especially in basal skull and rib fractures where the bones are often superimposed on one another and appear misleadingly similar to fracture lines. Otherwise obvious fractures catch the attention of the examiner. The practicing forensic medical specialist knows that diagnosis of fractures of the nasal bone and ribs are often in error, and in a part of these cases repeating the x-ray reveals that the nasal fracture was actually the line of a vessel and the fracture line of a rib was in reality an artifact caused by superimposition of another rib. Sometimes the original picture gives no indication of the exact diagnosis. In these cases the course of healing can help decide whether there was a break or not by taking another x-ray a few days later. The formation of callus unambiguously shows the diagnosis. To

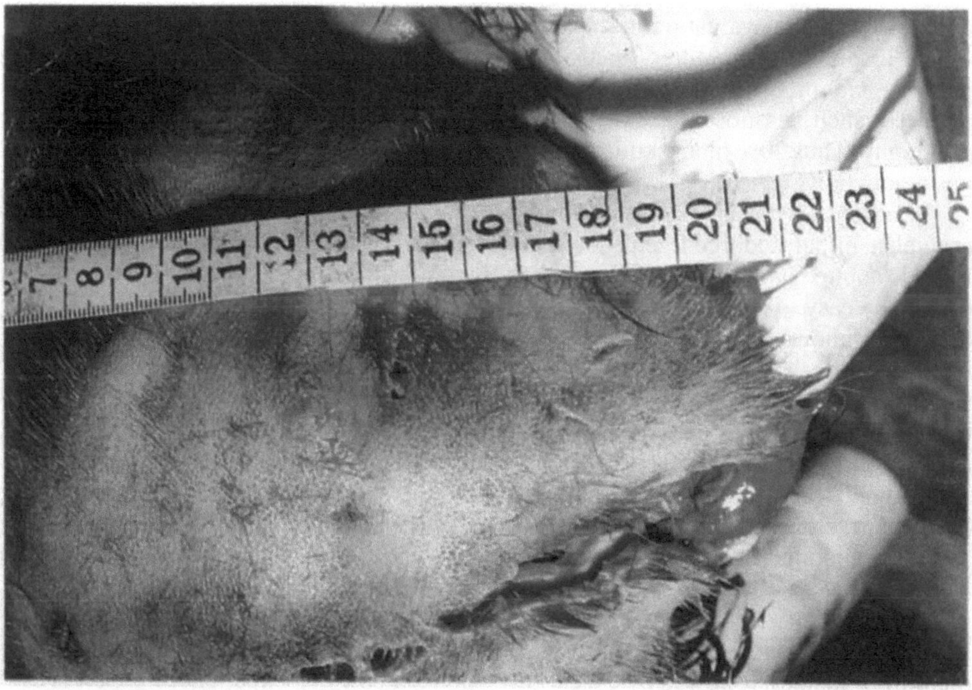

Fig. 45. Laceration injury to the scalp caused by a length of chain: the open parts correspond to the distance between the links interspersed with intact skin bridges

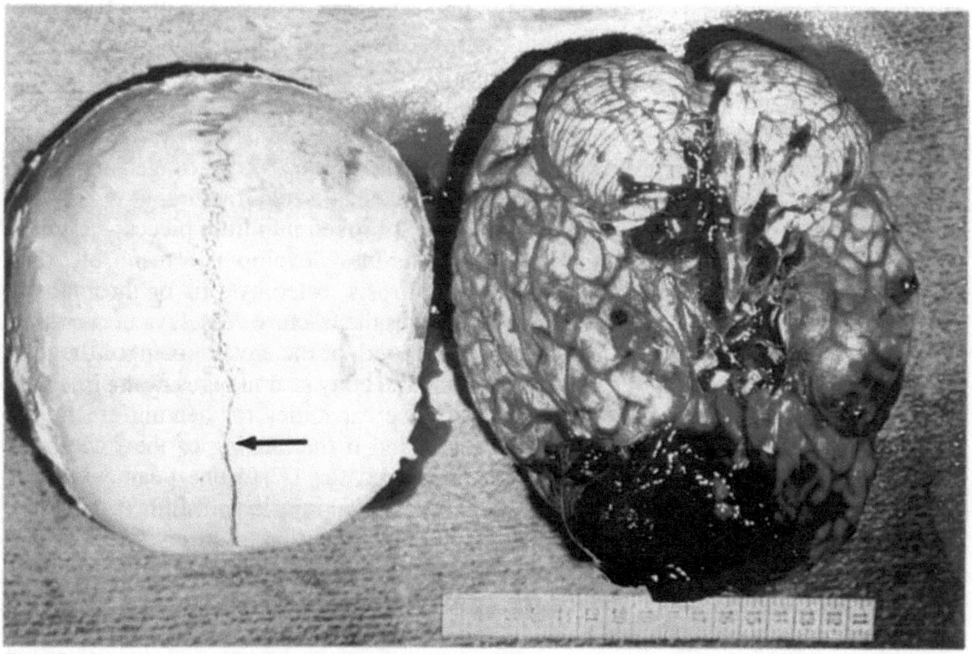

Fig. 46. Linear fracture of the skull with cerebral contusion

avoid the dubious evaluation in the differential diagnosis of fractures, special exposures and preparation techniques are required, such as fluoroscopy or xenoradiography. Thus 20% of all skull fractures go unnoticed *(Fig. 46)*.

The autopsy is not an easy matter for the specialist, either. In large fractures a great force is applied and the mechanism is occasionally easy to clarify, and the fracture can bring about an infiltration of blood into the soft tissues. At other times a fracture may go unrecognized during autopsy in the absence of external signs, especially if no X-rays are made.

We will deal with the more common types of fractures to various body areas and the alterations caused by blunt instruments.

The healing of a fracture is similar to the healing of the wounds. The periosteal hematoma organizes, followed by the callus, consist of connective tissues, later the formation of the bony callus, take on the characteristic trajectorial structure and create the osseous scar on the weight-bearing bones. The course depends on the location of the fracture, the age and naturally on a complication-free process. A nasal bone fracture has the ability to heal the quickest, 3-4 weeks. Rib fractures consolidate within 4-6 weeks, and fractures of bones of the extremities, the phalanges, metacarpals, and bones of the foot usually heal without functional damage within 6-8 weeks. An exception is a fracture of the navicular bone, after which in numerous cases due to bone resorption or formation of pseudoarthrosis, can cause later complaints.

The care the fracture receives modifies its healing appropriately. The regenerative capacity of fractures to the weight-bearing bones rests with the ability to form the callus, and if this comes about, we consider it as being healed, from a forensic viewpoint and if the function is unimpeded, this further supports our opinion. We must deal with those pathological fractures which can result from previous illnesses. A fracture resulting from a tumorous alteration can be recognized without any doubt, in that the previous course has created a special condition in which even without the application of force (spontaneous fracture), or with very little force, a break can occur and healing is doubtful. It is improper to trace a tumorous disease back to a previously applied force. In other cases, osteoporosis in the aged can predispose to fractures from the application of very little force. Such cases are known of where even coughing has resulted in rib fractures in the elderly. The recognition and rendering of an opinion concerning fractures is not a simple task. The opinion derived from the special examination performed by an experienced expert is especially counted on concerning the signs involving skull fractures and rib fractures. In our local experience, skull and rib fractures are sometimes misdiagnosed.

Healing in most cases is without complications, and the physiological functions are restored completely. At other times the healing process is prolonged and in the case of shattering fractures – when the bone is broken into little pieces – complications may develop as a result of pseudoarthrosis, osteomyelitis or thrombosis. Besides the fracture vessels or nerves may be injured, or the envelopment of the nerve in the bony scar may result in paralysis. If these capacities for healing are modified, and if the healing of the fracture is prolonged for 1/2 to one year, we don't speak of appropriate healing processes, but emphasize that a serious deterioration of health has accompanied the fracture. After a serious deterioration of health regardless of whether associated with healing, sometimes the fracture heals leav-

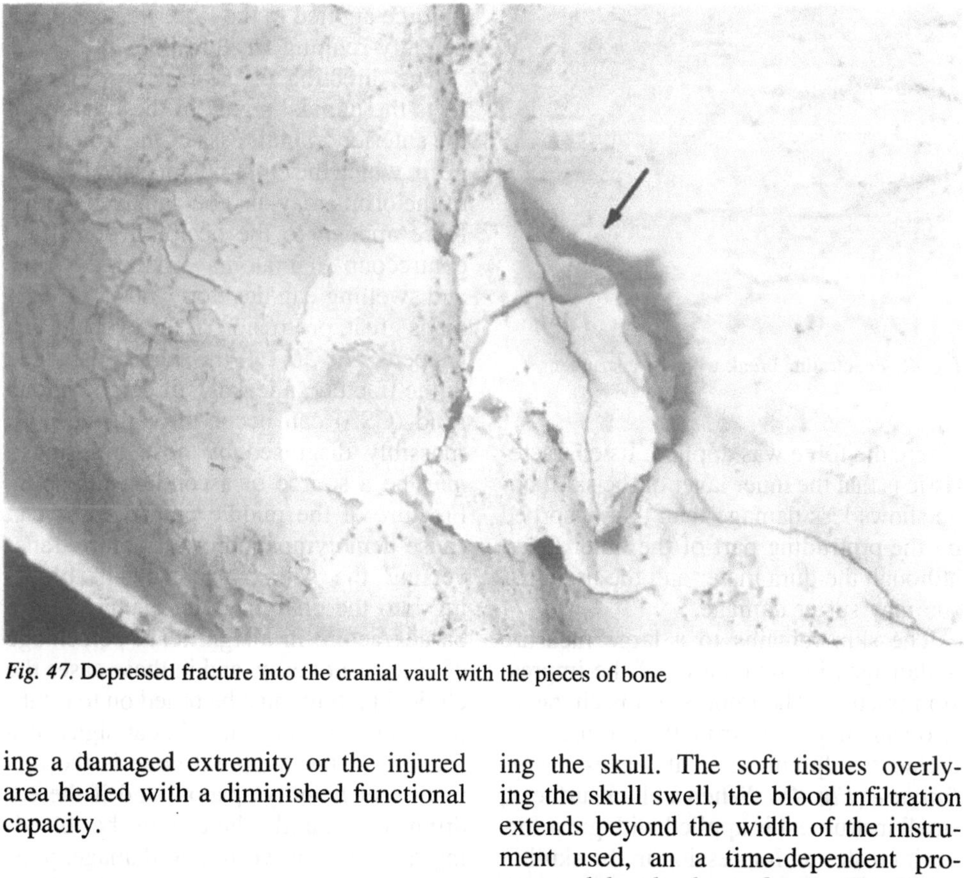

Fig. 47. Depressed fracture into the cranial vault with the pieces of bone

ing a damaged extremity or the injured area healed with a diminished functional capacity.

Head injuries

Skull fractures

Skull fractures can occur to the cranial roof, base and face. Fractures to the roof may be line fractures in which the application of force is to protruding part. If the sutures aren't ossified, the borders of the bones are not overlapped and the instrument isn't of the long kind – rubber baton, piece of cable, etc. – isolated bone fractures will occur, especially in newborns and children. If we find fractures covering more area in infants or newborns – skull roof and base – we have to consider the possibility of a strong force used in crushing the skull. The soft tissues overlying the skull swell, the blood infiltration extends beyond the width of the instrument used, an a time-dependent pronounced local edema forms. The linear fracture to the base and roof of the skull which can occur as a result of a fall has a characteristic appearance on the occipital region of the head.

Strong force with a broad surfaced instrument can cause a *spider web fracture.* The lines of the fracture radiate outward from a center in which we find a mildly indented fracture or one shattered to pieces leaving a star-like pattern. If further force was applied, the ensuing injuries occur along the lines of the previous breaks. From this we can follow the effects of the successive attacks.

The *impression fracture (Fig. 47)* occurs in the area of the previous fracture in the center, or in a circumscribed part

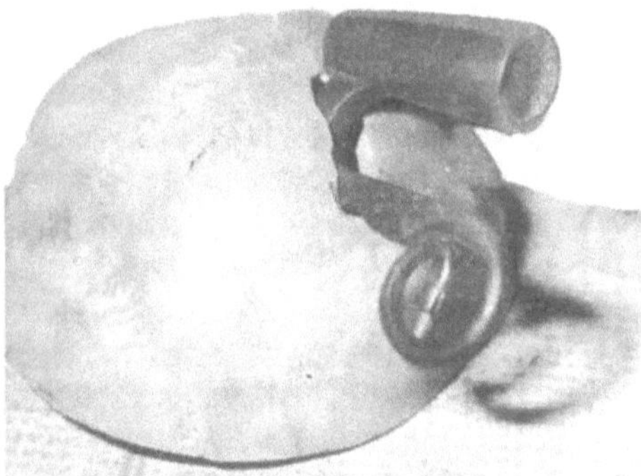

Fig. 48. Penetrating break with the instrument

where the force was applied. Its characteristic is that the inner layer of the skull bone shows less damage than that absorbed by the protruding part of the outer layer, although the dura mater and the brain tissue may suffer damage.

The skin remains to a large measure undamaged in some cases of the impression fracture. The impression is characteristic and important from the forensic medicine standpoint when it leaves a *hole fracture (Fig. 48).* When a blunt surfaced, small instrument is applied with great force, it creates an impression in the skull in its own shape, which can be of immense value in identification of the instrument.

Skull base fractures (Fig. 49) are the result of either roof fractures that extend to the base or of a specially applied force which causes them without calvaria fracture. They represent 24% of all head injuries. Force plays a role in the formation of the fixed skull, in which the propped up part of the skull is moved in the opposite direction. The force shortens the fixed parts of skull and here forms the fracture. The lines of the fracture run between the poles of the force, thus causing the sagittal fracture lines alone the sagittal suture, or in force applied to the side, we see a horizontally-running fracture line.

The direction of the fracture lines affects the clinical signs. In the fracture of the anterior cranial fossa of the frontal bone, in which the ethmoid bone and the area of the orbits may also be damaged from a force applied to the occipital bone as a contrecoup, hematoma around the eyes and swelling can develop, and if the edema is great, protrusion of the eyeballs can happen *(Fig. 50.).* If the dura is damaged in the fracture, a leakage of cerebrospinal fluid (CSF) can occur through the nose (possibly disguised by nose bleeding!), may be a source of ascending infection. Fracture of the middle cranial fossa can cause hemotympanon or a fracture transversing the sella can result in bleeding into the pharynx. The diagnosis of a basal fracture in a significant percentage of cases is not easy, and in these cases the clinical picture must be relied on to establish them. Among the clinical signs of a fracture of the temporal bone is the formation of hemotympanon, and if the ear drum is injured, there will be bleeding from the ear, vestibular damage, peripheral facial paresis, and occasionally a leakage of CSF from the ear. If the ear drum is intact, the liquor can reach the nose via the Eustachian tube. The sphenoid, ethmoid or temporal bone fracture can result in anosmia, bilateral periorbital bleeding or leakage of CSF. With the presence of these signs we can diagnose basal skull fracture even in the absence of positive X-ray findings. Pneumocephalus can result from fracture of the anterior fossa, the air coming in through the paranasal sinuses and with the increase in pressure reaching the subarachnoid area through the fracture.

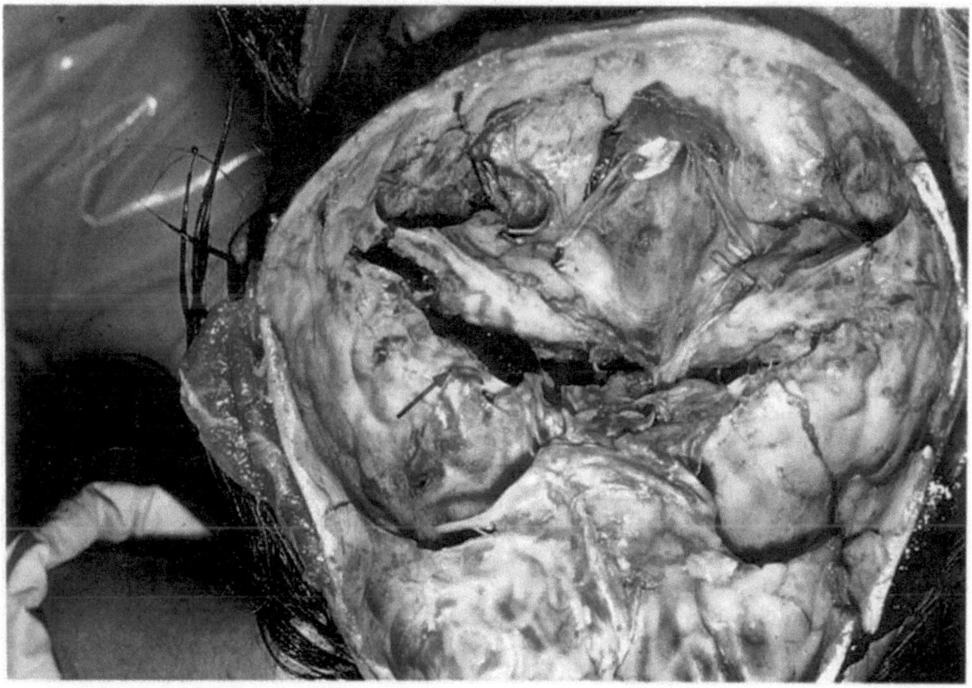

Fig. 49. Fracture of the base of the skull with lateral compression of the skull

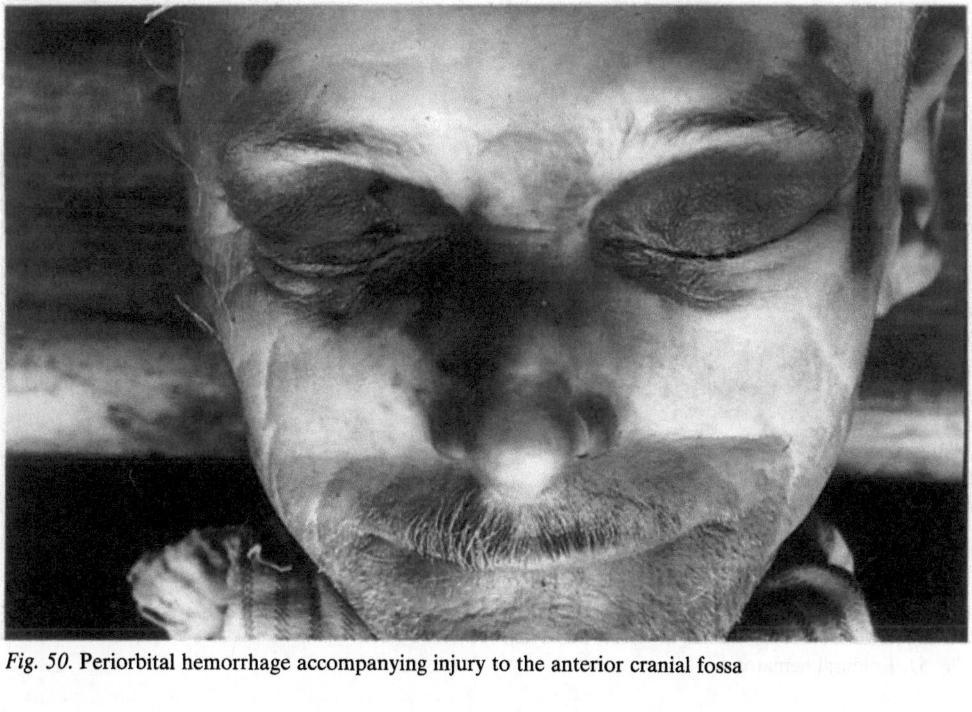

Fig. 50. Periorbital hemorrhage accompanying injury to the anterior cranial fossa

Intracranial hemorrhages

Epidural hematoma

Epidural hematoma is a relatively rare consequence of head injury, making up 0.2 – 4.6% of all head injuries. The greatest number of these occur in traffic accidents. The age of the patients is disparate, although occurrence in the elderly is rare. In this the gradual adhesion of the dura may play a role. In the 20-30 year age group these injuries are more common. Damage to the arteries of the dura are the primary cause in formation, and the reason is usually a skull fracture. The area of predisposition is the region of the temporal bone, in the area where branches of the medial meningeal artery run *(Fig. 51)*. A significant number of cases show a fracture recognized from the X-ray or during management of the patient, or occasionally at autopsy, but epidural hematoma can occur by vessel injury without skull fracture. The bleeding from the injured vessel forms a circumscribed separation between the dura and the inner layer of the bone of the skull and forms a characteristic lens-shaped hemorrhage. The separation of the dura and the size of the bleeding depends upon the age of the victim and the size of the vessel ruptured.

A well-adhered dura only separates a little bit and the epidural bleeding compresses the injured vessel preventing further bleeding. A widely spread hematoma can come about with an injury to a larger vessel and a poorly adhering dura, in which the expansion of the collecting blood may reach several centimeters. Venous injury can also result in epidural bleeding – the medial meningeal vein, the

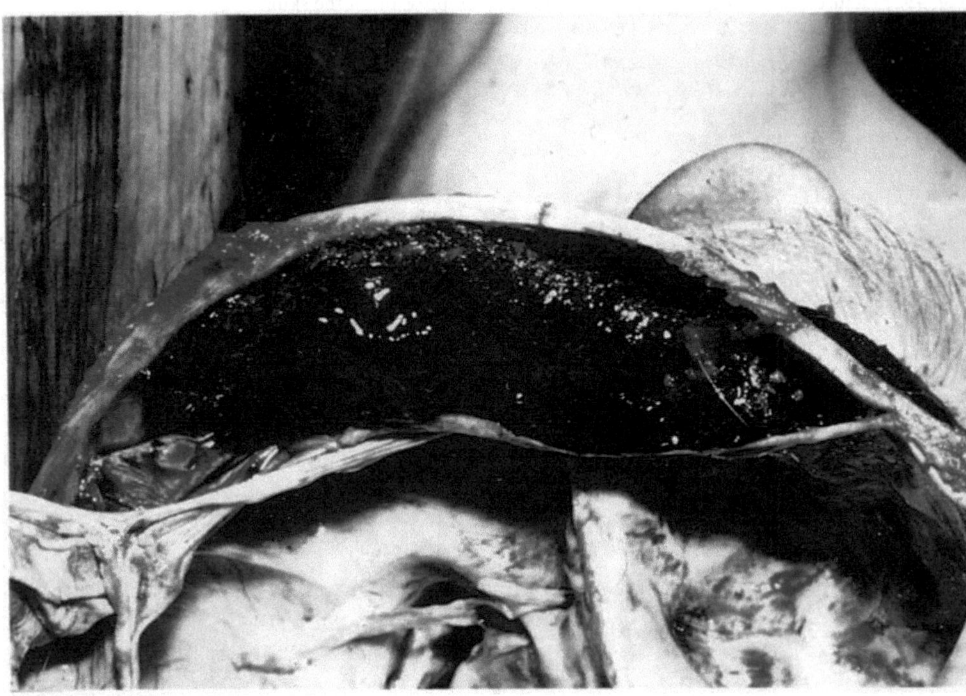

Fig. 51. Epidural hematoma

diploe veins, or dural sinuses –, but the low pressure in the venous system prevents a significant spread. The most common places of occurrence are the areas of the middle meningeal artery, the temporal bone, parietal bone and occasionally the occipital bone in areas where protruding parts are found under the dura.

The occurrence of the *subtentorial epidural hematoma* is more rare, but the diagnosis is even more problematic. The clinical presentation is not characteristic. It depends on the time that has elapsed since the occurrence and the speed of development of the hematoma. Epidural hematoma is not the only injury with a short period of unconsciousness followed by a symptomless period and another period of unconsciousness. The lucid interval may accompany other expanding intracranial processes, but in the epidural hematoma the free interval usually is not longer than 24 hours. The formation of papillary edema can be noticed in other compressive processes causing increasing intracranial pressure, as well as bradycardia, one or two-sided pupillary dilation, decerebration signs, or hemiparesis. The character and intensity of the intradural injuries naturally make the diagnosis difficult. In a significant part of cases serious contusions may accompany the application of force. We have already indicated the usefulness of X-ray examination, but its importance and indispensability emphasized by the neurosurgeon. A computer tomograph examination significantly aids in the diagnosis of developing or developed epidural hematoma, and in its absence, angiography is necessary. Mortality is variable. Depending upon the age of the patient, the localization of the hematoma, the time between the injury and appearance of symptoms, and first and foremost of all the extent of the intradural injury. Mortality figures lie between 5-43%.

Subdural hematoma

Acute traumatic intracranial bleeding, which tend to occur in an older age group – over 40 years – than the epidural hematomas, are more commonly encountered. From the mild application of force, to those caused by serious accidents, the rupture of the emissary veins play the main role. A strong application of force to the skull or the displacement of the brain by sudden movement can result in tearing of the veins draining the cerebrum and the veins connected with the sinuses. The localization of the bleeding is most commonly at the protrusion of the parietal and occipital lobes, and less commonly in the area of the falx cerebri and the bleeding usually covers the cerebral hemispheres. The bleeding, especially if great force caused the rupture of the emissary veins, can be accompanied with contusions on the side of impact and at the opposite side as a contre coup. These basically differentiate the clinical signs (the subdural hematoma complicated with contusions carries a relatively high mortality). The severity of the injury and the intensity of development of the subdural hematoma determines the clinical picture. After diffuse brain damage, the victim loses consciousness, and in the case of injury of a large bridge vein the hematoma increases rapidly and about 99% of the victims die.

In less serious injuries consciousness is not always lost immediately, or the free interval is variable, and the case of acute subdural hematoma may tend for a longer period to be described as an epidural hematoma, but the chronic subdural hematoma may afford a symptomless period of weeks to months. Anisocoria, motor disturbances and the results of any other central nervous system injury may shed significant light onto the question of which side the injury occurred. Ipsilateral pupillary dilation and contralateral hemiparesis indicate post-traumatic cranial vault injury processes. Subdural hematoma can cause motor signs due to traction on the contralateral cerebral peduncles, and injury to the midbrain with hematoma can cause contralateral pupillary dilation. The diagnosis is made from the previous data – head injury – and central nervous system injury, in which the processes of localized compression create the respective signs. (With intoxicated patients – alcoholics represent 40% of the cases – the differential diagnosis can be difficult, and a quick blood alcohol content determination can be decisive). Among the diagnostic possibilities available for aiding in the diagnosis, an X-ray of the skull only shows fractures and their revelation is occasionally decisive. Of much greater significance is computer tomography and carotid angiography and most recently, MR examination.

Lumbar puncture in the suspicion of both types of hematoma, epidural and subdural, is contraindicated due to the danger of herniation.

At the autopsy on the affected hemisphere we find a cap-like pool of blood which caused the gradual increase in intracranial pressure and is more expressed on the injured side, but on the opposite side we may find a decrease in the depths of the gyri with a flattening of the vessels and a crease left by the herniation of the hippocampus and cerebellar tonsils the signs of increased intracranial pressure. A large number of cases show the signs of contre coup injury on the opposite side, that is, we see contusion of the brain with hypoxic peduncular bleeding.

In the formation of *chronic subdural hematoma* in the practice of neurosurgery is considered if the symptoms begin to occur beyond 20 days after the injury. The process is subacute if 3–20 days elapse between the injury and the appearance of symptoms. They tend to occur in elderly patients with the average age being 50–60. In a high percentage of the cases the patient doesn't mention any previous traumatic event, but as we have pointed out, the acute form can come about by a rather mild force. Chronic alcoholism plays a role in part of the cases and epilepsy or coagulopathies in others. So-called *minor trauma* is stressed primarily in the cases of alcoholics. In the pathogenesis of the clinical picture mild subdural bleeding plays such a mild role that the injury may be passed over as symptomless. After the bleeding a small amount of blood collects and on the inner surface of the dura, following the organization the so-called aspecific granulation tissue forms which is capillary and fibroblast rich and in which a large amount of siderophages can be found. (Long ago the process was considered to be inflammatory and was given the name *pachymeningitis haemorrhagica interna.*) Today the mechanism is considered to be a new hemorrhage resulting from the hyperosmotically altered territory due to the growth of the granulation tissue after the organization of the original bleeding *(Fig. 52, 53)*. The progress of organization of the granulation tissue results in a scar, but in the meantime a spontaneously occurring or slight trauma induced rebleeding can happen, and thus form the next layer. Over time a 3-4 cm scar can build up on the dura mater by a process characterized by a large number of siderophages. Due to the prolonged period of time over which this all takes place, the affected cerebral hemisphere can compensate for the changes and the alterations caused by slowly developing hemorrhagic processes result in a remarkably low manifestation of symptoms and indeed there may be no complaints caused at all.

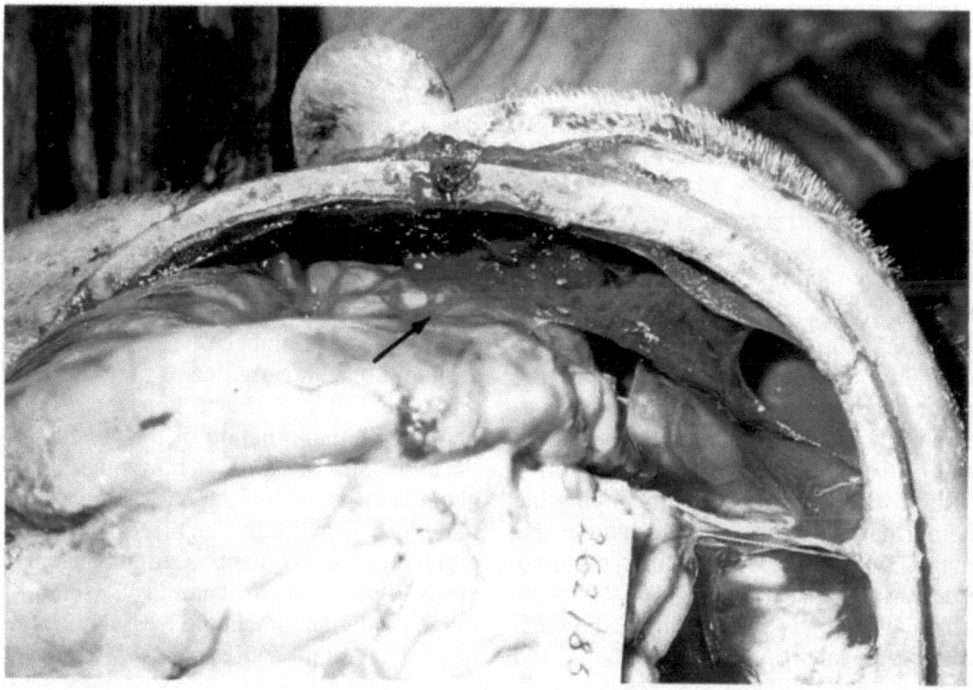

Fig. 52. Subacute subdural hemorrhage

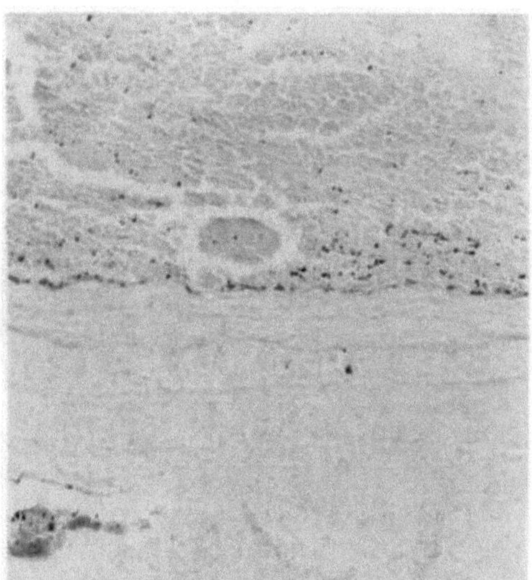

Fig. 53. Subdural hemorrhage with hemosiderin-containing macrophages, signs of fresh bleeding

● One of our cases involved a 72-year-old female patient who was admitted for neurological care in an unconscious state following a deterioration of health, who died before the treatment could begin. At autopsy we found on the right cerebral hemisphere a significantly compressed, 5 cm thick, organized, pinkish-brown, layered subdural hematoma. According to the next of kin, she had fallen and suffered a head injury more than a year before, but it had been completely symptomless.

On the other hand the hemolysis of the blood from the hemorrhage causes osmotic changes which play a role in renewed bleeding. During autopsy besides the previous mentioned, a thick granulation tissue with an extreme compression of the ipsilateral hemisphere could be found. The histological examination can shed light on the age of the process, within certain limits.

Subarachnoid hemorrhage

We divide them into traumatic and spontaneous forms. *Traumatic subarachnoid bleeding* is a characteristic consequence of brain contusion, most pronounced at the place of contre coup, but with the application of a great force, it may appear at the site of the blow. There are various forms of intracranial damage accompanying the hemorrhage, such as diffuse axonal damage, which cause clinical symptoms. The early characteristic sign of subarachnoidal bleeding is blood in the CSF which can be revealed by the presence of red blood cells in the centrifuged liquor sample. Over time the red cells deteriorate, and the CSF turns pinkish-brown in color, xanthochromic and this process verifies the subacute signs. (The differentiation of the origin of the bleeding as artificial or due to injury by distinguishing between bloody or xanthochrom liquor is important from the standpoint of the age of the injury.)

The greater number of cases of subarachnoid bleeding are due to injury to the circle of Willis. In the background of the hemorrhage is a dilation of the vessels at the base of the brain which may have come about as a result of trauma or developmental abnormalities. The bleeding due to either injury or spontaneous rupture can be easily distinguished at autopsy. Hemorrhage of the subarachnoid vessels at the base of the brain causes a massive, conf-

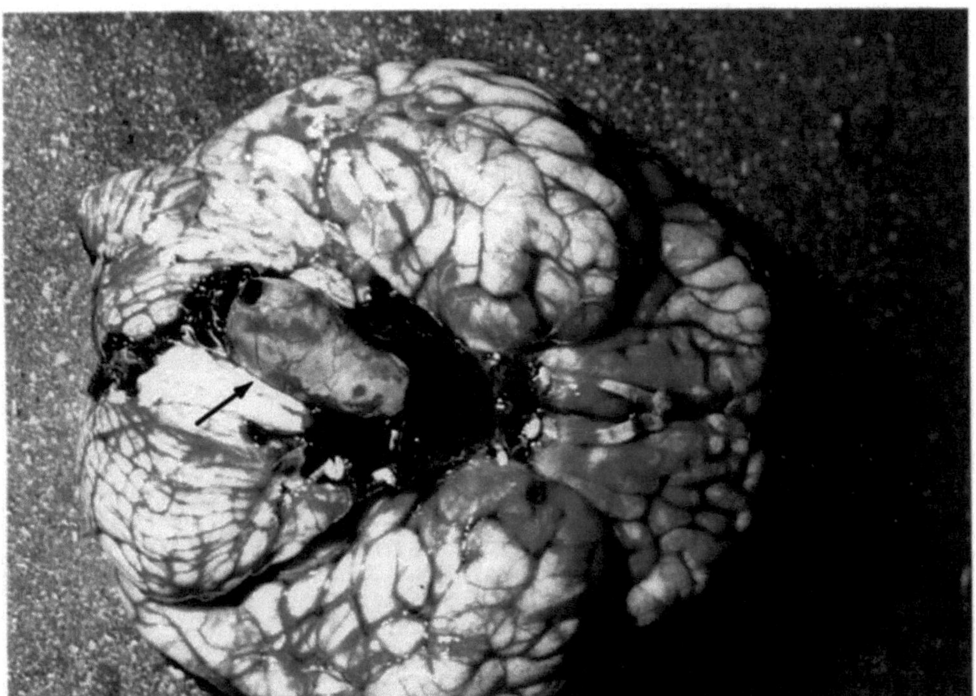

Fig. 54. Subarachnoid hemorrhage from an aneurysm of the posterior cerebral artery

luent pool of blood *(Fig. 54).* To find an injured vessel in this, – which is indispensable in the examination, especially if we want to clear up the etiological factors – requires a great deal of experience and thoroughness. Such attempts, which are recognized in the literature, as filling the internal carotid artery or the vertebral artery with contrast material and seeking the point of leakage by X-ray, show promise. Differentiating subarachnoid hemorrhage caused by post-traumatic, so-called minor traumatic, bleeding from ruptured aneurysm is not an easy task. Rupture of dilated vessels can occur due to elevation of blood pressure in absence of any externally applied force. Determination of a connection between an occasional light trauma and the rupture of an aneurysm is impossible.

● In our practice a 16-year-old boy was hit in the face by a companion while playing soccer. Shortly afterward he lost consciousness. He was taken to the local hospital, from which he was discharged and sent home, since he regained consciousness at the hospital and was lucid. At home after a short while, he lost consciousness again, and was returned to the hospital where he died. At autopsy we found a 4 mm diameter ruptured aneurysm deep in a branch of the left vertebral artery with quite massive subarachnoid bleeding and signs of increased intracranial pressure. In our opinion rupture occurred in two parts and a vessel injury resulting in bleeding occurred in which the previous injury played no part.

We usually accept that vessel injury has occurred as a result of trauma:

1. if the vessel had not been previously injured, and

2. if the vessel wall was found to be intact by histological examination.

In the consideration of damaged vessel walls, besides the above-mentioned aneurysm, the presence of angioma is possible.

A *pseudoaneurysm* is more likely to be the result of an injury. It is not a common alteration, but it can accompany penetrative head wounds, closed cranial alterations, and surgical intervention. The circulatory system of the brain is responsible for its origin. In the opinion of some, the walls of the arteries that cross the dura become thin and the number of their elastic fibers significantly decreases and injury to the vessel wall can easily occur in predisposed areas along the line of a basal skull fracture. In the area of the injured intima and internal elastic membrane a protruding vessel macroscopically resemble a true aneurysm, but circumscribed bleeding from the injured vessel may form the wall of the pseudoaneurysm, following organization. About 40% of all traumatic brain base aneurysms rupture, and cause massive subarachnoidal hemorrhage. The rupture of the traumatic aneurysm occurs in 90% of the cases within three weeks of the injury.

The most common place of the aneurysm is the middle cerebral artery followed by the anterior cerebral artery and the internal carotid. Congenital aneurysms tend to occur most commonly at the sites of vessel bifurcation. At autopsy following the special fixation of the brain the circle of Willis can be prepared and the vessel ruptures more easily demonstrated than in areas where fresh bleeding has taken place. Besides the subarachnoid hemorrhages, the post-traumatic aneurysms of the cortical arteries can cause bleeding into the cortical substance, and finding the injured vessels is almost impossible. Differentiation of a spontaneous cerebrovascular accident is possible because of the localization, although rupture of a congenital aneurysm gives similar symptoms.

Concussion of the brain

This a post-traumatic condition characterized by loss of consciousness and vegetative signs due to blow to the head. Nausea, vomiting and dizziness following an injury rouses the suspicion of concussion if loss of consciousness cannot be verified. Loss of memory often accompanies this condition in which not only the circumstances of the accident, but events before and after it cannot be remembered. The loss of memory is short and transient. A loss of memory lasting for a longer time is not due to concussion but to a more serious damage to the central nervous system. Thus the lucid interval following the epidural hematoma may be accompanied by symptoms of concussion. The morphological background is known only from animal experiments. The neurological dysfunction can appear without permanent anatomical damage due to force since if following the damage the electrochemical function returns, connections between the cerebral hemispheres and brain stem also return, and the victim regains consciousness.

Diffuse axonal injury (DAI)

Animal experiments and human autopsy reports verify that diffuse axonal damage can follow injury. (The classical form of DAI is considered those injuries which render the victim unconscious at the moment of injury and there are no CT signs of mass lesion. SAHUQUILLO et all published a study of 24 patients who suffered severe head injury and the postmortem examination demonstrated unequivocal signs of DAI. One group (15 cases) included the injured persons, in whom there were no signs of alteration with CT scan. In the second group the DAI was together with mass CT lesions, from 9 patients 6 acute subdural haematomas, 2 intracerebral and 1 extradural haematoma were demonstrated. The injuries were the results of traffic accidents and falls from height).

The number of axons damaged depends upon the severity of the injury. In clinical practice these can be divided into mild, moderate and severe cases with appropriately well described clinical signs. In especially severe cases of DAI the clinical signs resemble brain contusion or primary brain damage. Nowadays these signs of autonomic dysfunction – hypertension, hyperpyrexia, hyperhydrosis – are considered signs of axonal damage. Morphologically, in the tissue of the brain we find tiny hemorrhages appearing in certain areas which manifest macroscopic axonal damage. Areas of predilection include the corpus callosum, the rostrum and the superior cerebellar peduncle. Early damage to axons following an accident can only be seen with the electron microscope, but after 12 hours light microscopic alterations can be seen in the injured area and the so-called *"retraction balls"* form which on the injured axons are characteristic of Wallerian degeneration. Two to three weeks following injury in the place of the retraction balls proliferation of microglia signify the focal injury, and months later with the completion of the Wallerian degeneration, the so-called *long-path degeneration* develops in the cerebral hemispheres and spinal cord. (DAI accompanies serious brain injury, and is especially common in traffic accidents and falls from heights.)

Cerebral contusion

If a prolonged loss of consciousness follows an injury, or if focal signs appear, a brain contusion has been caused by a blunt force. A contusion can occur in the cerebral hemispheres or in the cerebellum, at the *place a blow (coup)* was delivered, or at the *opposite side (contre coup injury).* In other cases we can find a contusion to the brain caused by a mild application of force, and if primary symptoms are not recognized, later complications – epilepsy, atrophy and later vegetative signs – verify the injury. The injury does occur on the non fixed skull, in the form of an isolated contusion, when the application of force causes a sudden acceleration or deceleration, the brain – because of inertia and mass – doesn't follow in phase, and its motion causes it to strike the bony features inside the skull. Most commonly injuries arise at the protruding temporal pole and the anterior and inferior areas of the frontal lobe. Due to the fixation of the tentorium, the brachium conjunctivum is tractioned at the pons and a cerebellar contusion results. The mechanism of the contre coup injury is explained in that just as the brain hits the inside of the skull due to its inertia upon receiving the blow, a contusion can just as likely occur by its sudden collision with the other side. The mobility of the material inside the skull provides its vulnerability to damage caused by sudden accelerations. The movement of the head shows an external acceleration positive to the applied force, while the brain experiences a deceleration negative to it. This can produce a pressure seven times that of normal that lasts 0.3 – 6 milliseconds. The compliance of the liquor in the formation of a contusion in the brain means that if the thicker layer of liquor absorbs the energy, then a serious contusion will not develop. This supports the idea that in the case of an atrophied brain the seriousness of the contusion is lessened or avoided altogether. In an impulse-type force – a fall from a height or a traffic accident – in which the difference between the primary speed and the following deceleration is quite pronounced, the contre coup injury will occupy a large area, and the contusion will extend deep into the brain tissue, or lacerations will develop which may not be matched by the injuries seen on the other side *(Fig. 55).*

We use the *contusion index* to establish the severity of the contusion, which de-

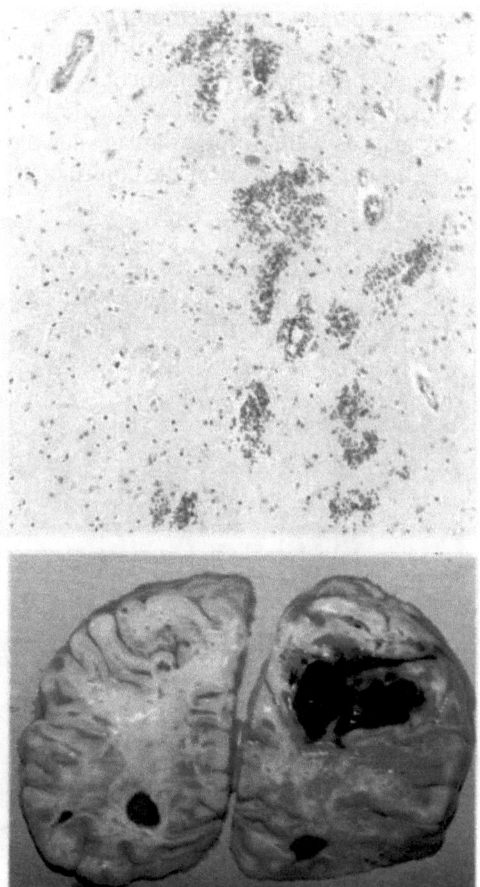

Fig. 55. Microhemorrhages, and hemorrhage-following contusion

pends on the extent, localization and depth of the injury. Especially important areas are the frontal and temporal lobes. A contusion to these areas are commonly much more severe and often are accompanied by skull fractures, loss of consciousness after the injury and difficulty in regaining consciousness. The signs depend on the localization with small contusions even being symptomless, and motor or sensory dysfunction resulting depending upon the area. The formation of edema around the contusion area can exacerbate the symptoms. The complaints may spontaneously subside, or residual signs may remain, especially in the temporal lobe.

Macroscopic morphological contusion changes come about, which not only affect the cortical substance, but the medullary substance as well. Similar damage can also be found in the area of the contre coup *(Fig. 56)*. The contusion injury is accompanied by circumscribed subarachnoid hemorrhages. The fresh hemorrhage appears blackberry-red in the subarachnoid spaces as stripes and spots. In rougher injuries, the hemorrhagic areas appear as confluent softening with the bruise extending into the white matter, so that bloody, soft areas of brain tissue are formed around which characteristic tiny hemorrhages can be seen. In the area of the contusion the red blood cells first escape into the perivascular space, and with the developing edema spread further along with the plasma flow. About two hours later leukocytes begin to migrate into the hemorrhage and can be demonstrated for up to four weeks. Monocytes appear first within 14 hours of the injury but stay for years in the damaged area. Siderophage activity can be demonstrated as in other

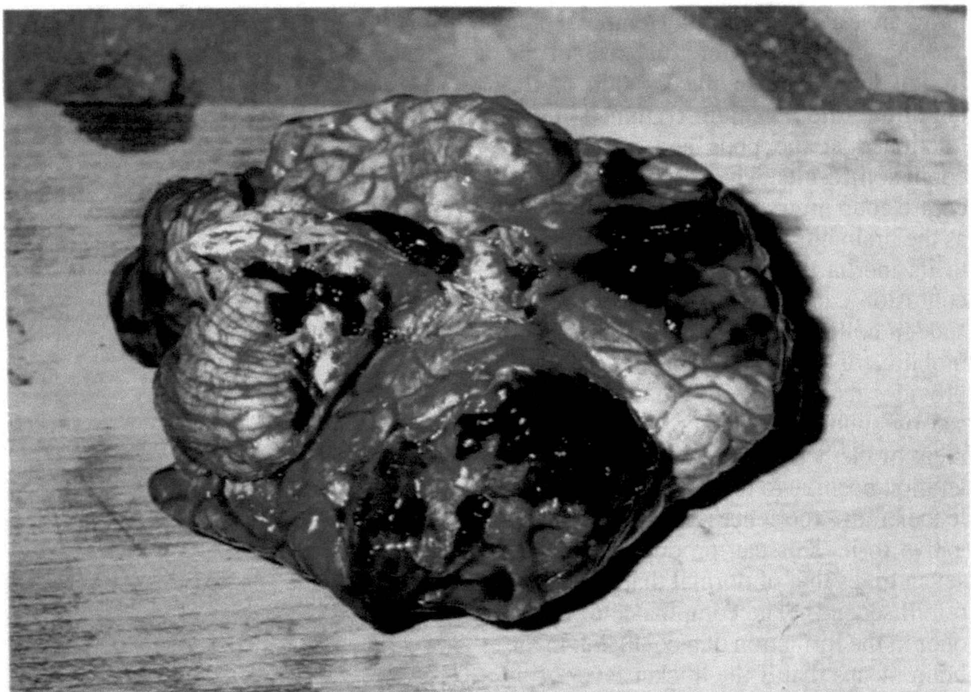

Fig. 56. Traumatic crush hemorrhage in the contre-coup location

injuries over a 3-4 day course, and remain visible for decades. Neuronophagia develops within hours with axonal swelling over the first days and continues to exist for years. Fibroblasts appear six days after the injury, but this is already a permanent state mesenchymal sign associated with glial cells. Healing of a circumscribed glial scar from a mild application of force leaves a larger, soft cyst.

Traumatic cerebral hemorrhage

In the practice of forensic medicine the condition known as *traumatic apoplectic alteration,* which occurs a few days or weeks after the injury, is a rarity. The patient shows the characteristic signs of apoplexy, and as much as the previous history reveals arteriosclerosis or hypertension, the connection of the alterations with a previous trauma is debatable. It is much harder to judge those cases in which trauma immediately preceded or the injury developed from a previous cerebral hemorrhage and during the resulting loss of consciousness a head injury was sustained. For this reason it is necessary to differentiate between traumatic and apoplectic hemorrhages. While the apoplectic hemorrhage in a significant number of cases develops in the internal capsule, those who perform autopsies on cases of sudden death know well that they can appear in other areas – cerebellum, pons, or other regions of cerebral hemispheres – as well. There is not a background of arteriosclerosis or hypertension in every case, either. Rupture of congenital aneurysms also play a prominent role.

In one kind of *traumatic cerebral hemorrhage* it is quite easy to verify an origin from application of force. Here we note an impression fracture which causes damage to the tissue of the brain. A similar mechanism is seen in penetration injuries of the skull (stab, gunshot), which are accompanied by cerebral hemorrhage. Every alteration at the site of application of force which causes injury to the vessels of the brain brings with it bleeding, and if the injury occurs to a large vessel, a large globular-shaped blood filled cavity forms, the size of which is variable, and typically can be found in the dorsolateral part of the brain. After healing a cystic alteration remains. With bleeding from a wound penetrating the cranial vault one must differentiate whether the deep tissues of the brain were also injured and whether the ventricles of the brain were opened causing an internal hemocephalus. We have already in part dealt with the situation of cerebral hemorrhage accompanying a blow from a blunt object under the section concerning contusion injuries of the brain. Nevertheless the characteristics of this group merit review, especially in the case of traffic accidents and falls from heights, if the mechanism of injury is such that an apoplectic form of hemorrhage can develop and from the etiological factors it is not clear which one happened first.

Forensic medicine literature commonly uses the Courville classification of traumatic cerebral hemorrhage as does the discussion of brain injuries in the handbooks. The classification of major injuries is quite useful in the practice of forensic medicine as well. In a brain injury resulting from a blow to the skull there may be a *primary white matter hemorrhage* and possibly *secondary alterations* which involves contre coup injuries. Hemorrhages may form in the frontal lobe, the temporal lobe, and in the area of the basal ganglia. The traumatic frontal lobe hemorrhage most commonly occupies the lower medial quadrant of the white matter, between the gyrus rectus and the orbital gyrus, extending to the anterior horn of the lateral ventricle, which it occasionally penetrates. The second group of hemorrhages lie deep in the frontal lobe, and may touch the corpus callosum forming cortical petechiae medially in the brain tissue touching the falx cerebri, which are the characteristic alterations of this case. Rarely the superior dorsolateral superficial frontal hemorrhage appears which is globular-shaped and not greatly spread. More expansive are the frontal alterations which result form a moving head suddenly meeting a solid object, and the bleeding may cover the entire frontal lobe, disperse along the corpus striatum and breach the lateral ventricle as well. (This kind of bleeding more closely resembles apoplectic hemorrhage.) We have already discussed the characteristics of *secondary hemorrhages* accompanying brain contusion and cerebral hemorrhage may accompany subarachnoid bleeding and extensive laceration of brain tissue, usually in a basal location.

Primary traumatic bleeding in the temporal lobe can be distinguished from the above cases in that it lies very close to the cortical substance. The characteristic form is a hemorrhage occurring in the uncinate fascicle. This expands backwards in the temporal lobe and little circumscribed, confluent hemorrhages from lacerative damage appear and the probability is greater of penetration into the subarachnoid or lateral ventricle as in a frontal lobe hemorrhage. Secondary hemorrhages of the temporal lobe can likewise also occur as contre coup injuries.

Primary traumatic hemorrhage in the basal ganglia is rare, but similar to the injuries described for the frontal lobe, can be mistaken for acute apoplectic hemorrhage. With careful examination, however, apparent primary hemorrhages turn out to be secondary ones resulting from contusions found at the base of the brain.

Edema of the brain

One of the acute complications accompanying injuries to the head is edema of the brain. The post-traumatic form can occur locally – in the surrounding area of a contusion – but may be generalized. The manifestation depends upon the etiological factors, the place of the edema and the time of the course. Influential factors that alter the metabolism in the brain are such biochemical processes which disturb the structural and functional integrity (hypoxia, drugs, toxins, injuries) and altered physiological circumstances which damage the blood brain barrier allowing plasma to efflux. The formation of edema is dependent upon many factors:

a) increased intracranial pressure, which results in a disturbed perfusion of nutrients and metabolism,

b) disturbances in liquor reabsorption,

c) alterations in the blood brain barrier.

Whether diffuse or local or perifocal, an increase in the weight of the brain or affected area is characteristic – the brain may be 1600–1800 grams – the gyri flattened out, and the sulci shallower. Around the cerebellar tonsils or in the area of the hippocampus a pronounced crease tonsillar, hippocampal herniation may be found. The cut surface is shiny, oozing blood from the cut vessels, and the substance of the brain adheres to the knife. In determining status spongiosus, microscopic alterations are suggestive of the process.

Edema of the brain may be vasogenic or cytotoxic in origin. *Vasogenic edema* is primarily the result of endothelial damage. Plasma crossed the vessel wall, causing edema mainly in the white matter. The plasma filtrate, having a high protein content, yields a PAS positive reaction which appears histologically in the extracellular space first. The Virchow-Robin spaces are dilated, filled with PAS positive material.

The processes of the astrocytes are swollen and show degenerative signs, staining less strongly with myelin-specific stains and the vessels are dilated. Due to the effects of trauma, infarct, intracerebral hemorrhage or tumor may develop.

The *cytotoxic form* results from acute osmoregulatory or electrolyte transport disturbances. In the later stages it may be combined with the vasogenic form. It is caused by poisons that result in hypoxia, asphyxia, hypercapnia or acidosis. Disturbances in vessel wall permeability play the leading role in its development, and may appear in either the cortex or medulla. The development of edema by ultrafiltration is not combined with early vasogenic alterations and the extracellular spaces are not dilated.

Death from an intense edema occurs due to the herniation of cerebellar tonsil or hippocampus causing damage to vasomotor and respiratory control centers.

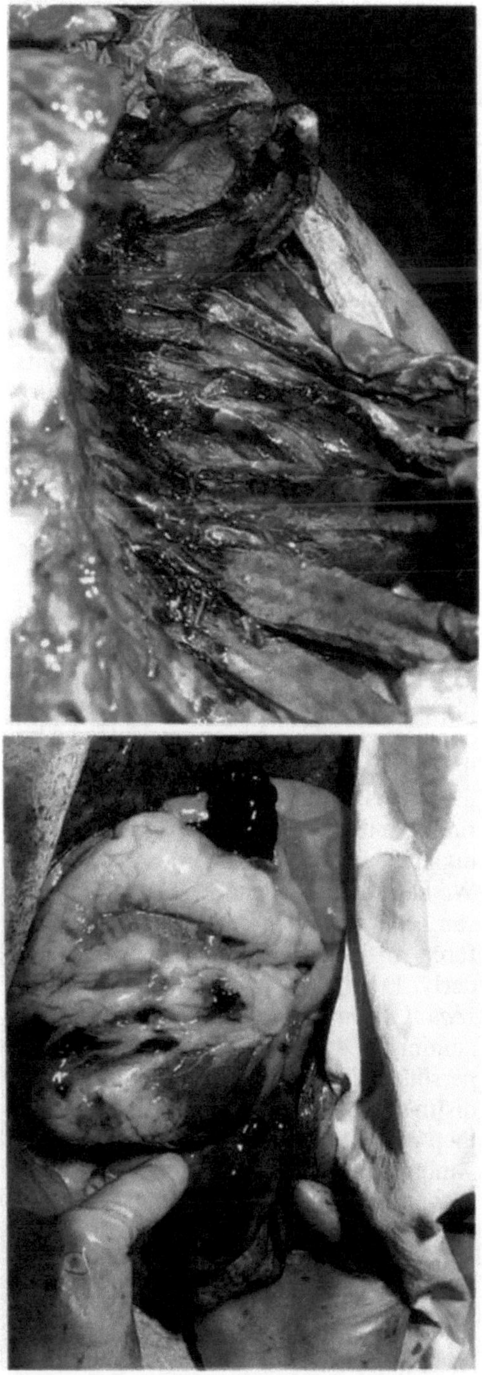

Fig. 57. Direct fracture of the ribs with penetration injury to the heart

Injuries to thoracic organs

Force applied from a blunt instrument can damage the thoracic wall and organs. The result of such force is most commonly broken ribs. The form of rib fractures, the location of the broken ends can provide insight into the causal mechanism during examination of the living patient, but even more so in autopsy. If the force is applied to a circumscribed area and the ribs in the contact area are broken, we speak of a *direct fracture*. It is characteristic that the fractured ends are moved in towards the thoracic cavity, and can damage the parietal pleura, even often injuring the lungs resulting in pneumothorax and hemothorax, and the presence of these signs support the suspicion of direct fracture. Besides injury to the lungs, the broken ends of the ribs can pierce the heart resulting in the so-called *pseudostab wound (Fig. 57).* The fracture can be the result of a kick, punch, or blow from any small surfaced blunt instrument, but a fall on a protruding object may also produce such a break.

If the force is dispersed over a wide area, the ribs may suffer a characteristic *bending fracture.* The location of the break occurs at a place distant from the point of impact and fractures the bone in such a way that the jagged edge points outward to the skin surface and thus injury to internal organs do not usually take place. Such fractures can happen from trampling or application of any compressive force to the thorax. Compression alterations in which fractures fail to occur due to the elasticity of the ribs are the most characteristic injuries to the thoracic wall and thorax suffered by young people. The sternum can be compressed all the way to the vertebral column, but of course serious contusions and lacerations are suffered by the internal organs. Besides the injuries to the organs, at the location of the impact we find contusions and streaks of bleeding in the fibers of the intercostal muscles. We have already mentioned that fractures can occur *spontaneously* or by very little force in the osteoporotic ribs of the elderly. In other cases it may result as the *sequel of cardiopulmonary resuscitation* administered by medical or paramedical persons. The forensic pathologist has to distinguish whether the rib's fracture was the result of injury or resuscitation. Among the *complications* that can surface are pneumothorax or internal bleeding, which may be a sign of injury to the lung. At other times, due to thoracic adhesions, the appearance of not pneumothorax but subcutaneous emphysema may indicate injury in the thoracic cavity. With injuries to the ribs from many directions – direct, indirect or fractures to various locations – we may consider the possibility of multiple attacks.

Powerful blunt impact may cause damage to the heart and great vessels as well as the lungs, and often occur in conjunction with falls from a height or traffic accidents.

Among *injuries to the heart,* rupture of the pericardium is not common, but its diagnosis is important because early recognition dictates the course of treatment. It can be an overlooked cause of death in the victim, at autopsy.

● A 22-year-old male traffic accident victim was taken to traumatic surgery for treatment of injuries to the extremities. While being examined, he was turned on his side and sudden cardiac arrest developed and attempts to resuscitate were unsuccessful. At autopsy rupture of the pericardium was found from which the heart protruded and death ensued after torsion of the great vessels.

Such cases are also to be found in the literature.

Concussion of the heart can be caused by relatively light thoracic injury. With a larger application of forces sudden reflex cardiac arrest can occur. In 15% of the cases of extensive thoracic injury cardiac damage takes place, contusion of the heart, from which circumscribed hemorrhages, petechiae and myocardial rupture can originate. Myocardial damage has been described in a deceleration from 36 km/hour. At other times fractures of the sternum, ribs and occasionally the clavicle can result in angina-like complaints, but 24–72 hours may pass between the injury and the clinical manifestations without a sign on the ECG. Two-dimension echocardiography has been used in early diagnosis with good results. Patients with se-

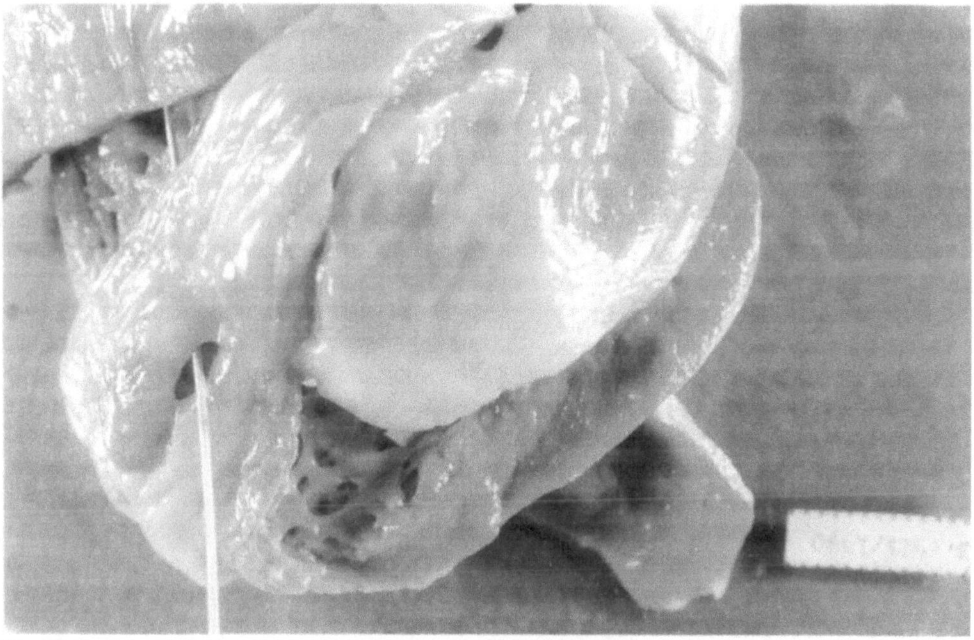

Fig. 58. **Rupture of the heart on the course of attempted resuscitation**

rious thoracic injury examined by echogram show almost 50% occurrence of irregularities which indicate perivascular hemorrhage or focal ventricular disturbances. For this reason anginal pain following an injury, especially in the young, should raise the possibility of heart concussion. Cardiac shock, asystole or cardiac rupture may cause death. It may follow immediately after injury or years later. Morphologically, a mild injury may result in serious microscopic alterations. Histological results may resemble the alterations of infarct, although the demarcation is not so pronounced. There is bleeding between the fibers of the myocardium, tears of the muscle fibers, and later – if the patient survives – the appearance of leukocytes with siderophages turning up 2–3 days later and the damaged area becomes scarred. In this case the alteration cannot be distinguished from an infarct.

An even rarer complication of thoracic trauma is *coronary occlusion* The most common location is the anterior descending branch, which is more vulnerable to injury and which from the various possibilities may result in subintimal bleeding or intimal rupture, both of which are more predisposed in the presence of atherosclerosis. The possibility of posttraumatic coronary occlusion in the young must be emphasized, in which a great compression can have been applied to the thorax without leaving external signs. It is rarely diagnosed clinically, only at autopsy.

A direct compression to the thorax, as mentioned above, may cause internal injuries without fracture of the ribs in young people. One form is heart rupture, which happens when a force is applied while the heart is in diastole *(Fig. 58)*. Usually the thinner right ventricle or atrium bursts

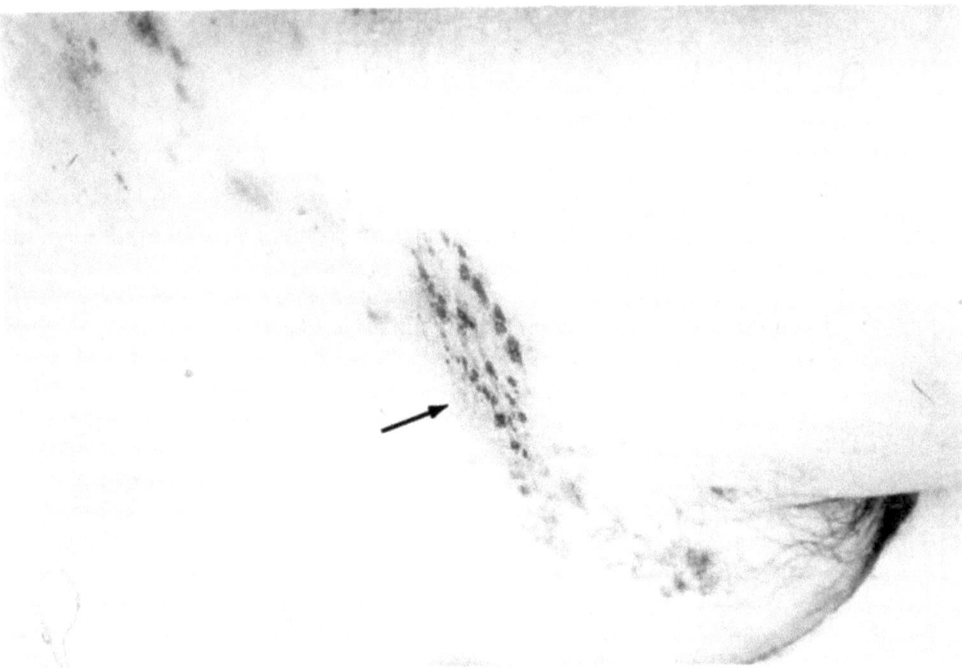

Fig. 59. Mechanical stress injury to the skin of the groin following trampling of the abdomen

causing pericardial tamponade. Falls from a height may cause not only cardiac concussion, but contusion as well, and the heart may be torn from the great vessels. Damage to the great vessels by direct blunt force happens relatively rarely. With very great force, we may encounter rupture of the pulmonary artery or aorta, but more commonly damage to the aorta is caused by a sudden deceleration or shearing force applied by vertebral fracture.

Injuries to the lungs can result in the form of contusion or serious laceration. In milder thoracic trauma *subpleural petechiae* from application of force can develop into *subpleural suffusions* which can be well distinguished from the surrounding healthy tissue. We find subpleural blood vesicles on the cut surface, and bloody infiltration can be followed deep into the tissue. (Pulmonary hemorrhage must not by confused with infarction, in which V-shaped hemorrhagic necrosis limited by the borders of the lobes and embolism or thrombus in the vessels feeding the lobules can be found!) In the case when force is applied while the lungs are filled and the glottis closed, we can count on finding injury to the pleura and pneumothorax. In falls from heights blister-like hemorrhages form around the hilus and the lung is even torn. Most commonly the left main bronchus and lung are injured.

Blunt injury to the abdomen

A large number of deaths among young people are attributable to accidents. The injuries are generally polytraumatic, but among these injuries those to the abdominal organs play a relatively large part. Of the sources of injury, traffic accidents play the leading role, but falls from heights or direct impact – kick or blow – also make up a part in the formation of abdominal injuries *(Fig. 59)*. The diagnosis is made difficult when the victim has severe alcoholic intoxication. According to an account given by Cox in a traumatic surgery department, of 870 cases of abdominal injury, 22.9% were drunk. A significant proportion of these were traffic accidents and only a small amount of them were from accidents around the home or injuries of unknown origin.

Any organ in the abdomen can be injured, but from a practical standpoint, *splenic injuries* are considered the most important. At 42%, of the traumatic abdominal injuries, the spleen is at the top of the list. Splenic injuries can be acute, with profuse hemorrhage or delayed. In the former case a blow is delivered to the area of the left costal margin and injury is caused to the spleen directly from that force, with immediate bleeding which can in a short time result in hemorrhagic shock. In delayed rupture of the spleen the tissue of the spleen is damaged, the bleeding occurs within the confines of the capsule and if the capsule ruptures from the pressure, intra-abdominal bleeding will occur within a short time or up to several days later. The delayed form of splenic rupture causes significant diagnostic difficulties in clinical recognition even at the hospital.

- In our experience an elderly man received an injury, he was bitten with a club by his wife. After a transient period of discomfort, his fitness returned. The general practitioner examined him. He wasn't referred to hospital, and two days after the injury he suddenly got worse and died. At autopsy we found a delayed rupture of the spleen. Due to the extensive adhesions around the spleen, the bursting was rather unusual. We could only follow the injury to the spleen under the costal margin. The histological examination verified that there had been an injury to the spleen at least two days before and the rupture of the capsule had occurred only later.

In examination of splenic rupture, we must turn special attention to the physical status of the victim, since some diseases carry with them enlargement of the spleen, which is more easily ruptured. In chronic congestion, lymphomas, malarial splenic changes, the spleen can be easily injured by a small force applied at the costal margin to the enlarged spleen.

Rupture of the liver is the result of a greater blunt blow, and usually acute bleeding occurs while two-phase injury to the liver is relatively rare. In childhood there is a characteristic form in which the child falls while riding a bicycle and injury to the spleen occurs as a result of falling on the handle bars.

- A nine-year-old boy suffered an injury while riding a bicycle, fell down and two hours later died. At autopsy we found an extensive bleeding into the abdominal cavity caused by injury to the liver, although in the hepatic tissue and area of the hemorrhage extensive hemangioma were also found *(Fig. 60)*.

The morphological picture can also explain the mode of origin. Direct application of force causes a star-shaped injury with lacerations deep within the hepatic tissue, which can occur from a fall from a height, and tearing the supportive tissue of the liver resulting in subcapsular bleeding.

The *diagnosis of intra-abdominal bleeding* is not always simple. Contusion around the kidneys from an injury to the mesenteric root or fracture of the pelvis

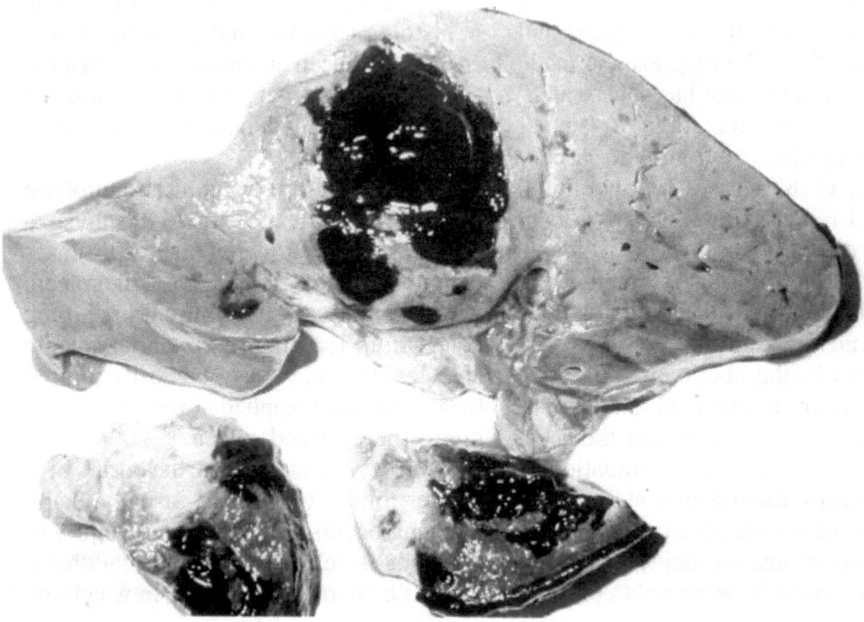

Fig. 60. Rupture of the liver due to hepatic hemangioma following a bicycle injury

often carry with them injury to vessels and retroperitoneal bleeding. Due to the expansion, the signs of severe blood loss appear, however the usual diagnostic modes – peritoneal lavage, laparoscopy – do not reveal abdominal bleeding. Only careful observation of the patient shows a probability of retroperitoneal processes. (88% of deaths due to abdominal injury are due to blood loss.)

Injury to the diaphragm is a common consequence of fall from a height. We most often find a rupture of the left diaphragm. The stomach and the small intestines may be found in the thoracic cavity and with the pulling on the mediastinum a torquation of the heart or great vessels can cause sudden death. At other times the loops of the small intestine trapped in the injured diaphragm may necrotize and result in the death of the victim. Application of force may also cause a right diaphragmatic hernia with extensive liver injuries, or may be accompanied by thoracic perforation and abdominal alterations *(Fig. 61)*.

Injury to the gastrointestinal tract may result in opening of the cavities of these organs, or bleeding into the wall of the intestines causing necrosis, and peritonitis. The root of the mesentery may be injured, especially by abdominal compression, and even torn. If the stomach or the intestines are full, they can also be injured. Injury to a full stomach or intestinal tract is much more common. In the empty state they move easily out of the way of the force. Injuries to the stomach and intestines are usually easy to follow, occasionally with air in the abdominal cavity and the signs of peritoneal irritation, but injuries to the pancreas and duodenum in numerous instances remain hidden, even though tearing of the duodenum because of its retro-

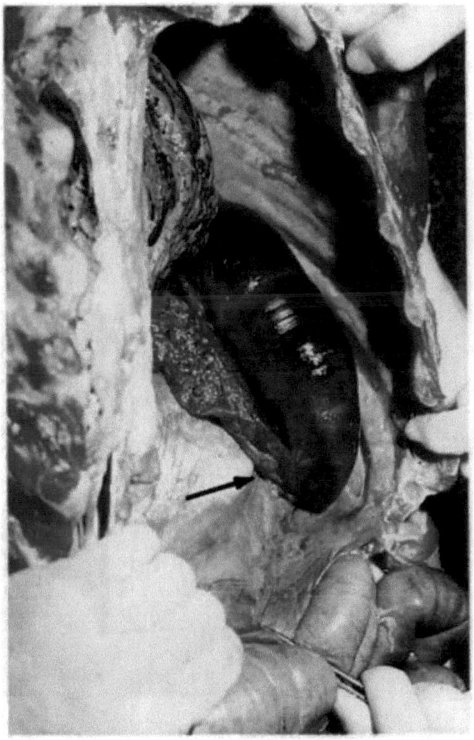

Fig. 61. Traumatic rupture of the diaphragm. Strangulated section of the intestine pushed through the diaphragm into the thoracic cavity showing hemorrhagic necrosis

peritoneal situation are some of the most common intestinal injuries *(Fig. 62)*.

Ultrasound examination of the abdomen can give significant diagnostic aid.

Renal injuries are mostly the result of traffic accidents. Falls from heights don't bring about more serious injuries, but a blow applied to the small of the back causes injury to the kidneys in almost every case. The blow causes lacerations to the tissue. *Bladder injury* usually accompanies fracture of the pelvis, especially if the full bladder was elevated up out of the pelvis. A blow to the lower abdomen can cause an injury to the fundus of the bladder. Compound fracture of the pelvis may damage not only the bladder, but the *urethra* as well.

A blow to the pregnant uterus elevated up out of the pelvis may rarely cause damage to the fetus, or interruption of the pregnancy. Following a very great application of force resulting uterine contractions may bring a premature delivery or abortion *(Fig. 63)*.

Traffic accidents

Together with the increasing of motorization the number of traffic accidents is growing steadily. In those countries in which the number of motorized vehicles is great, traffic accidents cause 44% of all deaths in young people. The injuries are of the polytraumatic type, and after even milder impact we can count on injuries of various kinds and later complications. Some of the modes of origin are characteristic of the circumstances of the accident, the injury revealing the kind of instrument and sometimes the type. The examination of the traffic accident is a combined team work. It requires great cooperation at the scene between the traffic expert conducting the examination, the investigator, the medical specialist, and the motor vehicle specialist. Only their concerted, circumspect labors can produce results that will clear up the circumstances of each accident. For this reason the early phases of the investigation at the scene must be purposeful on the part of the experts *(Fig. 64)*.

In a traffic accident the effects of numerous factors appear, and every circumstance, every injury and every accident victim plays a role. Among the *circumstantial or external factors* is the weather as one of the more influential factors. In rainy weather driving on a wet road is a risky situation, even under ideal

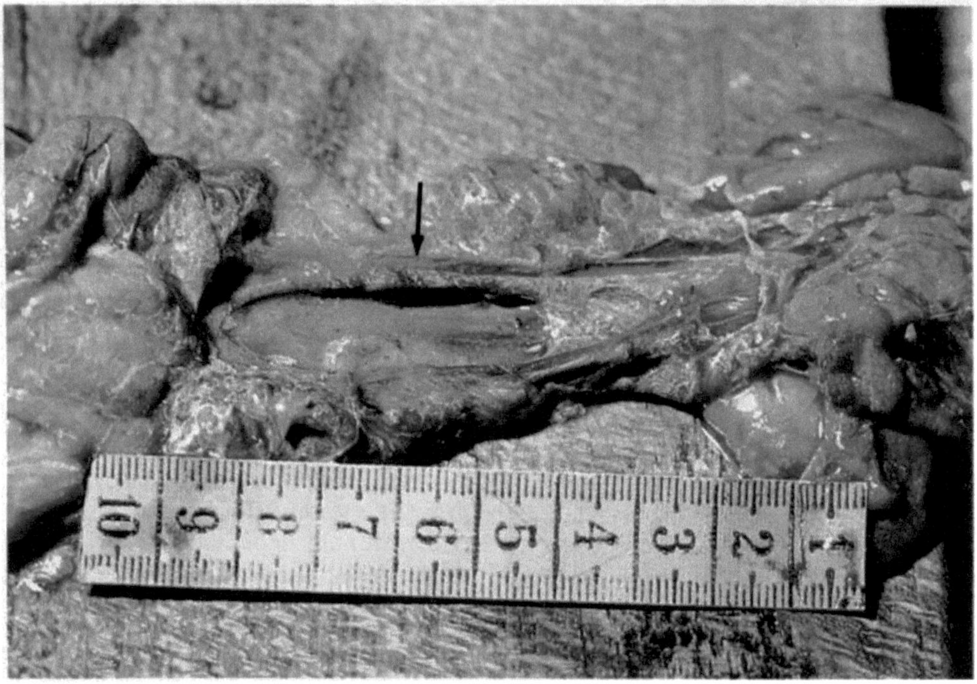

Fig. 62. Intestinal rupture. Collapsed wall of the injury

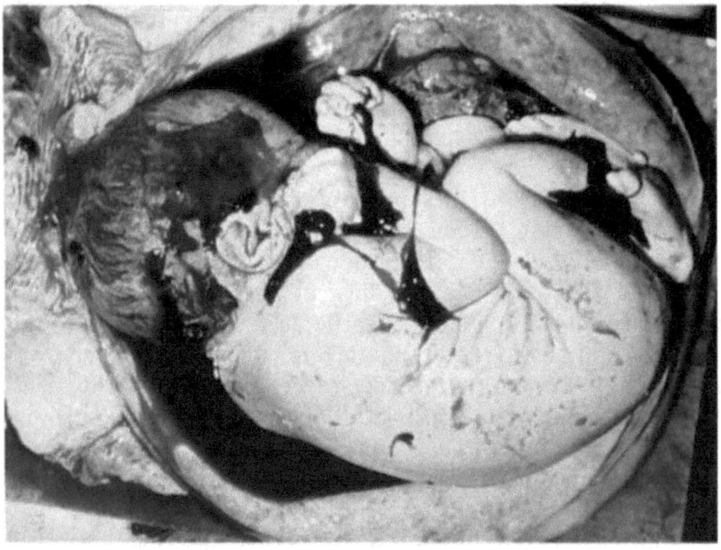

Fig. 63. Intrauterine hemorrhage, injury to the placenta, death of the fetus in a traffic accident

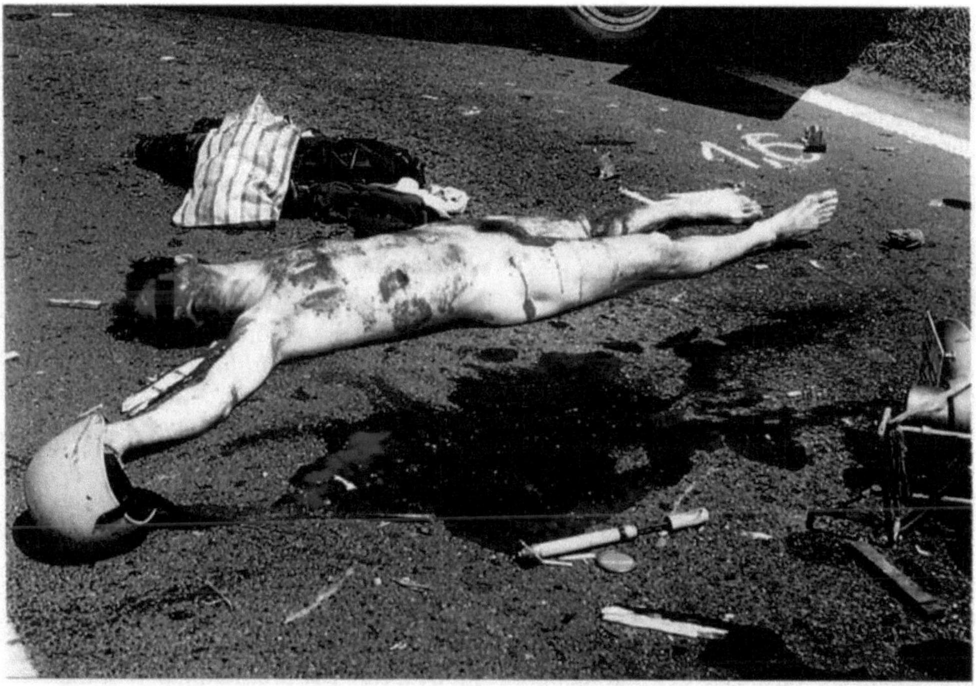

Fig. 64. Examination of the victim of a traffic accident at the scene

conditions – driving at the proper speed with a vehicle in optimal mechanical condition – and is especially dangerous if the safety factors are compromised. At high speeds when a car hits a wet patch of road, aquaplaning takes place – when a thin film of water forms between the tires and the road and the vehicle is for all practical purposes sliding – which makes the vehicle less steerable. A similar situation occurs with sudden one sided seizing of the brakes or improper use of the steering wheel which can result in an accident. The increase in traffic accidents in the fall due to muddy or icy roads attests to this. Among the environmental effects is the condition of the road. Long, straight stretches of road make the driver sleepy and tired and these understandably help cause accidents. Signs warning of bends in the road and providing other information can not help but increase the safety in driving. Frequency of accidents specified by the time, is highest between 0–6 o'clock a.m..

The *internal factors* are numerous. Starting with diseases, we can list the various intoxications. We should deal with the most common of them in detail. In first place stand those alterations which cause sudden loss of consciousness. Among these *epilepsy* or a special form, the so-called *photoepilepsy,* is worth mentioning. In the latter case, the person is sensitive to rapid changes in light and dark, which precipitate an epileptic seizure. The epileptic driver must be cautiously restricted and provided he does not withhold from the examining physician the fact of his illness, he may drive under restricted circumstances. Similar regulation apply to the *diabetic* driver. Despite this, in many cases the drivers have been unable to remember the circumstances of the accident because they became ill right before it. In many cases they remember experiencing symptoms which are characteristic of hypoglycemia. These possibilities are hard to cast aside or verify, and only the appearance of clinical signs make the condition probable. We also count among the internal factors the so-called negative effect of the *weather front.* Those who are more sensitive to the weather fronts and drive in a careless manner, may only recognize the presence of danger too late. There are such diseases of the *cardiovascular system* in which sudden loss of consciousness occurs – arrhythmias, serious coronary sclerosis, ischemic myocardial changes – which show up in traffic accidents in a significant percentage.

Not last on the list of safety compromising factors are various *drugs and alcohol* and occasionally both together. These days numerous drug groups are recognized which cause deterioration of the reflexes and orientation, and they are therefore forbidden to be consumed under such circumstances as would cause danger. This includes the driving of motor vehicles, but also of bicycles, horse-drawn vehicles or pedestrian traffic, too. The victims or perpetrators of traffic accidents are showing a use of these drugs in a rising percentage of traffic accident statistics. The *postalcoholic syndrome* which was not widely recognized until recently, is becoming known among alcoholics. Inasmuch as drunk driver accidents only count the cases in which alcohol was consumed, the postalcoholic group that causes accidents is just as significant, only the customary examination in which the general practitioner measures the alcohol level doesn't verify them.

Monitoring of the blood alcohol level in traffic accidents is imperative! (Even in a negative breath test, it is worth while to take a blood sample as well to catch the possible presence of drugs!)

The significance of *psychiatric diseases* are especially quoted in relation to traffic accidents. In people with certain personality traits, who are more irritable, less tolerant, prone to immature behavior, and hyperactive, tend to have more accidents. Especially affected is the so-called sociopathic group. According to some, there are those victims in this group who take the accident, or the circumstances of an accident, as an opportunity for suicide. One may say that a person drives as he lives.

A traffic accident may involve a pedestrian, bicyclist, motorcyclist and passengers.

The injuries to the *pedestrian* show a characteristic formation, if the person is hit by a car. The protruding part of the vehicle first hits the standing or walking victim, and the alterations are the result of the speed. At great speed the moving vehicle first causes significant fractures at the place where the vehicle struck – in cars it is usually the bumper or hood – which indicate the direction of impact *(Fig. 65, 66).*

Besides the fractures, serious *injuries to soft tissues* also form in that area with crushing of muscles, tearing of vessels, extensive bleeding into the soft tissue areas, and the formation of blood filled cavities. Collision by a car or motorcycle causes fracture of the tibia or fibula while collision by a truck or larger vehicle causes impact higher up, commonly producing injuries to the buttocks or back as *primary injuries* in which pelvic fractures and kidney ruptures may result. Following the primary impact, the victim may be thrown to the ground causing *secondary injuries* often facial and skull fractures. The body thrown forward or sideways to the ground

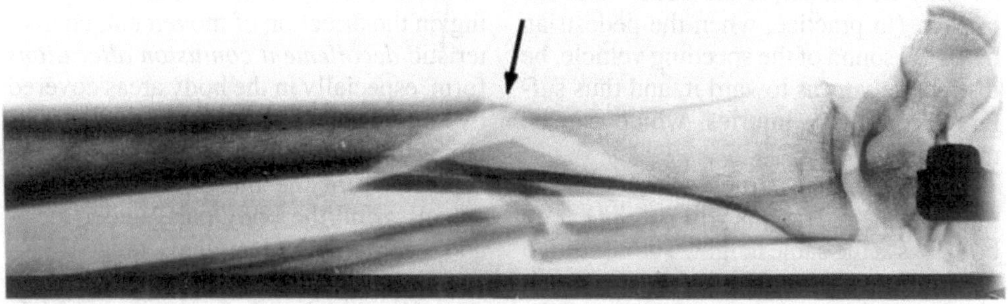

Fig. 65. Tibial fracture following a traffic accident. The arrow indicates the direction of the impact

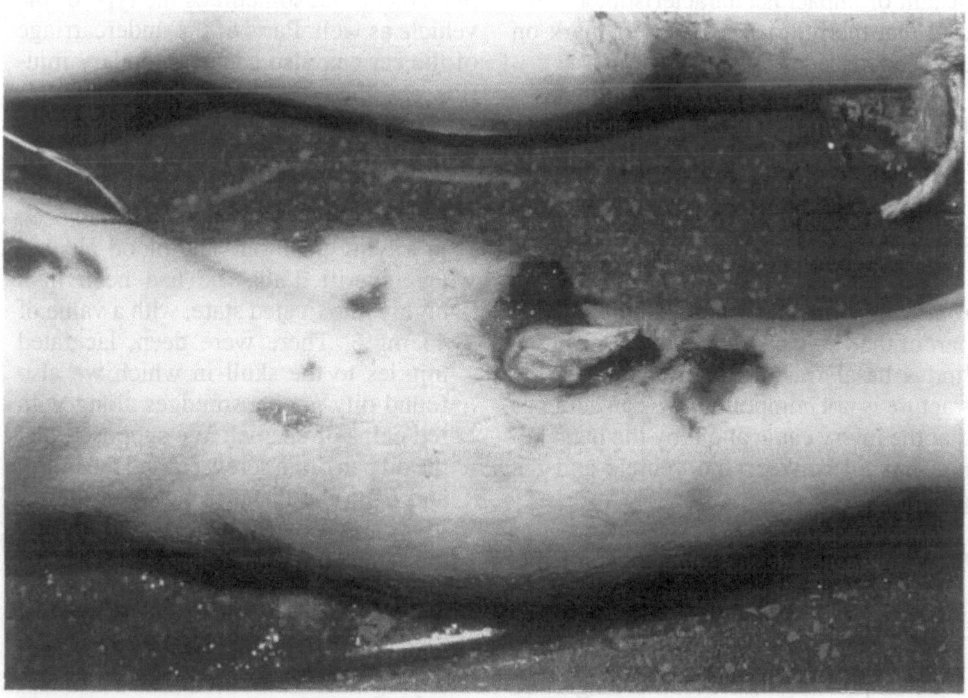

Fig. 66. Open fracture of the lower extremity, caused by the bumper of a car

can suffer contusions. Following the impact, the pedestrian may slide along the hood striking the windshield or windshield flange and fall off to the side. Whiplash fractures may form. The hood of the car can cause contusions or fractures to the high parts of the body it hits. A fracture impression in the form of the windshield flange may be created on the skull, and on the sides with great force the body may suffer residual injuries, most commonly injuries to the thoracic organs, skull injuries and damage to the upper extremities.

Clarification of the primary injuries is an important task of the medical specialist.

From the injured parts of the body, occasionally we can derive the direction of the impact. (In practice, when the pedestrian hears the sound of the speeding vehicle, he instinctively turns toward it, and thus suffers the primary injuries, which can be misleading).

In a pedestrian struck while walking midstep, the alterations will not appear on both legs at the same height. The condition of the footwear can provide important information, in that the appearance of the sole that was in contact with the road at the instant of impact is characteristic, and we find that the injuries leave their mark on the road surface.

- In one case, deep and fresh skid marks left by the boots of the victim were found several meters from the body, marking the point of impact.

The injuries of the *person lying on the roadway* come about according to which part of the vehicle struck the victim. If we find a basal fracture of the skull, if the fracture is not compound, we can suppose that the injury came about by the head being pressed between the vehicle and the ground.

- We surmised that it was a probable hit-and-run accident when a head injury was caused by a car almost stopping right before the victim with the front wheel pressing the head into the ground from the side and causing a fracture. At the place of contact of the tire small soft tissue injuries were found, with similar contusions on the opposite side and a basal fracture running between the two poles. Later the suspect confessed that he had stopped on the head of the victim who was lying on the ground, and saw only the superficial injuries. Being drunk, he fled the scene.

Injuries are often caused by a vehicle *running over a lying victim.* Depending on the direction of movement, characteristic *decollement contusion alterations* form, especially in the body areas covered by larger layer of soft tissue – thigh or upper arm. The skin and the fatty tissue separate from the muscle tissues as the wheels grind the body parts under them, and here bloody fat-filled, ragged sacs appear. Injuries and fractures dependent upon the weight of the moving vehicle form and not only show the direction of movement, but sometimes the type of the vehicle as well. Parts of the undercarriage of the car can also cause secondary injuries, and these can be characteristic.

- We examined the corpse of a young man after a hit-and run accident. The injuries indicated that the man had been in a lying position. The blood alcohol level verified that he had been in a highly intoxicated state, with a value of 45 mg%. There were deep, lacerated injuries to the skull in which we also found oily-greasy smudges along with red chips of enamel. We supposed that the oil pan drain screw caused the injury and from the distance between the injury caused by the wheels and that by the screw, the vehicle expert advised us we could look for a Shiguli (a common Russian car in Hungary) as the vehicle which had run over the man. The next day the man who had hit the victim was arrested and found on the screw of his car blood and hair.

A car rolling over a person can cause serious thoracic and abdominal internal injuries which are dependent upon the weight of the vehicle. The alterations caused by a *train or tram* is characteristic. Especially in the young a train which runs over the victim leaves abrasions and con-

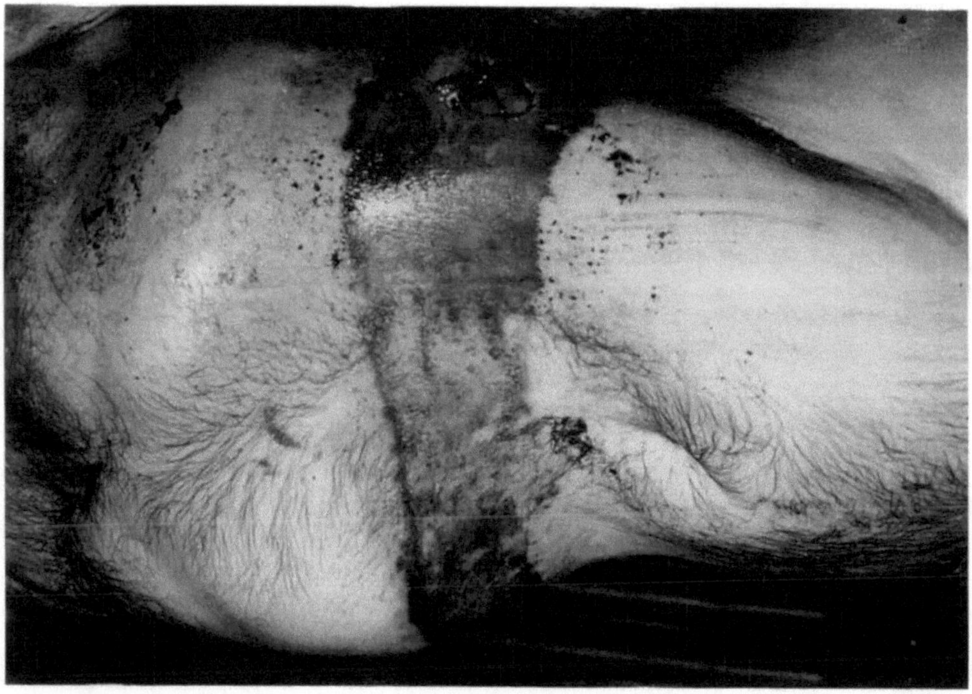

Fig. 67. Imprint of the wheel of the railway on the abdominal skin

tusions on the skin, depending on the width of the wheels, and the soft tissue and bones at the point of contact are ground to bits *(Fig. 67)*.

The specialist in practice must answer an essential question – whether the victim was hit while standing or lying – described characteristics basically are not simple. The alcohol level of the victim, the examination of the clothing, the traces found on the vehicle (textile or biological traces) and the characteristics of the injury can help us.

The *bicyclist* can suffer such an accident that, due to a tumble or sudden braking, he may land on the handle bars. The injuries can be so severe that they arouse the suspicion of being hit by a car. Sometimes in the examination of a bicyclist who has been in an accident it is difficult to decide whether he has been hit or not. We have already dealt with abdominal injuries suffered by children in bicycle accidents, the most common of these being liver injury caused by hitting the handle bars. A *fall from a bicycle* can result in serious head injuries and broken bones. In sudden braking, the forward-moving body can suffer such injuries as though it had been hit from behind. The injuries characteristic for almost every bicyclist *hit from behind* with great force is not found. If the bicycle absorbs first the impact, the vehicle which suddenly lurches forward between the legs can cause a characteristic bruises or tears to the scrotum in men *(Fig. 68)*.

Extensive contusion injuries to the small of the back can happen when a bicycle is hit, with kidney damage and fractures of the vertebrae. Often a primary injury to the left lower extremity caused

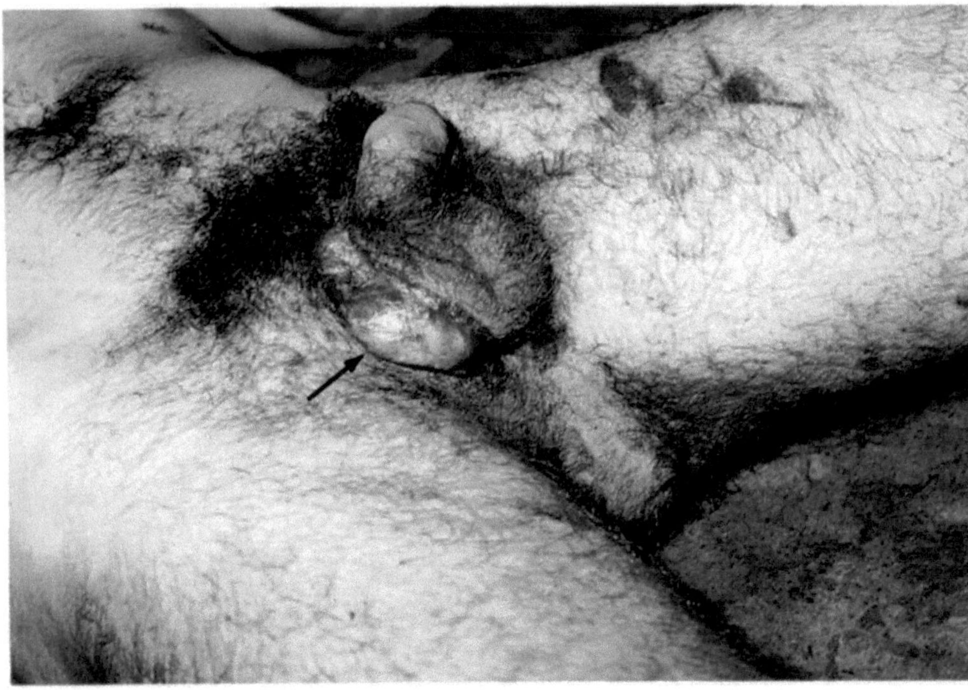

Fig. 68. Characteristic injury to the scrotum of a bicyclist when hit from behind

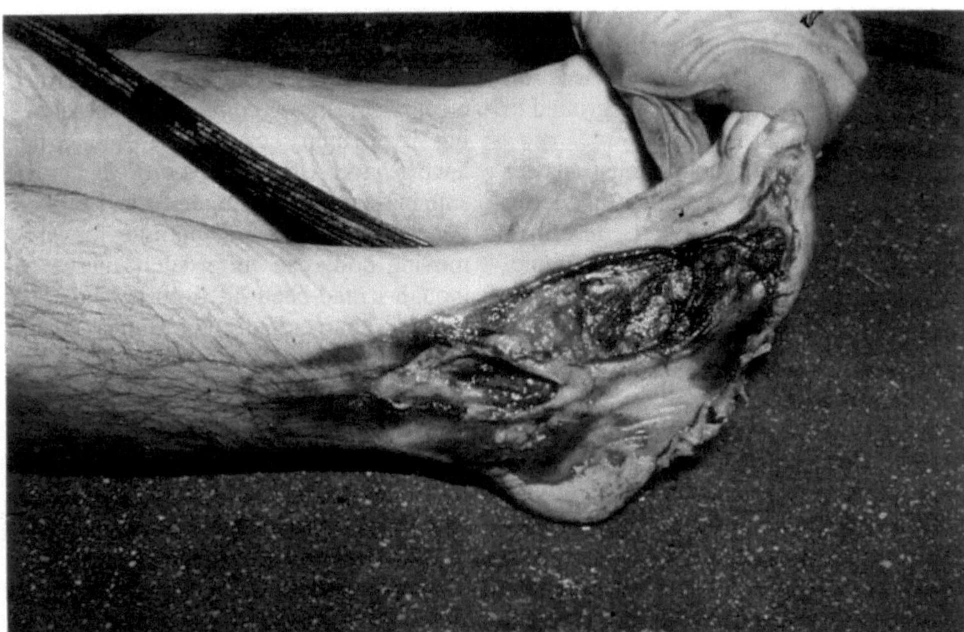

Fig. 69. Flaying injury to the foot. The cyclist was hit from the side by the motor vehicle

by a *passing vehicle* may fracture the ankle in pieces while leaving the bicycle undamaged. The victim falls to the opposite side and suffers secondary injuries. A similar situation develops if the bicyclist is bending forward or hangs over the vehicle. Here as well the lower extremity closest to the on-coming vehicle suffers the primary injury and the falling body is injured on the side where it hits the front of the vehicle or the hood of the car *(Fig. 69)*. In any case of the examination of an injured bicyclist found in the roadway, the scene must be considered as a possible site of collision.

- A 56-year-old man was found dead on the side of the road next to his bicycle. Two and a half hours before being found, he had left a nearby liquor store in a severely intoxicated state. There were laceration injuries on the top of his head and abrasions on his face. Hit-and-run was considered, but the examination by a specialist suggested that a blow by a blunt instrument was more probable, and the fall from the bike after the blow gave rise to the facial injuries. Within a short time the investigation turned up the perpetrator, who had followed the victim after he had left the liquor store and struck him down, to get revenge for an insult.

Injuries to *motorcyclists* are numerous and fit every significant category of injury. A speeding vehicle in a collision or fall results in extensive injuries. In a collision, the *forward parts* of the body of the motorcyclist receive the most serious injuries. Contusions to the thorax, rib fractures and damage to internal thoracic organs accompany them. On the face, if the helmet did not provide protection, we find abrasions, contusions, and fractures to the facial bones. On the gripping surface of the hands abrasions and contusions with fractures are seen, which are similarly present on the knees and tibial surfaces of the lower extremities. In an accident the most serious injuries are those to the head and neck. The wearing of helmets does not significantly decrease the number of injuries, especially at high speeds. In a great impact the helmet is not capable of protecting and in numerous instances the helmet was also broken above the impression fractures that were found. In helmet-wearing motorcycle accident victims the characteristic injury is the so-called *ring fracture*. The ring fracture occurs when a backward pulling force is applied to the base of the skull, connected with the angular acceleration of the head, and in this case there is no injury to the scalp or blood infiltration. A *torsion fracture* forms on the skull, the fracture of the base of the skull being asymmetrical with respect to the base itself. The fracture always brings with it tears to the pons or medulla. Head injuries without fracture can cause central cerebral bleeding, rupture of bridge veins or subarachnoid bleeding from contusions. A *fall onto the side,* besides the primary injuries to the respective side, abrasion injuries resulting from the continued rolling can appear with serious internal injuries. In the clarification of the mechanism, the clothing examination in this case also can add relevant data.

Polytraumatic injuries are characteristic of *automobile accidents*. The injuries of the front seat passengers are caused by the seat belt. The deformation of the vehicle and the speed yield the force of the impact in the car to the passengers.

$$G = \frac{K \cdot v^2}{d},$$

G = acceleration, v = speed of the vehicle, K = constant (0.0039), d = stopping distance of the car.

The shorter the so-called passive safety distance of the car, the greater the deceleration affecting the passengers and from that comes the injuries.

In *frontal impact*, if the victim was not wearing a seat belt, he goes with the movement of the car, and is thrown forward with injuries occurring to the face and head. The victim in the driver's seat may acquire injuries from the steering wheel, with the imprint of the wheel being visible on the skin and contusions to the thoracic organs, rib fractures, concussion to the heart, lung contusions and rupture of the thoracic aorta being manifest. The unguarded head is thrown against the windshield and contusions and fractures are incurred. The broken bits of glass cut the soft tissues of the face. The safety-layered glass breaks into angular pieces and usually cuts sharp bordered abrasions, but cases have also been described where the survivor breathed in tiny bits of safety glass. The forward moving body may also hit the edge of the dashboard fracturing the patella or the tibia. Head, face and knee injuries are characteristic for the driver of the vehicle as well as the passenger beside him. The recoil of the forward moving body may also result in spinal fractures.

The *wearing of seat belts* results in fewer injuries to the face and head, but at the same time results in more thoracic injuries. The properly worn seat belt flexibly retains the forward-thrown body while itself being irreparably damaged. (A seat belt that has been through an accident cannot be used again!) The injuries suffered by a person wearing his seat belt can be characteristic, and later can show which side the victim was sitting on. At the areas of contact of the belt, pinpoint hemorrhages form on the skin, abrasions mark the area of impact verifying the localization of the position of the belt. Wearing seat belts has raised the number of fractures of the clavicle, the one sitting on the left side suffering a fracture of the left bone and the one on the right fracturing his right clavicle. Rib and sternum fractures, and heart contusions have also risen, and the sudden deceleration can cause tearing of the aorta. In those accidents where such injuries were caused by the wearing of seat belts, there would have been heavy shattered injuries to the face and head injuries had the belts not been worn. Undoubtedly, when the seat belt is worn properly, the injuries to the passengers and the seriousness of the accident are positively altered. An *improperly worn seat belt,* on the other hand, does not prevent injuries, but raises the number of unusual types of damage. The too loosely worn seat belt does not retain the body of the passenger at the moment of impact, and it is thrown forward resulting in the injuries described above. The too loose belt can slide up and if he slides under it, neck injuries may be suffered. Such a case has happened where the too loosely worn seat belt has decapitated its wearer. The special case of where the seat belt is worn under the arm pit has been considered. During impact abdominal injuries can occur, but the trunk can be thrown forward and face and head injuries can be caused.

The injuries that can occur to the *back seat passengers* include a frontal blow to the head and thoracic damage. Commonly, when the body is thrown from the back seat, it hits the car's roof and we can notice contusion injuries on the temples, and sometimes with hitting the upholstery, injuries to the cervical vertebrae can occur *(Fig. 70)*. The body thrown out the open door also suffers further injuries.

When *hit from behind,* the car is thrown forward, the body is pressed backward into the seat, and if the neck is not supported by a headrest, the cervical spine can suffer a strain injury. In the mild form of this

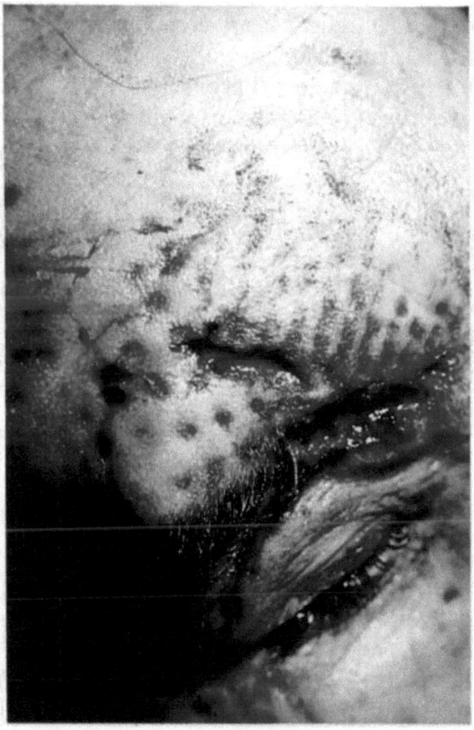

Fig. 70. Impression of the ceiling upholstery on the skin of a victim who was sitting in the back seat and suffered an injury to the forehead

traction on the spinal cord, a temporary dizziness and paralysis develops, and in more serious cases, fracture to the vertebrae, contusion or tearing of the spinal cord can happen. In such collisions we can count on the manifestation of long-lasting complaints such as paraesthesia of the upper extremities and balance disturbances.

In the *examination of the victim of a traffic accident* – if performed with proper technique and care – many questions can be answered, which an inexact description and inappropriate examination in the future would be unable to answer. In the examination at the scene, the autopsy or the examination of the injured victim, it is important to determine the primary injuries. The position of the body at the moment of the accident can also provide some indication of the make and type of the car. (In a collision with a motorcycle, the handle bars or the foot rest can cause injury. On a lying person run over by a motorcycle, we can find one, or two very close, tyre prints left by the wheels in which place the seriousness of the injuries do not compare to the injuries caused by being run over by a car. Injuries left by a passenger car first of all are more likely to be those left by the bumper, and therefore the primary injury depends upon the height of the bumper off the ground). The distance of the injury from the plane of the sole must be taken in every case during the examination of traffic accident victims. The characteristic wedge shape of the compound fracture indicates the direction of impact and the speed. The examination of the clothing of the victim hit by a car is critical. On them we not only find the impressions left by the vehicle, but in many cases the exact identification of the vehicle can be made from the paint imprints and occasionally from broken bits of the car left behind. In the examination it must be decided whether the victim was hit by a car or whether the injuries could have been caused by something else.

In those accidents which occur with a vehicle in technically unimpeachable condition and a good driver, it must be clarified whether the driver suddenly falling ill caused the accident. Many times an instant of unconsciousness can be mentioned, the subsequent verification or exclusion of which requires careful judgement. With similar accidents of fatal outcome it is easy to clarify morphological signs of sudden unconsciousness that accompany diseases. Among these ischemic heart damage can be indicated by a severe coronary sclerosis and narrowing, sometimes the swelling of the coronary plaque may cause acute occlusion, ruptured aneurysm or apoplexy caused by intracranial bleeding can lead to the accident. Sometimes the carbon monoxide level of the hemoglobin must be determined in case the morphological alterations might not explain the sudden unconsciousness. A leak of gas from a broken exhaust system into the passenger compartment of the car can bring in a large amount of carbon monoxide unnoticed, making the passengers unconscious.

If we do not find such alterations which point to an occasional unconsciousness – the so-called "accident of unknown cause" – we can begin to suspect suicide. Frontal collisions especially indicate this, whether head-on with another vehicle or into an object by the side of the road, evidence of braking or skid marks just prior to the impact are missing, and the crash occurs with the vehicle travelling at great speed.

In the examination in many cases it must also be decided *who was driving the vehicle.* We have already commented on the characteristics of the injuries. The injuries caused by the seat belt can be of help, and sometimes the injury caused by the steering wheel can be characteristic. Injuries on the passenger sitting on the left side of the car tend to occur on the left side and in more than one instance, blood stains found on the left door or surrounding area have decided the question. Imprints of the gas or brake pedal may be left on the footwear of the driver.

We have already discussed the significance of testing for blood or urine alcohol in the victims or perpetrators of traffic accidents. The samples not only shed light on the alcohol level, but can identify or exclude the consumption by the driver of medications influencing driving safely.

The *examination of traffic accidents,* as we have already indicated, requires the teamwork of several qualified experts, indispensable among which is the medical expert. In recent years computer modelling has been tried for traffic accidents, but the human factors (unconsciousness, driver experience, mental disposition, etc.) are not easily programmable.

Electrical injuries

Electrical injuries make up only a small part of the huge number of unusual deaths, nevertheless the significance of electrocution, the difficulties in diagnosis, and the extended complications endured by the survivors make this form of injury an active constituent in the practice of forensic medicine. Among the more commons forms of these injuries are the household or work place accidents and the improperly attended or repaired instrument, or the jury-rigged electric appliances can play a role. Among these the hair drier used in the bath, the 380 volt industrial cement mixer with a bare wire, or the welding tools always turn up. Electrical injuries from attempted suicide rarely occur, though in many articles one can find cases of homemade devices used for autoeroticism causing lethal injury. (There was published a male nurse's case who attempted suicide applying cardiac defibrillator to his head).

Electrical injuries vary with the strength of the current, voltage (tension), frequency, type (AC or DC), tissue resistance, the course through the body, and individual sensitivity of the victim.

The strength of the current is one of the most important factors from the standpoint of the manifestation and severity of the injury. Some differential between weak and strong current injuries in that the tissue damage from the current passing through depends on the strength of it. According to Joule's law the damage caused by local heat cannot be neglected, especially in applications of electricity with high amperage. The strength of the current depends upon the voltage and tissue resistance. Household appliances of 110–220 volts vary between 1–2 A and 15–20 A. Ten mA are rarely dangerous, although as little as four mA can cause lethal damage in children. Ten to 20 mA causes a tingling sensation, but muscle contraction may also result from it. At a level of around 50 mA the victim is still conscious but incapable of making a sound and crying for help. Death results form tetany of the thoracic muscles and asphyxia, not directly from electrical damage. Fifty to 100 mA can cause *ventricular fibrillation.*

Voltage is divided into *micro-, low-, and high-tension* (below 42 V and above 1000 V). Regardless of the way the injury happened, the strength of the current plays an important role, moreover there are cases known of where less than 60 V have caused fatalities. The greater percentage of electrical injuries occur from low-tension currents of less that 1000 V. Micro-tension voltages can cause injuries in children, their sensitivity to electric current being greater that was previously realized. The household 110–220 V can physiologically induce ventricular fibrillation, and burn injuries from the heating effect of the high voltage. Ohm's law in respect to *tissue resistance* determines the character of injury. At the instant of application of electric current, the resistance of the skin is significant and it ensures a period of protection. The resistance of the skin reduces the power of the current, but if it "breaks through" the skin resistance, the strength of the current comes back. The break-through point happens where there are superficial blood vessels or where the channels of the sweat glands penetrate. The resistance of the different tissues is variable. The blood vessels, in which the blood behaves like electrolytes, conduct current well, similar to nerves. Muscle tissue also behaves well as a conductor. If the current touches the body at the surface of the skin, the electrical power that breaks through the initial resistance continues its way on the above path. The superficial resistance of the mucous membranes is negligible, generally 100 Ohm/cm^2. The skin resistance varies between 200–2000 Ohm, depending on whether the skin surface was dry or wet. The bones, ligaments and adipose tissues are poor conductors with significant resistance, and if touched by a high voltage current, they melt in the heat evolved from it. In the neighborhood of the bones *"bone pearls"* form. In longer applications of current the alterations of bone tissue, is preceded by damage of periosteum. Occasionally, damage to the deeper muscle tissues may be more significant than that of the superficial muscle fibers at the place of application.

The *type of power* also determines the nature of the injury. Direct current (DC) is less dangerous than alternating current (AC). *DC current* causes simple muscle contraction, while *AC current* with a frequency of 50–60 Hz can cause tetanic muscular contraction, due to the periodicity of the current. In the current touches the hand, the flexor and extensor muscles both contract, and with the flexors being the stronger, it appears as if the victim has grabbed the source of the current, and he cannot let go. Due to the more pronounced polarization of DC current, metalization changes take place in which material from the source appears on the surface of the body. Aluminum causes a silvery-white, copper a yellowish or green, and iron a black galvanization.

The role of *individual sensitivity* in the examination of the consequences of electrocution cannot be neglected. We have already mentioned the sensitivity of children. Similarly, a low voltage or low strength current can cause fatalities in those suffering from circulatory disorders, especially cardiac diseases, but the hyperthyroid patient is similarly sensitive. Some count in individual sensitivity an increased sweating as well, in that in such people the resistance of the skin is, like that of the child, negligibly shallow.

In a significant number of *fatal cases* an especially low voltage has caused irreversible ventricular fibrillation, while in higher voltages asystole is common. If cardiac arrest does not occur in the patient, the various forms of *arrhythmias* may develop (with the signs of disturbance of the interventricular conduction system, and ST segment changes). At other times the ECG shows signs of coronary ischemia which are hard to differentiate from an acute myocardial event. The current conducted by the great vessels also carry a consequent heat damage to the myocardium. The role of the vessel constricting effect of electric current cannot be neglected. Current applied to the head will also result in *damage to the brain* The development of edema with the increase in intracranial pressure can cause death, but it is caused by paralysis of the vital centers. Execution by electrocution is carried out in the electric chair by application of 1600 V and 150 Hz. The victim loses consciousness immediately, the electrodes burn at their points of contact, and the temperature in the brain rises to 63 ⑤C.

Death by electrocution is currently categorized into four separate types, by JELLINEK:

1. *exitus momentaneus,* the current causing instant death,

2. *exitus retardatus,* the victim living for an extended period after application of current,

3. *exitus·dilatus,* in which the victim may live for several hours,

4. *exitus interruptus,* the victim losing consciousness regaining consciousness and ability to act, but then suddenly dying.

With the direct effect of the current, *mechanical injuries* cannot be neglected since in many cases they may disguise the original effects of the electric shock. For this reason in cases of falls from heights under circumstances where electric shock cannot be ruled out, or when there is evidence that points to it – power station workers, electric devices, electricians, etc. – the coroner's inquest and autopsy must be carried out with great care looking for the signs of electric shock.

● A power station worker suffered an accident falling from a transformer. The circumstances of the accident and the nature of the work he was doing were unknown. Indications at the coroner's inquest that pointed to electric shock were absent. During the autopsy cratery tissue alterations characteristic for electric injury were found on the sole of his feet. These came about as the result of the electricity being introduce along the metal hobnails in the heels of his boots *(Fig. 71).*

Skin alterations in electric shock are due to Joule temperature. The character and extent of the alterations depend on the size of the contact through which the electricity was introduced. At broad areas of contact, we hardly find any changes, especially if the surface of the skin was wet and the resistance, and therefore the resulting rise in temperature, is negligible. Electricity can cause heat effects at pinpoint or small areas of contact. The alterations that appear are characteristic of the heat effect.

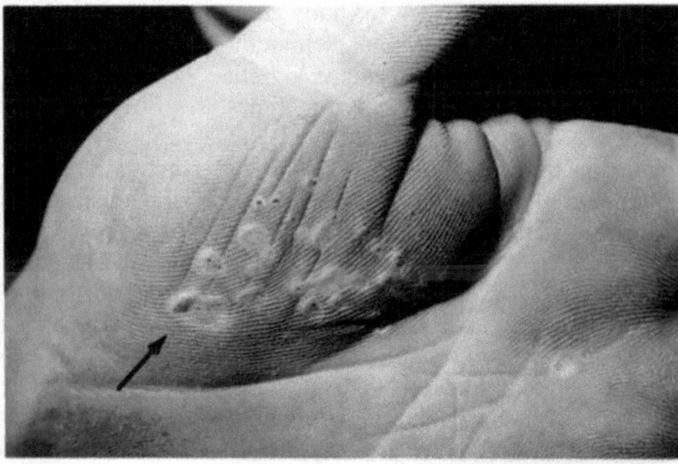

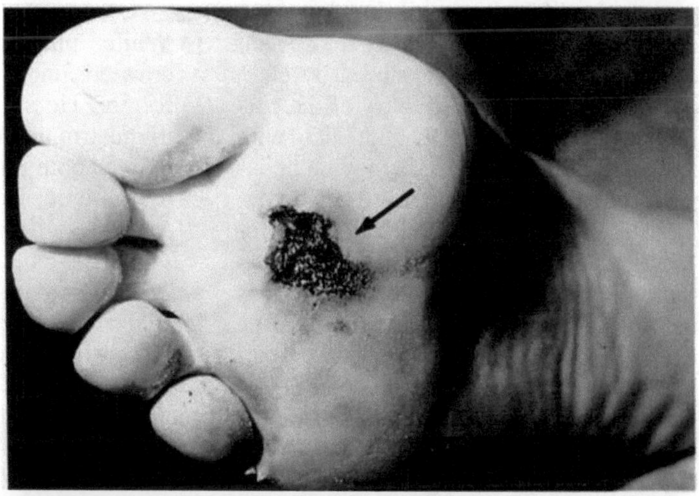

Fig. 71. Electrical current injury on the palm and location of the exit of the current on the sole

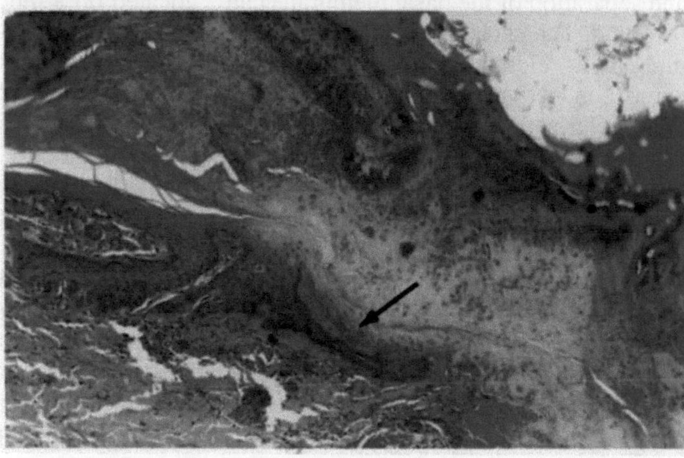

Fig. 72. Histological picture of electrical injury. Nuclear elongation. Crater-like impression of the stratum corneum into the basal cell line

We see on the surface of the body greyish-white, swollen alterations with crater-like depressions in the center and built up areas around the rim which sometimes reflect the form of the wire or the conducting instrument *(Fig. 72)*. Histologically, the injury just shows the characteristic effects of heat. The basal cells form in a palisade, the cells and nuclei becoming spindle-like, vacuoles forming in the plasma, the stratum spinosum rising up and forming pseudovesicular cavities. Similar alterations take place, in heat-caused injuries thus the local signs at the point of entry must be evaluated critically. These diagnostic difficulties call for those examinations which can identify the special characteristic alterations caused by electric shock. In the area of entry of the current, especially with DC, but also with AC, material from the wire may be deposited (galvanization) and these can be demonstrated by microchemical or histochemical techniques. To identify microimpressions from histological sections the so-called Energy Dispersing X-Ray (EDX) microanalysis can be put to excellent use. Tests for local and general morphological changes are linked with the name of Somogyi et al. In the area of the current markings damaged mitochondria, and separation of the basal membrane can be found. The chorium is raised, the Malpighi cells elongated and the subcutaneous connective tissue is homogenized. With polarization optical techniques hidden electric current marks can be demonstrated.

The pathological alterations in the heart and conduction system may be due to a fatal arrhythmia. In the heart muscle we can see widespread focal necrosis, involving the myocardium, and specialized tissue of the sinus and atrioventricular nodes. Contraction bands, and the smooth cell's necrosis of the wall of coronary arteries also occur. The alterations are more explicit in the persons suffering chronic heart failure.

Beside the above-mentioned circumscribed heat-induced alterations, electric shock can also cause *extensive burns* which can be the effect either of arcing or the explosion like ignition of combustible material in the electric machinery. In mild cases first or second degree burns appear, but an electric arc applied for an extended period especially under high voltage can cause third and fourth degree burns even with amputation of limbs *(Fig. 73)*.

- While playing a 7-year-old child crawled under a high-tension transformer. He suffered an electric shock to the arm and thigh which almost amputated both limbs at the line of contact by the wire. He bled to deat.

The most common point of *entry of electricity* is the skin on the palm of the hand. Here we usually find the injury if we look carefully. An electric source may accidentally meet another part of the body such as when a wire falls on someone or when one bumps into a frayed extension cord, etc. In such instances, if the injury is located on a hidden part of the body, for example the hair-covered skin of the head or the surface of mucous membranes, finding the point of entry of the current is practically impossible. Occasionally when the electric lead lies over a large area of the body recognizing the point of entry can be problematic. If the place of exit of the current had the appropriate requirements as in the case of entering current – a wire lying on a small area of high resistance – here we can find the same kind of heat alterations as at the entrance point, only the metalization is missing *(Fig. 74)*.

We often feel the effects of *static elec-*

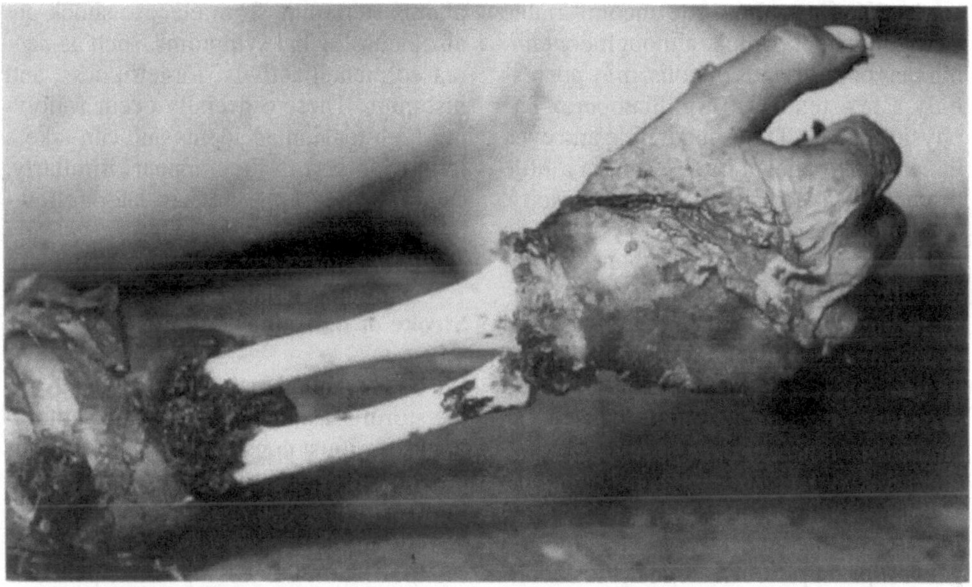

Fig. 73. Extensive soft tissue injury following high tension electrical injury

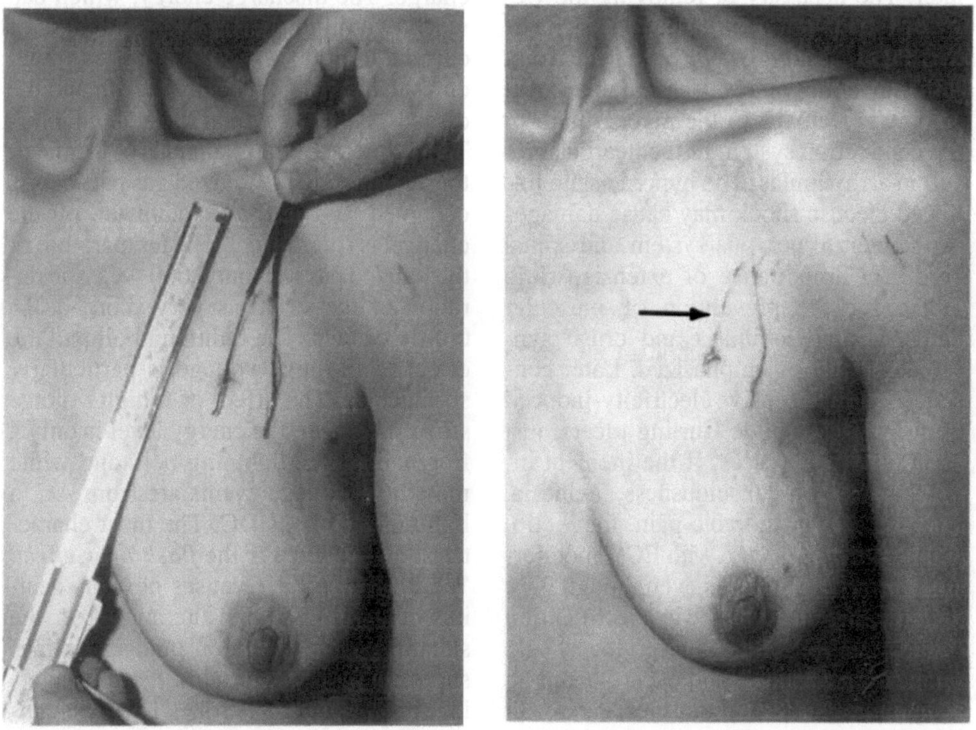

Fig. 74. Electrical current injury to the thorax (homicide attempt). The electrical circuit was closed by the thin skin between the two electrodes

tricity. We feel only a little uncomfortable snap of a shock which, although containing tens of thousands of volts, may possess only a few tenths of a milliampere. The physiological effect is negligible and even in sensitive patients it only causes a little momentary discomfort. Static electricity, although causing no injury by itself, in those places where inflammable or explosive material can be found can be dangerous. In the old days when ether was used for anesthesia in the operating room or in such places where coal dust or flour gets into the air, static electricity caused explosions.

The *care of electric shock victims* is described in the field of emergency care. In forensic medicine we must know the general principles of care and those consequences which can bring on complaints later. The necessity of removing the victim from the source of the electricity is obvious, but not always easy, and if not carefully done can result in endangerment to others. Damage to the myocardium or the conduction system of the heart can result in arrhythmias. The hypoxic state followed electric shock may cause damages of the central nervous system and spinal cord. The importance of extensive fluid intake for the prevention of muscular damage, myoglobinuria and crush syndrome should be emphasized. Later consequences of extensive electricity-induced burn injuries include Curling ulcers, just as in other burn cases. If the incident involved loss of consciousness, amnesia, burn injuries or thoracic pain, the victim requires intensive care with ECG monitoring for at least 24 hours even though 97% of the arrhythmias caused by electrocution happen within minutes after the shock. Myocardial damage, and even damage to the peripheral skeletal muscles, can result in a rise in serum CK, especially the CK MB isoenzyme fraction. Among the complaints stemming from electric shock are also neurological symptoms, such as decreased mental activity, forgetfulness, and insomnia. These especially occur following high tension accidents and can take a long time before they appear. Similarly, cataracts may appear years later following electric injury.

Stroke of lightning

If a body is found in the field, especially in the storm season – May through September – one must consider the possibility of the victim being struck by lightning. This injury is not as common as generally believed, and only 30% of those cases are fatal. The clouds act as a positive pole and the ground as a negative pole in the discharge. The discharge energy, which can reach two billion volts and the strength of current 100,000 A, ionizes the gas molecules that happen to be in the path and the discharge follows this ionized channel. The diameter of the channel is 6–8 cm, but the aura around the ionized gas particles is occupied and the true diameter of the channel is fragmented. The temperature of the ionized gas is about 8,000 ⑤C. The duration of the stroke is very short, 0.01–0.001 seconds. The lightning bolt and the effect of the high voltage is particularly spectacular. The effect of a high voltage stroke is longer, the energy level is only a fragment of the lightning bolt, and while most high voltage events are from AC, a lightning stroke is DC. The most characteristic difference is the *flash over effect*. While high voltage causes obvious heat-induced changes, the alterations on the skin are not unambiguous and sometimes superficial. These provide the characteristics of a lightning stroke. The mechanical effect of abrasion injuries and discontinuities of the skin can take any form.

Rarely, the effect causes loss of material resembling gunshot entry wounds, but the injury channel ends blindly. Tears in clothing and occasionally loss of material can happen. At the scene, examination of the surroundings can reveal damage to other objects, for example a split tree trunk, or melted quartz crystals indicate that lightning has struck. The heat effect melts metal objects or magnetizes them and cloth may be shredded. Extensive burns are rarely found on the victim. They are more likely to be superficial burned alterations to the skin or hair. At the point of entry of the current we may find porcelain-hard greyish-white areas on the skin which are the characteristic manifestations of the histological changes induced by the heat effect. The most typical alteration caused by lightning is the so-called *"lightning figure"* left on the skin. These pine bough shaped branching red stripes can be seen on the skin, on the effect of the paralysis of the innervation and concomitant dilatation of the superficial vessels of the skin which can be seen for several hours on both live and dead bodies. The mechanical effects of being struck by lightning that can be listed include damage from the shock wave. The rapidly expanding ionized gas at the beginning, according to other explanations, caused by a high temperature in the bolt channel suddenly cools causing an implosion with a shock wave. Thirty percent of the injured die. Those who live develop amnesia after having lost consciousness, similar to the effects of electroconvulsive therapy. At other times paralysis remains, which may be of a temporary character or occasionally resembling the clinical picture of ALS (amyotrophic lateral sclerosis) and may develop even a year after the event. Cataracts often follow being struck by lightning like they do following electric shock. The shock wave may cause damage to the eardrum. Some skull fractures have been described as a result of the heat effect. Death may result from cardiopulmonary insufficiency. The lightning stroke can cause, as any high energy DC shock can, asystole. The mechanism is like the consequence of application of direct current in that after a short time the normal frequency of the heart beat returns, but hypoxia may result from respiratory damage which can cause secondary damage to the heart and fibrillation.

Radiation damage

Radiation energy mediated processes may include:

1. ionizing radiation, among which the most important are radioactivity and X-radiation
2. longer wave radiation (lesser energy) and electromagnetic radiation (ultraviolet, microwave radar, diathermy etc.)
3. ultrasound radiation.

Ionizing radiations are all those which contain sufficient energy to ionize the atoms and molecules of the tissue they pass through, meanwhile their energy decreased. The biological effects are expressed in the tissues absorbing the energy, and those radiations which deliver no energy to the tissues have no effect. The *biological effects* of radiation on the organs and tissues is due to the induction of ionization of their molecules. The penetration ability of the radiation depends upon the decreasing of specific energy it possesses, as does its ionization ability.

The most common types of *corpuscular radiation* are alpha, beta and neutron radiation. *Gamma radiation* is a high energy electromagnetic radiation which usually originates when an unstable atom in an excited state as a result of corpuscular radiation returns to ground state. *X-radiation* is likewise electromagnetic radiation (its spectrum and energy content overlap that of gamma radiation), which originates from the electrons of the atom *(characteristic radiation),* with the braking of high energy particle (Brehmstrahlung).

The biological effect of ionizing radiation is to a large extent dependent upon its penetration ability. The ionizing ability of alpha and beta radiation is great without significant penetration ability, so radiation from the outside has mainly a superficial effect. The penetration ability of the uncharged neutron is significantly greater than that of the formerly mentioned charged particles. Gamma and X-radiation lose their energy by similar mechanisms (photoelectric absorption, Compton effect, and with an energy of more than 1.02 MeV, gammaphoton pair formation) and cause ionization in the tissues.

Inasmuch as the biological effect of radiation above all depends on the energy absorbed, which means the amount of ionization, the units of radiation dosage are the amounts of energy absorbed by units of mass, are defined based on the original charge load.

Absorbed dose: The absorbed energy by a unit of irradiated mass. The unit is the Gray (Gy), which is one Joule/kg of energy absorbed. Older unit: rad = 100 erg/g absorbed energy.

Irradiation dose: SI unit is the Coulomb/kg; older unit: the röntgen (R). (1 R = the amount of radiation that produces in 1 cm^3 of air one unit of electrostatic charge, either positive or negative.) One C/kg dose of irradiation is roughly equivalent to an absorbed dose of 37.7 Gy.

Equivalent dose: The biological effect of the radiation on the radiation dose depends on the type of radiation and the circumstances of irradiation. The equivalent dose takes into account the factors affecting the absorbed dose and the biological efficiency. The unit is the Sievert (Sv). A dose of one Sv has the same biological effect on a human being as a dose of one Gy. of absorbed X-radiation.

A population related dosage unit was formulated as the genetically *significant dose* (GNS). In 1970 it was 0.2 μGy.

Radiation applied to living tissue may:

a) be ineffectual,

b) cause latent chromosomal damage which doesn't affect the cell, but the damage is manifested following a latency period,

c) cause such chromosomal damage which does not result in the destruction of the cell, but inhibits its division or destroys the cell at the moment of division (so-called *reproductive cell death,* the cell damage which is the purpose of tumor irradiation therapy),

d) cause immediate cell death.

Among the primary effects of ionizing radiation and the secondary effects due to the protons or charged particles released is the formation of unstable ions. These short-lived ion pairs often cause *free radicals,* which are of equally short lives. The reactive free radicals are capable of breaking chemical bonds and this causes the permanent damage of the ionizing radiation. They damage whatever molecule they hit in the cell, including the purine and pyrimidine bases, and thus have a significant effect on the DNA which may even result in breakages of the strand. The effect of radiation is dependent upon the dose, but also depends on the tissue tolerance. Actively dividing cells, such as the bone marrow and testicular tissue are significantly more sensitive than the cells which seldom divide or that are fixed in a postmitotic state.

Ionizing radiation may be natural, the so-called *background radiation,* (natural or artificial) which consists of *cosmic radiation* and perhaps *industrial,* so called *induced radiation,* which is called *artificial radiation* as well. Recent measurements indicate that the natural and artificial radiation depend on each country's degree of development. A significant part of the load of artificial radiation is from medical sources, and only a small part is made up of radiation from industrial, work place (mining), atomic power stations, radiochemical materials, accidents etc. The occupational radiation load since 1960 has grown rapidly worldwide. The largest group affected is the health profession followed by atomic plant workers. The judgement of damage caused by artificial radiation must be established in the light of occupational injury, accidents in the work place or inappropriate therapeutic intervention. In the estimation of radiation load and damage, we must also consider that besides cosmic background radiation, other sources may contribute to the load on the organism. These sources continually tend to limit the margin of safety in decreasing the radiation load. Often those who deal with fossils and the radioactive carbon content which gets into the air when it is burned, or deal with stone building material encounter a higher background radiation. The background for uranium miners is higher, as well. Exposure to radon predisposes one to tumor formation. The WLM (Monthly Working Level) gives the load, in which in one month 1.3×10^5 MeV of alpha energy emission in one liter of air results. The collective rate of lung carcinoma is significantly higher in examined miners.

Location plays an important role in population load of radon exposure, where in some places the level may reach 0.2 WLM. A similar effect may be achieved in exposure to different objects painted with radionucleotides or TV-generated radiation load, although the 40 µGy load is low. The ^{210}Pb and ^{210}Po content of tobacco smoke is held to be more significant, which directly affects the bronchial epithelia.

Radiation load associated with *medical activity* are categorize as:

a) from diagnostic radiological examinations,

b) from radiopharmacology,

c) from therapeutic radiation.

a) Diagnostic X-ray examinations do not give a large dose radiation load, and in intervention the whole body is not irradiated, but rather a circumscribed area receives the treatment. Since the greatest part of artificial radiation load is from medical intervention, not only the effective dose, but the genetically significant dose (GSD) must be considered.

b) The use of *radiopharmacology* is growing and with it environmental pollution. Among other procedures, thyroid disease examination uses ^{131}I and a myocardial scan Thallium-201 isotopes. The use of technecium-99 is a break-through in the decrease of radiation load.

c) Radiation therapy is used mainly in malignant transformation, although also in *benign lesion therapy* (keloid), in combination with radiopharmacology. The treatment dose depends on the changes in the tissue, malignant processes receiving 50–70 Gy and benign processes 10–20 Gy. In prolonged treatment, which is common with chronic tumorous diseases, the carcinogenic potential must also be taken into account.

Radiation load may cause:

a) Genetic damage,

b) tumorous diseases,

c) direct tissue damage.

a) The genetic effect on DNA in mutation is obvious. If the mutation occurs in a germinative cell, the damage is passed on to the progeny. If a somatic cell suffers a mutagenic effect, the effect can be individually assessed. The damage can be well seen in chromosomal changes, with abnormal chromosomes being seen. In the a tests for genetic damage of the population came to the fore and the connection with environmental radiation load. Naturally spontaneous chromosomal aberrations independent of radiation damage are recognized. Sex chromatin abnormalities, trisomy or structural autosomal euploid abnormalities are possible. Some genetic abnormalities are associated with predisposition to tumor formation, radiation sensitivity is especially amplified and the following diseases must be treated with greater care:

- xeroderma pigmentosum,
- ataxia telangiectasia,
- Fanconi anemia,
- Bloom syndrome,
- Cockayne syndrome.

b) Tumor formation is one of the most relevant somatic effects of ionizing radiation. Even one Gy (100 rad) can induce a tumor. The age plays a significant role, children being significantly more susceptible than adults. One of the essential aspects of the induced tumor is its latency period, which is the time between the radiation exposure and manifestation of the tumor. The latency period can be divided into two phases. In the first phase, the damaged cell grows without constraint. In the second phase the proliferation of the tumor tissue and the possibility of diagnosis are characteristic. The minimal latency period for leukemia is usually 2–3 years, for bone tumors 3–4 years, and the solid tumors require 10 years. The age and size of dose can modify the latency of the tumor formation. For example thyroid tumors develop in children in an increased number in those who have received only 0.1 Gy (10 rad) radiation therapy. There is debatable the connection between the penetration of the radiation and the frequency of tumors in newborns. The relationship which was described by English workers had not been supported by those in Japan. In the former, the mothers received 2–46 mGy. The Japanese based their observations on the children of women who were pregnant at the time the atom bomb was dropped. The damage to exposed workers also significantly grew according to certain sources. Among workers in power plants, leukemia, pancreatic and pulmonary carcinoma appeared in increasing numbers. Others are of the opinion that exposures, in the power plants, of less than 2.78 rem exhibit no tumor-generating effect. Among occupational diseases, the tumorous diseases of English radiologists has been worked up. In two time periods, before 1921 the tumorous diseases – skin, lung, pancreas carcinoma, leukemia – was significantly higher in radiologists, while after 1921 the difference between radiologists and other groups of physicians disappeared.

c) The *direct form* of radiation effect may be acute – the damage appearing within 6 months of the application – subacute – when symptoms develop soon after 6 months have passed – chronic – clinical symptoms within 5 years – and when symptoms appear after 5 years we speak of late clinical manifestations. X- and gamma radiation, especially particle radiation produced by orthovoltage devices, beta or neutron radiation can bring about effects. Skin damage often used to accompany orthovoltage radiotherapy, but with megavoltage irradiation (2–40 MeV) skin damage is negligible. The acute direct effect to rapidly proliferating tissues brings necrosis, especially affecting the mucosa of the gut, the bone marrow, the germinative cells, and the embryonic tissues. Later progressive damage to the stroma with scar formation follows which brings tissue edema and fibrin deposits organization after the damage. The characteristic manifestation of radiation damage is proliferation of the myointima of the vessels. The growth of *chronic radiation ulcers* on the skin are early stage changes. Likewise, *radiation dermatitis* is also described in the early stage. A single exposure to 6–8 Gy (600–800 rad) can result in skin erythema within 1–2 days, the background being dilation of skin capillaries and for three weeks following the treatment the skin will be red, warm and edematous. After a single dosage of 20 Gy (2000 rad) blisters, moist desquamated areas form on the skin in which, if the dose was large, appears under the basal layer, developing into a 2nd to 3rd degree burn. The subacute presentation – 6 months – the skin turns hyperpigmented due to the activation of melanocyte enzyme activity by the radiation, with the result of a consequent hyperpigmentation. (At high doses, the melanocytes can also be damaged.) In the area of the damaged skin over the next six months telangiectasia, skin atrophy, fibrosis and induration of the skin develop. Whole body irradiation has not only happened with the atomic bomb experiments, that is as a result of the Hiroshima and Nagasaki bombs, but in the last decades also with accidents at atomic plants or place of work. (1958, Los Alamos; 1958, Yugoslavia; 1986, Chernobyl; and also included could be accidents involving the storage and transport of atomic waste.) The resulting alterations can be divided into three main groups:

a) central nervous system,
b) gastrointestinal mucosa,
c) hematopoetic system damage.

With exposure to 3–8 Gy (300–800 rad) death ensues within 60 days without treatment, due to hemorrhage, infection and damage to the hemopoetic system and anemia.

With exposure to 10–30 Gy (1000–3000 rad) damage to the mucosa of the gastrointestinal tract, septicemia, fluid and electrolyte loss brings death within two weeks.

With an exposure of 30 Gy (3000 rad) or more death comes within 48 hours, but central nervous system symptoms, dizziness, ataxia, etc. are averted.

Fanger and Lusbaugh published two cases of high dose radiation damage pathology in which the injured received 88 Gy (8800 rad) of gamma and neutron radiation to the whole body. Death occurred in 31–49 hours after exposure.

On the surface of the skin subcutaneous and interstitial edema was pronounced in which the edema of the muscle tissue was also evident. Upon section of the edematous tissue a scarlet fluid flowed out. In the thoracic cavity and in the pericardium fluid had collected and the amount of ascites was negligible. The cardiovascular system exhibited characteristic changes, serofibrinous pericarditis, fine fibrin deposition on the epicardium composed of polymorphonuclear lymphocytes and fibrin, and leukocytes scattered among the cardiac muscle fibers. Around the capillaries was a mild interstitial edema, and in the subepicardial cardiac muscle fibers a fine granulation and intracellular edema could also be found. Around the vessels of other organs a mild infiltration of leukocytes had formed. In the airway and esophagus the submucosal capillaries were engorged and fragmented red blood cells could be seen in the obvious and stasis vessels. In the airways, with the swelling of the tracheal and bronchial mucosa, in the lung tissue an intraalveolar and interstitial edema was described. Microscopically, the mucosa of the airway was desquamated, the basal membrane was irregularly widened and hyalinized. In the mucosa, macrophages with vacuolized plasma, and in the alveoli, macrophages with brown cell fragments in the cytoplasm were found.

The mucosa of the gastrointestinal tract revealed the most characteristic changes. From the cardia to the colon the mucosa showed a pronounced edema, the mucosa of the stomach built up with thick folds marked by hemorrhages. Microscopically the mucosa was desquamated to different depths from the esophagus to the rectum. In the mucosa mitotic activity of the cells could not be found. Histiocytes, neutrophils, eosinophils and large lymphocytes appeared, but in small numbers in the mucosa, and the complete absence of small lymphocytes was striking. In the lymphoid follicles of the intestines besides damaged lymphocytes, the reticulo-endothelial skeleton contained only nuclear fragments. In the fibers of the smooth muscle of the gut wall intercellular and intracellular edema could be noticed, signs of pronounced vacuolar degeneration, which besides the muscle fibers also reached the intramuscular ganglion cells. In the lymph nodes the follicles consisted largely of hypertrophied reticulo-endothelial cells, among which were scattered, shrunken, pyknotic lymphoid cells and nuclear fragments. The reticulo-endothelial cells were basically intact, although in the sinusoids were few neutrophils or eosinophils. In the spleen besides signs of massive blood loss, the Malpighian corpuscles practically disappear and lymphocytes cannot be found. The central arterioles were conspicuous and well defined, and hypertrophies reticulo-endothelial cells were described. Only a few shrunken or damaged lymphocytes were there among the pyknotic, broken nuclear fragments. Scattered eosinophils, neutrophils, plasmacytes, histiocytes and reticulum cells were visible. Phagocytosis was mildly variable, and signs of erythrophagocytosis were not found. In the sinusoids and red pulp was a very small quantity of cells, partially in the areas of hemorrhage. Neutrophil leukocytes appeared in relatively large numbers in the red pulp and larger blood vessels. The bone marrow in the sternum, ribs, vertebrae, and femurs was examined. The bone marrow was scanty, jellied and pinkish. In the formerly erythropoetic areas only fixed reticulum phagocytes remained, which had phagocytized some nuclear fragments. The nuclei of the megakaryocytes were pyknotic, the erythrocytes were found in the dilated sinusoids and edema in the interstitium. Some cells looked like primitive stem cells with pyknotic nuclei, and signs of mitosis were not seen. The alterations found in the pancreas were atrophy of the acinar cells, vacuolar degeneration and necrosis of the ductal epithelium, lymphocyte infiltration, direct radiation damage could be discerned and similar changes were described in the pancreas of such patients who had received large doses of radiation to the epigastrium a few weeks before death.

The subject of *damage to the embryo by radiation load, radiotherapy,* and *radiological examinations* must be dealt with separately. The embryo is very sensitive to radiation in the organogenesis period, and the result may be retarded growth, teratogenic alterations and occasionally death in uterus. The reaction depends on the stage of pregnancy and the amount of X-ray or ionizing radiation. If the mother receives the radiation shortly after implantation, the embryo may die. Radiation applied later may result in developmental abnormalities which will be manifest in the newborn or in the retarded growth of the child, in microcephaly, mental retardation, and retinal pigment disturbances. In the anamnesis of the mother such treatments may be found in which radiation was applied for dysmenorrhea, metrorrhagia, arthritis or sacroiliac joint tuberculosis. In some cases these occurred when the radiologist should have been aware of an active pregnancy. Besides therapeutic radiation treatment, there are mixed opinions over the danger to the embryo posed by diagnostic radiological intervention, some holding to the view that even a low dose of radiation can cause, besides serious genetic damage, a higher incidence of leukemia when the load to the mother was 0.5–5 rad. Others deny this possibility, since a large number of diagnostic X-ray procedures so not touch the pelvic area and the amount of scattered radiation is so little that it does not endanger the fetus. It is especially noted that the results of those who exhibit fetal damage are from animal experiments extrapolated to apply to humans, and this must be viewed with precautions. Their opinions are based on the follow-up studies on the women who were pregnant at the time of the Nagasaki bombing, whose newborns and children show no greater incidence of tumors than the rest of the population. So diagnostic radiation examinations are never desirable in pregnant women, and especially in the early phase of pregnancy, since one cannot be certain the fetus will not be damaged or a tumorous disease will not result.

Damage related to *ultraviolet radiation* over a long period of time on outdoor workers may result in skin cancer. We rarely meet with it in the occupational diseases. However, such genetic damage is recognized, in which the patients being radiation sensitive have responded with tumorous transformation after exposure to either ionizing radiation or UV radiation. The probability of tumor development is significantly inclined toward population susceptibility. Among the diseases associated are xeroderma pigmentosum, Fanconi anemia, ataxia telangiectasia, and Cockayne syndrome. Among these xeroderma pigmentosum is the foremost in susceptibility to tumor induction by UV radiation. Both gamma and UV radiation are carcinogenic in Fanconi anemia. In ataxia telangiectasia chemical and physical challenge can provoke atypical cellular reactions, and in Cockayne syndrome molecular biological defects do not accompany UV sensitivity. The molecular biological basis of damage is alteration in the DNA. whether by UV or gamma radiation, pyrimidine dimmers may be formed which alter the biological function of the DNA in both radiation resistant and radiation sensitive cells. In the latter, however, the formed dimmers break down into monomers with the help of the cells photoreactive enzyme system, which normal photoproduction does not damage. (Since the material for the model of radiation damage comes from animal experiments and these data are extrapolated to imagine probable human alterations. Examination of the above listed genetic damage cases gives the possibility to observe and check the accuracy of the extrapolated data regarding radiation-induced mutagenic cell damage and carcinogenic effects.)

Besides UV radiation, the *electromagnetic radiation* of different wave lengths can cause injuries. Not only household appliances – microwave ovens –, but *telecommunication radar, radar navigation, radar meteorological, medical physio-*

therapy and industrial applications use devices that produce such waves that can increase the possibility of injury. Occupational hazards are in the forefront. Clinical observations have confirmed that radio waves of low intensity can cause functional and morphological changes. In these the intensity-dependent heat effect is the primary cause of nervous system, cardiovascular, or neurohumoral complaints. *Microwave* devices work with 300–300,000 Mhz and heat production is dependent upon the wave length, as is tissue penetration. While the shorter waves of electromagnetic radiation only evolve heat superficially and guarantee a penetration of only a few millimeters, the increase in the wave length and intensity can damage deeper tissues. Thus the usual 2500 Mhz frequency of the microwave oven penetrates a few centimeters and with a 25 mWatt power supply can cause a mild hyperthermia (the household device is designed for power in the kWatt range). The larger wave diathermy devices can cause deeper tissue damage. The organs are sensitive to the heat effect of microwave radiation, but radiation at these wavelengths beyond the heat effect cause no malignant or mutagenic effect.

The use of *diagnostic ultrasound* machines has multiplied greatly over the last decades. Their use does not cause ionization in the tissues. Indeed, their use often makes X-ray examinations unnecessary. In view of the current agreement on the absence of biological effects, risk factors of ultrasound examination are not present.

Gunshot wounds

Injuries caused by firearms make up a relatively small proportion of all injuries in the work of the local forensic medical specialist. Their screening and recognition is sometimes the responsibility of the specialist.

- A 47-year-old male suffered a gunshot wound from a police officer whom he had attacked. The wound was mortal. An investigation was ordered because of the use of a firearm, and the medical specialist first established that the shot had entered from the back and exited the front of the victim. Therefore the lawful use of a weapon was in doubt. The officer who had used the weapon and a witness also testified that the wound had been inflicted on the victim during the attack. A second autopsy established that the medical examiner had mixed up the entry and exit wounds and thus given a false direction of the shot.

Although the events surrounding the injury can unequivocally indicate the nature of the wound, sometimes after an isolated accident it is difficult to recognize the nature of the wound without knowing the original circumstances. (After hunting accidents it often happens that the origin of the wound misleads the doctor, and only during treatment the finding of a pellet of birdshot reveals the wound's true nature). Tsuda et al published statistical data about fire arm injuries. 3.4% all of the injuries were caused by gunshots. Almost 10% of firearm injuries was accidental caused by wrong use of hunting guns.

With gunshot wounds a few characteristic alterations must be kept in mind from the view point of the responsibilities of forensic medicine.

The gunshot wound is unique among other injuries in that an object of relatively *small mass* – 4.5–11.2 g – hits the body with *great energy.* The speed of the projectile represents its great energy and this is ranges from 300 m/sec for shotgun pellets to 700–1000 m/sec for rifle bullets. In these projectiles the muzzle energy is significant, E_0=4000 Joules, V_0=1200 m/sec. The energy is derived from the explosion of the *gunpowder.* The gunpowder in ancient weapons and ammunition was traditionally the so-called *"black powder"* which is used even today in certain circles. The composition – 15% carbon, 10% sulfur, and 75% saltpeter – also means that the combustion is incomplete, a significant amount of the gunpowder grains not being burnt up, and the muzzle flash and smoke were pronounced. A so-called *"smokeless powder"* is used in modern cartridges, which is made of nitrocellulose or a nitrocellulose-nitroglycerin combination. Various granulated forms are in use, each of which has its own outstanding characteristics and from that the source of manufacture can be discovered. Among the many advantages offered by a fast burning time is a significant gas-producing capacity, the burning being practically complete so that is a very small amount of the powder fails to participate in the combustion. The muzzle flash is smaller, and the amount of deposition in the barrel is less, as well. Smokeless powder was a vast improvement over the previous gunpowder, an equal amount of smokeless powder producing three times the gas produced by black powder. The gunpowder gas is mostly carbon dioxide, carbon monoxide, nitrogen and methane in small traces, with the content of the unburned part being high in nitrite and nitrate. In many cartridges a powder is used with is an 80% black and 20% smokeless mixture.

The construction of the *cartridges* used in firearms are designed to fit the weapon's intended use with attention given to its ballistic characteristics and target it is meant to defeat. Thus *completely jacketed* rounds bring about only a little laceration in the wounds they cause. Likewise the so-called "hollow point" or soft-point projectiles change shape radically after impact and thus have the ability to inflict more laceration. The unjacketed projectiles can also change their form such that after impact small pieces often break off.

The so-called *"explosive-tipped"* projectiles have a truly outstanding laceration and shock producing effect from the explosive charge. Their structure also shows that detonation occurs beneath the entry wound after impact and causes much more pronounced injury than the normal projectile does.

The casing of the cartridge is constructed of metal, usually brass, because of the great pressure caused by the ignition of the powder. The length of the cartridge and shape for each type of weapon is characteristic, being given in mm or inches. The form of the cartridge also accommodates extraction during use of the weapon, the base of its holding the rim of the cartridge and the detonator cap.

The construction of *shotgun shells* is different. While in the case of rifle cartridges, the tamping is performed by the bullet itself, due to the many small pellets that make up the projectiles of a single round, the gas could not be sealed behind them, so a wad is usually placed between the gunpowder and pellets to serve as tamponade and seal. In modern shotgun shells the pellets are contained in a plastic cup which holds the pellets together for a certain distance after leaving muzzle. The shell is made of paper, or more recently, of plastic with a brass base with a rim for extraction and an detonator cap. The diameter of the pellets is given on the shell's cup *(Fig. 75).*

The *classification of firearms* is based on practical reasons. In general we divide them into rifled bore and smooth bore. The *rifled bore* weapons have a barrel

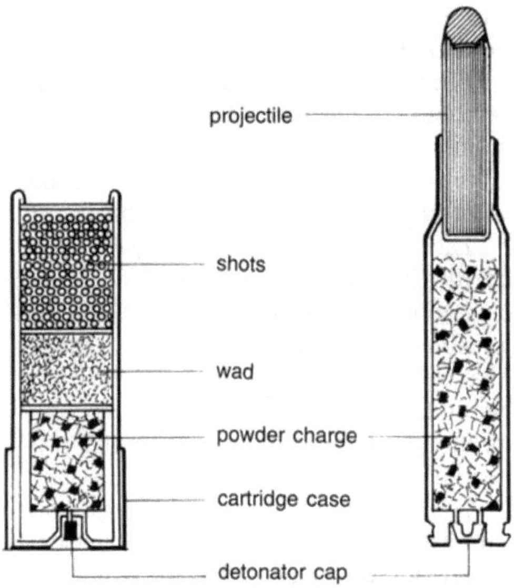

Fig. 75. Diagram of rifle and shotgun cartridges

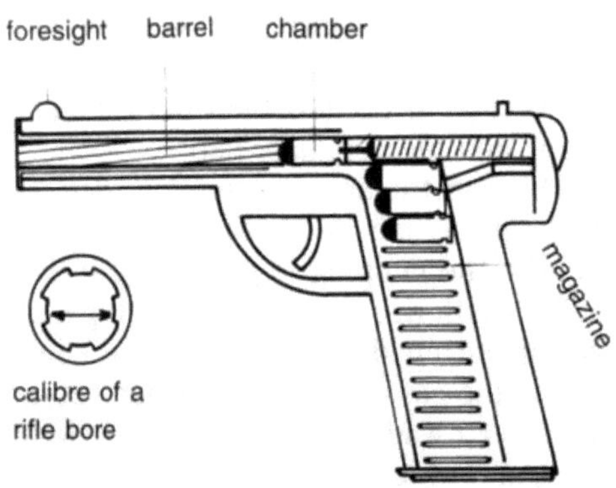

Fig. 76. Cross-section of a weapon with the functional components labeled. Cross-section of a the barrel of a rifled weapon

with spiral grooves running the length of the interior surface – rifling –, and we see the same measurement between the grooves of the barrel on the projectile that was fired from it, giving the projectile a rotation around the long axis for the purpose of stabilization and accuracy *(Fig. 76).*

The distance between the two raised ridges gives the weapon's *calibre,* which is written on the casing in millimeters, or inches.

Rifled weapons make up the greatest portion of firearms. *Short barreled* weapons are the revolvers or pistols. The barrel length varies. These are the so-called *handguns,* made for self-defense. The common characteristic is the relatively short barrel with a 6–14 round magazine, and usually semi-automatic action.

The construction of the two groups are different, as can be seen from cross-section. In the *revolvers* the cartridges are kept in the cylinder, and with each shot the cylinder revolves to move a new round into position. In semi-automatic pistols the recoil of the round operates the gun. In the moment of discharge a significant part of the energy propels the projectile down range, while the backward-directed force, the so-called *recoil,* moves the slide of the weapon backwards. With this the empty casing is extracted from the chamber, ejected to the side, and the firing pin is cocked. After this the spring under the slide kicks the slide forward, stripping a round off the magazine, feeding it into the chamber and the weapon is ready to be fired again. Pulling the trigger will result in another shot being fired.

The second category of rifled weapons is the long-barreled repeaters or automatic weapons. They are used by soldiers, hunters or target shooters. The barrel length is variable, some small calibre but high rate of fire automatic weapons having barrels barely longer than self-defense weapons, but in general the long-barreled weapons have barrels around 60 cm in length. The longer barreled weapons are more accurate. The construction of the weapons are outlined in the illustrations. The round and the method of discharge distinguish the description. In repeating weapons the bolt opens after every firing, the spent cartridge is extracted, a new cartridge is fed into the chamber, and then it is locked again. Automatic weapons are capable of the so-called *"single shot"* when they operate as a repeating weapon, or *automatic fire,* when the loading and extraction occurs much as was described for the pistols with the difference that as long as the trigger is pulled, the firing continues.

Airguns make up a special group of firearms, in which a carbon dioxide cartridge or compressed air propel the projectile. The weapon's barrel is rifled with an average diameter of 4.5 mm, firing soft lead pellets, which can inflict serious, even lethal injuries at short range, a few meters. The change of shape of the projectile upon impact is not as significant as in the above cases, due to the low muzzle energy.

● In one of our cases there was examined an air gun injury. We found 4 entry wounds in the right temple of the victim, with 1 cm diameter hole in the bone. Three of the bullets lacerated the cerebrum, and 1 was embedded in the bone. It was a self inflected injury. The victim survived 6 hours.

Hunting weapons may be single, double or even triple barreled, which may be both shotgun, both rifle or combinations. The double barrels may be side by side, which is the most popular form for bird shotguns, or one on top of the other, the so-called "over-under" *(bock) type.* The barrels are smooth bore and the shot cup holds the pellets until it leaves the muzzle in various degrees of tightness, the so-called "choke" regulation. We measure the effect by how many percent of the pellets strike within a one meter circle at 30 meters range. The pellet scatter at a given distance per unit area depends on the tightness. Hunting weapons are repeaters or semi-automatic.

We must discuss separately the so-called *"home-made"* weapons. These are made of various barrels and the chambers are made to fit the desired cartridge. The internal surface of the barrels are also irregular, and cause significant deformities in the projectile. There is no safety system, and the chance of an accident is great not only from accidental discharge, but the barrel made of various materials may blow up. The lack of tamponade behind the chamber can result in a back blast which may leave a large deposit on the hand of the user. The combustion of the round is incomplete with many unburnt grains, and if a shotgun is used, the shot scatters in an irregular pattern.

● A 22-year-old male was brought into the Urology Clinic with a gunshot wound. The entry wound was below the umbilicus on the left and the channel of the projectile lay under the skin reaching the scrotum and exiting between the two testicles, falling into the victims boot where it was found. The victim said that he was grazing his cow when he felt a blow to the abdomen, heard a roar, and then noticed that he was bleeding. The lie of the channel of the projectile and the projectile's unusual location didn't fit with the story, and examination of the clothing revealed that the shot had been fired at close range. Afterwards he admitted that he had intended to shoot deer with a home made gun which, loaded with a 4.5 mm cartridge he had hidden under his coat. The weapon had no safety and went off causing the injury.

The *sequence of firing* is made up of *separate phases* with which it is necessary to become briefly familiar with in order to understand what follows. The sequence is the same for just about every kind of weapon. The cartridge is seated in the chamber where at the moment of firing it is locked by the bolt, or with shotguns, the closing of the breach. At this time the extractor also hooks the cartridge rim. After locking the weapon can be put on safe automatically (as is the case with many hunting weapons), or the safety can be set so that the trigger cannot be drawn back. After taking off the safety, the weapon is ready to fire. After pulling back the trigger, the firing pin can be struck forward, striking the detonator cap on the base of the cartridge, igniting a special explosive which in turn ignites the gunpowder in the cartridge. The burning of the powder is such a chemical reaction which produces a significant amount of gas-and the burning, as mentioned above, almost completely consumes the contents of the cartridge. At the moment of the explosive-like burning the chamber and the pressure grow and the projectile flies out of the barrel and the pressure in the chamber suddenly stops. With the projectile the so-called *"residue of munitions"* the compressed air column ahead of the projectile, the projectile, the gas from the spent powder, the heat, the unspent powder grains and the flash. The following phases are the so-called extraction phase, in which the spent casing is extracted from the chamber and the so-called ejection phase, in which the casing is ejected to the side. A new cartridge can then be chambered and the process repeated. With repeating weapons these phases are followed in sequence, and with automatic-semiautomatic weapons the repetition occurs automatically after firing as was outlined above. The process that occurs at the moment of firing belongs to the realm of *internal ballistics.* A projectile leaving the barrel of a weapon is affected by drag and gravity. The shape and weight of the projectile affect both processes, and not least of all, the starting velocity. The path of the projectile from the muzzle to the target significantly deviates from the horizontal and begins to follow a ballistic path and a certain distance later takes the path of a dropping object. This path is characteristic for each type of round and the manufacturers publish these ranges with the positive and negative deviation from the ideal trajectory. *(External ballistic)*

From the standpoint of the forensic medical specialist, the terminal state of the ballistics holds significance. The *terminal ballistics* means when the projectile hits the target, what form did the path of the projectile take, what is the condition of the target and what are the characteristics of the wound. In terminal ballistics the influence of the first two processes, the initial velocity of the projectile – which depends on the powder charge and the weapon type – and the internal ballistic relationships, and even the influence of external ballistics as well, bear on the fact that a projectile covering a long distance may not only vary widely from its volley path, but its energy significantly decreases, too. Another important aspect of terminal ballistics is the variation of a projectile from the usual. (The terminal ballistic effect of a fully jacketed round is different form that of a so-called soft-point or an explosive-tipped round!)

A projectile hitting the body causes significant injuries. The entry wound at the point of impact, a channel, and an exit wound are formed.

In the area of the *entry wound* the effect of a high energy projectile the skin contacted by the projectile is destroyed in the center and a round hole is formed.

At the sides where the projectile touched the skin abrasions appear which may

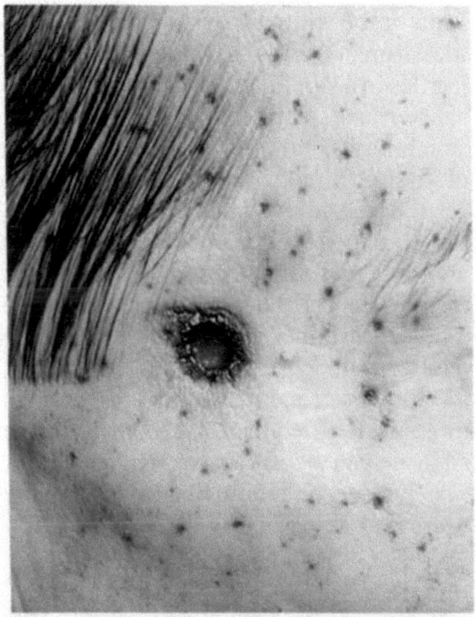

Fig. 77. Typical entry wound in gunshot injuries. The abraded open edge reveals the direction of the shot, the powder burns indicate the distance

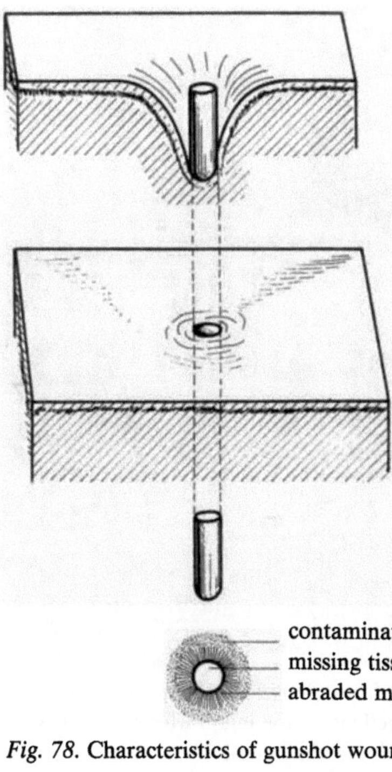

Fig. 78. Characteristics of gunshot wounds

be concentrically situated around the hole, depending on what angle the projectile entered the body. With angles close to perpendicular the hole is regular with the abrasions forming evenly around it, while the elongated abrasions of an obliquely produced impact point in the direction from which the projectile came *(Fig. 77).*

Smudges left by the projectile in the tissue is penetrated can be wiped up. This creates the so-called *contaminated zone,* in which, if the projectile carried with it a good quantity of deposits from the barrel of the weapon – primarily projectiles, gunpowder, gunsmoke, burnt oil, or corrosion remnants – stick together and can be so extensive that they may cover the abrasion marks as well. The three elements of a gunshot wound are the hole, the abrasion marks, and the contaminated zone *(Fig. 78).* The size of the entry wound through the skin depends on the area of the body. Because of the skin's elasticity, the hole is smaller than the actual diameter of the bullet in every case, but when the tissues are rich in elastic fibers, such as the palpebra and scrotum, pinpoint holes are all that can be seen, while the wound in the skin of the back is hardly smaller than the projectile itself. From the area of the entry wound, depending on the distance of the shot, the residue of munitions can more or less deduced.

The gunshot wound makes a peculiar form if fired from the immediate proximity – a muzzle in contact, or at a 0.5–1 cm distance – into a place where at a small depth under the soft tissues bone can be found *(Fig. 79).* A typical place is the scalp. In such a wound, the hole, the abrasion marks, the contaminated zone, and formation of the residue of munitions affect the skin and the skull together, separating the skin radially from the bony base by the gases inflating the skin and the imprints left by the barrel of the weapon.

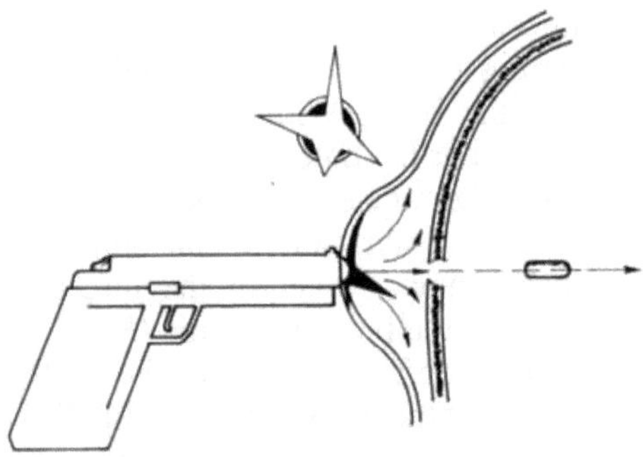

Fig. 79. Entry wound of gunshot wounds when the muzzle is in contact with the skin bullet accompanied by subcutaneous inflation due to the blast

The great pressure developed in this way blows the soft tissues to pieces. The residue of munitions applied to the area prior to the explosion creates a significant number of little pouches which can be found in the area. The soft tissues may be bright red due to the high amount of carbon monoxide with unburned grains of gunpowder embedded in them, which due to the effect of the explosion are shattered in a star shape which, if the tears are reunited, show the characteristic parts of the above described gunshot wound *(Fig. 80).*

The mounded skin and the imprints left by the contact points – the front site, the mark of the shotgun's other barrel – are the characteristic impressions, the so-called *stamp* left behind, in which abrasion injuries may be found. Pouches from the explosion are left behind in areas cushioned by soft tissue, and the residue of munitions can be found with a much smaller possibility of skin lacerations!

Estimation of the extent of alterations caused by the different types of wound takes a lot of practice. Projectiles that have lost much of their energy from being fired at long range or for other reasons – ricochets, travelling through a thick material, old projectiles etc. – cause dissimilar entry wounds. In these cases an important property responsible for the characteristic form of the wounds caused by the projectiles – great energy – is missing. The projectiles in a significant portion of the cases cause round, stab-like wounds, or contusion injuries, but there is no missing patch of tissue. Similar entry wounds can be seen in gunshot wounds caused by weapons equipped with silencers. The silencer not only deforms the projectile, but in many instances the wound does not create a hole, but rather resembles a rupture alteration with a bruised area at the place of the abrasions, and if the shot is made with the muzzle in contact, the imprint of the silencer can be seen around the wound. The residue of munitions are noticeably decreased as well. The form of the entry

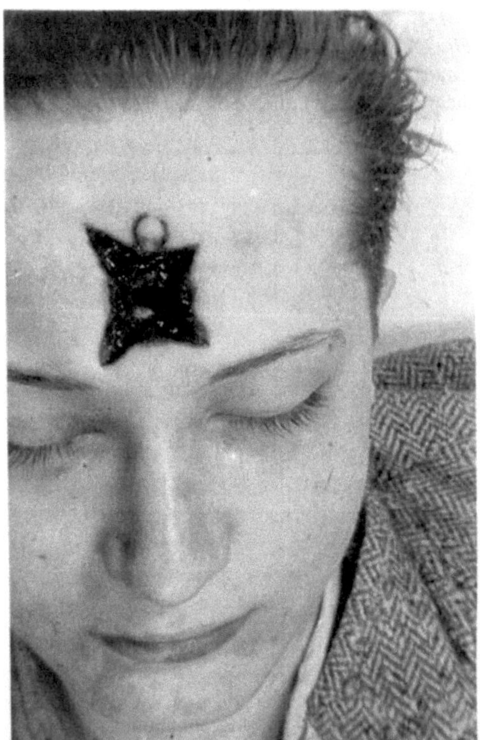

Fig. 80. Shot from a muzzle in contact with the skin. The starshaped laceration injury with missing tissue and the imprint of the muzzle

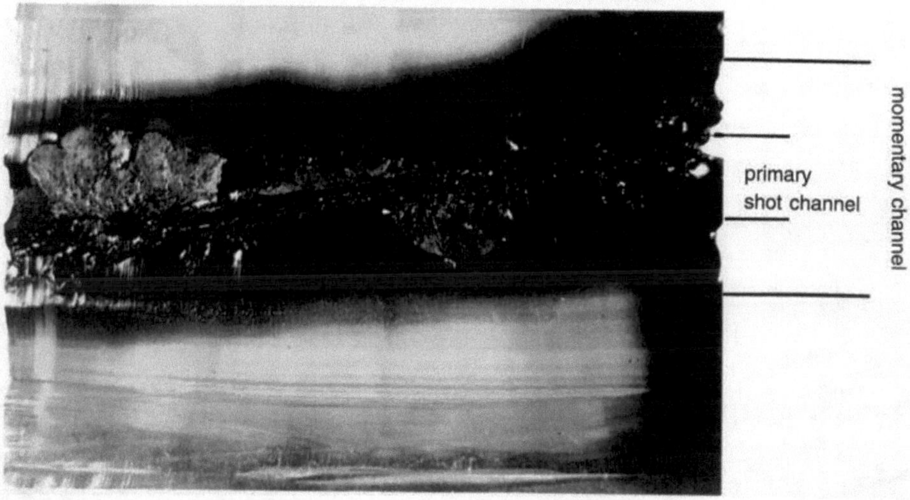

Fig. 81. Momentary and primary shot channel in gelatin

wound is variable due to the instability of the projectile and may not follow a straight course. Entries caused by deformed, fragmented projectiles cause bizarre forms which may even be multiple if the energy is significant, and the abrasion marks beside the hole are not missing. With atypical entry wounds in many cases it may be questionable whether it is a bullet hole at all. To confirm this lead or copper microimpressions should be sought in the area of the wound, the presence of which depends on the type of projectile, whether soft lead or copper jacketed.

The *shot channel* follows from the entry wound. The form it takes from the entry wound can in like manner be attributed to the projectile's great energy. At the moment of penetration the energy of the projectile not only describes a forward-pointing vector, but *lateral effects* are also manifested. The latter effect caused by a projectile traversing a section of the body extends as a multiple of the diameter of the projectile (10–20 times) for how far the tissue is destroyed and thus forming the so-called *temporary shot channel.* (This can be especially well visualized in an ultrafast film of a projectile piercing 20% gelatin.) In the temporary channel bleeding and cellular damage occur, – the border of the bleeding can be especially seen around shot channels through lung tissue, – and after the passage of the projectile the channel collapses, and the so-called *primary channel* is formed, the size of which depends upon the resilience of the tissue, just as does the entry wound *(Fig. 81).* (In lung tissue it is pinpoint sized and in compact parenchymal organs it almost matches the diameter of the projectile.) If the victim survives the wound, the territory of the primary channel will be demarcated by necrobiotic tissue, the damaged cells phagocyted, and in this stage we speak of the *secondary shot channel,* which is bigger than the primary channel and the diameter of the projectile, but it doesn't reach the size of the temporary channel. Later scar formation marks the place of the original injury.

Certain organs are more significantly injured in the area of the shot channel. The

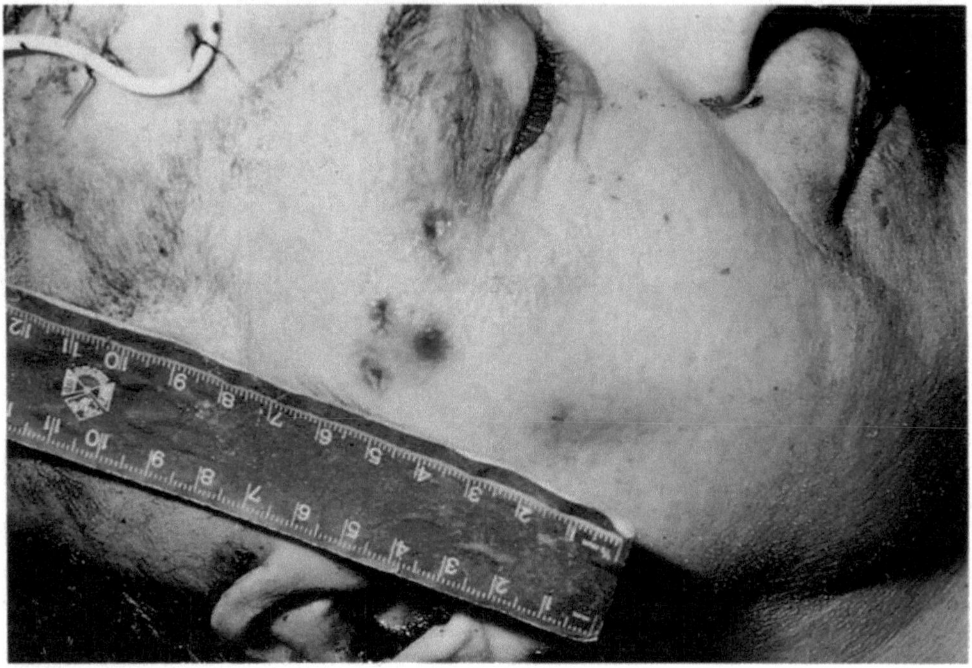

Fig. 82. Multiple airgun wounds to the right temple Suicide case

diastolic heart, the full stomach and intestines burst, and diaphysis of the long bones are shattered. The shattered fragments of bone absorb a great deal of energy from the pieces of the projectile broken off from impact, and the surrounding area is torn to shreds from the effect of this energy caused by the so-called *secondary injury particles.*

Characteristic alterations are found in the *shot channel of the flat bones.* The skull bones are most illustrative, in which a spongy layer is situated between the external and internal layers. At the entry wound the projectile causes inward compression on the external layer and an inward-directed expansion through the internal layer, thus the shot channel, because of the firmness of the compression and expansion forces on the bone, it expands in a direction related to the direction of the shot.

The *exit wound* similarly forms so that the hole in the internal layer is smaller than that exiting the external layer. The hole left in flat bones can reveal the precise diameter of the projectile – because of the bone's low resilience the diameter will be no more than 0.1 mm smaller. In measurement such special instruments must be used which lie concentrically flat against the edge of the hole, since other instruments give inaccurate data. Due to the deformation of the projectile, it isn't fruitful to measure the diameter at the exit wound. The pelvic bones and the sternum suffer similar injuries *(Fig. 82, 83).*

The bulk of the cases of *exit wounds* resemble lacerations, the projectile mounding up the skin and in the highest place tearing out a discontinuity in the form of an X or H. If the projectile shatters the bone it carries with it to a great degree, the exit wound may be greatly enlarged. The

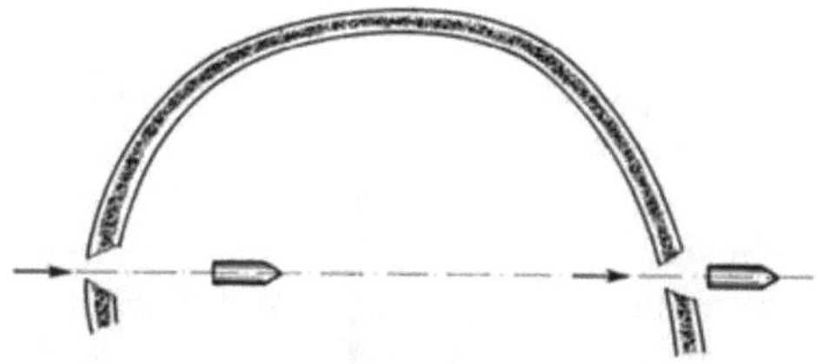

Fig. 83. Exit and entry wound in flat bone is expanded by the projectile in the appropriate direction

injuries, mentioned previously are different from those injuries produced by high energy projectiles. These form a hole like the at the entry wound, but not abrasion marks or contaminated zone can be found. At other times the exit wound of a lower energy projectile may result in an absence of material. If in the area of the exit the skin is bound up, be it by a waist belt or a wallet, etc. the central area of the skin is mashed to a pulp, and occasionally we see abrasion marks, but we do not find the contaminated zone.

- A 76-year-old night watchman suffered a gunshot wound. The exit wound also showed a hole with missing material caused by a weapon of medium energy. The investigation on the scene unambiguously judged that the victim has suffered the wound while leaning against a wall, since there were no abrasion marks around the hole.

Only an experienced specialist should perform the *autopsy of a shooting victim.* Very important cases have not been solved because the doctor performing the autopsy did not take proper care. The primary task starts at the scene. The necessity of the clothing examination we have already discussed, but it bears reemphasizing that the residue of gunpowders must be sought first of all on the clothing of the victim, the omission of which may make it impossible to establish the range of the shot. The appropriate packaging of the clothing is the responsibility of the medical specialist for the later weapons specialist examination.

During the autopsy, before describing the injury, examination of the hands is essential. In suicide, microtraces – from the gunsmoke – may remain on the hand that used the gun which unambiguously indicate self-inflicted injury. Besides the usual paraffin test, the surface of the skin should be wiped with dilute HCl or HNO_3 soaked cotton and the wiped up contamination examined for traces of antimony or barium, which can be detected in quantities less than 5 micrograms. The scanning electron microscopy/energy dispersing X-ray analysis (SEM/EDAX) gives excellent results in determining gunshot residue.

The precise description and measurement of the entry and exit wounds is imperative. Besides in the typical injuries, the known examination procedures can be of help, but we must deal especially with the establishment of the *direction of the shot.* After taking the coordinates of the entry and exit wounds the next step is to measure the distance from the plane of the sole and from the midline. We describe the character of the wound, especially noting any residue of munitions we find, the extent of contamination around the area of the wound by gunsmoke traces, and lodged, burnt grains of gunpowder. It is important that the scale of the injuries be included in the photograph! We dissect the *shot channel in layers,* with special care directed toward the tissue alterations beneath the wound and the contaminations. (In questionable cases shreds of cloth or other material from the outside, or skin or hair residues from the surface inside the area of the entry wound can be of significant help.) Sometimes residue of munitions can be found either by macro- or microscopic examination. The layered dissection of the shot channel and description of the direction of the shot is essential, in that the path of the projectile may change inside the body. In such instances the straight first part of the channel indicated the direction of the shot.

- Police officer shot an assailant. The bullet entered the left chest, of the level VIII. rib in the middle axillary line. The exit wound was right side also in the middle axillary line of the level II. rib. Thus the path of the projectile was steep. From that we can suppose that the policeman fired from the ground. At the autopsy we saw that the first part of the bullet channel was between the thoracic wall and spine. The bullet penetrated the VIII. vertebral body, lost energy, on the other side of the thorax it changed its direction at the VI. rib, and travelled up under the skin, exiting at the higher level, this given the impression of an angled shot. The first part of the path of the bullet was horizontal.

Finding the pieces of a projectile which broke up inside the body is of special significance. In this process, X-ray can be of great help, especially in those instances where the projectile finds its way into "hidden" body areas or body cavities.

- A 34-year-old male was autopsied after being shot. The police officer who had been attacked and used the weapon testified, and the autopsy verified a shot at close range, but no bullet could be found in the abdomen. Only after a lengthy examination it turned out that the projectile had penetrated the disc between the first and second lumbar vertebrae, got into the spinal canal and had slid down the cauda equina into the lower parts.

Searching for the projectile is essential if it remained in the body, and it requires care or a later examination to produce useful results. With wounds piercing flat bones, if the projectile cannot be found, the section of bone must be removed and checked.

Differentiation between *self- or other-inflicted wounds* is one of the cardinal points in gunshot wounds. The places of predilection – the right temple, oral cavity, chest, heart area – distinct alterations do not unambiguously point to suicide. Sometimes unusual form of suicide occurs. It was published the case of suicide by gunshot while the person driven the car, following the fatal traffic accident the gunshot wound also was found in the thorax of the deceased. Many cases are known in which, because of the location of the wound, suicide was judged when someone else inflicted the injury. A close range shot does not unambiguously mean suicide. In these cases an acquaintance may have been able to come close to the victim without arousing suspicion *(Fig. 84, 85)*.

- G. J. gunned down three fellow workers with all shots being at close range and the victims being unable to protect themselves due to the rapidity of the event.

After analytical study of several cases the opinion has evolved that the frequency of accidents is rare, and many times suicide is hidden by that mistaken idea. With suicide the demonstration of the above-mentioned microtraces is useful, for which numerous procedures have been worked out. Among these neutronactivation analy-

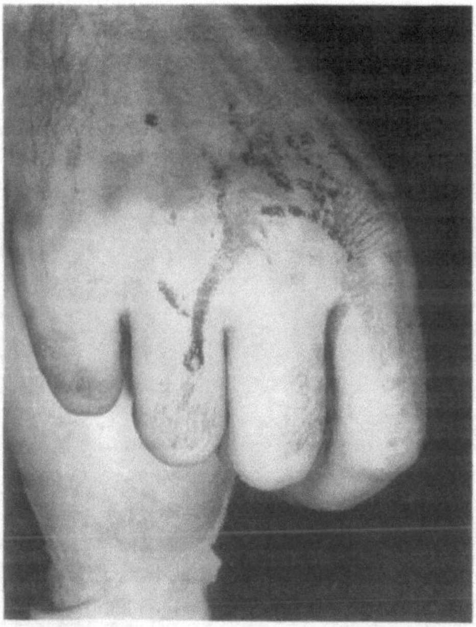

Fig. 84. Spattering of blood on the hand of a suicide shooting victim

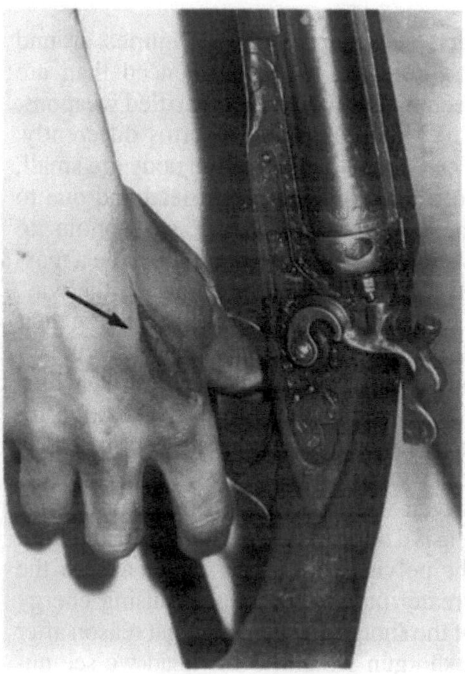

Fig. 85. Contusion to the soft tissue between the thumb and forefinger in a suicide shooting victim

sis and optical emission spectroscopy, can be mentioned which are able to demonstrate the presence of the above-mentioned contaminations, lead, barium etc. in μg amounts. To these procedures in recent years scanning electron microscopy or energy dispersion X-ray analysis have been added.

The roles of the medical examiner conducting the autopsy and the examination at the scene in the establishment of suicide must not be neglected, since in many cases the question can be settled there, such as in the case where in the use of a semiautomatic handgun, the backward motion of the slide can injure the skin between the thumb and the index finger, or blood or brains splattered back on the skin can guide the direction of the examination.

- Gy. Z. – the county chief attorney – was found dead in a patch of woods near his apartment, the cause of death being a gunshot to the skull. The possibility of murder was raised since the previous events didn't support a suicide. A judgement of suicide was justified by the finding of an injury between the right thumb and index finger of the deceased which had been caused by the backward moving slide.

Multiple gunshot wounds usually suggest attack by another, but Introna published 9 cases of suicide with more than two gunshot wounds. The victims suffered 3-5 wounds. The most common site for the injuries was the precordial region, the left chest, the head and the abdomen. Such alterations are also known in suicide where weapons of differing calibers were held in both hands.

- Sometimes bizarre cases of suicide emerge. The above mentioned case of using two weapons is outdone by the one where the person attempting suicide shot with old cartridges which had lost their energy. He tried to pull out the projectiles which had wedged into the bone of the skull with a pair of pliers, and failing that, he pounded them in with a hammer. After that he drank a nicotine-containing solution.

With *shotgun shootings* besides the small pellets, slugs can be fired from the weapon. The former involves a mass of the lead pellets of varied diameters, and the latter means a larger diameter lead or plastic sheathed projectile, the wound which it causes being very similar to a bullet wound. The pellets begin to spread a certain distance from the muzzle of the weapon, depending on the choke of the weapon and the type of munition. The amount of spread cannot be neglected in the establishment of the range of the shot. The shot cloud stays in a group for a certain distance, over which – as has already been described – it causes a hole, abrasion marks, and a pronounced contamination zone, in which besides the residue from the barrel, a great amount of residue of munitions make up the contamination, since with shotgun shells traditional gunpowder has been used for a long time. This can only be so pronounced in the use of home loaded shells, where the neighborhood of the hole is covered by a wide margin which hides the abrasions marks as well. The scattered pellets create wounds as individual projectiles, but with the increase in distance, their energy, which cannot be compared with that of projectiles from rifled weapons, decreases significantly and after causing superficial skin injuries wedge in the subcutaneous connective tissues. In short range shootings, however, we see the same hole left by the pellets as in the above-mentioned case. In shooting with the muzzle in contact, star-shaped tearing injuries around the hole are more pronounced than are seen with those caused by rifled weapons. The shot channel also forms differently. The pellets that pierce the body are small, soft, malleable pieces of lead and due to their small energy are susceptible to change in direction should there be a massive internal organ or a bone in the way. The deformed projectiles in changing their directions can cause numerous secondary projectiles from the bones as well, which can cause deformation and laceration injury. It has happened that deep in a shotgun wound many splinters of the ribs were driven widely into the body causing extensive injuries into the abdomen and even the pelvis. The thicker bones absorb the greater part of the injury-causing energy of the shotgun pellets. For that reason after a shotgun wound to the head we see numerous piercing pellets, but on the opposite side of the skull injury we can hardly

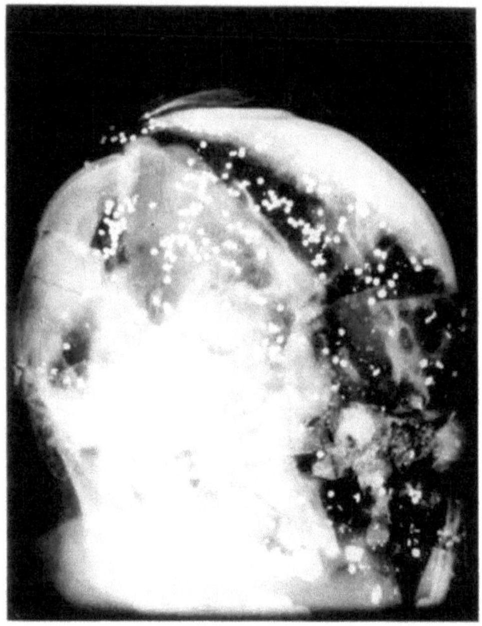

Fig. 86. Injury by shotgun pellets to the head

see any alterations to the skin and the group of pellets are scattered between the injured bone and the scalp, wedged in the soft tissue. At other times with a shot from point blank range the top of the skull with the soft tissues is literally blown off from the force of the blast. The simultaneous discharge of both shells from both barrels may produce single enterance wound *(Fig. 86)*.

With gunshot wounds the *following questions* must be answered:

1. From which direction came the shot?
2. At what range?
3. From which weapon?

ad 1. The lie of the shot channel gives the *direction the shot* came from. For this the line between the entry and exit wound must be measured, which in an ideal situation is also the direction of the shot. The measurements are taken at the autopsy for this specific purpose. The measurement from the plane of the sole and the distance from the midline yields the required coordinates. In a significant number of cases the establishment of the direction is easy. With non exiting gunshot injuries, or the alterations, in which the projectile deviates from its original path, the straight segment at the start of the shot channel indicates the direction of the shot. Sometimes may be difficult to distinguish between the entry and exit wounds. In a progressed decay of the corpse or water soaked injuries the entry and exit openings are not clear. To decide this we must examine the surroundings of the wound and the shot channel. Foreign material – textile, residue of munitions – found in the soft tissues of the area of impact indicate definitely the entry wound. The examination of the shot channel and the establishment of the direction of the shot are the most simple in shots that have pierced flat bones. The bullet hole in the bone widens as a cone shows the direction of the projectile's path. Other times we must histologically examine the shot channel if it passes through several organs. Thus a shot passing through lung, diaphragm, and liver leaves microscopic traces of the organs through the length of the channel.

With a *shotgun wound the direction* taken from the entry and exit wounds leave no doubt. The entry wound is characteristic in both close and long range shots. Identifying the exit wound, if present, is simple. Precise establishment of the direction is sometimes relevant, especially if it must be decided how many shots the victim received.

- In one of our cases we examined an elderly female victim who had suffered a shotgun wound. The pellet group was so scattered that it covered both buttocks and the area around both hip joints – as if having been shot around. Thus the possibility of a double wound surfaced. The suspect maintained that only one shot had occurred. The victim only heard one shot. In the examination of the area around the scene it turned out that the victim who was just then pouring out water when the shot occurred turned around in the shot cloud.

Among the various possibilities for establishing the direction of the shot, placing probes in the shot channels to demonstrate the direction should be mentioned. Due to the changes in direction of the pellets, sinking them deep into the wounds to find the direction is not productive.

ad 2. The *range of the shot* is relevant in establishing whether the wound was inflicted in suicide or by someone else. Studying the use of the weapon merits

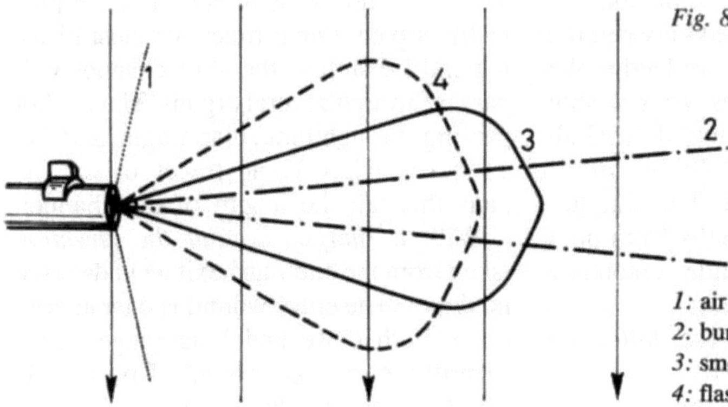

Fig. 87. Gunshot residue

1: air column in front of the projectile
2: burning gunpowder grains
3: smoke effect
4: flash effect

special significance. The shot may be from absolute close range – with the barrel in contact to 0.5-1 cm range –, close range – with short barreled weapons 30–40 cm, with long barreled weapons 60–100 cm, and long range – at distances beyond those just mentioned. The character of a shot produced at absolute close range is distinctive. Recognizing it is the most simple. With close range shots munition residue be found *(Fig. 86, 87).* We have already discussed the residue of munitions. These leave the muzzle of the weapon in a cone shape and the distance determines the dispersal. The greater the distance from the muzzle, the rarer the residue (mostly lodged, burnt granules of gunpowder) concentration, which disperses from an area of 1 cm^2. In close range shots of smokeless powder munitions, we may not even find residue (in shots to clothing covered body parts, the cloth will absorb practically all the residue, which further emphasizes that examination of the clothing is imperative). Examination of the weapon in question and test firing yields the range, and the range-dependent alterations caused by the residue must be studied. The answer in shotgun shootings is easy. If we know the type of cartridge used and the weapon – both have significant effects on the dispersal of the shot group, as we have mentioned – we can tell the distance with relatively good accuracy after a test firing *(Fig. 88, 89).*

To illustrate just how much the cartridge influences the nature of the wound, an example will be mentioned:

- K. S. gunned down his brother-in-law, two sisters-in-law and wife with a shotgun. The three women died at the scene, and the man received a wound to the arm. The shots – except for the injuries to the wife – were shown by the

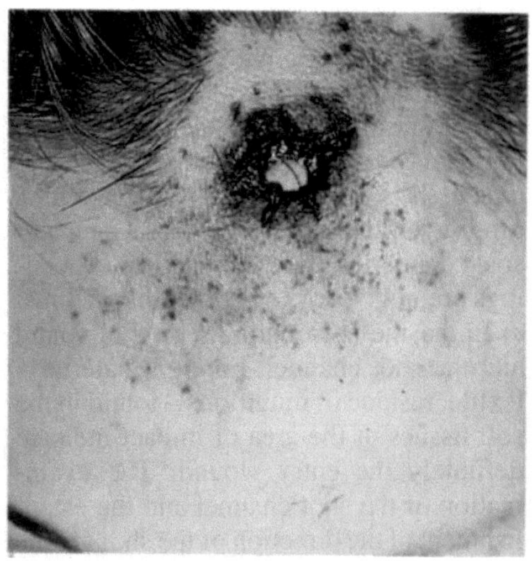

Fig. 88. Short-range shot. Gunpowder tattooing and star-shaped hole with lacerated edges

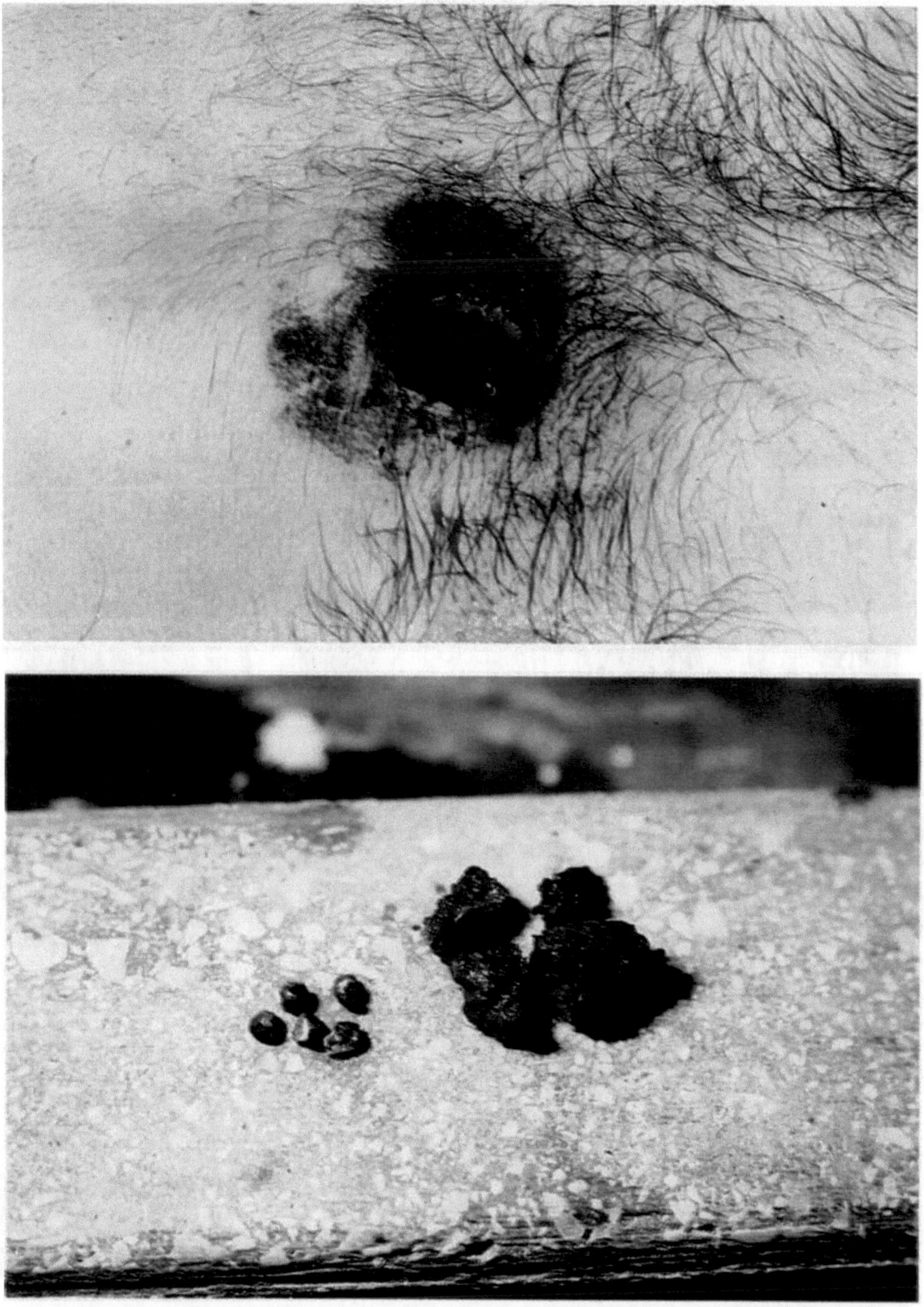

Fig. 89. Extensive gunpowder contamination, single hole, in a close-range shotgun wound. (Pellets and wadding from the shot channel)

a)

b)

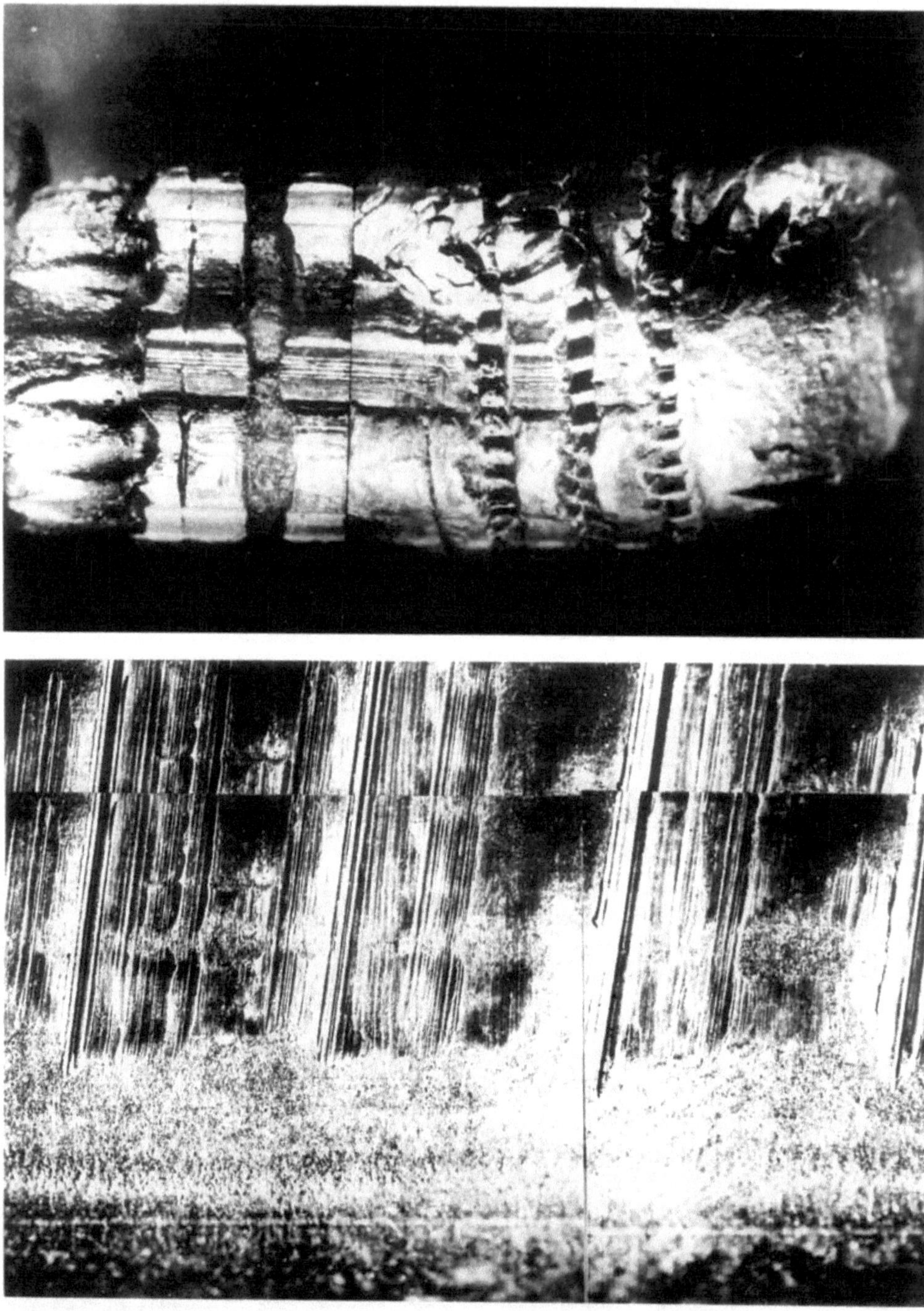

Fig. 90. Possibility of comparison in gunshot wounds. Grooved impressions on the surface of a soft lead bullet *(a)* impressions in a steel jacketed round *(b)*, comparison microscopic picture (from the ORFK Crime Laboratory)

cartridge type to have been taken at several meters range, since the plastic shot cup held the pellets together. The range was such that had traditional ammunition been used the pellets would have already been dispersed. Two of the victims received two shots, each shot hitting its target with a plastic cup lodging deep in the shot channel, so that the pellets held together by the cup formed a wound like a single projectile would.

ad 3. The most important question is *which weapon the shot came from.* This positive identification procedure of the weapon used, even if the circumstances are conducive, is less than certain. The rifling leaves markings on the projectiles, just as the chamber, the firing pin, the extractor, the ejector and the magazine all leave markings on the casing. The name of Balthazard, who in 1912 studied the markings left on projectiles by weapons, is associated with identification of firearms. Examination of the projectile ensures unambiguous identification *(Fig. 90).* If the projectile is found on the scene, whether in the corpse, it should be removed, and treated with such care that the wound remains in its original condition as much as possible. It is wrapped in cotton to protect it for further examination. The identification of the weapon is performed by a specialist on the following principles:

a) visual examination of the projectile,
b) the projectile's diameter and weight,
c) examination of the surface alterations,
d) comparison with the test fired projectile.

a) The projectile to be examined will be *soiled* or *damaged.* The contamination, the dried blood, remains of tissue, and various other things, must be removed from the surface and examined further. For this soaking in 10% perchloric acid followed by ultrasound treatment in distilled water should be performed, which removes not only the dried remains of a recent shooting, but the corrosion from a projectile that has been resting in a decaying body for a long period. (The carbonization of the surface of soft lead projectiles makes identification inconvenient.)

b) The *diameter* and *weight* of certain projectiles and projectile types is characteristic. Occasionally it may reveal the manufacturer. The diameter shows the caliber of the weapon. There are proposed radiographic method for estimating bullet weight and caliber of deformed and undeformed bullets.

c) The *surface of the projectile* – only of those fired from rifled barrels – the rifling of the barrel – ridges and creases – leave marks. In Balthazard's original description the width of these could be compared and reveal the weapon in question. The rifling of the weapon is a unique characteristic. In the reaming of the barrel, every weapon gets such individual markings which make it possible with complete certainty to establish the condition of the projectile – intact, not exploded, surface not significantly damaged – and after its examination, to identify the weapon. The number of rifle grooves must be counted and that may indicate the type of weapon. Here the most commonly used hunting weapons have four rifling ridged, but the military weapons are constructed with 5–6 ridges and grooves. The direction of the rifling may be characteristic: from right to left or left to right. The width of the rifling also depends on the weapon type. It may also happen that the elevated and depressed parts are not of the same width.

d) After finding the projectiles – or the cartridge – *test firings* of the weapons are performed. Sometimes this means firing a large number of weapons. The superficial markings caused by the tested weapon on the projectile are compared with those of the original. The test firing thus protects the surface of the projectile as much as possible by impacting into cotton or oily sawdust or a specially filled vessel or ice bank. Comparison of the micro and macro markings on the surfaces of the projectiles is required. Rifling leaves marks on soft lead clearly visible to the unaided eye, which by aid of a magnifying glass and microscope lead to the possibility of identification.

A special, so-called *comparison microscope* is used in the microscopic examination. The damage to the surface is photographed, and such identifying marks are sought which are characteristic of the barrel of the weapon, and if the appropriate signs match, it can be said that the two projectiles were fired from the same gun. This examination is so specific that subsequent changes to the barrel of the weapon are incapable of erasing the characteristics of the rifling.

Among the further possibilities for identification of the weapon is the *examination of the cartridge* (the only possibility for identification in the case of shotguns). Among the markings left on the cartridge, the print of the firing pin may be unique, the examination of which takes place as previously described with a magnified picture of the location and shape of the firing pin print being examined. This doesn't narrow our possibilities for weapon identification by much (since the same firing pin may for different marks and different pins, the same looking mark!). The extractor leaves a mark on the rim of the cartridge, the value of which is mentioned above as it later makes it easy to alter the surface of the extractor, and sometimes especially home made guns a rough characteristic mark is left on the side of the cartridge. Some weapons are not equipped with extractors.

Ejectors are a part of semiautomatic and automatic weapons, and their identification value is small since we don't in every instance find marks.

The magazine markings come from the metal parts of the magazine and may sometimes be characteristic, but are rarely useful in identification of weapons.

Injuries due to explosions

Of the numerous types of alterations – explosion of gas at home or boilers being the most common – those caused by explosive material are the most significant. A part of the injuries may appear in any for, each having its individual alterations which make differentiation more easy.

Explosive-caused injuries may be from an explosive mixture of nitrocellulose, nitrocellulose-nitroglycerin mixture, dynamite, or gunpowder. The container for the explosive may play a role when, if with the explosion it breaks into pieces and the pieces cause serious injuries. These injuries are similar to gunshot wounds, being high energy containing particles, they cause perforating and lacerating injuries, which due to the irregular tumbling tendency cause irregular shaped holes or large injuries to soft tissues, but larger pieces may cause amputations. Death occurs from shock or bleeding to death due to injury to vital organs. Among the later complications, soft tissue injuries are the most important and gangrene from infection by anaerobes is a possibility. Massive pieces of metal and metal bits or residue of the explosive may show the source of the injury. *(Fig. 91)*

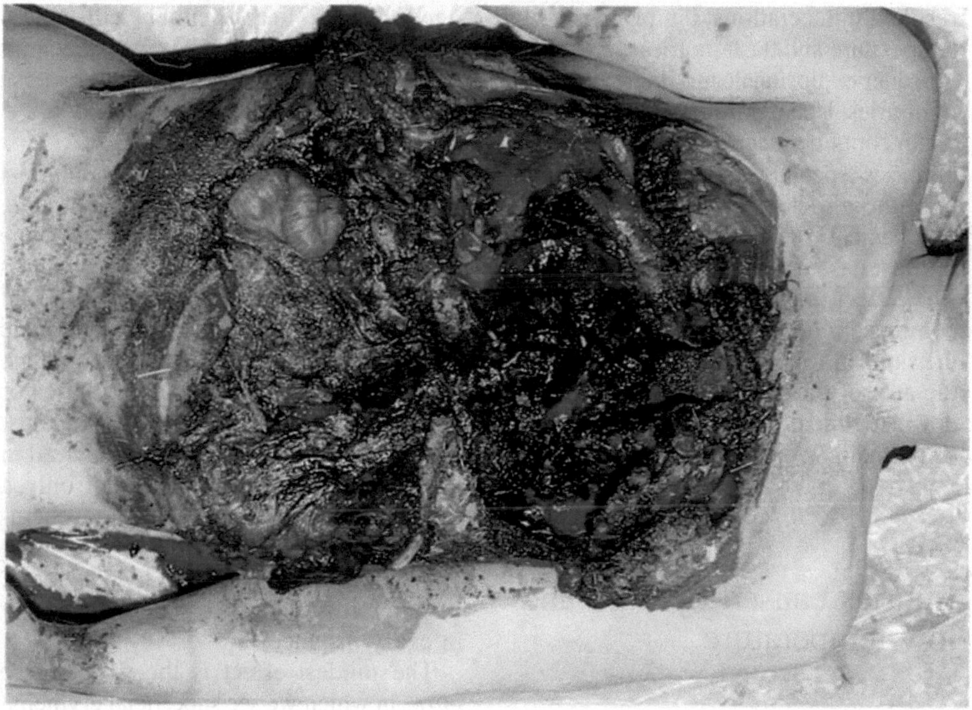

Fig. 91. Blast injury. The suicide victim detonated one kilogram of TNT on his chest

Explosion injuries caused a *shock wave* as an increased blast wave accompanying the explosion (with 20 kg of explosives the time of the increased pressure is about 0.006 seconds) and the following negative pressure finished the result, so that behind a positive compression wave a negative pressure follows. The effect of the negative pressure is longer than the positive pressure bearing in mind the amount of the previous charge exerting its effect in 0.03 seconds. The victim may fall from the effect and in larger explosions may be hurled against nearby objects, which may cause injuries. The air pressure wave may also cause injuries to internal organs, such as hemorrhages in the lungs and emphysema. Three factors play roles in the origin, one being the effect of high pressure, another the effect of negative pressure with alveolar capillary rupture, and the positive pressure may injure the thoracic wall. Victims injured in the water will suffer abdominal organ injury, intestinal and stomach perforation, and experimental data has shown that underwater explosions can cause extensive fat embolism.

Explosion of a gas appliance burn injuries stand out primarily from among the foregoing. The dispersed inflammable gases in appropriate concentrations can form an explosive mixture which with ignition burns with great speed. These are usually propane or butane, or natural gas. The latest several cases explosions occurred when gas escaping for the injured gas pipe drifted through the ground floor with its characteristic odor, filling the basement of each building and blowing them up. The shock wave of the explosion with pieces of the building or containers resulted in lacerations, but primarily high temperature and flash injuries were caused.

Boiler explosions cause more rare forms of injuries. Usually injury from the boiling water container occurs. While in the former cases special injuries were obvious, here the effect of hot steam is primary. Mechanical injury may also occur, which in most cases may be the cause of death. The effect of hot steam, especially if combined with high pressure when it hits the skin, may elevate the epidermis, and in the area of the surface of the blisters fine dew like fluid drops can be seen at the ends of the hairs.

Injuries caused by high and low temperature

Burn injuries

The effect of heat on the organism is the result of several factors. The resulting injury depends on the *thermal capacity* which is made up of the heat conductance capacity, the density of the material and the specific heat. Thus it is understandable that hot metal causes much more damage than materials with lesser conductance. The capacity of the body surface contact to transmit heat depends on the time and the temperature, so that 60 °C for one second only causes discomfort, but after 10 seconds causes reversible damage. The temperature which if applied for a few seconds causes alterations starts at 80 °C, but with 90 °C only a few tenths of a second are needed to cause damage.

The form of the damage depends on the surface of the affected area and its *heat conducting capacity*. If, for example, the microcirculation of the skin is not damaged by the heat, neither will alterations appear in the deeper parts because of the ability of the circulation to disperse heat.

The effect of heat may become manifest in the application of so-called *dry heat,* this being contact by a hot object. Damage may also be caused by *wet heat,* which is not only by steam but from the effect of any hot liquid. The most characteristic form of *radiant heat* is the *flash effect,* which is the result of exploding gases or ignition of explosive material. We must list separately the burn injuries incurred in burning buildings, which are not only a combined form of injury, but show chemical effects as well.

Whatever heat effect is encountered, certain forms of injury can be encountered in every instance.

The mildest effect is the *first degree burn,* in which we see superficial erythema and spread no further than the epidermis. This is caused by temporary dilation of the superficial vessels and heals in 5–7 days. Histologically the vessels running in the skin show dilation and stasis.

In *second degree burns* blisters appear. The process spreads to the superficial epidermis and to the underlying dermis. The vesicles are formed from raised epidermis, but under them a circumscribed erythema can be seen. The fluid in the vesicles is a protein-rich exudate with numerous leukocytes. The cells of the basal layer become spindle shaped, their nuclei elongated and simultaneously appearing arranged. Due to the mild edema, the damaged area is raised when the blister is removed. Within several hours leukocytes migrate to the area under the vesicles, but the alterations to the deeper layers of the skin doesn't occur so it will be healed without residual alteration. If the papillary layer is also affected the injury heals with a scar within 14–28 days depending upon the extent and depth.

With *third degree burns* the damaged area is darkly discolored, dense, and indurate, relatively sharply separated from the surrounding less damaged areas, and the injury affects the deeper layers. Due to coagulation of the blood in the vessels, necrosis appears in the neighboring tissue areas, with stasis in the marginal vessels. The muscle fibers become homogeneous, the cross striations disappearing, and in the margins of the injured area the characteristic elongated nuclei from the effect of heat can be seen. In this group of injuries a general toxic effect and the later formation of a tough, keloid-like scar can be expected which if in the area of a joint can result in diminished function of an extremity.

In *fourth degree burns* carbonization of the injured area develops as the result of a great heat effect and its application over a longer period of time. The characteristic form can be seen on the extremities, the limb due to the damage remaining back on the torso. If a high heat is applied to a single isolated body part, the carbonization will form there and the bone pearls from the melted bone will form. The protein in the bone burns up in the heat and the remaining dark mass consists of the mineral content of the bone, which easily breaks and crumbles.

We *divide the injured body surface* by percent using the "rule of nines." The head is 9%, the front and back of the trunk are 18% each, the upper extremities are 9% each and the lower extremities are 18% each. We give the groin area 1%. Mortality is related to the seriousness of the burn and the age. Thus 10% of all 20-year-olds with 30% of the body surface burned will die, whereas 100% of all 60-year-olds with the same 30% will. Moreover damage to 57% of the body surface is lethal to 60% of the young people, but to 100% of those over 45.

We have already dealt with the factors related to damage. These individually cause the characteristic injury groups.

With a *hot surface,* sometimes the *mark on the body surface* left by the object can be well seen. If the injury is circumscribed – for example, a cigarette burn – a deeper second or third degree burn may develop which is practically round in shape with sharp borders. At other times the mark left by the hot instrument may be indicative.

Damage caused by *radiant heat* affects larger areas. Usually these are those which form second or third degree burns or with a longer application, more serious injuries. One form of radiant heat is the flash effect, which originates from either low flash-point inflammable materials like gasoline, alcohol, etc. or the ignition of explosive gases. Besides the different degree skin alterations, characteristic damage is caused. With an explosion the hair, eyebrows and eyelashes are singed, and with unexpected explosion the victim instinctively closes his eyes and that is why the wrinkles appear around the eyes in the characteristic "crow's foot" burn form *(Fig. 92).*

Explosion injuries, especially from the explosion of high specific heat gases, not only damage the superficial areas, but the mucous membranes of the airways. Alterations from the inhalation of hot gas are most pronounced in the upper section of the trachea, but the bronchial epithelium may also be damaged. This shows up as both macroscopic and microscopic damage, but the most important are the pathophysiological consequences which accompany it. Sixty-five percent of those suffering from flash injuries are lost. The background to the injury is not only the role played by the heat effect, but of special importance are the nitrogen oxides,

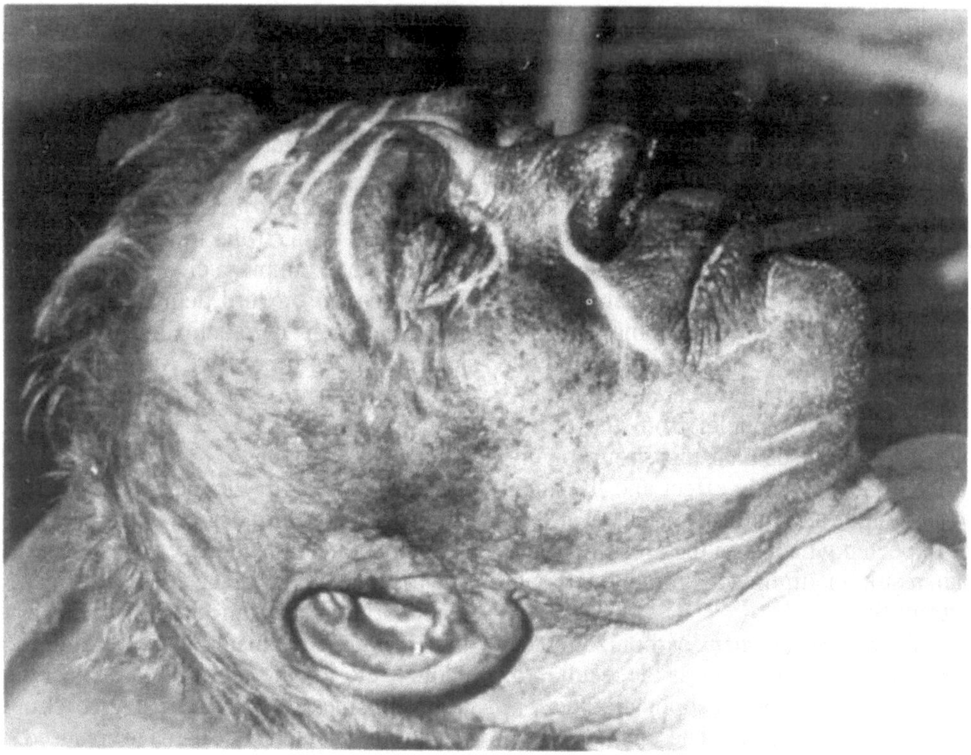

Fig. 92. "Crow's foot" pattern, flash effect

chlorinated compounds and carbon monoxide created by the burning. These have the effect of inducing spasms in the pharynx and pulmonary edema. In the background of pulmonary edema is an increased perfusion of blood in the tracheobronchial areas. The chemical and physical effect may cause this and the extravasation ten times normal and this is not only edema, but appears also as an exudate. With this such vasoactive materials are liberated from the damaged cells, like histamine and vasoactive proteins. The second relevant factor in the clinical alterations following inhalation injuries is the decrease in pulmonary compliance, which accompanies the decrease in surfactant activity. Similar changes have been described in patients suffering from acute respiratory distress syndrome.

The first pathological sign of inhalation of hot gases or steam is swelling of the mucous membranes and engorgement with blood. The damage to the mucous membranes of the trachea and main bronchi results in cellular detachment similar to the formation of a pseudomembrane which may narrow or even close the airway. The separation of the mucous membranes may affect only the superficial layer with swollen, eosinophilic staining vacuolized epithelial cells, nuclear damage, perivascular bleeding into the underlying areas of the mucous membranes, later leukocyte infiltration and bacterial invasion. This basal layer mucous membrane damage, pseudomembran like alteration does not reach the bronchioles, but peribronchial pneumonia may form. Edema in the alveoli followed by leukocyte invasion is the pathological sign of the flash effect. With the expansion of the interstitium stasis in the vessels occurs and in more serious cases hyaline membrane may form on the alveolar epithelium.

With *hot objects* as was mentioned regarding being touched by hot metal, the damage that occurs is dependent upon the contact time. Burns by *molten metal form* not only marks resembling running fluid, but occasionally the traces of the metal can be seen. Similar injuries can also be seen on the body surface when caused by molten glass. The molten material with a high specific heat damage the tissue by transferring its heat content and often cause quite deep holes.

Unfortunately, scalding by *hot liquids* is a common childhood injury. Not only the temperature of the fluid counts toward the severity, but the clothing worn, too. Scalding with close-clinging clothing cause more serious morphological changes, because the effect of the fluid is prolonged by being held in the cloth. The damage can be classified as previously into first, second and third degree burns, but fourth degree burns are never seen. The area affected is irregular, being scattered about the skin surface, and not uncommonly a child who has sat in hot water will show a "trousers-like" form to the damaged area of skin from below the waist.

We have already mentioned injuries caused by boiler explosions and steam. Their characteristic is the raising or the epidermis and formation of extensive patches of blisters, with shiny water drops forming of the ends of the hairs on the tops of the blisters, and the ability of the damage to spread deeply.

Death may occur in burn cases due to shock, airway damage, carbon monoxide poisoning, sometimes cyanide or hydrochloric acid poisoning. Complications in the survivors include pneumonia, sepsis, Curling ulcers, bleeding to death and kidney damage. Shock may be the primary immediate symptom of burns due to the increased sympathetic effect from the pain (nervous effect), or may be secondary to the increased fluid loss and metabolic changes. Changes in vessel permeability may result from burn injuries, and that means an increase in exudation of a protein-rich fluid and edema, especially in the area of a third degree burn impinging upon the active extracellular territory, significant hemoconcentration, a hypovolemic state, tissue hypoxia, and disturbances in myocardial function. Because of damage to the metabolism in the state of shock, edema of the brain, pulmonary edema, hemoglobinuria, and myoglobinuria due to serious renal insufficiency may form.

Carbon monoxide poisoning tends to occur in closed places in conjunction with burn injuries. The level of carbon monoxide may reach such high levels that a significant skin damage may not occur. If the victim survives the injury, the exclusion of carbon monoxide poisoning appropriately improves his condition. If this doesn't happen there is a high probability that the inhalation of hot gas with carbon monoxide will cause not only hypoxia, but damage to the respiratory epithelium as well.

A large quantity of hydrogen chloride is created with the burning of *pvc* or *other plastic polymer* materials, which has an irritating effect on the mucous membranes. The 100 ppm tolerance level may be exceeded by 10–20 times.

In the *autopsy of burn victims* the extent and seriousness of the injuries must by described. This is always by an estimation of the percentage of body surface burned

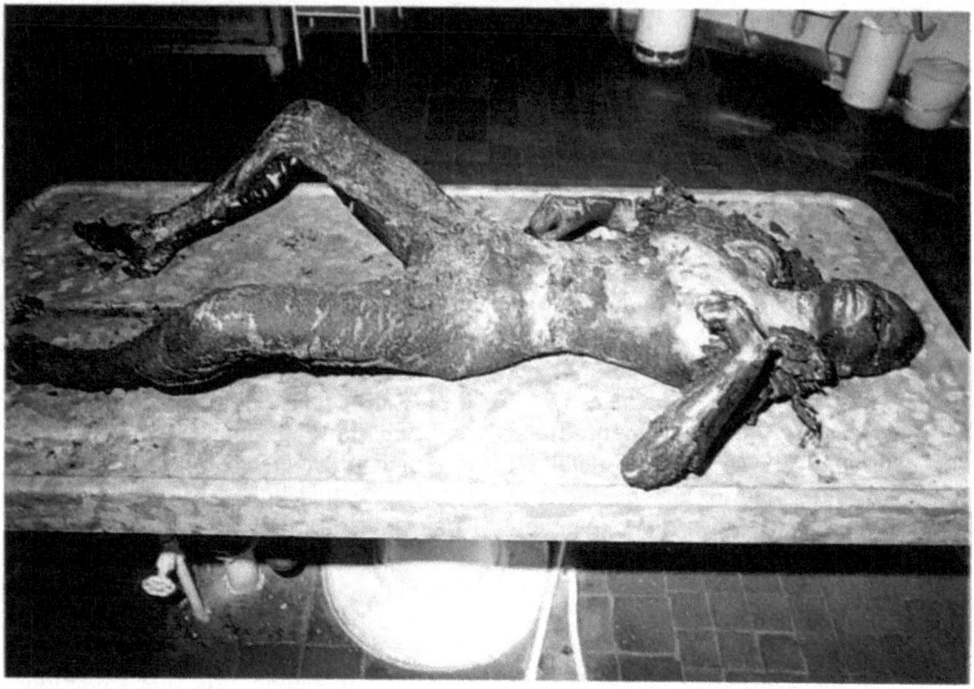

Fig. 93. Gladiator position in burn victim

and an attached schematic drawing. If at the edges of the injury or in the burned areas we find macroscopically regenerating areas or granulation tissue, the alteration is already several days old. Special care must be exercised with those characteristic alterations which signify the individual burn types, flash effect, scalding, or burning by being touched by a hot object. The coagulation of muscle proteins due to the high degree of heat in the appropriate places fixes the body in the so-called *gladiator posture,* which can be formed if the burns occurred in life or postmortally *(Fig. 93).*

Injuries affecting the head damage not only the outer layer of the skull, but the spongy layer, as well. Often the brain coagulates into a dust-like purplish mass. We have also seen such injuries to the skull bones, which due to the swelling of the brain and the uneven effect of the heat caused changes similar to skull fractures in the affected areas. Extensive "ruptures" in the skin of fatty tissues may occur which must not be confused with the vital injuries. With the internal examination the inhalation of particles of soot may be characteristic, which may be seen at the bifurcation of the main bronchi with the unaided eye *(Fig. 94).* Edema of the larynx is a sign of the flash effect. In every case we take a blood sample for determination carbon monoxide and alcohol level. More than once it has been necessary to determine whether the burn victim had been intoxicated previously. From the blood sample the necessary determinations of the presence of medications can be performed.

In the survivors pneumonia, a septic state, acute Curling ulcers in the duodenum may occur and result in bleeding to death *(Fig. 95).*

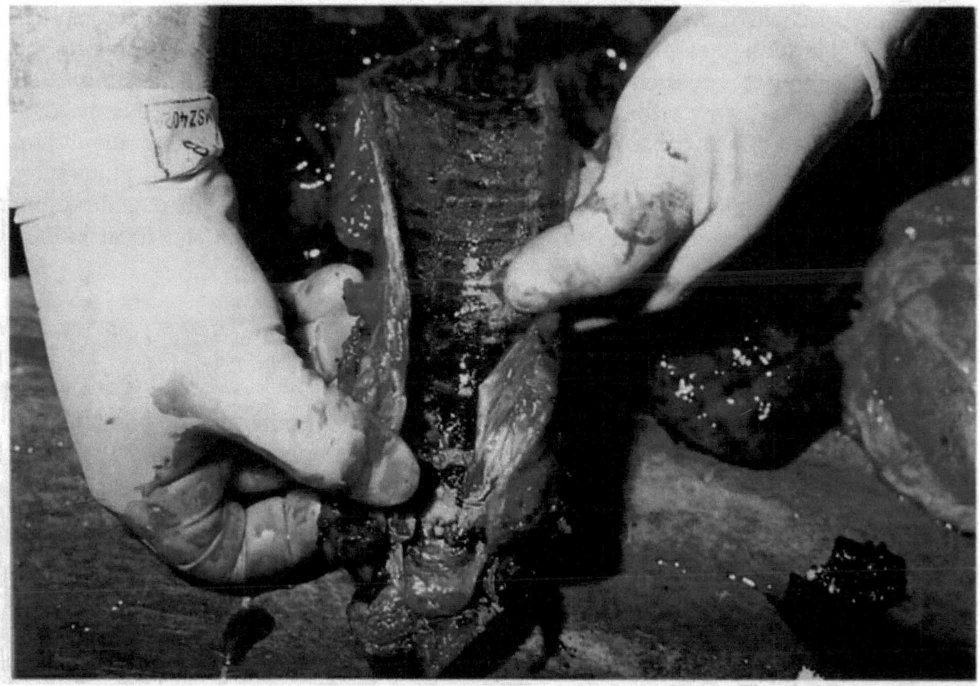

Fig. 94. Smoke inhalation, CO poisoning in burn injury

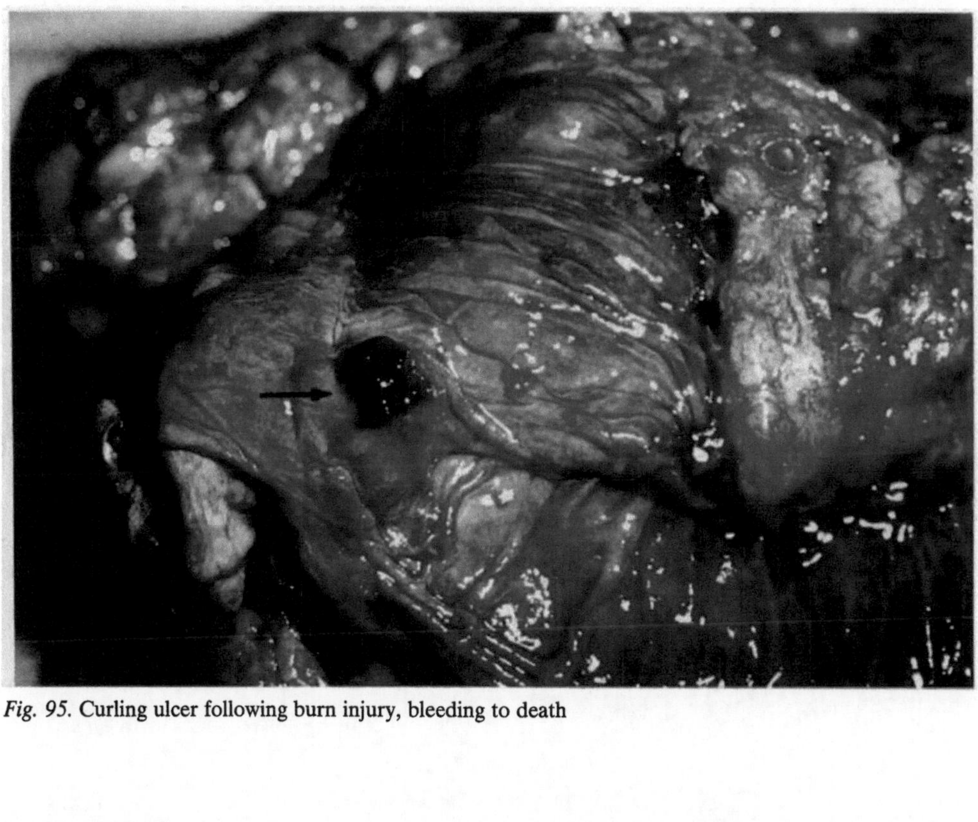

Fig. 95. Curling ulcer following burn injury, bleeding to death

With macroscopic examination the characteristic alterations can differentiate whether the injuries occurred in life or postmortally. The "crow's feet" accompanying the flash effect, because of their ocular reflex nature of origin, are taken as a vital sign, just as smoke or particles of soot found in the airways indicate that they arrived their during life. The histological examination can also unambiguously indicate the injury's origin. As mentioned previously, with first degree burns we see tissue signs, then the content of the vesicles at the base of the injury, with third degree burns the cellular reaction accompanying the injury is a vital sign. In quick death only the increased protein concentration of the blisters and the leukocyte content can help us and naturally the blood carbon monoxide hemoglobin concentration also indicated that the injury occurred in life.

Heat stroke

If the body temperature exceeds 42 °C we speak of heat stroke. The causes include a high external temperature and wearing heavy clothes while performing physical work. The effect and seriousness of the case are especially elevated if the air is humid. The clinical presentation of heat stroke is a red skin which is hot to the touch, a profuse sweating, cramps, vomiting, anuria and hemorrhages. The laboratory results point to serious tissue damage and renal alterations. Among the first signs of heat stroke is the hysteroid reaction. The possibility of heat stroke should be considered in behavioral deviations that suddenly appear following exposure to high temperatures. Among the provoking situations, a pronounced physical loading is the most important. Feverish states, alcohol consumption, and fluid loss are predisposing factors. The autopsy results and opinion which support the known prior information are accompanied by morphologically general edema, dermal hemorrhages, edema of the brain, pulmonary edema, interstitial pulmonary hemorrhages, myocardial degeneration, hepatocellular necrosis and focal kidney hemorrhages.

Death by cooling

In systemic hypothermia the human body drops to a temperature below 35 °C. The human organism is warm-blooded (homoiothermic), the body temperature being independent of the environmental temperature. Hypothermia therefore results when the body's loss of heat exceeds its production. The general cause is a low external temperature. We divide this into four categories:

1. The so-called environmental hypothermia, which comes about from a low environmental temperature and occasionally exhaustion.
2. Cold environment and toxic effect – alcohol or drugs – which damage the heat producing or storage capacities.
3. Such diseases in which the resistance of the organism is reduced.
4. Therapeutic hypothermia.

The damaging effect of the environment depends upon whether it is wet or dry. The increased loss of heat in a wet environment speeds the cooling process significantly. The wetting of the clothing is enough to significantly increase heat loss. The age of the victim also plays a role in that heat loss is relatively quicker in infants, whose body temperature regulating mechanism is still inadequate, and can develop hypothermia even in places of relatively high temperature. In young adults, physical exertion may result in exhaustion which destroys the thermal regulation system. In elderly persons inadequate nutrition is most often behind hypothermia.

The critical environmental temperature for a naked person is 27 °C, which is the level at which the organism is capable of regulating the body temperature at complete rest.

Early clinical signs of hypothermia point to central nervous system damage, when the body temperature is at about 30–32 °C analgesia, hallucinations and slowed reflexes can be noticed. At about 30 °C sleep ensues and reflexes and pupillary reactions cease at 27 °C and 26 °C, respectively. If the unconscious state is prolonged, permanent damage in the form of epilepsy and dysphasia develop. Besides the central nervous system, the heart and circulatory system are also sensitive and a drop in pulse volume is noticed most early. On the ECG the PQ interval is prolonged, depolarization slowed, repolarization disturbed, a negative T-wave develops, and at around 30 °C the so-called *J-wave* following the QRS complex appears. Under 30 °C there is often atrial fibrillation, and ventricular fibrillation develops between 28–25 °C. The breathing frequency and cardiac output decrease. The airway dead space may increase by 50% due to the increase in alveolar dead space. Pulmonary perfusion decreases and with it a relative right heart insufficiency. Later respiratory acidosis may develop. Hypothermic intestinal wall damage may also occur, and therefore hemorrhages in the gastric mucosa, erosions and the so-called *Wischnewsky ulcers* may be seen. These are caused by changes in the microcirculation of the mucous membranes and the release of the vasoactive amines histamine and serotonin.

The connection between hypothermia and alcohol and certain sedative-hypnotic drugs is important. Alcohol predisposes to hypothermia by dilatation the vessels of the skin and skeletal muscles increasing heat loss. An incapacitated state from heavy alcohol consumption can also lead to heat loss in a person inadequately clothed for the cold climate. Cooling to death in a heavily alcoholic intoxicated state ensues. According to the literature the average blood alcohol concentration level in these cases is around 16 mg%. In connection with freezing to death, among the sedatives and hypnotics, the barbiturates and chlorpromazine figure the most prominently. Occasional hypothermia is one of the characteristic signs of barbiturate intoxication.

The *survival time in cold* environments has been studied as well. A survival time of about two hours is given in 4 °C water, while in 0 °C water death from cooling occurs in under 1/2 hour. The danger of swimming in cold water merits attention since the dilation of the vessels in the working muscles also increases heat loss. This explains the drowning of some young athletes in cold water.

We must mention the special forms of cooling which often raise the suspicion of crime. The so-called *paradox reaction* in cases of cooling to death occurs when the person being cold undresses from a feeling of warmth. Several authors have mentioned such cases where the body of the cold victim was found partly or completely unclothed. To explain the occurrence, such pathophysiological changes were suggested which appropriately explain paresthesias. The effect of cold is peripheral vasoconstriction and paralysis of the nerves in the vessel walls leads to vasodilation, which brings a feeling of warmth. According to others the reflex vasoconstriction, which happens in the first stage of hypothermia, brings about a paralysis of the vasomotor center, and such a feeling arises as though the body temperature were higher than it really is and in a paradox reaction, the person undresses. All the authors call attention to the necessity of considering the paradox reaction in every case where a victim or body is found in the open with inadequate or no clothing.

The diagnosis of death by cooling today is based on the same classical signs which for the most part have been used by pathologists and practitioners of legal medicine since the last century. KENYERES in his book mentions the bright red patches of lividity, the purple changes formed on the skin, the dilation of the cardiac chambers, the brighter than usual red color of the blood, and the separation of the sutures of the skull. These signs are common in death by cooling, but not pathognomic. We have already mentioned the bright red color of the patches of lividity in wet environments which is explained by the postmortal diffusion of oxygen through the skin. A more livid discoloration of the hands, knees, and feet is a sign of mild freezing damage. In these areas histologically the skin is edematous, there is stasis in the vessels and in their neighborhood an infiltration of inflammatory cells can be seen. In hypothermia dilation of the right heart, bloody pulmonary edema, engorgement with blood of the pulmonary tissues, and liver and splenic congestion are characteristic, which are the signs of acute right cardiac insufficiency. For a certain time, survival is complicated by bronchopneumonia. Hemorrhages in the gastric mucosa, erosions and the so-called Wischnewsky ulcers can be found relatively frequently. These, according to some, occur in 90% of the cases, while others place the incidence significantly lower. In our experience of deaths by cooling damage to the gastric mucosa has been found only rarely. Acute pancreatitis also resembles death by cooling in some aspects, but in practice it is seen quite seldom. Likewise acute tubular necrosis of the kidneys is not characteristic, nor is lipoid deposit in the glomerulus. The urinary catecholamine level may be pathological since it has been reported that a significant number of the victims of hypothermia release catecholamines.

According to DALLOS the content of brown fat in the organism, being a special reserve material, plays a role in cases of cooling. The combined effect of hunger and cooling being lessened by the brown fat. The reticulum proliferates, separates crudely and in the cases of death by cooling lipoid can hardly be found in the brown fat cells.

Recently, in the diagnosis of the cooling besides the elevation of the level of MM creatine kinase isoenzyme, the BB isoenzyme fraction will also be elevated. In the cases of death by cooling – an increased creatine kinase value was measured and the enzyme activity surpassed significantly the increased CK activity at myocardial infarction or muscle damage.

The blood alcohol effect and the toxicological examination must never be omitted.

References

Injuries

[1] ADAMS, J. H., D. I. GRAHAM, L. S. MURRAY, G. SCOTT: Diffuse axonal injury due to nonmissile head injury in humans. Ann. Neurol. 12 (1982) 557-563

[2] ADKINS, R. B., J. E. KEYSER: Recent experiences with duodenal trauma. Am. Surg. 51 (1985) 121-131

[3] BERGQUIST, D., H. HEDELIN, B. LINDBLAD, T. MATZSEK: Abdominal injuries in children. Injury 16 (1984) 217-220

[4] BURIS, L., MESTER Gy.: A fej önkezűleg okozott vágott sérülései. Belügyi Szemle III. (1965) 118-120

[5] CASSON, W. R.: Delayed cardiac tamponade. Anaesthesia 40 (1985) 49-50

[6] CLIFFORD, R. P., K. S. GILL: Traumatic rupture of the pericardium with dislocation of the heart. Injury 16 (1984) 123-125

[7] COAST, G. C., D. J. GEE: Traumatic subarachnoid haemorrhage. J. Clin. Pathol. 37 (1984) 1245-1248

[8] CONTOSTAVLOS, D.: Massive subarachnoid haemorrhage due to laceration of the vertebral artery associated with fracture of the transverse process of atlas. J. Forensic Sci. 16 (1971) 40-56

[9] COPPA, G. F., M. DAVALLE, H. L. PACHTER, S. R. HOFSTETTER: Management of penetrating wounds of the back and flank. Surg. Gynecol. Obstet. 159 (1985) 514-518

[10] Costs and benefits of skull radiography for headinjury. Editorial. Lancet 2 (1981) 791-795

[11] COURVILLE, C. B.: Traumatic intracerebral hemorrhages. Bull. Los Angeles Neurol. Soc. 27 (1962) 22-38

[12] DEMETRIADES, D., B. RABINOWITZ: Selective conservative management of penetrating abdominal wounds. Br. J. Surg. 71 (1984) 92-94

[13] ESTRERA, A. S., M. J. LANDAY, R. M. MCCLELLAND: Blunt traumatic rupture of the right hemidiaphragm. Ann. Thorac. Surg. 39 (1985) 525-530

[14] FLEISCHER, A. S., J. M. PATTON, G. T. TINDALL: Cerebral aneurysm of traumatic origin. Surg. Neurol. 4 (1975) 233-239

[15] FLETCHER, T. B., H. SETIAWAN, R. S. HARRELL, H. C. REDMAN: Posterior abdominal stab wounds: role of CT evaluation. Radiology 173 (1989) 621-625

[16] FRAYER, D. W., J. G. BRIDGENS: Stab wounts and personal identity determined from skeletal remains J. Forensic Sci. 30 (1985) 232-238

[17] FREYTAG, E.: Autopsy findings in head injuries from blunt forces. Arch. Pathol. 75 (1963) 402-413

[18] FUKAMACHI A., K. KOHNO, Y. NAGESAKI, S. MISUMI, H. KUNIMINE, T. WAKAO: The incidence of delayed traumatic intracerebral haematoma with extradural hemorrhages. J. Trauma 25 (1985) 145-149

[19] FULLUM, T. M., S. M. SIRAM, M. RIGHINI: Stab wounds to the chest: a retrospective review of 100 consecutive cases. J. Natl. Med. Assoc. 82 (1990) 109-112

[20] GALBRAITH, S. L.: Age distribution of extradural haemorrhage without skull fracture. Lancet 1 (1973) 1217-1218

[21] GARZA-MERCADO, R., R. A. RANGEL: Extradural hematoma associated with traumatic middle meningeal artery pseudoaneurysm. Neurosurgery 5 (1979) 500-503

[22] GENNARELLI, T.: Cerebral concussion and diffuse brain injuries. In: Graham, D. I. and all.: Pathology of Brain Damage in Head Injury. P. R. Cooper Williams and Wilkins Baltimore (1987) pp. 72-88

[23] GILROY, D.: Death from blunt trauma. Injury 15.(1984) 304-308.

[24] GRAHAM, D. I., J. H. ADAMS, T. A. GENNARELLI: Pathology of Brain Damage in Head Injury. P. R. Cooper Williams and Willkins Baltimore (1987) pp. 72-88

[25] HARRISON, J. D., F. J. BRANICKI, G. S. MAKIN: Pancreatic injury in association football. Injury 16 (1985) 232-234

[26] HASEKURA, H., H. FUKUSHIMA, I. YONEMURA, M. OTA: A rare suicidal case of a ten-year old child stabling himself in the throat. J. Forensic Sci. 30 (1985) 1269-1271

[27] HEISKANEN, O.: Epidural hematoma. Surg. Neurol. 4 (1975) 23-26

[28] HOBIN, F. P.: Air embolism complicating percutaneous ultrasonic lithotripsy. J. Forensic Sci. 30 (1985) 1284-1286

[29] IRÁNYI, J., IRÁNYI J.-NÉ, SOMOGYI, E.: Az elektromos baleset és a villámcsapás klinikuma és patológiája. Akadémia, (1967)

[30] KALISKY, Z., D. P. MORRISON, C. A. MEYERS, A. von Laufen: Medical problems encountered during rehabilitation of patients with head injury. Arch. Phys. Med. Rehabil. 66 (1985) 25-29

[31] KAPUSZ, N., BURIS L.: Eszközmeghatározás jelentősége szúrásos sérülések esetén. Belügyi Szemle III. (1965) 97-100

[32] KEET, P. C.: Extradural haematoma. S. Afr. Med. J. 66. (1984) 193–196
[33] KELEMEN, E,: Significance of fat embolism in injuries. Acta Morph. Suppl. (1958) 57–
[34] KETTUNEN, P.: Cardiac damage after blunt chest trauma diagnosed using CK-MB enzyme and electrocardiogram. Int. J. Cardiol. 6 (1984) 355–371
[35] KIECK, C. F., J. C. DE VILLIERS: Vascular lesions due to transcranial stab wounds. J. Neurosurg. 60 (1984) 42–46
[36] KIRKPATRICK, J. B.: Forensic considerations in examining the brain. Semin. Diagn. Pathol. 1 (1984) 98–113
[37] KRANTZ, K. P. G.: Head and neck injuries to motorcycle and moped riders with special regard to the effect of protective helmets. Injury 16 (1985) 253–258
[38] KULSHRESTHA, P., B. DAS, K. S. IYER, K., K. A. SAMPATH, M. L. SHARMA, I. M. RAO: Cardiac injuries, a clinical and autopsy profile. J. Trauma 30 (1990) 203–207
[39] LAU, O. J., F. P. SHABBO, J. SMYLLIE: Acute left anterior descending coronary artery occlusion following blunt chest injury. Injury 16 (1984) 55–56
[40] LAWRENCE, R. D.: Inaccuracy of measuring wounds on autopsy photographs. Am. J. Forensic Med. Pathol. 6 (1985) 17–18
[41] LEADBEATTER, S., B. KNIGHT: Resuscitation artefact. Med. Sci. Law 28 (1988) 200–204
[42] LEE, W. C., J. F. UDDO, F. C. NANCE: Surgical judgment in the management of abdominal stab wound. Ann. Surg. 199 (1984) 549–554
[43] LINDENBERG, R., FREYTAG, E.: A mechanism of cerebral contusions a pathologic-anatomic study. Arch. Pathol. 69 (1960) 440–469
[44] MARKIEWICZ, W., L. A. BEST, S. BURSTEIN, H. PELEG: Echocardiographic evaluation after blunt trauma of the chest. Int. J. Cardiol. 8 (1985) 269–274
[45] McKISSOCK, W.: Subdural haematoma. Lancet 1 (1960) 1365–1369
[46] METTER, D.: Die Hypoglykamie als Ursache von Verkehrsunfallen. Blutalkohol 26 (1989) 185–194
[47] OEHMICHEN, M., G. RAFF: Timing of cortical contusion. Z. Rechtsmed. 84 (1980) 79–99
[48] PATTISAPU, J., R. R. SMITH, J. BEBIN: Traumatic decerebracy with preserved consciousness and voluntary movement. Neurosurgery 16 (1985) 71–74
[49] POLK, H. C., L. M. FLINT: Intraabdominal injuries in polytrauma. World J. Surg. 7 (1983) 56–67
[50] REECE, I. J., K. G. DAVIDSON: Emergency surgery for stab wounds to the heart. Ann. R. Coll. Surg. Engl. 65 (1983) 304–307
[51] ROBERGE, R. J., M. J. MORGENSTERN, H. OSBORN: Cough fracture of the ribs. Am. J. Emerg. Med. 2 (1985) 513–517
[52] ROMANOWSKI, U., E. WILHELMS: Vergleichende Untersuchungen zur Identifizierung des Tatwerkzeigs bei Stichverletzungen Krim. Forens. Wiss. 53–54 (1984) 89–93
[53] ROTHSTEIN, R. J.: Myocardial contusion. JAMA 250 (1983) 2189–2191
[54] SAHUQUILLO, J., J. VILALTA, J. LAMARCA, E. RUBIO, M. RODRIGUEZ PAZOS, J. A. SALVA: Diffuse axonal injury after severe head trauma. A clinicopathological study. Acta Neurochir Wien 101 (1989) 149–158
[55] SCHÖN, H., M. KUHN, J. ALLEMANN, R. RATTI: Traumatischer Myocardinfarkt. Schweiz. med. Wschr. 116 (1986) 218–221
[56] SHERMAN, K., J. MACKINNON: Motorcycling injuries in children. Br. Med. J. 289 (1984) 877–878
[57] SIMONSEN, J.: Fatal subarachnoid hemorrhage in relation to minor head injuries. J. Forensic Med. 14 (1967) 140–155
[58] SIVALOGANATHAN, S.: Traumatic subarachnoid haemorrhage as part of the NAI syndrome. Med. Sci. Law 30 (1990) 138–140
[59] SPERRY, K.: Anterior thoracic wall trauma in elderly homicide victims. The "CPR defense". Am. J. Forensic Med. Pathol. 11 (1990) 50–55
[60] STATES, J. D., D. F. HUELKE, M. DANCE, R. M. GREEN: Fatal injuries caused by underarm use of shoulder belts. J. Trauma 27 (1987) 740–745
[61] TENZER, M. L.: The spectrum of myocardial contusion. J. Trauma 25 (1985) 620–627
[62] Testi sérülések és egészségkárosodások igazságügyi orvosszakértői véleményezéséről. 2. sz. Módszertani levél, Bp. (1977)
[63] THAL, R. E.: Peritoneal lavage. Arch. surg. 119 (1984) 579–584
[64] THORNBURY, J. R., J. A. CAMPBELL, S. J. MASTERS, D. G. FRYBACK: Skull fracture and the low risk of intracranial sequelae in minor head trauma. Am. J. Roentgenol. 143 (1984) 661–664
[65] URBAN, R., J. EIDAM, W. KLEEMANN, H. D. TROGER: Isolierter Herzstich ohne Probierstiche-Suicid oder Tötung. Betr. Gerichtl. Med. 47 (1989) 272–277
[66] WASHINGTON, B., R. F. WILSON, Z. STEIGER, J. S. BASSETT: Emergency thoracotomy: A four year review. Ann. Thorac. Surg. 40 (1985) 188–191
[67] ZULCH, K. J.: Die traumatischer Spatapoplexie. Forstschr. Neurol. Psychiatr. 53 (1985) 1–12
[68] ZULCH, K. J.: Delayed post-traumatic apoplexy. Neurosurg. Rev. 12 (1989) 252–255

Traffic accidents

[1] ADEYEMO, A. O., A. O. ARIGBABU, O. ADEJUYIGBE: Thoracic injuries in road traffic accidents. Injury 16 (1984) 30–24

[2] AKANE, A., H. SHIONO, K. MATSUBARA, S. TAKAHASHI: Identification of the driver in an automobile collision. Am. J. Forensic Med. Pathol. 11 (1990) 246–251

[3] ALLEN, M. J., M. R. BARNES, G. G. BODIWALA: The effect of seat belt legislation an injuries sustained by car occupants. Injury 16 (1985) 471–476

[4] ASBUN, H. J., H. IRANI, E. J. ROE, J. H. BLOCH: Intra-abdominal seatbelt injury. J. Trauma. 30 (1990) 189–193

[5] BRINKMANN, B., G. SCHWARZ, E. STICHNOTH: Zur problematik der liegend überfahrenen Fussgangers. Arch. Kriminol. 175 (1985) 137–144

[6] BUDVÁRI, R.: Közlekedési balesetek áldozatainak oknyomozó boncolása. Belügyi Szemle V. (1963) 56–64

[7] CHI, M., J. VOSOUGHI: Engineering aspect of automobile accident reconstruction using computer simulation. J. Foren sic Sci. 30 (1985) 814–821

[8] COX, E. F.: Blunt abdominal trauma. Ann. Surg. 199 (1984) 467–474

[9] FÖLDES, V., HARSÁNYI, L., SZABÓ, Á: Tömeges közlekedési balesetek orvosszakértői vizsgálatának feladatai. Belügyi Szemle XI. (1965) 45–47

[10] FÖLDES, V., HARSÁNYI, L.: Kihantolással bizonyított közlekedési balesetek. Morph. Ig. Orv. Szemle 2 (1967) 150–153

[11] FÖLDES, V., SZABÓ, Á., HARSÁNYI, L.: A koponya és nyaki gerinc közlekedési baleseti sérülései a baleseti mechanizmus szemszögéből. Belügyi Szemle IX. (1971) 109–111

[12] Front-seat hazards. Editorial. Br. Med. J. 4 (1969) 63

[13] GILROY, D.: Death (144) from road traffic accidents occuring before arrival at hospital. Injury 16 (1985) 241–242

[14] HAMILTON, J. R., CH. DEARDEN, W. H. RUTHERFORD: Myocardial contusion associated with fracture of the sternum. Important features of seat belt syndrome. Injury 16 (1984) 155–156

[15] HANSOTIA, P., S. K. BROSTE: The effect of epilepsy or diabetes mellitus on the risk of automobile accidents. N. Engl. J. Med. 324 (1991) 22–26

[16] KERWIN, A. J.: Sudden death while driving. Can. Med. Assoc. J. 131 (1984) 312–314

[17] MURDOCK, M. A., K. WAXMAN: Helmet use improves outcomes after motorcycle accidents Wat J. Med. 155 (1991) 370–372

[18] NAGY, L.: Auf starke stumpfe Bewalteinwirkung entstehende Extension Ringfrakturen der Schadelbasis. Zbl. Verkehrsmed. 19 (1973) 129–136

[19] SAUTNER, D., W. SAEGER: Retroperitoneale Blutungen im Obduktionsgut: Haufigkeit und Ursachen. Pathologe 11 (1990) 101–102

[20] TSUANG, M. T., M. BOOR, J. A. FLEMING: Psychiatric aspects of traffic accidents. Am. J. Psychiatry 142 (1985) 538–546

[21] TSUDA, R., Y. ITO, T. INOUE, M. HARA: A statistical survey of medico-legal activities for the traffic accidental death. Igaku Kenkyu 59 (1989) 29–34

[22] VAN KIRK, D. J.: A scientific approach to documenting evidence for accident reconstruction. J. Forensic Sci. 29 (1984) 806–815

[23] WALLER, J. A.: Health status and motor vehicle crashes. N. Engl. J. Med. 324 (1991) 54–55

[24] WILD, B. R., J. KENWRIGHT, S. RASTOGI: Effects of seat belts an injuries to front and rear seat passangers. Br. Med. J. 290 (1985) 1621–1623

Electrical injuries

[1] ANDERSON, R. E.: Introductory comments. Pathology Studies of the Atomic bomb Causalty Comission. Human Pathol. 2 (1971) 461–470

[2] BRENT, R. L.: The effect of embryonic and fetal exposure to X ray, microwaves and ultrasound. Clin. Obst. Gynecol. 26 (1983) 484–510

[3] BROSS, I. D. J., N. NATARJAN: Genetic damage from diagnostic radiation. JAMA 237 (1977) 2399–2401

[4] BURIS, L., K. ZSIGMOND, M. SZABÓ: Histochemical examinations of electrical injuries. Acta Histochem. 28 (1967) 355–358

[5] CHANDRA, N. C., C. O. SIU, A. M. MUNSTER: Clinical predictors of myocardial damage after high voltage electrical injury. Crit. Care Med. 18 (1990) 293–297

[6] COOPER, M. A.: Electrical and lightning injuries. Emerg. Med. Clin. North. Am. 2 (1984) 489-501

[7] DIXON, B.: The biological and clinical effects of acute whole or partial body irradiation. J. Soc. Radiol. Pract. 5 (1985) 125–128

[8] Evolution of occupational and environmental exposures to radon and radon daughters in the United States. National Council an Radiation Protection and Measurements Bethesda M. D. 20814 (1984)

[9] FANGER, H., C. C. LUSBAUGH: Radiation death from cardiovascular shock following criticality accident. Arch. Pathol. 83 (1967) 446–460
[10] GRUMET, G. W.: Attempted suicide by electrocution. Review and case report. Bull. Menninger Clin. 53 (1989) 512–521
[11] GRUNDFEST, W. S., LITVACK F., FORRESTER J. S.: Laser ablation of human atherosclerotic plaque without adjacent tissue injury. J. Am. Coll. Cardiol. 514 (1985) 929–933
[12] HARM, W.: Biological Effect of Ultraviolet Radiation. Cambridge Univ. Press (1980)
[13] HOUSINGER, T. A., L. GREEN, S. SHAHANGIAN: A prospective study of myocardial damage in electrical injuries. J. Trauma 25 (1985) 122–124
[14] IRVINE, J.: Electric shock and associated injury. Practitioner 233, (1989) 1454–1457
[15] JABLON, S., H. KATO: Childhood cancer in relation to prenatal exposure to atomic-bomb radiation. Lancet 2 (1970) 1000–1003
[16] JAMES, T. N., L. RIDDICK, J. H. EMBRY: Cardiac abnormalities demonstrated postmortem in four cases of accidental electrocution and their potential signifi-cance relative to nonfatal electrical injuries of the heart. Am. Heart J. 120 (1990) 143–157
[17] JINDOP, P., J. ROTHBLATT, P. WEBBER: Radiation casualties in a nuclear war. Nature 313 (1985) 345–346
[18] METTLER, F. A., R. D. MOSELEY: Medical Effects of Ionizing Radiation. Grune and Stratton Inc. Orlando, Fl. (1985)
[19] MODAN, B., E. RON, A. WERNER: Thyroid cancer following scalp irradiation. Radiology 123 (1977) 741–744
[20] NAJARIAN, T.: Mortality from leukemia and cancer in shipyard nuclear worker. Lancet I. (1978) 1018–1020
[21] NEEL, J. V.: Genetic effect of atomic bombs. Science 213 (1981) 1205
[22] OPPENHEIM, B. A.: Genetic damage from diagnostic radiation? A critique of the Bross-Natarajan study. Jama 242 (1979) 1390–1393
[23] PIERUCCI, G., P. DANESINO: The macroscopic detection of metalisation in the latent current mark. Z. Rechtsmed 85 (1980) 97–105
[24] PÜSCHEL, K., B. BRINKMANN, K. LIESKE: Ultrastructural alterations of skeletal muscles after electric shock. Am. J. Forensic Med. Pathol. 6 (1985) 296–300
[25] RINSKY, R., R. D. ZUMWALDE, R. J. WAXWEILER, W. E. MURRAY, PH. J. BIERBAUM, PH. J. LANDRIGAN, M. TERPILAK, C. COX: Cancer mortality at naval nuclear shipyard. Lancet I. (1981) 231–235
[26] RUBIN, PH., G. W. CESARETT: Clinical Radiation Pathology. W. B. Saunders Co. Philadelphia (1968)
[27] RUSSEL, W. L., L. B. RUSSEL, E. M. KELLY: Radiation dose rate and mutation frequency. Science 128 (1958) 1546–1550
[28] SETLOW, R. B.: Repair deficient human disorders and cancer. Nature 271 (1978) 713–717
[29] SHAHEEN, M. A., N. A. SABET: Bilateral simultaneous fracture of the femoral neck following electrical shock. Injury 16 (1984) 13–14
[[31] SMITH, P. G., R. DOLL: Mortality from cancer and all causes among British radiologist. British J. Radiol. 54 (1981) 187–194
[31] SOMOGYI, E., RÓZSA, G., SÓTONYI, P.: Histochemische und fluoreszenzoptische Untersuchungen der Strommarke. Acta Morphol. Acad. Sci. Hung. XIII. (1965) 311–314
[32] SOMOGYI, E., SÓTONYI, P., RÓZSA, G.: A bőr kollagen rostjai elektromos áram hatására történt változásainak polarizációs optikai vizsgálata. Morph. Ig. Orv. Szemle 3 (1965) 186–191
[33] SOMOGYI, E.: Kísérletes áramjegyek szubmikroszkopikus vizsgálata. Morph. Ig. Orv. Szemle 4 (1965) 256–257
[34] STEVENSON, A. C., R. MASON, K. D. EDWARDS: Maternal diagnostic X irradiation before conception and the frequency of mongolism in children subsequently born. Lancet 2 (1970) 1335–1337
[35] SURREL, J. A., R. C. ALEXANDER, S. D. COHLE, F. R. LOVELL, R. A. WEHRENBERG: Effect of microwave radiation on living tissue. J. Trauma 27 (1987) 935–939
[36] SZABÓ, M., K., ZSIGMOND, L. BURIS: Identification quimica experimental de la marca producida por la descarga elctrica. Associacion Nacional de Medicos Forenses 51 (1966) 11–16
[37] TORRE, C., L. VARETTO: The ultrastructure of the electric burn in man. J. Forensic Sci. 30 (1985) 448–455

Gunshot wounds

[1] AGRAWAL, J.: Unusual chamber marks on plastic shells. Forensic Sci. Int. 19 (1982) 249–252
[2] ALFONSI, A., S. CALATRI, E. CERIONI, P. LUCHI: Shooting distance estimation for shots fired by a shotgun loaded with buckshot cartridges. Forensic Sci. Int. 25 (1984) 83–91
[3] AGUILAR, J. C.: Shored gunshot wound of exit. Am. J. Forensic Med. Pathol. 4 (1983) 199–204
[4] BERGMAN, P., H. EVEN, N. AGRON, A. KLEIN, E. SPRINGER: Estimation of a bullet U,s diameter

using bullet hole identification kit. J. Forensic Sci. 32 (1987) 866–879

[5] Bixler, R. P., C. R. Ahrens, R. P. Rossi, D. Thickman: Bullet identification with radiography. Radiology 178 (1991) 563–567

[6] Booker, J. L.: examination of the badly damaged bullet. J. Forensic Sci. Soc. 20 (1980) 153–162

[7] Booker, J. L., D. D. Schroeder, J. H. Propp: A note on the variability of barium and antimony levels in cartridge primers and its implication for gunshotresidum identification. J. Forensic Sci. Soc. 24 (1984) 81–84

[8] Bratike, H., W. Poll, B. Kader: Ungewöhnliche Handungsfahigkeit nach Kopfschuss. Arch. Kriminol. 175 (1985) 31–39

[9] Brihaye, Cl., R. Machiroux, G. Gillain: Gunpowder residues detection by anodic stripping voltammetry. Forensic Sci. Int. 20 (1982) 269–276

[10] Brissie, R. M., E. S. Collum: Shotgun wounds. Multiple probes and shielding effect as adjunct to determining position of the deceased at time of injury. J. Forensic Sci. 25 (1980) 228–232

[11] Copeland, A. R.: Accidental death by gunshot wound – fact or fiction. Forensic Sci. Int. 26 (1984) 25–32

[12] Dixon, S. D.: Determination of direction of fire from grease gunshot wounds of internal organ. J. Forensic Sci. 29 (1984) 231–235

[13] Donoghue, E. R., M. B. Kalelkar, J. M. Richaond, S. S. Teas: Atypical wounds of enterance; an empirical study. J. Forensic Sci. 29 (1984) 379–388

[14] Elisele, J. W., D. T. Reay, A. Cook: Sites of suicidal gunshot wounds. J. Forensic Sci. 26 (1981) 480–485

[15] Fackler, M. L.: Wound ballistics. JAMA 259 (1988) 2730–2736

[16] DeGaetano, D., J. A. Siegel: Survey of gunshot residue analysis in forensic science laboratories. J. Forensic Sci. 35 (1990) 1087–1093

[17] Hellmiss, G., W. Lichtenberg, M. Weiss: Investigation of gunshot residues by means of Auger electron spectroscopy. J. Forensic Sci. 32 (1987) 747–760

[18] Introna, F., J. E. Smialek: Suicide from multiple gunshot wounds. Am. J. Forensic Med. Pathol. 10 (1989) 275–284

[19] Jauhari, M., S. M. Chatterji: Automation in firearms identification. Forensic Sci. Int. 15 (1980) 259–264

[20] Jauhari, M., T. Singh, S. M. Chatterji: Primer residue analysis of ammunition. Forensic. Sci. Int. 19 (1982) 253–258

[21] Josselson, A. R., A. C. Johnson, W. D. Washington, G. N. Wagner, D. D. Garner, F. B. Johnson, D. R. Lundy: A study at .22 caliber in fire exploding bullets. J. Forensic Sci. 30 (1985) 760–772

[22] Kenyeres, I., Gerencsér, Gy.: Öngyilkosság egyedülálló esete. Belügyi Szemle 12 (1965) 118–123

[23] Kelemen, E.: Vadászbaleset vagy előre kitervelt szándékos emberölés kísérlete. Belügyi Szemle 8 (1963) 112–116

[24] Kijewski, H., S. Berg, R. Sprung: Suicid mit Luftgewehr. Z. Rechtsmed. 84 (1980) 209–220

[25] Medich, M. G., S. D. Cohle, M. Burritt, F. Davison: Single wound produced by simultaneous discharge of both shells from a double-barrel shotgun. J. Forensic Sci. 35 (1990) 473–476

[26] Menzies, R. G., R. J. Scroggie, D. I Labowitz: Characteristic of silenced firearms and their wounding effects. J. Forensic Soc. 26 (1981) 239–262

[27] Missliwetz, J.: Ungewöhnliche Handlungsfahigkeit bei Herzdurchschuss durch Schrotgarbe. Arch. Kriminol. 185 (1990) 129–135

[28] Missliwetz, J. W. Denk, I. Wieser: Shots fired with silencers. J. Forensic Sci. 36, (1991) 1367–1394

[29] Modi, J. K., C. Nigam, K. Kumar: Improvized firearms versus regulator firearms. Forensic Sci. Int. 26 (1984) 199–205

[30] Murphy, G. K.: Suicide by gunshot while driving an automobile. Am. J. Forensic Med. Pathol. 10 (1989) 285–288

[31] Nolte, K. B.: The tubular "cookie cutter" bullet: a unique projectile. J. Forensic Sci. 35 (1990) 1461–1467

[32] Petty, Ch. S.: Firearm injury research. Am. J. Clin. Pathol. 52 (1969) 277–288

[33] Pollak, St.: Zur Morphologie der Einschusswunden im Palmar und Plantarbereich. Z. Rechtsmed. 86 (1980) 41–47

[34] Randall, B., R. Jaqua: Gunshot enterance wound abrasion ring width as a function of projectile diameter and velocity. J. Forensic Sci. 36, (1991) 138–144

[35] Rudzitis, E.: Analysis of the results of gunshot residue detection in case work. J. Forensic Sci. 25 (1980) 839–846

[36] Steinberg, M., Y. Leist, M. Tassa: A new field kit for bullet hold identification. J. Forensic Sci. 29 (1984) 169–176

[37] Stone, I. C., C. S. Petty: Interpretation of unusual wounds caused by firearms J. Forensic Sci. 36, (1991) 736–740

[38] TSUDA, R., Y. ITO, T. INOUE, M. HARA: Statistical survey of medico-legal activities for the murderous and accidental death (40 cases) by use of fire arms. Igaku-Kenkyu 59 (1989) 23–28
[39] TWIBELL, J. D., L. TURNER, K. W. SMALDON, D. G. HIGGS: The persistence of military explosives on hands. J. Forensic Sci. 29 (1984) 284–290
[40] WOLFENSBERGER, M., R. STEIGER, P. LÜTHI: Instrumentalanalytische Charakterisierung zwekkentfremdeter Treibladungspulver (Nitrocellulose). Arch. Kriminol. 182 (1988) 167–174
[41] YINON, J.: Analysis of explosives by negative ion chemical ionization mass spectrometry. J. Forensic Sci. 25 (1980) 401–407
[42] ZACKERMAN, S.: Experimental study of blast injuries to the lungs. Lancet 2 (1940) 219–224

Heat-induced injuries

[1] ASSIA, E., Y. EPSTEIN, Y. SHAPIRO: Fatal heatstroke after a short march at light. Aviation, Space, Environ. Med. 5, (1985) 441–442
[2] BURIS, L., L. DEBRECZENI: The elevation of serum creatine phosphokinase (CPK) at induced hypothermia. Forensic Sci. Int. 20 (1982) 35–38
[3] BURIS, L., M. FODOR, L. BURIS, JR., L. DEBRECZENI: Veranderungen der Kreatinkinase (KK) bei Todesfallen durch Unterkühlung. Krim. Forens. Wiss. 65 (1987) 57–61
[4] CHEN, W. Y.: Effect of Na+ pump suppression on reactive of rat tracheal to cooling. Clin. Exp. Pharmacol. Physiol. 16, (1989) 375–381
[5] CRAPO, R.: Smoke inhalation injuries. JAMA 246 (1981) 1694–1696
[6] DALLOS, GY.: A barna zsírszövet igazságügyi orvostani jelentősége. Morph. és Ig. Orv. Szemle 10, (1970) 252–256
[7] DRESE, G.: Unterkühlung Todesursache oder Wesentlicher nebenbefund. Krim. Forens. Wiss. 55–56 (1984) 184–189
[8] ECKERT, W. G.: The medicolegal and forensic aspects of fires. Am. J. Forensic Med. Pathol. 2 (1981) 347–357
[9] ENDRIS, R., R. BERRSCHE: Farbenwandel der Zahnhartgewebe als Zeichen thermischer Schadigung. Z. Rechtsmed. 94 (1985) 109–120
[10] FISHER, D. A.: Cold diuresis in the newborn. Pediatrics, 40 (1967) 636–641
[11] GRABER, CH. D., R. B. REINHOLD, J. G. BREMAN, R. A. HARLEY, G. R. HENNIGAR: Fatal heat stroke. JAMA 216 (1971) 1195–1196
[12] HERNDON, D. N., P. B. THOMPSON, M. BROWN, D. L. TRABER: Diagnosis pathophysiology and treatment of inhalation injury. In: Boswick, J. A.: Burn care Aspen Publ. Inc. Rockville, M. (1987) pp. 153–161
[13] HIRVONEN, J.: Necropsy findings in fatal hypothermia cases. Forensic Sci. 8 (1976) 155–164
[14] HIRVONEN, J., R. ELFVING: Histamine and serotonin in the gastric erosions of rats dead from exposure to cold. A histochemical and quantitative study. Z. Rechtsmed. 74 (1974) 273–276
[15] HIRVONEN, J., P. HUTTUNEN: Increased urinary concentration of catecholamines in hypothermia deaths. J. Forensic. Sci. 27 (1982) 264–271
[16] LINTON, A. L., I. M. LEDINGHAM: Severe hypothermia with barbiturate intoxication. Lancet 1 (1966) 24–28
[17] MANN, T. P., R. I. ELLIOTT: Neonatal cold injury due to accidental exposure to cold. Lancet 1 (1957) 229–234
[18] MANT, A. K.: Autopsy diagnosis of accidental hypothermia. J. Forensic Med. 16 (1969) 126–129
[19] MANT, A. K.: Taylor,s Principles and Practice of Medical Jurisprudence. Churchill-Livingstone Edinburg (1984) pp. 249–281
[20] MATSUBARA, K. A. AKANE, C. MASEDA, H. SHIONO: "First pass phenomenon" of inhaled gas in the fire victims. Forensic Sci. Int. 46 (1990) 203–208
[21] MCDANIEL, J. E. DEVINE: Elevations of creatine kinase izoenzyme CK, in patients with exposure induced hypothermia. An. Clin. Labor Sci. 10 (1980) 155–160
[22] MOLNÁR, G. W.: Survival of hypothermia by men immersed in the ocean. JAMA 131 (1946) 1046–1050
[23] PATON, B. C.: Accidental hypothermia. Pharmac. Ther. 22 (1983) 331–377
[24] PRESCOTT, L. F., M. C. PEARD, J. R. WALLACE: Accidental hypothermia, a common condition. Br. Med. J. 2 (1962) 1367–1370
[25] SIVALOGANATHAN, A.: Undressing and hypothermia. Med. Sci. Law 26 (1986) 226–229
[26] STEFFEN, J. M.: Glucose, glycogen, and insulin responses in the hypothermic rat. Cryobiol. 25 (1988) 94–101
[27] TREVINO, A., B. R. RAZI, B. M. BELLER: The characteristic electrocardiogram of accidental hypothermia. Arch. Intern. Med. 127 (1971) 470–473
[28] YONG CHIH-CHUN, HSU WI-SHIA, SHI TSI-SIANG: Treatment of burns. Springer Verlag Berlin (1982) pp. 23–40
[29] ZAWACKI, B. E.: The local effects of burn injury. In: Boswick, J. A.: Burn care. Aspen Publ. Inc. Rockville, M. (1987) pp. 25–36

Vital injuries

One of the most important questions in the description of an injury is whether it occurred before or after death, and to estimate the age of injury. examination of vital signs answers this question. We differentiate between vital signs and vital reactions.

We understand *vital signs* to be those alterations whose presence could only have occurred in each injury during life. Among those are bleeding, bloody infiltration, the ability to form blisters around the mark of hanging, aspiration of foreign material, the various forms of embolism, and edematous swelling in soft tissue areas.

The *vital reaction* means the microscopic alterations in cells and tissues which occur only during life.

Orsós lists the difficulties encountered in differentiation in his description of the subject. Orsós emphasizes the basic differences between injuries and cell death. The differences are:

1. intravital reactions occurring during life,

2. agonal reactions which occur during the death throes,

3. those reactions happening at the moment of death,

4. postmortal reactions occurring after death.

Differentiation between the vital and postmortal injuries is made more difficult by the fact that there is no sharp boundary between the antemortem and postmortal state of injuries. The physical signs of death do not appear in certain tissues so that their living functions immediately cease. Metabolism in tissues and organs continue after death – *intermediate life* – depending on their sensitivity to lack of oxygen. Thus the oxygen-sensitive central nervous system suffers irreversible damage shortly after death, and its life functions stop completely. In contrast to this, the tissues of other organs – muscle, cartilage, and cornea – are capable of showing alterations similar to vital reactions for a time after death which can misleadingly appear as though they occurred before death.

Hemorrhage occurring in the area of the injury is held to be one of the most important vital signs even today. Bloody infiltrations into soft tissue areas depends upon blood pressure, and the general opinion is that blood entering the tissues after death can be easily washed away with a water spray. The evaluation is made more difficult by the fact that blood infiltrating the tissues from injuries inflicted during the agonal state can also be easily washed away like that of postmortal injuries, since at this point bloody infiltration is not pronounced due to the low blood pressure. Professional experience, however, shows that an autopsy performed without proper care can produce postmortal blood similarly infiltrating soft tissues and water spray can hardly remove it, so it may be mistaken for bloody infiltration that occurred in life. Postmortal infiltration may similarly occur in the areas of hypostasis if adequate compression is applied and the blood is pressed from the vessels into the tissues.

The *amount of bleeding* is held by many to be a vital sign. A more pronounced bleeding may indicates that the injury occurred during life. Bleeding from the areas of hypostasis injured postmortally can be substantial, especially if the blood remained fluid after death, as in cases of suffocation and sudden death. At other times following injury to hollow organs we see a more expressed postmortal bleeding (thus in a heart stopped at diastole and filled with blood from left chamber, to which is administered an intracardial injection during the agonal period may release a large amount of blood into the pericardial sac).

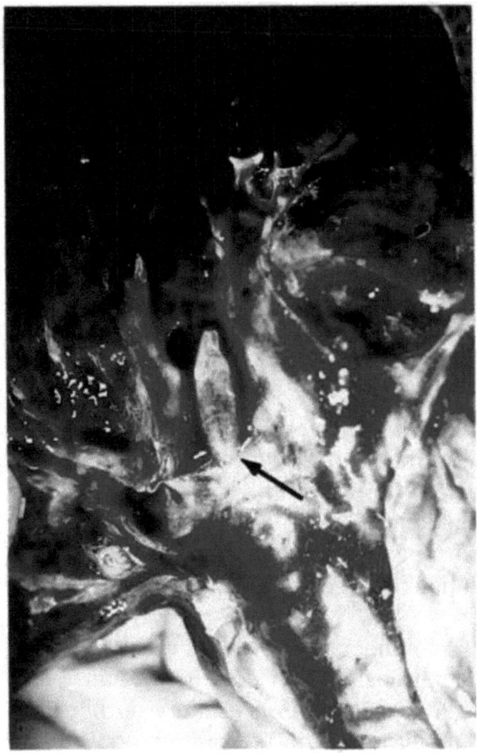

Fig. 96. Aspirated tooth at the bifurcation of the trachea

Among the *embolisms,* tissue embolism, air embolism and blood clots released into the circulation, are valued as vital signs. *Aspiration* is considered a vital sign only in the case where the aspiratum reaches the terminal bronchioles, or if finer particles, the alveoli, although such instances have occurred where aspiratum forced with a greater pressure has been shown to reach the terminal bronchioles. (In these cases extensive acute emphysema shows the forced inspiration.) *(Fig. 96)*

Although invisible to the naked eye, the inhalation of *carbon monoxide* in the cases of explosion and burn injuries with the formation of carbon monoxide hemoglobin, the *dilution of the blood* in the left chambers of the heart in fresh water drowning victims, and the finding of *diatoms* appropriate to the location of drowning in the victim are considered vital signs.

Among the *vital signs* we must list those microscopic signs which are not connected with active cell functions. The formation of *fibrin* following bleeding in the area of the injury belongs here. Many consider a prolonged ability to form fibrin to be a vital sign. Several have, on the other hand, verified that the ability to form fibrin can appear in the agonal life, especially in those instances where the blood remains fluid for a short period after death.

If bleeding can be demonstrated in regional lymph nodes, *erythrophagocytosis* verifies that the injuries occurred during life. This can be shown after a short period following the injury, about 20 minutes.

The *wound healing* stage follows bleeding from injury and tissue damage. Leukocytes migrate among the injured fibers, which appear in the injured tissue in great numbers about six hours after the injury, and macrophages are the first of these to appear. The first signs of repair are held to be the appearance of fibroblasts, which can be demonstrated six hours after injury *(Fig. 97)*.

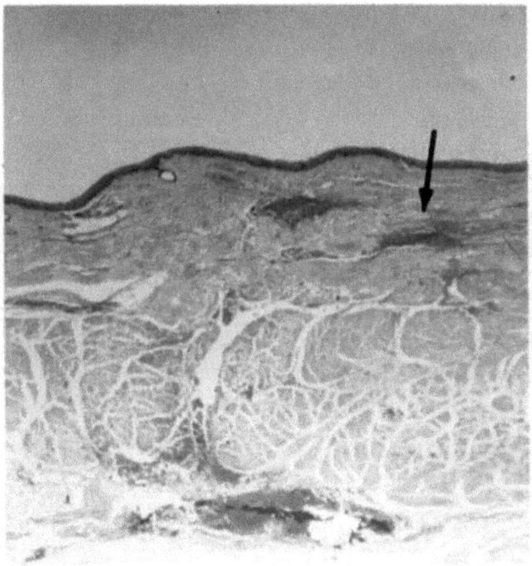

Fig. 97. Fresh contusion, hemorrhage into the tissue

The formation of *hemosiderin* in the area of the injuries is a vital reaction. The decay of the red blood cells and the phagocytosis of the iron containing pigments plays a role in its formation. According to some, the formation of hemosiderin can first be demonstrated nine days after the injury. The pigment in detectable quantities can be found in the histiocytes participating in the decay within 48-72 hours, which a few days later shows up with increased intensity in the cells and later fill the cytoplasm of the cells with a diffuse mass *(Fig. 98)*.

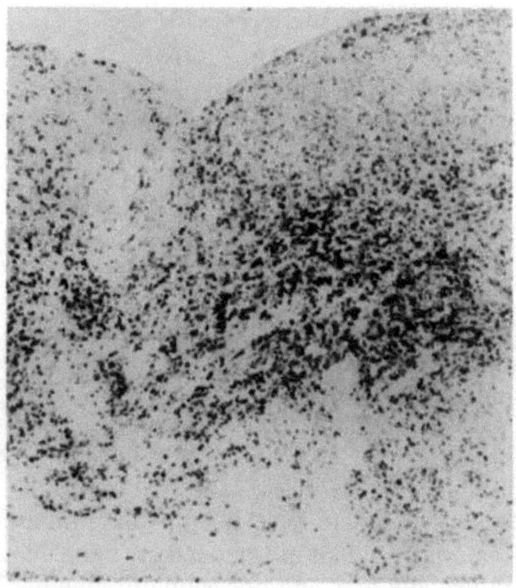

Fig. 98. Massive formation of hemosiderin in the territory of subacute hemorrhage

Many include the *enzyme histochemical alterations* following injury as vital reactions. The name of RAEKALLIO is associated with these examinations. These do not so much concern the question of whether the wound was antemortem or postmortal, but rather the time elapse from the occurrence of the injury. According to his examinations, the injury can be divided into two zones, the internal, which is about 300 microns in width and in which the decrease in the all enzyme reactions can be found, and an area extending for another 300 microns toward the intact tissue in which increased enzyme activity is described. The enzyme activity can be followed in relation to the time lapsing from the injury. In the inflammatory phase vasoactive substances proliferate in the injury, which include proteolytic enzymes and from a few seconds to several hours they can be found in the area of the injury. Development of glucose-6-phosphate dehydrogenase activity signals the increase in phagocyte activity, which reaches a maximum in 12-14 hours after the injury. The author also emphasizes that it is not

Table 2.
Establishment of the age of the wound based on histochemical signs

Enzymes	*Time in hours*
RNA proliferation	1
Glucouronidase	1
Peptidase	2
Hydrolases	4
DNA proliferation	6
Esterase	8
Protein proliferation	12
Glucosyl transferase	12
Succinate dehydrogenase	128

Table 3.
Establishment of the age of the wound based on histochemical and morphological signs

Characteristic	*Time*
Appearance of leukocytes minutes	15-45
Erythrophagocytosis	20 minutes
Large numbers of leukocytes	6 hours
Macrophages	from 6 hours
Fibroblasts	from 6 hours
Thrombosis in the small vessels	12 hours
Hemosiderin	from 48 hours
Epithelial migration	from 48 hours
Uniting of wound edges, formation of aspecific granulation tissue	5-6 days
Scar tissue	from 2 months

easy to compare experimental and human materials, which are dependent upon the injury and age, and occasionally whether following brain injury as well, the enzyme reaction time may vary. Thus the establishment of the age of the injury cannot be made from the observation of one histochemical reaction, and many histochemical reactions together are required to establish the time of the injury.

FAZEKAS and coworkers described the release of *histamine* in the area of the *ligature mark of hanging.* An increase in free histamine content in the area of the ligature mark which appears within a few minutes after injury was discovered with hanging that was performed while the victim was alive. A similar elevation of *serotonin* level was also demonstrated.

After the injury *repair processes* begin which result in a significant increase in the amount of DNA, RNA and protein. The increase in RNA can be demonstrated 10–15 minutes after the injury, and in two hours it significantly exceeds the average level. Raekallio also noticed the proliferation of DNA as an unambiguous sign of an inflammatory reaction reflecting the migration of cells into the area of the injury.

According to our knowledge to date, *there are no vital reactions which would verify an injury of a few minutes occurring in life.* The healing processes which begin after injury that would be of primary use in determining whether the injury occurred during life and that can be detected by modern means unambiguously appear only after 1/2–1 hours after the injury. The determination of the age of the injury in part depends on the migration of cellular elements, and in part on enzyme histochemical reactions. We have already discussed the importance and possibilities of the vital signs. Sometimes the vital signs take us much closer to the accurate determination of whether the injury occurred in life or postmortally than the vital reactions *(Table 2, 3).*

References

[1] Buris, L.: Histochemical examination at vital and postmortem injuries. Acta Histochem. 38 (1970) 65–69

[2] Buris, L., S. Tatár-Kiss: Electronmicroscopical examination at the early period of the wound healing. Verh. Anat. Ges. 68, (1974) 507–512

[3] Buris, L.: Autoradiographic examinations in the early period of wound healing. Acta Histochem. 48, (1974) 286–290

[4] Buris, L.: Vizsgálatok vitalis és postmortalis sérülésekben és a regeneratio korai szakában. Kandidátusi értekezés (1974)

[5] Buris, L.: Untersuchungen über vitale und postmortale Verletzungen and über das Anfangsstadium der Wundheilung. Kriminal. Forens. Wissensch. 32 (1978) 55–61

[6] Fazekas, I. Gy., E. Virágos-Kis: Der Gehalt der Erhangungsfurche an freiem Histamin als vital Reaction. Z. f. d. ges. Gerichtl. Medizin 56 (1965) 250–260

[7] Hallermann, W., Illchmann-Christ: Über einartige Strangulationsbefunde. Z. f. d. ges. Gerichtl. Medizin 38 (1943) 97–128

[8] Jankovich, L., J. Incze: Blutungen in den lymphoknoten des Halses beim Erhangungstod. Z. f. d. ges. Gerichtl. Medizin 20 (1933) 122–139

[9] Krauland, W., H. Bratzke: Verletzungen der grossen Hirnschlagadern und vitale Reaktion. Z. Rechtsmed. 99 (1987) 1–33

[10] Maxeiner, H.: Zur lokalen Vitalreaktion nach Angriff gegen den Hals. Z. Rechtsmed. 99 (1987) 35–54

[11] Oehmichen, M., T. Lagodka: time dependent RNA synthesis in different skin layers after wounding. Experimental investigations in vital and postmortem biopsies. Int. J. Leg. Med. 104 (1991) 153–159

[12] Orsós, F.: Die vitalen Reaction und ihre gerichtlichmedizinische Bedeutung. Beitr. Path. Anat. 95 (1935) 163–237

[13] Ökrös, S.: Gerichtlich-medizinische Bedeutung des elastischen Fasersystem der Haut. Z. f. d. ges. Gerichtl. Medizin 29 (1938) 485–500

[14] Piedelievre, R.: Les ecchymoses en medicine legale remarques sur la coagulation du sang. Verch. I. Internat. Kong. ger. u. soc. Med. 5 (1938) 584–586

[15] Raekallio, J.: Histochemical studies on vital and postmortem skin wounds. Mercatorin Kirjapaino Helsinki (1961)

[16] Raekallio, J.: Histochemical distinction between antemortem skin wounds. J. Forensic Sci. 9 (1964) 107–118

[17] Raekallio, J.: Enzyme Histochemistry of Wound Healing. In: Progress in Histochemistry and Cytochemistry. Gustav Fischer Verlag, Stuttgart (1970) pp. 51–151

[18] Robertson, I., R. A. Mansfield: Antemortem and postmortem bruises of the skin. J. Forensic Med. 4 (1957) 2–10

[19] Robertson, I., P. R. Hodge: Histopathology of healing abrasions. Forensic. Sci. 1 (1972) 17–25

[20] Somogyi, E., Gy. Rózsa, T. Varga: Histochemische Untersuchungen zur Regeneration von Verletzungen durch elektrischen Strom. A. Histochem. 35 (1970) 28–31

[21] Strassmann, G.: Formation of hemosiderin in the lungs. Arch. of Pathol. 38 (1949) 76–81

[22] Walcher, K.: Über vitale Reactionen. Z. f. d. ges. Gerichtl. Medizin 15 (1930) 16–57

Chapter 3

The extent of wound healing

In the description of injuries, we will deal with those according to the characteristics of the previous chapter. The extent of healing of the wounds must be sought and this depends on the nature of the damage, its characteristics, the degree of force applied and such other factors which carry a positive or negative effect on the healing processes. (An injury in an inflammatory state, the later possibility of infection, inappropriate wound care, the individual characteristics of the injured person – advanced age, certain diseases – etc). We shall return to the role of the factors influencing the healing processes later. Such modifying factors must be presented not only in the medicolegal certification but in the opinion of the examining medical specialist as well.

The medicolegal certificate

The instructions for the exposition of the medicolegal certificate is regulated. The regulation states that if the injured person or next of kin request exposition of a medicolegal certificate, the medical department, or the primary care physician who treated the injured person must exhibit a medicolegal certificate in connection with the injuries in question. It is required to prepare the medicolegal certification on the official form printed for that purpose. The physician or the leader of the health care institution for the question of the police, the court, or the forensic medical specialist may request in writing the information related to the injured person by completing the form entitled "Medicolegal certification and opinion" and filing it with the appropriate office. The treating physician fills out the certification, or if not possible, the physician closest involved. A copy must be made of the certificate.

In *filling out the certificate* the personal data must be taken from the appropriate documents, perhaps using the injured person's identification card, driver licence which may also be useful in establishing the identity. It is also essential to include the exact time and means of arrival for medical care. It is also necessary to get the name and particulars of the person accompanying the injured person. Filling in the preliminary data is the responsibility of the physician preparing the certificate. The precise collection of the preliminary information provided by the injured person, or accompanying person can be of great help later in the establishment of the origin of the injuries. At such times outside sources or concerns may aid in relating the complaints of the victim and information

. . . .

. . . .
(The preparing physician, health institution name and address)

MEDICOLEGAL CERTIFICATE AND OPINION

Name of the injured person . . . .
Place and date of birth . . . .
Mother' maiden name . . . .
Occupation . . . .
Address . . . .
Employer' liability name and address . . . .
Date and time medical care was sought: 19 . . . year . . . . month
. . . . day . . . . time

Mode; walking – ambulance or,

. . . .
Name and address of accompanying person: . . . .
. . . .
Circumstantial information (the time, place and circumstances, time the victim was unconscious, presence and amount of intoxicating substances e. g. ethanol consumed, according to the injured person or accompanying person): . . . .
Present condition (general physical, medical condition).
. . . . RR; . . . . Hgmm. P; . . . . min.
Nervous condition (reflexes, Romberg sign, pupils etc.), signs indicating concussion (loss of consciousness, amnesia vegetative signs) . . . .
. . . .
Physical signs of alcoholic state (odor of alcohol, condition of facial skin and conjunctiva etc.) and psychological signs (speech, behavior, orientation, memory etc.): . . . .
. . . .
External markings (wounds) location, form, length, width, depth (if possible exactly in mm or cm), description of the shape, edges, sides, base, and area (contamination) in the case of gunshot or stabbing, the distances of the entry and exit wounds from the plane of the sole (in the case of multiple superficial marks, they should be listed in order from a fixed anatomical point or body area: . . . .
Details of special medical findings (X-ray etc.): . . . .
. . . .
Care administered to the injured person (medical treatment, bandaging, operation, referral to out-patient department or hospitalization etc.) . . . .
Diagnosis: . . . .
. . . .
Opinion: Healing time approximately . . . . days.
Remarks: (for example, can any permanent physical disability or serious deterioration in health be expected):

. . . ., 19 . . . year . . . . month . . . . . day

. . . .
signature

regarding the circumstances of the injury. The time spent in an unconscious state and the amount of alcohol consumed and the degree of drunkenness must be emphasized.

In the presents status a detailed medical and neurological examination must be carried out. In head injuries the possibility of compression processes in the cranial vault must always be kept in mind.

We must pay special attention to the *description of the injuries.* From the standpoint of wounds, we record the size, the character – discontinuity or missing material – and the location. With some injuries – stabs, gunshot wounds or traffic accidents – the precise distance from the plane of the sole must be specifically measured. We describe the wound with two coordinates or in relation to a fixed anatomical point, so that it can be easily located. If characteristic alterations are found, we must make a suitable photograph. The measurements must in every case be included in mm or cm, and we must refrain from inexact descriptions such as finger-breadths or palm-widths, etc. We describe individual injuries at certain points, except when characteristic of a large area, e. g. burns or abrasions. The mentioned scheme should also be used specifically to depict injuries to the head, neck, trunk, and upper and lower extremities.

We can when necessary send the injured person for special examinations (radiological, dental etc.). These cases must be described exactly in the appropriate section of the certificate. Likewise, we must indicate whether we referred the patient to a health care institution. In the description of signs we summarize the alterations and give an opinion as to the healing time. (If we prepare the certificate immediately after the injury and the healing of the injury is uncertain, the injured person should be re-examined in seven days and the expected length of healing time then given.) It should also be indicated whether later complications can be expected to result in serious deterioration of health or permanent disability.

In the establishment of *healing time,* according to law, in Hungary, the healing times must be divided into those healing within eight days and those taking more than eight days. Those taking longer than eight days are considered legally as serious injuries, while those healing within eight days are considered as light physical injuries. The law justifies considering physical injuries which heal within eight days as light since lighter injuries or operational incisions heal within eight days under suitable conditions. Injuries that take longer than eight days to heal are required to be reported by the facility or the physician.

Differentiation between the injuries healing within eight days and those taking longer is not indifferent from the standpoint of healing time. The healing of injuries is affected by anatomical and functional considerations and the two modes of healing differ significantly from each other. The importance of differentiating between the anatomical and functional healing time is shown by the position of the Supreme Court Council (Hungary) that the legal classification of actual healing time must be kept in mind in the criminal prosecution of bodily injury. The actual healing time is the anatomical healing time, which must in every case be indicated.

We understand *anatomical healing* to be if the injured tissues connect in their anatomical position, so the sides of the wounds to soft tissue areas rejoin, the beginning repair shows granulation tissue connecting the sides of the wound, the wound no longer secretes anything, epithelium covers the surface of the wound, the scab is removed or in the process of falling off, and in the case of broken bones, the fractured part is capable of bearing weight through the bridging callus.

We consider the *functional healing* to be the time it takes for the injured part to regain its function. In the area of the injury, complete repair means: in contusion injuries, the spilled blood is completely reabsorbed; in joint injuries the joint regains its motion without pain; in damage to the nervous system, the residual signs have disappeared and the complications which accompanied the injury have been healed. In general principle it can be said that the functional healing time in almost every case exceeds the anatomical healing time.

Permanent disability is examined in the question whether the injury brought about such alterations as the lost of a body part, or a complete functional disruption. Did organs or organ systems suffer similar alterations? Are the residual signs related to the injury and does the damage cause a decreased capacity to work? (Cosmetic injury causes a decreased capacity to work only in certain professions – performing artists, public personalities etc. –; nevertheless if it causes deformation in the place it occurs, it can be considered as permanent damage).

Serious deterioration in health may be the result of damage or complications of the injury which prolong the usual healing time of the injury, and these require a prolonged healing process:

1. if the complication of the injury prolongs the healing, for example a bone marrow infection following a fracture, the formation of a pseudoarthrosis, temporary impairment of joint function,

2. if the injury causes a deterioration in a previous illness (a traumatic injury to the spine of a person with spondylosis, or a patient with varicosities or post-thrombotic syndrome receiving a blunt injury to the lower extremity, in which the soft tissues develop a slowly healing ulcer.

Serious deterioration of health is such a condition which is of temporary character and appearing in connection with the alterations caused by the injury, which represents a decline from the original state of health, but exceeds the usual healing time for such an injury and occasionally results in no permanent damage.

Among the injuries healing within eight days are these: "...epithelial flaking and peeling on the surface of the body and mucous membranes; slight bleeding; the superficial incision, cutting, contusion or laceration wounds whose sides can be reapproximated; superficial stabs or stabbing incisions which reach the muscle tissue but do not require multiple muscle stitching; first degree burns of limited extent, scalds, frost-bite or chemically caused corrosive injuries; strains; loosening or loss of up to three teeth; breaking of the crown of a tooth or loss of a tooth without fracture of the alveolar process; ruptured eardrum (without bleeding from the middle ear). An eight day healing time can only be established in those cases of mild degree, without loss of consciousness or – medically verified – a very short loss of consciousness and quickly passing concussion with vegetative signs, a mild toxic process, and also in case of primary healed gonorrhea."

The above-listed cases naturally heal within eight days only in the absence of complications.

The injuries, which heal over a period longer than eight days are: "...confluent hemorrhages which occur over larger territories of the body (e. g. body areas); bleeding into the testicular tunics which cause pain and difficulty in walking; confluent epithelial flaking and peeling over larger areas (multiple or connected body areas); incision, cutting, contusion or laceration wounds whose edges cannot be reapproximated; stabbing, incision or cutting wounds piercing a body cavity or resulting in significant blood loss (hemoglobin and hematocrit!); gunshot wounds; injuries to the tendons and joints; sprains; injuries to vessels and nerves (especially if requiring stitches); second degree or more severe burns, scalds, frost-bite and chemical injuries from corrosives; moderate and serious concussions; organic injury to the central nervous system, the brain and other internal organs and their complications; injury to sensory organs (functional damage exceeding eight days must be verified); all bone fractures (including nasal fractures even in the case of healing without complications); serious poisonings; sexually transmitted diseases (except primary healed gonorrhea)."

In the description of the actual healing time, we have mentioned the various groups of injuries.

Healing is influences by several factors, from which the anatomical healing time is calculated, and these together yield the actual healing time. It is, however, necessary to note what is responsible for deviation from the average healing time, the occasional complication, which is independent of the patients attitude and behavior toward the injury, or the prolonged healing caused by inappropriate behavior on the part of the patient. We have already briefly discussed the factors influencing the healing time.

There are data mentioning circumstances under which the healing time is prolonged, so if surgical intervention is required in the case of an injury which opens a body cavity, opening of the cavity is necessary, the healing time is that typical of the operative procedure and the occasional complications.

The role of the so-called *special physical conditions* must by specially mentioned since each application of force causes a more serious than average injury. Thus a dental injury is far more serious and extensive in those who have periodontal and alveolar diseases due to the damage to the ligaments fixing the teeth and the consequent loosen of the teeth. Likewise the more easily broken thinner than average skull and the osteoporotic bones must be considered and bleeding into arthritic joints and bruising. The effect on the healing time carried by some diseases is recognized (the prolonged healing of a diabetic's injuries, the scar-forming capability of susceptible injuries to reform into rough keloid).

In the Supreme Court's 15th Directive appear the revisions in the specific questions in connection with healing time and the positions taken on bodily injury: "The notion of a threat to life appears from an actual possibility of death, but is not identified by a possibility of certain death. The former comes to attention when in the course of bodily injury a causal process ensues which may lead to death, but as a matter of course the disappearance of the threat to life may arise, or the possibility of averting death by suitable intervention."

Thus an injury can be considered life-threatening:

1. if the possibility of death may appear in connection with the injury,
2. vital organs are injured,
3. the function of vital organs is impaired by secondary processes,
4. acute external or internal bleeding results,
5. it causes shock,
6. body cavities are opened with it,

and all of these are subject to the condition that death can be averted by treatment. (An under eight day healing time does not exclude the possibility of a life-threatening injury!)

The law differentiates between indirect and direct threats to life. Indirect threats to life are those which even without medical intervention do not cause certain death. Direct threats to life are those which result in death in the absence of medical intervention.

The revisions deviate from the list of injuries resulting in direct threats to life, however, these consist only of generalities. The establishment of these depends on the practice of the physician or medical specialist. Besides the listed injuries, numerous cases can be found which may be either directly or indirectly threatening to life.

Direct threats to life according to the revisions:

1. injuries to vital – circulatory – organs,
2. vessel injuries resulting in loss of blood,
3. state of shock from the injury or loss of blood,
4. opening of body cavities which may result in injuries causing bleeding of the internal organs (here we can list the perforation of hollow organs into the abdomen which without treatment causes a direct threat to life from infection),
5. hemothorax or pneumothorax, if a distorsion of the heart or great vessels may result from the pressure,
6. serious brain injury, an injury which penetrates the skull, or piercing projectiles, or injuries causing an increase in intracranial pressure.

We speak of *indirect threat to life* when:

1. significant bleeding does not accompany internal injuries,

2. alterations opening the thorax in which insignificant amounts of air or blood collect.

The classification of indirect threats to life by regulations is unfortunate. Here as well such injuries not fitting the appropriate criteria of the revisions can come about which are indirectly threatening to life since in the absence of treatment they do not always cause death. (For example, injury to the hollow organs of the thorax, opening of abdominal organs, gastrointestinal injuries, or septic complications of cavity injuries which in the opinion of the practicing surgeon constitutes a direct threat to life.)

The Supreme Court bulletin is much more practicable when it states, "The life-threatening status of an injury is a special matter which the medical specialist must necessarily establish. The medical specialist must declare in the matter whether the injury was directly or indirectly life-threatening." Each injury must by listed as it is known in medical biology so as to avoid erroneous classification and provide the possibility for misunderstanding. Thus in the answering of this question the characteristics, findings and results of the preliminary information, the diagnosis and the surgical intervention are absolutely desired.

The medical certification

The medical certificate may be prepared by full time forensic pathologist for official or private request. Expert medical opinion may be given regarding injuries, work disability, alcohol consumption, mental status, etc. These certifications are different and answer different groups of questions, so regardless of their format, their structure is the same, so that, except for the official questions, the medical specialist in practice must answer the technical questions in connection with each case.

The *medical certificate has three parts.*

The *first part* consists of the personal data of the examined persons (presentation of the identification number), the authority ordering the examination and the list of general questions posed by the authority.

Anamnestic data: consists of the events leading up to the injury or data concerning previous illnesses, details about the injured person or statement of the condition of the patient, and also the list of medical documents and their origin.

In the *findings section* we begin with the general medical and neurological examinations. We record the complaints of the patient, following which the medical and neurological examinations, along with other appropriate examinations necessary to the case, are completed. (The name of the person performing the special examinations and details of the findings must be recorded.) We describe the injuries from the viewpoints already mentioned, precisely recording those locations, measurements, characteristics of the injuries and degree of healing, with attention to the age of the injuries.

The findings section may also play a role in the examination of instruments being important in criminal activity. Signs of criminal activity may be instrument caused injuries on the victim or possibly the clothing of injured persons. We have already discussed the aspects of the clothing examination, likewise the manner of description of the injury-causing instruments, so detailing them in this section is unnecessary.

Sometimes by the way of clinical data we must give evidence of the healing time of the injury or the amount of alcohol consumed in the examination for criminal activity. In these cases we place the description in the preliminary data. Naturally for our purposes we must include those examination results – findings, data from completing examinations, occasionally X-ray pictures, instruments – which are indispensable to the formulation of the opinion. The basic document of the opinion cannot provide, however, an opinion concerning the permanence of an injury.

The preparation of a medical opinion requires care. *Medical opinions,* as already mentioned, must be state in accordance with the body of medical biological knowledge, for such persons who are not familiar with these matters. It is therefore expected that the opinion be clear and understandable, with the questions appropriately answered, and the construction of the expert medical opinion in accordance with the prescribed format. The diagnosis, the answers to the appropriate questions and the data beyond the questions which are relevant to the practice of the expert in connection with the examination must be included.

The opinion may be:

definite, if the data obtained supported by a natural scientific basis supports the conclusion (for example, death in association with an unambiguous pathological picture, pulmonary embolism, coronary occlusion etc.),

probable, if the explanation of the signs – and the biological processes in large part – do not give an unambiguous answer. A probable opinion may be very probable, probable with limited evidence, or indefinite.

In the expert medical opinion special technical questions must be answered. The directions from the Supreme Court can offer help in these.

The Supreme Court Bulletin number 4

lists such factors, modus operandi, assessment of abuse, direction, force applied, character and location of the injury, the instrument – which are necessary in the formulation of the expert medical opinion. The medical specialist must keep the following in mind:

1. the seriousness of the injury,
2. the anatomical particulars of the injury location,
3. the amount of force applied,
4. the characteristics of the instrument causing the injury (its capability of inflicting serious injury),
5. the direction of the applied force.

In the opinion it must be emphasized whether the characteristics of the instrument allow for the possibility of infliction of more serious injury.

The direction of the applied force can be decided only in those cases when the instruments had been emplaced in a given location, since direction cannot be established from scattered injuries covering several body areas. Judgements of absolute certainty are not the task of the medical specialist.

The assessment of injuries and the answering of the technical questions require great expertise and are tasks of the highest responsibility.

Chapter 4

Examination of biological traces

The examination of biological traces is one of the most important matters in connection with criminal activity. Procedures for examining blood stains in the solving of mysteries beginning in the last century today have reached such a level where a miniscule amount of material can with great certainty yield the biological origin.

In 1911 KENYERES – the famous Hungarian forensic pathologist – wrote: "Although the decree of the minister of justice in 1888 directed that the examination of blood traces should lie within the area of responsibility of the court chemist, newer stipulations allow that the justice leadership should not exclude medical specialists from performing these examinations." From this establishment by KENYERES and the displaying of biological traces began the long and tiring road from uncertainty until when by the use of recombinant DNA techniques and DNA fingerprinting methods in blood samples we can identify with certainty the origin of every blood sample or biological material. This is not only the task of the forensic medical specialist, but also requires a well equipped laboratory and occasionally the employment of an experienced expert, or team of experts. The performance of justice can only be carried out with appropriate experience, due criticism and great certainty preceding the formation of the expert opinion in bringing about a decision. Those special examinations which are based on uncertain methods of determination show, or the opinion reflecting the inexperience of the one making the determination shows, that it is fitting that decisions regarding the origin of each biological material be made with the necessary certainty.

Procedures for testing blood stains

Questions to be decided in the examination of blood stains:

1. Is the stain really blood?
2. Is the blood of human or animal origin?
3. If human blood, what group?
4. How and when did it get there?

1. In the *identification of blood stains* orientation and verification procedures can be used. Although the first determination is the TEICHMANN demonstration of haemin crystals which belongs to the category of verification procedures, even since 1856 – when Teichmann described the method – numerous similar articles

have appeared which serve in the orientation testing of blood stains.

In 1863 SCHÖNBEIN described how when *hydrogen peroxide* is dripped onto a stain suspected to be blood, the tissue peroxidase evolves water and oxygen and stain on which the hydrogen peroxide dripped bubbles. For this 1-3% hydrogen peroxide is used, but the background of the experiment is, above all else, a hydrogen peroxide releasing material. Thus rust, various metal oxides, bacteria, etc. react similarly, and moreover, old dried blood stains don't give a positive reaction.

SCHÖNBEIN also developed the *guaiac test.* Positive results can be obtained even from highly diluted blood (1:20,000). The essence of the test is a dilute guaiac resin in alcohol in the presence of hydrogen peroxide shows the effect of tissue peroxidase by coloring a colorless solution – guaiac test blue – by the production of oxygen. Similarly as for the previously mentioned test, numerous false positives can result. Any kind of material which can release nascent oxygen in the above mentioned tests can give a false positive, even fresh plant fibers.

In 1904 using a preparation from the *Merck* factory *(p-diaminodiphenil),* experiments with *benzidine* found that in great dilutions (1:300,000) it could detect the presence of blood. The basis of the test is similar to the aforementioned color production in the presence of hydrogen peroxide due to oxidation. Today it is one of the most widely used tests to detect the presence of blood. The reaction brings an intense coloration which can be easily recognized. The positive greenish-blue color reaction is not stable for long, being quickly oxidized in the air and turning brown. The benzidine test suffers from the same drawbacks as the previous tests, with many possibilities for false positives.

Among the orientation type procedures for examining blood many methods can be listed, among which the *phenophthalin* test can be mentioned, the execution of which is extremely simple, which gives a positive result even in very large dilutions, but according to several authors gives no false positive reaction in the presence of vegetable matter.

We would like to mention separately among the orientation tests the *luminol test.* In the presence of blood contamination 3-aminophthalic acid hydrazide with hydrogen peroxide gives a chemoluminescence. The *chemoluminescent effect* can be seen only in the dark, but the intensity of the luminosity is so obvious that it can be used to uncover *latent blood stains.* It is especially useful in examining a wide area, since the appearance of a glow effect in the area suspected to be stained by blood sprayed with the aerosol and this test – according to the one describing it – isn't so damaging to the blood stains as to render them unusable for later tests.

The tests mentioned so far are all orientation tests, and can only indicate that the material examined may be contaminated with blood, but for precise identification, further tests are needed.

Among the described testing methods we will mention the most commonly used ones in detail.

Benzidine reaction: (The proportions are not important.) Dissolve a pea-sized quantity of aggregated benzidine in 1/3 of a test tube of glacial acetic acid, then add 0.5-1 ml of hydrogen peroxide. The positive reaction immediately forms a dark greenish-blue color.

Phenophthalin reaction: For the reaction we use a phenolphtalein reduced product, phenophthalin. For the reaction we add 2.5 g NaOH to 20 ml 96% ethanol into which we dissolve 0.2 g phenophthalin, and then we add 0.5 ml concentrated hydrogen peroxide. Thirty ml of distilled water are added to the solution with separated precipitate. The reagent prepared thus can be preserved under refrigeration for several weeks. We apply the reagent which has been strained by filter paper to the suspected blood contamination, in alkali's agent the oxidation effect of phenophthalin shows as a brick-red on the filter paper in the shape of the blood stain.

One gram of the *luminol test* reagent – 3-aminophthalic acid hydrazide – is mixed with 50 g sodium carbonate and 50 ml hydrogen peroxide, and then filled with distilled water to make 1 liter. We perform the test in a dark place with a brush or dusting if a wide area is to be examined.

The orientation tests only indicate the possible presence of blood stains. Identification requires further testing.

The oldest blood examination procedure is based on the *Teichmann haemin crystal* test. We put dried blood on a microscope slide, add a few crystals of sodium chloride to the dried blood, mix it with a few drops of acetic acid and cover it with a slip cover. In the microscopic examination we see the characteristic rhombus-shaped rods of haemin crystals.

Likewise the *Takayama hemochromogen* crystal method is an identification-type procedure. The Takayama reagent is made up of 3 ml of 10% NaOH, 3 ml of piridine, 3 ml of saturated glucose solution, and 2 ml distilled water. The solution can be preserved for 3-4 weeks. For the reaction we put a little of the material to be examined on the slide, drip 1-2 drops of the reagent onto it, and within 20-30 minutes raspberry red crystals form, which are the haemochromogen crystals *(Fig. 99)*.

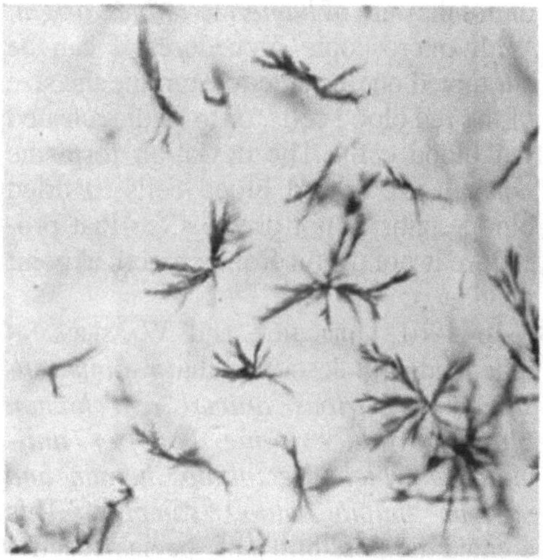

Fig. 99. Hemochromogen crystals in the Takayama reaction

The procedure in which the *spectroscopic properties of oxyhaemoglobin* are used in the examination of blood stains is associated with the name of FELLETAR. The characteristic spectrum of oxyhaemoglobin (541-576 nm) can be seen in the microspectroscopic examination of diluted blood stains, and after reduction the two absorption bands blend into one wide band (536-596), signifying reduced hemoglobin. Recently such factory made preparations, – Hemo-Quant[R] – have been made available for blood examinations, which also make the application of a specific probe much easier. Although used to demonstrate the clinical presence of occult bleeding, they emphasize that it can be used to demonstrate any fresh or digested blood. Since they detect the reduced heme, the porphyrin, content of the blood trace, it seems the procedure is specific for the examination of blood.

2. If the identification procedures for demonstration of blood stains yield a positive result, it must be decided whether

or not they are of *human or animal origin.* With microscopic procedures it can be attempted on one side to examine the size of the red blood cells, or to find nucleated red blood cells. The deviation form the normal size of red blood cells in dried blood stains is not obvious, so that procedure is not useful from a practical point of view.

In 1901 UHLENHUT and WASSERMANN independently described that *rabbits sensitized to various animal and human bloods produce some kind of anti-material which precipitates human and various animal blood samples.* This created the possibility of species-specific differentiation in criminal serology. The procedure can produce results not only in fresh, but dried blood samples as well. In the majority of cases it is only necessary to determine whether or not the blood is human, so anti-human serum is used and if positive, further examinations are not necessary. More recently various *immunological methods* have been employed to determine the nature of biological traces, so that with direct and indirect immunofluorescence procedures, and due to the great sensitivity of the *RIA* and *ELISA* methods, type specificity can be determined. For the identification of human blood pigments, these are among the most widely used and most specific procedures, which can obtain results from even 4-week-old blood stains.

Certain circumstances make the determination of type-specificity more difficult, so that *decay alterations,* which are due to the deterioration of the proteins, may make it impossible to determine the type. The other influential factor is the *age of the biological trace,* although with the more sensitive methods an examination of a blood stain several weeks old or biological trace can be performed. Heat may exert a significant influence on the examination results. *Heat denatured* proteins are unsuitable for determination, although in some cases even heat-denatured samples can be examined and yield type-specific results. Material containing *diluted proteins,* whether blood pigments or other biological traces can yield false negative results.

3. If the biological trace has been determined to be of human origin, the next task is to determine *from whom it originated.* LANDSTEINER in his 1901 article "The agglutination properties of normal human blood" indicated the applications in criminal blood group research, too. In 1903 LANDSTEINER and RICHTER emphasized the significance of the properties of blood groups in criminal investigation, and mentioned that the examination of the properties of blood groups was a significant development in the identification of blood stains. The determination of blood types by RICHTER and later LATTES was for their time significant, but it had numerous drawbacks, which could not be neglected in criminal group determination. On one part the determination of agglutinins from dried blood samples, with which LATTES is associated, in many instances gave misleading results, since the agglutinin titers in the dried plasma could decrease independently of each other and this influenced the group determination. On another part the contamination of the blood stain was a significant factor which also caused a decrease in the titer. A change came to the field of blood stain determination from the research of HOLCZER in 1931 with absorption blood group determination, which took almost three decades before it was adapted for the practice of forensic serology. The essence of the method: The blood stain is treated with a known titer of *anti-A* and *anti-B* plasma, which, depending on whether it

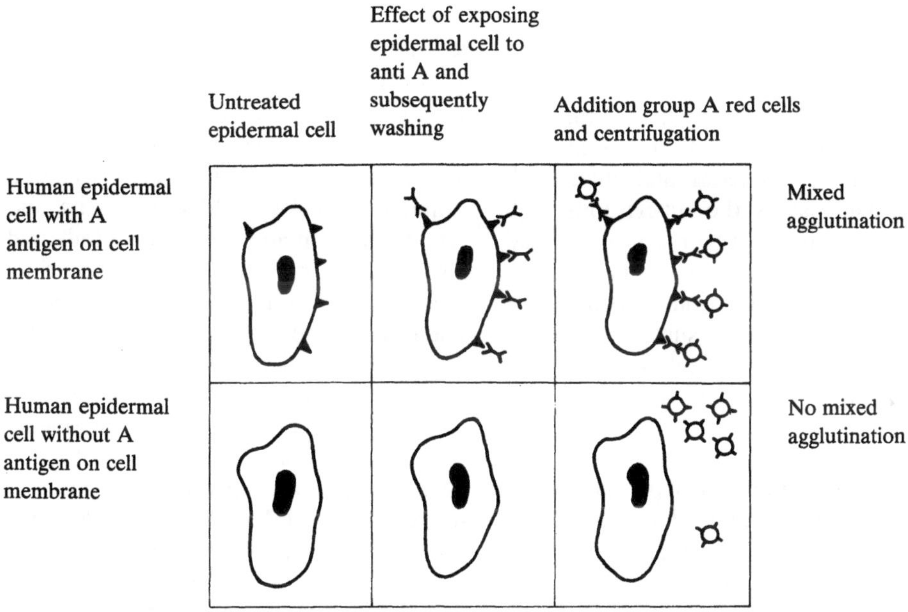

Fig. 100. Mixed erythrocyte—epidermal cell agglutination reaction for detection of the A antigen on epidermal cells. (COOMBS et al)

belongs to group A or B or both, decreases the plasma titer. From this follows the group properties. The disadvantage to the method was that a large sample of blood was needed for the determination of the blood group, and the contamination of the sample influenced the test results in that it caused aspecific decrease in titer. But the methods biggest drawback, however, came from the fact that it was not suitable for the establishment of the other group properties beyond those of the classical AB0 system. Later, with a modified absorption procedure, first the properties of the MN and then the Rh factor could also be distinguished. Thus the possibilities of blood group differentiation from blood stains has significantly grown.

In 1956 Coombs' article appeared in which it was shown that human epithelial cells produce antibodies with such a structure which can be of assistance in identification. The procedure was called *mixed cell agglutination.* In essence it can be summarized that if the epithelial cells originate from a blood group A person, they contain the A antigen, and furthermore, are capable of pulling together these epithelial cells in the presence of a high enough titer of anti-A in the plasma, the antibodies bound to their surface also binding the type-A red blood cells. Moreover, the type-A red blood cells show a specific affinity toward the epithelial cells of the type-A person whose epithelial cells have been pre-treated with anti-A serum. Likewise, the epithelial cells of the type-B people only absorb anti-B serum. The original Coombs reaction can be followed schematically in the accompanying diagram *(Fig. 100).*

In 1960 Kind published a new procedure for examining the group characteristics of dried blood stains, which was called the *elution blood group test.* This was based on a description of an older method in which the agglutinin were stripped off the surface of the red blood cells and differentiated. High titers of anti-A, anti-B, anti-0, anti-M, anti-N and anti-D immune plasma are dripped onto the unknown blood stain or material and incubated. After rinsing away the superfluous high titer antiserum, the residue is processed further and the essentials are that following elution after the final washing, the antibodies come off the surface of the red blood cells by running physiological saline at 56 °C over them and the control. Thus the agglutinins can be redissolved and from the solution with a suspension of blood of a known group, the blood group's properties can be determined. The method has many advantages over the previous ones. For one thing, it requires very little blood stain to obtain a determination of the blood group. Aspecific reactions hardly ever occur, "thus the rendering of a definite opinion has become possible with respect to a blood stain originating from a certain person" (BUDVÁRI). The properties of such subgroups can be determined, which further refines the possibilities of blood stain identification.

The group determination and the identification of biological traces, aside from the demonstration of the group properties on blood, can be performed on bodily secretions – saliva, sexual secretions, tissue fluids – and parts of tissue. About 76% of the population belong to a group which carry the A, B, or AB properties. In the 0 blood group people who are secretory type, H-substance can be found, which is not group specific, since it can be demonstrated in small quantities in the other blood groups. To determine whether one is a secretory or a non secretory, the *Lewis group system* examination is useful.

JEFFREYS and co-workers published procedures useful for the identification of biological traces in 1985, which point beyond the determination of the properties of blood groups and, according to the authors, make possible "...this technique can be used for forensic purposes; DNA of high relative molecular mass (M_r) can be isolated from 4-yr- old bloodstains and semen stains made on cotton cloth and digested to produce DNA fingerprints suitable for individual identification." Their procedure has been called *DNA fingerprinting,* and promise such advantageous tests which will bring significant changes to the practice of forensic medicine in the identification of biological traces. Thus with their tests, the authors suggest that the DNA sequence of a sperm cell found in vaginal secretions can be identified by such a treatment which involves anti-sperm, and moreover that a two year old sperm stain can be examined with DNA fingerprinting methods, compared and identified. The DNA fingerprint comes from the fragments of genetic material which can be differentiated by centrifugation according to their disparate concentrations, the so-called satellite DNA. Satellite DNA make up about 15-20% of genetic material. About 15-20 fragments of mini-satellite appear, with hypervariable regions, which in connection with amino acids, order the joining for replication, the base pair sequence being of individual character, and so the same only in identical twins. With the examination it can be verified that the characteristics of these mini-satellite regions can be used in identification, their genetic line being greater than that of other genetic markers, thus individually varied. If, for example, each region contains 20 alleles, we can find 400 possible combinations in each person. If several mini-satellite fractions can be examined, each of which consists of various types of alleles, the exclusivity significantly grows. Thus with the examination of 10 mini-satellite regions the chance is 1:10^9. This is why JEFFREYS could assert that mini-satellite regions are identification markers being individual from one person to the next. Researchers believe that, aside from identical twins, there are no identical persons in whom the DNA fingerprint is exactly the same.

In the original description, the use of the procedure in forensic medicine was not referred to, but three years later it was used in the determination of the origin of biological material. The use was unlucky in that the re-examination of some cases verified such technical deficiencies which raised basic doubts concerning the use of the DNA fingerprint procedure in criminal investigations.

This underscores the need for attention to the changes which DNA undergoes postmortally. Although DNA has been isolated from a 2000-year-old mummy, such a test has also been published which found rapidly occurring damage to the DNA following death. Within days of death such damage was found in the area of the tissue sample which showed short-chain, 3.5 kb shorter fragments had been created. In these neither a string of base pairs nor an allele string could be found to amount to enough which would have been satisfactory for identification. (Fixation should be performed in pure alcohol or acetone to inhibit autolysis). The restriction fragment length polymorphism analysis of human DNA also may be useful for blood as biological traces examinations, especially pYNH24 and CMM101 probes.

The genotypes Hp2, Hp1F, Hp1S also were distinguished from dried blood stains up to 15-18 month old.

Another procedure useful for identification which reflects individual characteristics is the demonstration of autoantibodies *(individual specific autoantibodies IS)*. The IS antibodies are definitive in serum concentrations of 1-10 μg/ml and can be found in other bodily fluids. It should be pointed out that the IS antibodies cross the placenta and maternal antibodies can be found for several months after birth. The individual characteristics which do not change through the course of life can also be used in the determination of biological traces.

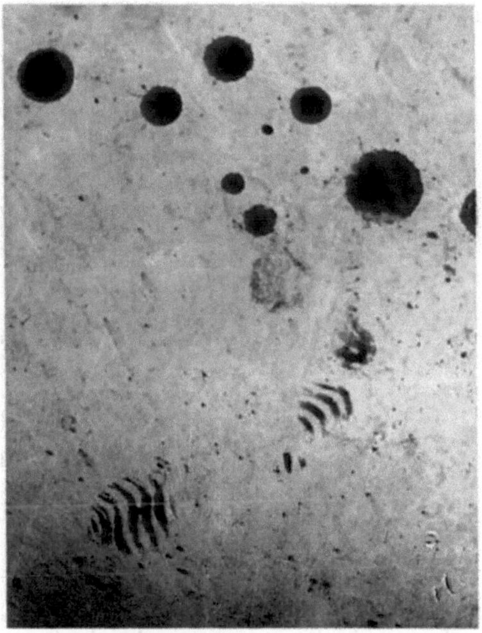

Fig. 101. Drops of blood and shoe sole prints on a linoleum covered floor

4. The *characteristic shape of the blood stains* indicate which manner they came about. The so-called *dripping blood stains* fall almost perpendicularly to the surface of the trace-bearing surface and their shape varies with the distance they fell *(Fig. 101)*. Blood drops falling from a short distance are practically round in shape, and with increasing distance begin to take the so-called corona form. This

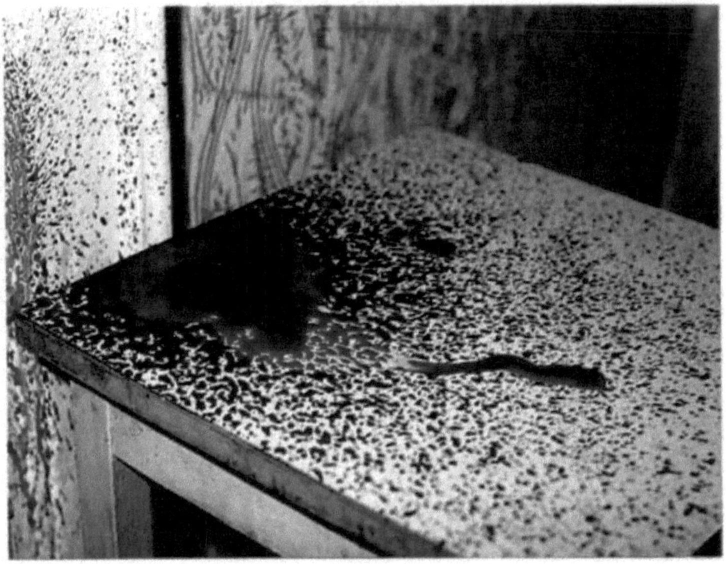

Fig. 102. Spattered blood with the formation of rivulets

means that the larger blood drop outside edges with the increase in height form more like a ring, so that with 0.5-1 meter distance side drops form around the main drop which with the increase in height separate further and further in a circle from the main drop. Drops falling onto a slanting surface or spurting blood stains give a characteristic exclamation mark spot where the tail of the blood stain indicates direction of the spurt or slant of the surface. The blood stain forms similarly in those cases where blood has dripped from the injuring instrument in the area and alters the direction of the spurting injury if the instrument strikes a bloody surface. In these cases we see the characteristic exclamation marks stains not only the immediate area, but also on the injury-causing instrument *(Fig. 102).*

With more significant bleeding, depending on the surface of the corpse, *blood streams* may form. These flowing, stripe-like bleedings dry after a time, and with a restarting of the bleeding should the body be moved, may cross the first dried blood stains and reach the dried patches of blood, widening them slightly, flowing a little further to the side.

The histological examination of the blood traces sometimes can indicate the *source* as well. With *nose bleeds* a smear prepared from the blood – a smear can also be made from dried blood dissolved in physiological saline – containing ciliated epithelium indicates the source of the bleeding. With *menstrual bleeding* a large amount of vaginal squamous epithelial cells and elements of the functional layer of the uterine mucosa can be seen.

The color of the blood stain shows the *age of the spilled blood.* The color of a dried blood stain in the beginning is dark red, then gradually becomes more brown, brownish-black and greyish-green. Determination by semi-quantitative spectrophotometry measures the change of oxyhemoglobin from reduced hemoglobin, which can differentiate the younger from the very old blood stains.

In numerous instances it is also necessary to determine what *quantity the blood sample* was. The difference between dried blood and fresh blood is a ratio of 21.2:1000, so the comparison and relative measurement can be well approximated. Otherwise, if we must state the amount of bleeding which has gotten into a body fluid, or environmental fluid, the concentration of hemoglobin in the fluid can give a valuable indication.

Examination of hair

Of the biological traces left at the scene for examination, hair is common. There is good reason to discuss hairs in identification, as they can be used to construct a relationship. Hairs found on the victims of rape or the perpetrator, hairs that have fallen or been pulled out at each scene or on each victim today provide useful information in the formulating a picture of the their origin. In the above-mentioned cases we must very carefully search the clothing and the victim for foreign hairs.

After *unaided visual examination* of the scene, *light* and *scanning electron microscope examinations* follow in a laboratory environment, which determine whether the hair was human or animal in origin, and to recognize certain diseases as well. The group properties of this formation give further indication as to their origin, while DNA fingerprint procedures or neutronactivation analytical tests unambiguously establish the certainty of the evidence. The keratin formation, like the hairs, are fairly resistant not only to processes of decay, but to the effects of chemicals as well. This property gives the possibility of performing toxicological examinations even decades after death using the hair. The processes of decay affect the hair by changing its color, and even darkly pigmented hairs fade, turning reddish-brown.

Hair begins to appear from the third gestational month. The fine hair covering the body of the fetus, the lanugo from the fifth to the sixth month of intrauterine life begins to change significantly on the scalp with the fuzz-like hairs becoming stiffer and stronger. The number of follicles is permanent at the time of birth, and their number does not increase during life. After birth the lanugo is of a fine fuzzy character, differentiating later into the body hair, eyebrows and eyelashes, which are already formed during the embryonic life, into their terminal state. The terminal body hair consists of the pubic, axillary and facial hair.

The *structure of the hair and body hair* are the same. The hairs grow from the follicles, the lower end being thick and knobby, pushing into the connective tissue papilla, which is rich in vessels. The hair follicle is cell-rich, largely consisting of cells of the basal layer of the skin and this nurtures the hair. The hair being pushed up dries out, so the keratogenous zone is formed by soft keratin making up the core tissue of the hair, while the hard keratin parts form the cortex and cuticle layers. Division in the germinative layer is a cyclic process, a consequence of growth. The hair follicle may have an active and resting phase. In the active phase the germinative layer divides, characterizing hair growth, while in the resting group the germinal cells are inactive and atrophic. After this the hair separates from the matrix and the hair follicle moves it upward, finally falling out. Meanwhile in the follicle over the papilla, the downward growth of the external root sheath envelops the papilla, which is renewed or completely rebuilt. Then from the new germinal matrix the growth of a new hair begins. The growth cycle for scalp hair is the longest, the active phase being possibly 2-3 years, while on other parts of the body the active phase is shorter, 1-2 months following a longer 3-4 month resting phase. On some areas a high percentage of the hair follicles are in an active phase and only a small number are in the resting state, so that the scalp hair in active state may reach 80-90%. The *daily growth of a hair is 0.4 mm.*

We examine the structure of the hair to determine whether it is of animal or human origin. The core is surrounded by the cortex, which is enveloped by the outer layer, the cuticle. The core is made up of soft keratin which in human hair may be missing or thin, or distended, containing air spaces. (The core of animal hair is wide, making up a significant percentage of the width of the hair, but is atypical for the location on the body, similar to the core material of the body hair of a human.) If the hair is strongly pigmented, it may cover the core tissue and so making it visible only by cross-section examination by microscope.

The cortex is made up of hard keratin, with the pigments dwelling in its cells giving the hair its color. The pigment or the form of the granules may be arranged diffusely. In a cross-section of dyed hair the artificial coloring can be well seen in the outer layer, since the original pigment around the core or inside the hair can be easily differentiated. (Similarly, we derive the time of dye application from the length of the undyed hair.) The natural color of the hair can be seen a few days after dying in the area around the hair bulb, so an examination must be intentionally made in this area!

The outermost layer of the hair is the cuticle, a very thin, flattened, with a surface covered by scaly cells also made up of hard keratin. The cells lie open on the hair all the way to the end, and are like the external root sheath, but in the other direction the open-lying cells stick together,

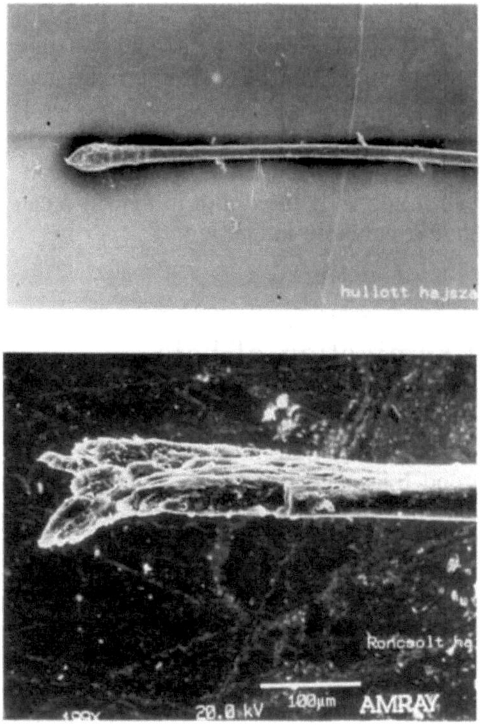

Fig. 103. Upper picture: club-shaped end of a naturally fallen hair. Lower picture: broken end of a hair pulled out by force. Scanning electron micrographs

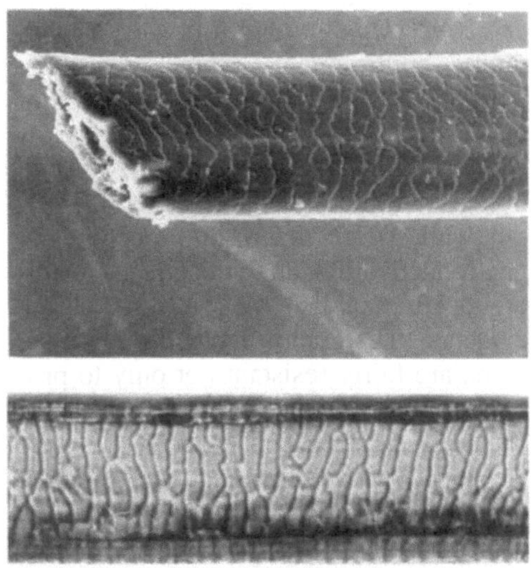

Fig. 104. Scanning electron micrograph of a cut hair showing the surface pattern (above) and the impression of a hair set in gelatin (below)

fixing the hair in place. This connection gives the plucked out hairs their individual morphology. The plucked out hair pulls with it part of the internal root sheath, while a hair that falls out by itself comes out with its rounded, knob-like end *(Fig. 103)*. The exterior cuticle layer gives the hair its individual superficial form and this can shed light on the origin of different hairs *(Fig. 104)*.

The exterior pattern of human hair is fine with showing almost parallel rows of cells which hardly rise from the surface *(Fig. 105)*. The surface of animal hair is rough with the cells standing up, and the impression they leave when examined under scanning electron microscope is that of a scaly pattern *(Fig. 106, 107)*.

In the hairs various signs of injury may be left. Blunt injury may leave a ground up impression with the ends brush-like (similar to the split ends of long hairs that have been subject to frequent pulling). With incising injuries the end of the hair is cut off sharply, with flash burns the hair is singed, kinked and friable with air spaces appearing *(Fig. 108)*.

Whether the scalp hair or the body hair is to be examined, samples should intentionally be taken from several areas. Hair samples from the temples, the forehead, the crown, the nape of the neck should all be taken. We cut the hair close to the root, or even better, pull out hairs with the roots intact. We package the samples separately, marking them with their place of origin. For microscopic examination, whether light or scanning electron microscope, the hairs must be prepared. We wash them in acetone followed by rinsing with distilled water, which yields better

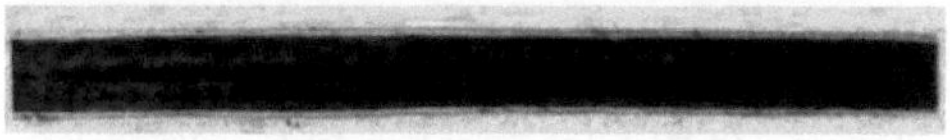

Fig. 105. Light microscopic picture of a human hair. The medullary cavity is thin, semi-patent

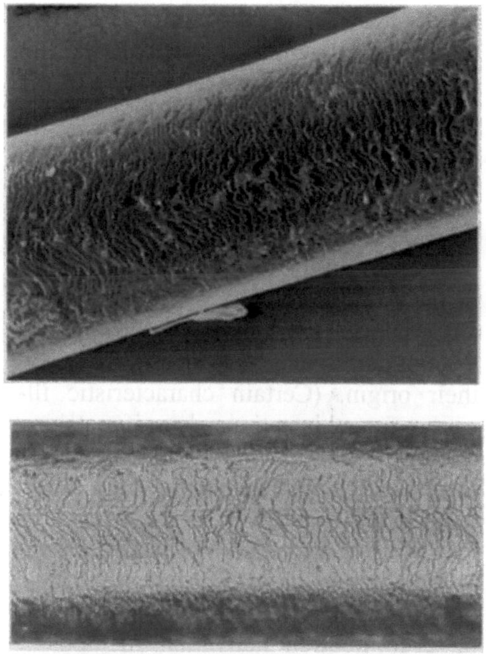

Fig. 106. Animal hair (pig) picture by electron micrograph (above), gelatin impression (below)

Fig. 107. The medullary cavity of animal hair is thick, covered by a thin cortical layer

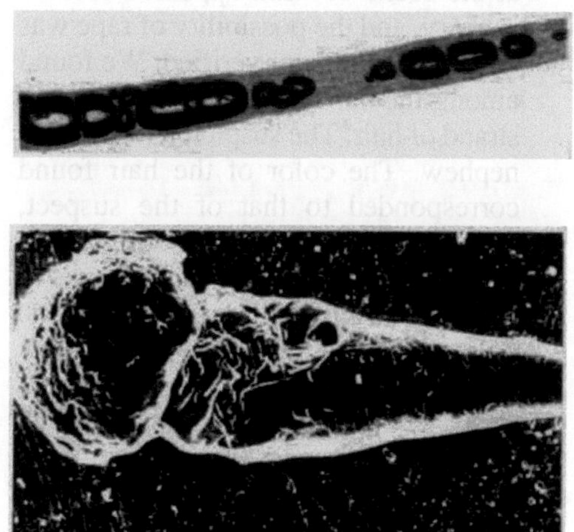

Fig. 108. Scanning electron and light microscopic pictures of a burnt hair

results than detergent washing. For light microscope examination the hairs are set in paraffin, while for examination of the hair surface we place the hair in gelatin on a microscope slide, and after the gelatin hardens the hair can be pulled off leaving behind the impression of its surface. These examinations are appropriate only for determination of the human or animal origin of the hair.

Certain effects may point to injury, though not suitable for determination of their origin. (Certain characteristic illnesses, fungal infections, dyes, if matching one of the suspects, may allow a positive identification, but in practice this rarely happens.)

Modern examination procedures, whether the demonstration of group properties, or the use of DNA fingerprinting methods, or even neutron activation methods – which make the appropriate identification possible – require only a small sample, but performing prior examinations should be avoided, because they jeopardize the success of the later procedures.

- The body of an elderly lady was found at the scene of what appeared to be a robbery, and the possibility of rape was uncovered and later verified. We found among the hair of the victim a foreign strand of hair. The suspicion turned to a nephew. The color of the hair found corresponded to that of the suspect, further morphological examinations were attempted, so the strand was set in Canada balsam and brought no results. A later examination by neutron activation analysis was no longer possible due to the contamination of the hair. The suspect was freed due to lack of evidence.

Examination of seminal stains

Examination of seminal stains as one of the evidences of rape is a part of the practice of the forensic medicine. Such requirements arise which demand not only the verification of the nature of the stain, but that the specialist unambiguously declare whether or not it is the semen of a man. If so, then he should estimate approximately how long ago it arrived at the place of discovery and, if possible, determine the group properties and reveal the suspect. Keating, who is especially prominent and whose work in the above questions is widely accepted calculated that between 1975-1985 the incidence of rape doubled.

The *examination of the stain,* which we will discuss in the chapter on rape, requires a microscopic evaluation of the sample taken during the gynecological examination following rape. Otherwise identification of the tissues or contaminating substances taken from the surface may be considered.

The determination can be made with orientation procedures, some of which methods can be applied to a wide area. The application of a positive orientation examination may expose not only semen, but determine the group properties as well. One of the main preliminary examinations is that of the clothing or a wider area with an analytical quartz lamp, which shows suspicious areas with a sharp bluish-white light. (False positive reactions can occur from vaginal secretions or fecal contamination on the clothing!)

In the layered examination of seminal stains, or in such cases where aspermia or oligospermia is suspected, *acid phosphatase (AP) activity* should be shown or measured in vaginal secretions. (There is data which suggests that 1.9-12.5% of the perpetrators are azoo- or aspermic. Similar considerations can be made with cases of hypospermia resulting from repeated rape.)

The two procedures differ essentially in that with the former only the high AP activity with the former can be exhibited, and is useful as an orientation procedure, whereas the measurement of activity or the isoenzyme picture can differentiate the origin of the secretion. The measurement of a high AP activity suggests prostatic fluid. The test can yield results not only on fresh samples, but we can obtain a quick, intense reaction in dried stains five years old. The principle of the demonstration is the known phosphatase reaction from a histochemical examination which produces a color reaction in sodium alpha-naphthyl phosphate and tetrazolium salt. The procedure is more of an orientation test for the examination of larger areas by spraying. The kit produced by the Sigma company is a simpler determination, which also makes quantitative measurement possible. The results are expressed in Sigma units:

above *138 Sigma/U/ml* means the intercourse occurred within the previous 24 hours,

between *50-138 Sigma/U/ml* shows a great probability of intercourse around 24 hours previously,

20-50 Sigma/U/ml indicates intercourse around 48 hours previously,

a sample showing under *20 Sigma/U/ml* did not enter the vagina within the previous 24 hours.

After intercourse the AP activity quickly and significantly declines in a time dependent manner.

The highest values for prostatic secretions according to the literature are between 9-272 Sigma/U/ml. The AP activity of the vaginal secretions never exceeds 20 Sigma/U/ml. (interesting that a determination of AP activity with positive sperm findings from the mucosa of the rectum or its contents can be made with quite low enzyme measurements – 2-10 Sigma/U/ml). Likewise, an instance is recorded where a measurement of 220 Sigma/U/ml of AP activity was made from a saliva sample from the oral cavity in a rape and murder case.

We have mentioned that not only the AP activity of the prostatic secretions can be demonstrated from the vaginal secretions, but the vaginal AP activity influences the values as well. This must be taken into careful consideration when values of around 20 units are found. This is close to the maximal values for AP activity in the vaginal secretions, and may also signify earlier intercourse. Electrophoretic examination of the secretion unambiguously establishes the origin since the electrophoretic mobility of prostatic AP is different from that of vaginal AP. Similarly the migration distance and the optimum pH of body fluid and plant origin AP are different in electrophoresis. (Another property of prostatic AP activity is the inhibition by L-tartarate, which doesn't inhibit vaginal AP activity.)

Besides the demonstration of AP activity, among the orientation tests, the Florance test is used to demonstrate the choline content of the sample. After ejaculation, choline phosphate is quickly hydrolyzed to choline and phosphate. The process is aided by AP. The choline phosphate concentration of fresh ejaculate is 0.4-1.4 mg/ml. It is especially important in the determination of oligo- or aspermia. The *direct determination of choline* is a good deal more sensitive than the Florance test, since in one survey of 201 samples, 171 showed a positive choline determination, and only 81 by the Florance test. (Care is warranted, since there is a large content in, for example, tomatoes.) With the orientation examinations we can also mention the demonstration of spermine and leucine aminopeptidase, and seminal LDH, as well as the demonstration of the presence of $F_{1\,alpha}$, $F_{2\,alpha}$ prostaglandin level.

Since almost no orientation test – aside form the extremely high AP values – unambiguously verifies the presence of semen, even today we must hold the exhibition of sperm as definite proof.

The sample may be taken from the surface of clothing or something worn. We soak the section cut out from the suspected area of the clothing in physiological saline, which can be preserved under refrigeration for 6-12 hours. We soak out the greater part of the contamination from the piece of clothing. It has been reported in some articles that more of the contamination can be obtained if the soaking material is mechanically shaken than by previous methods. The stain is purposely scraped off of smooth surfaces with a sharp blade and soaked. Cellular elements can be identified from the precipitate of the centrifuged solution, and type determination can be attempted from the supernatant. Other and various procedures are applied and suggested for the examination of the victim. Removal of suspicious contamination from the body surface should include the pubic hair, being wiped from the skin surface with cotton soaked in physiological saline or distilled water. In this country they preferentially use a vaginal douche and demonstration of cells from the centrifuged sample. By the calculations from centers surveying rape cases, a significantly decreased incidence of sperm found in the fluid of vaginal douches has been described. A sample must be intentionally taken from the vaginal entrance, the vaginal vault, and the cervical canal (where the sperm can be demonstrated the furthest) axilla and buttocks area *(Fig. 109)*.

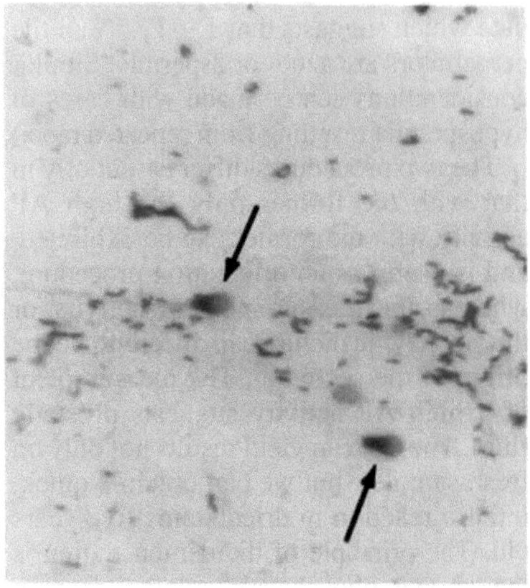

Fig. 109a. Sperm and sperm fragments in vaginal secretions

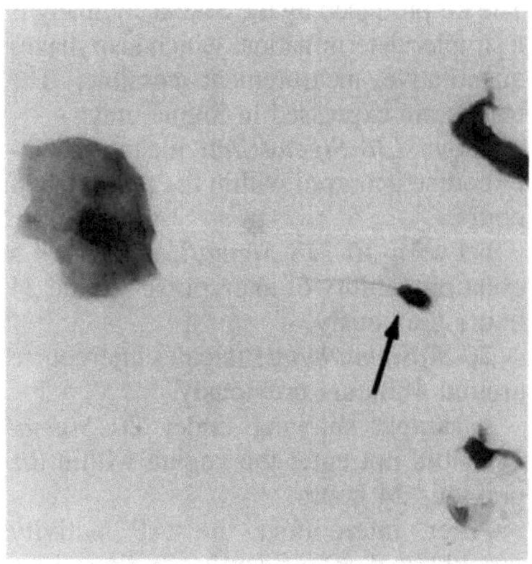

Fig. 109b. Artifact in preparate, spermlike elongated nucleus of epithelial cell

Good results can be obtained from the emplacement of a tampon, which absorbs a significant amount of the vaginal secretions. The authors not only recommend a vaginal examination, but the taking of rectal and oral samples, as well. The tampon emplaced and then removed from the vagina should be cut into four parts, one part put in 1 ml distilled water to extract the cellular elements, the extraction being aided by agitation of the sample, and then drops removed from the cotton piece places on a microscope slide. Another part should be measured for AP activity, and the remaining half should be used to attempt group determination. The values are suggested according to the *DAVIES-WILSON scheme:*

- ++++ numerous sperm visible in every visual field,
- +++ many sperm in most visual fields,
- ++ some sperm in some visual fields, but easy to find,
- \+ sperm difficult to find on the smear,
- 0 no sperm on the smear.

It is also necessary to differentiate the sperm fragments, the heads and tails, but recognition of these requires lots of practice!

Taking *samples from dead bodies* requires the same amount of care. Blood smears should be prepared with the same methods from the vaginal entrance, the vaginal vault, the cervical mucosa, the cervix, the surface of the uterine mucosa, and the area around the anal opening. If oral or anal sex is suspected, samples must be taken from the mucosa of the rectum and ampulla or of the ampullar contents, the oral cavity mucosa, and the pharynx. For possible group determination, samples should be taken of the above areas with a cotton tampon kept under refrigeration until examined.

The motility of the sperm in the examination of a native smear soon after intercourse can determine the time that has elapsed. We can heat fix the preparation and *stain* with *hematoxylin-eosin* or *May-Grünwald Giemsa.* These two staining procedures better reveal the sperm cells than the methylene blue stain does. Even appropriately stained smears can give false positive results, since some of the vaginal squamous epithelial cells may be mistakenly diagnosed as sperm cells. Depending upon the cleanliness of the vagina, on the smear we may find cellular elements, bacteria, – masses of Döderlein-type rod shaped bacteria – squamous epithelia, which appear in large polygonal form, leukocytes, and sperm cells. The examination is begun first at low magnification. With this the sperm can be recognized, with the artifacts of the preparation and the staining being easily differentiated. Human sperm cells are 330-350 microns long and the heads take up about 30 microns. The ejaculate contains only a small percentage of damaged forms, so the greater amount of the sperm cells are healthy and easily recognized. Over the process of evolution due to the differentiation of the acrosome, the front of the sperm head stains more darkly, being a carbohydrate-rich part which caps the seed part of the sperm cell. The neck of the sperm cell contains a high amount of mitochondria, and in the tail we find microtubules wrapped in filaments. The latter are obvious in electron micrographs. The scanning electron microscopic examination is a more damaging procedure than the light microscopic examination, and it naturally requires a properly equipped institution and personnel experienced in such examinations, but with this method the sperm fragments can be identified with certainty even on the surface of the worn material *(Fig. 110).*

There have been studies which were made of tampon examinations by volunteers which either showed poor results or were unable to demonstrate sperm. If sperm can hardly be recognized in the vi-

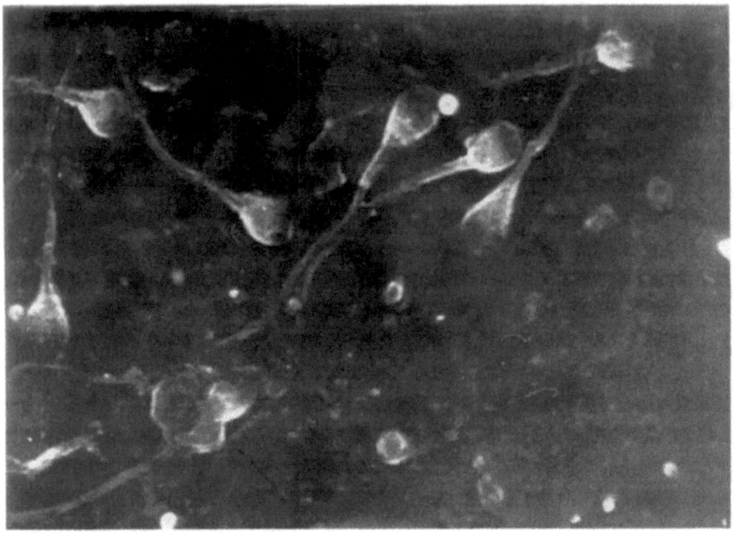

Fig. 110. Sperm cells from a sample of a superficial trace by scanning electron micrograph

sual field (Davies-Wilson classification +) the intercourse occurred at least five days earlier. The form of the sperm not only depends upon the time elapsed – as already noted – but may result from a faulty sampling, a washing after the intercourse, or from incomplete intercourse, about which we have very little data. The sperm may fall victim in great part to phagocytosis. In the female reproductive system leukocytes and mononuclear cells play the main role, the speed of the process depending on the location, whether in the cervical or vaginal cervix and individual factors. For these reasons we can count on a deviation in the vaginal survival times of the sperm cells. During phagocytosis the main parts of the sperm, head and tail fragments appear in the vaginal and cervical secretions and smears prepared from here show the parts in the leukocytes and phagocytes.

On of the questions in the examination of the secretions is *who produced the contamination.* We have already mentioned the possibilities of exhibition with secretory type, the mixed cell agglutination procedure, or the elution test, which are well applicable to clean, unmixed stains. Mixed samples of body fluids and vaginal secretions cannot be examined for group properties in a simple manner, since the deviant group properties make this impossible. According to the literature that deals with this, the AB0 system can be successfully determined from seminal stains, along with the Lewis property Gm, the PGM, glyoxalase and peptidase systems. The examination of mixed secretions, especially in the differentiation of mixed vaginal secretions and sperm, has been succ(ssfully performed by colloidal silica gel differential centrifugation, in which cells of differing densities can be separated and thus today opening the possibility of application of DNA fingerprinting methods which require only quite small amounts of material.

Examination of bite marks

Bite marks are found not only on the sufficient materials at the scene of the crime, but on the person of the victim as well. The latter are mainly found on victims of sexual assault. Among the impressionable materials which can bear bite marks quite well are chocolate, hard fruits, apples, pears, etc., but also such things with a consistency which can be altered by the temperature of the surroundings, and consequently the impressions as well may be altered or even destroyed. The character of the impressions depends on the quality of the impression-carrying material and its capacity to preserve them.

Impressions left on the victim must be immediately preserved photographically so that the picture also reflects the dimensions. The standard photometric procedures which we can find in just those articles which deal with the commonly occurring sex crimes, especially emphasize the photographed impression and the dimensional scale often yield parallax errors. Photographs taken under electric light are also held to be unsatisfactory, recommending the use of special lighting for a detail-rich picture. A photograph fixes the static state. More recently by the use of video recording the dynamics of a bite on the body surface by the suspected set of teeth can be studied. To find the less visible bite marks, lighting by a fluorescent lamp has been employed, the saliva marks left behind showing a shiny effect in the examination. Such fixation procedures must be begun in the examination which leave the injured area intact. The first of these is the taking of a sample of the saliva perhaps left behind for serological examination. This is performed by wiping the area with a piece of cotton soaked in distilled water, taking care not to touch the other contaminations, as these may influence the results. The sample is kept refrigerated until used. After taking the sample, we must fix the impression by any of several methods, the fixation of barely visible marks on the body surface making use of dusting techniques used in the taking of fingerprints and cellophane sheets for the purpose of taking samples, the details of which, if transferred to microscope slides, can be magnified, or the microscopic tooth impressions obtained. Thus the finer construction of the biting surface can also be evaluated. It is considered a good idea to fill the bite mark with a dental sample-taking material, or prepare a sample with elastomer material. These in part suffer alterations during polymerization, but on the other hand make quite good impressions.

The difficulties in support are also to be mentioned since from the start of the examination an experienced forensic dental specialist is required, or at least a dentist to do the examination, upon whom the success of later identification depends.

Bite injuries into the surface of the body – depending upon the amount of force applied – may bring about injuries ranging from the superficial wounds with tissue damage to separation discontinuities. The fixation of milder injuries does not tolerate procrastination since the hyperemia following a small application of force rapidly dissipates.

The bruising accompanying injuries from the front teeth are superficially narrow and straight, those of the eye-teeth are pointed, while those of the premolars and molars leave wide, characteristic marks. Now and then the increase of the blood infiltration of the injuries, with bloody infiltration in the corpse, can be better seen 12-24 hours later due to the discoloration. (Bite injuries must purposely not be examined after removal, since the skin suffers such alterations after incision which can make the precise identification impossible.)

Bite marks may be:

1. *"bite into" marks* (the mark-bearing materia carrying visible impressions of both rows of teeth),

2. *"bite out of" marks* (the marks of the incisors being left behind, with a part of the mark-bearing material bitten out of the surface).

The alterations resulting for mild application of force leave signs of pressure anemia being lighter than the surroundings. Shortly after the injury the area becomes hyperemic and a measurable edema forms, the they disappear in 1-2 hours.

In forceful applications abrasions form with bleeding depending on the force of the bite, edema, and the possibility for identification. During life the measure of the disappearance of the edema varies while the corpse suffers from shrinkage and changes in dimension with drying out, so early examination of the injury is essential. The front and eye-teeth sinking in may cause soft tissue injury, perhaps even reaching the musculature. In these injuries the skin separates depending upon the line of force, so identification is not possible in every case. The injuries generally do not heal well, and often become infected and take longer than eight days to heal. Bites that remove tissue are the most serious form. In their manifestation, the incisors play a tearing and rending role; in practice the biting off of ears and noses is encountered most often *(Fig. 111)*. The characteristics of the set of teeth is exceptionally reflected in the injuries *(Fig. 112)*.

Examination by scanning electron microscope is held to be superior to examination with the naked eye or magnifying glass, emphasizing that the appropriate magnification and depth of field dictates the proper method for the examination of injuries in more than one plane. Not only the bite marks on the body surface, but those on the surfaces of other materials bearing impressions offer excellent examination possibilities, remembering that cheese, apples, margarine, marzipan leave identifiable impressions, and with the help of the surface characteristics, mainly the cutting surface of the front teeth are reflected *(Fig. 113)*.

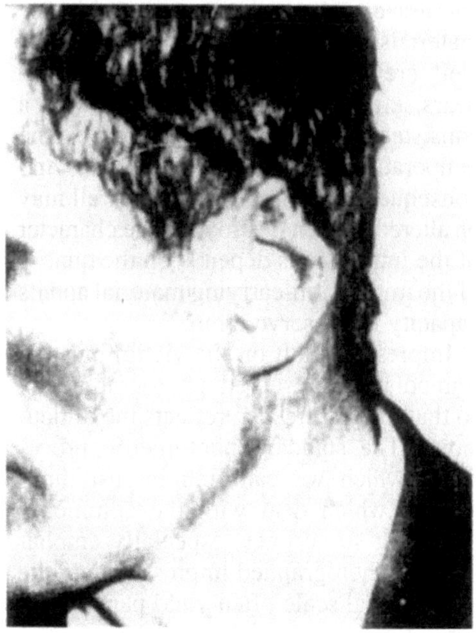

Fig. 111. Ear injury. Part of the ear was bitten off during a fight

Injuries from sexual assault most commonly are found on the areas of the breasts, the face, the arms, thighs and buttocks, but we have examined a case of sexual assault where the nose was bitten off, too. Bite marks in association with sexual assault may extend from superficial alterations to deep injuries and are completely independent of the age of the victim. (Very great care is necessary in the examination of the impressions. There has been an account a of pendulous breasted, elderly woman inflicting bite wounds on herself in the area of the breasts). It is very difficult to differential bite marks occurring during normal intercourse or those previously mentioned from those incurred during sexual assault.

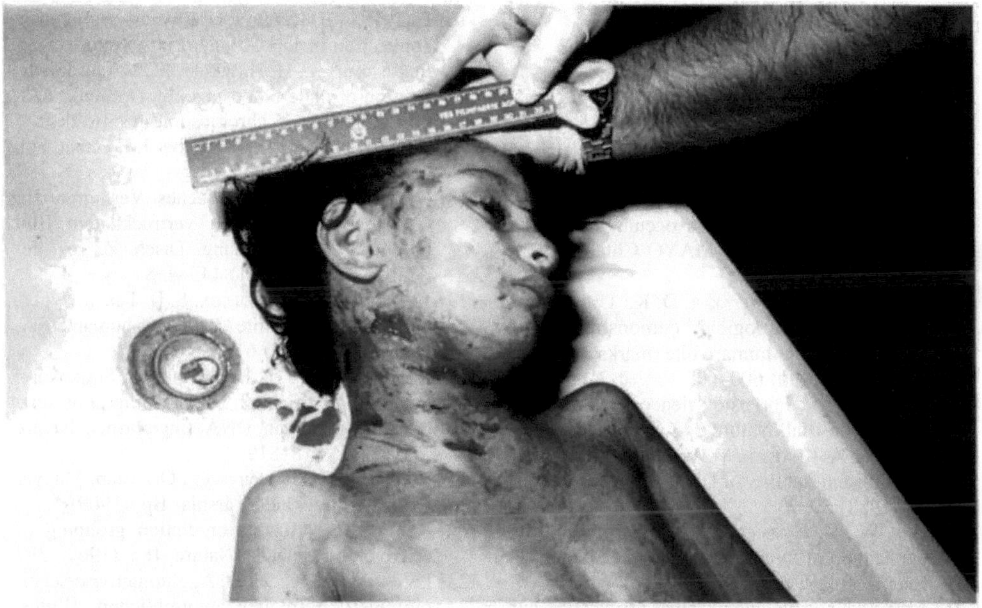

Fig. 112. **Bite marks on the neck region. The victim was bitten by a dog**

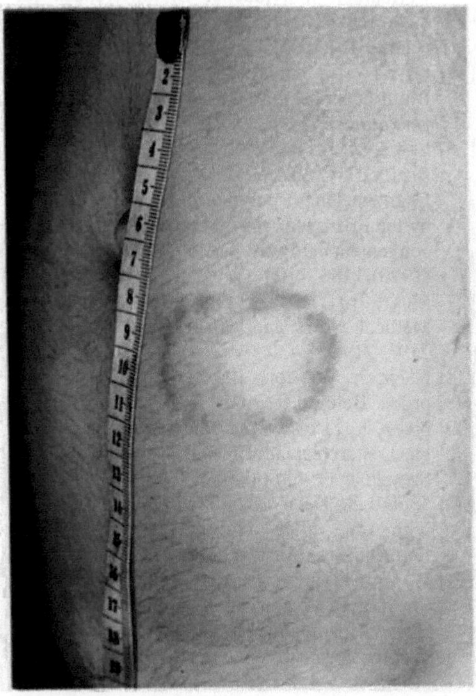

Fig. 113. **Bite marks on the skin can be measured for identification matching**

In the absence of other injuries the possibility can be accepted that the bite marks may not necessarily have occurred during rape.

After the examination of the marks, it must be clarified from whom they originated. If from among the suspects there is one whose bite can be demonstrated by some arrangement, and the impression of his teeth examined in the mark-bearing material, then the identification is easy. In other cases basic special equipment and procedures are called for, which means a special examination by a dental expert. If it is possible to photograph the prints and identify the impressions, dental impressions prepared from the suspects can be used which can be examined by the appropriately fashioned phantom surface or superimposed photograph procedures. In identification, attention must be drawn to the size of gaps between the teeth, the width of the teeth, and arch of the line of the teeth. Exclusion is much easier than making a positive identification.

References

Blood stains

[1] Ahlquist, D. A., V. F. Fairbanks, R. D. Ellefson: Hemo-Quant test for occult blood. The Sherlock Holmes test? MAYO Clin. Proc. 59 (1984) 766–768
[2] Allison, R. T., Whittaker, D. K.: Use of benzidine for histological demonstration of haemoglobin in human bite marks. J. Clin. Pathol. 43 (1990) 600–603
[3] Anderson, A.: Forensic science: DNA fingerprinting on trial. Nature 342 (1989) 384
[4] Bar, W., A. Kratzer, M. Machler, W. Schmid: Postmortem stability of DNA. Forensic Sci. Int. 39 (1988) 59–70
[5] Bar, W., K. Hummel: DNA fingerprinting, its application in forensic case work. Experientia-Suppl. 58 (1991) 349–355
[6] Beer, a Untersuchungen Über Vorproben auf Blut in der forensischen Medizin, unter besonderer Berücksichtigung der neuen Blutvorprobe mit Luminol. Inaugural dissertation. Buchdruckerei Friedl und Co. Bern (1940)
[7] Budvári, R.: Vérfoltok azonosításának új módszere az elúciós vizsgálat. Belügyi Szemle 1. (1963) 40–84
[8] Bugawan, T. L., Saiki, R. K. Levenson, R. M. Watson, H. A. Erlich: The use of non-radioactive oligonucleotide probes to analyse enzymatically amplified DNA for prenatal diagnosis and forensic HLA typing. Biotechnology 6 (1988) 943–947
[9] Butt, R. W.: Identification of human blood stains by radioimmunoassay. J. Forensic Sci. Soc. 23 (1983) 291–296
[10] Coombs, R. R. A., D. Bedford, L. M. Ruillard: A and B blood group antigens on human epidermal cells. Lancet I. (1956) 461–463
[11] Eckert, W. G., S. H. James: Blood Evidence in Crime Scene Investigation. Inform Publ. Wichita, Kansas (1987)
[12] Editorial: DNA and the law. Lancet I. (1990) 381–382
[13] Evett, I. W., D. J. Werrett, P. Gill: DNA fingerprint on trial. Nature 340 (1988) 435
[14] Francoeur, A. M.: Antibody fingerprinting: a novel method for identifying individual people and animals. Biotechnology 6 (1988) 822–825
[15] Francoeur, A. M.: Biotechnology in forensic medicine: new ways of fingerprinting. J. Biotechnol. 10 (1989) 203–208
[16] Gill, P., A. J. Jeffreys, D. J. Werrett: Forensic application of DNA fingerprints. Nature
[17] Fukushima, H., H. Hasekura, K. Nagai: Identification of male bloodstains by Dot hybridization of human Y chromosomespecific deoxyribonucleic acid (DNA) probe. J. Forensic Sci. 33 (1988) 620–621
[18] Holzer, F. J.: Ein einfaches Verfahren zur Gruppenbestimmung an vertrocknetem Blut durch Agglutininbindung. Dtsch. Z. ges. gerichtl. Med. 16 (1931) 443–458
[19] Jeffreys, A. J., V. Wilson, S. L. Thein: Hypervariable "minisatellite" regions in human DNA. Nature 314 (1985) 67–73
[20] Jeffreys, A. J., J. F. Brookfield, R. Semeonoff: Positive identification of an immigration test-case using human DNA fingerprints. Nature 317 (1985) 818–819
[21] Kenyeres, B.: Törvényszéki Orvostan. Magyar Orvosi Könyvkiadó Társulat Bp. (1909)
[22] Kind, S. S.: Absorption-elution grouping of dried blood smears. Nature 185 (1960) 397
[23] Landsteiner, K.: Über Agglutinationserscheinigungen normalter menschlichen Blutes. W. Klin. Wochenschr. 14 (1901) 1132
[24] Landsteiner, K., M. Richter: Über die Verwertbarkeit individueller Blutdifferenzen für die forenzische Praxis. Arch. für Medizinalbeamte 16 (1903) 85
[25] Lattes, L.: Praktische Erfahrunger Über Blutgruppenbestimmung in Flecken. Dtsch. Z. ges. gerichtl. Med. 9 (1927) 402–410
[26] Lewis, M. E., R. E. Kouri, D. Latorra, K. M. Berka, H. C. Lee, R. E. Gaensslen: Restriction fragment length polymorphism DNA analysis by the FBI Laboratory protocol using a simple, convenient hardware system. J. Forensic Sci. 35 (1990) 1186–1190
[27] Merz, B.: DNA fingerprints come to court. Medical News and perspektives 259 (1988) 2193–2194
[28] Nagy, J., Zsigmond K.: Kemilumineszcenciás próba. Belügyi Szemle 1. (1963) 52–60
[29] Nagy, J., Zsigmond K.: Phenolphtalein előpróba, kristályreakció Takayama szerint. Belügyi Szemle 1. (1963) 60–65
[30] Nanko, S.: Decrease of Y chromatin frequency with time after fixation of blood smear. Forensic Sci. Int. 15 (1980) 1–2
[31] Waye, J. S., L. A. Presley, B. Budowle, G. G. Shutler, R. M. Fourney: A simple and sensitive method for quantifying human genomic DNA in forensic specimen extracts. Biotechniques 7 (1989) 852–855
[32] Webb, P.: DNA and the law. Lancet I. (1990) 608–609

[33] Wiener, A. S., M. Shapiro: Advances in Blood Grooping II. Grune and Stratton N. Y. (1965) pp. 245–247
[34] Yokoi, T., K. Sagisaka: Haptoglobin typing of human bloodstains using a specific DNA probe. Forensic. Sci. Int. 45 (1990) 39–46

Examination of hair

[1] Bate, L. C.: The use of activation analysis in procedures for the removal and characterization of the surface contaminations of hair. J. Forensic Sci. 10 (1965) 60–72
[2] Camps, F. E.: Gradwohl US Legal Medicine. J. Wright and Sons Bristol (1968) pp. 221–230
[3] Choudhry, M. Y, C. R. Kingston, L. Kobilinsky, P. R. De Forest: Individual characteristics of chemically modified human hairs revealed by scanning electron microscopy. J. Forensic Sci. 28 (1983) 293–306
[4] Clegg, M. S., C. L. Keen, B. Lünnerdal, L. S. Hurley: Influence of ashing techniques on the analysis of trace elements in animal tissue. Biological Trace Element Res. 3 (1981) 107–115
[5] Cortivo, P., M. Biasiolo, C. Scoretti, P. Benciolini: The detection of A and B antigens on human hair by the absorbtion-elution technique using LISS and papain treated test cells. Z. Rechtsmed. 91 (1984) 195–199
[6] Forshufvud, S., H. Smith, A. Wassen: Arsenic-content of Napoleon's hair probably taken immediately after his death. Nature 192 (1961) 103–105
[7] Ham, A. W., D. H. Cormack: Histology. J. B. Lippincott Co. (1979) pp 626–632
[8] Jervis, R. E.: Neutron Radioactivation Helps Solve Crimes. Canadian Nuclear Technology Winter (1962) pp. 21–24
[9] Moore, J. E.: A key for the identification of animal hairs. J . Forensic Sci. Soc. 28 (1988) 335–339
[10] Peabody, A. J., R. J. Oxborough, P. E. Cage, I. W. Evett: The discrimination of cat and dog hairs. J. Forensic Sci. Soc. 23 (1983) 121–129
[11] Riggott, J. M., E. H. Wyatt: Mensuration of Scanning micrographs. A possible means of hair identification. J. Forensic Sci. Soc. 23 (1983) 155–160
[12] Somogyi, E.: Scanning electronmicroscope studies of human hair. Krim. Forens. Wiss. 53–54 (1984) 40–50
[13] Wickenheiser, R. A., D. G. Hepworth: Further evaluation of probabilities in human scalp hair comparisons. J. Forensic Sci. 35 (1990) 1323–1329

Seminal stains

[1] Adams, E. G., B. G. Wraxall: Phosphatases in body fluids the differentiation of semen and vaginal secretion. Forensic Sci. 3 (1974) 57–62
[2] Allard, J., A. Davies: Further information on the use of p-nitrophenyl phosphate to quantitate acid phosphatase on vaginal swabs examined in cases of sexual assault. Med. Sci. Law. 19 (1979) 170–172
[3] Blake, E. T., CH. E. Cook, J. S. Bashinsky: Evidence that "vaginal peptidase" is a bacterial gene product. J. Forensic Sci. 32 (1987) 887–889
[4] Clausen, J., B. Oulissen: Lactate dehydrogenase isoenzymes in human semen. Biochem. J. 97 (1965) 513–517
[5] Concheiro, L. A. Carracedo, F. Guitian: The use of scanning electron microscopy in the examination of seminal stains. Forensic Sci. Int. 19 (1982) 185–188
[6] Davies, A., E. Wilson: The persistence of seminal constituens in the human vagina. Forensic. Sci. 3 (1974) 45–55
[7] Davies, A.: A preliminary investigation using p-Nitrophenyl phosphate to quantitate acid phosphatase on swabs examined in cases sexual assault. Med. Sci. Law. 18 (1978) 174–178
[8] Davies, A.: The appearance and grouping of mixtures of semen and vaginal material. Med. Sci. Law. 22 (1982) 21–30
[9] Goldberg, E.: Lactic and malic acid dehydrogenases in human spermatozoa. Science 139 (1963) 602–603
[10] Keating, S. M.: The laboratory US approach to sexual assault cases. Sources of information and acts of intercourse. J. Forensic Sci. Soc. 28 (1988) 99–110
[11] Kind, S. S.: The Acid Phosphatase Test in A. Curry: Methods of Forensic Science Interscience Publ. London (1964) pp. 267–288
[12] Noppinger, K., R. Morrison, N. H. Jones, H. Hopkins: An evaluation of an enzyme choline determination for the identification of semen in casework samples. J. Forensic Sci. 32 (1987) 1069–1074
[13] Piner, S. C., M. S. Sanger: Lewis grouping of human secretion stains. Forensic Sci. Int. 15 (1980) 87–92
[14] Randall, B.: Persistence of vaginal spermatozoa as assessed by routine cervicovaginal (PAP) smears. J. Forensic Sci. 32 (1987) 678–683
[15] Takatori, T., T. Sasaki: Isolation of spermatozoa in vaginal contents by centrifugation in a colloidal silica gradient. Forensic Sci. Int. 15 (1980) 61–65

[16] WILLOTT, G. M.: Frequency of azoospermia. Forensic Sci. Int. 20 (1982) 9–10
[17] WILLOTT, G. M., J. E. ALLARD: Spermatozoa-their persistence after sexual intercourse. Forensic Sci. Int. 19 (1982) 135–154

Bite marks

[1] BENSON, B. W., J. A. COTTONE, T. J. BOMBERG, N. D. SPERBER: Bite mark impressions. A review of techniques and materials. J. Forensic Sci. 33 (1988) 1238–1243
[2] GOLDSTEIN, E. J.: Infectious complications and therapy of bite wounds. J. Am. Pediatr. Med. Assoc. 79 (1989) 486–491
[3] GUSTAFSON, G.: Forensic Odontology. Am. Elsevier Publ. Co. N. Y. (1966) pp. 140–165
[4] HYZER, W. G., T. C. KRAUSS: The bite marke standard reference scale. ABFO 2. J. Forensic Sci. 33 (1988) 488–506
[5] RAO, V. J., R. S. SOUVIRON: Dusting and lifting the bite print. A new technique. J. Forensic Sci. 19 (1984) 326–330
[6] ROBINSON, E., J. WENTZEL: Toneline bite mark photography. J. Forensic Sci. 37 (1992) 195–207
[7] SOBEL, M. N., J. A. PERPER: Self-inflicted bite mark on the breast of a suicide victim. Am. J. Forensic Med. Pathol. 6 (1985) 336–339
[8] SOLHEIM, T., T. I. LEIDAL: Scanning electron microscopy in the investigation of bite marks in foodstuffs. Forensic Sci. 6 (1975) 205–215
[9] STUCKER, F. J., G. Y. SHAW, S. BOYD, W. W. SHOCKLEY: Management of animal and human bites in the head and neck. Arch. Otolaryngol. Head Neck Surg. 116 (1990) 789–793
[10] WEST, M. H., J. FRAIR: The use of videotape to demonstrate the dynamics of bite marks. J. Forensic Sci. 34 (1989) 88–95

Chapter 5

Sudden death

The examination of cases of sudden death make up a significant part of the practice of the forensic medical physician. We speak of sudden death when it happens to a person of healthy appearance in the absence of the usual clinical preliminaries or outside influence. Inasmuch as clinical signs do not accompany the case, the possibility of foul play or poisoning can be considered. At the same time, cases appearing to be sudden death may conceal criminal activity. In the examination of sudden death, at the scene the answers to the following questions must be sought:

a) was death by natural causes?
b) what information indicating illness do the surroundings provide?
c) was some occupational injury instrumental in the sudden death?
d) had a previous accident occurred?

Only a small percent of the cases of sudden death involve foul play, but their significance is great.

● A district general practitioner was called on to examine the body of a 70-year-old man, and upon superficial examination established that the elderly man had died of natural causes. According to the statement of an eye-witness, "... the doctor just looked at the body from the door." The relatives dressed and laid the body in state. During the night watch a curious neighbor noticed that the shirt of the body lying in the coffin was bloody. Immediately after making the discovery, she notified the local police. After that a police medical examination took place. It then turned out that the deceased had received a stab wound to the back left side of the thorax. The son-in-law of the deceased had stabbed him.

Cases of sudden death belong to the so-called *unnatural death* category. Basic practical skill is required of the physician in the autopsy and examination. Inexperienced physicians, or those unfamiliar with the examination of cases of sudden death can make serious errors if they don't keep in mind the causes of natural death, especially if in the course of the autopsy, their evidence is destroyed. (Thus making the subsequent diagnosis of bolus death impossible.) It is similarly uncorrectable if the signs of foul play are misinterpreted or unrecognized. For these reasons, the examination of sudden death is one of the most important matters in practice and deserving of the greatest professional experience. (It merits special importance if the body is cremated after the autopsy and further examinations are made impossible.) Inasmuch as the cases involve pathology to a significant extent – degenerative changes, inflammatory diseases, tumorous pathological pictures – it is expected of the physician that familiarity with pathology must accompany the knowledge of the forensic medical specialist.

Various examinations must be performed in the course of most autopsies, among which most commonly are the histological examinations, which may have documentary value in the judgement of the cause of death as well. At other times bacteriological, occasionally toxicological or other laboratory examinations may be of help in the diagnosis. If doubt remains with the autopsy with respect to the cause of death, it is proper to call upon the help of an experienced specialist or specialists. In cases of sudden death a coroner's inquest is performed in most cases by a practicing physician. Here we direct the attention of the coroner's inquest to the defined aspects and to whether they provide an indication of whether the death was natural or due to violence.

Unnatural death must be differentiated from sudden death in such cases when a previous illness or illnesses which were not considered come into the picture.

The grouping of sudden death cases can be by age, but it is more practice to group them by organ systems.

Alterations in the circulatory system causing sudden death

A significant part of the developmental abnormalities of the circulatory system are of a nature which manifests itself early in neonatal life, or are incompatible with life. Thus only the hidden changes can cause sudden death. The predominant portion of developmental abnormalities are *septal defects.* Ventricular septal defect is an easily recognizable auscultatory finding, but the diagnosis of the small or circumscribed atrial septal defects may remain hidden and although their significance in sudden death is low, they can cause a fatal brain or coronary occlusion if even a mild embolization gains access to the systemic circulation. The place of predilection for atrial septal defect is the area around foramen ovale. In this area the alteration in blood flow and an increased "whirlpool effect" creates a place of predilection for the formation of endocarditis. The bits of built up vegetations that break off can just as easily cause embolism. If the ventricular septal defect is larger, the left ventricular shunt and the resulting right ventricular hypertrophy may cause pulmonary hypertension, dilation of the pulmonary artery and an acute right heart insufficiency, as in chronic cor pulmonale, causing sudden death. Rarely we may come across such developmental abnormalities which are not common, and pass unnoticed, remaining undiscovered.

The *origin and course of the coronaries* may be abnormal. Multiple coronary orifices are not common, but may develop a double coronary ostium with hypoplasia of the branches resulting in disturbances of nutrition to the myocardium. The coronary may arise from the pulmonary trunk, leading to hypoxic damage to the myocardium due to the channeling of venous blood *(Fig. 114).* More common are the abnormal origins of the right coronary branches. Compression of the vessel branches originating from the left aortic sinus may result in sudden death.

Transposition of the great vessels rarely cause sudden death and have more of a pathological significance than a forensic medical one. Among the *developmental*

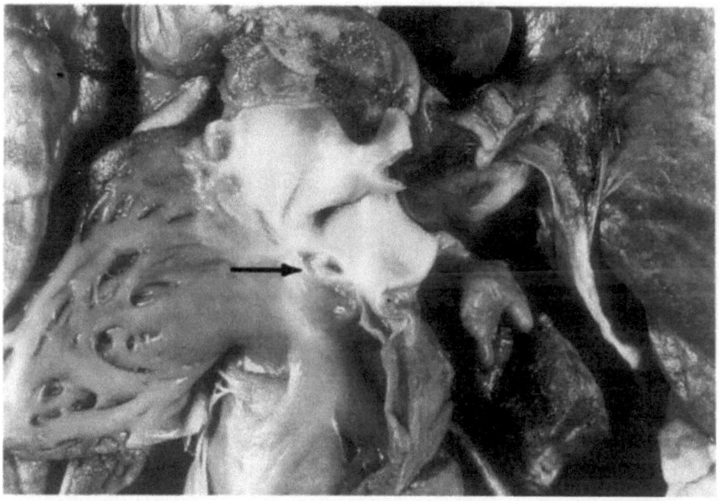

Fig. 114. The origin of the coronary artery from the trunk of the pulmonary artery

abnormalities affecting the aorta, *persistent duct of Botall* (ductus arteriosus) can be found physiologically for the first three months of life. After this, due to the postnatal circulatory changes, it is obliterated by sterile inflammation. If it does not close, a shunt between the pulmonary and systemic circulation will result in pulmonary hypertension and chronic cor pulmonale which may lead to sudden death. With the closure of Botall's duct, an aortic stenosis may arise, which appears proximally in the infantile form between the left subclavian artery and the opening of Botall's duct, and may cause sudden death in children and infants. Anatomically, a persistent ductus arteriosus means the possibility of a bypass, the circulation passing through it instead, avoiding a completely closed or significantly narrowed aorta section. Without correction soon after birth the patient dies at the age of a few months. The adult form appears distal to the duct of Botall, and may be symptomless and only diagnosed if complications, such as, hypertonia, dissecting aneurysm, stroke bring about sudden death.

The *peripheral vessels,* especially circumscribed dilations in the area of the *circle of Willis* may arise in the angles of the dividing arterial trunks. The immaturity of the internal elastic membrane may play a role in their formation. Besides on the vessels of the base of the brain *(Fig. 115, 116),* they may form on the internal carotid. Rupture of a distended vessel may cause sudden death. The dissecting aneurysm of the coronary artery may cause cardiac tamponade.

First place in sudden death statistics is held by *ischemic heart disease.* In Hungary the number instead of has declined, but has even risen over recent years. Death occurs suddenly in most cases and the pathological backgrounds in most cases are disturbances in coronary circulation. The conduction system of the heart is illustrated in *(Fig. 117).* The topological acquaintance with these cannot be disregarded, indeed when examined, many "inexplicable" instances of sudden death are elucidated.

Disturbances in myocardial nutrition may result from coronary insufficiency or low oxygentension in the circulating blood. Of the alterations causing these, the following may be mentioned:

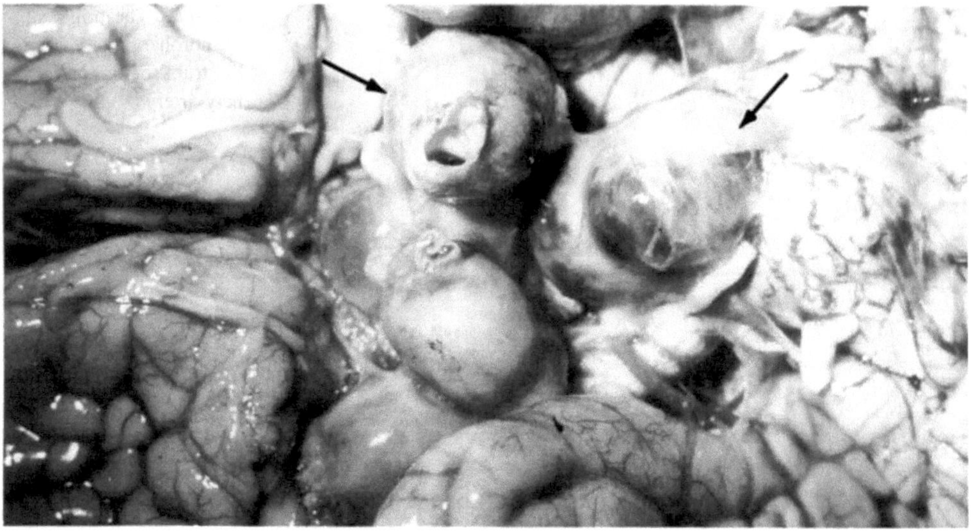

Fig. 115. Multiple aneurysms at the base of the brain

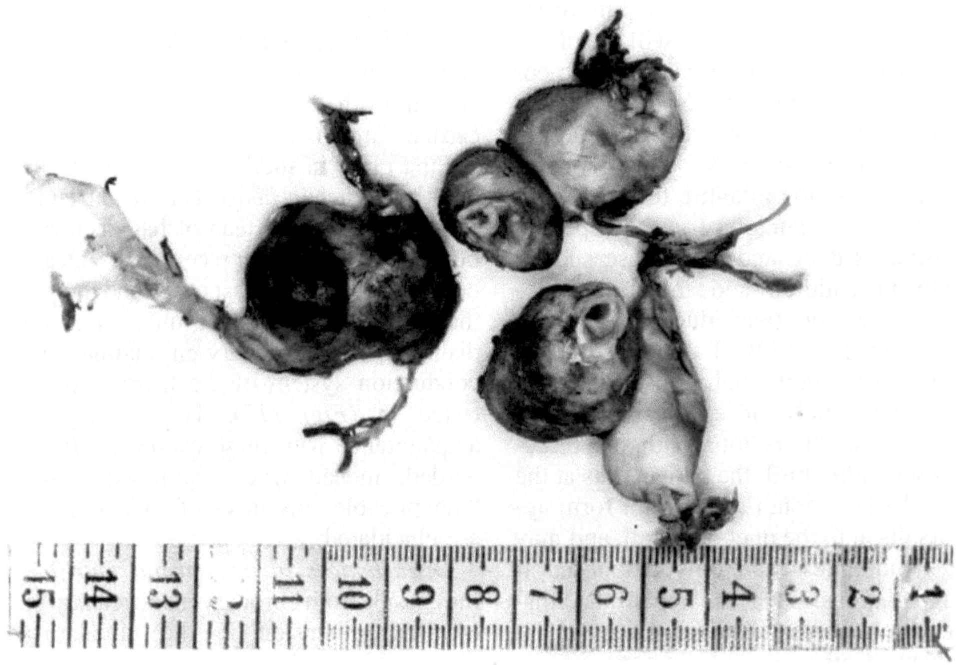

Fig. 116. Localization of aneurysms in the Circle of Willis

a) coronary atheromatous alterations,
b) functional coronary stenosis – coronary spasm, connecting muscle fiber bridges,
c) narrowing of coronary orifices,
d) relative coronary insufficiency (hypertrophic myocardium),
e) coronary thrombosis,
f) subintimal hemorrhage, edema,
g) faulty origin of coronary branch,
h) chronic hypoxic state.

Atheromatous coronary lesions appear with advancing age, the development of which may reflect not only a familial tendency but nutritional habits as well. The appearance in youth by age 20 is not rare, and not only the large branches of the coronaries affected, but the small epicardial vessels as well. The small arteries and arterioles among the muscle fibers, however, are not damaged. The deposits eccentrically narrow the coronary branches. At autopsy this can be better demonstrated in cross sectioning of the coronaries, and the measurement of the narrowing can be made. The narrowed coronary in youth histologically shows hyaline degeneration and we see an evenly stained subintimal endothelial proliferation with edematous swelling which could lead to the occlusion of the vessel. In the narrowed areas later in life a lipoid, cholesterol-rich material forms under the intima surrounded by fibrotic tissue. These deposits or plaques cause a chronic narrowing of the vessel lumen, leading eventually to a chronic disturbance in myocardial nutrition, which also leads to anginal complaints. If the affected plaque should swell or subintimal bleeding develops acute occlusion may occur. At other times a thrombus may form on the surface of the exulcerated plaque and cause acute obstruction. In old age in the area of the atheromatous plaque calcified deposits form and the coronaries become stiff, pipe-like form.

The penetrating muscle branches of the

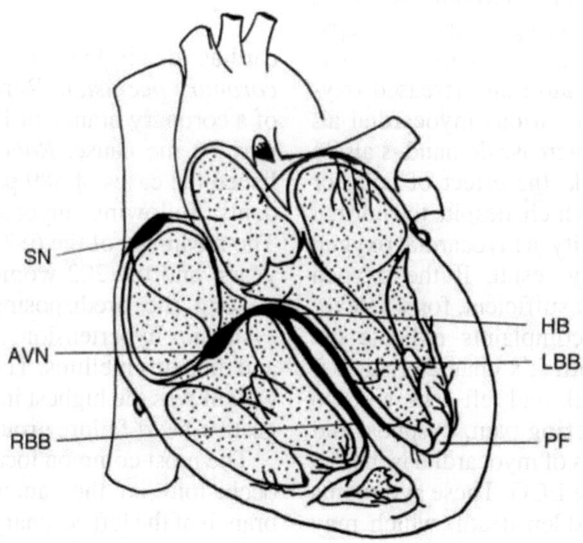

Fig. 117. Topography of the conduction system of the heart. SN – sinus node, AVN – atrio-ventricular node, LBB – left bundle branch, PF – Purkinje fibres, RBB – right bundle branch, HB – His bundle

coronaries may develop a relative insufficiency along with significant myocardial hypertrophy. Chronic nutritional disturbances of various etiologies cause similar consequent damage. In the myocardium a diffuse focal fibrosis appears, and if the fibrotic part also affects the conduction system, we can count on functional disturbances as well, and the paroxysmal tachycardia or arrhythmias often lead to sudden death, sometimes with quite sparse signs at autopsy.

Similar alterations in the myocardium can accompany those *coronary diseases* which are localized to the coronary orifices and by progressive obstruction cause the so-called *ostium barrier* with hypoxic damage. Syphilitic aortitis or an extreme atheromatic aorta may be accompanied by a significant orificial narrowing, but a similar effect may occur by the abovementioned developmental abnormalities of the coronaries when the coronary originates from the pulmonary trunk carries venous blood causing a hypoxic state. A similar case is the alterations resulting from a decreased oxygen carrying capacity caused by grave anemia. Hyperthyroidism may cause an increased oxygen demand with various myocardial alterations, but an increase demand is also a sign of hard work, the effect of cold, or serious injury in which, despite the normal O_2 carrying capacity, a myocardial oxygen insufficiency may result. If the oxygen supply becomes insufficient, for whatever reason, anginal complaints indicate the hypoxic state, with it's characteristic radiation to the neck and left arm, and the retrosternal squeezing pain, dyspnea, and tachycardia. Signs of myocardial ischemia can be seen on the ECG. These symptoms often precede sudden death, which may follow either ventricular fibrillation or coronary occlusion.

A significant part of the cases of sudden cardiac death have occurred following *coronary occlusion.* Rarely an embolism of a coronary branch or Buerger's disease may be the cause. *Robertson* et al published the cases of 889 patients, died suddenly following myocardial infarction. The mean age of the 687 man was 60 ± 11 years, and the 202 women 68 ± 13 years. Among the predisposing factors where systemic hypertension, angina pectoris and diabetes mellitus. The increased heart weight was the highest in the chronic congestive heart failure group of the patients.

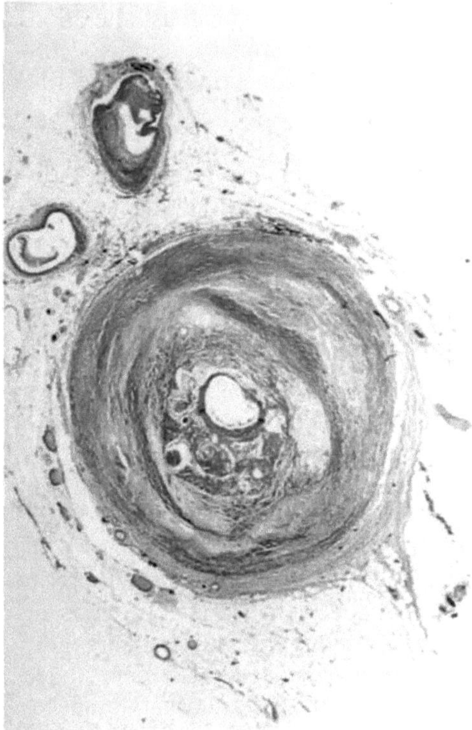

Fig. 118. Recanalization signs in a chronically obstructed coronary artery

The most common location of coronary occlusion is the anterior descending branch of the left coronary followed by the right circumflex artery. More rarely the left circumflex branch is occluded. Closure most commonly occurs over an exulcerated atheromatous plaque. When newly formed it causes a deep red, friable clot which can be easily extracted from the vessel lumen, or may fall out during a careless autopsy. For this reason it is necessary to section the coronaries at 2–3 mm. intervals. Later the clot turns greyish-red and shows signs of organization, vessel buds and fibroblasts from the surface of the intima begin to penetrate the area of the thrombus, fixing it to the vessel wall, and recanalization processes ensue *(Fig. 118)*.

One may often find such chronic thrombi in the areas of fresh occlusions, as well. Depending upon the location of the closure of the coronaries, an infarct may occur in various locations in the heart. In the case of an anterior ventricular or interventricular septal infarct, we will find the occlusion in the left anterior descending branch. A right coronary occlusion results in a posterior wall infarct, and the closure of the left circumflex branch results in myocardial infarction at the side of the left ventricle. With a fresh occlusion *(Fig. 119, 120)* which causes a significant portion of sudden death cases we often can not see any significant morphological alteration with the naked eye, in the cases of early death. Even with submicroscopic examinations we may not be able to differentiate postmortal muscle damage. Six to eight hours following the occlusion, with a macroscopic histochemical enzyme examination – decrease in lactate dehydrogenase, succinate dehydrogenase activity – the area of damaged myocardium can be demonstrated *(Fig. 121)*.

The first sign of an *infarct* is the swelling and due to the anemia, the damaged myocardium appears greyish-brown, more compact than the surrounding areas, this occurs 18–24 hours following the damage. This gives the infarct its characteristic pathological picture, sometimes the pathological age of the myocardial infarction can

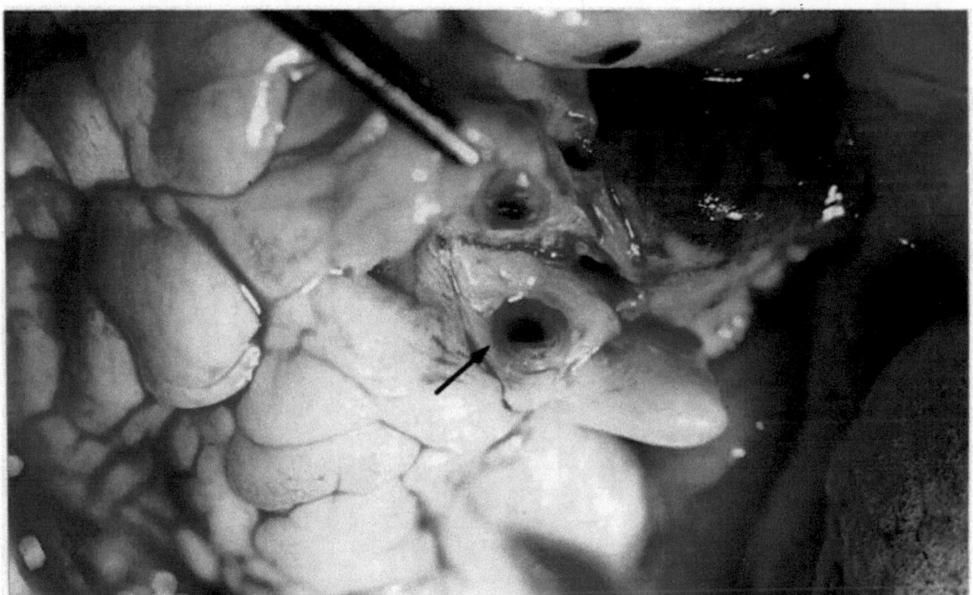

Fig. 119. Acute coronary obstruction

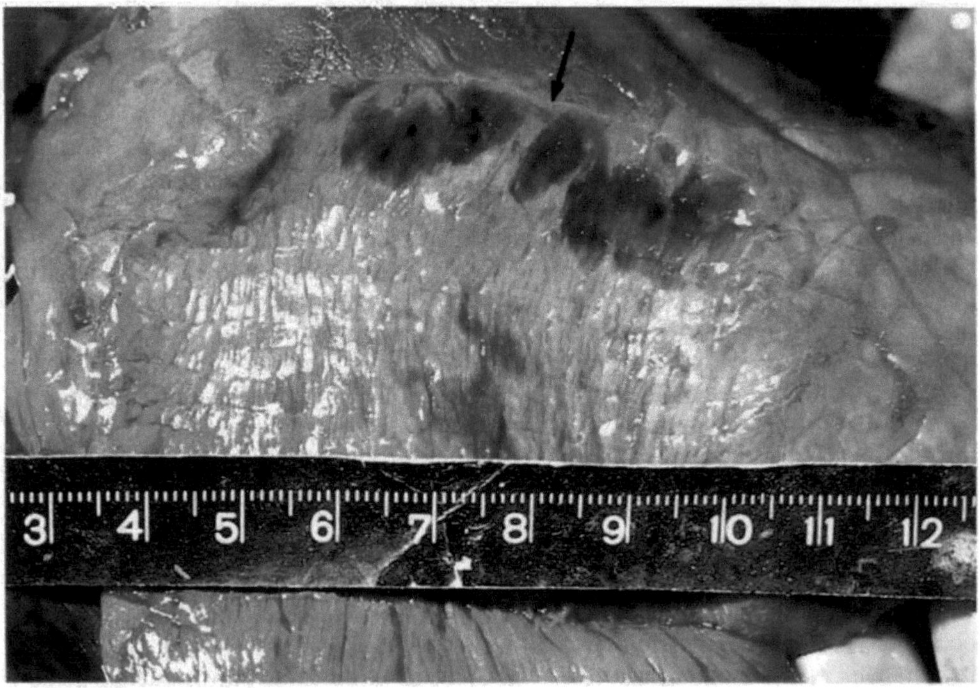

Fig. 120. Recent myocardial necrosis, clay-yellow necrotic area with marginal hemorrhages

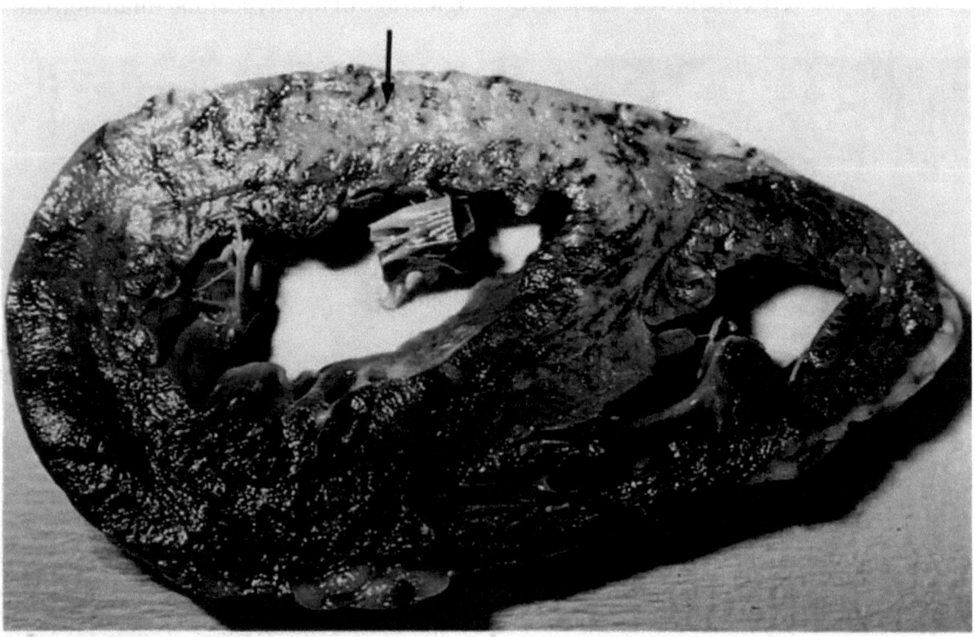

Fig. 121. Myocardial necrosis. Macrohistochemical reaction. Succinate-dehydrogenase staining. The light area indicates the necrotic myocardial tissue

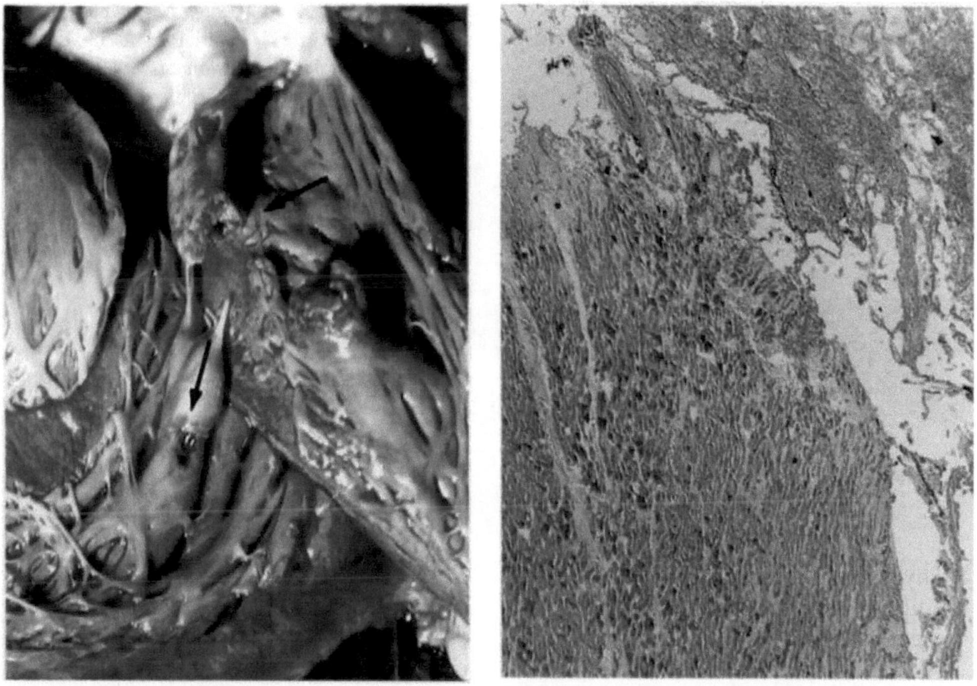

Fig. 122. Papillary muscle rupture. In the histological picture the necrotic myocardial tissue with homogeneous staining along with Endes trichrome staining the surface fibrin network, homogeneous necrotic myocardial fibers

not correlate with the clinical age. The clinical signs appear younger then the age of pathological alterations alone.

The damaged myocardium is clay yellow, marginated by a hemorrhagic zone. The surface of the infarcted area is covered a thin layer of fibrin. Histologically, the muscle tissue of the infarction undergoes coagulative necrosis, hemorrhage may appear in the peripheral areas, with numerous leukocytes. A few days later macrophages appear and fibroblasts begin to invade from the periphery, showing organization of the damaged area. The myocardium is replaced weeks or months later by a scar tissue. In the infarcted area after a few days leukocytes and macrophages phagocyte the damaged muscle fibers, and in the course of proteolysis (myomalacia cordis) the heart or a papillary muscle may rupture, causing pericardial tamponade, and/or sudden cardiac failure *(Fig. 122)*. Following a fresh myocardial infarction, the resulting ventricular fibrillation may be responsible for the sudden death. At other times cardiogenic shock or left ventricular insufficiency may be behind the sudden death and acute pulmonary edema may accompany the death. Later complications may be; aneurysm, mural thrombosis, embolisation, late conduction disturbances and reinfarction causing sudden death.

Myocarditis

Inflammatory changes to the myocardium may lie behind part of the incidences of sudden death with previous arrhythmias or

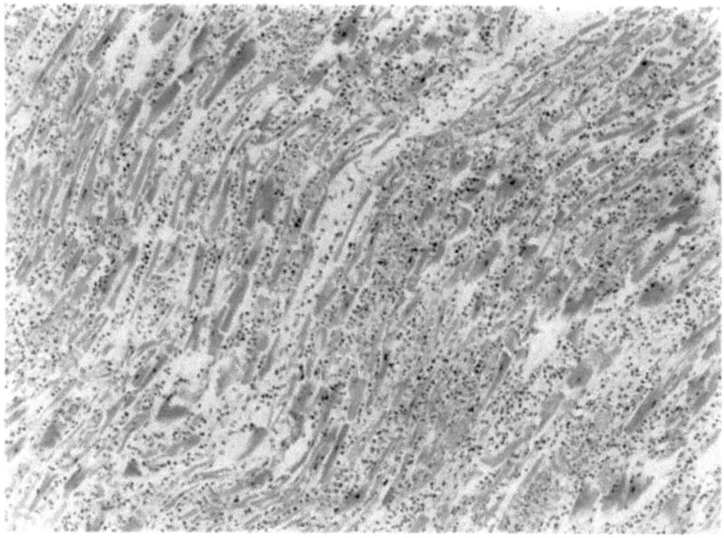

Fig. 123. Autopsy material of a 33-year-old women with viral myocarditis. Extensive infiltration by lymphocytes and macrophages

tachycardia. Myocarditis is not a common finding in general autopsies. It occurs in sudden death cases with an incidence of 7–9.2%. Besides bacterial and viral infections, various toxic processes can bring about inflammatory changes as well. In cases of sudden death all acute and chronic forms must be considered. Acute myocarditis, like other inflammatory processes, is characterized by myocardial necrosis and leukocyte infiltration. It may be the result of a general bacteremia or pyemia, or may spread directly from an inflamed valve to the cardiac muscle. Isolated inflammatory alteration is a rare form which may bring about focal myocardial necrosis and an infiltration of macrophages, eosinophilic leukocytes, lymphocyte plasma cells with giant cells *(Fiedler type giant cell myocarditis)*. Over the last decade there has been an increase in the number of such publications which suggest the possibility of viral infections and their consequences in the cases of cardiac death of unknown causes *(Fig. 123)*.

These occur more commonly among health workers who deal with Coxackie or Echo viruses caused diseases. In the myocardium, besides interstitial edema, lymphocyte and macrophage infiltration can be found, and later, due to the damage of the conduction system, the appearance of arrhythmias can be expected. Myocardial damage is known to accompany certain infectious diseases. Of special significance are the forms following diphtheria or pneumoccocal pneumonia, but toxic myocardial damage can be expected following a serious bacterial infection. Coagulation necrosis is the characteristic histo- morphological picture with leukocytes, macrophages and lymphocytes seen around the damaged area. The healing may occur with focal fibrosis, commonly with damage to the conduction system resulting in functional disturbances.

Cardiomyopathy

In a part of the cases of sudden death, aside from hypertrophy and dilatation of the heart, other findings of value are not uncovered. Hypoxic myocardial damage, hypertension, pulmonary hypertension, valvular disease or toxic damage may be behind the cardiomyopathy. In the other cases the hypertrophic obstructive cardiomyopathy may be familiar condition with a risk of sudden death. Similarly the familiar occurrence of the right ventricular dysplasia in the surviving members of the families was observed ventricular arrhythmias with the left bundle branch block.

The myocardial changes may be hypertrophic, which asymmetrically enlarge the heart. Besides the above-mentioned causes, the factors which disturb of cardiac output – subvalvular aortic stenosis, chronic embolism of the pulmonary artery – may also play a role. The alteration often appears as a cause of sudden death.

- A 58-year-old male foreigner had been a patient in the Cardiology Department in his country two years before his death due to a "myocardial infarction". For two years he had been practically symptom-free when suddenly he died. Autopsy revealed an organized chronic thrombus situated at the junction of the first branching of the pulmonary artery, an enormously enlarged right ventricle with a hypertrophic musculature and diffuse focal fibrosis. The infarct which had been diagnosed two years before had actually been an acute embolism.

If the heart dilatation is significant, we can count on a relative valvular insufficiency, congestion of the upstream areas, with induration. The alteration shows a familiar pattern. Besides the diffuse focal fibrosis, the histological findings reveal a hypertrophic hyperplasia of the myocardial fibers with an increased glycogen content.

In the case of *congestive cardiomyopathies,* a similar familiar occurrence is also found. Among the etiological factors, events leading to thromboembolism can be mentioned. A dilated ventricle dominates the autopsy findings, with the myocardium appearing paler, friable, edematous and with fine fibrosis and with the formation of mural thrombi. In numerous incidences previous alcoholism plays a role.

Obliterative cardiomyopathy caused mostly by endocardial alterations, with the myocardium being less affected. In the case of endomyocardial fibrosis there are connective tissue changes in the endocardium, together with the underlying muscular layer also being affected by fibrosis, damaging the myocardial function resulting in an incomplete ventricular emptying, thus results an atrial dilatation without accompanying ventricular hypertrophy. Subendocardial fibroelastosis causes a similar alteration which occurs in infants and children. A milky-white thick opaque endocardium in the area of the left ventricle and on the valves can be seen *(Fig. 124).*

Idiopathic hypertrophic subaortic stenosis is an uncommon developmental abnormality. A fibrotic ring, or a built up thickened muscle pad, or some combination of the two, impairs the emptying of the left ventricle. Bacterial endocarditis may cause not only cardiomyopathy, but hemodynamic changes as well. A major portion of these changes have gone undiagnosed during the life of the patients.

Disease of conduction system

In those instances of death in which the autopsy findings do not explain the cause of sudden death, a special macro- and microscopical-examination of the conduction system is warranted. As already mentioned, in sudden death, a significant

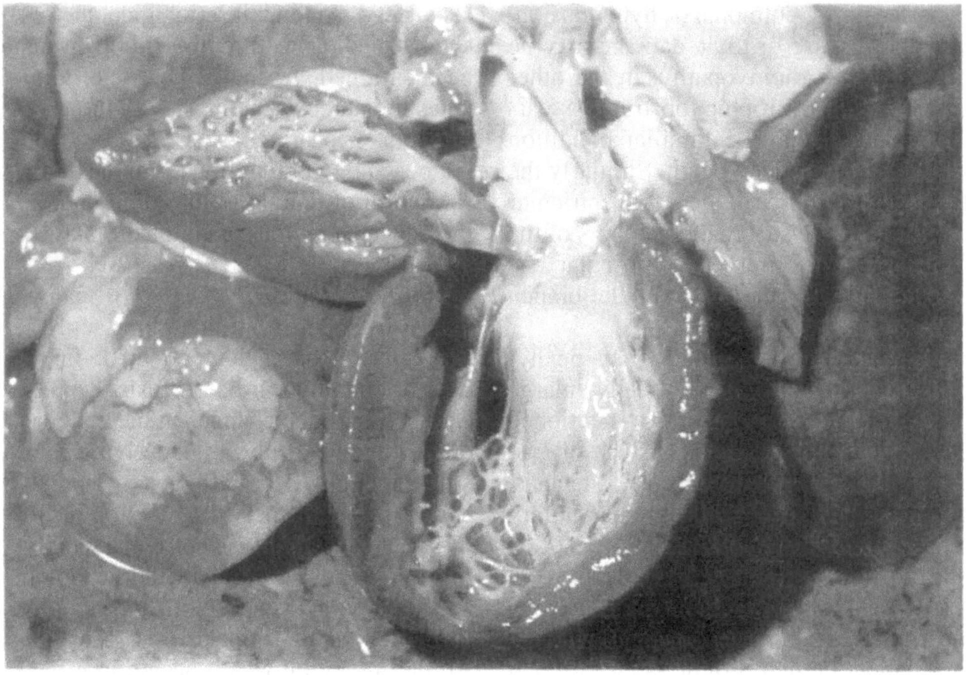

Fig. 124. Result of subendocardial fibroelastosis with ventricular septal defect (case of sudden infant death)

number of the cases stem from rhythm disturbances or conduction blocks which are fatal. These deaths often occur in the absence of any clinical signs or complaints, so there is no preliminary data to rely on. *Hypoxic damage,* whether from sclerotic coronary disease or insufficient blood supply to the sino-atrial node, will result in scarring of the impulse-generating node, which can be easily seen histologically. A similar scarring may form in the atrio-ventricular node or in the area of the bundle of His. Not uncommonly do the above pathological pictures figure into cases of sudden death in young people. Besides the scarring, functional disturbances may also result from the *edema* or *fatty infiltration* in these areas. In the cases of sudden death in young athletes, more than one instance has been explained by the *chronic narrowing or embolism of sino-atrial artery.* In scarring of the sino-atrial node in youth, sometimes hyperplasia of the media of the nodal artery and intimal proliferation can be seen. Embolism may often originate from the microembolisation of the coronary artery, which later in life may develop from a subintimal atheromatous plaque, or may originate from similar alterations in the aorta.

The repolarization changes are commonly occurred following cerebrovascular alterations, after stroke, subarachnoideal haemorrhage, or epilepsy. Behind these forms of cardiac arrhythmias is the insula controlled cardiac chronotropic organization, involved in the genesis of arrhythmias.

The circadian rhythm occurs not only in various biological phenomena, but it have also been noted in cardiac and cerebrovascular diseases e.g. sudden cardiac death or stroke.

Damage to the impulse-generating center or the conduction system may be the result of an *accident.* A strong blunt force to the thorax may result in a heart concussion and contusion, with consequent hemorrhage, the healing of which may occur with scarring. If the impulse-generating center or the conduction system lie near to the area, the temporary edema around the injury may result in arrhythmia lasting up-to several months, or various conduction disturbances, or AV-block.

- A 41-year-old man was the victim of a traffic accident as a passenger on a bus. Contusion injuries were inflicted about the thorax and a rhythm disturbance developed eight days following the accident which necessitated the implantation of a pacemaker. The cause of the arrhythmia was a complete AV-block.

Cases of delayed damage resulting in sino-atrial node degeneration *(fatty infiltration)* have been recorded years after the accident. Their connection can be traced back to the accident.

Scarring of the sino-atrial node may be not only from the above-mentioned reasons, but also as a result of focal *inflammatory alterations.* Sudden death may ensue in the acute stage of inflammation as well. At other times tumorous infiltration of the impulse-generating center or the impulse-conducting bundles has been the cause of sudden death.

Sudden death due to vascular disease

Vascular alterations dictate the outcome of a significant portion of cardiovascular diseases. Of the etiological factors tabulated to date, nutritional disturbances hold first place. The *narrowing of the vascular lumen,* whether from sclerotic disease or the consequence of inflammatory changes not only results in damage to the tissue fed by the vessel, but also exerts general or distant effects, such as embolization or "liberation" of toxic substances from necrotic areas. The most common alteration is sclerosis of the vessels. The pathological details and characteristic picture on autopsy is well- known. We have discussed the role of coronary sclerosis in sudden death in detail. In the great vessels, the formation of small plaques can be demonstrated in young people, which then consist of hyaline connective tissue and subintimal proliferation of smooth muscle with lipoid deposits between the fibers. Later deeper necrosis forms where here, next to unstructured tissue debris, deposits of lipoid and cholesterol appear and then calcium deposits, which cause the stiff, pipe-like form of the vessel. Around the alterations leukocytes and macrophages may also appear, the latter containing phagocytized lipid droplets and cholesterol crystals. Due to the damage to the internal elastic membrane, the process may spread to the media. Macroscopically, plaques of exulcerated debris can be seen on the internal surface of the aorta, which may form mural thrombi in their neighborhood. These may sometimes result in complete obliteration, or the closure of a distal narrower vessel due to an embolism from a broken off mural clot. If the vessel feeds a vital structure (coronary or brain vessels), it may cause sudden death. In the territory of the *weakened vessel,* an *aneurysm may develop* which differs from those due to developmental abnormalities partly histologically and partly because of its localization and form. *Rupture of the dilated vessel* wall can cause bleeding to death. Places of predilection are the abdominal aorta, which causes retroperitoneal bleeding, and the thoracic aorta. Similar aorta aneurysms may form due to *syphilitic damage* to the aorta. Here the damage affects the media in which extensive scarring and chronic infiltration of inflammatory cells are seen, while in the area of the vasa-vasorum obliterative inflammatory proocess can be seen. The most pronounced alteration is seen in the ascending aorta and it is the common place the arteriosclerotic aneurysm. In the sac of the aneurysm mural thrombi may form which may cause embolism *(Fig. 125).*

Dissecting aneurysms may appear on the ascending portion of the aorta, their etiology, besides hypertension, includes degenerative changes to the media (medianecrosis idiopathica cystica) or Marfan's

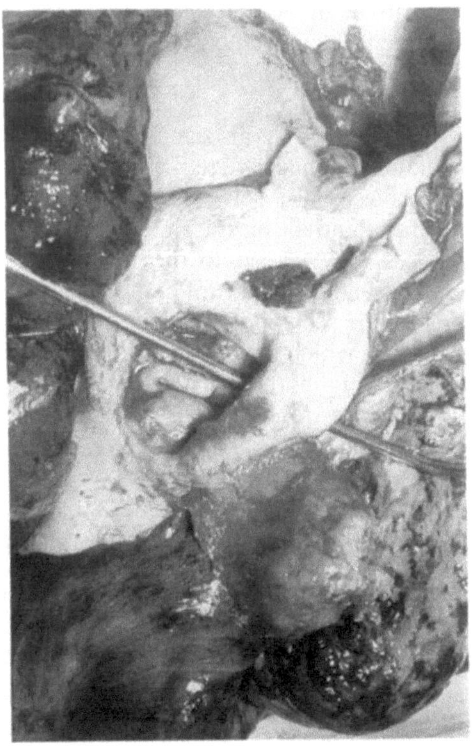

Fig. 125. **Sudden death due to rupture of a dilated sclerotic aorta**

syndrome. In the damaged area the aortic wall is damaged such that blood in the depths of the media separates the layers of the aorta so that a double channel forms which can be followed usually in the abdominal, and more rarely, in the femoral arteries. Death occurs either from compression of the coronary branches, or from shock or bleeding.

We have already discussed the aneurysm alterations of the vessels of the brain and their consequences of subarachnoidal hemorrhage.

Among the diseases of the vessels which can cause sudden death, we could mention periarteritis nodosa, which when localized in the coronaries may cause sudden death.

Thrombosis in the venous system and the accompanying pulmonary embolism plays a role in 5% of the cases of sudden death *(Fig. 126).* Places of predilection include the deep veins of the lower extremity and the periprostatic venous network in men, but after delivery, thrombosis may originate from the pelvic vessels of women, too. We may meet a discrete pulmonary embolism from the thrombotic hemorrhoidal plexus, as well. Sometimes the first sign of peripheral venous thrombosis is a pulmonary embolism. Finding the place from which the thrombus broke away is not always easy. In the elderly, in chronic congestion illnesses requiring lengthy bed rest, fractures of the extremities or occasionally rough soft tissue injuries we can count on their appearance. If the embolization stems from a branch of a large vein, a so-called *saddle thrombus* may close the pulmonary artery at a main bifurcation causing acute right heart insufficiency. The closure of smaller branches of the pulmonary artery may be relatively symptomless, but if congestion of the systemic circulation is avoided, a so-called red infarct forms.

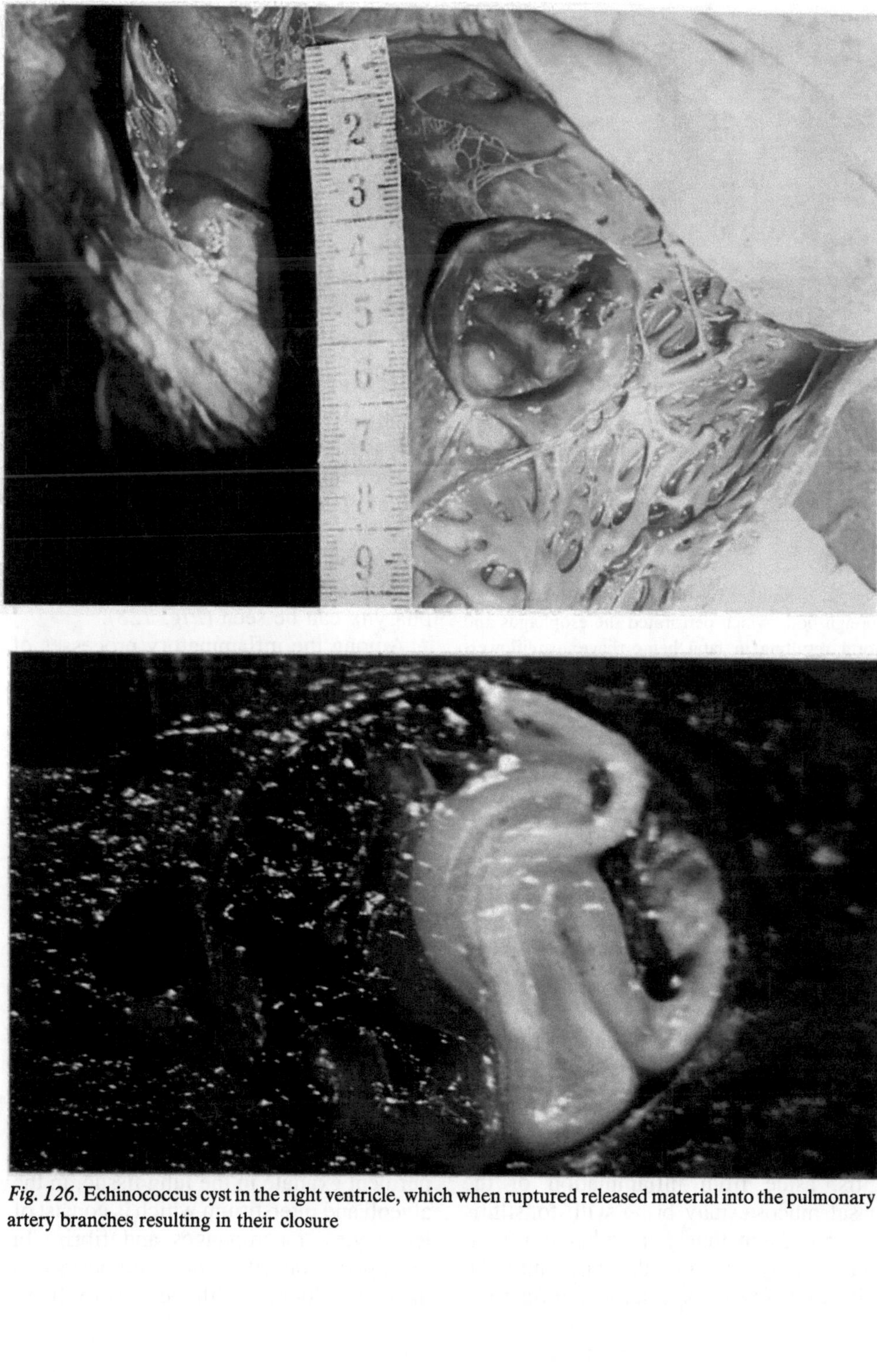

Fig. 126. Echinococcus cyst in the right ventricle, which when ruptured released material into the pulmonary artery branches resulting in their closure

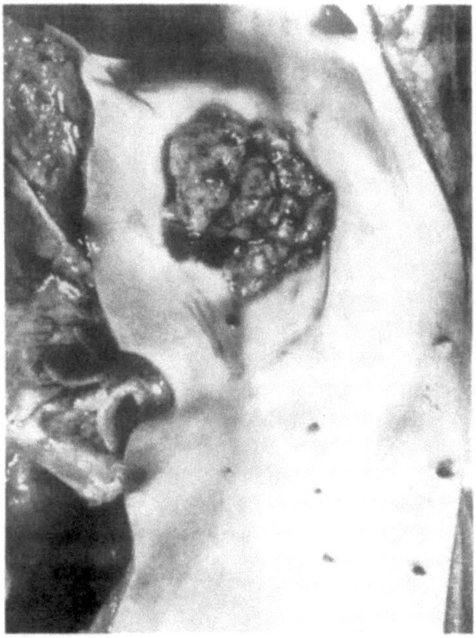

Fig. 127. Sudden death due to swallowing of a foreign body which perforated the esophagus and aorta resulting in fatal hemorrhage; cauliflower-shaped thrombus in the intima of the aorta

(Thrombosis or embolism in the area of the portal vein cause the so-called *Zahn infarcts.*)

Alterations of the respiratory system causing sudden death

Alterations of the respiratory system causing sudden death may be of inflammatory origin, caused by acute upper airway obstruction, processes obstructing excursion of the lungs, and the inhalation of foreign substances. Among the *inflammatory diseases,* infantile nasopharyngitis, aside from inflammation of the nasal mucosa, may bring with tonsillitis as well. Edematous, hemorrhagic inflammation may constrict the nasal mucosa, with high fever, especially if inflammation of the tonsils is the salient feature of the process. Owerfeeded-obese children often precedes sudden death in infants. In autopsy it is necessary to intentionally open the sinuses to examen of the nasal mucosa according to Genersich. With *Haemophilus influenzae* infection tracheitis subglottica develops relatively rarely, but its occurrence and recognition is still important because its rapid progress can bring about death in a matter of hours. Not only the local effects, but the serious toxicosis is also a part of the disease's course. The autopsy picture is one of a swollen pharynx, inflammation of the mucosa of the epiglottis with hemorrhages in the lung tissue, micropneumonia foci and an intense edema of the brain. Histologically, an intense edema and diffuse acute infiltration of inflammatory cells into the epiglottis and the area of the pharynx can be seen *(Fig. 128).*

Among the inflammatory processes of the lung, *bronchopneumonia,* and rarely *lobar pneumonia,* can be found in cases of sudden death. Lobar pneumonia is a frequent, intercurrent disease of alcoholics or chronic drug users, and those in very poor condition. Of the bronchopneumonias we often see confluent bronchopneumonia. In the lung tissue we find a diffuse dark red massive friable area not confined to the borders of the lobes, in which the various stages of inflammation can be demonstrated. On part may be abscessed while another part on the periphery may show the early signs of inflammation. Pus may press out from the bronchioles. In the central part of the alteration, a bronchus or bronchiole containing acute inflammatory elements may be seen surrounded by a purulent exudate in the lung tissue, in the alveoli and interstitium which is consist of leukocytes, macrophages and fibrin. In lobar pneumonia the process is confined to the lobe or lobule. With the age of inflam-

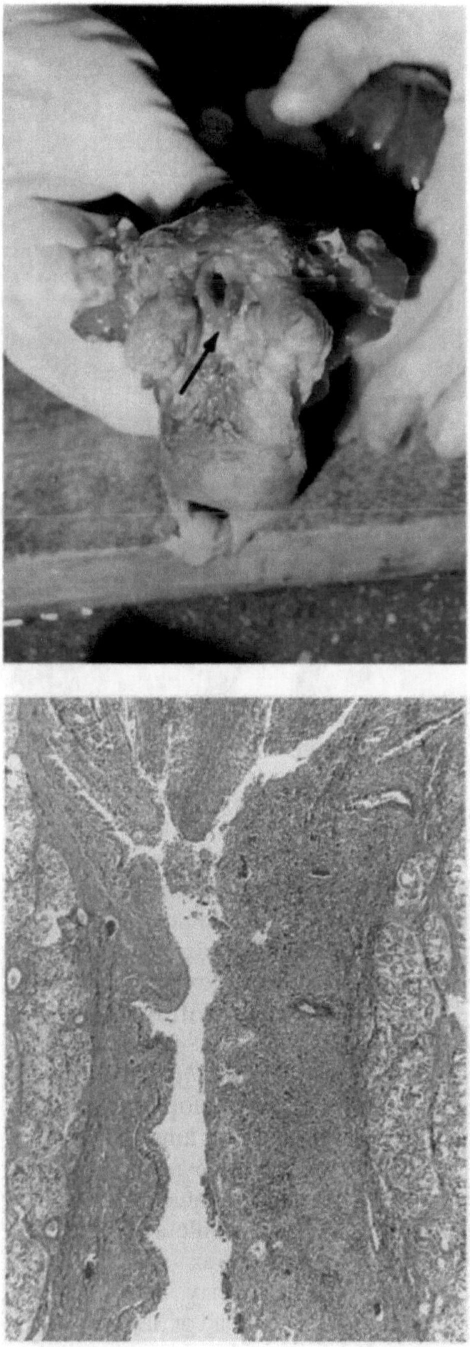

Fig. 128. **Diffuse, acute infiltration of inflammatory cells; subglottic tracheitis; edematous constriction of the tracheal opening**

mation the morphological picture of the inflammatory process is variable. In the early stages – 1–2 days – the lung tissue is heavy, reddish, bulky and friable. Microscopically in the pulmonary capillaries are stasis, edema, leukocytes and erythrocytes are seen in the alveoli. After 2–4 days the lung changes to a liver-like texture with a fibrinous exudate on the pleural surface, and upon section the lung appears dark red, friable, airless and finely granulated. In the alveoli, red blood cells, many neutrophilic leukocytes and a fine fibrin meshwork appear. After 4–8 days the process continues into the so-called *grey hepatization stage.* The lung is heavy, bulky, with an expressed inflammatory process on the pleural surface. On section the tissue is greyish-red, friable, homogeneous, and finely granulated. In the alveoli we can see fibrin, leukocytes and alveolar phagocytes. After eight days the inflammatory macrophages appear in great numbers, phagocytizing the fibrin which is subsequently digested by fibrinolytic enzymes. The lung is greyish-red and friable, and healing can take place within 20–30 days. The process may resolve without destruction, with the rare consequence of exudative organization. Due to the carnification process the lung may contain parts with a texture like that of muscle, with homogeneously staining fibrous tissue seen in the alveoli in place of the exudate. The process may cause sudden death years later as a result of chronic cor pulmonale.

The inflammatory processes due to *influenza infection* begin with necrotic, hemorrhagic alterations in the trachea and bronchi. At the place of necrosis, a lymphocyte infiltration of the mucous membranes and submucosa can be shown, mixed with few leukocytes. If the process spreads further, macroscopic hemorrhages in the tissue of the lung may be seen.

Edema, bleeding and fibrin forming inflammation signify influenzal bronchopneumonia, which is mainly accompanied by alveolar and interstitial infiltration of leukocytes and macrophages. The process often leads to sudden death. At other times, infection by *Staphylococcus or Streptococcus* leading to necrotizing tracheobronchitis may cause bronchopneumonial complications. We may find the more rare forms of inflammatory alterations in the practice of forensic medicine. Thus we have seen cryptogenic fibrotic alveolitis and desquamative interstitial pneumonia, although infantile interstitial pneumonia is not a rare finding in the autopsy material in sudden death.

Among the alterations causing *acute upper airway obstruction,* of the greatest significance is laryngeal edema. The loose connective tissue of the laryngeal submucosa in the area of the vocal cords is capable of accumulating significant quantities of interstitial fluid. Trauma or allergic inflammation and other related factors may trigger a mild inflammatory process localized to this area. The development of acute edema may cause acute airway obstruction and suffocation. Postmortally, the edema "disappears" quite rapidly and in many cases the wrinkled, slack condition of the mucous membranes is all that marks the previous process. The edema is recognizable in the vocal cords for a relatively longer period of time, histologically the submucosa is loose with eosinophils among the fibers in the extracellular fluid.

Although acute airway closure may happen, it is much more likely that sudden death will result from a reflex effect when a piece of food is inhaled *(bolus death) (Fig. 129).* The bolus – a piece of a swallowed food – lying in the piriform recess stimulates the vagus nerve which can then cause cardiac arrest. If the appropriate care is not administered during the removal of the neck structures at autopsy, the inhaled foreign body may fall out. Especially common is the bolus death in an alcoholic intoxicated state, due to the reduced gag reflex.

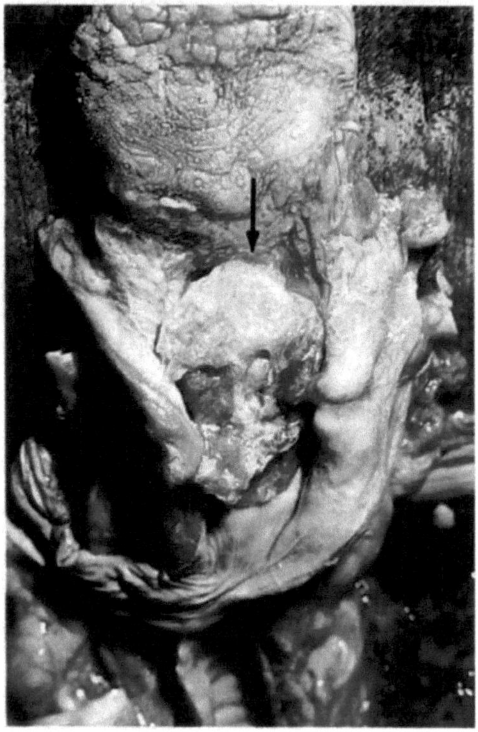

Fig. 129. Impaction of a bite of fodd

Restricted excursion of the lungs may come about as a result of unilateral or acute bilateral *pneumothorax* (PTX). It may appear due to developmental abnormalities – i.e. polycystic lung -, or in adult or old age bullous emphysema. If the alteration is bilateral, a quick *suffocation* may result in death, while a spontaneous unilateral pneumothorax with previous circulatory disease may cause sudden death due to the overload of the circulatory system. If we consider this a possibility during autopsy, we should purposely introduce water into the thorax by use of a thick needle and syringe. The bubbling air signifies the presence of PTX. (Caution! The process of decay may give a false positive.) Another clue is if the lungs are found collapsed by the sides of the spinal column at autopsy. It can especially be seen if we fill the thorax with water, inflate the lungs and look for escaping bubbles at the place of the injured pleura. Thus it can be differentiated from the similar-looking spontaneous pneumothorax from collapse due to senile atrophy of the lung tissue.

Sudden death may also be caused by *aspiration* of material into the lung tissue. Aspiration of stomach contents or vomit while in an unconscious or alcoholic state is a common occurrence. Not only the closure of the airway and suffocation, but a reflex cramp of the glottis in response to the acid material can not be neglected as causes of sudden death. Aspiration of stomach contents carries a characteristic morphological picture *(Fig. 130)*. The lung tissue is edematous, and hemorrhagic, with necrotic areas visible, rapid leukocyte infiltration develops and in the later stages of inflammation foreign body giant cells appear, signifying aspiration pneumonitis. Aspiration of blood may accompany tuberculosis of the lung or tumors, but it may also result in the rupture of dilated esophageal vessels. At other times the aorta may rupture into the airway.

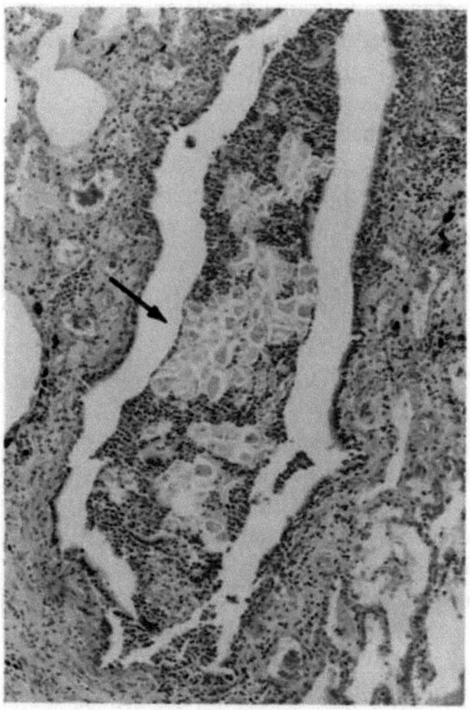

Fig. 130. Bronchiolitis following aspiration of a foreign body, areas of incipient micropneumonia

Asthma plays a role in some cases of sudden death in youth. Death may occur in the course of asthmatic status or chronic cor pulmonale due to acute right heart insufficiency. During an asthmatic attack in the case of sudden death the autopsy picture may be characteristic. The lung is inflated, and fills the thorax, and on section a tough, glassy, mucoid substance press out. Histologically, the bronchioles are filled with a mesh-like basophil staining mucous substance in which, besides fragments of degenerated bronchial epithelia, eosinophil leukocytes can be seen. In the bronchial submucosa a similar infiltration of eosinophilic cells can be seen together with engorgement of blood.

Diseases of the abdominal organs causing sudden death

A profuse hemorrhage and death can occur from rupture of *dilatated* esophageal *veins* – most commonly the result of portal hypertension due to cirrhosis of the liver –, *esophageal ulcer,* or swallowing of a foreign body. Similar hemorrhage can cause sudden death in alterations accompanying acute gastric ulcer and the *opening of an irregular artery* in the mucosa or in the area of a chronic ulcer because of the *arrosion* a vessel lies superficially *(Fig. 131).*

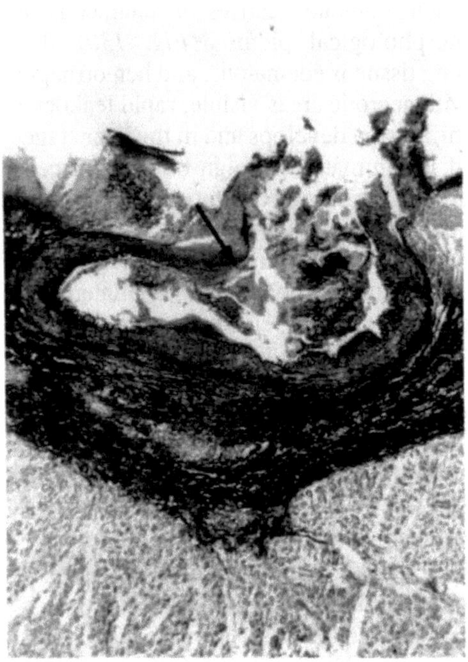

Fig. 131. Sudden death due to rupture of the caliber persistent artery of the gastric mucosa

Thrombosis or embolism of the artery or branches of the mesenteric vein in the territory of the small or large intestine can cause sudden death, depending on the location. Most commonly a thrombosis or embolism occurring in the area of the superior mesenteric artery can result in *small bowel hemorrhagic necrosis.* Sudden death can be explained partially from shock, partially from the absorption of toxic material released from the necrotic parts. Later peritonitis can develop from the effect of the bacteria crossing the necrotic bowel wall.

Sudden death can result form acute enteritis during infancy with *Salmonella paratyphi* infection, but it can similarly result from electrolyte loss due to the vomiting and diarrhea from common *E. coli* infections. At other times sudden death may result from *intestinal twisting* due to volvulus or invagination. Of the abdominal organs whose alterations can lead to sudden death, *acute hemorrhagic pancreatitis* must be mentioned. Previous alcoholism, gall stones and obesity play roles in the bile reflux into the duct of Wirsung. Rarely, a previous trauma is postulated. In the autopsy findings upon opening the abdomen a bloody ascites is found on the peritoneum, the mesenterium is yellowish-white with soapy areas to be found which give a positive Benda reaction (the area turns blue on exposure to copper acetate). The pancreas is edematous, hemorrhagic, enlarged, bulky, and the tissue can hardly be recognized on section due to the bleeding. Histologically, necrosis and acute inflammatory infiltration can be seen.

Bleeding from *rupture of the spleen* can cause sudden death, the *spontaneous* form being quite rare, however in diseases associated with enlargement of the spleen – malaria, typhus, leukemia – a mild previous trauma can be a probable cause. With bleeding into the retroperitoneal space especially in the elderly we must consider rupture of the abdominal aorta.

Diseases of the central nervous system causing sudden death

Alterations in the central nervous system make up one of the largest groups of the causes of sudden death. The natures of the diseases are differentiated into those causing sudden death in *youth* and those of *older age. Increase in intracranial pressure* in the young may stem from congenital hydrocephalus internus or may be a result of Arnold-Chiarri malformation. Death may result from tonsillar herniation with damage to the respiratory and vasomotor centers, or may follow a mild fever state as well. For similar reasons we may find sudden death in diseases with early ossification of the sutures of the skull. The characteristic autopsy sign of which is the ossification of the sutures at the age of around 16-18. On the internal layer of the skull the impressions of the vessels and gyri are pronounced, and in the process the so-called compensatory area is significantly restricted and sudden death may result from compression of the medulla during a rather mild fever. (The *compensatory area* is the liquor-filled territory between the brain and the skull, which due to either extracerebral or intracerebral expansive processes, allows a certain area for the growth of a tumor, bleeding, or edema. As the liquor area becomes restricted, the amount of partly the ventricular and partly the subarachnoid liquor decreases, and is due in part to the decrease of the blood volume of the cerebral veins. If the compensatory area becomes restricted, a slight infectious process or feverish state can lead to death by tonsillar herniation.)

Stroke is the most common condition of the central nervous system that leads to sudden death. The bleeding occurs in the area of the internal capsule from the rupture of the arteria lenticulo striata, or from its microaneurysm. Hypertension or arteriosclerosis plays a preliminary role. In elderly patients it is more common for the hemorrhage to be damaging in character, forming a cavity filled with blood and damaged brainfragments in the cavity around which edema and streaked hemorrhagic infiltrations can be seen. The affected hemisphere is swollen with the gyri over the hemorrhage flattened out, and the brain fluctuates. The hemorrhage often breaks into the lateral ventricle causing haemocephalus internus, and may escape into the subarachnoid space as well. Death comes from either destruction of vital areas or increased intracranial pressure and tonsillar herniation. The hemorrhage may also be localized to the territory of the pons or the cerebellum. With a mild pontine hemorrhage hyperpyrexia may ensue affecting the pyramidal tract and death follows quite quickly *(Fig. 132)*.

The spontaneous form of *subarachnoidal*

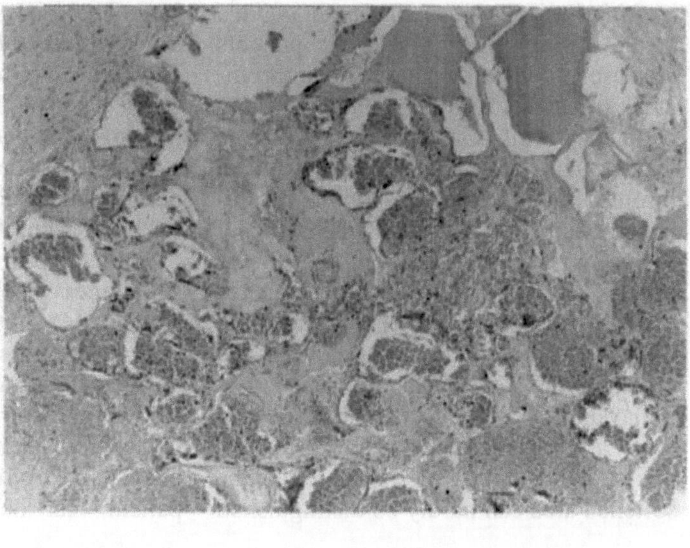

Fig. 132. Hemangioma in the brain

hemorrhage may be explained by arterial *aneurysm* alterations. The most common location is at the division of the middle cerebral artery. Bleeding into the area of the fossa Sylvii is the most significant, the effect of the middle cerebral artery being followed by the anterior cerebral artery and the posterior cerebral artery. Hemorrhage breaks into the subarachnoidal space forming a thick perivascular mass at the base of the brain, and finding the distended vessel in there is not always easy. The hemorrhage may intrude into the substance of the brain as well, mimicking an apoplectiform picture. Death is often due to the follows compression of the medulla. Sometimes the connection between subarachnoidal hemorrhage and trauma may cause problems for the examiner. The cases of sudden death from a ruptured aneurysm following a blow or the sudden rise in blood pressure from excitement cannot be left out. The rise in blood pressure may be a reason for rupture of previous aneurysms. Establishing the connection requires great care, if we emphasize in the opinion the previous special physical state.

Thrombosis of the vessels of the brain or *embolism* play a small part in sudden death. Mainly elderly, sclerotic patients are susceptible, but we have found thrombosis in cases of sudden death of young people as well. ÖKRÖS emphasized the significance of sudden death from a thrombosis of the carotid syphon. Thromboembolisms to the area of the circle of Willis most often find their way to the middle cerebral artery. The consequence of the occlusion may be emollient brain tissue, there may be bleeding into the emollient area, red malacia forms, and so it may appear similar to a stroke. *Cerebral infarction* as a result of thrombosis or embolism of the cerebral arteries the start of the softened area can hardly be distinguished from its surroundings, with it becoming more pronounced after 24 hours and histologically well delimited. Around the infarcted area edema forms which may raise the intracranial pressure. Sometimes *embolism* occurs during a heart operation, air embolism having been described, but tissue embolism can also occur. Recognition of the alteration at autopsy is simple in the case of red malacia. The fresh occlusions sometimes it is easier to recognize in fixed brain tissue *(Fig. 133)*.

Sudden death following *inflammation* of the pia mater is relatively rare. The infection that spreads from an *inflammation* of the sinuses or the inner ear to the pia mater may be of bacterial or viral origin. With meningococcus infection previous inflammations of the nose and throat may be the source and with meningococcus sepsis death may ensue within hours. The autopsy picture is characteristic, with diffuse pinpoint hemorrhages on the skin and bleeding into the adrenal cortex being manifest. In the early stages a cloudy exudate appears in the subarachnoidal space which turns purulent. In this stage death occurs due to increased intracranial pressure. The process in the inner ear sometimes results only in circumscribed meningitis, but may also form an abscess in the brain. Sudden death due to tuberculous meningitis is hardly found these days.

The sudden death of an *epileptic patient* deserves special attention. It constitutes 1.22% of natural deaths. (The blood level of antiepileptic medications may vary, sometimes reaching a toxic level, and sometimes subtherapeutic.) Death occurring due to status epilepticus may be accidental during the course of the seizure (drowning, aspiration of vomit, fall from a height etc.). Another group of the cases we understand from the personal data of the patient that he was epileptic, but at

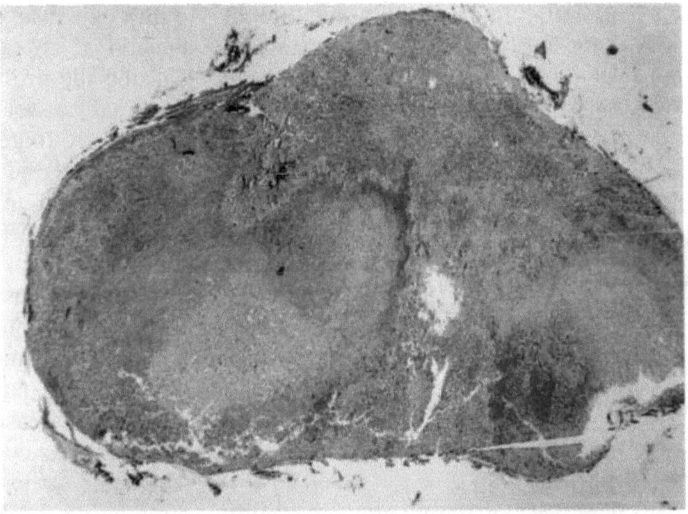

Fig. 133. Extensive hypophysial necrosis in a case of sudden death

autopsy of an acute occurrence we find no abnormalities. According to the literature this previous group makes up about one third of all epileptic cases. In the establishment of death the clinical preliminaries with a negative autopsy findings and negative toxicological examinations should be referred to. A large number of the cases of death occur while the patients are asleep. EEG examinations have verified that in the dreams of both grand mal and petit mal sufferers the spike and wave discharges grow at the beginning of dreams, continuously grow "to the stage of slow wave dreaming" and a pronounced decrease in discharge rate at the start of REM. The seizure can alter numerous autonomic functions, like the number of heartbeats, blood pressure, frequency of breaths, and vasomotor tone, so that bradycardia or transient cardiac arrest may occur. When death occurs during a grand mal epileptic seizure, the signs of death by suffocation dominate, with conjunctival hemorrhages, petechiae on the skin of the face and neck, bite injuries to the tongue, bloody saliva running from the mouth, the blood still fluid, passive engorgement of blood in the viscera, bleeding under the serous membranes, the lungs hyperinflated with edema, and edema of the brain. Histologically in the hippocampus the number of neurons is decreased, and fibrosis increased and the area macroscopically appears more massive with anassymmetry caused by scarring.

Tumors of the central nervous system are not a common cause of sudden death. Meningeoma, which are often an incidental finding on autopsy, do not cause an increase in intracranial pressure due to their slow growth rate. An ependymoma of the IV ventricle can lead to sudden death if it affects the respiratory and vasomotor centers. Sometimes the bleeding of metastatic tumors may cause tonsillar herniation.

Sudden infant death syndrome (SIDS)

This occurs in a previously healthy infant between the ages of one month and one year. According to the literature it is most common at three months between May and October. It is more rare in firstborns.

The infant is by definition healthy or almost healthy and the death remains a mystery even after a careful autopsy and histological and toxicological examination. The syndrome touches on heterogeneous diseases, each of which are capable of causing sudden death. Since the greater part of the infants die in their sleep, the syndrome is also known as *crib death.* It has an occurrence of 1.5–2 per thousand live births among newborns.

SIDS is more likely in infants in whom the following prior conditions exist:

a) retarded intrauterine development, small birth weight,
b) manifest developmental retardation following birth,
c) being the second or later birth,
d) the mother smokes,
e) the infant is restless, tachypnea, tachycardia, prone to vomiting.

But it is held to be relevant in selecting the infants prone to sudden death that an occasional sign of value on the ECG is the lengthening of the QT segment, a prior apnoea state and cyanosis. Acute dehydration – diarrhea and vomiting – can lead to SIDS as well as electrolyte disturbances. Among the etiological factors an allergy to cow's milk, infections, parathyroid hypofunction, regurgitation of stomach contents, idiopathic prolonged apnoea states, and the mother taking barbiturates have been mentioned. The diversity of prior data and etiological factors do not make a pathological examination possible. According to Naeye the deviations found on autopsy can be grouped as the following:

a) In the pulmonary vessels, hyperplasia and hypertrophy of the media of the small arteries and arterioles occurs in approximately 60% of the cases. The process accompanies chronic hypoventilation of the lungs and a vicious circle develops with right heart hypertrophy and hypertension of the pulmonary arterial system causing the proliferation of the media of the small vessels.

b) A prolonged brown fatty degeneration around the adrenals, which can be demonstrated in 50% of the victims of SIDS, and an effective hypoxia for a prolonged period of time prior to death is one sign. Several instances have been accompanied by an abnormal enlargement of the adrenals with an elevated epinephrin level.

c) The hypoxic state explains the large number of cases in which persistent erythropoesis could be found in the liver. The state is explained by the hypoxia stimulating the kidneys to release erythropoetin.

d) A pronounced proliferation of astroglia in the reticular formation which is a consequence of chronic hypoxia.

A portion of the deceased show a hypoplasia of the glomus caroticum. The role of the glomus in the regulation of breathing is known. In infants with the poorly developed glomus caroticum, after a prolonged apnoea episode the infant is not capable of restarting breathing.

It is difficult to judge what comprises the alterations of sudden infant death syndrome, since each of them are characteristic of other individual diseases. Together with various examinations it is possible to satisfactorily define sudden infant death syndrome.

Sudden death in youth

Sudden death in youth can be comprised of various groups, the importance of which is not explained merely in that it affects young, apparently healthy individuals, but the cause of death occasionally has its own characteristics. Division by age may be misleading, as shown by the work of LUKE and HELPERN who dealt with analysis of the pathological findings in sudden death between the ages of 20–45, two decades later than the literature concerning those who died between the ages of 1–20. The cases of sudden death in young people tend to happen most commonly around the age of two, and least commonly around ages 10–12. They increase again between ages 15–20. Recognition of the autopsy material is best seen on a pathological basis rather than one of age, as the material of LUKE and HELPERN deals with the alterations more associated with age: coronary sclerosis, coronary occlusion, pulmonary embolism, pancreatitis, etc. and not mentioning those pathological pictures usually associated with the age at which sudden death in youth is characteristic. Among the cases of sudden death in youth we could list such diseases in which death occurs within 24 hours of the appearance of the first symptoms, but here such cases are also tabulated in which the patient died days after the first symptoms appeared, but was unconscious to the end. The decisive majority of the cases of sudden death in youth involve cardiovascular alterations followed by central nervous system diseases, then alterations of the respiratory system and finally damage to the gastrointestinal tract.

In the cardiovascular group the most common alteration is the acute-subacute myocarditis, but in a significant number of cases cardiomyopathic alterations also appear. Prolapse of the mitral valve is more frequent than believed and plays a role in several instances of sudden death associated with physical overwork or sports. The alterations not only involve lengthened chordae tendineae with the development of incomplete closure of the valve leaflets, but also ventricular arrhythmias caused by damage to the conduction system which can be verified histologically. Among the *developmental abnormalities,* anomalies of the origin and course of the coronaries can cause sudden death, but a role is also played by circulation loading caused by the juvenile form of *coarctation of the aorta.* Occasionally quite mild previous pathological alterations can result in serious clinical signs. Damage to the conduction systems lies behind numerous cases of sudden death of unknown, or from the autopsy picture hardly explainable, origin and sudden death can result from a ventricular tachyarrhythmia caused by a multifocal ectopic focus.

Among the alterations of the central nervous system in cases of sudden death in youth, one part belongs to the *rupture of aneurysms* of the vessels of the brain with a subsequent subarachnoidal hemorrhage. The process of inflammation of the pia mater, whether by pneumococcus or meningococcus sepsis, has a partial, though frequent significance, especially in childhood from an unrecognized infection of the inner ear. *Premature ossification of the bones of the skull* in young people can cause sudden death from restriction of the compensatory area.

Among the alterations of the respiratory organs in cases of death in youth, the number of cases of fulminate *tracheobronchitis* and *bronchopneumonia* is high, but a more frequent cause of sudden death is an asthmatic attack.

Sometimes such diseases can cause sudden death which by virtue of their rarity are overlooked at autopsy.

References

[1] Anderson, R. C.: Idiopathic mitral valve prolapse and sudden death. American Heart J. 100 (1980) 941–942

[2] Anderson, J. R.: MUIRU'S Textbook of Pathology. Edward Arnold LTD London (1985) pp. 15.1–15.45

[3] Arminger, L. C., W. M. I. Smeeton: Contraction-band necrosis: patterns of distribution in the myocardium and their diagnostic usefulness in sudden cardiac death. Pathology 18 (1986) 289–295

[4] Baccino, E., D. Le Goff, G. Lancien, M. Le Guillou, D. Alix, D. Mottier: Exploration of acid gastrooesophagial reflex by 24-H pH metry in infants at risk of sudden infant death syndrome. Forensic Sci. Int. 36 (1988) 255–260

[5] Bergevin, M. A., C. C. Daugherty, K. E. Bove, A. J. McAdams: The internal carotid artery syphon in children and adolescents. Hum. Pathol. 22 (1991) 603–606

[6] Bernier, R. H., J. A. Frank, T. J. Dondero, P. Turner: Diphtheria-tetanus toxoids-pertussis vaccination and sudden infant death in Tennessee. J. Pediatrics 101 (1982) 419–421

[7] Buris, L.: Oesophagus-Aorta Perforation durch einen Fremdkörper. Dtsch. Z. ges. gerichtl. Med. 56 (1965) 97–100

[8] Buris, L., Gy. Mester, T. Fülöp: Über die Spontanruptur des Papillarmuskels. Zacchia 41 (1966) 3–11

[9] Buris, L., Kiss S., Poczkodi S.: Hirtelen halál a koszorúsverőér ritka fejlődési rendellenessége miatt. Morf. és Ig. Orv. Szemle 19 (1979) 32–35

[10] Buris, L., S. Poczkodi, A. Gömöry: Embolism of hearth tissue to the middle cerebral arteriy as a complication of heartsurgery. Z. Rechtsmed. 83 (1979) 87–89

[11] Buris, L., Törőcsik I.: Primer pulmonalis hypertonia. Morph. és Ig. Orv. Szemle 22. (1982) 215–218

[12] Buris, L., P. Takács, M. Varga: Sudden death caused by hydatid embolism. Z. Rechtsmed. 98 (1987) 125–128

[13] Cabin, H. S., W. C. Roberts: Comparison of amount and extent of coronary narrowing by atherosclerotic plaque and myocardial scarring at necropsy in anterior and posterior healed transmural myocardial infarction. Circulation 66 (1982) 93–99

[14] Fernando, R.: Sudden unexpected death due to familial hypertrophic obstructive cardiomyopathy. Forensic Sci. Int. 46 (1990) 285–288

[15] Fowler, N. O.: Classification and differential diagnosis of the myocardiopathies. Progr. Cardiovasc. Dis. 7 (1968) 1–16

[16] Furlanello, F., R. Bettini, F. Cozzi, A. Del Favero, M. Disertori, G. Vergara, G. B. Durante, M. Guarnerio, G. Inama, G. Thiene: Ventricular arrhythmias and sudden death in athletes. Ann. N. Y. Acad. Sci. 427 ( ) 253–279

[17] Goodwin, J. F., H. Gordon, A. Hollman, M. B. Bishop: Clinical aspects of cardiomyopathy. Brit. Med. J. 1 (1961) 69–79

[18] Gormsen, H., A. Lund: The diagnostic value of postmortem blood glucose determinations in cases of diabetes mellitus. Forensic Sci. Int. 28 (1985) 103–107

[19] Guntheroth, W. G.: The QT interval and sudden infant death syndrome. Circulation 66 (1982) 502–503

[20] Hirsch, Ch. S., D. L. Martin: Unexpected death in young epileptics. Neurology 21 (1971) 682–690

[21] Hogg, J. C.: Pathology of asthma. Clin. Chest. Med. 5 (1984) 567–571

[22] Houghton, J. L.: Pericarditis and myocarditis. Which is benign and which isn't? Postgrad. Med. 91 (1992) 281–282

[23] Huser, C. J., J. E. Smialek: Diagnosis of sudden death infants due to acute dehydration. Am. J. Forensic Med. Pathol. 7 (1986) 278–282

[24] Iscovich, A. I.: Sudden cardiac death due to hypoglycemia. Am. J. Emerg. Med. 1 (1983) 28–29

[25] James, N. T.: Anatomy of human sinus node. Anat. Rec. 141 (1961) 109–141

[26] Kaplan, D. W., A. E. Bauman, H. F. Krous: Epidemiology of sudden infant death syndrome in american indians. Pediatrics 74 (1984) 1041–1046

[27] Lewin, D. C., J. T. Fallon: Significance of the angiographic morphology an localized coronary stenosis. Histopathologic correlations. Circulation 66 (1982) 316–320

[28] Luke, J. L., M. Helpern: Sudden unexpected death from natural causes in young adults. Arch. Path. 85 (1968) 10–17

[29] Metter, D.: Agonale Verletzungen beim plötzlichen naturlichen Tod. Beitr. Gerichtl. Med. 42 (1984) 139–142

[30] Miller, D. D., D. D. Waters, J. Szlachcic, P. Théroux: Clinical characteristics associated with sudden death in patients with variant angina. Circulation 66 (1982) 588–592

[31] Molz, G., H. P. Hartmann: Plötzlicher Sauglingstod, epidemiologische Erhebungen bei nicht, Teilweise oder hinrechend erklarbarer

Todesursache. Helv. Pediatr. Acta 39 (1984) 395–404

[32] Moore, A.: The sudden infant death syndrome. Br. J. Hosp. Med. 26 (1981) 37–45

[33] Mork, S. J., I. Morild, J. Chr. Giertsen: Subependymoma and unexpected death. Forensic Sci. Int. 30 (1986) 275–280

[34] Naeye, R. L.: Pulmonary arterial abnormalities in the sudden infant death syndrome. N. Engl. J. Med. 289 (1973) 1169–1170

[35] Naeye, R. L.: Sudden infant death. Scientific Am. 242 (1980) 56–62

[36] Neuspiel, D. R., L. H. Kuller: Sudden and unexpected natural death in childhood and adolescence. JAMA 254 (1985) 1321–1325

[38] Roberts, C. S., W. C. Roberts: Aortic dissection with entrance tear in the descending thoracic aorta. Ann. Surg. 213 (1991) 358–368

[38] De Sa, D. J.: Isolated myocarditis as a cause of sudden death in the first year of life. Forensic Sci. Int. 30 (1986) 113–117

[39] Sapire, D. W.: Sudden cardiac death in adolescents. Tex. Med. 81 (1985) 55–59

[40] Schwartz, C. J., W. J. Walsh: The pathologic basis of sudden death. Progress in Cardiovasc. Dis. XIII (1971) 465–481

[41] Schwendler, L. A., J. C. Troncoso: Evaluation of sudden death in epilepsy. Am. J. Forensic Med. Pathol. 7 (1986) 283–287

[42] Shem-Tov A., A. Schneeweiss, M. Motro, H. N. Neufeld: Clinical presentation and natural history of mild discrete subaortic stenosis. Circulation 66 (1982) 509–512

[43] Shiono, H., N. Tabata, M. Fujiwara, J. Azumi, M. Morita: Sudden infant death syndrome in Japan. Am. J. Forensic Med. Pathol. 9 (1988) 5–8

[44] Siboni, A., J. Simonsen: Sudden unexpected natural death in young persons. Forensic Sci. Int. 31 (1986) 159–166

[45] Szabó Á., Kádas L.: Üzemi balesetet utánzó hirtelen halál. Morph. Ig. Orv. Szemle 3. (1963) 16–21

[46] Szabó I.: A koszorúsérrendszer ellátási tipusa és a hirtelen szívhalál közötti kapcsolatok kimutatása post mortem coronarographiával. Kandidátusi értekezés (1975)

[47] Takeichi, S., C. Wakasugi, I. Shikata: Fluidity of cadaveric blood after sudden death. Am. J. Forensic Med. Pathol. 5 (1984) 223–227

[48] Topaz, O., J. E. Edwards: Pathologic features of sudden death in children, adolescents and Young adults. Chest. 87 (1985) 476–482

[49] Torvik, A.: The pathogenesis of water shed infarcts in the brain. Stroke 15 (1984) 221–223

[50] Towbin, A.: Pulmonary embolism. JAMA 156 (1954) 209–215

[51] Valdes-Dapena, M.: Sudden infant death syndrome. Morph. update for forensic pathologits. Forensic Sci. Int. 30 (1986) 177–186

[52] Van der Hal, A. L., A. M. Rodriguez: Hypoxic and hypercapneic arousal responsens and prediction of subsequent apnea of infancy. Pediatrics 75 (1985) 848–854

[53] Varga, M., L. Zsonda: A simple method for postmortem detection of acute myocardial infarction. Forensic Sci. Int. 37 (1988) 259–263

[54] Varga, M., S. Kiss, L. Buris: A caliber-persistant artery of the gastric wall resulting in fatal haemorrhage. Z. Rechtsmed. 96 (1986) 141–144

[55] Warner, J. A., W. E. I. Finlay: Fulminating epiglottitis in adults. Anaesthesia 40 (1985) 348–352 [56] Wilson, A. J., V. Stevens, C. I. Franks, J. Alexander, D. P. Southall: Respiratory and heart rate patterns in infants destined to be victims of sudden infant death syndrome, average rates and their variability measured over 24 hours. British Med. J. 290 (1985) 497–501

[57] Wink, K., H. Schmitz: Cytomegalovirus myocarditis. Am. Hearth J. 100 (1980) 667–673

Chapter 6
Death by suffocation

In the simplest case, anoxia results from interruption of circulation. Consciousness is lost within seconds of interruption of the brain's blood supply and within one to two minutes irreversible damage to the brain due to anoxia develops. If the lack of oxygen lasts only a few seconds after loss of consciousness, the injured person or patient regains consciousness on his own. Hypoxia endured over an extended period may not result in damage and may only cause a loss of consciousness if the alveolar O_2 tension falls below 33 Hgmm. The clinical symptoms of hypoxia (headache, dyspnoe, difficulty in concentration, occasionally euphoria) are manifestations of lack of oxygen and can be caused by an alveolar O_2 tension below 50 Hgmm within hours. A hypoxic state accompanies not only some diseases such as severe anemia and processes causing airway obstruction, but poisoning (CO, CO_2, CN) and some injuries can cause a hypoxic state as well. The distinction between acute and chronic hypoxic states is relatively simple. The *acute oxygen deficient state,* whether by poisoning or by airway obstruction, is easy to discover. Morphological changes which are the consequence of low oxygen content, such as a rise in the number of red blood cells, an increase in erythropoesis, and hypoxic fatty degeneration of the myocardium, make it easier to recognize the *chronic hypoxic state.* They are the possible consequences of a lower level of PO_2 in the inspired air, insufficient pulmonary ventilation, a decreased diffusion capacity of the alveolar membrane, insufficient circulatory capacity or poisoning.

The *anoxemia of suffocation* typically carries with it a lowered blood O_2 level, chemoceptor activation, increase in pulse and ventilation rate and cyanosis due to insufficient oxygen. *Anemic anoxia* due to CO poisoning or drug intoxication may result in a low arterial O_2 level although the PO_2 is normal with neither accompanying cyanosis nor chemoceptor stimulation. In *histotoxic anoxia* with cyanide poisoning we see depression of the cellular oxidation system resulting in metabolic anoxia.

The following may cause suffocation:

1. Closing of the airway openings by fluid or solidmaterial,
2. Airway strangulation,
3. Restriction of thoracic expansion,
4. Pneumothorax,
5. Inhibition of tissue respiration.

Autopsy findings in the case of death by suffocation are only occasionally (as in CN or CO poisoning) pathognomic. Many indications from the autopsy may point to

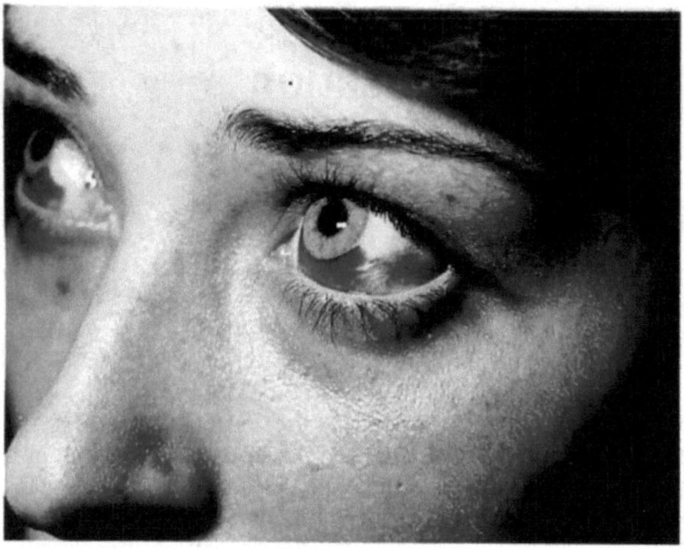

Fig. 134. Hemorrhage into the sclera following strangling at the neck with covering of the nose and mouth; characteristic scratch marks on the area of the nose

a sudden death. At other times the characteristic hypoxic bleedings, extravasation due to vessel wall damage, may form. Thus to establish death by suffocation one must indeed make a careful comparative appraisal of the findings. The hypoxic state has a special presentation in the case of prolonged suffocation. The expanding cadaveric hypostasis or lividity following death must be appraised within hours since the patches turn light pink due to postmortal oxygen uptake. Otherwise, because of the blood's fluid character, the dark red patches of settling blood over many days may be misleading. The increasing vascular wall permeability and fragility seen in the dermal bleeding of prolonged suffocation accompanies the hypoxic state, especially in the case of thoracic restriction and is noticeable to a great extent in manual strangulation *(Fig. 134).*

Subconjunctival petechiae and subcorneal suffusion are also accompanying signs in prolonged suffocation. In rapid death by suffocation we never, or hardly ever, find bleeding from the integument, nor from the usual place under the serous membranes. Otherwise the presence of petechiae which are not related to the recent hypoxic state may be misleading. In the toxic state, and even after infections, we can often see bleedings due to damage to the more fragile vessel walls. A characteristic example is the multiplex skin bleeding accompanying Waterhouse-Friderichsen syndrome. We have already discussed in the chapter on signs of death the postmortal origins of ecchymotic patches, and how petechia-like bleedings may form mainly in dependent areas to which the patches of blood settle.

One of the signs of death by suffocation is the appearance of blood engorgement of the viscera. *Congestion* is one of the signs of prolonged asphyxia. The visceral veins and capillaries are filled with blood. Because of asphyxia the *blood reservoirs,* including the spleen, become empty. At autopsy the congestion of the liver and the kidneys with the engorgement of the vessels of the brain is manifest. Similar signs also develop in the case of sudden death or after a chronic septic state. Blood engorgement of the lung tissue and the formation of edema is associated with prolonged suffocation. In the case of manual strangulation often bloody edema will exude from the sectioned lung surface.

The *autopsy technique* in the case of death by suffocation should reveal the injuries, which serves to clear up the original circumstances. Attack to the neck leaves characteristic markings which can, with carefully chosen techniques, be investigated and their origin be deduced. On the body we seek such injuries to the neck which are characteristic of their origin. The impression left by a cord or an unusual mark and its direction are relevant findings. We must examine the ligature mark's character, width, impressions within the crease which reflect the impression of the instrument used, and the area surrounding the ligature mark. We measure from the mental protuberance and mandibular angle to derive the true distance to the highest point of the mark. On the hands we search under the fingernails for the fibers of material from which the instrument was made. We take an impression of the fingers with scotch tape and stick it on a microscope slide for the specific purpose of looking for foreign fibers.

We search for fingernail imprints on the skin of the neck *(Fig. 135)* and scratches from self defence or struggle on the upper and lower extremities. If sexual motives have played a role, we examine the thighs and external genitalia carefully, taking samples from the relevant secretions. Froth at the naso-oral area or foreign material (sand or mud) may point to the circumstances surrounding suffocation. (Carp bites in a decayed drowning victim have been mistaken for gunshot wounds!)

The internal examination is a great exercise and merits caution. Bleeding into the soft tissues of the neck can point to the

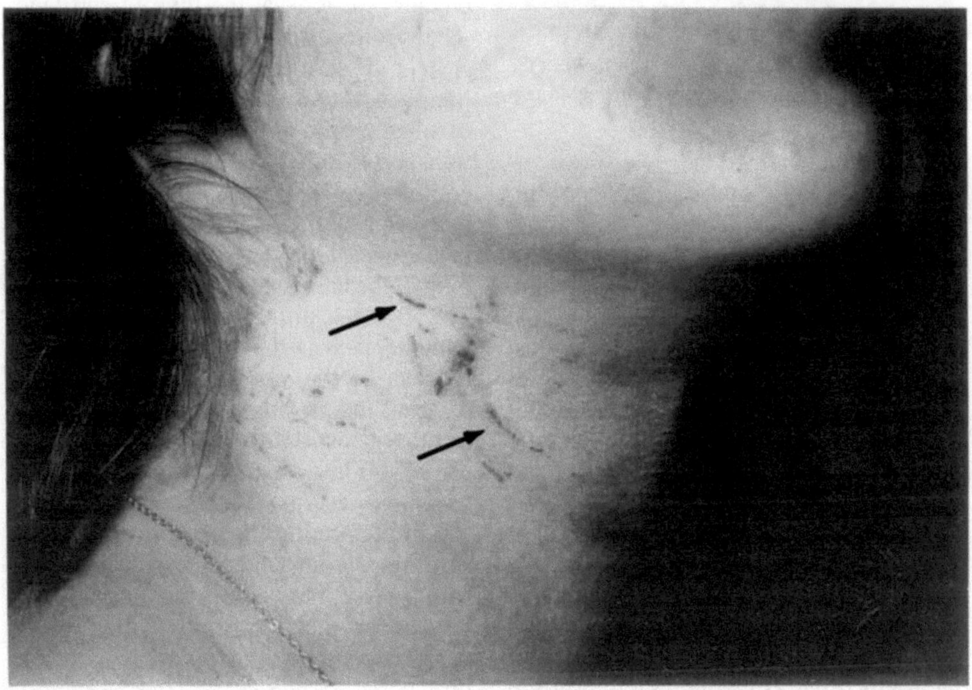

Fig. 135. Grip marks on the neck

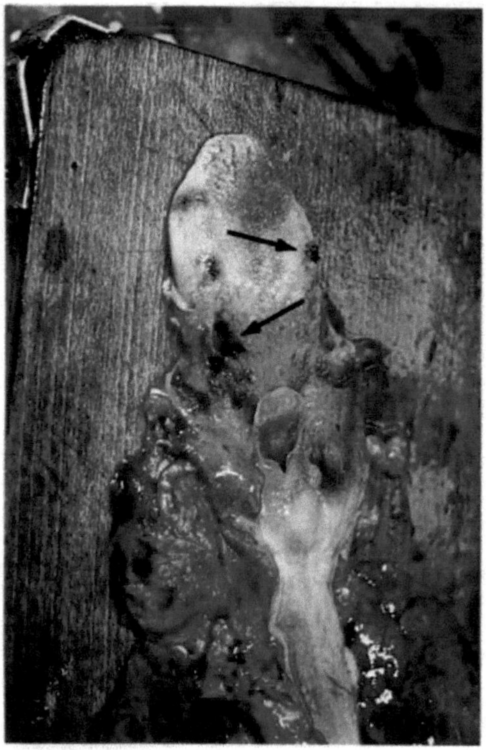

Fig. 136. Blood infiltration into the substance of the root of the tongue and tongue itself following strangling

use of force, but may originate from improper autopsy technique as well. It is not easy to distinguish between pre and postmortal bleeding or infiltration of blood. The possibility of postmortal imbibition of the congested organs of the neck must especially be taken into account. Therefore the first task is to drain the neck organs of blood which is one specific reason for prior removal of the brain and heart. This can be done by the so-called "layered" dissection. *Layered dissection* means the separate preparation of the overlying and deep muscles of the neck. Blood infiltration of the neck muscles the rupture of the muscle fibers are the sign of the use of force. (In hanging the insertion of the sternocleidomastoid at the clavicle as well as the muscle fibers will show infiltration of blood.) We continue with the examination of the soft tissues of the neck and the dissection of the cartilaginous skeleton of the throat *(Fig. 136).* Fracture of the hyoid bone by application of direct force as in, for example, hanging or finger pressure, or indirectly by traction of the thyrohyoid ligament in hanging are relevant. Injury to the cartilaginous skeleton of the larynxis more likely to be the result of strangling by a cord or by hand. Bleeding into the esophageal or pharyngeal mucous membranes is evidence of the application of force. (Sometimes the laryngeal bleeding occures following intubation during reanimation.) The special types of submucosal bleeding are symmetrical with respect to the vocal folds, and the elastic conus, under the points of airway obstruction. After examination of the esophagus, we look at the thyroid cartilage, the thyroid cartilage horn, the cricoid and arytenoid cartilages, and open up the joints of throat, the thyroid and cricoid cartilages and the cricothyroid joint. A transverse split in the intima of the common carotid artery *(Amussat's sign)* is caused by hanging. Manual strangling of the neck almost always involves grabbing of the nasal and oral openings as well. This causes chafing and bruising wounds which appear in the oral mucosa or in the mucosa of the vestibule along with the external lacerations and bruises. In other instances, especially with strangling by use of soft instruments (gloved hands) external injuries may not be seen, but application of force in the periorbital areas or soft areas around the nose will cause infiltration of blood into the fatty tissues and under the periostium which is revealed upon peeling back the skin of the face.

In *drowning,* if the signs of decay have

not appeared, we perform a special test to compare the blood of the right to that of the left heart. In drowning in fresh water, the blood in the left heart is diluted and the decrease in dry weight is well seen. For this test we take blood samples from the right and left ventricles with a special dry(!) syringe at the beginning of the autopsy. Diatoms in the marrow or kidneys may also be demonstrated.

Potassium, sodium and chloride concentrations in the aqueous humor of the eye are beginning to be used for the determination of the time of death in drowning. These tests are still in the experimental stages.

In death by suffocation the blood is fluid. This explains the wide expansion of the settling blood forming the hypostasis, but the settling may disturb the later determination of the organ blood content. This develops similarly in the case of sudden death the organ blood content and the blood's fluid character. In experimental circumstances postmortal acidosis brings about active fibrinolytic activity. The acceleration of endothelial plasminogen activator also helps explain the increased fibrinolysis.

Hanging

Hanging is one of the most common forms of suicide. Though rarely occurring by other than the victim's own hand, we must consider the possibility of murder both in the coroner's inquest and in the autopsy. Hanging requires the use of an instrument of suspension, wrapped once or several times around the neck of the victim. The body weight provides the tightening force. The body may hang on the ligature either touching the ground or completely suspended. It requires relatively little force to close the vessels of the neck, the carotid artery, being closed by 5 Kp, (49 N), the jugular veins by 2 Kp (19 N) and the vertebral arteries by 30 Kp (294 N) respectively. The instrument of suspension usually causes injury to the neck, the character of the ligature imprint depending upon the nature and direction of lie of the material of the ligature and the applied force. In the typical case the mark is situated between the hyoid bone and the thyroid cartilage largely equidistant from the angle of the mandible on both sides and tractioned at an angle backwards and upwards toward the highest point, the external occipital protuberance.

The *atypical mark,* which shows a distinctly different pattern from this, although nevertheless characteristic, deviates upward from the horizontal appropriately suspending the body. With an open crease the imprint shows up lighter on one side and soon disappears. Hanging in the lying position shows an almost horizontal trace and can be completely mistaken for the mark of the strangulation. Among the common conditions around the impression into the skin are a fresh red chaffing injury deep in which fine raised splinters of skin can be noticed. A few hours later they will be dried and parchment-like and discolored brownish yellow. The impression left by the instrument of suspension, if it had a surface pattern such as a cord, chain or belt, can be examined with the naked eye. Using a magnifying glass allows for a more detailed examination of the impression, which sometimes helps elaborate the comparison of the ligature with the mark left by it. If the hanging was performed delicately or with a smooth-surfaced material, we won't find any typical signs in the crease. The situation of the mark not only causes difficulties in analysis, but sometimes in the diagnosis of death by hanging if the

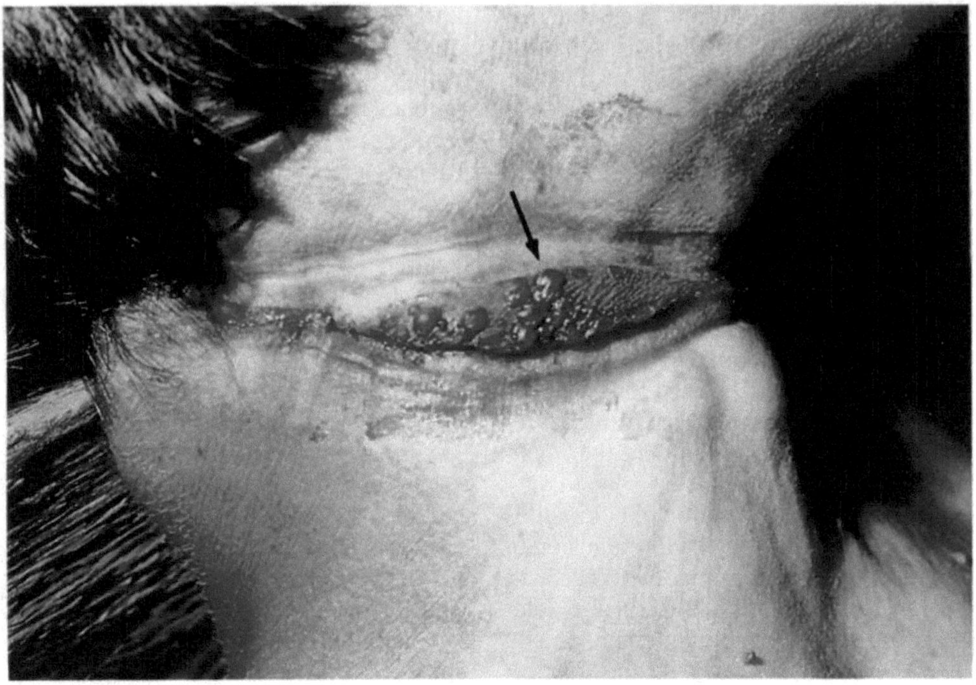

Fig. 137. Blister formation between the intact skin along the hanging ligature mark

hanging is done with a broad ligature, as in the case of the so-called *"padded hanging."* A soft, wide, protective material placed between the instrument of suspension and the skin leaves hardly any trace of injury, or none at all, and the mark is missing. If the instrument of suspension is wound several times around the neck pieces of skin may be pinched in the coils and the crease will show separated or torn crests. Pinpoint hemorrhages may form in the swollen skin wrinkles and fine vesicles can be made out on the edges of the ligature *(Fig. 137).*

Among the external signs of hanging is *congestion* which may be found beyond the ligature such as also accompanies suffocation. If the compression of the neck vessels was complete, congestion does not develop above the ligature. The face and connective tissues are pallid. If the compression was incomplete, whether in the area of the vertebral arteries or the carotid, and only the jugular vein was closed, we will see the signs of expressed congestion. Due to edema of the retrobulbar tissues, the eyes bulge out, the conjunctiva becomes edematous, subconjunctival and subcorneal petechiae form and the skin of the face becomes livid and swollen along with the soft areas of the face as well. The tongue protrudes between the teeth. At autopsy we rarely find bleeding in the superficial muscles of the neck, this being more a consequence of the so-called *"drop hanging"* (when the victim jumps from some height), but in this case we also find bleeding together with the muscle tears. Commonly we find striolate infiltrative bleeding at the clavicular insertion of the sternocleidomastoid or subperiosteal hemorrhage. The hyoid bone is broken between the body and the greater horn in 10-20% of the cases and infiltrative bleeding forms in the neighboring soft tissues. The superior horn of the thyroid cartilage is rarely broken, though it may be fractured by the protruding knot of the noose, or broken off in the fall. Infiltration of blood into the root of the tongue doesn't accompany hanging injuries. Transverse splitting of the intima of the common carotids may form as the so-called *"Amussat cracks."*

Death from hanging may be due to:

a) Reflexogenic, whether by vagal traction or stimulation of the glomus caroticum, can cause cardiac arrest even without finding alterations of the vagus trunk or the glomus caroticum unrelated to the ligature mark. In the case of reflex-caused death, the signs of death by suffocation are weakly developed, the blood infiltration is missing, the internal organs are severely congested and there is edema of the brain.

b) Due to spinal cord injury, especially in drop hanging, the sudden force causes the dislocation of the 2nd and 3rd or 3rd and 4th cervical vertebrae and injury to the spinal cord and/or the myelencephalon. The victim loses consciousness immediately.

c) Due to anoxia in the brain which is the most common cause of death. Besides compression of the neck vessels, compression of the airway plays a role and the root of the tongue being forced back may block the inlet of the throat. However, due to the cessation of the cranial circulation, these factors don't matter. The critical importance of the cervical vessels is granted inasmuch as the carotid artery can be occluded by so slight a pressure which takes effect at the moment the ligature is tightened. This causes immediate loss of consciousness, and thus it is understandable, that so-called *"self-rescue"* is not possible. Of all the methods of suicide, hanging is top on the list of final acts.

Hanging is generally considered a single suicidal act, but it may be combined with other factors so that the victim may also be drugged, weakened or unconscious. Also, unusual hanging methods and accompanying injuries point to foul play. It may happen that prior violence inflicted by someone else may be tried to be made to look like a suicide hanging. It cannot be determined from the ligature mark whether the injury occurred before or after death. Also in the area of the ligature mark dermal hemorrhages may develop if the hanging can be performed immediately after death. The appearance of visible vesicles at the edge of the ligature mark is a sign of life, demonstrating unambiguously that the mark occurred while the victim was alive. Tamaki and al. suggested the examination of thyreoglobulin level in plasma following the compression of the neck. By the ELISA method the plasma thyreoglobulin level without the external compression of the neck or neck injuries was lower then 200 mg/ml but following the neck compression the Tg level increased 2190 mg/ml. The increased Tg content of plasma was suggested by the authors as a vital sign in strangulation. Erythrophagocytosis can be demonstrated in the regional lymph nodes. The diagnostic value of follicular hemorrhage in the regional lymph nodes is uncertain because erythrocytes, siderophages were encountered in the lymph node sinuses both in neck trauma and without mechanical injuries.

Examination of the *instrument of hanging* is an indispensable part of the coroner's inquest and the autopsy. The instrument must be removed in such a manner that the knot can be examined. At the same time the palms and spaces under the fingernails of the victim must be examined for pieces of the ligature material. We have already discussed previously the particulars of the ecchymoses indicating the hanging and change of body position. Hypostasis in the legs brings about the ecchymoses, but early moving of the body (within the first six hours) may cause these to wander and only the superficial cutaneous hemorrhages mark the previous areas of ecchymosis.

In the autopsy blood and urine samples and tests for possible alcohol intoxication are necessary in every case. At the scene of the incident, a doctor examines the position of the body (if the site can be considered in its original condition), the manner of hanging, height, and whether the deceased could have reached the place from which he was hanged. Of special significance is the exact recording and observation in the case of the above-mentioned padded hanging. The superficial marks which may have been visible at the scene of the hanging may disappear by the time of the autopsy. Unusual manners of hanging which may be part of a combination suicide must be examined with special care. Examination at the scene can provide indispensable data.

- The duty police medical examiner was called to the coroner's inquest in the case of a hanging suicide of a 56-year-old man. The examination revealed that the ligature was bloody, but the palms of the deceased were unstained by blood. On the beam which held the noose could be seen such marks as though the rope had been pulled under weight. The victim's son had strangled him the previous morning and tried to mask the crime as a suicide.

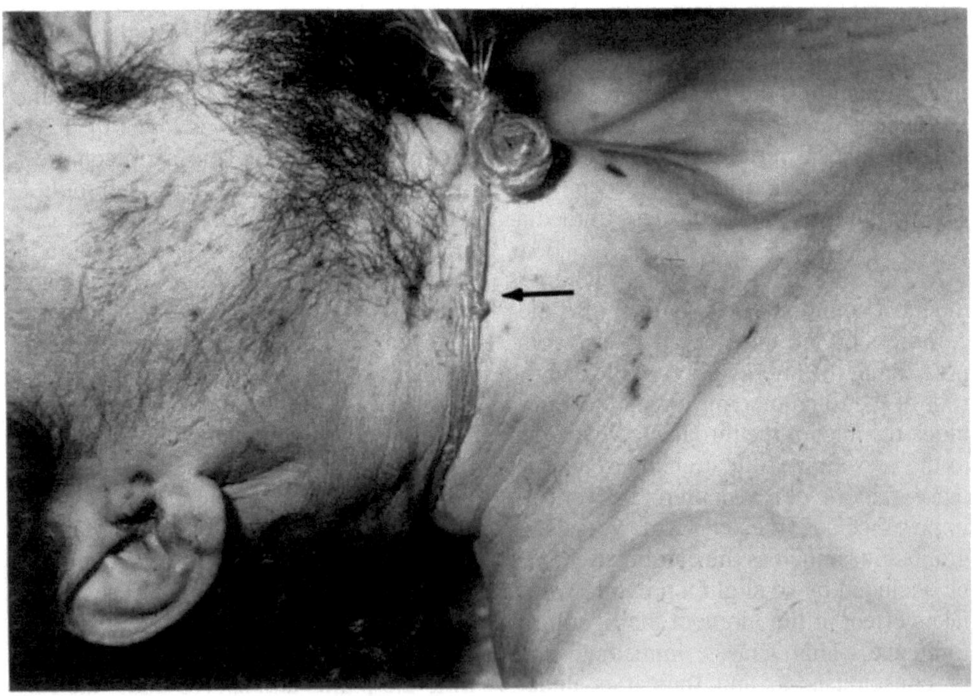

Fig. 138. Strangling by ligature. Horizontal crease and ligature. Superficial chafe marks in the area

Strangulation by ligature

Inasmuch as the weight of the body makes for the force on the ligature in hanging, so in strangulation the force comes from manual pull. This does not ensure a swift and effective compression of the vessels, and also yields telltale alterations. It occurs relatively infrequently and makes up only a small proportion of all deaths by suffocation. The instruments tend to be similar to those used in hanging and when the neck is squeezed a mark is left. The *garotte mark however (Fig. 138)* is different from that left by hanging being practically horizontal and more deeply seated. It is often dragged under the laryngeal cartilages. Since the compression is prolonged and incomplete (the vertebral arteries are never closed), congestion is more expressed and this is obvious from external examination as well. On the face the soft areas swell, the face and neck above the mark are engorged with blood and livid and pinpoint hemorrhages can be seen on the skin while petechiae and suffusions can also be found in the subconjunctiva and gums. The strangulation mark, if the instrument was thin, is well shown, and especially resembles the mark of hanging. If a knot was tied in the ligature, chaffing similarly widens the mark and makes it more expressed. If foreign material such as a shirt or hair or the victims fingers come between the garotte and the skin, the mark will appear interrupted or hardly recognizable as if the strangling were performed with a broad material such as a belt or nylon stocking.

Upon external examination congestion and hypoxic injuries are more pronounced, the areas of injury to the neck showing bleeding into the muscles more often which is more obvious than in hanging. Bleeding may be seen at the throat and pharynx as well as in the area of the submucosa of the vocal cords. The great horn of the thyroid cartilage is more often fractured, and suffusion of blood more vigorous. In the elderly because the thyroid cartilage is more calcified, fracture of the thyroid cartilage is more commonly encountered. If the instrument slides up during the struggle, it may break the hyoid bone also. In the viscera the prolonged hypoxia causes petechiae under the serous membranes, bloating of the lung tissue with bloody edema, and the liver and kidney tissues are found to be severely congested.

Suicide by self garotting is very rare. SZABÓ records two instances in which hospital patients committed suicide. The rarity is explained by the fact that when the cord is tightened by the victim's efforts, he passes out, but then the loop slackens and the victim regains consciousness. In self garotting, if a material with a rough surface is used, the noose won't slip, or if the material is stretchy and stays tight to the neck, it will keep the vessels closed.

At the scene the doctor must note well the positioning of the cord and its direction of lie and the removal of the cord is done as in the case of hanging.

The accidental form of strangulation also occures. In childhood the dangers of losse wires, cords or other potential ligatures are emphasised.

Manual strangulation

The soft tissues of the neck can be gripped and compressed. In violence the hand or pads of the little finger can compress the throat against the vertebrae thus closing the pharynx and the upper opening of the airway while partially closing the vessels of the neck as well. A similar mechanism functions if the forearm, or a stick is used. A grip of the neck by one hand can cause partial closure of most of the vessels of the neck and this can bring about a swift loss of consciousness, inasmuch as the hand squeezing the neck in most cases takes hold under the mandible, presses on the root of the tongue and obstruction of the pharynx increases the hypoxic state. A two-handed grip to the neck largely succeeds in compressing the airway. The thumbs over the throat exert the pressure if the victim is attacked from the front. An attack from behind results in a grip that is more likely to close the vessels. Occasionally grip to the neck can cause a quick *reflex death.* Traction on the *vagus* can cause cardiac arrest even without the presence of noticeable external or internal injury.

- During an argument, a 43-year-old woman grabbed hold of her son's neck. The victim immediately died. There were no discernable injuries on the surface of the neck, but around the right vagus we found a fingertipsize hemorrhage ensheathing the nerve. The results of the autopsy were negative, as were the toxicological tests. Stimulation to the tenth cranial nerve had caused the heart to stop.

A sudden death also occures due to mechanical irritation of the *carotid sinus.* This region is a reflexogenic zone and the compression of the sinus may cause acuta cardiac arrest. The histological analysis of stepwise mode slides of the carotid arteries from the region of sinus may be informative e.g. hemorrhage infiltration.

Manual strangulation is possibly the most variable form of all the methods of strangulation ranging from the most severe injury to hardly detectable alterations. The typical case shows on the skin characteristic scratches and bruises where the neck was attacked *(Fig. 139).* The scratches which can be seen on the skin as brownish, crescent-shaped dried areas are caused by the nails and lie just under the fingertip impressions which appear as 7-10 mm wide bluish-red bruises. In an attack by a right-handed man facing the victim we find the impressions of four fingers on the left and a thumb on the right sides of the neck. However, commonly the injuries to the neck only partially fit this typical picture. In the majority of cases bruises or scratches and chaffing are evident in which the crescent-shaped marks or round bruises are hardly discernable. The absence of these characteristic injuries can be attributed to the struggle of the victim to protect himself as the attacker again and again grabbed at the neck and his hands changed positions. The typical surface marks to the neck are therefore more commonly seen on victims who are weak or disabled. If the compression of the neck is performed by application of a soft instrument (if the attacker was wearing gloves or used the forearm to squeeze the soft tissues), wounds will be hard or impossible to find although severe internal injuries may be present.

A significant proportion of the cases of strangulation include grabbing at the nose and mouth of the victim, on the one hand to close the airway and on the other to keep the victim from crying out. In the areas of the nose and mouth we will find the same above-mentioned scratches and bruises such as we find on the neck and more expressed around the bridge of the nose.

At *autopsy* in the soft areas of the neck we find injuries proportional to the force used. If cardiac arrest has occurred as a result of the vagus reflex, the area of the vagus must be dissected out in search of blood infiltration around the nerve. A general dissection, however, reveals that

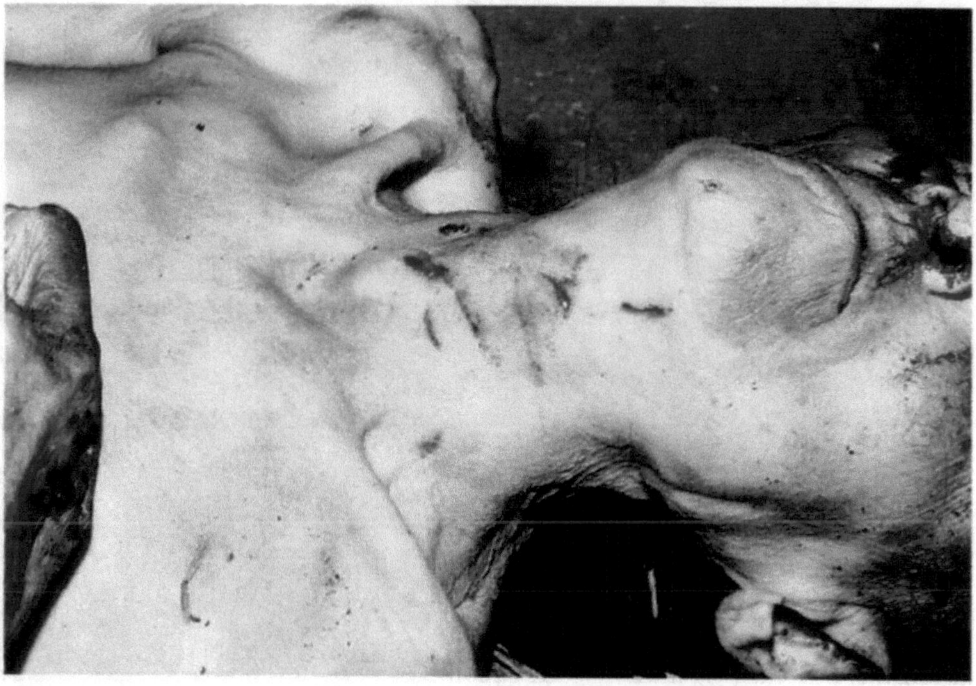

Fig. 139. Scratch injuries, bruises in the neck on a victim of manual strangling

attack to the neck with compression injuries most seriously to the soft tissues and throat has occurred. We find bleeding in the superficial and deep muscles of the neck histologically evident by the tearing of the fibers. Pressure to the root of the tongue not only causes striolated infiltrative bleedings to the muscles of the tongue but to its tissues as well. Often the hyoid bone is fractured along with the superior horn of the thyroid cartilage. A fracture of the right superior horn points to a right-handed assailant where he gripped the victim with his thumb injuring the victim's hyoid and throat. If the neck was gripped by two hands, or if the neck was compressed by the forearm as mentioned above, along with the infiltrative bleeding of the soft tissues, the thyroid cartilage may also be broken in pieces.

In youth the thyroid cartilage may remain uninjured although bleeding in the tissue of the thyroid gland and subcartilagenous membranes may become evident. Compression to the throat applies stress to the joints of the throat, such as the cricoarytenoid and cricothyroid joints. In the joint capsule bleeding may occur into the joint space. The soft tissue hemorrhages, the injured hyoid bone, cause map-like infiltrations of blood into the soft tissues surrounding the cartilages of the throat, but well-visible bluish red bruises also appear at the inlet of the throat and in the esophageal mucous membranes *(Fig. 140)*.

Besides the external injuries to the periorbital soft tissues caused by gripping the nasal and oral openings, subperiosteal injuries also occur. Injuries from the victim's own teeth can happen as a result of pressure over the mouth, and the mucous membranes in the mouth will be bruised and lacerated, and even injuries to

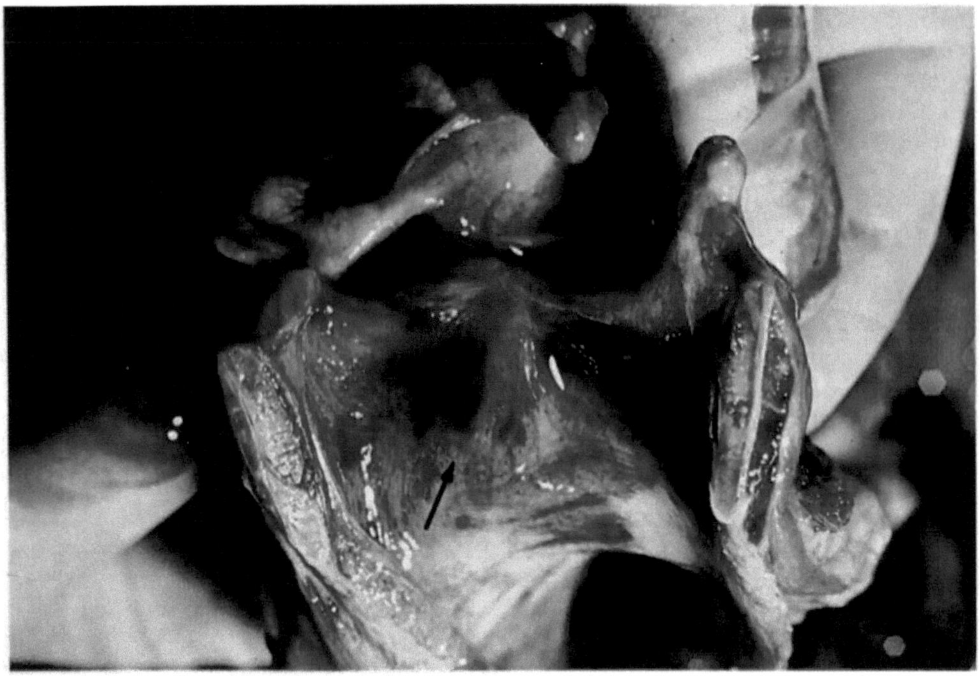

Fig. 140. Injuries to organs of the neck – thyroid cartilage, cricoid cartilage – infiltration of blood into the soft tissues following strangling

the teeth themselves may occur which can be seen at the examination of the body *(Fig. 141)*. If the cervical vessels and soft tissues were discontinuously compressed, the suffocation is prolonged.

The signs of congestion and hypoxia are even more pronounced than the previously mentioned injuries. Bleeding under the connective tissue along with subcorneal suffusions can be found. The most dramatic are the pulmonary alterations, in which acute emphysematic areas form, and "pearl string" air bubbles appear in the subpleural and interlobular septae. The lungs swell with air (volumen pulmonum auctum acutum), and bloody edema oozes from the cut surface. The pulmonary edema is the morphological

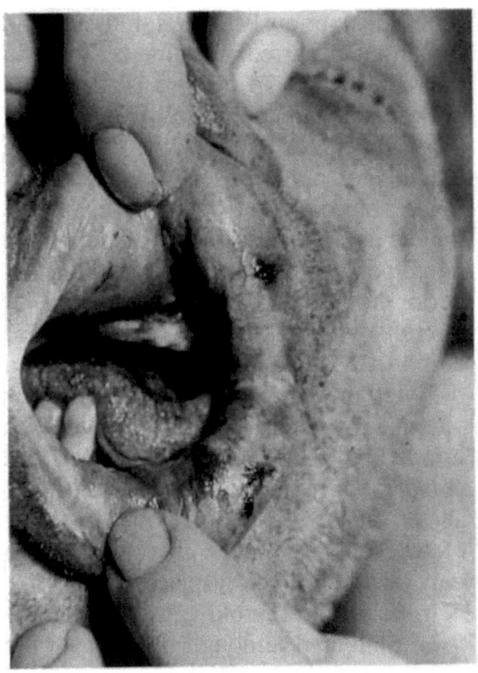

Fig. 141. Injuries to the mouth, mucosal bruising following gripping of the mouth

changes in asphyxia. Its case, the endothelial cells have abundant pores and intracytoplasmic vacuoles. In the case of asphyxia the histamin content of the lung tissue increases. The increased histamin concentration induces an enhancement of the endothelial permeability. There will be subpleural and subepicardial hemorrhages. The right heart will be dilated, the blood uncongealed and the organs engorged.

The neck wounds must be observed critically and with appropriate circumspection in the examination at the scene of the crime, since not every neck wound is evidence of some attack and not all attacks leave externally visible markings. In case of general suspicion or doubt, an autopsy should be performed without delay to clarify the cause of death and the necessary arrangements should be made right away. Inasmuch as manual strangling often involves some sexual consequences, the appropriate trace samples must be taken as quickly as possible.

Injuries to the neck occur in the course of the struggle between the victim and the assailant. There may be marks on both. Under the fingernails of the victim samples can be removed (we look for skin, hairs, or other material), but on the arms and hands we can also find injuries caused during attack or defense.

Drowning

Drowning, usually in water, is one of the most common manners of death by suffocation. Every year 150,000 die this way. Naturally, the countries with a coastline have more cases. The role played by alcohol and drugs cannot go unmentioned. The whole course of drowning takes place within a few minutes starting with cerebral hypoxia, then the continued production of CO_2 causes hypercapnia, and finally brain death, although spasms in the throat or reflex cardiac arrest may also develop.

Drowning can take place in very little water and the amount of fluid is unimportant since infants, unconscious, injured or sick people can drown in shallow water.

The so-called *"dry drowning"* is a unique form in which a small amount of fluid makes its way into the airway. Death ensues due to a spasm in the throat or reflex alterations in the airway which give rise to anoxia. The obstructive effect of froth production from mucus and air may also play a role. The entering fluid is blocked from descending further by the froth and bronchospasm. This type of drowning is seen more commonly in adults.

The first *stage of drowning,* on the basis of animal experiments, is *apnoe.* This is accompanied by bradycardia, dermal and abdominal shunting of blood, so that it can be reserved primarily for the brain and coronaries. Blood pressure immediately rises, the reflex processes and independently the baro- and chemoreceptors and part of the trigeminal sensors begin to increase their activity. Apnoe lasts until the PCO_2 level reaches the critical 55 Hgmm. Then the *deep breathing* stage starts with tachycardia and quick arterial hypoxia. A large quantity of water also gets into the airway and the stomach. This triggers the vomiting reflex before unconsciousness sets in and fluid, or rather vomit, may be aspirated. The cramping inspiration stage brings *apnoe* again and *terminal breathing* efforts develop. The time the whole course takes is age-dependent with children better tolerating the hypoxic state.

Water in the airways causes peripheral airway obstruction and the osmolarity of this fluid plays a more important role than the quantity. Experimentally, inspiration

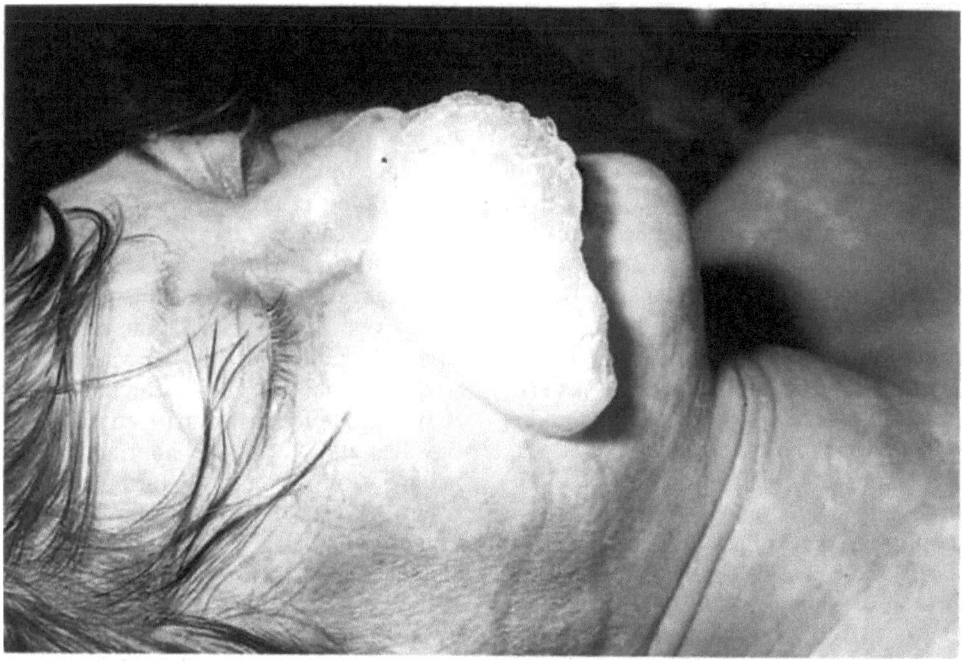

Fig. 142. Foam formation in drowning

of as little as 1 ml/kg of fresh water can cause pulmonary vasoconstriction and immediate pulmonary hypertonia. The larger quantity of fluid managing to get in due to the vasospasm decreases the ventilated area which is further decreased by the dilution of the surfactant factor and results in further alveolar collapse. After the introduction of fluid the originally reduced diffusion areas of the lungs show a three-fold relative increase. The fluid crosses the alveolar wall and diffuses into the capillaries, damaging the alveolar epithelium in the process and the injury to the type I and II pneumocytes is considerable. The most important consequence of this is the decreased production of surfactant. The fluid crossing into the capillaries exerts a *hemodiluting effect* primarily in the left heart (which is of diagnostic significance!). The damage to the pneumocytes with the decreased production of surfactant by the survivors is significant in that widespread atelectasis develops in the lung tissue resulting in *"secondary drowning"* with well visible morphological changes. Along with formation of hyaline membrane a protein-rich, cell-poor exudate appears in alveoli. In the partially diluted blood the red blood cells are damaged and the large amount of potassium released causes ventricular fibrillation. A lowering of serum fibronectin levels also accompanies the disturbance in circulation which may cause coagulation irregularities following rescue.

The *autopsy findings* in drowning is only slightly pathognomic. There may be quite a lot of foam at the nose and mouth which is formed created by the inflowing water, with a large quantity of mucus and air *(Fig. 142)*. (Similar foam may be produced in pulmonary edema as well.) Wet clothing or sodden skin only indicates submersion, but doesn't verify drowning. The sodden skin, or so-called "washerwomen's hand" which may be a result of submersion in water either before or after drowning, appears relatively quickly as the skin of the fingers will begin to wrinkle within 20-30 minutes and shriveling of the palms, depending on the degree of keratinization, occurs within 100-150 minutes from the start of submersion. We can find mud or plant fibers in the sack of conjunctiva which may also arrive postmortally. In drowning in cold water, the body will be pale grey due to the vasoconstriction in the skin and the livor mortis slightly reddish and rather restricted. Drowning in warmer water shows more characteristic signs which are obvious upon external examination. With a body that has been in the water for a long time the process of decay occurs more quickly due to the wrinkling of the skin. In warm weather the decay that can occur within a day may render the body unidentifiable and the identification of fine external injuries impossible. The autopsy findings are variable depending upon whether early reflex death occurred or not. In this case the small amount of inspired water causes no characteristic alteration. At other times the lungs display an acute emphysema, filling the thoracic cavity with ballooning, are "dry", light grey discolored lungs and may press no fluid from section surface. In the airway is whipped, foamy mucus. Under the serous membranes scattered petechiae can be seen. Most of the fluid which gets into the alveoli causes the lung to appear more massive and bloated on the sectioned surface being dry due to the absorption of that fluid. The right heart is dilated. In the stomach a large quantity of fluid may be found which may indicate the kind and quality of water where the drowning took place (containing water plants, sand or other material).

Drowning in *mud or muddy water* presents a special picture. The alterations are due to the presence of large quantities of sand or suspended bits of clay in the water. We find in the airway and alveoli a large amount of muddy water which is similar to that found in the stomach. Sand causes a quartz-induced fibrotic inflammation to occur in the survivors with interstitial and alveolar damage, granulomatous pneumonitis and diffuse fibrosis. In the macrophages material which refracts light can be demonstrated and X-ray microanalysis can play a significant role in diagnosis. The course of pathological events develops quickly and carries a bad prognosis.

The autopsy data are weak in establishing death by drowning. The rapid course of decay makes diagnosis especially difficult. The demonstration of dilution of blood in the left heart is of use only if the death was recent. Possibly the most useful information is provided by the diatoms which float in the water. In 1941 INCZE demonstrated the significance of *diatoms* in the establishment of death by drowning. Since that article, numerous subsequent examinations have appeared raising arguments both in favor and against the procedure. The inspired diatom-containing water traverses the airway into the lungs, crosses over into the pulmonary capillaries gaining access to the circulation and thus make their way to the fine capillaries of the reservoir organs, the kidneys and bone marrow. With appropriate techniques they can be demonstrated in the kidneys and bone marrow and be characterized as well. Demonstration of the same diatoms from the bone marrow and the water where the body was found establishes that the drowning took place there. The appropriate diatoms demonstrated in the lungs or left heart blood is not of diagnostic significance because they can arrive there by gradual seepage over time. Only the demonstration of the appropriate kinds of diatoms in any organs is significant in the establishment of drowning and the place it occurred. Diatoms can be demonstrated in the kidneys and bone marrow even if drowning didn't occur since diatoms can be found in dried pond and stream beds which the wind can stir up and be introduced into anyone's airway by normal breathing. A quantitative diatom analysis also may be useful for diagnosing death by drowning.

Thoracic restriction

Whether in a mass disasters or in any accident in which the injured person finds himself *under a heavy weight* and the thorax is under pressure the signs of death by suffocation may form in their entirety. While upon external examination the spread of dark red hypostasis is apparent on the face, neck and shoulders, sometimes we also find pinpoint hemorrhages on the skin of the chest which demonstrate the presence of suffusions under the subconjunctival tissues. The palpebral conjunctiva is swollen. The congestion in the head and neck veins bring the above mentioned hemorrhages. On internal examination besides the organs being engorged with blood, the lungs appear severely emphysematous, there are interstitial and subpleural air bubbles, and we find spreading, pinpoint bleedings under the serous membranes.

The autopsy findings are similar to those cases where suffocation occurred while *being buried alive.* Besides the above findings in the palpebral conjunctiva fine material can be found in the nose, mouth and throat and as far as the terminal bronchioles. The stomach will also reveal swallowed material of the same type inhaled which establishes that the victim was buried alive.

Similar results follow the *inspiration of vomit* which may have found its way into the airway either as death ensued or postmortally, and from the stomach contents it can be distinguished that it has reached as far as the terminal bronchioles. Foreign material can also be found clogging the nasal or oral openings. In the case of BRINKMANN the demonstration of pieces of cotton serving to block the nasal cavity established the presence of homicide.

External occlusion of air

This is one of the more rare forms of death by suffocation. It often occurs in combination with manual strangulation when the nose and mouth are covered. Another rare case is that when a child covers his face with a plastic bag and suffocates. There are also known instances of a child hiding inside a refrigerator or washer or drier and suffocating. Unusual suffocation cases were pulished by HISS and ARENSBURG due to misuse of gas masks during the Gulf war. The autopsy picture is typical of prolonged suffocation and the presentation is characteristic.

References

[1] ATLEE, W. L.: Report of a Series of Experiments made by the Medical Faculty of Lancaster, upon the body of Henry Cobler Moselmann, executed in the Jail Yard of Lancaster County, Pa., on the 20th of December, 1839. Am. J. Med. Sci. LI. (1840) 2–32

[2] AUER, A.: Suicide by drowning in Uusimaa province in southern Finland. Med. Sci. Law 30 (1990) 175–179

[3] AUER, A.: Qualitative diatom analysis as a tool to diagnose drowning Am. J. Forensic Med. Pathol. 12 (1991) 213–218

[4] BRAY, M.: Chemical estimation of fresh water immersion intervals. Am. J. Forensic Med. Pathol. 6 (1985) 133–139

[5] BRINKMANN, B., G. FECHNER, K. PŐSCHEL: Identification of mechanical asphyxiation in case of attempted marking of homicide. Forensic Sci. Int. 26 (1984) 235–245

[6] DAVIS, J. H.: Bodies found in the water. Am. J. Forensic Med. Pathol. 7 (1986) 291–297

[7] FUNAYAMA, M., Y. AOKI, I. M. SEBETAN, K. SAGISAKA: Detection of diatoms in blood by a combination of membrane filtering and chemical digestion. Forensic Sci. Int. 34 (1987) 175–182

[8] HANSEN, L. K., BRANDSLUND, I., D. JOHANNESSEN, P. K. ANDERSEN: Low plasma fibronectin after drowning. Intensive Care Med. 11 (1985) 100–102

[9] HISS, Y., B. ARENSBURG: Suffocation from misuse of gas masks during the Gulf war. BMJ. 304 (1992) 92

[10] INCZE GY.: Diatomák vízbefúltak ereiben. Jankovich László Emlékkönyv, Debrecen (1944) 69–94

[11] INCZE, G., L. TAMÁSKA, J. GYÖNGYÖSI: Zur Blutplanktonfrage beim Tod durch Ertrinken. Dtsch. Z. gerichtl. Med. 43 (1955) 517–523

[12] KARCH, S. B.: Pathology of the hearth in drowning. Arch. Pathol. Lab. Med. 109 (1985) 175–178

[13] KITA, T., FURUYA, Y.: Histamine effects on pulmonary blood vessels in strangulation. Z. Rechtsmed. 103 (1989) 85–91.

[14] KRAUS, J. F.: Efectivness of measures to prevent unintentional deaths of infants and children from suffocation and strangulation. Public. Health Rep. 100 (1985) 231–240

[15] LIN, C. Y.: Circulatory functions during immersion and breath-hold dives in human. Undersea Biomed. Res. 11 (1984) 123–128

[16] LUKE, J. L., T. R. DONALD, J. W. EISELE, H. J. BONNEL: Correlation of circumstances with pathological findings in asphyxial death by hanging. J. Forensic Sci. 30 (1985) 1140–1147

[17] MAXEINER, H.: Weichtelblutungen im Kehlkopfinneren nach Strangulation. Z. Rechtsmed. 94 (1985) 127–135

[18] MAXEINER, H., V. SCHNEIDER: Zum Erstickungstode beim Verschluss der Atemöffnungen durch Sand. Z. Rechtsmed. 94 (1985) 173–189

[19] MAXEINER, H.: Schleimhautblutungen des Larynx in Strangulation und anderen Todesursachen. Beitr. Gerichtl. Med. 47 (1989) 429–435

[20] MODELL, J. H., M. GAUB, F. MOYA: Physiologic effects of near drowning with chlorinated fresh water, distilled water, and isotonic saline. Anesthesiology 27 (1966) 33–41

[21] MODELL, J. H., J. H. DAVIS, S. T. GIAMMONA: Blood gas and electrolyte changes in human near-drowning victims. JAMA 203 (1968) 99—105

[22] NOGUCHI, M., V. KIMULA, O. TAKESABURO: Muddy lung. Am. J. Clin. Pathol. 83 (1985) 240–244

[23] OECHMICHEN, M., V. SCHMIDT: Erythrozyten in Halslymphknoten des Menschen als Folge einer Stauung und/oder Lymphdrainage. Fragliche diagnostische Bedeutung bei Strangulation und mechanischer Verletzung in Kopfbereich. Z. Rechtsmed. 103 (1989) 33–41

[24] PEABODY, A. J.: Diatoms and drowning. Med. Sci. Law 20 (1980) 254–261

[25] PEARN, J.: Pathophysiology of drowning. Med. J. Aust. 142 (1985) 586–588

[26] PLUECKHANN, V. D.: Alcohol and accidental drowning. A 25 years study. Med. J. Aust. 141 (1984) 22–25

[27] PUSCHEL, E., K. HADJIRAFTIS, B. BRINKMANN: Ungewöhnliche Aspirations-Todesfalle. Beitr. Gerichtl. Med. 42 (1984) 47–56

[28] REH, H.: Über den frühpostmortalen Verlauf der Waschhaut den Fingern. Z. Rechtsmed. 92 (1984) 183–188

[29] REITER, C.: Zum Nachweis des Ertrinkungstodes mittels ins Herzblut eingeschwemmter Raucherzellen. Z. Rechtsmed. 93 (1984) 79–88

[30] ROTENSTEIN, D. O., D. C. STONESCU: Oronasal obstruction lung volumes and arterial oxygenation. Lancet 4/16 (1988) 889–890

[31] SHEPERD, R. T.: Accidental self-strangulation in a young child. Med. Sci. Law 30 (1990) 119–123

[32] Sigrist, T., K. Meier, U. Zollinger: Zum traumatischen Karotissinus Reflextod. Beitr. Gerichtl. Med. 47 (1989) 257–266

[33] Sodeman, W. A., T. M. Sodeman: Pathologic Physiology. W. B. Saunders Co. (1985) pp. 1059–1082

[34] Suzuki, T., N. Ikeda, K. Umetsu, S. Kashimura: Swimming and loss of consciousness. Z. Rechtsmed. 94 (1985) 121–126

[35] Tamaki, K., Y. Katsumata: Enzyme-linked immunoabsorbent assay for plasma thyroglobulin following compression of the neck. Forensic. Sci. Int. 44 (1990) 193–201

Chapter 7
Infanticide

Infanticide makes up about 10–12% of all homicides in Hungary. In recent years it has decreased, but each year we can see an almost seasonal increase.

In the 1878 V. Act the killing of children was defined as a separate crime and punished less severely than murder. The mother who bore a child out of wedlock and during birth or immediately afterward intentionally killed the baby could be punished by up to five years in prison. The criminal law codes today do not list it as a crime separate from homicide, but with penal practice emphasizing the circumstances of the perpetrator and the changes in the social situation regarding an unwanted birth, in general the lower limit of the penalty is not exceeded – five years – in punishing the perpetrator.

The crime of infanticide is especially prominent, in those countries having reached and reaching a significant percentage, where the question of birth control has not been resolved and abortion is prohibited. Thus in the 50's and 60's in Hungary there was not only a large number of illegal abortions with all their consequences, but a significantly higher percentage of newborn corpses came in for autopsy.

The investigations in infanticide, in most cases, are conducted against unknown perpetrators, since generally the body is found in abandoned places, usually in garbage dumps and due to this reason the results of an investigation and legal studies initiated are doubtful. At other times it may be reported because of the complications, with a heavily hemorrhaging woman after giving birth being brought into a medical institution and the institution making the report discovers the fact of delivery.

The question of over which spread of time *infanticide* should be considered child murder varies from country to country. In Hungary the practice prevails of considering it infanticide if it occurs during birth or immediately after. At the same time in other countries under the title of child murder are listed those cases where a child is killed up to 12 months of age, as it is in the United States, while in literature collected from Japan about child murder, attacks on children up to 15 years old are included. A large amount of statistical data has been amassed concerning child murder. Child murder makes up 10–24% of the autopsies in forensic medicine, of which a significant part, according to the statistical data, are infants between the ages of 8 days and 12 months.

In Hungary the rarest cases of child murder happen to several-day-old newborns, and the most common happen during birth or immediately afterward within a few hours. It is surprizing that although in our country the birth regulations and legal abortion are widely recognized, despite this the number of cases of child murder according to published data does not constitute a negligible part of the total homicides. Among the perpetrators a large part are young girls giving birth outside of wedlock, but it also occurs even with those who become pregnant while married or living with a partner, and sometimes the woman who has had two or three children will kill the newborn baby.

Japanese authors studying serial child killing, recount one case of a mother who killed eight of her newborns in a row. In this country 2–3 killings in a row of a woman's own infants has been rarely reported. In the report of CHATTOPADHYAY was mentioned previous infanticide cases from India, originated from socio-cultural and religious tradition. (In India the female child is unwelcome in the families). To prevent the crime the prenatal diagnosis of sex was proposed by the way amniocentesis.

The perpetrators may be women living in relationships with partners for various periods, or not living with them at all, and it cannot be ignored that the lack of sex education may play a significant role. In many instances health workers were investigated for their child killings have found cases where pregnancy could be considered impossible not to be recognized and obviously knew about the possibility of abortion. It is true that these pregnancies originated out of wedlock. The statistical data indicates that the about half of the perpetrators suffer from personality disorders or are mentally deficient. Those with a disturbed personality show personality disorders, labile lifestyles, hypothymia, infantilism, etc. Most of the mothers keep the pregnancy secret, even those perpetrators who are married.

Child murder is, like any other murder, an act committed local event, and the investigation of the scene must purposely include not a general practitioner, but a forensic specialist. In one part, the investigation of the scene may give certain information about the origin of injuries e.g.

- Medical specialists examined and autopsied a newborn who was partially packed in a nylon bag and covered by a straw pile, on the face and neck could be found superficial injuries resembling to manual strangulation, without which, in the absence of blood infiltration into the soft tissues of the neck, would have called attention to these injuries being caused postmortem, by scratches from the straw incurred while being covered under the stack.

At other times, interrogating the mother may add relevant information and help to decide such questions which may come up during the autopsy, but due to the progress of decay, cannot be answered.

- A young girl after giving birth buried her newborn at the edge of a forest by a farm. A few weeks later, the neighbor's dog was found playing with the head of the baby. After being reported, the rest of the remains of the baby could not be located, since the area where the mother had buried the baby had been plowed. According to her confession her pregnancy corresponded to a fullterm pregnancy, and the birth occurred when she was alone at the farm. The most important point was that she remembered that the amniotic fluid was greenish. This made it probable that prior to birth an intrauterine asphyxia developed with the discharge of meconium, perhaps inhaled, and if that were not tenable, the infant would have been born in a viable condition.

With the *autopsy of the newborn,* the examination of the superficial injuries and evaluation of the findings deviating from normal require much practice. The autopsy of the newborn, (see Special Autopsy Techniques) requires a special autopsy technique, and interpretation of the findings requires much experience. An inexperienced specialist may overlook such important autopsy findings which may have influence on the viability of the baby, and with the improper technique may not for example. notice the injury of the tentorium cerebelli, or at other times subependymal hemorrhages of the cerebral ventricles. Sometimes the signs of a live birth, may not be properly evaluated, since as mentioned above each investigation requires much experience from the forensic pathologist *(Fig. 143).*

- The body of a mature newborn baby boy was found in an out-of-the-way place in a nylon bag, and the forensic specialist conducting the autopsy established that he had been born alive, and properly instigated proceedings and an investigation. According to the description of the histological examination of the lungs, it was definitely established that there had been intrauterine breathing movements and extensive inhalation of amniotic fluid, which signified non viability.
From the autopsy record it turned out that the required examinations at autopsy, the lung floating test and the stomach-intestine floating test had been improperly carried out and could not be evaluated. Neither was the section of the superficial autopsy any better, since in the autopsy report the signs of maturity had not been listed.

Death of the newborn may occur due to:

a) an intentional act of the mother,

b) a consequence of negligence (e.g. hypothermia),

c) natural causes.

At the examination and autopsy of a newborn the medical specialist must *answer to the following questions:*

1. Was the newborn born dead or alive?
2. How long did the newborn live after birth?
3. Was it mature; in which month of pregnancy was it born?
4. Was it viable?
5. What was the cause of death?
6. What injuries could be found on the body, and what instrument could have caused them?

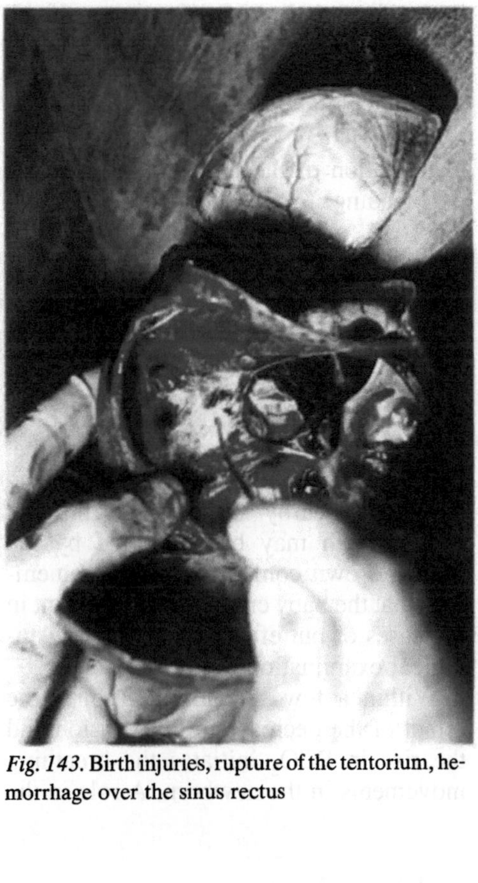

Fig. 143. **Birth injuries, rupture of the tentorium, hemorrhage over the sinus rectus**

7. If it had been delivered under proper medical guidance, could it have been kept alive?

8. Do the injuries found correspond to self assistance marks incurred during birth?

9. What is the blood group of the newborn?

10. Can traces of intentional care be seen on the newborn?

Questions concerning the woman who gave birth:

1. Did she in fact give birth?

2. When did she give birth, and the newborn was born by her?

3. During or immediately after birth did she suffer a pathological mental state?

1. The question of *live birth* is essential in the formulation of the opinion. If the baby is stillborn it can not be the subject of homicide.

The external signs of live birth are not obvious. It can only be decisive in the examination of the newborn if the signs of bleeding from some significant injury (e.g. exclamation mark traces) can raise the suspicion of injury caused while alive.

In the establishment of live birth the alterations may serve as proof which signify, and are created in relation to, the transition from fetal life. Following birth the newborn starts to swallow and breathe, move and cry. The last two are obvious to the people nearby. Occasionally the fact of live birth may be supported by the mother's own confession, if she remembers that the baby cried. This is relevant in the cases of putrefaction, in which histological examination are of no value.

Within a few seconds after birth the effect of the decrease in PO_2 tension and the rise in PCO_2 initiates the breathing movements in the newborn. A role in the initiation of breathing is also played by the sudden expansion of the thorax upon exit of the birth canal. Air enters the airway due to breathing movements and enters the stomach, small intestine and eventually the large intestine due to the swallowing movements, depending on the passage of time. The swallowing movements press air into the inner ear through the Eustachian tubes, and thus the tympanic cavity fills with air. The breathing movements partially alter the lungs of the newborn, and the changing hemodynamic relationships alter the fetal circulation. In the fetal circulation a negligible portion of the blood from the right ventricle enters the vessels of the lungs. From the right ventricle the blood does not enter the pulmonary circulation due to the pulmonary arterial shunt, and the oxygen-rich blood nourishes the brain and the upper extremities. The circulation passes through the ductus arteriosus and the foramen ovale thus circumventing the pulmonary branches. The changes due to breathing air after birth simultaneously changes the distribution of circulation and functional opening of the pulmonary vessels, and weeks later the shunt, the foramen ovale and the ductus arteriosus are obliterated. Unhindered respiration is a sign of maturity of the newborn, since it is a sign of the physiologically operating lung functions. The type II alveolar pneumocytes produce a surfactant substance which consists of phospholipids and its primary role is to decrease the tension resulting from molecular interactions between the water molecules and those of the tissue fluids. Thus with the decrease in surface tension, gas exchange across the alveolar walls can take place and the alveolar opening is assured. This is of special significance in the newborn, where the appropriate amount of surfactant ensures gas exchange and the opening and ability to retain air in those alveoli which during fetal life were filled with fluid.

In *fetal life the lungs* are in a collapsed state, found to the side of the vertebral column, are grey in color due to the paucity of blood supply, and with a texture like that of the spleen. *Histologically* the lungs have a glandular appearance, the alveoli being collapsed, lined with cuboidal or cylindrical epithelium, the bronchioli are star-shaped and little fluid being found in either the alveoli or the bronchioles, a small part of which may be amnionic in origin and the greater part being fluid from the capillaries of the lungs *(Fig. 144)*. Because of the amnionic part, we may find a few squamous epithelial cells and lanugo in the fluid, but the quantity of these does not even approach that found when intrauterine premature breathing begins with the accompanying inhaled histological elements found in the amniotic fluid.

With threatening *intrauterine hypoxia* the fetus begins respiratory movements and empties meconium into the amnionic fluid. With a large amount of meconium, the amnionic fluid becomes a thick, pea-soup green and stains the surface, body hair and vernix caseosa of the fetus, which is visible even on external examination! A mild emptying of meconium only discolors the amnionic fluid, but if the woman giving birth or anyone else present sees the amnionic fluid, they notice the color. The pulmonary circulation also changes with intrauterine respiratory movements. The branches of the pulmonary artery open and fill with blood, so that the lungs become larger and almost fill the thoracic cavity. They become blackberry red in color with a spleen-like texture, and if a large amount of meconium is inhaled, greenish areas appear through the visceral pleura and as a sign of death by suffocation extensive subpleural hemorrhages are seen. *Histologically* the tissue of the lung is airless and thick, greenish meconium can be seen in the alveoli, bronchioli and bronchi, which in stained preparations appears as formless, brown masses. If the passage of meconium was not significant, the premature respiratory movements results in the inhalation of a large amount amnion containing the characteristic fetal squamous epithelial cells and hairs which can also verify the cause of suffocation *(Fig. 145)*. Besides this, the open branches of the pulmonary artery fill with blood and give the lungs of the fetus dying of premature intrauterine respiration their dark red color.

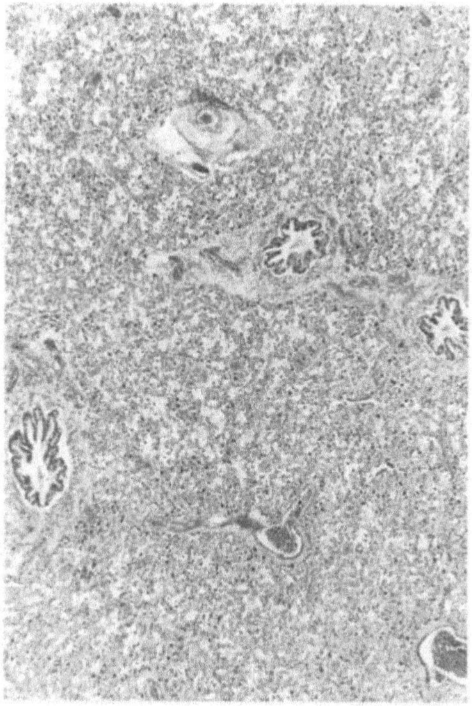

Fig. 144. Glandular picture of a lung that never breathed showing collapsed alveoli and star-shaped bronchioli

The *lungs of a live born* baby fill the thorax, are "pinkish red" in color, spongy in texture and light in weight, so that if

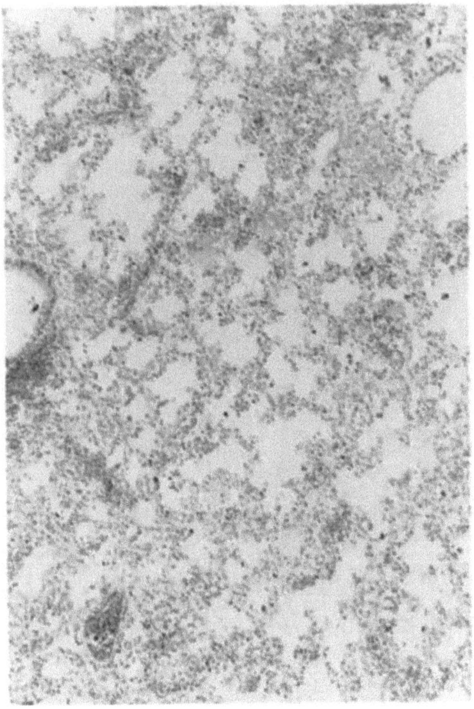

Fig. 145. Expanded alveoli, flattened respiratory epithelia and rounded bronchioli in a lung that has drawn breath

placed in water, either whole or in pieces, they float. The float test was developed by a doctor from Pozsony (Bratislava) named REYGER in 1670 as a means of determining live birth, but a positive test only means a decrease in specific gravity, and there are possibilities for error stemming from the autopsy technique. *Histologically* the ventilated lung is evenly filled with air but small sections of atelectasis may appear in the days following birth. The alveoli fill with air, the alveolar epithelia flatten out into the form of respiratory epithelia. The bronchioles stiffen and become rounded with free lumens *(Fig. 145)*. The interstitial vessels open and fill with blood and the argyrophilic fiber network of the lung stretches out. These together make up the histological picture of the ventilated lung and signify the live born status of the newborn, so to omit the histological examination of the lung in the autopsy of a newborn is a technical error on the part of the forensic specialist. The histological samples must purposely be taken from each lobe of the lungs, since occasionally a decreased respiratory movement may explain an inconstant aspiration of meconium or amnion in each lobe *(Fig. 146)*.

The *judgement of a live birth* based on the histological findings is not always unequivocal. In numerous cases we have experienced, – especially when an examination has been made of samples of each lobe –, that a ventilated lung had been diagnosed as unventilated and vice versa. False negative cases may occur in those newborns born with respiratory distress where the areas of lung containing very little air are absorbed postmortally, since after the cessation of breathing the heartbeat continues for a few minutes, and due to the pulmonary circulation, the air is reabsorbed. The alveoli of the ventilated areas collapse. An insufficient amount of surfactant also plays a role. At other times the evaluation of the histological findings in a stillborn may be erroneous due either to artificial respiration or the processes of decay. It may not be simple an inexperienced examiner to diagnose inhalation of amnion or meconium. Sometimes recognizing even dense appearances may cause problems. It is all the more difficult if artificial respiration or mild decay processes have resulted in air in the lungs of the newborn. Postmortally introduced air distributes evenly, breaks through the alveolar walls and large emphysema-like alterations may develop, but the alterations of the alveolar epithelia and the rounding out and stiffening of the bronchioles do not take place *(Fig. 147, 148, 149)*.

Among the signs of live birth are such

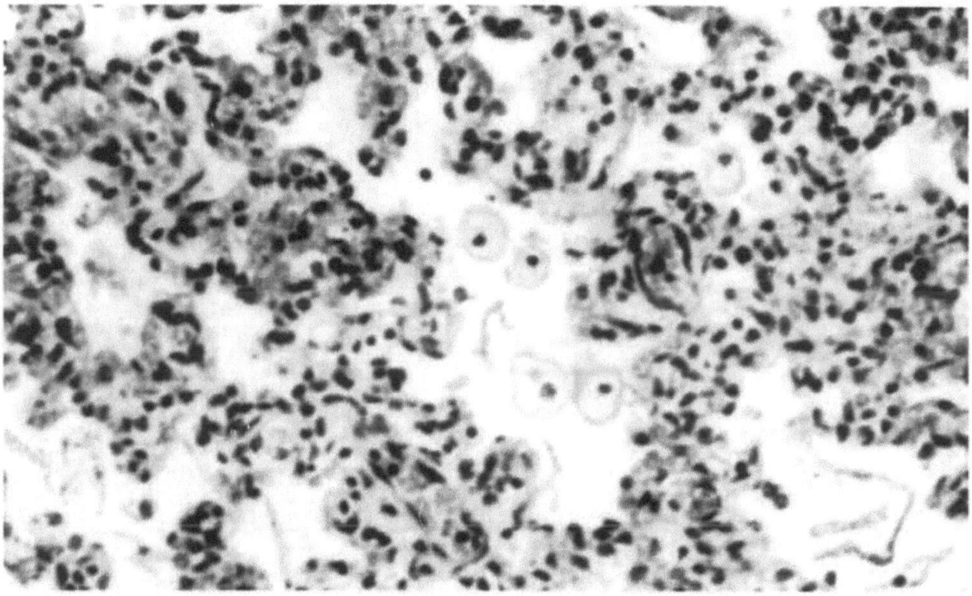

Fig. 146. Amnion aspiration, amnion squamous cells, lanugo in the alveoli (medium magnification)

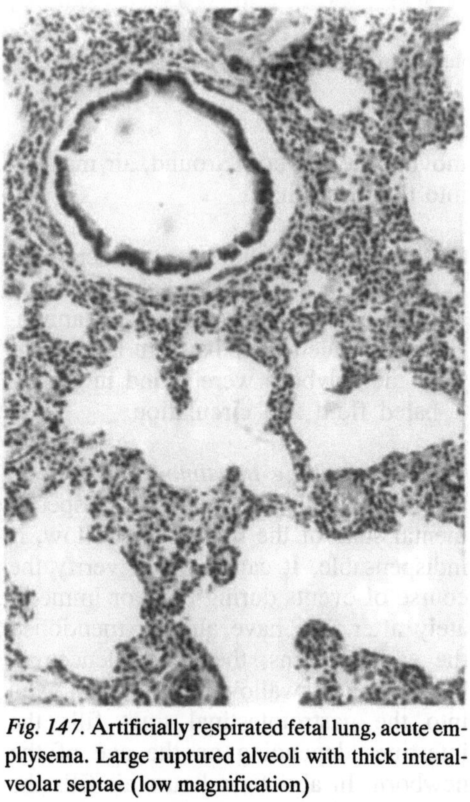

Fig. 147. Artificially respirated fetal lung, acute emphysema. Large ruptured alveoli with thick interalveolar septae (low magnification)

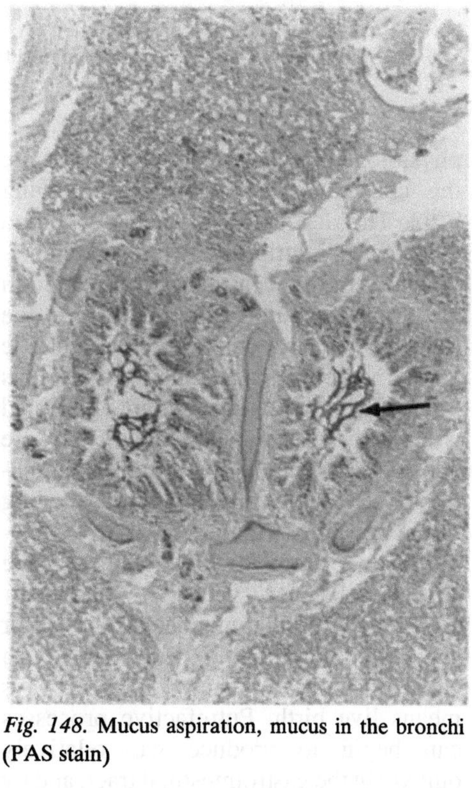

Fig. 148. Mucus aspiration, mucus in the bronchi (PAS stain)

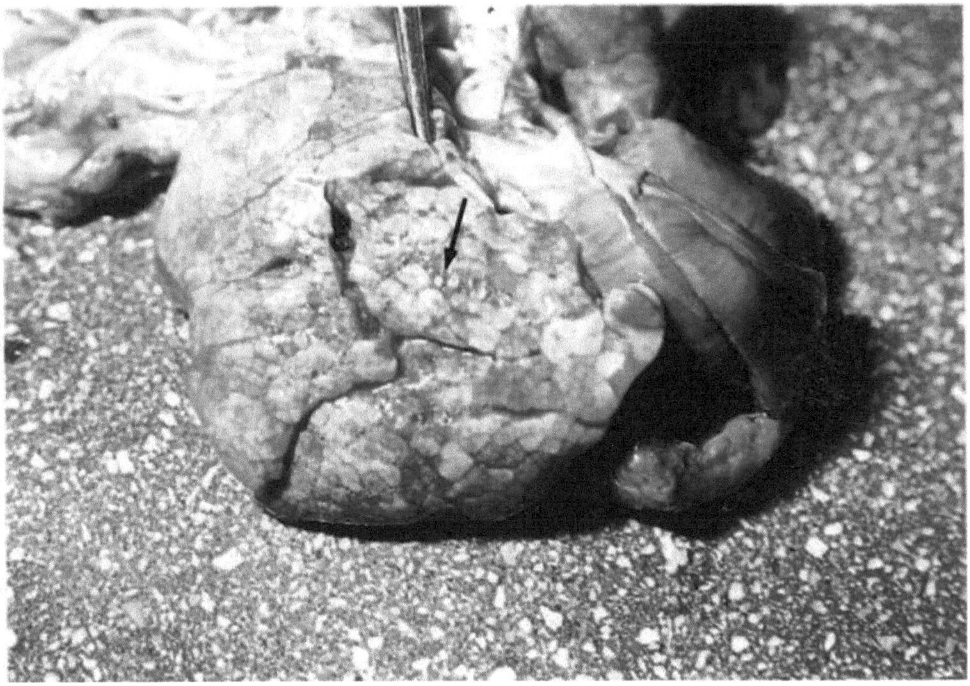

Fig. 149. Artificially respirated newborn lung, with ruptured alveoli, inflated lung tissue

physiological manifestations which are the consequences of events following birth. The destruction of fetal red blood cells releases purines which results in elevation of the concentration of uric acid in the urine, and urate salts deposit in the kidney tubules, causing characteristic golden yellow streaks. One to two weeks following birth the urate salts are eliminated without a trace, but until then, they are considered a sign of live birth. Examination of the gastric contents verifies feeding of the newborn. Mother's milk in the stomach is a whitish, cottage cheese-like stringy substance, which is easily differentiated for the mucous aspirated or swallowed originating from the birth canal. Air in the stomach does not always means live birth. Putrefactive processes can begin to produce gas relatively quickly in the gastrointestinal tract, and by moving the newborn around, air may get into the stomach.

- A forensic pathologist rendered an opinion of a live born baby who was born in to the water since the examination revealed diatoms from the organs of the newborn were found in the inhaled fluid and circulation.

2. *Determining the time elapsed from the birth,* to the extent that the special mental state of the mother will allow, is indispensable. It can serve to verify the course of events during birth or immediately after. We have already mentioned the earliest signs, the consequences of breathing and swallowing. Air swallowed into the gastrointestinal tract fills the intestines depending on the age of the newborn. In about six hours air fills the

small intestine, and in the next six hours it fills the large intestine. These values are rather uncertain. (One must not mistake the gas production of autolytic processes, which fills the bowels in segments, while swallowed air fills the bowels evenly.) Meconium is eliminated from the large intestine within about two days. We have already mentioned the formation of the so-called *urate infarcts* in the kidney tubules. The demarcation of the umbilical cord starts in newborns after about 12–14 hours, dries out, and 36 hours later, the skin is swollen and red, and on the sixth day the umbilical cord detaches, while the scab is visible for 12 days.

With the changes in fetal circulation, the closure of the shunts take place in varying stages. The ductus venosus is obliterated by sterile inflammation 5–10 days after birth, the foramen ovale after 4–8 weeks, and the ductus arteriosus after 8 weeks.

On the head serosanguineous infiltrations (caput succedaneum) may appear as circumscribed edematous, hemorrhagic swellings in the scalp, the edema of which is absorbed within a few hours, followed by the decay of red blood cells. Bleeding at the borders of the bones results in cephalhematoma located under the periosteum. It's organization requires weeks to complete, and sometimes organizes into an exostosis-like ossification.

3. The *newborn may be considered mature* if it has reached the 37–42nd week (259–293 days), a body weight of 2500 g, a cranial circumference of 36 cm, and a body length of 52 cm. Besides measurements, certain external signs can verify newborn maturity: some vernix caseosa found on the body surface, and intertriginous areas, developed subcutaneous fatty tissue, nails exceeding the fingertips, testes palpable in the scrotum of male infants, and labia majora covering the labia minora in girl babies. At autopsy the cranial bones are stiff and fragile, the brownish color of the fetal fat tissue differentiates it from the usual yellow, and in the distal epiphysis of the femur a 5–6 mm diameter ossification center can be found.

A premature newborn may exceed 2500 g, but the external signs of premature birth are obvious in this case. The body surface is covered by a thick, downy lanugo (fine hair), the fontanels are wide, the cranial sutures are well-palpable and wide open, the bones are flexible, the nails soft, and the umbilical cord is attached close to the symphysis.

The *stage of the pregnancy,* the age of the fetus, the time elapsed since conception can be indicated within certain limits.

4. *Viability* also depends on maturity. The viability of premature infants is significantly decreased, with the possibility of survival significantly decreasing with greater time remaining to full-term. In the past newborns under 1000 g have been considered as abortions and were considered to be non-viable – and in pathology this view is still maintained. Today with intensive perinatal care we can now keep a larger percentage of these small weight premature infants alive. In the forming of medical expert opinion it must be emphasized that the chance of survival of prematures infants is smaller, even with appropriate intensive care.

Viability is influenced by developmental disorders and birth injuries, which would cause either inability to adjust to life, or death soon after birth.

5. *Death of the newborn may result from:*

a) natural causes,
b) maternal neglect,
c) criminal acts.

The greater part of *deaths by natural causes* results from developmental disorders which either make adjustment to life immediately after birth impossible – i.e. malformed fetus, anencephaly, other disorders of closure of the spinal canal, severe meningocele, ectopic organs, serious developmental disorders of the heart, etc. – or they may be such which, without the appropriate treatment within a few hours or days of birth, may cause the death of the newborn, such as esophageal atresia, esophageo-tracheal fistula, bilateral absent kidney, or significant diaphragmatic hernia.

Among the birth injuries, intracranial injuries are those which, cause an increase in intracranial pressure, therefore causing the death of the newborn shortly after birth. Hemorrhage may originate from rupture of the emissary vessels, causing typical subdural hemorrhage, or more commonly with rupture of the tentorium cerebelli with accompanying subtentorial hemorrhage. If this occurs even to a small degree, it may cause death. The cause of tentorial rupture may be due to the configuration assumed in the birth canal and especially often it occurs in a hypoxic state or in premature infants due to the fragility of the tissues.

Especially in newborns we see subependymal hemorrhages rupturing into in the lateral ventricles.

During birth, traction of the spinal column may result in epidural hemorrhage in the spinal canal. ÖKRÖS pointed out the significance of this. In forced birth or precipitate labor, injuries are more common and, especially in precipitate labor, the fetus practically tumbles out of the birth canal, and the anterior parts may suffer serious injuries often resembling violent, foreign hand injuries. Among the birth injuries are listed rupture or subcapsular hemorrhage of the liver, which may result in bleeding to death if the capsule ruptures later.

Depending on the mechanism of birth, injuries such as fractures of the clavicle or humerus may also appear. The practical significance of these lies in that they raise the suspicion of abuse.

In newborns of secret pregnancies we find a greater number of birth injuries resulting in non-viability compared to those born in medical institutions. This may be due not only to the very poor condition, but also to the possibility that in many cases care of the newborn immediately following birth is delayed, and thus mild respiratory difficulties, which normally would not be significant in a medical institution, can be fatal. The inappropriate birth process, – i.e. unassisted birth – may also carry numerous consequences. (We examined a case of birth without professional assistance in which the newborn suffocated in its mother's amnion-soaked flannel underwear.) The care and chance of survival of an infant in a state of respiratory distress is uncertain even under appropriate institution. We have found histological alterations, due to distress syndrome, in a large number of cases of birth outside of hospitals against whom charges were pressed on the basis of alterations suggesting infanticide.

The examination of the case of natural death, either to verify or exclude, is one of the forensic medical specialist's most important tasks.

Maternal neglect makes up a relatively rare part of the examined cases. We may expect it mainly when the birth takes place in a cold environment, and the mother after birth becomes too weak, for example, due to loss of blood, and the infant dies of hypothermia. The relatively large surface area to body weight ratio together with the immaturity of the temperature regulating center increases the possibility for the newborn to suffer hypothermia even in a relatively warm external environment.

Hemorrhage to death through the umbilical cord is not likely due to the altered hemodynamic condition unless there are any developmental abnormalities which result in an increased venous blood pressure.

Suffocation of the newborn appears relatively frequently if the infant of the woman giving birth alone gets its face into the amnion-soaked cloths, or if the thighs of the mother block the airway of the baby. These are the cases which require special care in examination of the motives and ability of action of the mother, in other words, considering the special mental or psychological state.

Actions directed against the life of the newborn may be quite variable. National statistics indicate that strangulation is the most common mode of infanticide, however, in our practice death by suffocation seems to dominate. Manual strangulation rarely occurs, and suffocation following giving birth into a toilet makes up the largest percentage.

FÖLDES and coworkers compiled 25 cases taken from the same county as our material. Thus the killing of newborns by various modes can be followed over the last 20 years. In FÖLDES' material manual strangulation held the first place and relatively many – 6 – were death caused by rough trauma, i.e. trampling and smashing the head. In our material between 1971–1988 we examined 34 cases. The leading cause of death was already mentioned (suffocation), but traumatizing acts remained surprisingly low.

Among the methods of killing, besides those mentioned above, *obstruction of the airways* by hand or by a soft material may also occur *(Fig. 150)*. At other times an infant may intentionally born into a water filled vessel or a toilet or into an outhouse.

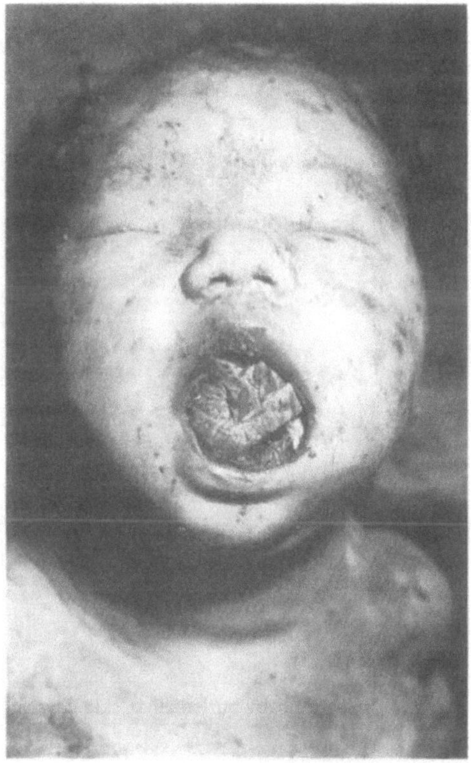

Fig. 150. Infanticide. Blocking the mouth

- An average sized infant born into a toilet bowl could not be flushed down the toilet because its head exceeded the diameter of the spout. Thus this possibility was excluded in the criminal action against the health care worker who, noticing labor pains, sat on the toilet and gave birth to the baby. At autopsy, local emphysematous alterations in the lungs indicated that intermittent airway obstruction had taken place, and fetal elements were not found in the airways. Later the mother confessed that she had flushed the toilet several times and thus drowned the baby.

It is rare, to examine a brutal attempt to hide or "disappear" an act of infanticide.

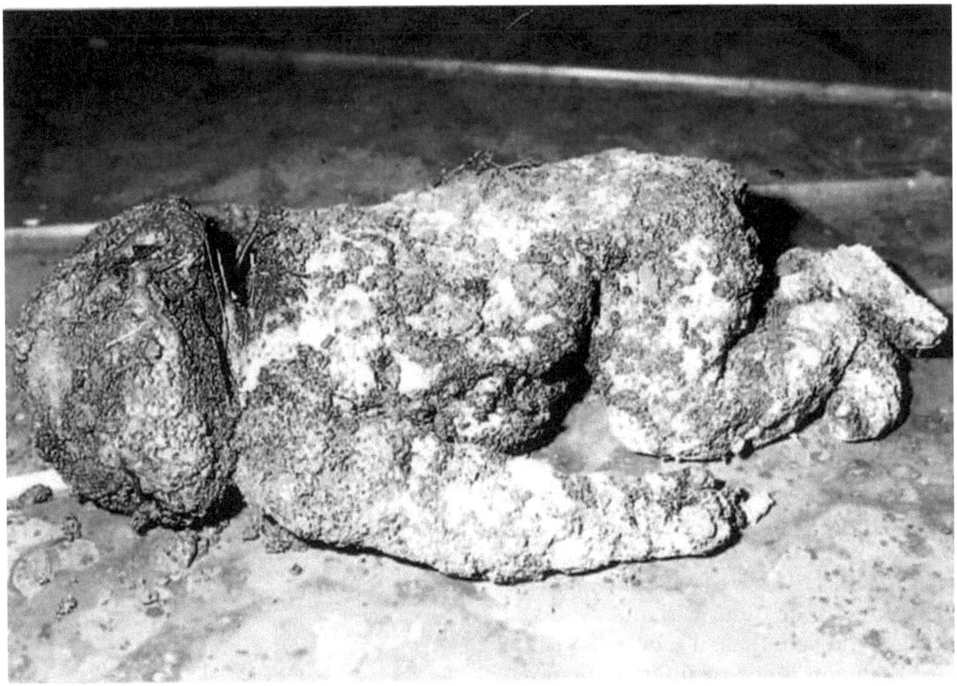

Fig. 151. Newborn baby buried alive, skin covered with clay

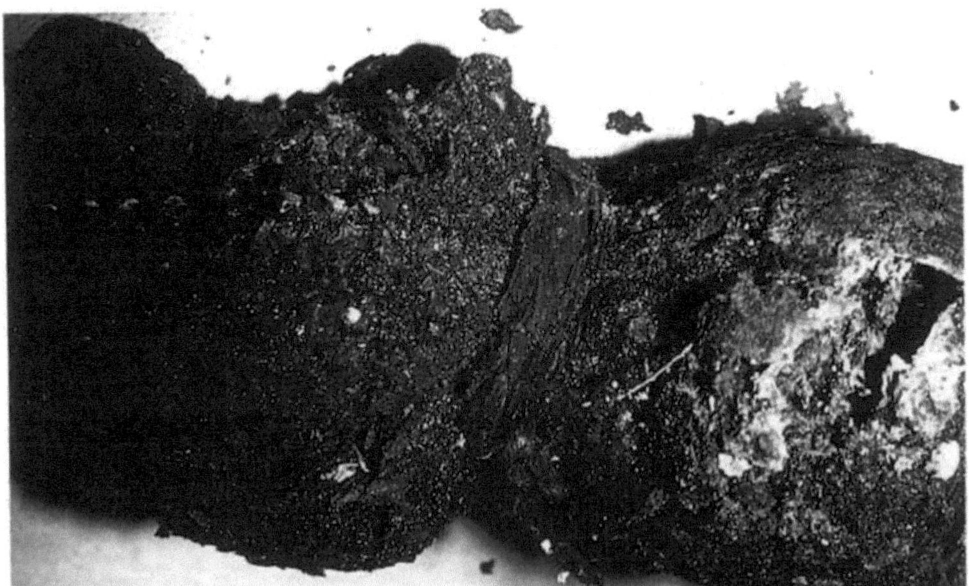

Fig. 152. Body of a burned baby after strangling. The strangling instrument can still be identified around the neck

In our practice a case occurred where the mother of a woman who gave birth, without the knowledge of her daughter, first strangled the unwanted baby and then tried to burn it up *(Fig. 151, 152)*. At the autopsy we found the strangling cord around the corpse's neck and were also able to establish that the infant had been born alive.

The above listed methods make up only a part of the killing methods used to free oneself from unwanted newborns.

5. Injuries of the newborn may result while passing through the birth canal or after the parturition and afterward. (Sometimes alterations caused by amnion strips can look like and be judged as injuries which may even cause amputation of the extremities.) We have already discussed injuries originating in the birth canal, such as the fracture of an upper limb which is not necessarily a sign of violence. In the case of speedy birth, the leading part may suffer bruising and laceration injuries with fracture of the skull often occurring. Skull fracture in the newborn characteristically appears as breaks in the bone radiating outward from the point of applied force, with the fracture lines extending outward from a center to the border of the same bone and may only extend beyond the sutures if the applied force reached there as well. Thus a multiple fracture in the base of the skull or fracture lines crossing several bones cannot be the consequence of a fall to the floor during the course of a speedy delivery. It is more likely the result of a compression force to the head of the newborn. Injury to the umbilical cord has often been described in the speedup birth. According to the general consensus, the umbilical cord rarely breaks in speedy birth, the 40–60 cm umbilical cord being long enough so that the newborn can hit the floor. At other times it ruptures at the skin-umbilical border and rarely leaves a longer umbilical section behind, rupturing at the end nearest the body.

Grip marks in the areas of the face, mouth and neck are not always the marks of intentional harm. During delivery the woman may grasp the presenting part and pull on the baby to facilitate the birth. These injuries belong to the de-finition of the "self-assisted" delivery. They are always found on the leading part of the newborn and may appear as rough injuries, whether as bruises or contusions around the eyes or crushing injuries around the nose and mouth. Injuries rarely occur to the neck. These injuries must be differentiated from intentional criminal acts.

6. Injuries to the newborn may originate after its death. Due to the delicate state of the skin, a relatively mild application of force can result in a superficial removal of epithelium which if dries, resembles external injury. We have described similar drying out in the area of the mouth, scrotum and genital labia of the newborn, due to loss of fluid across the thin skin. If the injuries are on the mouth or neck, and there are fine postmortal scratch-like areas, they may be often mistaken for grasp injuries to the neck. The absence of hemorrhagic infiltration in the soft tissues of the neck and face or other obvious signs of other causes of death help to direct the examination onto the right path.

7. The question especially arises in the autopsy of the abandoned newborn or newborn with a decreased viability of whether, with the appropriate conduction of the birth or presence of proper facilities, the baby could have been kept alive. Often at the onset of labor the woman to give birth hardly, or mistakenly, interprets the early labor pains as an urge to urinate or defecate, especially if she is a young first-

timer. It also occurs often that she couldn't get to a proper institution quickly enough even if she wanted to. (Infanticide does not always happen intentionally with secret pregnancies. The Hungarian Supreme Court 15th directive says: "The circumstance where a perpetrator does not prepare for birth, and does not arrange for medical treatment and care, does not in itself constitute a preplanned intentional negligent manslaughter."

Many factors may influence the woman keeping a secret pregnancy, such as shame, fear of loss of job, etc., but neither is the secret birth unknown in the practice of obstetrics.

- The Hungarian Supreme Court judged in a different manner the case of young mother who bore a child of a secret pregnancy. The newborn died abandoned with early intrauterine breathing movements – uterine asphyxia – playing a role in the cause of death, and the medical specialist reckoned the newborn to be of decreased viability. In the judgement the Supreme Court emphasized that a medical worker – the defendant was a certified perinatologist, working in an obstetrics institution – must have recognized the process of birth from the elements of her profession, the possible consequences, the importance of education of the pregnant woman and its significance. In her case, the Supreme Court judged that the child was not properly cared for. The fact was that at the onset of labor pains, the room mate did not even get up and walk the 150 m to the obstetrics institute where there was a realistic possibility of saving the baby's life, and this was also judged to constitute intent. The professionally qualified defendant was judged by the Supreme Court guilty with criminal intent.

The above case proves that the repercussions of professional birth assistance in keeping the newborn alive demands much experience and expertise, and the answering of these questions especially calls for the expert advice of an obstetrician.

The *search for traces of intentional acts* at the same time serves to clarify the capability of action and mental state of the woman following delivery. Directed activities testify to a series of acts meant to keep the newborn alive and care for it. The cutting of the umbilical cord to separate it from the placenta is part of an intentional series of actions. They can be unambiguously verified upon examination of the newborn. The removal of the dried blood and mucus from the body surface of the baby by washing, the little vernix caseosa on the mature newborn and its lack in the body creases indicate that the newborn was bathed and cared for previously. The swaddling and covering of the newborn are also intentional attempts for care. Naturally, these acts do not exclude the possibility of a later crime, or of a death by natural causes *(Fig. 153).*

The autopsy of the newborn must be performed as described in the chapter on a special autopsy techniques. At autopsy a specially taken blood sample, as already discussed, verifies the blood group characteristics that are already present in fetal life, and in one case Szabó identified the father through a successfully performed evaluation during the autopsy of a newborn.

Part of the *questions applying to the mother* can be answered in the course of the obstetric examination. Even if a long time elapsed between the finding of the newborn and the examination of the suspect, we can at least still find out whether or not she gave birth. Stretch marks on the abdominal wall and a healed scar in the

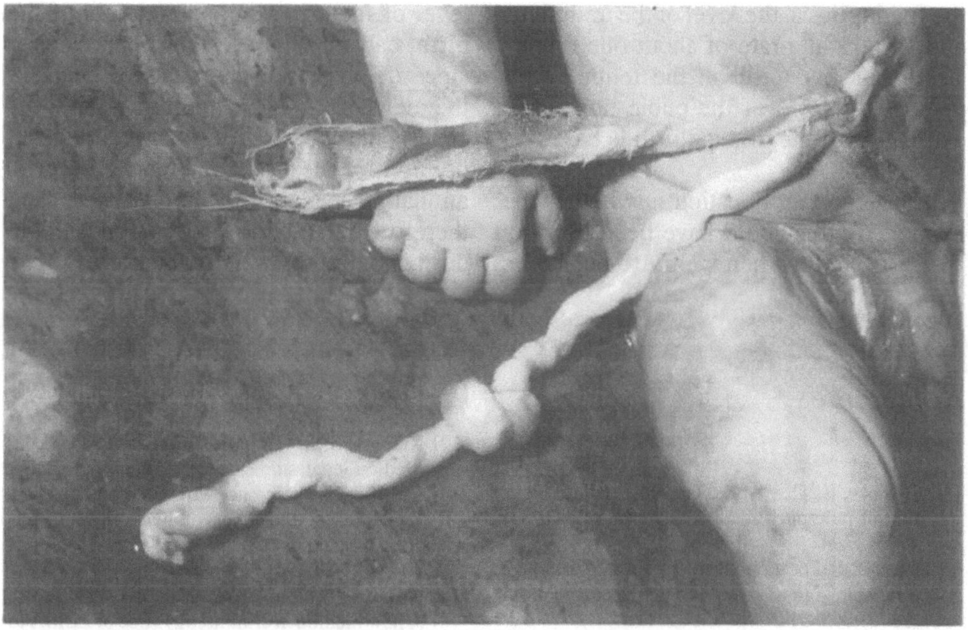

Fig. 153. "Home birth", cut end of the umbilical cord. Knotted umbilical cord tied with a rag

perineal region indicate a pregnancy and a delivery. With the internal examination, transverse scars from stretch tears in the vaginal mucosa are noticeable while the external part of the vaginal cervix is deformed by a transverse tear.

We can also indicate not only the processes following birth but the amount of time that has elapsed as well. The state of the external and internal genital organs immediately after birth, the shrinking of the uterus back to normal and the "discharge" of pregnancy can be indicative. These are detailed in textbooks on obstetrics, so we will give only a rough outline of them. After birth the fundus of the uterus can be found shrunken under the umbilicus. The cervix is flabby, and later contracts. The breasts are glandular with colostrum able to be expressed and the areolar areas are strongly pigmented. The internal examination reveals a dilatated, open and lacerated uterine cervical canal with oozing hemorrhages. In the vagina and perineum there may be lacerations. The surface of the uterus is irregular, especially where the placenta was attached. We may see areas of hemorrhage and histologically, remains of the decidua and trophoblast can be found in the basal layer. The surface of this gradually decreases and a few days following birth it has reduced itself to 6–8 cm in diameter.

With the healing processes, leukocytes and macrophages migrate into the superficial hemorrhagic, fibrin-filled depositions which are then discharged in a secretion – lochia – depending on the puerperal recovery time. The discharge in the first week is sanguineous, then turning serosanguineous. In the second week it is brownish, then yellowish-white, changing to serous in nature in the third week and disappearing completely after six weeks. The return of the uterus to normal after birth can also be observed. The first day the fundus lies at the level of the umbilicus and shrinks at a rate of about one fingerwidth per day until on the tenth day it reaches the level of the pubic bone. The estimation of the time of birth is based on these data.

The important question is whether the examined fetus could have been born by the suspected women we try to decide its level of maturity, the examination of the birth canals injuries, the time elapsed since delivery, and the signs of death in the newborn. As mentioned above, recently the possibility of rendering an opinion on the basis of blood group examination has been demonstrated, and therefore the taking of a blood sample during the autopsy is mandatory.

References

[1] BONHAM, E., CARTER R.: The architectural function of pulmonary capillaries. Lancet 1 (1957) 1292–1294

[2] BURIS, L., S. POCZKODI: Is the aeration of the lungs a reliable sign of live birth? Z. Rechtsmed. 83 (1979) 303–312

[3] FÖLDES, V.: Szakértői bizonyítás gyermekölés esetén. Kandidátusi értekezés (1958)

[4] FÖLDES, V.: A köldökzsinór test köré csavarodásának törvényszéki orvostani vonatkozásai. Orvosi Hetilap 93 (1952) 1068–1071

[5] FÖLDES, V.: Az arc és nyak szülési sérüléseinek igazságügyi orvostani vonatkozásai. Orvosi Hetilap 95 (1954) 771–772

[6] FÖLDES, V.: Szokatlanul súlyos szülési agysérülések. DOTE Tudományos ülésének évkönyve (1953–1954)

[7] FÖLDES, V., SZABÓ Á., HARSÁNYI L.: Újszülöttkori erőszakos halálesetek. Belügyi Szemle 4 (1964) 39–48

[8] FUNAYAMA, M., K. SAGISAKA: Consecutive infanticides in Japan. Am. J. Forensic Med. Pathol. 9 (1988) 9–11

[9] HIRVONEN, J., R. TIISALA, U. UOTILA, H. ARKO, E. TAHTI, K. LAIHO, A. MARTTILA, M. TENHU: Roentgenological and autopsy studies on the gas content of the lungs and gastro-intestinal tract in living and stillborn infants, and sources of error in resuscitation. 65 (1969) 73–86

[10] JASON, J., M. M. CARPENTER, C. W. TYLER: Underrecording of infant homocide in the United States. Am. J. Public Health 73 (1983) 195–197

[11] KENYERES, I.: Törvényszéki orvostan. Magyar Orvosi Könyvkiadó Társulat (1911) 438–507

[12] KURODA, S., H. NAGAMORI, M. EBE, M. SASAKI: Medico-legal studies on the fetus and infant: with special references to histological characteristics of the lungs of liveborn and stillborn infants. Tohoku J. exp. Med. 85 (1965) 40–54

[13] KURUCZ, E., F. KÓSA, É. MONOSTORI, I. ANDO: A new method in criminology: Use of ELISA to detect AFP on different materials with monoclonal anti-fetoprotein. Z. Rechtsmed. 93 (1984) 117–121

[14] LÖKÖS, B.: A gyermekgyilkosságról 32 elmeorvosszakértői vélemény elemzése alapján. Diplomamunka Debrecen (1989)

[15] Olson, C. J., D. J. Gee, B. Knight: The Essentials of Forensic Medicine. Pergamon Press Oxford (1985) pp. 514–531

[16] POCZKODI, S.: Gyermek élveszülöttségének megállapítása diatoma lelet alapján. MIOT esetbemutató (1987)

[17] PROKOP, O.: Zur Brauchbarkeit der elastischen Fasern der Lunge im Rahmem der Lebensproben. Z. Rechtsmed. 69 (1971) 177–184

[18] SHANKARAN, S., E. ELIAS, N. ILAGAN: Subcapsular hemorrhage of the liver in very low birthweight neonate. Acta Paediatr. Scand. 80 (1991) 619–619

[19] SCHMIDT, V., CH. BAEDEKER, E. KELLER: Tod eines Zwillings Kindestötung oder intrauteriner Fruchttod? Arch. f]r Kriminologie 176 (1985) 7–16

[20] SZABÓ, L.: Apasági vizsgálat magzatrészek és maradványok alapján. MIOT esetbemutató (1988)

Chapter 8
Sexual life in relation to the law

Rape

The Penal Code Section 197 "Whoever coerces a woman outside a permanent relationship, or by threat to life or health, to engage in sexual intercourse, or takes advantage of a state of the woman where she is incapable of expressing her will or of self-defense, commits a crime..."

The victim of such a crime can only be a woman, with whom the relevant element is that she is not in a permanent relationship wit the perpetrator. The act is considered to have been committed if the man at least touches the woman's genital organs with his genitals with intent to have intercourse. Thus the victim of the crime can also be a young girl who is physiologically incapable of sexual intercourse. The cases of rape have risen world wide. The ages of the victims are variable starting with little girls a few years old in whom we see serious injuries with sexual intercourse, but we have also examined a very shameful case of an old lady over 80. The perpetrators in a great many of the cases are drunk and males in the prime of life. In examination of the victims, numerous questions must be answered:

1. Did sexual intercourse occur?
2. Are signs of rape visible?
3. Was the victim incapable of expressing her will in self-defense?
4. What are the consequences of the crime?

Proof of rape may be established by:
a) loss of virginity,
b) injury of the genitals,
c) the presence of sperm,
d) pregnancy.

If the rape occurs with a virgin, the *loss of virginity* may prove sexual intercourse. Damage to the hymen with easily seen anatomical alterations occurs in a high percentage of cases. The hymen is a double layer of mucous membrane emplaced at the vaginal entrance which may appear in various forms *(Fig. 154).*

In the recognition of the intact hymen, its characteristic anatomical variability often provides opportunity for erroneous deductions. If the hymen has a small opening and is elliptical, then the possibility of the usual sexual intercourse normal cannot be entertained without injury. The various types of hymens can sometimes mislead even the practicing gynecologists regarding the status of virginity.

● We examined an 18-year-old mentally deficient girl who accused her brother

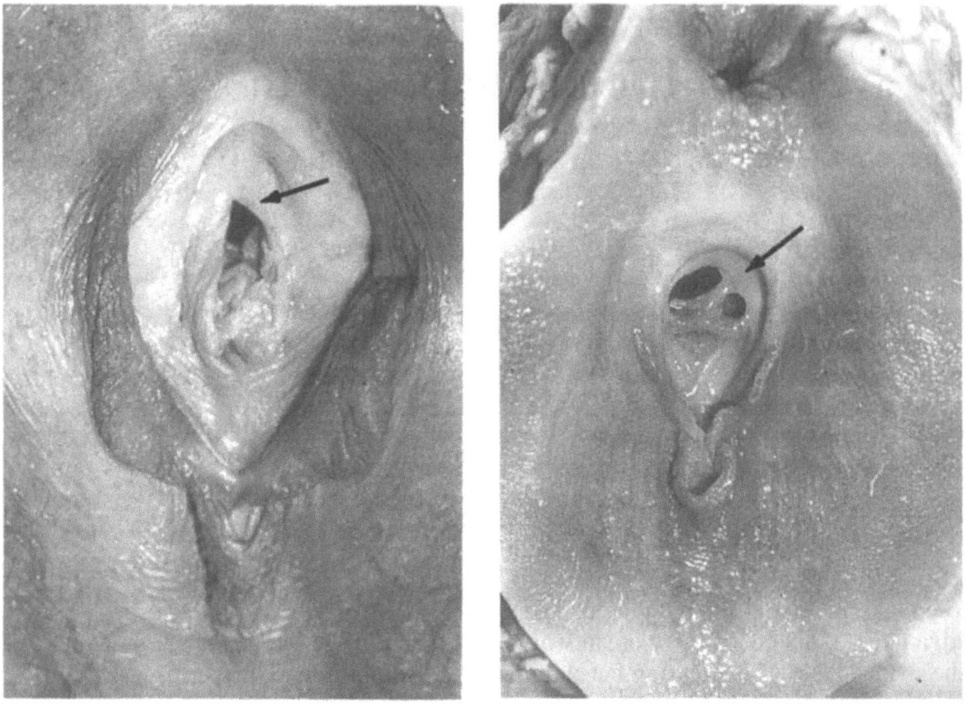

Fig. 154. Septate and annular hymens (from the collection of Prof. Ökrös)

and father of using her as a sexual partner. The preliminary gynecological examination described a "torn" hymen at the vaginal entrance. A repeated specialist and gynecological examination revealed an intact, lobulated hymen of a diameter admitting entrance of one finger, which would have been injured had sexual intercourse actually occurred.

The individual characteristics of the hymen are such that they can be evaluated only with individual examinations. Among the basic types, sexual intercourse without injury is possible with the low, elliptical hymen. In the lobulated hymen, the notch may extend into the vaginal mucosa as well, and in many cases had been evaluated as previous injury. Fresh injury to the hymen is not hard to identify. The injury usually develops within 5–7 hours with shallow bleeding, although sometimes the bleeding may be significant. Healing is rapid, as is the case for mucous membranes, and within 2–3 days evidence of a previous injury cannot even be seen. If it extends deeply, there may also be injury to the mucous membranes of the entrance of the vagina, and thus the healing may be prolonged to 7–10 days. After healing, the double mucous membrane is bound with scar tissue, the scarified area being poor in vessels, greyish-white, and incapable of becoming engorged with blood. (With rubbing the area around the scar will become engorged, but the scar tissue remains greyish-white). But differentiating from a physiological notching of the hymen requires a great deal of experience, an that is why it is better to examine the victim together with an experienced gynecologist. Magnification by use of a colposcope can be useful in doubtful cases. Care is very important in the examination so that the doctor himself does not cause damage to the hymen.

Injury to the hymen, as mentioned previously, is not always a sign of sexual intercourse. It can be caused by the introduction of a foreign object, and injury caused by the fingers, either from masturbation or prior to the sexual intercourse, is not rare. Due to its being relatively protected, isolated damage affecting only the hymen doesn't happen in accidents.

After loss of virginity, sexual intercourse may cause *injury to the external genital organs.* Alterations to the entrance of the vagina and the vagina itself may occur not only in rape, but also in normal sexual intercourse. In sexual intercourse, with unprepared women, introduction of the male organ may cause difficulty and we can expect the development of rough injuries. In the less supple sexual organs of elderly women, injuries are more common and serious. There may be superficial injuries to the vaginal mucous membranes, or deep ones with lacerations to the mucous membranes resulting in nearly fatal hemorrhage. In these injuries spatial disproportion is not necessary, and often a forcefully applied entrance into a woman with an inappropriate physical condition can cause injury. The appearance of such injuries in sexual intercourse that are caused by the male organ are especially common, but manual injuries are not rare, either. (Most cases of injuries to the sexual organs of small children are caused by fingers.) The injuries may extend particularly to the perineal region, where lacerations with acute and profuse bleeding may occur and become a threat to life. Healing may occur with such scarification that may be a problem to intercourse in the future. In mature women, sexual intercourse may cause only superficial injuries to the mucous membranes which may not even be visible to the naked eye. In the early stages there may be bleeding into the mucosa and the development of swelling, but these disappear within hours following intercourse.

The simplest and most definite proof of intercourse is the *demonstration of sperm* in the vaginal swab. One single intact sperm cell is sufficient. Sperm cells can be demonstrated in the vaginal swab for 2–3 days after sexual intercourse. In the corpse, sperm cells have been demonstrated a week after death. For this reason by examination of a vaginal smear it is not possible to tell when before death the sperm got in. In every case which we find a large number of heads and tail fragments with few intact sperm cells on the smear, intercourse did not take place immediately before death or the examination. In the corpse we can search for sperm cells not only in the area of the entrance to the vagina or in smears taken from the vaginal vault, but we should also examine the cervix, scrapings from the fundus of the uterus and the openings of the fallopian tubes as well. Within a few minutes following sexual intercourse the sperm cells can make their way into the cervical canal and into the uterine cavity, and here they are preserved for the longest period.

In considering whether it is truly sperm we are examining, the macroscopic signs can only give an indication, and demonstration by microscopic examination establishes the fact beyond doubt. Semen, examined with the unaided eye have a crusted texture and appear with a lobulated border, depending on the character of the surface on which they are found – a mat grey color on a dark base, or soaked into the cloth of a moisture-absorbing material. In the area of the genital organs a dried greyish-white stain can be seen. At other times on the body surfaces or materials "slug trails" can be seen standing out as greyish-white, dried patches.

The demonstration of motile sperm verifies sexual intercourse within the previous 12 hours. The demonstration of sperm only means that previous sexual intercourse occurred, but provides very little data as to how and when they arrived in the vagina. Many have dealt with the changes in sperm count and the characteristics of morphology over time in the period following intercourse. The findings are variable. And that is not surprising since, as we have elaborated previously, the sperm count can be influenced by many factors, and individuality may play a role in the destructive processes taking place in the vagina or cervix. The previously mentioned motility time – under 12 hours – only shows the average, and according to the literature sperm motility can be preserved in the vagina for 3–24 hours and 110 hours to 7 days (!) in the cervix. Sperm cells can be found, although in decreasing numbers, for days in the vagina, cervix and uterine cavity. It is worthwhile to once more discuss the significant decrease in sperm number found in examined samples taken from a vaginal douche. In the experimental data, sperm could be demonstrated in 64% of the vaginal tampons taken in the first postcoital day, and a similar ratio was to be found seven days later as well. In 10-day material positive results were rarely found. Others report a 25% positivity, and they ascribed the significant decrease in cell number in the experimental material to the alterations of the vaginal milieu caused by oral contraceptives. Sperm can be demonstrated from the cervical secretions of the corpse several days after death – in one case 110 days. Due the variations in the data, estimating the time of introduction of the sperm must be approached with great caution. The data concerning morphological alterations also varies, with some authors describing the appearance of heads and tail fragments in secretions 1–2 days old, and others not believing that the ratio of head and tail fragments can be a definite index of the time elapsed since sexual intercourse. However, it is generally accepted that if the tails of the sperm are fragmented, intercourse could have occurred 72 hours before.

Pregnancy is one of the proofs of sexual contact (if artificial insemination has not occurred!). Pregnancy does not necessarily mean that the male organ has penetrated and that virginity has been lost. We have seen pregnancy following sexual intercourse with an intact hymen. Following rape the victim must be followed up closely. We would call your attention to the possibility either of pregnancy – the cessation of menstruation – or of signs of sexually transmitted diseases, with the admonition to call a doctor should any unusual symptoms develop.

2. *The signs of violence:*

In general we consider physical violence a part of it. Many deny that a man of similar condition to the woman is capable of successfully raping her. In a large portion of the cases it is not a matter of only one man committing the crime, and in these the injuries are not so pronounced as they would be if only one perpetrator were involved where a prolonged struggle precedes the act. During the struggle characteristic injuries may occur with grip marks on the arms, bruises on the breasts, and at other times bites can be found on the face and even all over the body *(Fig. 155, 156)*.

Forcing the thighs apart causes bruises and clawing injuries to the lower extremities, and these are most pronounced on the surface of the thighs and external

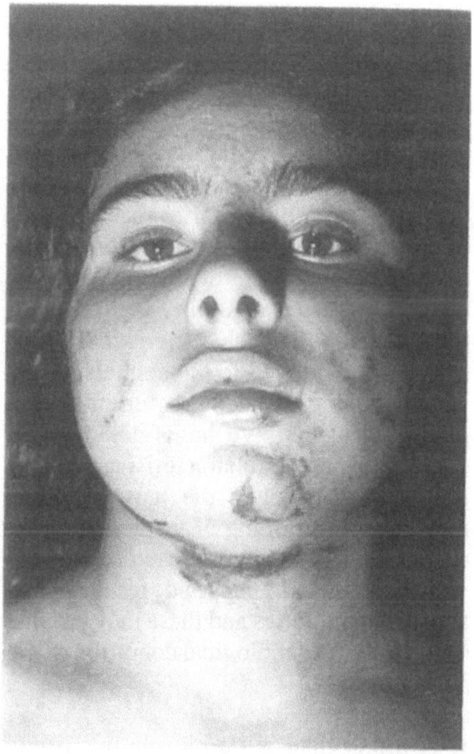

Fig. 155. **Bite marks on the face, scratch marks from gripping on the neck. After being gripped by the neck the victim lost consciousness and was incapable of self-defense**

genitalia. We must also search for such injuries which indicate that the woman put up a struggle, that she may have been choked, or very prominent injuries to the face, neck, hemorrhages into the sclera and conjunctiva, although there may have been an attack of such force that rendered the victim unconscious (knocked the victim down).

If we do not find such injuries, as in surrender, or if the prolonged struggle was sufficient to tire the girl out to the point of being unable to put up a fight, shallower injuries will be the only indication of attack. In these cases it is imperative, along with the examination of the victim, to examine the suspect and measure the physical strength between the two of them. It has happened more than once that after sharing a few drinks together, intercourse followed, and later the man was accused because he didn't pay the previously agreed price, or the mother of the girl coming home late alleged rape by way of excuse. In these cases the absence of injuries is conspicuous. At other times some have tried to produce the usual intercourse injuries associated with rape as proof. Both of these require delicacy and an expert forensic pathologist should perform the examination as soon as possible after the crime was committed along with the gynecologist. It is a fact that if we do not find external injuries on the victim, it does not mitigate against the occurrence of rape, in light of the fact that if life or

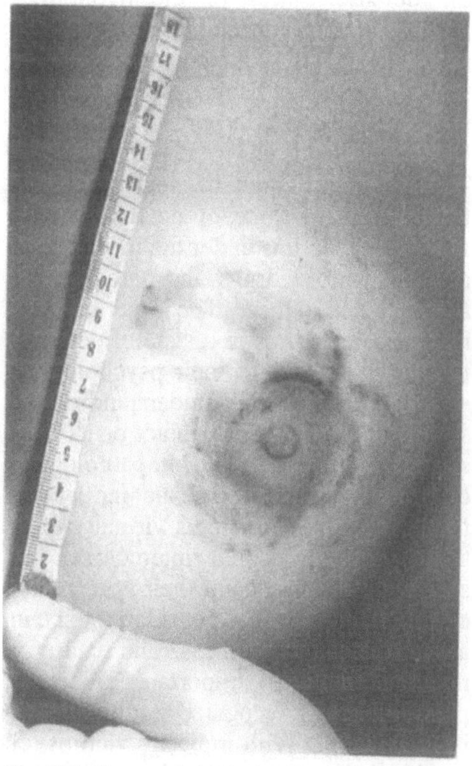

Fig. 156. **Characteristic bite injuries on the breast of a rape victim**

physical health were threatened the law considers it rape, emphasizing that with threat a "serious fear" must be involved.

3. The judgement of a state of *defenselessness* is the responsibility of the medical specialist in some cases. This may be the result of illness, and rape has been reported to be committed when the victim was unconscious following an epileptic attack. We examined a case involving an ambulance medic who tried to rape a sedative intoxicated patient. A woman under heavy influence of alcohol is likewise considered to be in a defenseless state. We must take serious precautions, however, in accepting that a woman was taken advantage of while sleeping and awakened while the act was in progress. Similarly, the defenselessness of the hypnotized person is also unacceptable. Children under the age of 12 are considered defenseless. The state of being unable to express one's will depends in part on the state of the patient, that is, the psychological basis. The first group cannot be clearly differentiated from the state of defenselessness since those victims under the influence of alcohol, various drugs and narcotics are also included in these. The larger group is made up of victims in a state of defenselessness who, due to their psychological state, are incapable of understanding the significance of sexual contact or its consequences. In some psychopathological conditions an increased sexual inclination is prominent. The patients virtually offer themselves for sexual intercourse, but since the significance of their acts are not clear to them, they are considered to be in a state of defenselessness. The nature of the illness is also important, since the perpetrator must recognize that his partner is mentally ill. With imbecile victims, or maniac patient the problem is not obvious. The judgement of a state of inability to express one's will is the proper task of a psychiatrist.

The most serious *consequence of rape* is death. It may be the result of attacking the victim. The external signs may point to the nature of the applied force, but it may also be the result of injuries received during intercourse. The verification of the connection between death and rape is primarily the responsibility of the forensic specialist. The characteristics of the injuries, the injuries to the genitals, or the verification of sexual intercourse make the picture clear-cut. We have already indicated earlier the characteristics of the injuries, nevertheless the most common may be from gripping of the neck or covering the mouth to stifle the cries of the victim. Often the applied force brings about rough injuries and these may provide a clue to the psychological condition of the perpetrator.

- A drunk man put a bicycle pump into the vagina of his partner and pushing it in caused injuries to the abdominal organs. Years later we came across a similar case when the naked, severely decomposed body of a woman found in the forest was brought in for autopsy. We found that she had been impaled through the vagina. The perpetrator, who was drunk, was incapable of performing sexual intercourse with the victim and impaled her with a near-by branch. The perpetrator was an imbecile *(Fig. 157)*.

Occasionally the motivation for the murder may be the fear of being discovered or identified.

Injuries may accompany sexual intercourse which damage the sexual organs so badly that they heal with permanent damage and lead to inability to have sexual intercourse, or later hinder the

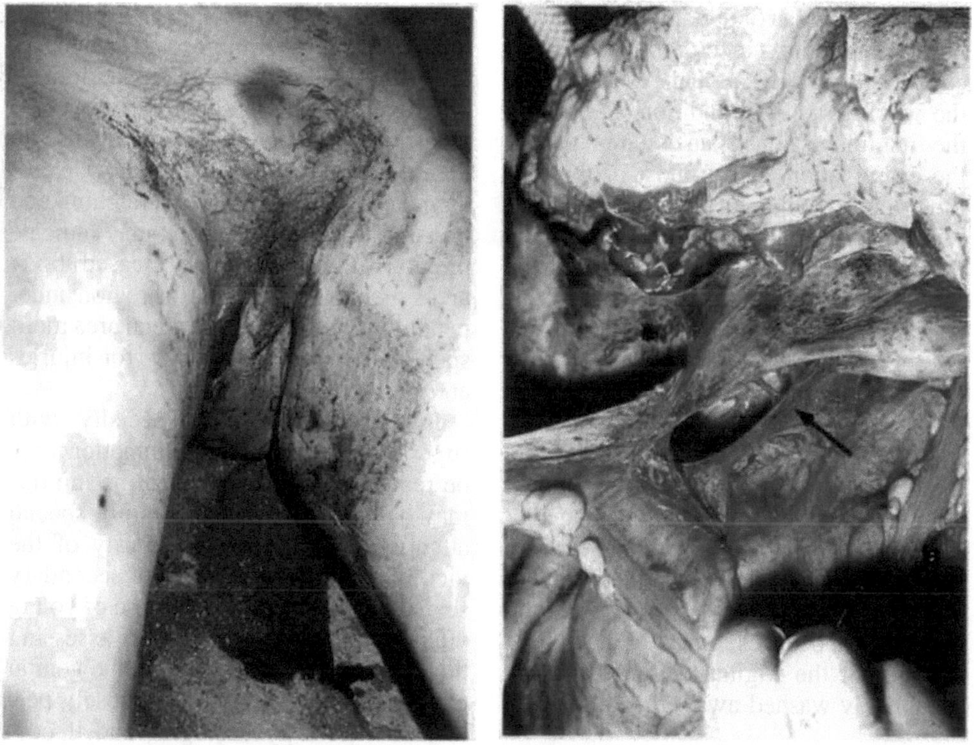

Fig. 157. Soiling in the area of the external genitalia following impaling, injuries to the mesentry, hemorrhage

normal process of birth. We have already mention pregnancy as a consequence of rape, the possibility of which must be emphasized to the victim.

Among the possibilities, the role played by transmission of sexual diseases must not be ignored. Not rarely it accompanies rape, and since it damages health, sometimes it must be decided who gave the infection to whom. If the process is acute in one person, and at a later stage in another, the decision is easier. In the case where the disease processes are close in their stages, we cannot render a judgement. It is necessary to consider the possibility of transmission of sexual disease in every case.

- A strange coincidence occurred when in one case, in which a girl was gang-raped, all the participants were infected by a very resistant strain of gonorrhea carried by the victim.

Examination of the victim

The victims of rape must be examined as soon as possible. Not just because of the transitory nature of the injuries (the swelling and hyperemia of the vaginal entrance and mucosa disappears in a few hours), but for the sake of demonstrating the presence of sperm. With procrastination comes the danger of the evidence being destroyed with the washing of the clothes and of the victim herself.

A basic principle of the examination is that another health worker be present besides the victim and the examiner. This does not necessarily pertain just to listening to the victim, since the facts and circumstances of rape are hard to recount in the woman's upset condition. Recording the first impressions is an essential part of the examination. Early, most of the victims being examined after the deed are worn out, and talk when pressed for the facts, which can be of as much value as the visual findings in untangling the preliminary data. By turning our attention in the proper direction, we may obtain such information which may later be relevant in the judgement of the case.

In the preliminaries, we must find out the time of the crime, what type of rape it was, whether the clothing was damaged or stained, whether the male organ achieved penetration, whether pain was felt or blood was noticed, whether ejaculation occurred, and if yes, where. Ejaculate at the area of the vaginal entrance may be completely washed away after rape.

- A 20-year-old girl alleged circumstantial rape by her teacher. After intercourse she cleaned herself up and washed out her pants. After filing the complaint neither rape nor sexual intercourse could be verified.

Did the victim clean herself after the action and in which manner? (The number of sperm cells in the vagina significantly decreases after vaginal douching!)

We perform the examination in a well-illuminated place and start with attention to the clothing. We search for evidence of rape, rips, wrinkles, stains which not only mark the discovery of ejaculate, but we describe every such trace which also occur, such as muddy contamination, grass blades, etc. After this we can put aside the clothing for later examination based on what we found.

On the unclothed victim we search for such injuries which may be grip marks on the arms, breasts or thighs and bite marks on the face or breasts (occasionally photographing these alterations next to a measuring rod may be of future use in identification of the perpetrator). Subconjunctival hemorrhages, scratching and bruising injuries to the neck may indicate previous throttling. (The creased body areas such as the arm pits, the region under pendulous breasts and the rectal area merit special attention in searching for injuries and biological traces.)

In uncertain cases, especially with superficial bruises, the examination may be repeated a day later when the injuries may be more prominent. We turn special attention to the general maturity of the victim, as the manifestation of secondary sexual characteristics in the case of young victims is very important. After assessing the general state of the victim, the genital examination follows. It is purposely performed with a gynecologist, and if possible, in a well-equipped gynecological consultation room. We look for injuries and contamination in the area of the external genitalia, and if we find contamination, it must be proved by further examination. Injury to the labia in youths is common, but in adults following intercourse they may be engorged and swollen only for a little while. We often find fingernail scratch marks. We must also take samples of swab from the vaginal entrance. This precedes the manual examination, and is performed by swabbing with a cotton tampon. Examination of the vaginal entrance also means examination and description of the hymen. We also make a smear of the vaginal mucosa, one from the lower section of the vagina, and another from the mucosa of the vaginal vault. The taking of both samples must precede the manual examination! With recent intercourse the vaginal mucosa may be swollen and hyperemic, but that may also be due to inflammatory processes. If we suspect sexually transmitted disease, we must take a sample for microbial culture.

Besides the examination of the victim, sometimes we must also examine the suspect or perpetrator.

- An elderly woman filed a complaint of rape. She claimed that the man had forced her to perform oral sex and during this, the victim bit the penis of the perpetrator. Upon examination of the suspect, we found fresh, parallel scratch injuries on the male organ, which were the imprints of the victim's single hollow tooth.

Examination of the suspect

As much as the possibility allows, we should examine the suspect as soon as possible after examining the victim. The same specialist who examined the victim may perform it since he is in a position to make a comparison with regards to the origin of the injuries. In this case, for example, he can closely examine the bite marks and their individual characteristics may make identification possible. With this examination we also start with the clothing, looking primarily for injuries and traces. We pay special attention to the front of the pants, for it is here we may find traces of ejaculate, pubic hair, or other contaminations. Similarly, we check the undershorts. We must clarify when the suspect cleaned himself up or changed his underwear or clothing and when he last had sexual intercourse. On the unclothed individual we look for injuries, for scratch marks on the hands, the forearms, the face, the chest and the back. With special care we examine the external genitalia and prepare a smear from the coronary sulcus. Here we may find glycogen-rich squamous cells from the vaginal epithelium. We may pick up a foreign strand in the pubic hair which may be used for identification. If the intercourse occurred before the examination, we look for sperm cells in the secretion pressed from the urethra. Examination of contamination from under the fingernails may be relevant not only in the case of the victim, but in the suspect as well. One must not forget to check the blood and urine for alcohol and perhaps drugs. Last but not least, it must be clarified whether the suspect in relation to the victim, was physically capable of committing rape.

- A 70-year-old man was accused of the rape of a mentally retarded girl of his acquaintance in a corn field outside the village. Proceedings were initiated against him for rape on the testimony of the mentally retarded victim. Upon examination we found neither injury nor ejaculate on the genitalia of the victim. Upon examination of the suspect we found a suspended, grapefruit-sized irreponable hernia which made sexual intercourse impossible.

Sexual deviation

Among the deeds of psychopaths, sexual aberrations figure prominently in the practice of forensic psychiatry. We can list a large number which are hardly distinguishable from each other in the deviant sexual behavior category, the evaluation of which are not only difficult for the psychiatrist, but not even completely agreed upon. The categorization is also fairly arbitrary, but embraces those cases which we most commonly encounter.

a) Such individuals in which sexual deviation would not be expected.

b) Sexually deviant persons which display illegal sexual behavior, but are fairly under control, and therefore not a criminal menace.

c) Sexually and psychiatrically deviant perpetrators, who are often of legal concern in sex crimes.

d) Psychiatrically deviant, but not sexually affected, persons with whom the committing of sex crimes can be traced not to sexual abnormality but to psychiatric alterations.

According to the above categorization, the significant part of those committing sex crimes do not suffer from pathological alterations in their sex lives. Deviant sexual behavior does not equal disease, so if other pathology does not accompany it, they cannot be evaluated according to pathological factors. The most common perpetrators are mature males in whom the influence of alcohol or previous central nervous system damage plays a role in a large percentage of cases. With respect to the personality level a high ratio of simple-minded, deformed or defective individuals can be found. In the analysis of sexually aberrant criminals, GUTTMACHER and WIEHOFEN mentioned the fact;

> "sex offenders are unique from other offenders, minor sex offenders later become major sex offenders sex offenses are increasing in frequency. '(Perhaps the most important is the establishment that in almost every case) all sex offenders are recidivists'!".

- A 40-year-old male criminal was released from prison where he had been doing time for rape. He was shucking corn with relatives. In the afternoon they noticed that the family's four-year-old daughter had disappeared. After a search they found the body of the child which had rough injuries to the rectal area and vagina, the distinctive marks of anal intercourse along with sperm found in the rectum. After the rape the perpetrator had strangled the little girl with a ribbon from her hair and then hanged himself *(Fig. 158).*

The necessity of experience in the judgement of such crimes must be especially emphasized for those who examine the perpetrators and not lastly stressed that a prolonged separation from society of the sexual deviant after committing a crime does not offer a complete solution to the problem of repeated offenses.

Disorders of sexual drive may manifest themselves in

a) their decrease,
b) their increase,
c) their perversions.

a) Decrease in sexual drive in men often occurs with impotence, while in women with frigidity. It may have an emotional basis due to the effect of upbringing or a previous experience (it may, for example, be the consequence rape), but it may also be organic due to the hypofunction of the endocrine system or spinal cord diseases. It is common in chronic alcoholics and drug abusers. The decrease in sexual drives does not bear much significance in the practice of forensic medicine, causing marital or paternity problems and divorce instead.

b) With increase of sexual drive the desire for sexual intercourse is not satisfied. With men who seek satisfaction over and over again, the danger of committing rape is great, while with women prostitution is common. It can increase with certain intoxications – mild alcoholic state, cocaine use – or with mental illness – mania, hysteria, schizophrenia. – The frustration may lead to other perversions, such as intercourse with animals or fre-

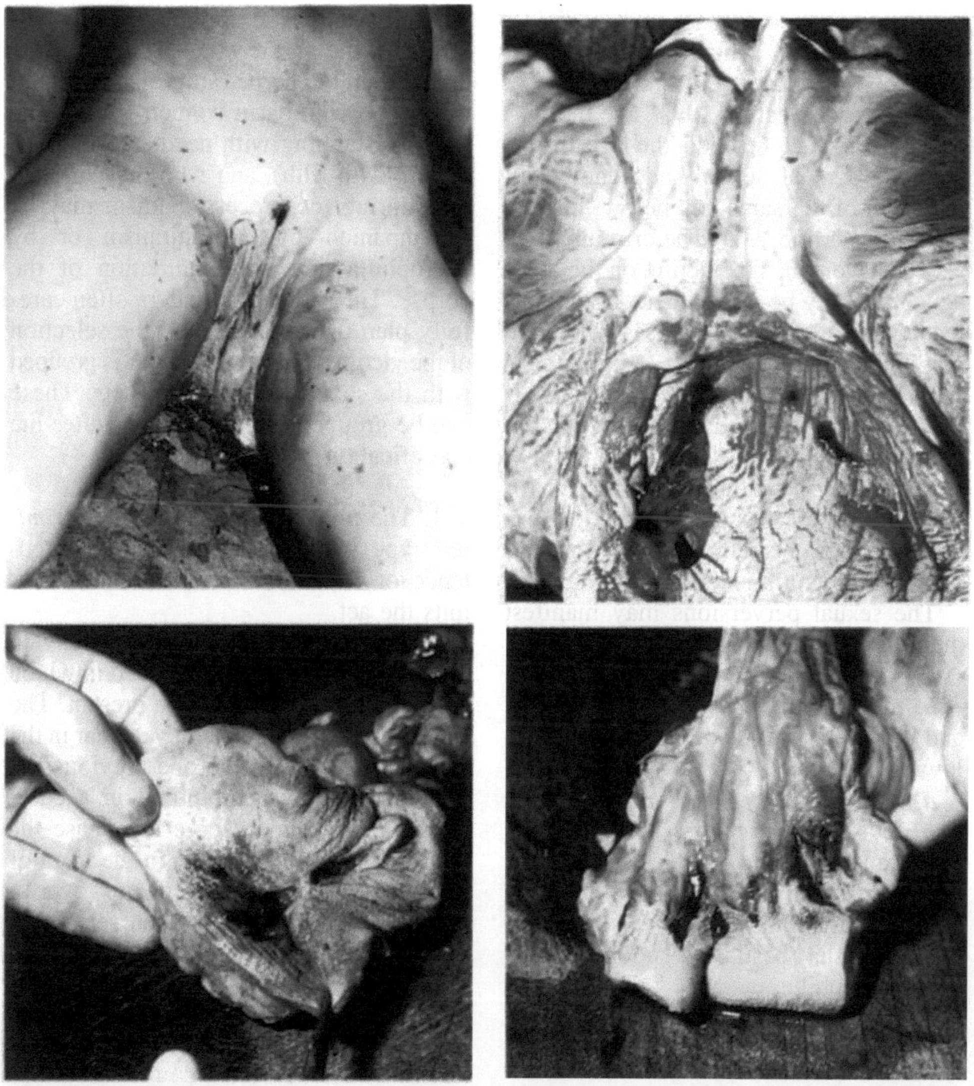

Fig. 158. **Perineal hemorrhage, extensive vaginal and rectal injuries in a 4-year-old child following vaginal and rectal intercourse**

quent masturbation. With hypersexual males, elevated testosterone level also was mentioned.

The largest group of disorders of sexual instinct are those disorders in which the *sexual behavior deviates* from physiological methods of intercourse in such a way that the deviant method serves as the primary form of the sexual life. It rarely occurs that methods of intercourse deviating from the normal are considered in every case to be abnormal, and are considered pathological only when they constitute practically the only method of satisfaction.

c) A small number of acts of perversion

have *significance in forensic medicine.* These are those which appear as the likelihood of crime.

Penal Code Section 199. "The individual, who having reached the age of 18, commits acts of sexual indecency with members of the same sex below this age commits a crime..." ("The criminal may also be a woman. The victim, on the other hand, can only be such a person who has reached the age of 14. In cases where the victim is under the age of 12, the crime is considered unnatural intercourse, and if the victim has reached the age of 12, but not 14, seduction must be established.")

Penal Code Section 208 "Whoever for the purpose of sexual satisfaction exposes him or herself indecently to another commits a misdemeanor..."

The sexual perversions may manifest themselves in acts of

a) sadism,
b) masochism,

and may appear as sexual acts in the following modes:

a) homosexuality,
b) fetishism,
c) transvestism,
d) exhibitionism,
e) voyeurism,
f) zoophilia (bestiality, sodomy),
g) necrophilia,
h) frotteurism,
i) paedophilia.

Sadism: Among the disorders of sexual drive, this carries the most serious consequences. Most of the perpetrators are men who in the sex act are otherwise not only the initiators, but during the act may cause small injuries to their partners. If more serious injuries come about, or if satisfaction cannot be achieved without harming the partner, and occasionally this alone creates the satisfaction even without intercourse, we speak of sadism. The most extreme form involves killing of the partner, the so-called pleasure murder, but perpetrators also belong to this group who harm women without the sex act (stabbing with needles or knives, soiling with filth), and who may masturbate during the process. Sadism may be accompanied by exhibitionism or by necrophilia and with mutilation of the corpse. The sadistic offenders often carefully plan their crimes, and the selection of the victims. Sadistic behavior is grouped with the sexually aggressive acts. These can be grouped into three types after the classification by REVICH:

1. The *impulsive murderer* and *criminal* type who, either because of impotence or resistance of the victim, commits the act.

2. The *convulsive criminal* type who kills out of a driving sexual need in which a sex act may or may not be present. The act may be repeated and may appear in the same ritual form as the one previous.

3. Sadistic acts committed in a *catathymic crisis* which serve to release the pent-up tension. It may be in the form of the release of stress built up over a prolonged period or a sudden release of destructive emotions.

In all three criminal modes the features of the schizoid personality are prominent.

Masochism: This is the opposite of the sadistic aberration. Satisfaction can only be achieved, either with or without the sex act, through suffering. Earlier women were unequivocally placed into this category saying that women are the passive partners in the sex act and by this they endure suffering. This perversion afflicts women and men equally and is often found in combination with a sadist as a partner. These sadomasochistic acts may often remain hidden and only come to light when one of the partners is seriously injured.

We touch only briefly on the modes of the acts among the manifest aberrations which, upon rare occasions, have significance in the practice of forensic medicine, since neither the seriousness of the acts nor their frequency merit detailed familiarity.

Voyeurism: Watching for others in the sex act brings satisfaction. Although it is a rather frequent aberration, and the perpetrators harmlessly lurk in the forests hidden off to the side or actively seek out couples making love. The deed is often accompanied by masturbation.

Zoophilia: Besides the mentally disturbed perpetrators, this was earlier described most commonly in shepherds and men cut off from society. Intercourse with animals may be performed by women as well as men. Besides goats, dogs and cattle, "sexual acts" have also been described with birds. Besides the filth the perpetrator may soil himself with from the animal, injuries, bites and claw wounds may be incurred. Occasionally a sadistic feature may be found in these acts.

Necrophilia: Sex acts with dead bodies appear in small number. In the sadistic form, mutilation of the body may also occur along with intercourse with the corpse. The perpetrators are seriously mentally retarded or, according to others, this does not even belong in the realm of sexual disorders and should be placed with mental disease, in which we may also find sadistic or fetishistic features.

Frotteurism: These are mainly male perpetrators who with their bare or clothing-covered sexual organs rub up against members of the opposite sex, most commonly in crowded public transportation vehicles.

In the next group we will deal with those sexual aberrations which are *more common* and which occasionally require a criminal judgement, emphasizing those that tend to come to examination by the forensic specialist.

Homosexuality: This means the achieving sexual satisfaction through contact with a member of the same sex. In the etiology, both genetic and environmental factors are mentioned. It is considered a crime only under certain circumstances (Penal Code, Section. 199.). It is known in women *(lesbianism)* as well as in men. To be mentioned with its genetic forms is the homosexual individual who looks like a member of the opposite sex. The homosexual man has a feminine shape while the woman looks more masculine. (Sometimes this is emphasized in both sexes, not only in behavior, but with an external manifestation in the features of a transvestite.) The role of the family environment is emphasized in the aquired form. (The boy reared by dominant, strong willed mother may be succeptible to homosexuality.) At other times in closed society, homosexual features in the same sex are intensified or brought out. Here in educational institutions, penal institutions or prisons, the sexual desires may be compensated, if only temporarily, but after a prolonged period become fixed in the partner of the same sex. The person may be capable of both hetero- and homosexual relations. In these bisexual persons, sexually transmitted diseases are of a particular danger, lately with the spread of AIDS. With lesbian lovers the sexual relations are manifested by cunnilingus, kissing and masturbation. In other cases the woman in the masculine role may, with the help of an appropriate device, imitate normal intercourse with her partner. With men the contact with a partner of the same sex is manifested not only in kissing and mutual

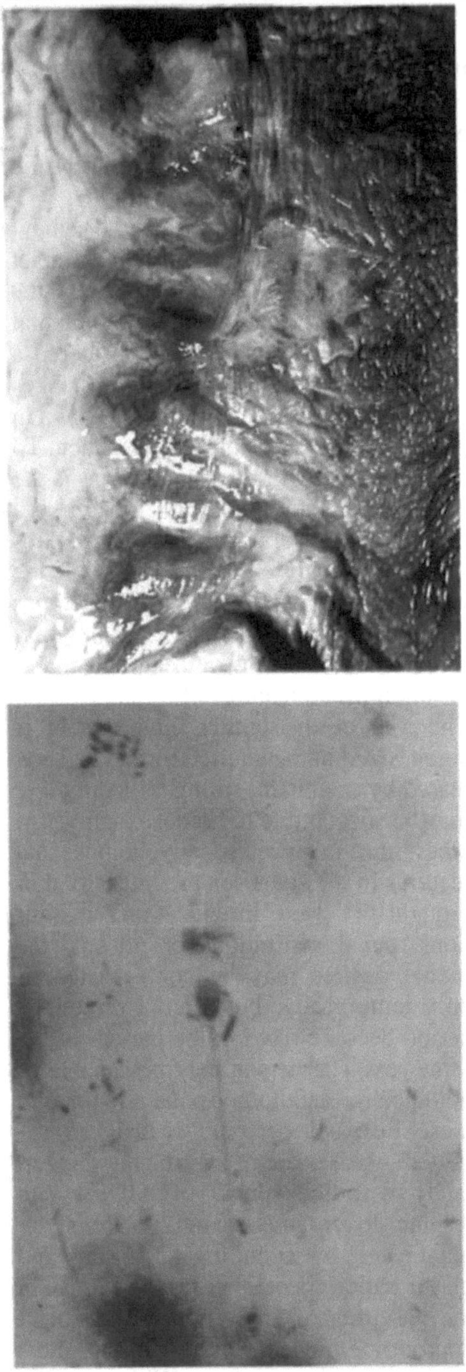

Fig. 159. Injuries to the rectal mucosa following anal intercourse (above); sperm from a sample taken from the surface of the rectal epithelium (below)

masturbation, but more commonly, with interfemoral or anal intercourse. Verification of homosexuality is easy only in the case of anal intercourse. Those alterations which are the consequence of frequent anal intrusion can verify a suspicion when found either in the living or dead body. In recent cases we may find not only superficial injuries to the male organ, but the presence of blood and fecal remains as well. In the passive partner we may find fresh abrasions and bleeding at the anal opening. The extent of the injuries naturally depends on the size of the organ, speed of the intrusion and "experience" of the passive partner. The first time, or in the case of rape, the injuries to the anal area are obvious even on external examination and may be pronounced. In chronic cases, due to the relaxation of the anal sphincter, the individual being examined may have an unpleasant odor from the continual leakage of fecal matter from the incontinent rectum. In examination of the corpse along with the inspection of the external genitalia, an inspection of the anus must not be left out. If traces indicating injury are found there – bruising, mucous tears, bleeding – with removal by the appropriate dissection technique we describe not only the extent of the injuries and seek their origin, but from the intestinal contents by preparation of a mucous smear we try to find sperm cells, which indisputably verify the previous act *(Fig. 159).*

● We dissected the body of a 50-year-old man who had not been examined in the anal area at the preliminary examination on the scene. The external examination revealed dried blood in the anal area, and upon exposure, mucous injury as well. Death had been by strangulation. The culprit had been a renter of the bed-ridden, incapacitated man, who, as

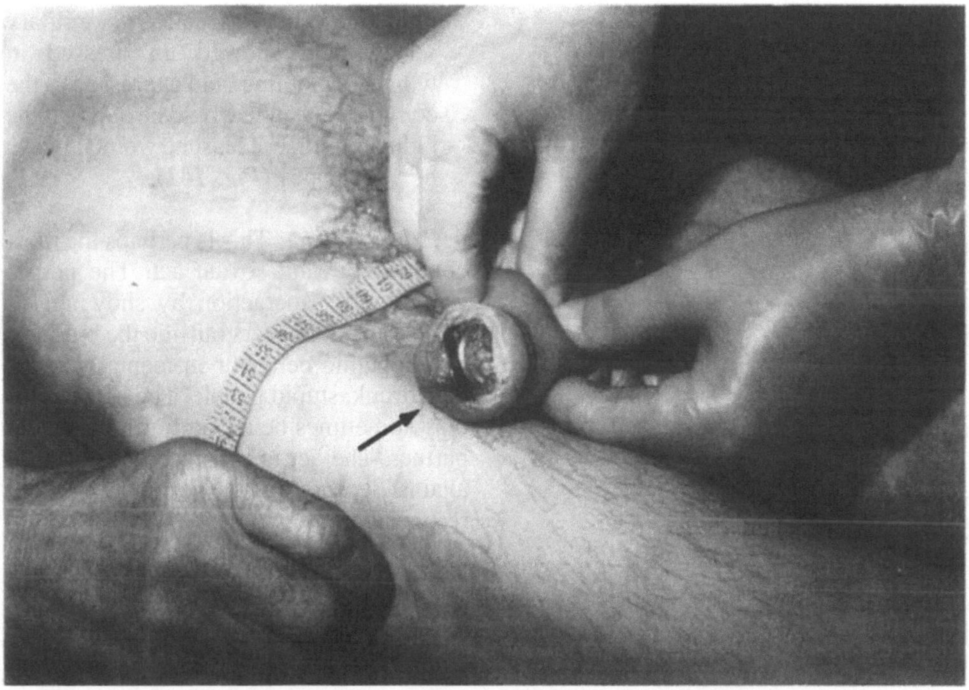

Fig. 160. **Woman's hair and beer bottle cap visible under the foreskin of fetishist**

he later admitted during the examination by the forensic specialist, had strangled his landlord following an argument, but when he kneeled behind him, he "wanted him" and had intercourse with him. Sperm demonstrated in the sample taken from the rectal mucosa verified completed intercourse.

Fetishism: This is when pieces of clothing or a collection of other objects belonging to the partner, such as a lock of hair or pubic hair, when viewed or touched to the sex organs result in the kindling of desire and can bring satisfaction. In its independent form of sexual pleasure, we speak of fetishism. Obtaining the objects has revealed the perpetrator of some crimes who stole them from their partners.

- A 71-year-old man was found dead in his apartment with strands of a woman's hair around his penis which hung out of his undershorts and to which a beer bottle had been emplaced under the foreskin, while his shorts were stuffed with a collection of female pubic hair *(Fig. 160)*.

Transvestism: Although mostly observed in homosexual individuals, it has been described as a part of some hetero- and bisexual relations as well. It appears in early childhood. Essentially, a man displays himself as a woman or vice versa, tries to make sexual contact, and if they try to pick up a member of the same sex, in more than one case they have been offended and attacked the offender.

- A 19-year-old young man in Budapest for more than a year and a half used to offer himself as prostitute at Rákóczi square. He only dealt with men and

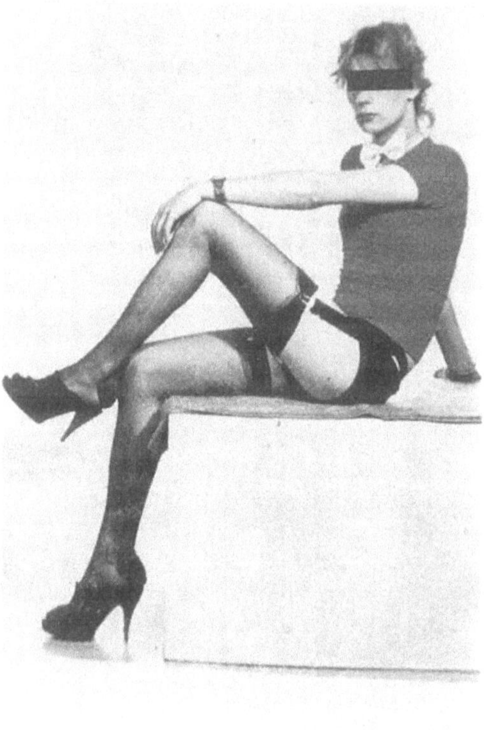

Fig. 161. Homosexual transvestite

claimed to be menstruating to every one who picked him up and could only offer fellatio. Many pictures had been taken of him. His true status only came to light when he was called to military service and showed up dressed in women's clothing, and expressed to the committee that he would be happy to be inducted, since at least he would always be with males *(Fig. 161).*

Exhibitionism: This is perhaps the most common deviant sexual act. The perpetrator seeks satisfaction by showing his sex organs. It appears outside the realm of psychopathic behavior in mentally retarded, drunk, stupid people. The perpetrator may sometimes be trying to find a sexual partner. The act is considered an offense against decency and the perpetrator is held responsible.

Paedophilia: Stupid, mentally deficient individuals sometimes attempt sexual contact with children. Some have tried to have intercourse with children while drunk. In the inebriated state, the loss of inhibition is responsible. These attempts can occasionally result in serious injuries to the anogenital area with bleeding, and not caused in every instance by the penetration or attempts at it by the sex organ of the perpetrator. There was a case in which the perpetrator caused serious injury to the rectum with his fingers.

Abortion

Penal Code. 169. Section: "Who performs an abortion commits a crime..."

"The woman who has performed an abortion, or causes herself to abort, commits a misdemeanor..."

The penal code separately emphasizes the qualified forms of the crime, among which are listed: for profit, without consent of the woman, serious physical injury, life-threatening, or lethal abortion. The law in justification stresses that interruption of pregnancy even by a physician is a dangerous intervention from which numerous complications can be expected in absence of the appropriate circumstances and if performed by a charlatan instead of a medical specialist.

The subjects of an abortion are the pregnant woman and the fetus. It is not inconsequential that pregnancy be verified. With an abortion or suspicion of such, the medical specialist must determine that the woman:

a) was pregnant,

b) that abortion occurred and with what effects,

c) what connection can be made, if any, between the possible intervention and the abortion,

d) the complications appearing after the intervention.

1. The *recognition of pregnancy* on the basis of the signs of suspicion or the signs of probability of pregnancy is possible, but in the practice of forensic medicine the demonstration of the certain signs of pregnancy are decisive.

Among the symptoms of *suspected pregnancy* are morning sickness, vomiting, cravings for certain foods, or aversions to them, (pica). These are just signs of changes in the organism and do not necessarily belong to pregnancy.

Among the *probable signs* of pregnancy, first of all cessation of menstruation should be mentioned. During reproductive age, women should first think of pregnancy, but it may be a hormonal effect as well. Bleeding irregularities have also been found with starvation and psychological distress. The breasts and the internal and external genital organs also change significantly. The breasts enlarge, become nodular to the touch and feel tense to the woman while the nipples become more darkly pigmented. Colostrum can be expressed from the breast. The external genitals, the labia minora and the vestibule, become engorged with blood and their lividity is obvious upon external examination along with an increase in production of mucus and vaginal secretions. The tissue of the uterus and its size also change. In the early stages of pregnancy the cervix softens and following this the consistency of the body of the

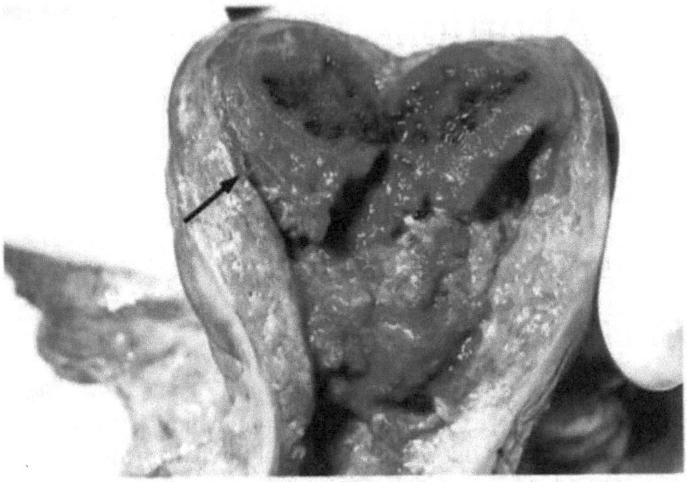

Fig. 162. Placental retention following abortion. Hemorrhagic, homogeneously colored necrotic tissue in the uterine fundus

uterus changes with its substance softening and becoming rounded and bulging at the site of implantation *(Piskacek's sign).* With the progress of pregnancy it grows to the size of a man's fist by the 12th week. The hormonal changes in connection with pregnancy can be detected either with biological tests or with special immunological reactions. These examinations only serve as signs of probable pregnancy, since other hormonal changes can cause a positive reaction. It is important to note that these pregnancy reactions can remain positive for 5–7 days following the interruption of pregnancy.

Only the *positive signs of pregnancy* are used in the practice of forensic medicine. This means demonstration of the fetus or placenta or amniotic sac. Ultrasound is the most modern non-invasive method of examination which can be used demonstrate pregnancy by the 6th week. We can register the fetal heart beat from the 12th week. From the 20th week the body parts of the fetus may be palpable. These examinations serve to verify an on-going pregnancy and exclude the so-called *false pregnancy* (pseudocyesis).

● (A 24-year-old after murdering her husband attempted a theatrical suicide in which a head injury was sustained. In jail she complained of menstrual disturbances and later cessation, mentioning the appropriate signs of early pregnancy. Her abdominal girth also started to grow and four months later in court, she had the appearance of a pregnant woman. The gynecologist excluded the pregnancy and diagnosed it as false pregnancy, the hormonal alteration caused by a later verified damage to the hypothalamus.)

In forensic medical practice, the verification of previous pregnancy is more important, especially in the cases of suspicion of abortion. The pregnancy reaction which remains positive, for days can provide the basis for suspicion of pregnancy while we search for definite signs by histological examinations. Menstrual disturbances are a consequence of almost every abortion. Placenta, decidua, or trophoblast parts demonstrated in the scraping carried out at this time are diagnostic *(Fig. 162, 163).* Only the decidual scraping may also be the result of hormonal alterations, and not in every case caused by pregnancy, but they may also be a sign of an extra-uterine pregnancy!

Verification of on-going or previous pregnancy in the corpse is also based on demonstration of the fetus or associated parts. If the abortion was not performed by curettage, after incomplete expulsion of the fetus or associated parts on the inner surface of the uterus, we can see macroscopically, parts of the placenta, fetal membranes, fetus, which unambiguously establish the fact of pregnancy. After abortion the adherence of the placenta to the uterine mucosa can be detected not only macroscopically, but microscopically as well. Pronounced trophoblast invasion accompanies decidual transformation of the uterine mucosa which reaches the myometrium, and serves to clearly verify previous pregnancy. We will discuss the injuries accompanying abortion below.

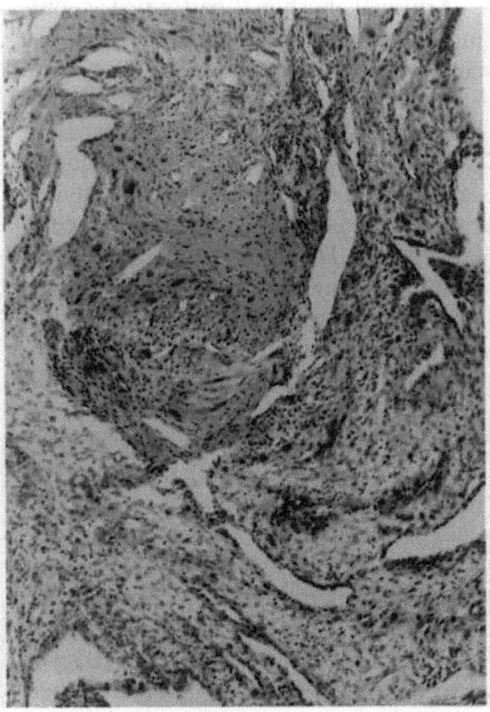

Fig. 163. **Trophoblastic invasion of the musculature of the pregnant uterus**

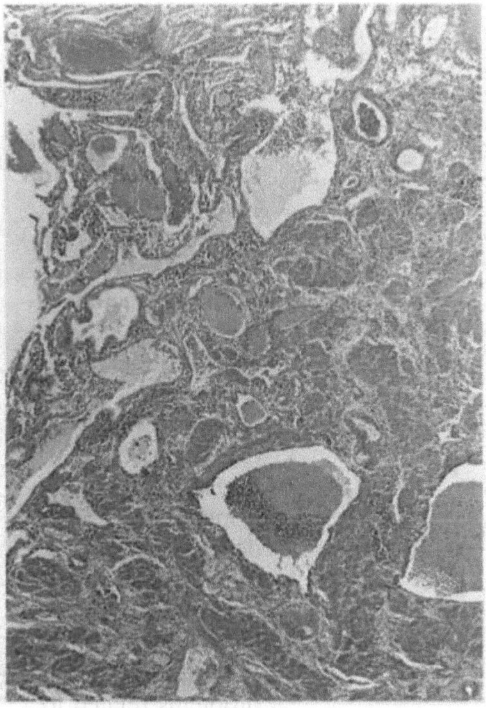

Fig. 164. **Endometritis and myometritis with canalicular inflammatory spread**

We consider *abortion* at week 20–22 as an interruption of pregnancy (a fetus of 500 g or less). It may be spontaneous, artificial, or criminal.

The causes of abortion

Etiology	*Provocative cause*
Maternal causes	
Genitally based	cervical insufficiency (trauma, connective tissue weakness)
	developmental irregularities
	tumors (e.g. myoma)
	endometrial damage (e.g. Asherman's syndrome)

	infection (endometritis, cervicitis)
	uterine irritability (psychological origin)
Extragenital origin	endocrin disease (diabetes mellitus, hyperthyroidism etc.)
	infections, fever, smoking, anemic
	trauma
Feto-placental causes	chromosomal irregularities
	disturbances of implantation
	disease of the trophoblast
	decrease in immunological tolerance
Paternal (sperm) causes	chromosomal irregularities
	problems related to sperm count, form and function
Iatrogenic and artificial abortion	drugs
	ionizing radiation
	vaccination
	interruption of pregnancy

[L. LAMPÉ: (Obstetrics and Gynecology] 2., 1981]

In *spontaneous abortion,* which very seldom comes to forensic medical examination – if its character suggests no outside reason, harm, accident or toxic effect –, numerous factors may be recognized which occasionally may be relevant to the medical specialist.

From the tabulated compilation it appears that even with the appropriate preceding events it is quite difficult to find the responsible preceding factor in each case of abortion, and the verification of traumatic precedents is especially open to question. For this, cooperation between the forensic specialist and the gynecologist is imperative. The signs and course of abortion are described in textbooks on obstetrics and gynecology. In real life their diagnosis is not the responsibility of the forensic specialist since the patient usually is examined by a general practitioner or gynecologist. We have already discussed the recognition of pregnancy in the corpse. With abortion, besides the described histological signs, we find a more or less inflammatory state at the beginning of the abortion in the endometrium and myometrium. With septic complications the characteristics of puerperal sepsis – abscessing myometritis, endometritis profunda, parametritis – can be seen, usually due to the retention of a necrotic piece of the placenta *(Fig. 164).*

Artificial abortion if performed according to regulations, produces few complications. With the regulation of artificial abortion, the previous high rate of illegally performed abortions for the interruption of pregnancy and their high rate of complications have decreased. The later modifications also emphasize the importance of prevention. The most modern methods employed show the improved conditions which entrust to the special institution the permission for abortion, instead of a committee, providing the appropriate conditions are met. (The signs of artificial abortion, the injury of tractioned cervix and the marks left by dilatation, are injuries which can be seen well for several days afterwards.)

The number of criminal abortions is dependent upon the permission or denial of medical abortions. In Hungary they peaked in the 1950's and from 1956 on gradually decreased, and with the liberalization of permission for artificial abortion, they are now only occasionally seen.

At the same time, in some other countries statistical data put the incidence of criminal abortion at 40% (!) of that of spontaneous abortion. Many show criminal abortion to be 10% of the rate of spontaneous abortion. For induction of abortion the following can be used:

a) drugs, chemical substances,
b) instrumental intervention.

Both groups provide the possibility for numerous complications.

Drugs, chemical substances. Even today we know of no usual substance neither hormones, nor drugs, which can cause an interruption of pregnancy by isolated damage to the fetus. Whether speaking of substances used generally or locally, the substance used to bring about fetal death and expulsion must be used in such high concentrations that it is also toxic to the maternal organism. During the early stages of pregnancy in the days following the missed period, menstruation can be induced by a prostaglandin preparation. This intervention is relatively free from complications, however, it remains questionable whether the woman was really pregnant. Its importance is negligible, since it is used only by clinics. At the same time, cases of abortion are known in which the use of a cytotoxic substance caused tumorous diseases in the pregnant mothers.

Certain drugs specifically affect the myometrium. These are also used in the practice of obstetrics. Prolonged uterine contractions develop with ergotamine preparations, but interruption of pregnancy only happens if toxic doses are used. Its toxic effects include arterial spasm with superficial necrosis of the skin of the ears and fingers, and a sequel of dry gangrene. Similarly, quinine is ineffective in inducing abortion, although its uterotonic effect can predispose and sensitize the uterus, especially increasing the effect of oxytocin, although in a healthy pregnancy neither alone is capable of inducing abortion.

Some of the substances which cause pelvic engorgement with blood are drastic purgatives. Among them, the herbal extracts, castor oil, podophyllin and aloe are significant. Some of these contain glucoretins which are broken down in the intestine to resin acid, causing stormy peristalsis by stimulating the intestinal wall, and pelvic engorgement develops along with intestinal and uterine bleeding. Certain drugs containing volatile oils, which are used for their laxative effect, are also popular abortives. Decoctions of parsley or juniper berries have been used since ancient times and were known as abortives. General poisoning and oral or local administration of heavy metals has been used to achieve interruption of pregnancy. Lead or mercury appear the most often with their characteristic signs. The locally applied abortives in part tend to cause local alterations and, according to some of the published data, these cause a deceptive bleeding which leads to an unjustified judgement of an emptying of the uterus upon superficial examination. Potassium permanganate tablets or crystals introduced into the vaginal fornix can cause a local erosion and bleeding, and with absorption, have a general toxic effect. Mercuric chloride has a similar effect.

Instrumental intervention. The previously mentioned procedures were unsuited for the interruption of a healthy pregnancy, without a harmful effect on the health or life of the pregnant women. The instrumental interventions include such forms in which a foreign object is introduced into the uterine cavity to achieve ejection of the blastocyst, or in other instances to attempt to dilate the cervix which may also injure the fetal membranes. Finally, intervention may be performed within the uterine cavity.

Foreign material introduced into the uterine cavity for the expulsion of the blastocyst is also employed in medical institutions. The material can be inserted either by lay personnel or medical specialists. Among those used for intervention are soapy water with iodine, potassium permanganate solution, mercuric chloride solution, or 70% alcohol. These are introduced with the aid of a special syringe or rubber balloon. Besides the local effects, even if the solution is considered "sterile", it can still cause not only extensive inflammatory consequences, but the absorbed substance may cause a generalized toxic effect. Lethal alcohol intoxication has been described following the introduction of 70% alcohol into the uterus. Dilatation of the cervix is a routine procedure in the practice of obstetrics and gynecology. Dilatation by use of laminaria for abortive purposes is not a common method in criminal repertoire because of the slowness. Dilatation of the cervix most commonly involves injury to the blastocyst, and thus induces abortion which is often accompanied by prolonged hemorrhage. Among the instruments suitable for this purpose, besides the members of the Hegar series, are the plastic or metal catheters, but any instrument is applicable which can be inserted into the cervix and damage the fetal membranes. Instruments which have been used for this purpose include knitting needles, hairpins, pencils, Hollyhock roots, etc. A completely evacuated uterine cavity or the traces of preparatory procedures, grasping of the cervix, signs of cervical dilatation indicate intervention performed by a medical specialist.

Proving the connection between intervention and abortion

The supposition that a pregnancy has been interrupted by external influence – a blow to the abdomen, fall from a height, bicycling – must be approached and evaluated with great care. In early pregnancy the uterus, due to its protected position in the pelvis, isn't usually harmed even by the application of a formidable force. With more advanced pregnancies the protective effect of the amnionic fluid is also considerable, and injury to the fetus or abortion only come about with lacerating injury to the uterus. Thus in the preceding events the connection between the alleged force and the abortion can only be investigated and evaluated with great circumspection.

Medications or chemicals are incapable of causing abortion without harming the mother. In the early and even few-day-old pregnancy prostaglandins applied to the cervix are capable of provoking bleeding, but the fact of the pregnancy is in question. Cases, investigating the mechanical effect, whether by dilating the cervix or by introducing a foreign substance or instrument into the uterine cavity, although infrequently have also been published as pertaining to the maintenance of pregnancy.

Consequences of abortion

Dilatation of the cervix can cause reflex cardiac arrest due to stimulation of the Frankenhauser ganglion. A consequence of interruption may be serious bleeding, which may not only be a consequence of the injury in the pregnant uterus, but in the cases of incomplete evacuation of the uterine cavity as well. Due to the pieces of the placenta which remain behind, the uterine contractions are imperfect. The most common consequence is infection. One type is ascending endometritis caused by the necrosis of the pieces of the placenta left behind from the incomplete abortion. The other can be traced to contamination by the instruments used. (Tetanus has been reported in an abortion performed using a Hollyhock root.) Behind septicemia may be an infection by E. coli, or more commonly Staphylococcus infection or at other times anaerobic infection. The course is rapid, and death may result within 24 hours as a result of the development of endotoxin-induced shock.

Air introduced into the uterine cavity with the solutions may result in air embolism as well. At least 100 ml of air is necessary to diagnose lethal air embolism. After the separation of the placenta, the air – even if only a circumscribed area has separated – may find its way into the circulation through an open vein, be whipped into a foam in the right heart chamber, enter the pulmonary circulation and cause acute right heart insufficiency. Late air embolism has also been described in which several hours transpired between the intervention and death. The mechanism is not known. (The possibility of air embolism must be considered in the autopsy of every case of suspected abortion and the appropriate techniques applied. We must in any case be duly cautious concerning the previous events, since air embolism has been described as a result of oral-genital sex with air being blown into the vagina during the act.)

Among the consequences of intervention, injuries also play a large part. Whether the pregnant woman attempts to perform the intervention or someone else, injury to the vagina, the vestibule and the uterus must be expected. The woman performing the abortion attempts to introduce an instrument into the cervix by guiding it with her fingers and during the process the vaginal vault may be perforated, although the softened uterus may also be perforated either in the area of the cervix or body of the uterus. If someone else controls the instrument, it may be by visual guidance, and the precervical injuries will be fewer. Injuries to the body of uterus may also develop, depending upon the anatomical knowledge of the abortionist. A specialist, taking into consideration the position of the uterus perforates the fundus, while a quack doctor causes injuries to the posterior wall of the uterine body. Serious hemorrhage can be caused by the injuries, but most commonly an inflammatory condition may result due to injury of the abdominal organs.

- One of our cases, which was performed in violation of the regulations of the profession, was a legal interruption of pregnancy being performed by the gynecologist with abortion forceps. Although he noticed that he had perforated the uterus, he continued the intervention and in the pocess caused multiple injuries to the small intestine.

References

[1] Bamford, F., R. Roberts: Child sexual abuse. Br. Med. J. 299 (1989) 377–382

[2] Benson, R. C.: Vacuum cleaner injury to penis. Urology 25 (1985) 41–44

[3] Bradford, J. M. W., D. McLean: Sexual offenders violence and testosterone. Can. J. Psychiatr. 29 (1984) 335–343

[4] Cohen, C., N. E. Matsuda: Sex crimes and forensic sexology, analytic study. Rev. Paul. Med. 109 (1991) 157–164

[5] Davies, A., E. Wilson: The persistence of seminal constituents in the human vagina. Forensic Sci. 3 (1974) 45–55

[6] DIVALL, G.: A new peptidase izozyme which may assist in the identification of vaginal debris. Forensic Sci. Int. 24 (1984) 239–246

[7] DONEY, I. E.: Sexual assault. Immediate detection methods. Police Surg. 27 (1985) 6–12

[8] ECKERT, W. G., S. KATCHIS, W. DONOVAN: The pathology and medicolegal apects of sexual activity. Am. J. Forensic Med. Pathol. 12 (1991) 3–15

[9] Editorial: A test to prove sexual assault. Emergency Med. 5.15 (1983) 115–116

[10] Editorial: Ano-rectal trauma. Inform Letter 20 (1988) 3–6

[11] EKE, F.: Child sexual abuse. Br. Med. J. 299 (1989) 742

[12] FATTECH, A., W. B. LEACH, CH. A. WILKINSON: Fatal air embolism in pregnancy resulting from orogenital sex play. Forensic Sci. 2 (1973) 247–250

[13] FRANK, E., B. D. STEWART: Passive symptoms in rape victims. J. Affect. Disord. 7 (1984) 77–85

[14] FREGIN, W., S. ROMMEIS, A. BERNOSOWSKI: Mikroskopische enzymatische und immunologische Untersuchungen an Vaginal-abstrichen. Eine Studie zur Zeitabhangigkeit des Nachweiss verschiedener Spermabestandteile post Coitum. Krim. Forens. Wiss. 55–56 (1984) 160–164

[15] FREUND, K.: Die Homosexualitat beim Mann. S. Hinzel Verlag Leipzig (1963) pp. 54–56, 82–85

[16] FRIED, P. H., A. E. RAKOFF, R. R. SCHOPBACH, A. J. KAPLAN: Pseudocyesis, a psychosomatic study in gynecology. JAMA 145 (1951) 1329–1333

[17] GORDON, I., H. A. SHAPIRO, S. D. BERSON: Forensic Medicine Churchill Livingstone N. Y. (1988) pp. 366–374

[18] HELWEG-LARSEN, K.: The value of the medicolegal examination in sexual offences. Forensic Sci. Int. 27 (1985) 145–155

[19] IMAMI, R. H., M. KEMAL: Vacuum cleaner use in autoeretic death. Am.J. Forensic Med. Pathol. 9 (1988) 246–248

[20] KEATING, S. M.: The laboratoryU,s approach to sexual assault cases. Part 1: Sources of information and acts of intercourse. J. Forensic Sci. Soc. 28 (1988) 35–47

[21] KEATING, S. M.: The laboratoryU,s approach to sexual assault cases. Part 2: Demonstration of the possible offender. Forensic Sci. Soc. 28 (1988) 99–111

[22] KNIGHT, B.: Fatal masochism – accident or suicide. Med. Sci. Law. 19 (1979) 118–120

[23] LAMPÉ, L.: Szülészet-nőgyógyászat. Medicina Bp. (1981) 335–344

[24] MACFARLANE, D. F.: Transsexual prostitution in New Zealand Predominance of persons of Maori extractions. Arch. Sex. Behav. 13 (1984) 301–309

[25] MAGNER, M. B.: Erotomania in man S. Afr. Med. J. 81 (1992) 167–168

[26] MARCINKOWSKI, T.: Death from an attempt to procedure an abortion by intra uterine injection of ethyl alcohol. Forensic Sci. 2 (1973) 245–246

[27] MORRISON, A. I.: Persistence of spermatozoa in the vaginal and cervix. Br. J. Venereal Disease 48 (1972) 141–143

[28] MESTER, H.: Zur aPhanomenologie und Enstekkungeschichte des Exhibitionismus. Fortschr. Neurol. Psychiatr. 52 (1984) 237–249

[29] NYÍRŐ, GY.: Psychiatria. Medicina Bp. (1961) pp. 12–130

[30] POLSON, C. J., D. J. GEE, B. KNIGHT: The Essentials of Forensic Medicine Pergamon Press (1985) pp. 496–513

[31] RAUM, B. A.: Rape trauma syndrome as circumstantial evidence of rape. J. Psychiatry Law. 11 (1983) 203–213

[32] REVICH, E.: Sex murderer and the potential sex murderer. Diseases of the Nervous System N. Y. 26 (1965) 640–646

[33] SADOFF, R. L.: Forensic Psychiatry. Ch. C. Thomas Publ. Springfield Ill. USA (1988) pp. 127–139

[34] SCHWERD, W., CH. KNEITZ, V. MÜLLER: Spermanachweis. Schnellnachweis und optimale Extraction von Flecken. Arch. Kriminol. 178 (1986) 76–81

[35] SILVERMAN, E. M., A. G. SILVERMAN: Persistence of spermatozoa in the lower genital tracts of women. JAMA 240 (1978) 1875–1877

[36] SIMPSON, K.: TaylorU,s Principles and Practice of Medical Jurisprudence II. Churchill Ltd. (1965) pp. 80–112

[37] SZABÓ, I.: Der röntgenologische Nachweis der Luftembolie. Kriminol. Forens. Wiss. 8 (1971) 167–173

[38] SZABÓ, M., BURIS, L.: Zur Analyse von Sexualdelikten unter besonderer Berücksichtigung Ihrer psychiatrischen Seite. Arch. Kriminol. 146 (1970) 26–32

[39] SZOBOR, A.: Affektív és voluntáris magatartásmódok igazságügyi elmekórtani értékelése. Medicina Bp. (1971) pp. 106–124

Chapter 9
Examinations for determining paternity

The legal status of the child within the family is regulated by the Family Law IV (1986). According to the law the father of the child must be considered at the one who, from the time of conception to the birth of the child, or at least during any portion of this period, was married to the mother. Nullification of the marriage does not affect the status of paternity [Section 35 (1)].

The *presumed date of conception* lies between day 182 and 300 inclusive, counted back from the date of birth. However, it is possible to prove that the conception occurred either before or after the presumed date (2).

If the mother was not married during any part of the time between the conception and the birth, the *father of the child must be considered to be,*

a) the man who by complete and open declaration acknowledges the child to be his, or

b) the one whom the court by valid judgement declares to be the father, or

c) who under the existing legal conditions marries the mother after the birth of the child (Section 36).

Section 38. (1) If the father of the child is not with complete certainty acknowledged by the mother, either in a state of marriage or by a marriage made later, paternity may be established by the court. There is no legal provision to establish paternity in cases of artificial insemination.

(2) The court declare that person as the child's father who had sexual intercourse with the mother at the date of conception and who, with thoughtful consideration of all circumstances, could be considered the one who through sexual intercourse fertilized the child, which was born following this sexual intercourse.

According to Familiar Law, not only the identity of the father may be disputable, but the identity of the mother may also have to be established.

Section 40. (1) The child may petition the court to establish that his mother is the one designated...

(2) Legal establishment of maternity may be petitioned by anyone who claims to be the child's mother.

Section 43. (1) The designation of paternity may be disputed if the one considered to be the father did not have sexual intercourse with the mother at the time of conception, or if due to circumstances, it would have been impossible for the child to be fertilized by him, if the origin were of artificial insemination and the husband of the mother gave no permission for the intervention.

The court may decide the paternity with a special process in the name of the minor, for the question of his/her mother or minor's guardian. Exclusion of paternity may be made by scientifically supported examinations and the court may accept the results of such expert opinion.

Exclusion of paternity may occasionally be made by:

1. examination for fertility,
2. the establishment of the time of conception and the maturity of the newborn,
3. examination of hereditary characteristics
   a) by blood group examination,
   b) by examination of hereditary serum factors,
   c) by examination of enzyme systems,
   d) on the basis of the HLA system,
   e) from hereditary anthropological signs,
   f) with chromosomal examination.

1. Examination for fertility

To establish the fertility of the putative father, we may request the opinion of an andrologist.

There are many possibilities of determining pre-existing (for months, even in some cases years) fertility prior to the birth of the child. In each case the appropriate criteria must be evaluated. The difficulties are increased by the fertility of the man from the clinical standpoint not being adequate in every case from a legal point of view. (With oligospermia, the man may be fertile, but it is emphasized in medical practice that the probability is slight due to the sperm count.) In many previous cases, paternity has been attempted to be legally established based on the results of unfounded andrological examinations, and it is a difficult task for the examining physician or the specialist, if he finds a normal andrological situation, to convince the court or the putative father his fertility. In other cases the transient damaging effects of various diseases, or decline in spermiogenesis can result in a decrease in fertility, which can make sometimes the exclusion or proof difficult.

The examination begins with taking the anamnestic data, which must turn attention to those diseases (parotitis, TB, varicocele etc.) which are capable of damaging spermiogenesis. In the examination, we inspect the genitals looking for such alterations which make sexual intercourse difficult or impossible, such as hypo- or epispadiasis, induration penis plastica, or a large irreponable scrotal hernia. Naturally, difficulties in sexual intercourse do not necessarily mean inability to fertilize. We examine the testes. Undescended testicles mean the severe disturbances of spermiogenesis, or infertility. Similarly, if alterations, cysts, tumors or varicoceles can be palpated in the testes or epididymis, they may be a cause of damaged spermiogenesis.

An external examination of the ejaculate is next. The ejaculate is produced through masturbation and we do not examine a sample brought in, partially because the motility of the sperm, the pH etc. in the ejaculate change rapidly over time and because spermicidal substances in condoms may damage the sperm cells. Since in practice the defendant may attempt to deceive the medical specialist, he may bring in a sample that was produced by someone else, and therefore we must purposely use fresh ejaculate and secretions expressed from the urethra to compare with the sample produced.

To the unaided eye, the ejaculate is a greyish-white, sticky substance of 3–6 ml in which sperm and secretions from the prostate and seminal vesicles are mixed. Fresh ejaculate is almost neutral with a pH of 7.2, and becomes more acidic upon standing. The consistency changes after 20–30 minutes and becomes fluid. Further examination turns to the morphology of the basic elements and their amount. The classification is made according to the recommendations by the WHO, which are:

a) normospermia
3–6 ml, sperm count above 40 million with at least 60% motile,
b) hypospermia
less than 3 ml ejaculate with a sperm count of 10–20 million/ml,
c) azoospermia
no sperm in the ejaculate,
d) necrospermia
the sperm do not react to intervention (supravital staining, warming),
e) asthenozoospermia
under 70% motile.

For morphological alterations and examination of damage, besides the supravital staining, we use May–Grünwald–Giemsa technique.

A damaged-looking state may also be created artificially. Overdose of estrogen may cause a hypo- or azoospermia, or in other cases taking cytostatics may harm spermiogenesis. Repeated findings of azoospermia in examination only establishes that at the time of the examination the defendant was sterile and extending the assumption to the time of conception opens the possibility of serious doubt. Testicular biopsy, which today is a routine intervention, can provide an explanation for decreased fertility or sterility. The biopsy material can verify a diagnosis which clearly excludes, even after treatment, the capability of fertilization – the biopsy findings in Klinefelter–Reifenstein–Albright syndrome belong here –, but a serious testicular atrophy, either from the degenerative effect of chemicals or following irradiation, chronic congestion or varicocele, may also have this result. If on the section we find testicular atrophy and hyaline degeneration in the spermatogenic tissues, we can unequivocally declare sterility. MOLNAR and PAPP especially call attention to the significance of the examination of the testicular biopsy material, and give particularly detailed data in this area for the correcting of spermatogenesis in men by medical treatment and restoring the ability to procreate, while in other cases unambiguously excluding the possibility based on the histological findings.

In classifying the material from the testicular biopsy, the findings may differ from normal by:

1. hypoplasia of the germinal epithelium with sperm precursors and normal Leydig cells,
2. tubular obstruction with normal spermatogenesis and azospermia,
3. damage to the germinal cells in which development to the level of spermatocytes can be seen in the germinal epithelium without spermatids or mature sperm cells,
4. only Sertoli cells visible and occasionally damage to a significant part of the Leydig cells,
5. hyaline degeneration of the tubular epithelium,
6. Leydig cell tumor.

Examination of the testicular biopsy can thus be a valuable indication of the previous fertilization capability over years, but the evaluation of the findings also requires the help of an experienced specialist.

Calculation of the time of conception

In the establishment of paternity in court, the stages between the presumed time of conception and time of birth can be investigated from the measurements of the newborn.

According to data from the WHO, the mature baby is born between the 37th and 42nd week – day 259–293 – of pregnancy, weighs 2500 g or more, is 53 cm in body length, and has a cranial circumference of 36 cm. We fin a wide variation not only in the time the fetus is carried, but in physical measurements of the newborn as well. Although the cranial circumference and the body length are fairly close in mature newborns and the variations at most are by a few percent, the newborns may show significant variation in body weight. The measurements and weight of the newborn may vary depending on the time of the pregnancy. Since the father of the baby must be considered to be the one who was living with the mother at the time of conception between days 192–300 before birth, the measurements of the newborn can be pivotal in determining the time of conception. On the basis of these measurements an opinion can be formulated concerning the most probable time and of the span of time the pregnancy was carried as well. In the observations of VARGA and coworkers, the probable time of conception and span of pregnancy with a mature newborn can be estimated to within 6–8 weeks, and with prematures, to within 8–10 weeks *(Table 4.)*. In the practice of obstetrics the "percentile curves" are not used in the estimation and determination of the stage of pregnancy, relying instead much more on the data derived from the weight, body length and cranial circumference.

No significant difference is found between n newborn boys and girls, so the tables can be used for the establishment of the time of conception for both sexes.

The duration of pregnancy with male neonates (postmenstruation time) relying on the weight at birth

Weight	Mean
1250 g	194 ± 14,0
1500 g	220 ± 18,0
1750 g	235 ± 20,0
2000 g	245 ± 23,0
2250 g	253 ± 20,0
2500 g	268 ± 19,0
2750 g	270 ± 17,0
3000 g	275 ± 15,0
3250 g	277 ± 14,0
3500 g	279 ± 13,0
3750 g	280 ± 11,0
4000 g	282 ± 13,0
4250 g	284 ± 11,0

The duration of pregnancy with female neonates (postmenstruation time) relying on the weight at birth
(Varga et al.)

Weight	Mean
1250 g	206 ± 18,0
1500 g	223 ± 23,0
1750 g	239 ± 21,0
2000 g	249 ± 24,0
2250 g	259 ± 21,0
2500 g	268 ± 18,0
2750 g	273 ± 15,0
3000 g	276 ± 14,0
3250 g	278 ± 14,0
3500 g	280 ± 13,0
3750 g	280 ± 13,0
4000 g	282 ± 14,0
4250 g	284 ± 13,0

Examinations of hereditary characteristics

Blood group examinations. Under the heading of blood group examinations we place all genetic examinations related to the description of all morphological and inherited biochemical characteristics. The biochemical methods consist of serological, isoenzyme, HLA and DNA sequencing techniques, and at present these are the methods most used in the exclusion or establishment of paternity and with serostatistical elements, are also considered for verification examinations.

For the establishment of paternity the examination performed must on a scientific basis exclude or confirm the putative father and the above-mentioned verification procedures provide the possibility that of 1000 uncertain fathers, exclusion will be unsuccessful in only one case.

In these procedures a familiarity with human genetics is necessary that far exceeds the scope of this book. Even so, the small amount of data which is necessary for the institution performing paternity examinations to understand opinions, or make opinions understood, in any case must be presented.

The above-mentioned inherited characteristics depend on the genes found on the chromosomes. At division, the chromosome pairs in the gametes separate and these gametes supply the owner with half of the chromosomal material and the genes found in it. With fertilization, two cells that have undergone meiosis find one another and the uniting of the sperm with the egg restores the normal chromosome number, of which half is paternal and half is maternal, and naturally along with the chromosomes, the genes. Thus it is understandable that the inherited factors derived from the unification of the gametes are obtained from the parents.

The genes on the chromosomes regulate heredity. During mitosis the genes may independently combine with one another, with the exception of those located next to one another, the so-called *linked genes.* These usually stay together even during mitosis, while at other times the linked genes may split, *cross over,* and thus recombinant chromatids may originate which consist of segments of the original chromosomes. Thus a gene inherited from the father may be on the chromosome originating from the mother linked to an original gene on the maternal chromosome. The genes are stabile, but under certain influences – chemical, radiation etc. – mutations may occur. Following mutation at certain places on the chromosome an alternative gene may be emplaced. These are called alleles and we may be able to differentiate two or more alleles at a given locus. The changeability of the alleles can result in such genetic polymorphism which may make evaluation of inherited traits either more easy or difficult.

As already mentioned, with the process of heredity, one member of the chromosome pair is maternal and the other is paternal, and thus the characteristics are passed on from the parents. Certain characteristics are typical at a given location on each chromosome and at this location certain genes or alleles are found. If these identical genes or alleles on the chromosome pair match, we speak of a homozygote, and if the genes or alleles differ from each other, we speak of a heterozygote.

Heredity may be dominant, recessive or intermediate. The *dominant form of heredity* means that when two genes are found together, only one phenotype is expressed. The other is not manifested, and a gene with this property of remaining hidden we call *recessive.* At other times several genes may behave so that they become manifest in the presence of each other, and the phenotype expressed is of the so-called *intermediate type.* The scheme of dominant heredity is simple. With the recessive property in heredity, the gene is ineffective by itself, and is only manifested when it appears on both members of the chromosome pair.

By heredity, the inherited gene pairs from the parents determine the individual genotype, including both the manifest characteristics, and those characteristics which remain hidden. Because of the hidden characteristics sometimes only the individual phenotype may be determined, and those genes which have a characteristically manifested property can also be demonstrated by certain methods. With paternity examinations the genotype can be determined only in certain cases, such as in the case of AB and 0 blood group when the phenotype is identical. At other times only the phenotype can be decided and the genotype, in which a recessive gene may be present, cannot be determined in every case.

In the scheme of heredity, those examinations have a great significance which divide the population according to the appearance of certain traits, based on such family examinations where the inherited trait can be identified. Family pedigrees make it possible to determine the origin of a trait when one of the parents are not available for examination, although an extended examination of the next of kin to the parent who is unavailable can be arranged for and it may serve to provide such data which can decide the paternity of the child. A publication appeared in which, following a kidnapping, the accused couple, their child (the one presumed kidnapped), and the mother of the child were examined. The father's group characteristics in this case were not known, and the blood group and inheritable enzyme trait examinations demonstrated the identity despite the numerous alternative possibilities. It made verification of the origin of the child possible and provided proof of a crime.

We have already discussed the properties of the blood group antigens. The blood groups are determined on the basis of antigens found on the surface of red blood cells. Since the discovery of the AB0 system, numerous blood groups have been described, a large part of which are useable for determination of paternity. The common – public – antigens can be found in a large portion of the population, and their usefulness is therefore meager (if only for exclusion). The significance of the private antigens on the other hand may be important, since outside of relatives, they cannot be demonstrated in anybody else. In the blood group system, the expression of alternative genes and their frequency provide a possibility for identification.

The genetics of the blood grouping is simply described in that:

a) the blood group, that is, the antigens on the surface of the red blood cells are hereditarily determined,

b) if a gene is present on the chromosome, with the help of an antiserum of the corresponding phenotype it can almost always be determined,

c) interaction between the genes is rare, and if present, detectable,

d) with respect to the allele pairs, the individual whose red blood cells react with one antiserum is homozygote and with two types of antiserum, is heterozygote.

Blood group systems

The heritable trait – the antigen on the surface of the red blood cells – can be demonstrated by serological reactions so that the phenotype and occasionally the genotype of the individual may be determined.

AB0 system:
The AB0 blood group is determined by the alleles found on one locus of the chromosome. The three genes are A, B, and 0. The AA trait is manifested in the A blood group, the BB in the B group, and the 00 in the 0 group. The A and B traits are dominant with respect to 0. This is of special value in the case of heterozygotic traits where the blood group determination is made on the basis of only one of the members of the allele pair. Thus it is not possible to differentiate whether the A group allele pair consists of A0, AA_1, AA_2 etc. Likewise the B trait is expressed with BB, B_3, B_m, B_x groups. Some of the members of the A subgroup may belong to an intermediate group, and the rarity of the A_3 variation makes it more valuable in verification of heredity. The numerous subtypes of A are so rare that, with those family pedigrees with the above-mentioned procedures, they can play a role not only in exclusion of paternity, but in verification as well. At the present state of knowledge, the B subgroup has no significance in paternity investigations.

The heredity pattern of the AB0 traits can manifest as A, B, 0 or AB blood groups. Besides these, the A and B groups can combine, as with the AB group, and can be inherited as dominant over 0. The A0 and AB trait simultaneously gives the genotype of the individual, while in both the 00 and AB cases, the phenotypic traits are also manifest. The A and B groups manifest only the phenotype, and by direct serological procedures the genotype cannot be determined. *(Possibility of exclusion 17.6%.)*

MN system:
For years the MN system was considered to be the simplest trait of the red blood cells which could be inherited in the MM and NN homozygote and MN heterozygote forms. The determination also revealed the genotype. It also had significance in examination for paternity, because it is none dominant and both genes are frequent, therefore the possibility for exclusion is rather large, and especially when combined with the AB0 system, the MN system is accepted as proof of exclusion. Two newly discovered antigens, S and s, complicated the system, and today we speak of the MNSs traits. The genes combine regularly and are inherited as MS, Ms, NS, and Ns groups. With determination the MN system and the Ss system can be investigated separately (SS-ss phenotypes are manifested). The system is complicated by the fact that rarely alleles of the MN system may rarely appear, as M_2, N_2 or M^g, M^c etc. Rare variations are of value only in expanded family pedigree examinations, but in these cases they have a validity as proof. SZABÓ considers the four gene system – the examination of four test sera – as one of the most powerful systems *(in the MNSs group exclusion is 32.1%).*

Rh group system:
The Rh group system has significance not only in obstetrics and transfusions, but in paternity examinations it has been one of the most valuable procedures which can absolutely exclude paternity about 28% of the time. The high percentage of exclusion is made possible by the genes being inherited on three linked loci on one chromosome. One is C-c, the second is D-d and the third, E-e. The connection is so close that crossing over has not been observed between them. Thus the linked gene may be transmitted in, for example, CdE form, but of the gene pairs at one locus only one can be expressed. The triplets are passed on from generation to generation, and thus may play a role in the family pedigree. In the fertilized ovum, the triplets of the

parents can be found, so that six genes may be expressed of which five can be determined by antiserum tests. Only the d trait is not expressed. The D trait gives the Rh positivity, which plays a role in the consequences of transfusion and, after the AB0 system, is the most significant and its obstetrical implications also are well known. The possibility of the triplets occurring in the gene complex and their expression can be represented according to the genes (FISCHER) or by an alternative symbol (WIENER).

FISCHER	WIENER
CDe	R_1
cde	r
cDE	R_2
cDe	R_0
Cde	r'
cdE	r''
CDE	R_z
CdE	r_y

In the absence of D antiserum only the phenotype can be determined in the triplets in which we can expect the inherited D trait. Thirty-six Rh gene types can be differentiated with antiserum, but in the genetic examinations of European populations only five genotypes are be listed.

(DCe) (cde) (DCe) (CDe)
(cde) (cde) (CDE) (cDE)
(cDE) (cde)

The rare occurrence of the variants and the appearance of the alternative genes emphasize the significance of the system, which makes the demonstration of positive proof of paternity possible. *(Possibility of exclusion 28%.)*

Duffy blood group system
We can investigate the manifestation of this two-gene system whose expression can be FY^aFY^a, FY^bFY^b or FY^aFY^b. For the examination we use FY^a and FY^b antiserum. As an antiserum reaction has not yet been found in blacks, a third so-called quiet gene is supposed to exist, thus among the blood group traits, the Duffy system shows the most conspicuous racial difference. *The exclusion possibility is 18%.*

Kell–Cellano system
The Kell group system was discovered in 1946 and the Cellano blood group system in 1949. The progeny of the individual giving a K^+ reaction can be either K^+ or K^-, but the K^- couple can only produce exclusively K^- children. The K^+ individuals have either one or two K genes. In the case of K^-, both are k genes, since K is inherited dominantly with respect to k. The possible genotypes are KK, Kk, or KKK. The exclusion percentage is low and due to its rarity it has a significance in positive proof of paternity *(exclusion 4.8%).*

Xg blood group system
The X-linked blood group traits are present in 66% of all men and 84% of all women. The system can be determined by two alleles in , Xg and Xg^a (dominant). The allele pair is carried only by women (XX chromosome), while men have only one allele (XY chromosome).
On the accompanying diagram the pedigree of inheritance can be easily seen as a typical X-linked dominant mode of inheritance.

Hereditary serum factors, and enzyme systems

In the biochemical examinations of proteins, the recognition of the line of inheritance of certain protein fractions and isoenzymes increases the possibilities in paternity examinations. Certain groups of serum proteins, such as haptoglobin, gammaglobulin and the $alpha_2$ protein (group specific component) can be distinguish into separate subunits by electrophoretic methods, which exhibit Mendelian inheritance characteristics.

The *haptoglobin system* was examined the earliest, in which three phenotypes can be differentiated, Hp 1–1, Hp 2–1, and Hp 2–2. With the examination of the haptoglobin trait, different variants and subtypes have been described, the significance of which in paternity examinations is low, the *exclusion possibility being 18%.*

Among the gammaglobulins the *Gm system* is examined. The present possibility of *exclusion is 12–13%.*

In the *Gc system* Gc 1–1, Gc 2–1 and Gc 2–2 types are differentiated and the *exclusion possibility is 16%.*

The examination of the *enzyme fractions* – isoenzyme investigations in which the isoenzymes are separated near their isoelectric points on a pH gradient – has provided numerous new results in heredity. The primary protein enzyme fractions can be separated into 3–4 phenotypes and further separation into 8–10 fractions, and this grows with the corresponding number of phenotypes. This significantly increases the exclusion possibilities as well. The isoenzyme systems of erythrocytes examined in paternity cases are: acid phosphatase *(AcP) with an exclusion possibility of 21%,* phosphoglucomutase *(PGM) with 24.5%,* adenylate kinase *(AK) with 4.2%,* adenosine deaminase *(ADA) with 4.5%,* glutamate-pyrofructate transaminase *(GPT) with 18.7%,* esterase D *(EsD) with 9.0.* When the above methods are used *together in combination, the exclusion possibility is 94%.*

HLA system

The introduction of this system in paternity examinations has significantly increased the exclusion possibilities and in serostatistical examinations it is positive proof of paternity. This makes it possible to find numerous cells in the organism besides leukocytes which carry the HLA antigens, and inasmuch as these tissue antigens play a significant role in organ transplantation, they are called transplantation antigens. Getting back to the place they occupy in paternity examinations, the polymorphism of the HLA system is quite large. Since in exclusion there are theoretically more than a million variations in genotype, by this method alone in phenotype examination the exclusion of non-fathers is 96%.

While keeping in mind Mendel's laws of heredity in the exclusion of paternity based on blood groups, Bernstein's principles are also presented:

1. a child cannot have such a blood group antigen which neither parent possesses (paternity examination is valid based on the Roman Law "Mater semper certa est" ("certainty of motherhood"), since the chracteristics of the child's blood group which are not found in the mother must have been inherited from the father. If, for example, both parents are 0–0, the child is 0, and an AB father must be excluded.),
2. if in the offspring the characteristic is manifested in homozygote form, then the opposite gene homozygote form in the either the mother or father is impossible (thus the parents of an MM child cannot have the NN trait).

The first rule means exclusion of the absent characteristic, while the other is based on the opposite homozygote.

The group traits, inasmuch as a great part of these may appear early in the development of the fetus, can be examined after birth. Among the protein traits, the haptoglobin system can be investigated even during fetal life. The inherited serum traits on the other hand appear after birth, and for that reason the child is examined at the age of one year. We have already discussed the inheritance of the group traits. These traits are unchangeable over the course of the life, and as mentioned previously, the genetics of the blood group is one of the best studied in heredity and a high percentage of them are the easiest examinations to perform as well. This simplicity also shows the pitfalls in the examinations and their evaluation. Since the classic blood group examinations – AB0, MN, Ss, Rh – were simple in the early stages of paternity examinations, their evaluation caused no difficulties either. Today no matter how pure the line of heredity, only a highly experienced institute especially equipped for this purpose can perform these examinations or have them performed. Thus the slightest possibility of error is avoidable, and these days the experienced blood group geneticist along with the numerous procedures applicable to the tasks and material available to him can pick out the responsible person in the pedigree. A particularly large amount of experience is required in the extended pedigree examination in such cases where the father is not shown. Sometimes in a genetic examination, factors can come to light which for a long time were excluded from the specialist's practice, such as the possibility of superfecundation.

In the bulletin of the Forensic Committee of The Scientific Committee of Ministry of Health (N^0 2/1969) on the basis of an examination of the Rh group system in a pair of twins, the father was excluded from having generated one of them!

The exclusion of paternity must be based on scientific proof. If paternity is excluded on the basis of blood groups, hereditary serum factors, enzyme or HLa systems further examinations are superfluous.

Proof of paternity

Genetic examination of the extended blood groups, enzyme traits and protein types have made it possible to, besides exclusion which under optimal conditions is above 90%, to determine probable paternity.

Mathematical calculations which are based on the occurrence of each blood group, enzyme trait and protein type in the population can serve in deriving positive proof, keeping in mind the ratio of the characteristic traits of the true father to those of the certain non-father. For this reason those traits are significant which rarely appear, especially when the trait is missing in the mother. The biostatistical examinations of these cases which do not absolutely exclude paternity must be specially performed, and such expanded group characteristics and hereditary traits should be available which support those which are obtained through probability calculations.

In Europe the Essen–Möller calculation is used, although the procedure was primarily worked out for the statistical evaluation of anthropological signs. Only with the discovery of blood group systems did serostatistical calculations start to be used, although then the small number of determinable hereditary traits did not allow for true proof. The Essen–Möller formula is the basis of Hummel gene statistic data which, was worked up on population group data taken from Central Europe. The data on the appearance of gene frequency values play a very relevant role in the calculations since the blood group geneticists aren't the only ones who emphasize that the serostatistical procedures can only be applied to individuals of the same ethnic groups from which the data came. Similar results are derived from those countries in which several types of ethnic groups with divergent gene frequencies invalidate the calculations. In these circumstances one can find critics of the Essen–Möller formula. Some such critics suggest that it was not even prepared originally for serostatistical, but for anthropological characteristics, and can be used only for AB0, MN and Rh systems. The paternity index (PI) is used more specifically, and probability statistical calculations are based on it which differentiate the true father from the non-father. At the same time it should be noted that probability statistics sometimes do not yield the appropriate results, since they also depend on the combinations of the phenotypes of the mother and the child. For positive proof it is necessary that such markers of the child and the supposed father be available which do not, or very rarely, appear in the general population. The more of such signs that are available between the two individuals examined, the higher the certainty of proof, since the chance that two very rare markers would coincide as a result of a mutation is negligible. The practical question is whether on the basis of the examination of some markers the paternity of the putative father can be excluded, or whether further tests are called for. Besides the objective possibilities – the possibility of determination, test serum support, etc. – theoretical considerations of these also have a limit. The investigations of Mickey and coworkers convincingly proved that examination of the HLA–A, B, AB0, Rh and MNSs markers exclude the putative father with a 97% probability and allows only 1% margin of error. These prove the practical value of the Essen–Möller serostatistical examination. In those cases where the possibility of paternity is less than 90%, the DNA fingerprinting method is called for. According to the author, probing the DNA minisatellites has immense significance in the establishment of paternity, and has been used in such instances of extended pedigree investigation when the putative father died in a traffic accident before the examination. The significance of DNA fingerprint tests together with the HLA system were emphasized for the exclusion in multiman cases.

In our practice, we constructed the following scale based on serostatistical evaluations according to the Essen–Möller formula:

99.75%	paternity practically proved
99.0–99.75%	paternity very highly probable
95.0–99.0%	paternity probable
5.0–95.0%	probability not able to be established
1.0– 0.2%	paternity highly improbable
0.2%	paternity practically excluded

Anthropological examinations

Anthropological examinations are likewise based on observation of heritable characteristics, descriptions and statistical evaluations.

True values have often been doubtful, and even today many consider the previous genetic examinations to be complementary and their value in proof not to approach the other methods. The newer tests, which are not regarded as classical anthropological examinations, are reported to be unambiguous procedures for proving heredity, among which belong the observation of the dominant signs and even more so, chromosome examinations.

The court usually orders the anthropological examinations together with the blood group examinations. The examination reports the comparison of such external signs which have been long used in for comparison in anthropology. Among the *morphological signs* examined are the hair color, the skull, the facial form, where here *anthropometric measurements* are employed, the form and size of the nose, the shape of the nasal openings, the shape of the brows, the eye color, the variety of the iris. In comparison of the mouth, the curve of the lips, the situation of the upper and lower lips, the form of the corner of the mouth, and the shape of the chin bear special significance. In the description of the chin, useful data such as their size and shape, whether the ear lobes taper in or hang free, and the situation of the auricle should be noticed. The form of the hands and nails found on general examination may be decisive. This information and these descriptions are the tedious tasks of the experienced anthropologist, and the compilation of an amount for approximation still does not provide the possibility of noticing the evaluation of the results. In Hungary for the mathematical evaluation of the anthropological points of measurement, the data of Somogyi and coworkers is applied. In this information biostatistical evaluation may be more useful than the statistical data of the previously described examinations, and the calculations do not reflect their opinion.

The recognized anthropological characteristics can only help other proofs, but by themselves do not establish proof of paternity.

We must specially mention the heritable characteristics which appear as the genetic characteristics of the disputed father, and these appear in a dominant expression in the offspring. These appear as morphological alterations or inherited diseases. With dominantly inherited characteristics the gene responsible for expression may originate from one of the parents or from a mutation.

Among the *dominantly inherited morphological characteristics* we can list arachnodactyly, brachidactyly, syndactyly, hypoplasia of the enamel, the appearance of Carabelli tubercle, which may appear in the offspring as a dominantly inherited trait. In general dominantly inherited traits can be found somewhere in the parentage, except when the genetic fault "skips" a generation. (For example, when the child's syndactyly is not found in the father, but in the grandfather.) In such cases examination of the family pedigree will reveal whether the trait was inherited through the mother or the father.

Dominantly inherited alterations may not be able to be traced back pathologically to the forebears. The faulty gene must have at some time originated from a mutation and been passed on. The same kind of mutation may originate, and the gene originating at this time is stable and passed on. The mutant gene occupies the same location on the chromosome. The one with the dominant defect originates from a heterozygote trait-bearer on the family tree who crosses with a healthy partner, but the defect may also be homozygotic, if both parents bear copies of the defective gene. A heterozygote trait-bearer or demonstration of a trait-bearer in the hereditary line unequivocally establishes the origin of the offspring, if the trait is found in the putative father.

In the opinion from the anthropological examinations the specialist must prepare a probability opinion. The probability opinion does not definitely establish paternity if only the above-mentioned detailed characteristic genetic traits are not carried by the offspring which were inherited from the putative father and appear very rarely in the population. A probability opinion means that the court must accept critically the anthropological examination and quantitatively-based determinations and not hold the procedures to be adequate in themselves to determine or exclude paternity. The anthropological examinations especially decrease the significance of the possibility of the blood group examinations and the serostatistical calculation which gives unambiguous proof, and a more certain opinion for the definite exclusion of the non-fathers. The further judgement by the court based on scientifically based examinations settles the issue and in practice these examinations occupy the forefront.

Chromosomal examinations

In Hungary the chromosomal examination by Bujdosó and coworkers is used in detail due to the usefulness of the method in the determination of paternity. In numerous cases its findings have been of help in the decision of the court. (They first reported A_2D translocation as proof in establishment of paternity.)

The basis of the chromosomal examination is in the heredity facts already mentioned, that one of the chromosomes of the pair is inherited by the offspring from the father and the other one from the mother. The possibility and application of morphological examination of the chromosomes unequivocally provides that the heritable traits can be described and used. Comparison of the morphological alterations, identification at the centromeres (this happens by description of the primary branching place on the chromosomes, the meeting of the arms, the secondary winding and description of the satellite localization. In the morphological description, the chromosomes are assigned numbers, 1–22, while the sex chromosome are labelled XX or XY. The goal of the morphological examinations is to observe any alterations from normal chromosomes. Missing chromosomes, duplications and structural alterations have been described.

The examination requires practice and the appropriate laboratory skills, since examination of chromosomes has to be done with chromosomes in metaphase and by inhibiting further progress of cell division, we obtain the customary chromosome picture. In this stage the two chromatids of the chromosomes can be seen, which are joined at the centromere. If a chromosomal abnormality is detected in a child and the putative father is a carrier, and the abnormality appears rarely in the population, it can be considered positive proof.

A chromosomal examination with the so-called chromosomal banding technique may also be performed. The staining may be stronger or lighter and the band forms appear. By use of the appropriate technique, G, C, or Q banding is possible and the band configuration is characteristic, with dark and light bands alternating one with another. With use of the banding technique various Q and C band polymorphism appears and these give much information about heredity *(Fig. 165)*.

Bujdosó and coworkers consider the banding technique useful in those cases which:

1. two or more men are examined with which neither blood group nor anthropological examinations have yielded results,

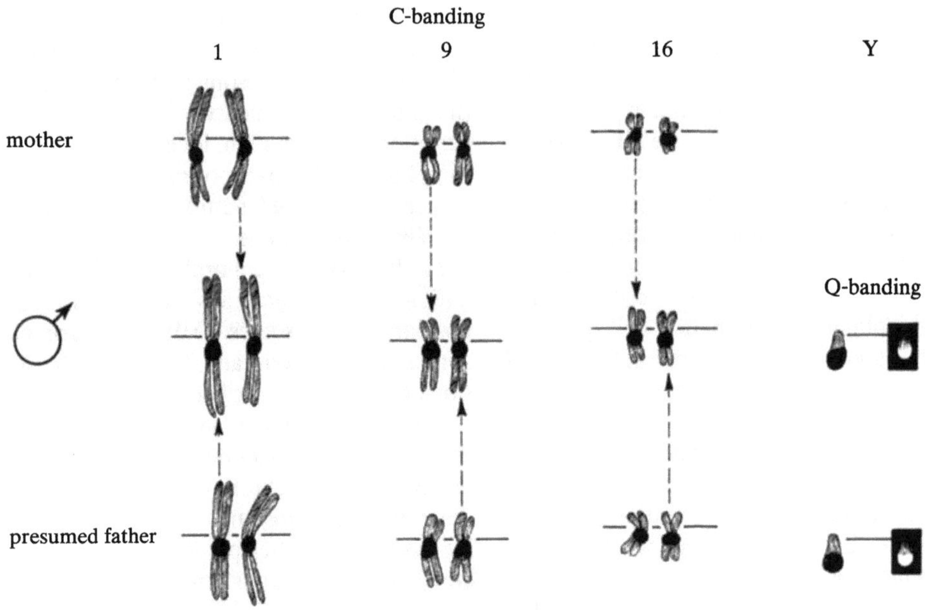

Fig. 165. With C-banding, the characteristic heterochromatin of chromosomes 1, 2, and 16 of the mother, child and presumed father.
The arrows, indicate which chromosome the child inherited from the biological father and which from the mother. In the case of the Y chromosome Q-banding is used in the determination. Under UV light the dark bands of the chromosome stained with C-banding fluoresce. With the help of the obvious polymorphisms and opinion of "very probable" was rendered. (from the material of dr. Györgyi Bujdosó)

2. in the case of two men whose sero-statistical values do not vary significantly from each other,

3. the blood group does not exclude the man designated by the mother, the sero-statistical examination yields an uncertain group and the anthropological examination is not convincing.

In all, the exclusion methods of paternity examinations based on blood group examinations are of primary importance in the cases of disputed paternity. The blood group examinations by serostatistical methods are considered as proof, although they carry the possibility for error.

One of the modern exclusion methods is the lack by a child of a trait characteristic on a certain chromosome found in the pedigree of the mother and father. The results of chromosomal examination are confirming and unambiguous, whether by morphological alteration or banding technique, if the alteration found in the father is passed on to the child. The results of those anthropological examinations may be confirmatory which are rarely found in the population and dominantly mask the trait inherited by the offspring from the father.

References

[1] AICKIN, M.: Some fallacies in the computation of paternity probabilities. Am. J. Hum. Genet. 36 (1984) 904–915

[2] BENCIOLINI, P., M. BIASIOLO, P. CORTIVO, L. CAENAZZO: Problems in probability of paternity interpretation. Forensic Sci. Int. 29 (1985) 199–206

[3] BERTRAMS, J., H. PREUSS: Ein Zwillingsfall mit wahrscheinlicher Superfetatio. Z. Rechtsmed. 84 (1980) 319–321

[4] BUJDOSÓ, GY.: A_2D transzlokációval bizonyított származásmegállapítás. Biol. Közl. XX (1972) 81–86

[5] BUJDOSÓ, GY., VINCZE I., BERGOU J., SOMOGYI E.: Morfológiai jellemzők biostatisztikai kiértékelése származásmegállapítási vizsgálati anyagban. Demográfia 1 (1982) 65–81

[6] BUJDOSÓ, GY., E. SOMOGYI, V. BERGOU: The use of chromosomes in paternity actions. Forensic Sci. Int. 25 (1984) 35–43

[7] BUJDOSÓ, GY.: X vagy Y. Apaság vizsgálat, igazságszolgáltatás. Medicina (1985) pp. 144–183, 198–212

[8] CHAKRABORTY, R., P. W. HEDRICK: Paternity exclusion and the paternity index for two linked loci. Hum. Hered. 33 (1983) 13–23

[9] CHAKRABORTY, R.: Paternity testing with genetic markers: Are Y-linked genes more efficient than autosomal ones? Am. J. Med. Genet. 21 (1985) 297–305

[10] DAVEY, F. R., C. A. HUBBELL, K. J. LAUENSTEIN, C. TINNESZ, J. B. HENRY: Analysis of paternity. The use of HLA and red cell antigens. Transfusion 24 (1984) 340–342

[11] DODD, B. E., P. J. LINCOLN: Testing paternity: traditional methods usually adequate. Br. Med. J. 295 (1987) 1435

[12] ELSTON, R. C.: Probability and paternity testing. Am. J. Hum. Genet. 39 (1986) 112–122

[13] ESSEN–MÖLLER, E., C. E. QUENSEL: Zur Theorie des Vaterschaftsnachweises auf Grund von Ahnlichkeitsbefunden. Z. f. d. ges. Gerichtl. Med. 31 (1939) 70–96

[14] GJERTSON, D. W., M. R. MICKEY, P. I. TERASAKI: Empirical paternity exclusion Rates. Am. J. Forensic Med. Pathol 8 (1987) 123–126

[15] KAISER, L., G. A. F. SEBER: Paternity testing. Likelihood ratio tests. Am. J. Med. Genet 20 (1985) 209–219

[16] KISHIDA T., Y. TAMAKI, C. WAKASUGI: A Japanese family with unusual segregation of GM phenotype: a GM silent allele? Hum. Hered. 41 (1991) 227–230

[17] LEWONTIN R. C., D. L. HARTL: Population genetics in forensic DNA typing Science 254 (1991) 1745–1750

[18] LI, C. C., A. CHAKRAVARTI: Basic fallacies in the formulation of the paternity index. Am. J. Hum. Genet. 37 (1985) 809–818

[19] MICKEY, M. R., D. W. GJERTSON, P. I. TERASAKI: Empirical validation of the Essen–Möller probability of paternity. Am. J. Hum. Genet. 39 (1986) 123–132

[20] ODELBERG, S. J., D. B. DEMERS, E. H. WESTIN, A. A. HOSSAINI: Establishing paternity using minisatellite DNA probes when the putative father is unavailable for testing. J. Forensic Sci. 33 (1988) 921–928

[21] ÖKRÖS, S.: Establishing of the genetic father by means of fingerprint identification. Zacchia, XL (1965) 1–39

[22] OROSZ, L.: Klasszikus és molekuláris genetika. Akadémia Budapest (1950) p. 20

[23] PAPP, Z.: Szülészeti genetika. Medicina Budapest (1986) pp. 65–99

[24] READING, P. L., E. G. REISNER: The effect of differences in gene frequency on probability of paternity. J. Forensic Sci. 30 (1985) 1130–1139

[25] ROBERTS, J. A. F.: Bevezetés az orvosi genetikába. Medicina Budapest (1968) pp. 129–151

[26] SALMON, D., C. SALMON: Blood groups and genetic markers polymorphism and probability of paternity. Transfusion 20 (1980) 684–694

[27] SHIONO, H., J. I. AZUMI, Y. SAKAMOTO, M. FUJIWARA, M. MORITA: Chromosome heteromorphisms and paternity testing. Am. J. Forensic Med. Pathol. 6 (1985) 199–203

[28] SMOUSE, P. E., R. CHAKRABORTY: The use of restriction fragment length polymorphisms in paternity analysis. Am. J. Hum. Genet. 38 (1986) 918–939

[29] SZABÓ, L.: Vércsoport vizsgálatok. In Bujdosó Gy.: Apasági vizsgálatok, igazságszolgáltatás. Medicina Budapest (1985) pp. 75–145

[30] VARGA, T., SUSA É., SZABÓ Á.: A fogantatási idő meghatározása a születéskori testméretek alapján. Anthrop. Közl. 23 (1979) 87–96

[31] VALENTIN, J.: Some fallacious thinking about the

paternity index. Am. J. Hum. Genet. 38 (1986) 582–585

[32] Valentin, J.: Exclusions and attributions of paternity: Practical experiences of forensic genetics and statistics Am. J. Hum. Genet. 32 (1980) 420–431

[33] Vydra G., Magasi P.: A herebiopsia. Orvosképzés 55 (1980) 315–320

[34] Wenk R. E., T. Houtz, F. A. Chiafary, M. Brooks: Two-man and two sibling paternity cases. Am. J. Forensic Med. Pathol. 13 (1992) 76–80

Chapter 10
Disability

The health of the population is connected with the economical and social systems of society and inseparable from certain customs, which may be dietary, behavioral and social in origin. By this the appearance of certain diseases in a given population or larger territory, even a country, can be explained. In some countries the diseases of the circulatory system are not only the consequence of the unhealthy diet, but can also be linked with an increase nervous load, the effects of excess stress and the increase in the so-called risk factors. Damage to the circulatory system not only leads in mortality statistics, but occupies first place in diseases that affect the ability to work and earn a living. A significant number of the diseases of the circulatory system can be ascribed to deterioration of the social situation. Because of a sedentary lifestyle and over-eating the number of people overweight is growing. Besides this nutritional ignorance, the number of people living on very low life-standard can explain subsisting on a diet deficient in essential nutrients. The unhealthy diet and the improperly equipped work place gradually affect the organism and damage not only the circulatory system, but the locomotor system as well. The improperly equipped work place, standing for long periods, lifting heavy loads on the job can explain the large number of spinal and joint complaints in the population, and with these come disability. In the last years the chronic pain means one of the most important factor of disability, especially for developed countries. Most of the cases chronic pain are of unknown etiology, other it may consequence of psycho-social distress, unemployment, etc. A special form of the disability the low back pain which may be the alteration of middle age persons, originated from occupational activities a heavy lifting at work, professional truck drivers etc. With the creation of the previous planned work places, from the viewpoint of labor health and labor psychology, a number of injuries in the work place were to be expected with a large number of these being locomotor disorders. The deterioration of health in Hungary can be traced back decades. We will list a few of the outstanding causes, but the tabulation by Makra unambiguously lists these and those claims which, supported or unsupported, appear in committee for judgement of disability.

Makra lists the following factors, among others, or deterioration of health:

1. The *low value* of human life and health. In this a significant role is played by the low level of education of the worker, and the low wages that accompany it, thus the overburdening of the worker in mak-

ing a living (special skills, harder physical labor etc.).

2. A depressed standard of living makes it necessary for the worker to adopt a *"self-exploitation"* lifestyle, either to avoid or achieve something. A sign of our times in Hungary is that the daily work period is strikingly long.

3. The increasing claims in judgements of disability the growing number of those unable to earn a living, and the lack of rehabilitation are all matters which provide unambiguous evidence of *social endangerment.*

The specialists of public health have for decades dealt with assessment and judgement of fitness for work and disability, and the policies that have been formulated provide guidance in the judgement of these situations. The governing institutions are responsible for framing the policy on health and a representative of each profession provides advice for the formulation of general policies which will be the basis of judgement of fitness for work, disability, and accident injuries or occupational diseases with respect to the various groups of illnesses. These policies have been modified in light of medical advances and with respect to not only domestic experiences but those of other developed countries, recognizing and bearing in mind those suggestions of value in rendering judgement in the above matters.

Deterioration of health may be temporary or permanent. *Temporary deterioration of health* is the case where the patient cannot perform his original job and becomes unable to work. According to the regulations, inability to earn a living applies to the type of work which the patient performed prior to the illness or injury. This usually means for a year, although with tuberculosis it may last two years. *During the period of disability* the worker cannot perform his original job, although his status may improve to such an extent that he could perform some other job without significantly endangering his health and his inability to earn a living must be judged in light of his original profession.

If the disability came about as a result of an accident – accident at the work place – the period of disability may exceed a year and unrestricted disability may be maintained until the status has improved to such an extent where he can perform his original job, or with permanent injury, undergo professional rehabilitation. Those claims and disabilities must likewise be judged which develop as a result of the profession and are considered hazards of the profession. *The judgement of inability to work* is the responsibility of the practising physician and is regulated by law, and if the judgement or verification of disability requires the facilities of a hospital, the primary care physician must refer the patient for admission according to the customary procedures. The appropriate procedures for handling a disability patient are regulated to inform the physician of how to deal with the patient, the necessary treatment and, not least importantly, the proper supervision. A committee of head physicians is arranged for the purpose of supervision.

After a certain period – when the period of disability has exceeded a year, or two years in the case of tuberculosis – either the patient or the employer may request a *determination of the severity of disability, the amount of work capacity lost and the amount remaining, and perhaps the possibility of rehabilitation.* This becomes due when the state of the patient following the disease or injury reaches the standard condition, further intervention is not planned, and the patient nears the end of his treatment. The medical specialist fulfills this area of responsibility. The work of this specialist requires much previous experience, since answering the special questions demands special training and a certain social and legal knowledge from the physicians chosen to serve on the committee. These committees work within the framework of the *National Institute of Medical Specialties (N.I.).* The first level committee is the forum, with which the patient or organization seeking an opinion must first meet, and against whose opinion is the possibility of appeal. In that case, the N.I.'s second level committee is that which decides whether to review the opinion of the first committee. The decision of the second level committee in individual cases may be altered by review by the Chief Executive of the N.I. Since 1988. the government gave the possibilities the redress of the decision of the second level committee. This is initiated by an appeal to the Civil Court. The *Civil Court* requests a medical opinion from the forensic medical specialist in the assessment of disability and poses such questions to the specialist which aids in the decision regarding the possibility if partial disability to a certain percentage, when deterioration of health ensues, how long the status will last, when a new examination is necessary, and what are the possibilities of rehabilitation.

These claims have significantly expanded the work of the forensic medical specialist, so we must deal with in more detail the supporting of such special claims of disability and every type of it.

The theoretical basis of the opinion of disability in social security is dealt with in the II. law of 1975.

Sections: 18. *Disability:*

a) that person who, due to illness, is unable to work,

19. Disability *compensation* is awarded at most however for one, or in tuberculosis, two years.

12. (1) Disability compensation expires for that person who, having been on renewed compensation status, if he becomes able to work, and following this verifiable performs work.

24. Disability *compensation may be withdrawn* for those who:

a) suffer delayed healing attributable to unsatisfactorily following the instructions of the physician,

b) do not appear for the arranged medical examination without an acceptable reason.

47. Disability *retirement is awarded* to those who:

a) have lost 67% of their ability to work, whether as a result of physical or mental defects, and the status is not expected to improve within one year (henceforth referred to as: disabled),

b) has fulfilled the required service time, and

c) does not work regularly and earns significantly less than he did before disability.

63. The award of disability retirement becomes valid on the day which is established in the opinion of the medical committee. If the medical committee does not specify a point in time, the time the disability begins is considered to be the date on which the claim was made.

50. The degree of disability retirement depends on the age at which the disability was claimed, the time served at the organization from which he is retiring, and the degree of disability. The degree of disability is appropriate

a) to the *III disability group* belongs

those who are disabled, but not completely incapable of working, may rehabilitate,
to the *II disability group* belongs those who are completely disabled, but are not cared for by others,
to the *I disability group* belongs those who are completely disabled and are cared for by others.

77. (1) an *industrial accident* is an accident which happens during the performing of an insured profession, or in connection with it, such as travelling to or from work.
(2) *Occupational disease* is such a disease which is incurred at a special risk by an insured profession. The laws regulating accidents applying to occupational diseases are established by the Government.

80. (1) *Disability compensation* is awarded to those who become disabled as a result of industrial accidents. Disabled is anyone who cannot perform his job due to an industrial accident and the physical condition accompanying by the appropriate medical treatment.
(2) Accident *compensation* – without time limit – lasts as long as the victim of the industrial accident is disabled.

83. (1) The degree of accident allowance awarded depends on the degree of disability incurred.

The degrees of disability are:
to 1. degree accidents belong those whose disability is .. 16–25%.
to 2. degree accidents belong those whose disability is .. 26–35%.
to 3. degree accidents belong those whose disability is .. 36–49%.
to 4. degree accidents belong those whose disability is .. 50–66%.

87. (1) Accidental disability retirement is awarded to those who suffer a disability of 67% mostly as a consequence of the accident and who do not regularly work, or earn significantly less than they did before disability.

Government Regulation establishes that the opinion of the N.I., I and II level committees can be challenged by the individual question and through legal procedures can request a new special medical examination. The special medical examination is performed by a forensic medical specialist and formulates the opinion of the patients status with respect to the previous examinations of I and II level committees. Formulation of the opinion with respect to the previous opinion of the committees implies such a specialized task in which can only be performed by a medical specialists practicing in a special institute.

Besides the supervision of the previous opinion, the courts can request an expert medical opinion in those cases where the insured person objects to the opinion of the insurance company's physician in connection with the disability, the permanent damage incurred, or the occasional establishment of allowances in connection with the injuries. Similarly the degree of disability of the injured person must be declared in such civil court process where not only the accidental injuries, but those due to carelessness require an opinion of the status of the injured person.

The court arranges for the formulation of an examination from the appropriate viewpoint. We will deal with these viewpoints as they apply to each group of claims. Sometimes the patient or the injured person requests the examination. The judgement of his status, the establishment of the degree of disability, if it was done by a previous special medical examination, the opinion of the I or II level committee can be arranged by the specialist. In these opinions the previous patient data is detailed, the complaints of the patient, a detailed internal medical examination is performed and those special examinations are ordered which apply to the patient's complaints. Complementary special laboratory examinations (for example, radiological, clinical laboratory, ECG) may be requested. The diagnosis is established on the basis of these along with the degree of disability.

Besides the above data concerning the *special medical examination,* it is necessary to collect all the medical documents of the patient which he brings with him to the examination, especially emphasized those medical findings and opinions which have been made in the time since the examination by the II level committee. such as hospital or institutional discharge papers.

We perform the examination so that the patient or injured person feels that the examiner is dealing with his problems. We must question the patient in detail about the previous circumstances, profession and previous professions, paying special attention to the previous job circumstances to which the opinion must refer, and deal with the possibility of rehabilitation. If we are forming an opinion concerning an accidental injury, we must also gather the data concerning the accident, the discharge papers of the primary care institution or outpatient papers. From the viewpoint of the medical specialist, the findings of the primary care physician who was the first to treat the patient are of decisive importance. This is usually a general practitioner. It is extremely important to record the circumstances in such detail that the mechanism of injury can be reconstructed. We have often experienced that the injured person, out of purely selfish interests (in order to obtain a 100% disability compensation, an insurance settlement etc.) will provide an entirely different story. The so-called *"first doctor findings"* and the data from the *traffic accident record* made on that day, however, in the vast majority of the cases spares him from the selfish tendencies. In every case we must strive to insure that the patient feels our care and concern. Those claiming disability come in part from a conflicting situation which is significantly influenced by attitude toward the examination. The complaints may by at times exaggerated, at other times a reserve may be exhibited at the examination. The specialist must try to estimate these factors carefully, perhaps exclude them, whether by careful interrogation of the patient or by physical examination. The objective complaints of the patient must be supported by the data and facts of the examination, since a the findings of a superficially performed examination may come back to haunt the examiner if the patient considers the examination to be unsatisfactory – especially if his claim is rejected – and a new examination and opinion will be requested by either the court or the chief inspecting physician of the Social Security Directorate.

Formulation of the opinion of disability by the medical specialist is sometimes made on the basis of recommendations found in the methodology literature. In the preliminary data section, the findings of the patient's previous examinations are described in detail, his complaints are emphasized, following the detailed examinations, and inasmuch as it is deemed necessary, special medical examinations are requested. (The appropriate medical specialist examination is especially requested for verification in that case when the percentage disability is changed from its previous percentage due to a change in its basic severity.) The examination and findings section of the medical specialist opinion must be completed in such thoroughness that the decision in the opinion section can be clearly indicated. A decision based on superficial or summary findings will not stand in the court of appeals.

In the opinion section the alterations are described, with diagnoses of the diseases, the amount of disability is assessed. Any improvement since the previous examination is noted or whether there has been a deterioration in the basic condition. An opinion must be given of when the next examination should take place (for individuals approaching retirement age – one or two years prior to retirement – the permanent condition must be described). For those reaching 50% disability, the rehabilitation possibilities must be described and in which areas of work they may participate.

Disability within certain disease groups deserve special attention. Complete or partial disability is described for a period of time and disability that exceeds one year must be that which in the opinion is a case of inability to earn a living. On the work place accidents or occupational illnesses do not necessarily have a time period. In such cases come to decision, then the ability to earn a living can be estimated as long as the injured status does not remain permanently, then the disability compensation may be cancelled and the percentage of damage due to the accident can be measured. Along with the estimation of disability, medical evaluation of accidental or occupational injury, it is also necessary to describe the patient's original status and to give the date of the following supervision.

In the estimation of the degree of disability, the status of the patient must be born in mind, since placing the patient in the *Class I group,* which means *total incapacity* although capable of taking care of himself with the help of others. In this category we put those who either due to their health status or their mental deficiency need care. This means help that without which the patient's life is endangered. To this circle belongs patient care, feeding, and adaptation of the environment. There are such cases in which the care is of a constant character, and others in which it can be interrupted for a short period, but must be considered as continuous care.

We put into *Class II* those who are *completely disabled* but can take care of themselves and therefore the abovementioned care is not needed.

We put into *Class III* those who are *67% disabled.* This means that they can take care of themselves and perform some other kind of work under so-called rehabilitation. They generally have a shortened work time and cannot bear physical stress. Developed countries provide social support for the occupationally disabled since successful rehabilitation is useful to society as well.

The literature dealing with *changes in disability* unambiguously points out that in numerous instances disability is the result of several diseases together. A certain percentage of these diseases or disease groups are also independently represented, however the percentage is not calculated together, but rather the collective work-limiting effect of the diseases must be considered in the evaluation of the percentage, since the diseases and the overall disability of the person must be born in mind.

Disability due to accidents is described as: "The accident inflicts on the human organism such external damage which, regardless of the will of the worker suddenly, or in a relatively short time, results in an injury, poisoning, or other deteriorations in health or even death."

After clarifying the circumstances of the accident, it must be declared how the accident caused the deterioration in health, whether the noticed deterioration in health could be in connection with the accident or with occupational illness, and what degree of deterioration could remain following the accident. If another natural illness is found which can also result in disability independent of the accident, it is important to describe what percent of the disability can be ascribed to the accident. We have already discussed the degree of disability and percentage. On the other hand, in the assessment of percentage in accidental disability, such practical guidance is provided for the specialists which can be used to explain and evaluate individual percentage values.

For accidental disability:

insignificant	1–15%
mild	16–25%
minor	26–35%
moderate	36–49%
significant	50–66%
major	67–99%

The specialist must also evaluate accidental injuries and occupational illnesses in cases resulting in death as well, whether there is a connection between the death and the accident or the occupation of the deceased. The examination by the forensic specialist clarified this. An opinion concerning the connection can be formulated on the basis of the previous data, the course of the illness and the autopsy findings.

The Public Health Law stresses the importance of *rehabilitation.* Rehabilitation is a process in which the disable person uses his/her knowledge necessary for optimal physical, psychological and social function. In Britain as a speciality concerned primarily with three groups (McLellan)

"1. those with multiple disability,
2. disabled people under going personal or social transitions, for example, school leavers,
3. those with disabilities requiring complex technical or medical solutions".

The patient who is a candidate for rehabilitation cannot perform his previous occupation without endangering his health, as noted in the Class III disabilities. Rehabilitation has special significance to those suffering accidental injury, where with the proper care or by transfer to another area of work, they can be completely rehabilitated. It is proper for the rehabilitation specialist not to describe in his opinion the area of work which the rehabilitated patient could perform, since he is not familiar with the details, environment and possibilities existing at the place of work. Thus purposely he describes which types of work the patient cannot perform. The appropriate regulation; the goal of employing the worker with altered work capability (occupational rehabilitation) in his condition following medical rehabilitation, is to ensure the training in the appropriate field of work. The area of work and the availability of work determine this while bearing in mind the previously mentioned facts and the practice of the worker. The committee formed for the purpose of rehabilitation considers the necessity and the committee makes recommendations and may help to create rehabilitation possibilities. It is most important point of view of the rehabilitation. To prevent the neurosis, the depression following the disability the specialist propose to start the rehabilitation process as early as possible.

Common conditions resulting in disability occurring in the practice of forensic medicine

Psychiatric diseases:

(besides the collection of the patient history, the special participation of the psychiatrist in diagnosis).

Arteriosclerotic dementia,
mild form 40–67%
serious dementia 100%
Alcoholic psychoses: alcoholic dementia, psychosis with memory disturbances, with internal medical alterations 67%
in serious cases 100%
Schizophrenic psychoses:
hebephrenic type 50–67%
cases of frequent active symptoms or serious personality changes 67–70%
catatonic type in good status 0–50%
with common recurrences, sequels 67–100%
Paranoid, symptomless or in good status 50%
in chronic form 67–100%
Oligophrenia, mild mental retardation 0–30%
serious mental retardation with personality disturbances, adaptation difficulties .67%
Anxiety states:
chronic fixation states 50–67%
Hysterical states, mild or transient cases 0–30%
serious fixation cases with personality disturbances 30–67%
Compulsive disorders:
compulsions, phobias mild cases 0–40%
psychotic state with serious personality regression 40–67%
Psychopathy: rarely decompensated, relatively well adjusted to society 0–50%
often decompensated, borderline mental illness with personality disturbances, serious regression 67–100%

Gynecological disorders:

Vaginal prolapse, with complete disturbances in urinary retention 67%
complete uterine prolapse 67%
with disturbed urinary retention 67–100%
Absence of both ovaries under age 20 50–67%
Removal of ovaries, tubes or uterus under 40 30–40%
Abdominal adhesions, without intestinal obstruction in connection with obstetrical operations 10–30%
adhesions with obstruction, subileal state 67–100%
Rectovaginal fistula 67–100%
post-operative fistula state, if the fistula could only be closed by routine operation 50–100%
Malignant tumors following modern treatment, without metastasis 67%

Internal diseases:

Heart disease: symptomless at rest, stress decompensation symptoms 67%

decompensation at rest 100%
Congestive cardiomyopathy 67–100%
Stenocardial complaints, with mild ECG signs 30–40%
Stenocardia with prominent ECG signs, extrasystoles with stress 67–100%
Postinfarct state, transient arrhythmia, mild circulatory insufficiency 40–50%
Angina with moderate stress, decompensation ischemia ECG signs 67%
Neurotic cardiac complaints (without cardiac alterations) 30–40%
Atrioventricular block 50–67%
Pacemaker 50–67%
Mitral disease, depending on compensation 50–67%
Aortic disease, depending on hemodynamic response 50–100%
Peptic ulcer pain, bleeding, stenosis 25–75%
Regular dialysis 67–100%

Surgical illnesses:

Gastric resection 50–67%
Post-operative gall stone state (depending on sequels) 30–40%
Splenectomy (due to injury) 15–25%
Prosthesis 75–100%
Obliterative vascular disease (necrosis gangrene) 50–100%
Stenosis of the subclavian artery 30–50%
Stenosis of the carotid artery 67–100%
Vertebral artery syndrome 30–50%
Postthrombotic syndrome 30–50%
Renal post-transplantation state (patient in renal balance) 50%
Renal stones: no disability
One kidney missing 30%
Mild chronic urinary bladder infection 10–20%
Varicocele 10–30%

Neurological illnesses:

Damage to cranial nerves 10–40%
Trigeminal neuralgia 30–50%
Meniere's disease 30–67%
Damage to vagal nerve, with disturbances in swallowing or vocalization 30–67%
Paralysis of brachial plexus 67%
partial paralysis 20–40%
Herniation of cervical disc, discopathy, with root complaints of the upper limb 50–67%
Spondylosis 20–50%
Epilepsy, with rare seizures (rehabilitation!) 40–50%
focal epilepsy 40–100%
petit mal epilepsy 40–50%
Herniated disc, post-operative state 0–30%
Herniated disc, post-operative state, with residual root symptoms 30–50%
Herniated disc, spinal fusion, with prominent root symptoms 50–67%
Herniated disc with prominent residual effects, reoperated state 67–100%

Permanent injuries resulting from accidents

Permanent damage resulting from accidents make up a distinct proportion of opinions on disability. This not only includes work place accidents, but various insurance companies may also request the opinion of medical specialists. We have already dealt with determination of the cause of accidents. The evaluation of permanent consequences of an accident, clarification of the circumstances surrounding the accident, whether the accident could have produced certain results, the evaluation of fractures of osteoporotic bones or the so-called pathological fractures, the injurious effect of alterations caused by new force applied to a previously injured body part, etc. is the responsibility of the medical specialist of the insurance companies, and in case of dispute, the opinion of a forensic medical specialist may be sought. The traumatology practice recommends the so-called neutral, zero-method and evaluation of the alteration from the neutral position. The individual examined is examined in the standing position with hanging arms with the thumbs facing forward, closed parallel legs facing forward. In principle the degree of motion should be noted from the zero position in the direction which the joint moves.

The motion of the joint in question should be compared to the opposite one and the difference expressed in degrees. If the examined body part cannot be compared to the other side, then the measurements must be compared to those of a person of comparable age and health status. The recommendation differentiates between extension and hyperextension. We speak of *hyperextension* when the motion of the joint exceeds that appropriate for its physiological function, for example, when the knee or the elbow joint can be extended beyond the straight position. Pain occurring with motion of the joint must be recorded as well as palpable alterations discovered over the joint (crackles and clicks). We use a goniometer for the measurement of joint motion in degrees form the zero position. The most commonly occurring joint measurements that appear in practice are listed below on the basis of the methodology recommendations.

Upper extremity

Shoulder joint, abduction and adduction. The arm can be *abducted* upward from the body from 0–180° in the frontal plane. The arm can be *adducted* past the midline of the body from 0–75°.

The arm can be *moved forward* in anteroflexion in the sagittal plane from 0–180⑤. Backward extension can be performed from 0–60°.

The motion of the arm in the *horizontal plane* is 0–135°, which means horizontal extension from a plane behind the back. The rotation of the shoulder is measured in two positions, with the arm in the hanging position next to the body and with the arm in 90⑤ adduction.

Elbow motion: The zero position is the outstretched straight arm and the wrist can be flexed between 0–150°. Extension of the wrist joint beyond 0° is called hyperextension. With forearm motion the freely hanging palm indicates the zero position from which in pronation can reach 80–90°, and in supination can reach 80–90° for a total range of motion of 160–180° .

Wrist motion: In examination, the zero position is with the palm facing inwards with the outstretched wrist lying in the same line as the forearm. Flexion is 0–80°, extension 0–70°, from the zero position in the ulnar direction 0–30° and 0–20° radially.

Hand motion: The zero position of the thumb is outstretched next to the index finger and with extension can reach 90⑤ in the radial direction and with flexion can reach the pad of the little finger. Sometimes the individual joints of the fingers must be measured. Along with the thumb, motion in the carpometacarpal joint, the metacarpo-phalangeal and the interphalangeal joints may be measured. Motion occurs in the distal interphalangeal joint (DIP), the proximal interphalangeal joint

(PIP), and the metacarpo-phalangeal joint (MP).

Along with the *motion of the fingers,* it is important to assess the ability to make a fist. The fingers must be able to reach the palm and if they cannot, the distance in centimeters from the palm they can be flexed must be recorded. Besides the ability to make a fist, the squeezing power of the hand, or decrease in power, must be evaluated along with that of individual fingers against the thumb. Along with loss of individual finger function, damage to the so-called complete function must be evaluated, which is not the additive measure of the individual functions.

Lower extremity

The ball and socket *joint of the hip* makes possible the appropriate flexion, extension, abduction, adduction and rotation.

The *neutral position* is in the supine position with outstretched legs and with bent knees, a flexion of the hip can reach 0–120°.

Extension is measured with the patient prone and with straight knees, the hip can be extended 0–30°.

With *rotation* both the knee and the hip are bent 90°. The lower extremity can be roteted internally 60° from the midline. External rotation with bent knee and hip can reach 45°. We perform *abduction* and *adduction* of the hip from the neutral position. With adduction the leg moves away from the midline and we measure the degree achieved; with abduction we move the leg across the midline with the other elevated so that the leg on the side examined passes under the other.

Examination of the *knee joint:* Flexion is the natural motion of the knee. The knee can be flexed 0–135°. Thin patients with loose joints can achieve 0–150°. With each joint, the motion is compared with that of the non-injured side and the difference in values is important. If the knee can extend beyond 0⑤, we speak of hyperextension. Along with the function of the knee we also examine the status of the lateral ligaments, the deviation of the medial and lateral femorotibial gap (varus-valgus), the quadriceps femoris and the crucial ligaments (desk drawer sign) and the stability of the patella (hydrops, crepitation).

With examination of the *ankle* we see the dorsiflexion and plantarflexion of the talocrural joint. Dorsiflexion is about 20°, and plantarflexion from the rest position with a bent knee is 50°. During the examination we should examine the motion of the tarso-metatarsal joint which is performed by grasping the heel and rotating the foot laterally.

With examination of the lower extremity, functional evaluation must be performed. In this the patient must squat, stand on tip-toes, and on the heels. Alterations in the hip, knee or ankle joints cause pain upon squatting, while pain upon standing on tip-toes or heels is the result of functional disturbance or injury to the tarsal joints.

Spinal column

In examining the *cervical vertebrae,* we observe flexion, extension and lateral flexion. Rotation occurs with turning of the head. The neutral position is with the head in the resting position, either standing or sitting. The comparison is measured in degrees, but we measure the flexion and extension by the distances remaining between the chin and the chest. With lateral flexion, we measure the distance from the ear to the shoulder.

With examination of the *thoracic and lumbar* vertebrae, the starting point is the straight standing position. With straight legs the patient bends forward and the distance is measured between the ground and the outstretched fingers. For the lumbar and thoracic spinal examination a tape measure is also used, since in a healthy patient under normal circumstances, when he bends over the increase in distance that occurs due to the spaces between the vertebrae opening up is about 10 cm. The decrease in distance that occurs with a straight back bending over is the result of the degeneration of the intervertebral ligaments as in spondylosis or spondylithis.

With lateral flexion motion we measure the ability of the patient to bend to the side. Under normal circumstances the normal person can reach the knee with the outstretched hand which means about 35° from the starting position on each side.

We examine *backward bending* either from the standing or the prone position. From the standing position, 30° can be achieved and from the prone, 20°.

In the spinal column examination we must describe the *presence or deformation of the physiological curves,* blow sensitivity, sensitivity at the points of exit of the nerves, and the defanse of the lumbar musculature.

Not only morphological but functional damage may be a permanent result of an accident, so damage to health can be expressed as a percent.

Categorization of injuries to the upper extremity

Amputation or functional loss of the upper extremity 70%
Dislocation of the shoulder, depending on the functional damage 15–20%
Irreparable dislocation 35–40%
Fracture of the surgical neck of the humerus with incomplete healing resulting in a mild loss of function of the shoulder joint 25–35%
significant loss of function of the shoulder in which loss of complete rotation is lost 35–50%
Closed fracture of the humerus depending on residual complaints 0–10%
fractures causing functional disturbance 15–35%
Fracture to the elbow causing functional disturbance depending on the amount 10–45%
Fracture to the forearm without functional disturbance or significant dislocation 0–10%
fracture healed by pseudarthrosis 20–45%
fracture causing stiffness to the wrist 25–35%
scaphoid bone fracture without loss of function 0–10%
scaphoid bone fracture with loss of function 15–35%

Upper extremity amputation damages percentages

	right	left
	in%	
Loss of both forearms, upper arms or hands	100	100
Upper arm	80	80
Lower arm	70	70
Hand	70	70
Thumb and metacarpal	35	35
I finger	30	25
II finger	20	20
III finger	10	10
IV finger or V finger	10	10
I finger end of digit	15	13
Nail section	5	3

Nerve damage to the upper extremity:

Paralysis to the axillary nerve	20–35%
Damage to the radial nerve	10–30%
Sensory damage with out motor damage	0–10%
Damage to the median nerve without sensory damage or loss of motor function	0–20%
with loss of motor function	20–45%
Partial sensory disturbance in the ulnar nerve	0–10%
Hand muscle atrophy, loss of grip power	15–25%
complete paralysis with trophic disturbance	30–40%

Damage to the lower extremity:

Among these fractures are those which destroy the stability of the *pelvis,* occasionally damage the pelvic organs as well. These may injure the urinary bladder or open the urethra. Most of the fractures are to the pubic bone or the ischium. Permanent damage is assessed at 30–40%.

With *acetabular fracture* damage to the surface of the joint can be expected. Residual reduced movement, pain can occur, as a consequence of in most cases, accompanying arthrosis. Damage is assessed at 25–50%.

Femoral fractures, for the most part and especially in the young, heal without lasting complications, but when mild arthrosis accompanies it, 10–20% damage to health can be assessed. In the serious cases, necrosis of the head can accompany. These are treated by implanting endoprostheses. With the implantation of an endoprosthesis, depending on the amount of weight that can be borne, 25–35% damage can be assessed. With a well-carrying but limited range of motion prosthesis, the damage may be 40–55%, while with a movable and uncapable prosthesis, it may mean complete disability (70%).

Femoral fracture healing without functional disturbance is 0–10%. If axial deviation exceeds 15_0, it is 15–20%, and axial deviation with shortening, hip or knee functional disturbance 20–35%.

With *knee injuries,* decreased range of motion, arthrosis, and joint instability may result. Depending on the seriousness of the case, damage is assessed at 10–40%. With secondary arthrosis accompanying patellar fracture, it is 10–20%, with partial removal of the patella, it is 10%, with complete removal of the patella with preserved function, 15–20% can be assessed. Among the injuries to the lower bones of the knee joint, fractures to the areas of ligamentous insertion can cause significant functional damage, arthrosis, and difficulty in walking. Damage is between 10–40%. Significant damage to cartilage can occur as a result of meniscus injuries or previous meniscus degeneration. It is important following injuries to the meniscus to wait at least a year before establishing the final assessment. A damage of 0–15% may be awarded. With multiple repeated cartilage injuries in which a serious arthrosis occurs, the damage is 20–35%.

With complete or incomplete *fractures to the leg,* some can be treated with a plaster cast while others require internal or A0 fixation. The resulting complications and the characteristics of the fracture determine the degree of damage. Thus leg fractures that heal with a 1–2 cm shortening without functional disturbance means 0–10% damage. A shortening of greater than 2 cm is 10–20%. If the fracture requires correction or is accompanied by disturbances in movement of the ankle or knee, or if arthrosis appears, the damage is 25–35%.

Ligamentous injury, especially separation of the tibiofibular syndesmosis, instability can occur without surgical correction. Thus even without fracture, arthrosis, ankle dysfunction and disturbed movement may remain. Stiffness in the upper tarsal joint is 25–30%. Stiffness to both the upper and lower tarsal joint with pes equinuus is 40–50%. Stiffness in the lower tarsal joint is 15–20%. Rupture to either the internal or external lateral ligaments of the ankle with resulting instability is 10–15%. Pain, arthrosis and ankle instability following rupture of the syndesmosis means 15–25% damage.

Lower extremity amputation percentages

One sided thigh amputation	80%
One sided lower leg amputation	70%
One sided foot amputation	40%
Amputation of the thigh at the middle and lower third	70%
Lower leg amputation with functionally damaged knee	70%
Amputation of both thighs	100%

Damage due to spinal column injury

Damage can affect the vertebrae, the intervertebral joints and the intervertebral disc.

We have already mentioned the points of the vertebral examination. From a medical expert's point of view, *vertebral degeneration (spondylosis)* is most commonly encountered and only seldom does a ruptured disc have to be evaluated. In the examination of spondylosis alterations the physiological range of motion of the vertebrae is described, the degree of decreased range of motion and in every case the alterations in the affected segment are verified by an X-ray picture. If the status following *vertebral fracture* is to be assessed, we must pay attention to the possible kyphosis formation above the fractured vertebra, damage to the nerve exiting at that vertebral level, the sensory decrease of the territories supplied by that nerve root, and paralysis. The specialists work is complicated by those cases where he must make an opinion regarding an accident type herniated intervertebral disc. A primary disc hernia occurs when the degenerative processes are advanced enough that a hernia can occur without the application of external force or when lifting or a wrong movement makes the patient's status worse. We can accept the accidental disc herniation when an application of force can be verified at the time the patient's condition got worse, and to such a degree that he became suddenly unable to work, or the so-called "bridge signs" connect a surgical intervention with the worsening of the patient's condition, which means that the disability following the accident or the operation suddenly started to deteriorate gradually and the process could be observed from the trauma.

Following vertebral fractures, especially if the vertebral body is fractured, a damage of 0–25% is assessed depending upon the permanent complaints. Development of a kyphosis, radicular signs, arthrosis or disturbances of movement may appear following the fracture which may amount to 25–50%. Transverse lesions of the spinal cord, if partial, may mean 50–70% disability, while urinary or fecal incontinence accompanying spinal cord injuries means 100% disability.

The role of the forensic medical specialist in compensation process

In the National Institute of Forensic Medicine's Methodology letter, "The Responsibility of the Forensic Medical Specialist in Tort Law" details the tasks of the forensic medical specialist in civil and occupational injury assessment and provides such perspectives in the judgement of medical insurance and civil law questions concerning the evaluation and judgement of non-financial damages and certain claims following injury.

The Civil Codes provide the principles for *civil compensation,* according to which, "Whoever causes illegal injury to another is required to pay compensation.".

Section 345 (1–2): "Whoever pursues an activity with increased danger is required to pay compensation for any damages incurred by it. He is freed from liability if it can be proved that the damage resulted from such an unavoidable cause that lay outside the activity pursued with increased danger. These regulations also apply to whoever causes injury to another while pursuing an activity with increased danger within human surroundings. Compensation need not be awarded is such instances where the injuries result from the misbehavior of the injured person."

The Civil Codes and civil law does not recognize the so-called *non-financial damage* and it is not acknowledged. The establishment of compensation is done in accordance with the establishment of culpability under civil law only in those cases where financial damages accompany personal injury.

In the 1974 IV. revision of the Civil Codes, Section 354. it is stated: "The injuring person is liable for non-financial injuries to the injured person if the injuring person causes a permanent or serious hindrance to the participation in social life, or the maintenance of life, or if that person negatively influences participation in earning a living."

This new change has been brought into tort law and carries with it the implication that judgement is the responsibility of the medical specialist. In the formulation of compensation, the law unambiguously emphasizes the necessity that participation by the injured party in everyday life, due either to injury or damage, must be permanently or seriously hindered.

The *concept of compensation* in civil law deals with the payment of such expenses which under certain circumstances only the opinion of a physician or medical specialist can judge. The injuries may be such that render certain work impossible either temporarily or permanently. In such instances a position must be taken on what percent of lost income is due to the decrease in health caused by the injury.

Judgement of non-financial damages

The law considers anything that hinders participation in social life or carrying on a normal life to be non-financial damages. Injuries must be such that cause the abovementioned consequences and effects.

Hindrance to social life touches on a wide area which means not only the things that happen in everyday life, but the creation and maintenance of human relationships as well. The question requires a special medical answer. The medical expert must express in detail what the injury affects in each case, how the injury hinders fitting in with and participation in social life, maintaining life, and what affects social function. Alterations causing a decrease in health lasting for a few months to a year temporarily hinder the maintenance of life of the injured person and does not correspond to the way the law is expressed, that the consequences of injuries should be a permanent process and state. The medical specialist should bear in mind the location of the injury, character, must clearly assess the non-financial damage in the opinion and must refrain from expressing the non-financial damages in the statement of total compensation as well. Included are the permanence and seriousness of the injury, when it occurred, its significance, and if the permanent injured state has not yet fully developed, when it is expected. It is the medical examiner's' responsibility to answer these questions.

- A specialist evaluated the non-financial damages of a 21-year-old girl incurred in a traffic accident, who as a result suffered serious damage to the hypothalamus and the damaged internal organs suffered diffuse injury, physical deterioration, bleeding disturbances and the cessation of menstruation. The status had not improved a year after the accident, as indicated by the hormonal investigations. The damage was considered as non-financial since the injury affected her participation in social life, especially permanently and seriously impairing her life.

A part of non-financial damage claims are the consequences of amputation accidents in which the injured person in many cases through further claims seeks compensation beyond the assessed percentage of damage to health, and these claims are in part non-financial damages which must be established. With amputation accidents, even bearing in mind the initial assessment, individual judgements is called for.

- On another occasion we judged the case of accidental injury to an internationally famous scientist at the threshold of a significant career in his specialty, who was paralyzed in both legs and as a result was compelled to almost completely give up his scientific work, as he could no longer manage the experiments.

The judgement of cosmetic injuries requires the same care of the forensic medical specialist. With women in some professions – public figures, actresses etc. – even small disfiguring scars can bring such psychological consequences which permanently and seriously hinder earning a living, while the same injury in a man would not cause an alteration that would be considered grounds for claiming damages.

- A 70-year-old man who suffered an injury to the mouth came for forensic medical examination. The non financial damage claim was that he couldn't feel anything in the mouth when kissing. The forensic medical specialist rejected the claim. On the other hand the claim was accepted of a girl who in a traffic accident had suffered non-financial damages for the many small superficial, but roughly healed scars from injuries to the face.

To the sphere of participation in social life belong such amusement activities as sports or other pastimes according to one's tastes which played a significant role in the life before injury. In these cases the forensic medical specialist must also judge non-financial claims that as a result of injury the former options have been made impossible, to what extent they have hindered the activities of the injured person and bearing these in mind declare the legitimacy of the claim.

In the concept of non-financial damage within the scope of the forensic medical specialist's work is dealt with not only in the insurance company guidelines, but by the . Methodology Letter of the National Institute of Forensic Medicine. The Methodology Letter not only provides general guidelines for the establishment of non-financial damages, but lists the kinds of injuries according to groups of post-injury states which, from the standpoint of forensic medicine, appear most often for judgement and on which damages can be based. The Methodology letter gives the following groups:

a) Lost expense, lost income or utility,
b) Expenses and disbursements,
c) Non-financial damages.

The forensic medical specialist's work in the liability court process is the judgement of questions involving damage claims which are the result of injuries. Thus the injured party may claim incurred damages due to injury, lost income or use expenses.

Loss of income, sick pay and total reimbursement of actual income appear among the damage claims, and the establishment of a connection is the task of the forensic medical specialist. He must examine how to establish the

1. time span of the sick pay allowance connected with the injury,
2. whether any previous illness was involved,
3. how much of a role the basic illness plays in the, seriousness of the injury and
4. to what percent could the injury have caused the seriousness of the status or the prolongation of healing.

If the forensic medical specialist finds such damage which affects the work capacity of the injured person, it must be evaluated and the disability expressed as a percentage. We have already mentioned that the expression of disability in percentages with each illness or injury group does not automatically mean the complete disability, but the effect of the injury on the entire organism and the overall effect on the injured person's ability to work must be kept in mind. If the injury affects such a person with whom the performance of his work requires a special accommodation, and he loss the work capacity in his special field, the medical examiner has to sign the possibilities of rehabilitation, and with this accommodation is still able to do his job, the possibility of rehabilitation must be mentioned, or if he can perform the same work, it must be declared whether under certain circumstances he could perform his previous task at the level of the average worker. The opinion of the forensic medical specialist must declare how long the status is expected to last, and if improvement occurs the measurement of the improvement must be reflected in the percentage of assessed disability. The medical specialists of social security and private insurance companies generally assess (not being bound to an established profession) disability or permanent damage. The loss of the third finger of the left hand of a professional violinist and an unskilled worker is the same 10% damage in each case, although the former can no longer play and the latter hardly notices the loss. In cases of liability insurance claims the forensic medical specialist assesses the actual losses incurred by the injured party.

With the judgement of a damage claim, in every case the connection between the claim, the injury and the lasting complaints must be examined. These must be extended so that the residual complaints in their entirety or in part can be traced back to the injury, occasionally whether other pathological factors could have caused the complaints, or whether they could have developed by themselves without external influence. Inasmuch as the greater part of the claims come to the forensic medical specialist for judgement months, and even 1–2 years later, obtaining the appropriate documents and information, and a thoughtful consideration of the connection between the basic injury and the sequelae are imperative.

In connection with the injured person with his injuries various claims may come up. Among these the judgement of damage affecting the wearing of clothing is not the task of the forensic medical specialist. But the task of the forensic medical specialist in connection with injury involves the judgement of such claims which appear in the form of incidental expenses. One of the most common claims is the establishment of an improved diet. Generally, an improved diet is accepted in the case of serious injuries which are accompanied by physical deterioration – the consequence of chronic osteomyelitis, injuries involving a great loss of blood, old age, or damage resulting in a lengthy bed rest. With improvement of diet we must remember that with prolonged bed rest, the lack of movement not only causes digestive and absorptive problems, but the organism requires an increased protein supply for recovery which must be supplemented and appears in the form of additional charges. The forensic medical specialist has the right to establish not only the period of home care improvement of the diet, but under the appropriate circumstances in certain instances to also declare the length of time of hospital care with a dietary improvement of such a character which hospital support can provide. (It is common that fractures of the jaw necessitate special meal requirements because of the splinting, and with a case lasting several weeks, claims for the feeding of the injured person may amount to a considerable sum.)

We have already discussed disability following injury, but we must mention separately those claims in connection with the injured person which appear during the convalescent period and bring the possibility of home care and later help in house and yard work.

Following hospital care, a large percentage of injured people require home care, some being bed-ridden, others due to care in connection with splinting of extremities, movement difficulties, etc. In the judgement of these it is the responsibility of the physician to take into account the seriousness of the injury and method of care when determining how long and for how many hours a day it should be allowed. The performance of housework especially affects women who are injured who formerly cared for their families and their absence naturally brings a greater need of help for the family. Bearing the above-mentioned point of view in mind, the forensic medical specialist must judge with appropriate care and measure the necessity and span of time.

The expense of medications and equipment in connection with recuperation may be claimed by the injured person, and such peculiar claims in which the added expense of visitors, increased wear and tear of bed linen, as well as increased heating and light expenses, and equipping the vehicle for use by a disabled person may appear. The judgement and evaluation of these claims requires an experienced forensic medical specialist, as we have already discussed previously.

The satisfaction of the claims of accident victims requires, beyond the normal work of the forensic medical specialist, such training and humane attitude which inspires trust in the injured person and after the appropriate judgement understands the capabilities of the specialist and his opinion in connection with his claim. For this, along with the appropriate handling of the injured person, the relation of the sequelae, the detailed familiarity with the claims, and discussion are necessary. By this we can avoid causing such psychological damage from a superficially performed examination and observation of symptoms which may later result in a practically untreatable neurosis.

References

[1] Az igazságügyi orvosszakértők feladatai kártérítési perekben. Országos Igazságügyi Orvostani Intézet 8. sz. Módszertani levele Bp. (1979)

[2] Aronoff, G. M.: Chronic pain and the disability epidemic. Clin. J. Pain 7 (1991) 330–338

[3] Kalabay, L.: Egymillió személysérüléses baleset orvosszakértői értékelése az ÁB statisztikájában. Biztosítási Szemle 22 (1976) 289–293

[4] Kalabay, L., I. Szabó: Die Entwicklung der Lebensversicherungsmedizin 33 (1981) 25–27

[5] Kalabay, L.: Balesetbiztosítási orvosszakértői útmutató. Állami Biztosító kiadványa (1969) és (1982)

[6] Kalabay, L.: Sportsérülések, sportártalmak orvosszakértői elbírálása. Állami Biztosító (1985)

[7] Kalabay, L.: Analyse der dauernden unfallbedingten Körperschaden anhand der Statistik der Staatlichen Versicherungsanstalt. Versicherungsmedizin 41 (1989) 200–203

[8] Kalabay, L., S. Bíró: The Practice of Insurance Medicine in Hungary and other East European countries. Journal of Insurance Medicine 22, (1990) 18–21

[9] Kalabay, L.: Analysis of 331,949 school accident claims in Hungary. Journal of Insurance Medicine 22 (1990) 46–49

[10] Kurucz, B.: A társadalombiztosításról szóló 1975. évi II. törvény és végrehajtási rendelkezéseinek egységes szerkezetbe foglalt hatályos szövege. Népszava, Bp. (1988)

[11] McLellan, D. L.: Neurology or rehabilitation medicine? J. Neurol. Neurosurg. Psychiatry 55 (1992) 47–50

[12] Loeser, J. D.: What is chronic pain? Theor. Med. 12 (1991) 213–225

[13] Millard, R. W., N. Wells, R. W. Thebarge: A comparison of models describing reports of disability associated with chronic pain. Clin. J. Pain 7 (1991) 383–391

[14] Paál, Gy.: Munkaképesség orvosszakértői vizsgálata, értékelése, véleményezése. Medicina, Bp. (1989)

[15] Paál, Gy., Zsiray, M.: Szakmai irányelvek a keresőképesség orvosi elbírálásához. Medicina, Bp. (1989)

[16] Ross, P. D., B. Ettinger, J. W. Davis, L. J. Melton, R. D. Washnich: Evaluation of adverse health outcomes associated with vertebral fractures. Osteoporos. Int. 1 (1991) 134–140

[17] Somogyi, E.: A biztosítási orvostan helye az orvosi felsőoktatásban. Biztosítási Szemle 11 (1979) 379–380

[18] Tait, R. C., J. T. Chibnal, P. N. Ducro, T. L. Deshields: Stable factors in chronic pain. Clin. J. Pain 5 (1989) 323–328

[19] Tate, D. G.: Workers disability and return to work. Am. J. Phys. Med. Rahabil. 71 (1992) 92–96

[20] Walsh, K., M. Cruddas, D. Coggon: Interaction of height and mechanical leading of the spine in development of low-back pain. Scand. J. Work Environ. Health. 17 (1991) 420–424

Chapter 11
Toxicology

The significance of toxicological examinations of poisonous substances is illustrated by their rapid numerical and environmental growth, among which we count, besides the medications, herbicides and food additives used in everyday life, other injurious materials, for example industrial pollution. The recognition, demonstration and quantification of these, among other things, constitute a part of the responsibility of toxicology.

The *three great areas of toxicology* are the *clinical, environmental* and *forensic toxicology,* within which legal toxicology, analytical chemistry and clinical toxicology have their own composition. The demonstration of poisonous materials and determination of their quantity, make up the *forensic toxicologist's* primary duties, and its notes those difficulties which is likely to be encountered with the determination of each unknown poisonous material (in the absence of clinical signs, insufficient preliminary data, biotransformation of the material which is decays rapidly, etc.).

Those responsibilities and requirements which toxicology demands of the specialist are made up of separately related disciplines. In the foregoing brief survey we have also listed those difficulties which can be expected from the demonstration of each unknown substance. The task of the toxicologist cannot be better stated that this, by A. J. LEHMAN: "...anyone can become a toxicologist in two easy lessons, each of which takes ten years."

Neither can we offer a clear-cut picture of the work of a toxicologist – toxicological procedures, the manifold toxic effects, the methods of determination –, but we must include those types of poisonings and demonstrative procedures which the forensic specialist should be expected to be familiar with.

The *toxic material* seriously injures or damages the vital functions of the organism, which is to say, it leads to death. With respect to their chemical natures, they could be such which damage various target organs (kidney, liver, hemopoetic organs), or have general effects. According to their mode of use they may be drugs, herbicides, solvents or food additives; according to their effects, carcinogens or mutagenic substances; according to their physical state, poisonous gasses, liquids, explosive materials, etc.; according to their biochemical effects, SH group inhibitors, a formers or influence of enzyme activities. Naturally, since any method of categorization is artificial, each toxin can belong to several groups due to its multiple effects. Each material has a dose-dependent effect, which we express in toxicology by the LD_{50}.

The formation of the *toxic effect* depends on numerous factors. A significant role is played by the site of application, which may be enteral, parenteral, percutaneous or inhalative. The toxic effect is most expressed if the material is introduced intravenously, followed by intraperitoneally, subcutaneously, intramuscularly and orally. Sometimes the method of introduction itself determines the toxic effect, so that if metabolism in the liver is carried out completely, a substance introduced *per os* will be less toxic due to the portal circulation than if it were introduced by inhalation. The industrial toxins are in numerous instances of an inhalatory character while in suicide cases the poisonous substance is most commonly introduced via the digestive tract. The absorption relationships decisively influence the introduction into the organism and the toxic effect, so that a dose of nicotine of 0.5 cg taken *per os* is deadly while many times that amount would be required for the same effect if absorbed across the skin.

Some toxicologists divide the *time of effect* into an acute, subacute, subchronic and chronic intoxications (toxins exerting their effects over 24 hours, one month, three months and longer than three months). Although this classification with respect to the clinical signs is debatable, and significantly stereotypes the toxin, even so the classification is accepted and generalized among toxicologists, especially regarding the types of poisons with acute and chronic effects (acute poisoning with benzol damages the central nervous system while chronic poisoning causes damage to the bone marrow). At other times a frequent intake of a poison in small doses decreases the effect. The adaptation of the detoxification system of the organism plays the role (for example, after ingestion of barbiturates or alcohol), of speeding the biotransformation or excretion of the ingested substance. The latter happens when the accumulation of a toxin ingested in small amounts begins to slow and the steady state is reached in which the toxin taken in equals the amount excreted.

The appearance of *side effects* must be expected from certain substances. Certain medications or chemicals can harm the organism if unexpected effects develop. These cases also demand attention. On other occasions unexpected reactions can lead to such side effects which could not have been predicted. Allergic reactions may result from the introduction of medications, chemical substances or other foreign materials. The hapten theory is generally accepted to explain the immunogenicity of small molecular weight chemicals. The reaction occurs due to the prior sensitization which may have gone unnoticed by the person who was poisoned, and the allergic reaction resulting from exposure to the hypersensitive person of a small amount of the substance can result in serious damage to his health. Numerous chemical substances are capable of, either in themselves or by formation of metabolic haptens, initiating the formation of antibodies (the effect occurring within 1–2 weeks), and through the antigen-antibody reaction caused by a new provocation, a typical allergic process follows in which there may be clinical manifestations. The recognition of these processes is one of the most difficult tasks in the practice of the forensic medical toxicologist.

Besides these we must take into consideration the *interactions of the toxic substances* as well. It is a well known fact that some toxins intensify, neutralize or inactivate the effects of each other. With the *additive effect,* two separate substances, but with similar effects enter the organism and perform their effects together. Thus, if multiple cholinesterase inhibitors enter the organism, the enzyme inhibition is additive depending upon the amount and effect of the substances. With some substances the effect is *synergistic* and not a matter of simple addition of the amounts of the toxin. In this case the effect multiplies and the damage essentially tends toward the effect the two have in common. (The combined effect of alcohol and sedatives.) A *potentiation effect* occurs in the organism with such substances which separately would not carry a toxic effect, or when the shallow effect of the one which alone would not damage the health of the organism increases the effect of the other resulting in intoxication. With *antagonistic effects* – most commonly in the cases of various antidotes – the toxic material ingested is neutralized, such as in functional antagonism (cholinesterase inhibition and the effect of atropine) or with the help of *chemical antagonism* (administration of BAL in metal intoxication), or in *competitive antagonism* when we use a common point of action (administration of ethanol in methanol intoxication).

Tolerance plays a significant role in the manifestation of poisoning, which is a known characteristic in the case of some toxic agents. The effects of some chemicals decrease or may be missed with repeated exposures. An example of the first is the increased tolerance of the chronic user of morphine or the alcohol addicts, and the disputed fact which has been observed in those who chronically ingest arsenic whose capacity for absorption has changed being manifested as tolerance, an example of the second.

Tolerance, a hypersensitivity toward some materials respectively augments the catabolic processes leading the metabolism of the toxic substances.

Metabolism of toxic substances

The metabolism of toxic materials takes place primarily in the liver. Here the process is carried out of selecting out the materials which can be passed through the kidneys by virtue of their water solubility, polar materials and passed through the bile being non polar lipid soluble compounds. From a toxicological point of view, the selection and change in structure of the foreign material may also decisively determine the direction of the toxicological examination. These materials are not usually biological in nature, but rather drugs, different organic or inorganic chemicals, and even in recent times the so-called *xenobiochemical examinations* have been given more attention than the metabolism of drugs, since in practice the effects of these, the effects and determination of the metabolites, elimination of the substances, etc. cause the most problems. Since most xenobiotic materials are more or less toxic, they tend to change the parent compound into chemical less toxic to the organism during the process of metabolism, but at other times the attempt is unsuccessful, and the less toxic original chemical over the process of detoxification process the metabolites may be more toxic or active. A lot of the foreign substances introduced into the organism can be sought by toxicological examinations, among which are the drugs, industrial chemicals, food preservatives, pesticides, but here also belong the toxins of bacterial metabolism.

It is a fact that harmful substances in the organism undergo a detoxification process, an observation which was made during the last century from the examination of phenol excretion. Phenyl sulfate appearing during metabolism became less toxic than the original material. This observation launched the research of metabolites *(Fig. 166).*

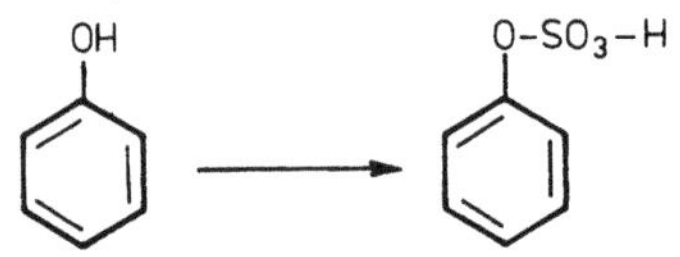

phanol phanolsulphat

Fig. 166. The metabolization of phenol

The original material usually becomes more water soluble during the process of metabolism, and can be carried via the blood stream to the kidneys and eliminated. A small portion of the metabolites are eliminated with the stool, or cast off in the expired air. Material that gets into the liver can be detoxified through numerous pathways by being conjugated, hydrolyzed, reduced or oxidized. But with materials undergoing hydrolysis, oxidation or reduction, they may be eliminated after the first phase, or be conjugated in the second phase.

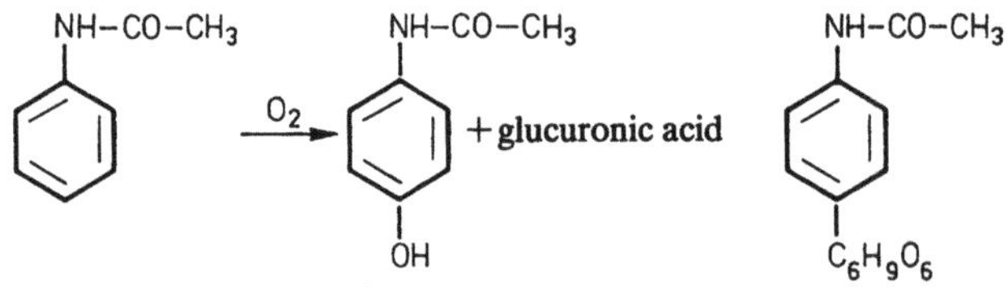

phase I. acetanilide — phase II. p-acetaminophenol — acetanilid p-glucuronate

Fig. 168. Drug metabolization

Phase I. reactions:

The common form of oxidative metabolism is in the elimination of drugs, oxidation taking place in the first step, and in the second step some group being conjugated to the chemical.

A significant role in the metabolization of drugs is played by cytochrome P_{-450} (CP_{-450}) *(Fig. 167).*

$$\text{NADPH} \xrightarrow{-e} \begin{matrix}\text{cytochrome } P_{450} \\ O_2\end{matrix} \qquad \begin{matrix}\text{drug} \\ \text{oxidized drug}\end{matrix}$$

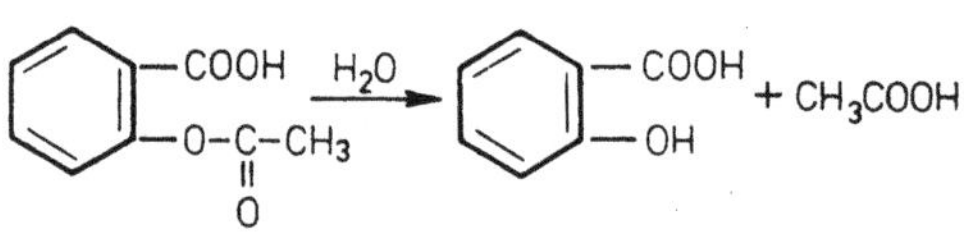

acetylsalicylic acid salicylic acid acetic acid

Fig. 167. The metabolization of acetic acid

Cytochrome P–450 plays an important role in the microsomal oxidation of xenobiotics, and another part in demethylation processes, as in the case of the hydroxylation of morphine, codeine and amphetamines and somewhat in the metabolism of steroids. In the processes the different forms of CP_{-450} may play roles, and takes a special role in the breaking down of certain materials.

The *reduction processes* are of lesser significance in selection than oxidative metabolism. Reduction may be nitroreduction (the reduction of an aromatic nitrogen group), azoreduction (the classic example being the reduction of prontosyl, in which a more effective substance is created, sulfonamide), and the reduction of halogenated groups.

The *hydrolysis* may be the first step in metabolisation of some foreign materials and oxidative process happens only following this. A typical example is that of the metabolism of salicylates, such as acetylsalicylic acid *(Fig. 168).* Hydrolysis also occurs in the decay of some epoxy chemicals, the process of which generates some truly reactive chemicals.

The phase II. reactions:

The conjugation may be a direct step in detoxification, with the goal of making a more polar molecule which because of its water solubility may be eliminated from the organism more rapidly. The conjugated metabolite is generally less toxic than the original substance, but it may become more toxic as well! Different molecules perform the conjugation, the most common being a binding with glucuronic acid, conjugation with glucose (glycosylation), or ribose (ribosylation). Different amino acids may be bound, such as glycine, glutathion, glutamine and certain derivatives may acetylate in connection with acetyl CoA. Among the many possibilities, the special selection and *conjugation with glucuronic acid* by the organism is much more common that happens with, for example, glucose. Conjugation is an energy-requiring process in which the original material or the conjugated agent may be the active chemical. With glucuronidation the conjugated molecule is active and this form of metabolism and metabolization of drugs is the most common.

Binding by glycine is one of the oldest known detoxification processes. It was described by Liebig in 1929. Glycine conjugation happens with many aromatic carboxylic acids such as benzoic acid and phenylacetic acid.

Conjugation with glutathion can be observed in several aromatic, halogenated, or nitrogen group containing substances. The starting reaction is often spontaneous, and later with the help of glutathion transferases the ingested material is bound to an electrophilic center, for example, for glutathion conjugation a large dose of phenylacetate is required, and results in a significant depletion of glutathion in the liver.

Methylation, conjugation by S-adenosyl methionine, is one of the important steps in detoxification. Methylated products are usually less toxic than the original substances.

Acetylation affects numerous amino group containing materials, and acetyl transferase plays a role using acetyl CoA. This has primary significance in the detoxification of drugs. (The simplest example is the formation of acetyloleate from the sulfonamide groups.)

$$\text{UTP} + \text{glucose 1 Ⓟ} \rightarrow \text{UDP} - \text{glucose} + \text{Ⓟ} - \text{Ⓟ}$$

$$\text{UDP} - \text{glucose} + \text{NAD}^{-} \xrightarrow[\text{dehydrogenase}]{\text{UDP} - \text{glucose}} \text{UDP} - \text{glucuronic acid} + \text{NADH}$$

$$+\text{ATP}$$

$$\text{UDP} - \text{glucuronic acid} + \text{X} - \text{OH} \xrightarrow[\text{transferase}]{\text{glucuronyl}} \text{XO-glucuronate} + \text{UDP}$$

We must also mention the *induction of drug metabolism.* Clinical observations verify that in some cases and with certain drugs the patient's tolerance changes, grows. Numerous drugs are capable of activating those oxidative processes which take part in the metabolization of drugs, and the increased enzyme activity can lead to a quicker break down of the drugs. Thus after treatment with phenobarbiturates for a few days a significant concentration of cytochrome P_{450} can be measured, and if the treatment continues, the level of cytochrome P_{450} increases. Numerous other similar inducing materials are known, such as insecticides as well. Among these are those which may accumulate in the fatty tissues and by their slow release an increase in the level of CP_{450} appears, simultaneously with the increased elimination of the substance *(Table 5).*

Table 5. The relative inductive effect of certain substances according to Wills

Anesthetics	N_2O_2	+
	ether	+
	halothan	−
Sedatives	barbiturates	+ + +
	thalidomide	−
	ethanol	+ −
Anticonvulsants	parametadion	+ +
	trimetadion	−
Tranquilizers	chlorpromazine	+ +
	promazine	−
Pain relievers	phenylbutazon	+ +
	amonopyren	+ +
Psychomotor stimulants	imipramin	+ + + +
Inselectides	DDT	+ + +
	dieldrin	+ + +
	aldrin	+ + +
Carcinogenic hydrocarbons	benzpyrine	+ + +
	methylchloranth-rene	+ + +

Metal poisoning

Poisoning by metals with a toxic effect including especially some compounds of copper, mercury, lead and arsenic must be discussed. Their common property is the ability to *form complexes,* the physical basis of which is that the inner electron shell is not full and they can form stable complexes with electron donors. In the *formation of a chelate,* the donor molecule binds at two places and forms a much more stabile compound than in the original complex. The NH_2 group of amino acids are typical chelate forming molecules, as are the SH-groups (cysteine) and the two O atoms of the salicylates. Certain metals show a particular affinity for binding, such as Hg^+ to CO and S-containing compounds, and the alkali metals for O ligands. If the metal holds a high affinity toward the ligand, the metal-protein complex formed causes such changes in the protein molecule – a chelate appears – that the change in the protein arrangement causes a change in biological effect – activity –, and indeed denaturation of the protein may even occur.

Copper and its compounds

In the organism cytochrome oxidase contains Cu^{++}, and moreover lysyl oxidase is also a copper-containing enzyme. Thus copper essentially belongs to the trace elements. A daily intake of about 2 mg is required matching the daily loss, but 0.6 mg is reabsorbed from the intestinal tract and finally 0.1 mg is eliminated in the bile. In the liver it is stored in the content of ceruloplasmin. A larger amount of copper intake can result in toxicity because of the above-mentioned capacity of copper to form chelates.

Among the copper compounds $CuCl_2$, CuO and $CuSO_4$ may have toxicity. A compound being given locally or absorbed through the gastrointestinal tract must be taken into consideration. A local reaction may appear on the skin, the alteration being papulovesicular or eczematous at the place of contact which may advance to necrosis. If coming into contact with the eye, it may cause conjunctivitis or a corneal ulcer. Inhalation of the powder form of the compound may cause swelling, inflammation and ulceration of the mucous membranes. After ingestion by mouth the first symptom is vomiting (in the past a 1% solution of copper sulfate was used to induce vomiting). With the vomiting, a significant portion of the toxin is removed. The vomit is at first green in color and later turns bloody. With this epigastric pain and serious occasional bloody diarrhea develops. The absorbed toxin turns the tongue, the mucosa of the cheek, esophagus and stomach green and causes bleeding of the gastric mucosa. In subacute cases damage to the kidney and liver are behind the clinical symptoms which may follow anemia. Finally coma and circulatory insufficiency lead to death.

Mercury and its compounds

Mercury is a silvery white metal which evaporates at room temperature and thus its vapor can be dangerous the organism. Mercury poisoning is primarily and occupational disease which affects people who work at such places where the mercury content of the air exceeds 100 mg/m^3 (dentists, dental assistants, thermometer and barometer makers, etc.). If a large amount acutely enters the air, the transport across the alveolar membrane results not only in a general effect, but local alterations and pneumonitis. Such cases have been described in which mercury entered the intestinal tract from the bursting of a mercury-containing rubber balloon and following aspiration into the lungs a serious fibrotic granulomatous inflammation developed, the center of which contained foreign body giant cells, epitheloid cells and peripheral fibroblasts around droplets of mercury.

The more important form of toxicity is the chronic effect, chronic mercury damage. If one is exposed in the work place over a period of months to the above air values, one may suffer from the characteristic alterations. After absorbing the finely dispersed metallic mercury, it crosses the blood brain barrier and accumulates in the brain tissue and cortex. Here it oxidizes to mercury ions which have a strong chelate-forming capacity and due to the binding to proteins has a non-specific inhibitory effect on the enzymes. Damage to the central nervous system results in intention tremor and mercurial eretism with psychiatric signs of poisoning (depression, an increase in irritability, emotional instability, and symptoms of regression). From the standpoint of differential diagnosis, the extent of these symptoms and anamnestic data determine the seriousness.

Inorganic compounds: $HgCl_2$ (sublimated), Hg_2Cl_2 (calomel), $Hg(NO_3)_2$ (mercury nitrate) had a primarily medicinal use (antiseptic, laxative, stain and gunpowder). One of the effects of organic mercury compounds is that of an antiseptic, and another use is that of a seed-dressing. Calomel is a poorly absorbed compound which used to be used as a laxative and with chronic used caused kidney damage, colitis and dementia.

With poisoning by inorganic mercury compounds, $HgCl_2$ carries the most significance. It can cause poisoning at a level of only 20 mg/kg body weight. The poisoning happens accidentally or as a result of a suicide attempt. Shortly after ingestion by mouth, the patient complains of a metallic taste in the mouth, and then acute gastrointestinal complaints develop among which are a pronounced cramping pain in the pharynx and stomach, bloody vomiting, salivation, the mucosa of the mouth turning greyish-white, coagulation. Diarrhea with a characteristically greyish-black stool from the mercury sulfide content. The clinical picture 24–48 hours later is dominated by the development of kidney damage, anuria, and uremia. The autopsy findings in acute poisoning are characteristic. The upper part of the gastrointestinal tract shows greyish-white areas on the mucosal membranes from the coagulation caused by the mercury chloride, and the gastric mucosa is swollen, with hemorrhages, a dysentery-like colitis develops in the colon, the stool is greyish-black from the mercury sulfide. The alterations in the large intestine can be traced back to the resecretion of absorbed mercury by the mucous membranes of the colon and the salivary glands. The kidneys are enlarged, the tissue greyish-white, the epithelial cells of the proximal tubules are destroyed, and if the patient survives longer in place of the deceased epithelial cells calcium is deposited, and the liver and myocardium show fatty degeneration *(Fig. 169)*.

Among the organic mercury compounds *methyl mercury* poisoning merits being the center of attention. Between 1953–1960 in Minamata Bay, Japan, a mass organic mercury poisoning occurred among the residents. Methyl mercury causes serious and irreversible damage, easily crossing the blood brain barrier and the placenta, causing both pre- and postnatal damage. The fetus or infant is especially sensitive to intoxication. In the poisoning that occurred at Minamata Bay between 1955–1959, 6% of the babies born had brain damage while their mothers suffered only mild paresthetic alterations. The red blood cells of the fetuses showed a 30% higher concentration of methyl mercury than the red blood cells of the mothers did.

Any mercury compounds that manage to get into the organism can be converted to methyl mercury and accumulated in the organism. About 90% of the amount entering is absorbed through the gastrointestinal tract and covalently bound to carbon atoms. Elimination occurs through the bile, and a significant enterohepatic circulation develops due to the reabsorption. Only 10% is eliminated in the urine. Swedish researchers have demonstrated that any kind of mercury contamination that gets into the organism can be methylated by the organism. The half-life in fish is long, about two years, and this is 2–5 times longer than the half-life of metallic mercury. In the human organism the biological half-life is 70–90 days. The decay is quiet slow and the muscle tissue primarily accumulates the compound. This explains the appearance of the poisoning, being enriched in the muscle tissue of the fish, a continuous build-up of mercury compounds can occur from the pollution and transformation. The clinical signs depend on the exposure time, the age of the patient and individual sensitivity. The atrophy of the granular layer of the cerebellum causes progressive incoordination, ataxia and dysarthria. The paresthesia and disturbances in palpation are early signs of poisoning. Mercurial eretism may develop as well. Atrophy and degeneration of the cerebral cortex has been described at autopsy. The exposure can usually be verified by examination of the liver, the blood and occasionally the brain. The lowest mercury level in the blood which can cause symptoms is 0.22 ppm, while a toxic effect has been noted with hair levels at 50 ppm. The weekly mercury load allowed by FAO/WHO in foods is 0.3 mg, of which 0.2 mg may be methyl mercury. This means 3.3 micrograms/kg body weight.

A similar effect can be found from other organic mercury compounds. In Iraq an alkyl mercury poisoning from a fungicide was recorded. Alkyl mercury is not so well absorbed as the previously noted mercury

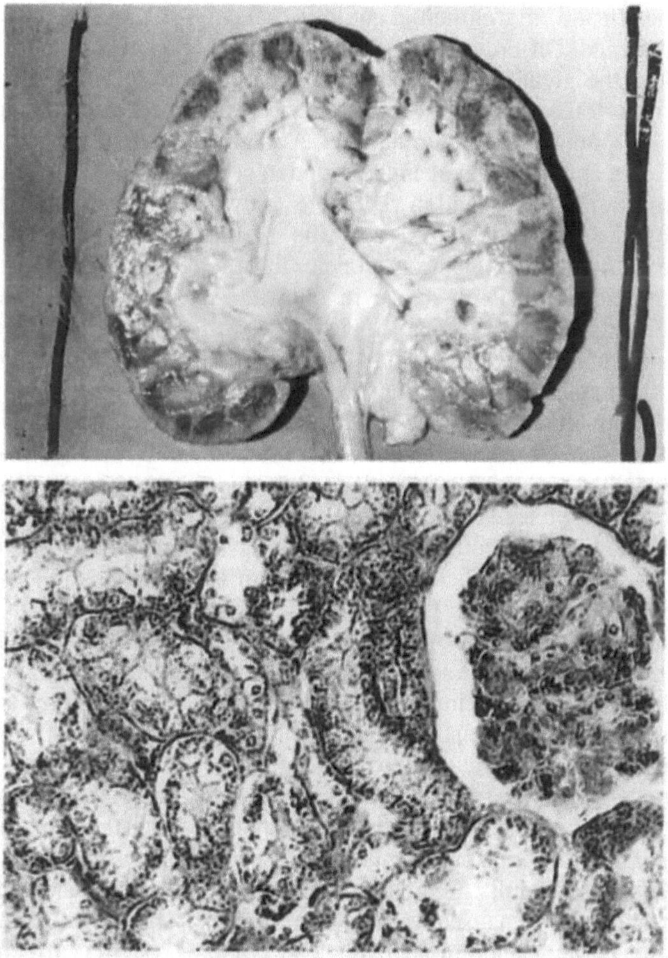

Fig. 169. Mercury poisoning. Macroscopic picture of the kidney (above); microscopic picture of damage to the epithelium of the proximal tubules (below) (material of Prof. Endre Somogyi)

compounds, and is not capable of a stable C–Hg binding. Due to the instability the mercury is mainly eliminated through the kidneys in the ionic form. Clinical signs usually develop within two months after exposure with cerebellar damage and disturbances in visual and sensation. In the fungicidal material contains phenyl mercury, intestinal and renal complaints similar to those caused by inorganic mercury compounds may develop. Organic mercury containing antiseptics are poorly absorbed and cause poisoning only in large amounts.

Lead and its compounds

Lead intoxication has always been one of the most common forms of poisoning even in ancient times. Among the sources, many maintain that lead-glazed vessels could have caused a chronic poisoning from a slow dissolving into the food, but lead acetate was used as a sweetener in wines even in the 18th century as well. Chronic lead poisoning can result from lead bullets left inside the body. Due to its significance and frequency in the last decades, examinations by the public health and environmental authorities have returned. Different lead-containing paints and the great rise in lead contamination from traffic are the biggest sources of environmental contamination. A significant amount of lead can be found in cow milk, fruit juices, and in vegetables grown by the road-side. It is the hope of the environmental protection agencies that the intoxication will decrease in our times.

It may reach the organism via the gastrointestinal tract or the lungs. Organic lead compounds can also be absorbed through the skin. It can gain access to the organism as a trace element, but is not an essential metal. About 10% of the daily 300 micrograms of lead is absorbed, and 15–20 micrograms is counted via the airways. The significance of childhood poisoning is shown in that 50% of the ingested lead is resorbed. The absorbed lead is accumulated in the blood, the soft tissues and finally in the bony tissues in the form of insoluble lead phosphate mostly in the areas where there is active bone growth. This shows up on X-rays as the typical *"lead lines"* in the tibia, radius and femur. Acute poisoning – from lead vapors, paints, plastics – usually happens to adults. In the mouth a metallic taste, dryness, nausea, vomiting, cramping and burning abdominal pain, lead colic, diarrhea (with black stools from the lead sulfide) develops. The single lethal dose is not known. Serious toxic damage can be expected with the ingestion of 2–3 grams of lead acetate.

The effect of lead in the organism is not easy to diagnose. Molecularly, the effect of binding to SH groups becomes manifest, with damage to those enzymes which are necessary to heme synthesis and the production of hemoglobin and cytochrome. Besides this, it damages the membranes of the red blood cells (through the Na/K–ATPase pump mechanism) and caused an increased fragility. Anemia develops from the affinity of lead for the red blood cells and in compensation for this the increased work of the bone marrow produces more erythrocytes and immature reticulocytes with their basophilic stippling begin to appear in the peripheral circulation. In children it often causes iron-deficiency anemia. Lead poisoning can cause Fanconi syndrome-like symptoms in the kidneys. Due to the damage to the myocardial fibers, a diffuse fibrosis can develop. A central nervous system edema and a damage to the peripheral myelin sheaths appears. The damage to the central nervous system can result in encephalopathy as the effect of chronic lead poisoning. With chronic ingestion in children a decline in IQ, disturbances of fine motor coordination and pica can develop.

The biochemical effect – the disturbance of heme biosynthesis – gives the possibility for early diagnosis through the determination of the qualitative urinary coproporphyrin level as the most simple procedure.

Poisoning by tetraethyl lead through both the gastrointestinal and dermal routes is common. Metabolization evolves triethyl lead and lead, the effects of which are toxic. Primarily the central nervous system is affected, with vomiting, nausea, irritability, insomnia, nightmares, then tremor, chorea and mania add to the picture. In serious cases, kidney and liver alterations develop.

Arsenic and its compounds

Arsenic poisoning is also one of the most common forms of poisoning known from ancient times. Properties contributing to its wide use include its watersoluble compound being a powerful poison, colorless and tasteless. Among the arsenic compounds arsenic sulfide or orpigment was known in ancient times and used by HIPPOCRATES as a medication for ulcerated areas. Because of its color – from which it gets its name – it was a favorite compound of the alchemists. Arsenic oxide is the anhydride of arsenious acid which is difficult to dissolve in water (3:100), but easier if the water is warm (1:10). The arsenic-containing poison used in 17th century Italy may have been an aqueous solution of As_2O_3. It was used later in Hungary and became a significant area of forensic medicine and toxicology, the Tiszazug murders having been committed by aqueous solutions of arsenic trioxide at the beginning of this century.

Metallic arsenic is not toxic and not absorbed by the gastrointestinal tract. It becomes poisonous in its compounds. Among these As_2O_3 had a practical significance earlier. Arsenic trioxide and arsenious acid(H_3AsO_3) are the trivalent form of arsenic. The pentavalent As_2O_5 is less toxic. Potassium sodium arsenate is more toxic than arsenic oxide due to its greater solubility. It used to be used as an insecticide. Arsenic poisoning may appear as an occupational disease in those metallurgical operations performing pyrite smelting containing a significant amount of arsenic. Such arsenic poisonings have been described in which the not only the level of arsenic was raised in certain key organ systems, but pathological alterations (cirrhosis) also followed as a chronic effect. These poisonings may also occur from ingestion of arsenic-containing medications available on the open market, and although these are no longer used in many countries, even so the so-called *homeopathic treatments* have resulted in numerous cases of poisoning. Arsenic oxide was used in these remedies which accumulated with chronic use. This fact may lead to a mistaken suspicion of arsenic poisoning.

- In our experience the autopsy of a 50-year-old woman uncovered liver alterations, fatty liver degeneration, which raised the suspicion of arsenic poisoning. Although the above-mentioned examination was unknown the previous history revealed that the deceased had for years been regularly taking large doses of Fowler solution as a tonic, an we could not exclude the possibility that the quantity of arsenic accumulated in the organism had entered by this route. The arsenic concentration of the liver was 39.6 micrograms% and of the nails 278 micrograms%.

After acute poisoning with arsenic trioxide a significant amount – 80% – is absorbed. In the organism the unbound arsenic is metabolized into the less toxic compounds of monomethyl arsenic acid and dimethyl arsenic acid. The unaccumulated half of the arsenic is eliminated in the urine. (After treatment with BAL the whole amount of ingested arsenic is eliminated in its methylated form). A significant toxicological role is played by the binding to SH groups and the SH groups are especially sensitive to the trivalent form of arsenic forming chelates and thus influence the oxidative processes of the cells. The water-soluble forms can be absorbed through the skin and mucous membranes and are eliminated only slowly, so repeated ingestion, as mentioned, results in accumulation in the organism. The lethal dose of arsenic trioxide is 120 mg, the measured concentration in the organism: liver 0.005 mg%, kidney 0.0048 mg%, hair 0.01 mg%, brain 0.0048 mg%. A short time after acute intoxication – 15 minutes – symptoms appear if the stomach was empty. If the arsenic was ingested in a powdered form on a full stomach, the symptoms may appear only hours later. Following ingestion of a lethal dose, death ensues after 18–36 hours and with children ingesting larger doses, one hour. Among the early signs are a burning retrosternal pain which spreads to the epigastric area and nausea with vomiting. The vomit at first consists only of the stomach contents, then watery mucous with pieces of the mucous membranes, rarely blood and often bile. Dehydration and collapse may occur in this stage. The intense gastrointestinal excitation causes tenesmus and a pronounced choleriform enteritis with dilute, grey, rice-water stools containing pieces of the mucosa being passed. Serious abdominal and cramping pelvic pain characterized the picture (with women it may be mistaken for extrauterine pregnancy!). Due to the increased loss of fluid the skin is dry and slack, the eyes sunken, and oliguria develops which may proceed to uremia.

The autopsy findings are not characteristic. Pinpoint bleedings on the gastric mucosa, mucus, swelling and erosions appear. If the poison was ingested in a powder form, greyish-white, half-dissolved remnants of the poison may be found on the gastric mucosa. The mucosa of the small intestine forms a picture of cholera-like enteritis, the kidneys are enlarged and swollen. The diagnosis can only be make from the toxicological examination of the gastric contents and urine. Thirty minutes after ingestion of a large quantity of arsenic, it can be demonstrated in the hair bulbs.

In chronic intoxication the poison accumulates. Primarily in the cornified tissues, the hair and nails, but the liver enlarges significantly and the bony tissues contain arsenic as well. Among the clinical signs the skin alterations can be noted, as the chronic effects of arsenic is the hyperkeratosis of the skin of the palms and soles. A characteristic yellowish-brown pigmentation appears in the skin as the so-called arsenic *melanosis* in the wrinkles, the abdomen and hands. At other times we may see papulovesicular alterations. The nails accumulate arsenic giving rise to the so-called *Aldrich-Mees lines* (greyish-white lines in the nail bed). The alterations of arsenic polyneuropathy have diagnostic value in which changes occur in the peripheral nerves with a characteristic picture of paralysis in the lower extremity, which may in many cases be the first sign of arsenic intoxication. Chronic liver alterations, cirrhosis, and jaundice may be later complications. Autopsy findings of arsenic melanosis, the Mees sign, hyperkeratosis, fatty degeneration of the liver suggest that if death does not occur for years following the ingestion of arsenic, cirrhosis may develop.

Of the arsenic compounds, it is worth noting AsH_3, which is very toxic, colorless gas with a garlicky odor. We must consider all cases where arsenic-containing metals are hydrolyzed or electrolyzed as possible sources. The symptoms are vomiting, abdominal pain, hemolysis, hemoglobinuria, jaundice, oliguria and anuria. The renal changes characterize the autopsy picture with hemoglobin cylinders visible in the collecting ducts.

Arsenic can be demonstrated as with poisoning by any metal-containing compound and will yield results years after death. The degenerative processes do not influence the concentration in the cornified and bony tissues. A determination made from the cornified tissues verifies not only the fact of poisoning, but of a chronic, prolonged exposure. Bearing in mind the growth rate of the hair (1 cm/month) the time of exposure can be estimated. Examination of the concentration of arsenic in the nails yields not only an estimation of the time, but a possibility for a quantitative determination as well (the nails grow 0.12 mm per day).

Carbon monoxide

Carbon monoxide poisoning used to be one of the most common forms of death from suicide and accidents. These days the significance has diminished, but under certain circumstances one must consider its possibility.

Incomplete combustion can result in a large amount of carbon monoxide. Earlier coal-burning stoves, furnaces and lamp gas (containing 14% CO) were used. Today the significant quantity of carbon monoxide in exhaust gas can cause acute or chronic intoxication. It may also occur with the incomplete combustion of propane or butane.

- In a rental apartment which was heated by natural gas where the hot water system for the bathroom also used a factory-made natural gas boiler, a five-year-old boy and his parents were found dead. At the inquest the medical specialist raised the possibility of carbon monoxide poisoning on the basis of the color and spread of the hypostatic patches. This was supported by the autopsy and laboratory findings. The source of the carbon monoxide poisoning was the incomplete combustion by the factory-made boiler in the bathroom, the exhaust chimney having been narrowed to a fourth of its diameter by a brick left in during construction. The blood level of CO-hemoglobin was 62% in the child.

Cigarette smoke contains 3–6% carbon monoxide. This explains the 1.9–3.0% CO hemoglobin levels found in the blood of smoking pregnant women which makes its way into the fetal blood at 1.8 times that amount.

The carbon monoxide hemoglobin content in an average blood sample does not exceed 1.0% and the endogenous production of CO may play a role in it from the metabolism of hemoglobin and tetrapyroles. Carbon monoxide causes tissue hypoxia. Two pathways lead to it: with one the oxygen binding in the red blood cells decreases causing tissue hypoxia, with the other the oxyhemoglobin dissociation is shifted to the left and that means that the partial pressure is lowered which slows oxygen diffusion into the tissues. Carbon monoxide reversibly binds to hemoglobin forming carboxyhemoglobin (COHb). This binding is approximately 240 times as strong as the binding of oxygen. Thus the inhalation of a relatively low concentration of gas can significantly influence the oxygen carrying capacity of the red blood cells. This means that a 50% COHb concentration can be reached when the environmental air has a CO concentration of only 1/240th the concentration of O_2, which is only 0.08% CO (800 ppm!). The hemoglobin-oxygen dissociation curve is sigmoid in shape and a left shift means that the curve becomes more hyperbolic and in the aforementioned situation oxygen can dissociate when the tissue oxygen demand is increased. If the hemoglobin molecule is bound to CO the oxygen available to the tissues decreases along with the partial pressure of O_2, and this situation causes tissue hypoxia. Besides binding to hemoglobin, CO also binds to myoglobin and to intracellular cytochrome oxidase which increases the tissue and cellular hypoxia. The blood COHb saturation depends on the CO content of the environmental air, the exposure time and the pulmonary ventilation. Numerous factors influence the blood carboxyhemoglobin saturation, infants or those suffering from diseases which raise the basal metabolism, anemia, and those suffering from cardiovascular disease are more sensitive to the toxic effect of carbon monoxide. The elimination of carbon monoxide from the COHb binding is slow, the biological half-life in healthy adults being 4–5 hours. This can significantly diminish the oxygen intake capacity.

The signs of acute poisoning are mainly the result of damage to the brain and heart.

0–10% COHb: no clinical signs.

11–20% COHb: mild headache and dyspnoe, dilation of the vessels of the skin.

21–30% COHb: headache, throbbing temples, mild weakness, occasional adynamia.

31–40% COHb: headache, visual disturbances, nausea, vomiting, adynamia, collapse.

41–50% COHb: collapse, syncope, rise in pulse and breath rate.

51–60% COHb: syncope, coma, convulsions.

61–70% COHb: coma, intermittent convulsions, circulatory and respiratory depression, death.

71–80% COHb: weak pulse, irregular breathing, death within hours.

81–90% COHb: death within one hour.

91– % COHb: death within minutes.

Among the symptoms headache is considered as a result of cerebral edema. The damaging effect on the central nervous system is well known, but less is known about the effect on the strength of the myocardium. Death often results from myocardial ischemia and in sensitive individuals a COHb level of 9% can cause noticeable irregularities in cardiac function, on the ECG, and occasional arrhythmias. After poisoning – if it was not a lethal exposure – within 3–4 days the patient's status may return to normal. A comatose state lasting more than 24 hours regularly leaves lasting central nervous system damage. Later damage to the central nervous system is a patchy demyelinization. The newborn is especially sensitive to carbon monoxide poisoning, and the gas can cross the placental barrier.

Of the autopsy findings, a bright pink color to the hypostatic patches is noticeable, and the musculature and parenchymal organs are also bright pink on section. The blood is bright red, fluid, the lungs are distended and edematous under the pleura, and under the external layer of the pericardium are pinpoint hemorrhages. The brain is edematous and hemorrhages can be found in the striatum and cortical tissue. After a few days survival these areas become significantly softened *(Fig. 170).*

Determination of the blood COHb content yields the unequivocal diagnosis (although the possibility of postmortal

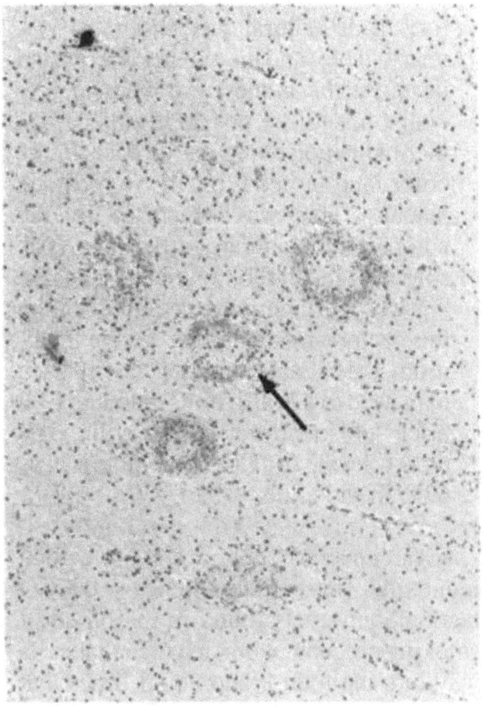

Fig. 170. Ring hemorrhages in the brain following carbon monoxide poisoning

origin has been raised in recent years). A postmortal formation can be expected in a body submerged in water for a prolonged period, originating from the microorganisms being in the water, due to the anaerobe decomposition of myoglobin and hemoglobin.

Among the clinical signs and symptoms of chronic poisoning headache, anemia, tachycardia, palpitations, precordial pain, depression and irritability are worthy of mention. With women the menstrual cycle may be altered. Chronic poisoning is a disease of those working in an environment containing carbon monoxide – traffic police and garage workers –, the blood level of carboxyhemoglobin of whom may exceed 3–5%.

Treatment depends on the saturation level of carboxyhemoglobin. The first step is the removal of the victim from the carbon monoxide-containing environment and then administration of oxygen. Movement should be avoided since the increase in muscular work increases the oxygen demand and the oxygen supply to the central nervous system will be decreased. If the carboxyhemoglobin level does not exceed 15%, it is enough to just give the victim fresh air. Administration of 100% oxygen should be arranged when the saturation level exceeds 15%. Above 40% carboxyhemoglobin, hyperbaric oxygen should be given.

Cyanide poisoning

Hydrogen cyanide (HCN), and potassium or sodium cyanide (KCN) poisonings are not frequent in the practice of forensic toxicology. Hydrogen cyanide is a highly volatile liquid (boiling point 26°C), with a characteristic odor of bitter almonds. The odor is noticeable at a level in the air of 1 ppm. The potassium-sodium cyanide are substances, which decompose in the open air, create hydrogen cyanide and potassium carbonate. Potassium and sodium are used in metallurgy, the exposure of hydrogen cyanide can occur in the chemical laboratories, but its formation must be expected with the burning of certain plastics (polyurethane and nitrocellulose). Many instances have been recorded in which cyanide poisoning has occurred with the ingestion of the pits of certain fruits. It is rarely used for the purpose of suicide, even in workers who are employed at such places where it is available. In recent times the mass poisoning that occurred in 1978 at Jonestown, Guyana – more than 900 members of a religious sect died – again brought attention to the possibility of cyanide poisoning.

The pathophysiological effect is the inhibition of the final step in the terminal oxidation system, by forming a complex with cytochrome oxidase. The result is that pyruvate is not oxidized further in the citric acid cycle, but rather reduced to lactate and this leads to a build up of that product. The patient actually suffocates, but not due to disturbances in oxygen transport, but because the transported oxygen cannot be used by the tissues. The lethal dose is 2 mg/kg, and blood level 12,4 mg/l, although it is often emphasized that not the blood level, but the intracellular concentration in the tissues is significant. The MAC of hydrogen cyanide is 10 ppm.

The bright red color of the blood, the patches of lividity, and the light red discoloration of the organs is the consequence of the saturation of the blood by oxygen and the significant decrease in its consumption by the tissues. Thus the oxygen saturation in the veins almost reaches the level of that in the arteries.

The ambiguity of the signs may make the clinical presentation and diagnosis difficult. The odor is characteristic, but only occasionally noticeable. The headache, tachypnoe and feeling of weakness accompany other types of poisonings as well. The fate of the patient depends on the dose. It is a very rapidly acting poison, with death that can occur within minutes. The first signs quickly progress to stupor, apnoe, then convulsions and death. The most characteristic early sign is lactic acidosis. The most rapid effect is achieved with an intravenously injected poison or by inhalation of hydrogen cyanide. A prolonged effect may occur following dosage *per os,* since after absorption it reaches the circulation after passing through the liver and due to detoxification processes in the liver a part is transformed reacting with thiosulfate (catalyzed by rhodanase), forming thiocyanate, which is less toxic. The other possibility for poisoning is the ingestion of cyanide-containing fruit seeds. In these seeds the cyanoglycoside amygdalin can be found which, with the help of hydrolysis by beta glycosidase, releases hydrogen cyanide (beta glycosidase can be found, for instance, in the nut of the bitter almond, in apple seeds, in apricot and plum pits, in various vegetables, in mushrooms, green peas, carrots, etc.).

The *chronic form* of poisoning is less known. Some articles have described chronic poisoning as an occupational hazard, but these were shown to be only moderate recurring acute forms.

The results of *autopsy* resemble the findings of carbon monoxide poisoning. The patches of lividity are bright red, the organs and tissues are light red as is the blood which is fluid. The gastric contents have the odor of bitter almond, the gastric mucosa is engorged with blood, swollen and showing a hemorrhagic gastritis.

The chemistry examination verifies the diagnosis, and since it involves a volatile substance, the organs and materials to be examined must be purposely kept in alcohol for the testing for the presence of toxin.

The specific part of the *treatment* can be traced back six decades. That is when the methylene blue treatment was formulated as a cyanide poisoning antagonist. Later the administration of nitrite came to be considered appropriate, and amyl nitrite was employed. Both form methemoglobin, and the cyanide ion in the Fe^{+++} cytochrome system did not allow the binding to take place. It is not worth while to raise the level of methemoglobin above 40%, since toxic signs begin to appear. These simultaneously yield potassium thiosulfate, which forms the above-mentioned thiocyanate with the cyanide rendering it less toxic. The process is slow, but thus the cyanomethemoglobin is just a transient binding on its way to thiocyanide. These observations are mostly the results of animal experiments. Another antidote to the poisoning is aminophenol, which forms methemoglobin more rapidly than nitrite does, and dicobalt EDTA, which forms cobalt cyanide $[Co(CN)_6]$ with cyanide (here the toxic effect of cobalt must also be expected). As a specific treatment with hydroxycobalamine was proposed, due to the low toxicity in which 400 micromoles/kg can be given, which binds cyanide in equimolar amounts forming cyanocobalamine (vitamin B_{12}).

Poisoning by corrosives

The determination of poisonings with corrosives is a broad field which contains the effects of acids, alkalis and corrosive metal salts. A common property to all members, and others besides, is tissue damage which to a certain extent may be characteristic of the applied substances.

Alterations may appear from household hydrochloric acid, sulfuric acid, ammonia and besides the above, industrial acetic acid, nitric acid, medicinal zinc chloride, mercuric chloride, chlorine bleach, silver nitrate, and potassium permanganate. The poisonous substance can cause damage depending upon the various concentrations and amounts. With children the ingestion of a small amount of caustic material can result in serious local and general signs and the accidental form of these poisonings appear in children in significant numbers, while with adults the number of accidental cases is lower and cases of suicidal intent higher.

With poisoning with corrosives, the external signs may attract our attention. There may be corrosions around the mouth left by the dribbling of the caustic agent which may quickly dry out, but these traces may be expected in children and women postmortem if the gastric contents came out around the mouth. Occasionally the perioral corrosions caused by acid poisoning raise the suspicion of homicide injuries.

Poisoning by acids appears with strong acids of a pH around 2. (The pH of some acids can approximate or reach this – lemon juice, carbon dioxide-containing carbonated drinks – but these have no toxic effect.) Numerous inorganic – sulfuric acid, hydrochloric acid, nitric acid –, and organic chemicals – oxalic acid and acetic acid – belong here. A common property of them is the corrosive effect, which results in coagulative necrosis, the denaturation of proteins. This has a local significance, the effect being external or on the mucous membranes. Orally ingested acid causes corrosions to the mouth and esophagus which passes relatively quickly through the esophagus and so leaves less damage. In the stomach the damage is more pronounced, the mucous membranes being discolored, coagulated, and the gastric wall stiff and compact in places depending on the acid. In the stomach one finds coffee ground-like deposits of blood (acid hematin). Perforation in the case of acid poisoning, on the other hand, is rare, compared to alkali poisoning. The damage is most pronounced on the lesser curvature and prepyloric areas. We rarely find damage to the small intestine. Following acid poisoning, among the general effects described is acidosis, which is mentioned only in poisoning by oxalic acid in the books dealing with emergency toxicological treatment.

Sulfuric acid (Oil of Vitriol(H_2SO_4)

Battery factories, laboratories, agricultural and industrial areas are where this is found. The *lethal dose* is 3 ml. We see brownish-black deposits around the mouth if ingested orally. There is a great pain in the throat and retrosternal areas, followed by nausea and vomiting of a black, acid hematin-containing vomit. The pulse races, the breath comes in gasps, and the victim collapses. The cause of death is perforation of the stomach, shock and respiratory insufficiency. At autopsy we find corrosion and brownish-black discoloration of the mouth, tongue, throat, esophagus, and gastric mucosa with the wall of the stomach stiff and compact.

Nitric acid (Aqua Fortis HNO_3)

It is used in industrial factories, laboratories, and the preparation of explosives. It is a colorless, or amber-colored fluid, the *lethal dose* of which is 3 ml. The clinical pictures carries signs similar to sulfuric acid poisoning, the coagulative form being characteristic, and the so-called *xanthoprotein reaction* effect of nitric acid appears forming a yellow-colored crust. The cause of death is shock. Perforation generally does not develop with this poisoning and at autopsy the mucous membranes are discolored yellow and we find edema of the lungs.

Hydrochloric acid (Spirit of Salts HCl)

Besides being used in industrial laboratories, this can also be found in household care, so accidental acid poisoning by hydrochloric acid causes the bulk of the damage. It is a colorless or yellowish, strong-smelling liquid. The vapor also has an irritating effect. It can cause glottis spasms, edema and pulmonary edema. The lethal dose is 4–8 ml. The gastric juice contains it in 0.2% concentration.

The alterations that occur depend on the mode of application. Inhalation of the vapors can cause an acute inflammation of the airways, pulmonary edema, glottis spasm, then pneumonia, collapse and shock. The signs appearing with poisoning *per os* match those of sulfuric acid and nitric acid poisoning. At autopsy we can see on the coagulated surfaces of the mucous membranes greyish-white, compact areas, acid hematin in the stomach, and perhaps perforation, but postmortal perforation (!) can also be expected.

Acetic acid (CH_3COOH)

Of the poisonings that occur with organic acids, acetic acid carries significance. Besides its use in industrial laboratories, its diluted form can also be found in housekeeping. It is a liquid with a characteristic odor, the lethal dose being 20 ml. In the concentrated form it has a corrosive effect, but diluted it also irritates. In poisoning, its characteristic odor gives it away. Vomiting, with the vomit having the typical odor and being bloody, with a bloody stool may occur. Hemoglobinuria and then oliguria develop. In chronic cases – which occurs with workers in vinegar factories – there is anorexia, gastritis and bronchopneumonia. At autopsy the characteristic odor, coagulated areas of greyish-white discoloration, and occasional renal damage aid in the diagnosis.

Alkalies

Earlier a significant percentage of the poisonings happening with corrosives were performed by alkalis, because of the characteristic properties (making soap from fat), it had a wide-spread household use. Thus it was common in accidents or suicide attempts and murder. Substances with a chemical effect at pH 11.5 and above belong here.

KOH (potassium hydroxide) and *NaOH (sodium hydroxide)* are used in the manufacture of soap, in laboratories, and in various household products (drain cleaners). They denature proteins, saponify fats, and therefore the areas of their effect are spread more deeply, causing a liquefaction, and occasionally penetrating corrosion. Among the clinical signs that can be mentioned are a burning sensation of the mouth and stomach area, the oral mucous membranes become soap-like slippery and discolored brownish (alkaline hematin), the vomit is bloody and containing broken off pieces of the gastric mucosa. The breathing is frequent with a racing pulse, and then collapse follows the poisoning. Death follows shock or glottis edema. Later intercurrent illnesses, pneumonia, mediastinitis and peritonitis develop 2–3 days after the poisoning. If the patient heals a later complication of esophageal stenosis may develop (ago decades among the etiological factors of various complications causing esophageal stenosis, a large percentage were childhood accidental ingestions of alkali.)

The gastric acid is unable to neutralize the alkali that gains entrance to the stomach, and so colliquative alterations develop, commonly with perforation. Alkali that touches the skin can cause injuries resembling I–III degree burns, depending on the concentration and time of exposure of the material. Material touching the cornified membranes cause a corneal destruction and scarring. The *lethal dose* is 3–5 g. Colliquative necrosis characterizes the autopsy findings, the mucous membranes touched by the alkali turning soap-like and slippery. The damage not only affects the superficial layers of the tissue, but reaches the deeper ones, too, and in numerous cases causes penetrating or perforating injuries. In those dying in the acute phase besides those mentioned above, we can find a separation of the esophageal mucous membranes, incipient mediastinitis, periesophageal edema, and occasional edema of the pharynx. Similar alterations can be found in the stomach with gastric perforation often accompanying the poisoning. Stenosis of the esophagus at the points of physiological narrowing develops later.

Corrosive metallic salts

We can list numerous compounds here which have as their common property the denaturation of proteins. For this reason they were used as antiseptics, and in small amounts as astringents. Mercuric chloride (see mercury poisoning), $KMnO_4$, $AgNO_3$ and $ZnCl_2$ are of practical significance. Their common property is protein denaturation and a discoloration of the affected area depending on the compounds in the denatured area.

Silver nitrate ($AgNO_3$). It has primarily a medicinal use, a caustic effect, and coagulates proteins in the affected area forming a significantly compacted greyish-black crust. Consumption of a *lethal dose* of 2–10 g results in death. When a small amount is ingested or occasionally following a repeated consumption argirosis may develop in which a local build-up of silver in the organism characteristically pigments the organs or tissues primarily in the areas exposed to the light, the conjunctiva, fingers and nails. In large quantities we find in the oral mucosa first greyish-white, then greyish-black colored compact areas, in the throat and stomach areas a burning pain, a black vomit and in serious cases convulsions and then coma.

Potassium permanganate ($KMnO_4$). This is an effective oxidizing agent, which besides being found in industrial concerns can be found in laboratories, and due to its antiseptic properties is also used in medical practice. The *lethal dose* is 5 g. It causes corrosion when concentrated, with severe tissue destruction. It may be involved in accidental poisoning or suicide. The signs depend on the concentration of the compound. A 1% solution causes a burning sensation in the throat, a purplish-red discoloration, vomiting and mild gastroenteritis. A 3% solution causes, aside from the above-mentioned signs, an edema of the pharynx. The patient cannot swallow or speak as a result of the damaging effect to the mucous membranes of the organism. A 5% solution is nephrotoxic, the sign of which is albuminuria. Due to edema of the salivary glands, salivation is decreased. Death occurs as a result of circulatory insufficiency (we see local corrosion in the vagina mucous membrane when potassium permanganate crystals are applied for the purpose of inducing abortion.)

Zinc chloride ($ZnCl_2$). This is a greyish-white or colorless substance which dissolves easily in water with a *lethal dose* of 30 g. Signs: burning pain in the mouth, nausea, vomiting, bloody diarrhea, then anuria and collapse. Liver and kidney damage develop. The toxic effect can be mentioned that it is rarely lethal since the emetic effect of the substance ensures that a significant portion of it will be eliminated. It has a fungicidal and antiseptic effect. At autopsy the gastric mucosa is swollen and erosions can be seen. The mucous membranes are discolored yellowish-grey, hemorrhages can be found in the submucosa, and similar alterations can be seen in the small intestine. The parts of the mucous membranes affected by the substance is coagulated and compact.

Pesticides

The use of materials with pesticidal effects can be traced back a thousand years. In the beginning sulfur, which when burned gives off sulfur dioxide, then various arsenic compounds were noticed to have antifungal effects and were used. In the 17th century the similar results of extracts of tobacco were described and these materials were used for centuries along with copper sulfate for the protection of plants. The growth in the number of pesticides may account for the rapid increase in production throughout the world following the second world war, but from this has also begun the growth of substances which cause environmental pollution with unexpected consequences, among which could be mentioned the "wonder chemical" *DDT* and its now known polluting effect on the environment, and although its use has been banned for decades, even today it is still detectable in organisms. The environmental pollution of pesticides can perhaps be better understood if we direct our attention to their properties, which with some groups includes their resistance to deterioration. Naturally, the heavy metal compound containing pesticides belong to this group, but it may be noticed that the organic chloride compounds and organic phosphate insecticides also persist a long time in the environment. They also break down slowly in the soil, and among other damaging effects, their ability to reach distance areas should be mentioned (pollution washed into bodies of water, chemicals absorbed into soil particles etc.) and unexpected effects appear.

The pesticides are biologically active compounds with toxic effects, not only with the possibility of poisoning humans, but domestic and wild animals as well. The modes by which they can enter the organism are varied. Examinations of those who work with these substances has verified that sometimes a significant amount of pesticidal material can be demonstrated on the surface of the skin. Thus the percutaneous mode of penetration is one of the most common forms of occupational hazards. The use of aerosols with their rapid absorption is an enhancement factor in poisoning via the airways. (The effect of aerosol exposure on pilots involved in crop dusting should be mentioned.) The most common form of poisoning not associated with occupational hazards is oral ingestion. A great part of these are ingestion with suicidal intent, and the remaining part are accidental introduction into the organism of the patient. Often the unintentional ingestion of a pesticide brought home from the work place occurs when it is mistaken for an alcoholic beverage.

- A 26-year-old man brought home from work an unknown "substance" and used it to treat skin diseases of his cows.

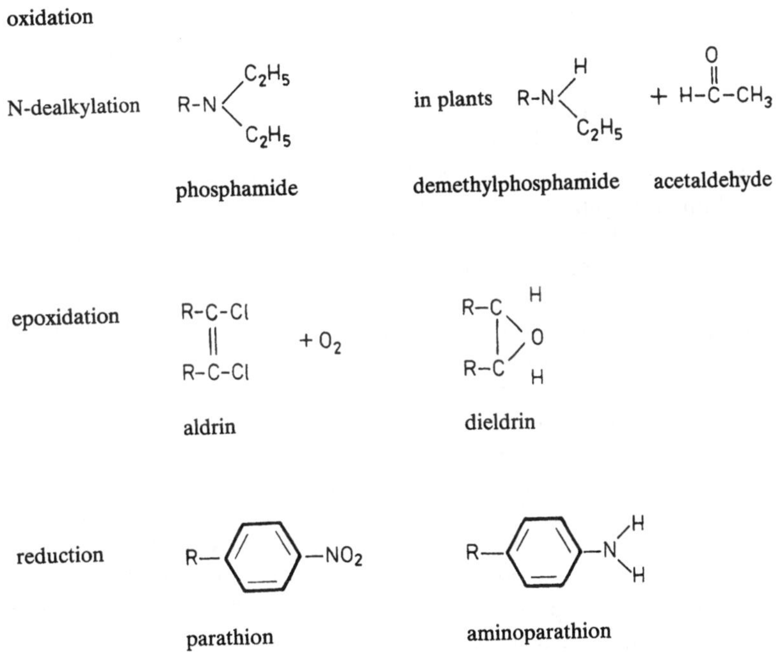

Fig. 171. Metabolization of the more common pesticides

A few hours after the treatment all of the animals were dead. The man who administered the treatment got sick himself. Vomiting and diarrhea developed, and the serum cholinesterase activity significantly diminished. The proper treatment stabilized his status, but the story continued because one of the patient of the hospital, thinking that the bottle containing the poison actually was orange juice, drank from it. He died. The doctor treating the patient was indicted for breach of professional regulations since the poison brought in was allowed to stand for hours in the emergency room contrary to the rules next to the clothes of the victim who had been brought in.

A significant part of it is metabolized in the organism. These metabolic processes must be recognized and the possibility of metabolization must not be neglected when interpreting the results of toxicological examinations *(Fig. 171)*.

Certain countries make a characteristic use of pesticides. Developing countries tend to make more use of insecticidal pesticides and the developed countries employ more herbicides.

Insecticides

The organophosphate group of compounds were prepared in the second world war by the Germans for the production of nerve gas, and their insecticidal effect was recognized early on. *Parathion* is one of the most common compounds with an effective insecticidal character, but it is also very toxic to humans. Today several thousand groups are synthesized and examined for insecticidal effects, though only a few eventually are put into use. All of these compounds have a similar toxic effect, although some are used as medications (physostigmine, neostigmine). These compounds cause the most common poisoning in human organisms, with only a few mg being lethal (parathion 3 mg/kg, malathion 1375 mg/kg, tetraethylpyrophosphate 1 mg/kg). Their effect is the inactivation of pseudocholinesterase in the plasma and the inactivation of cholinesterase at the synapses. With the inactivation of the enzyme, the level of acetylcholine rises, and inasmuch as the toxin binds near both muscarin and nicotine receptors of the central and peripheral nervous systems, this produces the characteristic clinical signs. Small dose organophosphate intoxication primarily stimulates the muscarine type receptors (postganglionic and parasympathetic). Large doses primarily affects the autonomic ganglia and the central muscarine receptors.

The reason for the enzyme inhibition is the complex-forming ability of the organophosphate compounds with the methyl and even ethyl groups of enzymes, but this binding is reversible and stable for a few hours. The binding with secondary or tertiary alkyl groups is strong and generally irreversible. For this reason 1–4 weeks are required for the regeneration of plasma pseudocholinesterase and from four weeks to several months for the regeneration of the RBC and synaptic cholinesterase to normal activity levels. Parathion is metabolized in the liver and paraoxon is formed, which is a stronger cholinesterase inhibitor than the original compound.

The signs of intoxication are those of the inhibition of cholinesterase at the respective receptor.

Muscarin type: tear production, myosis, sweating, salivation, vomiting, diarrhea, tenesmus, bradycardia, disiness, gasping for breath.

Nicotine type: exhaustion, weakness, muscle twitching, tremor, paralysis, dyspnoe, pallor, racing heart beat (ganglion stimulation), rise in blood pressure.

Central nervous system signs: anxiety, insomnia, restlessness, nightmares, neurosis, headache, ataxia, emotional instability, dizziness, babbling, halting speech, general weakness, seizures, respiratory and cardiovascular depression, and coma.

Sometimes there develop symptoms only at the site of exposure, so there may be myosis or cloudy vision if it gets into the eyes, perspiration in the affected area of exposed skin and muscle twitching.

Treatment of poisoning by organophosphate must be begun immediately when an early diagnosis or suspicion or exposure is made. There is no place for hesitation, as it puts the patient's life at risk. The preceding events and the clinical signs provide the diagnosis, but if possible the plasma pseudocholinesterase and even the erythrocyte cholinesterase activity should be determined (the erythrocyte cholinesterase activity also well reflects the central nervous system enzyme activity). The therapy in mild to moderate cases is to give 1–2 mg atropine intravenously, but as daily dose of 25–50 mg may also be given. Atropine blocks the peripheral muscarine activity, but does not protect against the development of neuromuscular paralysis in massive intoxication. In serious poisoning we give 2–4 mg of atropine intravenously. Pralidoxime is a specific antidote to organophosphate poisons, partly because it regenerates acetylcholinesterase, and partly because it hydrolyzes the accumulated acetylcholine (on the average we give a dose of 1 mg which can be repeated 20 minutes later).

Chlorinated hydrocarbons. Aldrin, dieldrin and DDT belong to this group.

The most well known and widely used compound used to be *DDT,* not only because of its insecticidal effect, but its pronounced effect against ectoparasites as well. It is poorly soluble in water, decomposes slowly, and remains in the environment for a long time. Its half life being about 10 years. It is very lipid soluble, and for this reason it accumulates in the fatty tissues and causes the signs of poisoning. In the human organism it can arrive via the food chain accumulating in the fat-rich organs and tissues. It easily penetrates the exoskeleton of insects but not the skin of mammals (the oral LD_{50} in rats is 118 mg/kg, and transdermal LD_{50} 2510 mg/kg). The toxic effect is primarily manifested in damage to the central nervous system. The sensory and motor neurons of the motor cortex are injured. The pathological alterations are very slight. Some animal experiments have mentioned liver damage, but it is reversible with cessation of exposure. The effect on the central nervous system can be explained by DDT blocking the Na^+ efflux across the membrane. The chance of fatal poisoning by chlorinated hydrocarbons is relatively slight. We see a toxic effect only after ingestion of a large dose of 10 mg/kg. In the human organism the LD_{50} is 300–500 mg/kg. A day after absorption we find the highest concentration in the serum, then appearing in the brain and musculature. It may be demonstrated from the fatty tissues for months, even years. The clinical signs are nausea, vomiting, lingual and oral paresthesia, insomnia, restlessness, then tremor, convulsions, respiratory disturbances and coma.

Due to its long half life, it has accumulated in the organisms even long after being banned throughout the world.

Aldrin and dieldrin belong to *chlorinated cyclodienes* and are more toxic than DDT, being absorbed across intact skin. Their toxic effect may be not only acute, but chronic as well. They are also terratogenic and carcinogenic compounds. The acute effect is primarily neurotoxicity, the biochemical background explaining that its effect is to alter the ratio of amino acids in the brain, and the ammonia concentration in the tissue increases. They are metabolized in the liver by epoxidation, and inasmuch as a product more toxic than the original form results, the metabolization can essentially be considered an activation reaction. Following intoxication the pupils are first constricted, then dilated. Hallucinations occur. Due to the constriction of the blood vessels the extremities are cooler, and muscle weakness, cramps, then muscle relaxation, coma, cyanosis and abdominal pain develops. The central nervous system is damaged. After poisoning, if the victim remains alive, the EEG may be pathological for months.

Herbal insecticides. In place of chemicals, herbal insecticides have been used not just from the viewpoint of protection of the environment, but from that of long experience. Numerous herbal insecticides are known and used.

Nicotine: An alkaloid of the tobacco plant (which contains 1–4%) in its purified form is colorless, odorless, strongly basic, and when left exposed to the air becomes oxidized and brownish with an unpleasant dottle odor. The *lethal dose* is 60 mg (1–2 drops!). It is formulated for insecticidal use in a 40% solution. It stimulates the autonomic ganglia – both sympathetic and parasympathetic – and the neuromuscular junctions, but also affects the central nervous system, the effect being to a certain degree similar to the picture of an elevated acetylcholine level: nausea, vomiting, diarrhea, perspiration, pupils first constricted and then dilated, the extremities cool due to the constriction of the blood vessels, muscle weakness, convulsions, then muscular relaxation, bradycardia, hypotonia, dyspnoe, and collapse. Death occurs due to respiratory paralysis which is the result of both the paralysis of the muscles of breathing and the respiratory center. It is a rapid poison which acts within minutes to hours. It can be absorbed across the skin, but the vapors are also toxic, and the absorption through the gastrointestinal tract after oral ingestion depends on the fullness of the stomach. After absorption it accumulates in the liver, kidneys and brain. A small part is eliminated unchanged in the urine, and the greater part is metabolized to biologically inactive compounds.

From the autopsy findings the corrosion of the mucous membranes of the mouth, and throat from the alkali affect can be mentioned. In the corroded areas are found thick, tough layers of mucus, and erosions, petechiae and edema can be found in the gastric mucosa with a reddish, tough mucus adhering to it. The effect on the stomach is that of an alkali.

- At the autopsy of a 21-year-old pregnant woman, the police surgeon found scratch injuries reminiscent of fingernail marks about the mouth and neck areas. This raised the possibility of homicide. The husband of the deceased admitted that he had previously beaten and kicked his wife, but denied any further assault and battery. After the beating his wife had disappeared. She was found in the vicinity of a corn silo. The autopsy did not support a manual strangulation. The injuries to the neck were only superficial scratches. In the stomach contents a faint odor of nicotine was detected without any morphological signs. The chemical examination verified nicotine poisoning, and after the autopsy a reexamination of the scene where the body was found turned up a few discarded, washed out boxes previously used for containing nicotine. The scratch marks to the mouth and neck originated from being thrown to the ground by the twitching.

Herbicides

Among the bipyridyl derivatives, *paraquat* is the most well known and toxic member of the group. Paraquat was developed as an oxidation-reduction indicator. In 1950 in England its herbicidal property was recognized and since then has been widely used in agriculture. The substance damages only the green leafy plants and is inactivated upon contact with the soil. It is distributed in different forms and under different names. The granulated form consists of 2.5% paraquat and 5% diquat. The liquid and aerosol forms contain 20–40% of the active substance. Although widely used, it presents few cases of occupational hazard, and tends to appear more in accidents or ingestion with suicidal intent. Mortality is given at 20–50%. According to our studies, a fatal outcome resulted within a few weeks of ingestion in 100% of the cases.

The clinical signs depend on the amount of poison. After ingestion of the concentrated substance local damage develops at the mouth and pharynx, the mucous membranes of the esophagus and in the stomach. Diarrhea is common. It damages the liver and kidneys. The victim becomes comatose, and soon after ingestion of the poison pulmonary edema develops and death ensues within days. Following the ingestion of a slight amount of poison the initial symptoms are mild, and sometimes the victim complains only of nausea. A day later pain at the mouth and throat develop. If the anamnestic data of the patient does not indicate ingestion of paraquat, the diagnosis is almost always in error! Kidney and liver damage appear on the second and third days, the urine amount decreases and the patient becomes jaundiced. Blood creatin, bilirubin and transaminase levels rise. If he survives this damage, the consequence which leads to death is the respiratory distress, which in days or sometimes weeks is noticed after ingestion of the poison, and in the background lies a progressive pulmonary fibrosis specifically caused by the substance.

- The picture is so characteristic that when the body of a 54-year-old man was autopsied, the possibility of paraquat poisoning was suggested on the basis of the pathological alterations in the lung tissue. The toxin determination was not performed, the patient had survived two weeks in the medical facility, but on the basis of the histological examination, the special forensic examination also supported paraquat poisoning. An investigation established that two days before being brought to hospital the wife of the deceased had given her undiscerning, alcoholic husband a 0.5 dl dose of paraquat in his daily rum and poisoned him *(Fig. 172)*.

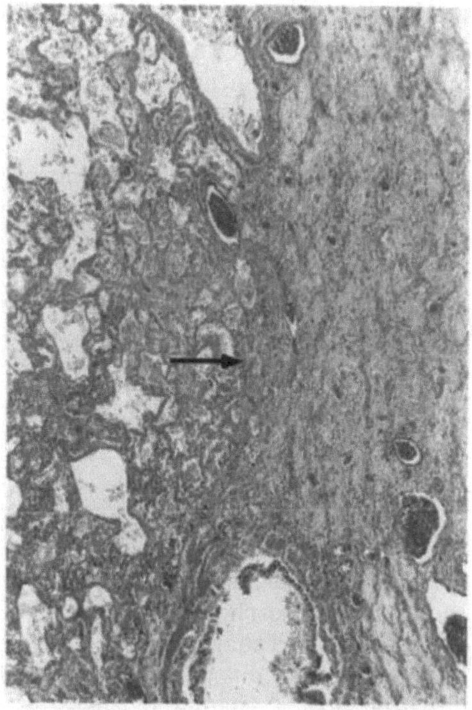

Fig. 172. Diffuse fibrosis to the lobular border. Besides the fibrosis hyalin membrane formation can be seen in the aircontaining portions of the lung, paraquate poisoning

Among the treatment possibilities, numerous procedures are used, over which the opinions on their effectiveness is strongly divided. They are: emptying the stomach after poisoning, forced diuresis, hemodialysis and hemoperfusion. Treatment by superoxide dismutase is recommended on the basis of experiments, by which the free H_2O_2 radicals which are the intermediates of paraquat are eliminated. Others recommend immunosuppressive treatment. We have not seen results from the above treatments in the clinics. The patient despite lengthy, careful treatment progresses to a state of respiratory distress.

At autopsy the pharynx and the mucous membranes of the esophagus is swollen, edematous, as is the gastric mucosa as well. The lungs are distended, heavy, compact, later having parts with a muscle-like texture. These are airless areas macroscopically reminiscent of carnificated pneumonia. Histologically the lung tissue is edematous with a large number of alveolar macrophages in the alveoli, hyaline membrane, organizing fibrin, with respiratory metaplastic squamous epithelia. Toxic myocarditis can be seen in the myocardium, centrilobular necrosis in the hepatic tissue, and acute tubular damage in the kidneys.

Rodenticides

The most widely varied chemicals are known for the extermination of rodents. HCN, strychnine sulfate, zinc phosphate, and elemental phosphorus have been used for a long time. Today coumarin derivatives are used for this purpose.

Warfarin is a vitamin K antagonist (structural analog), forming an inactive precursor in place of the bioactive precursor for the vitamin K dependent clotting factors (gamma carboxylation of the glutamyl side chain) thus inhibiting their formation and their de novo synthesis. Thus prothrombin synthesis decreases, due to the failure of carboxylation of the numerous glutamyl side chains, and a bioactive precursor to prothrombin is not formed. From this bioactive material bound to the surface of the thrombocytes, active thrombin is formed by limited proteolysis. Poisoning occurs with the ingestion of 0.5–1 kg (!?). Days later nose bleeds and dermal hemorrhages appear, anemia, bleeding into the joints, stools turning bloody, and blood in the urine can be demonstrated. Then stroke and hemorrhagic shock may follow. Pronounced decrease in prothrombin level which is correctable by vitamin K helps the diagnosis.

Narcotic poisoning

For decades the number of drugs used without medical prescription has significantly risen, and with these the combinations, whether medicines or other substances – for example alcohol – used to reach a dazed state. In recent years an increase in the use of the so-called *hard drugs* have come to be expected her in the European Countries causing serious economical, social and medical situations. The threatening danger is evidenced as well from previous data already collected showing that the seeds of narcosis-producing plants and weeds have been consumed as a substitute narcotic, a so-called cocktail of the exudate of the pod of the poppy which has a similar effect to morphine, can be expected from the East European Countries, which besides the narcotic effect, brings with it other medical problems (embolism with parts of plants, anaphylactic reactions etc.). The danger of habituation to these is also significant. Especially if hard drugs come into traffic, then they bring not only a medical but a criminal danger. "Of the various drugs, a dependency on narcotics is such a psychological and sometimes physical state in which the drug and the organism mutually affect one another, which is characterized a behavioral or other response, in which the person is always continually or periodically occupied by the compulsion to take the drug and the cessation of exposure produces uses an uncomfortable feeling." (WHO)

Habituation and dependency can develop with many drugs, such as opium and its derivatives, barbiturates, certain sedatives, diazepam, cocaine, amphetamine derivatives and certain organic solvents. Among these it is possible to formulate by common agreement a discrete group of drugs to which a dependence develops sooner or later after ingestion, and the cessation of administration brings with it withdrawal symptoms.

Cocaine

The alcaloid of Erithroxylon coca has been known for centuries as having a stimulating, sense-sharpening effect when chewed. It is used as a local anesthetic and is an excellent desensitizer of mucous membranes. This bitter, white crystalline substance is easily soluble in alcohol. The *lethal oral dose* is 1.2 g. It has a sympatheticomimetic effect, but interferes with the adrenerg nerve transmission, norepinephrine and causes such cardiovascular signs as tachycardia, sudden rise in blood pressure and vasoconstriction. When administered intravenously it immediately affects the myocardium and may cause sudden death. Cocaine is *sniffed as a powder* by 39% of the users, using the base for this since the euphoric effect is greater than that of cocaine hydrochloride, which can be administered intravenously. In poisoning the lethal blood level is 0.9–21 mg/l. In some cases values of around 1.06 mg% have been measured when the drug smugglers have swallowed balloon-containing drugs and the balloon burst in the digestive tract. Anaphylaxia and death from it has been described following cocaine ingestion, this being a reflection of the purity of the so-called street preparations. Cocaine is commonly taken with other drugs, especially heroin or other opiates *(speed ball)*. Cocaine significantly potentiates the effect of heroin. With acute poisoning: tachycardia, mydriasis, hypertension, hyperreflexia, tremor, convulsions, hallucinations, muscle spasms, doxogenic mental alterations develop. The intoxicated person in a state of cocaine paranoia may commit crimes.

With chronic intoxication euphoria, anorexia, personality changes, and mental deterioration occur. Habituation is not so pronounced as with morphine and heroin, although the physical dependency is strong. The withdrawal symptoms are not stormy; the patient complains of feeling chills.

In the organism *cocaine is metabolized slowly* in the liver, thus the intoxication is prolonged. Its metabolite benzoylecgonine is eliminated in the urine.

The autopsy findings are not characteristic, the organs are engorged with blood, pulmonary edema may develop, the mucous membranes of the nasal septum may be ulcerated, or the septum may even be perforated, this being explained by the local vasoconstrictor effect of cocaine on the vessels of the mucous membranes. A significant portion of the lethal cases are the result of intravenous administration. Gas chromatography, immunological methods and RIA can be used for the determination of cocaine, the limit of demonstration being 1.0–20 micrograms/ml. Lately EMIT (Enzyme, Multiplication Immunological Technique) has been used.

LSD (lysergic acid diethylamide)

This is a compound first synthesized in 1938 in Switzerland which is effective in small doses, colorless and odorless. A year later human experimentation was conducted in which the uterotonic effect similar to ergotamine was noticed. It is a hallucinogen (similar to mescaline and psilocybin). The half life is three hours. In fatal cases the plasma level is 9.5×10^{-9} g/kg. Pronounced changes in behavior can be produced by $25–50 \times 10^{-9}$ g. Its psychomimetic effect is explained by its being a 5-hydroxytryptamine (serotonin) antagonist. Auditory, visual and olfactory hallucinations and sensations occur in very colorful forms with geometrical and kaleidoscopic figures in motion with a rainbow of colors. Perception of distance, size and space is disturbed. A "trip", which is not always pleasant can occur with the ingestion of 200–400 micrograms. Hyperthermia, pyloerection, tachycardia, hypertension and hyperglycemia may accompany these "bad trips." Many have experienced a sudden returning "flashback" months after having used LSD. These manifest themselves in three forms:

perceptual; vivid, colorful visions and sounds,

somatic; paraesthesia, tachycardia,

emotional; panic reaction, depression, and later in more serious cases, suicide.

The substance, given intravenously binds to plasma proteins in the blood. It is rapidly metabolized almost completely in the liver chiefly by conjugation with glucuronic acid and is eliminated in the bile with only remnants being eliminated in the urine.

Marihuana

The resin of *cannabis sativa* or *cannabis indica* is known by many names, among which are marijuana and *hashish.* One of its active agents is tetrahydrocannabinol. Stupefaction upon the inhalation of the smoke from burning hemp was known by the ancient Greeks, but neither the Greeks nor the later European cultures made use of it. Its use appeared in the Far East cultures. Later in the American colonial period it came into use as a cultivated plant. Due to the extremely low toxicity the LD_{50} is unknown. Death following use is rare. A dried preparate of the raw flowering plant is used in cigarette form, and hashish used in the same way produces the same effect of marijuana with about one tenth the amount. The effect is variable depending not only upon the species of the plant, but upon the population, individual sensitivity and mode of use. When smoked like a cigarette, a small amount of the active agent is quickly absorbed. When chewed it is absorbed more slowly and produces a more intense and prolonged effect. Peripheral vasodilation is characteristic and the conjunctiva and sclera become blood-shot as one of the more obvious signs. Besides this, dizziness, insomnia, apathy, and fatigue develop as does an increase in the pulse rate, then euphoria and colorful dreams with dryness of the mouth, increased libido, depression, and at other times disturbances in alertness and behavior and unusual social behavior can be noticed. With chronic use inferiority complexes, hypersensitivity, irritability, insomnia, apathy, lethargy and deterioration of concentration and memory occur.

An increase in tolerance is not recognized, and indeed even the occurrence of "flashbacks" has sometimes been described. The half life is long and a cumulative effect is accepted. Its metabolization is not recognized.

Morphine

Opium is the greyish-white, resin-like secretion of the poppy capsule which has belonged to the group of medications and recreational drugs for thousands of years. Opium itself has been and is used primarily in the Far East, mostly by inhaling the smoke to achieve stupefaction. Morphine has the greatest practical significance among its alkaloids (morphine, narcotine, tebaine and codeine). The content of morphine in raw opium is 10%. Morphine is a basic alkaloid, a white crystalline substance with a bitter taste which is easily soluble in either water or alcohol with a therapeutic blood level of 0.01 mg%, and a toxic level of 0.1 mg%. The half life is four hours. It is well absorbed from the stomach, but its absorption is dependent upon the pH of the gastric contents. It also crosses the blood brain barrier and the placental barrier. The toxic dose is 60–100 mg. with 0.2–2,3 mg/l. blood concentration. Ninety percent of the ingested morphine is eliminated through the kidneys, partly in free and partly in glucuronic acid bound form, and 7–10% of the remaining quantity will be found in the stool.

Acute poisoning can occur with oral or parenteral ingestion. With oral ingestion the signs appear about 20 minutes later, while signs develop quite rapidly with parenteral and especially intravenous dosing. With acute ingestion due to the depressive effect on the central nervous system concentration diminishes while euphoria and tolerance to pain grow. The intoxicated person feels liberated. Perception of space and time decreases followed by feeling dryness in the mouth, narrow pupils, cyanosis, feeble and superficial breathing, pulmonary edema, cardiovascular depression, and coma. Before death the pupils dilate. The cause of death is respiratory insufficiency.

The autopsy findings in acute intoxication are not characteristic. Along with signs of acute congestion, the viscera are engorged with blood, cyanotic, the blood is fluid, and the pupils are occasionally narrowed to pinpoint size.

Parenteral administration is the common form of chronic intoxication. Needle marks from the injections can be found on the body and they are often extensively scarred. Due to the repeated use of improperly sterilized needles there will be inflammation and abscesses at the places of injection and on the body surface of the chronic user we find dermal alterations in various stages of development. Often we can find the signs of injections in the hidden skin surfaces such as the hairy areas of the head and the prepuce etc.

- Once a physician was admitted for chronic "depression" and the possibility of chronic morphine use was raised. Upon physical examination no trace of needle marks could be found on the surface of the body, but it turned out that the patient wore his socks continuously, even in bed, having mentioned that he caught cold easily. When this part of the body was examined as well the dorsal surface of the feet were discovered to be covered with syringe needle marks.

A general physical deterioration, dry and rough skin, alternating constipation and diarrhea, then irritability, apathy, and waning sexual function appear, and the previously active individual becomes inactive and disinterested.

From the autopsy findings alterations at the places of administration can be mentioned. Physical deterioration, infectious diseases (TB, hepatitis), nutritional disturbances may accompany the other changes, but there are no characteristic autopsy findings.

Withdrawal symptoms commence 4–8 hours after the last administration with watering eyes and runny nose, yawning, sweating, and restless sleep. After 20 hours appear pupillary dilation and agitated tremor. Within 2–3 days the symptoms become more pronounced: insomnia, weakness, pain in the extremities and muscles, a rise in blood pressure and pulse rate, sweating, dehydration and cardiovascular disturbances. Similar withdrawal symptoms have also been described in the newborn babies of addicted mothers!

The semi-synthetic morphine derivative of *heroin,* diacetylmorphine, is a white, water-soluble crystalline material which under the influence of esterase in the organism is metabolized to 6-monoacetylmorphine and then to morphine and normorphine. The greatest portion is eliminated in the urine as morphine or its conjugated form. Researchers have verified that the pharmacological effect can be expressed even after metabolization to 6-monoacetylmorphine. The effect is similar to that of morphine, but four times as strong (toxic level in plasma 0,12–0,25 mg/l) and shorter, with a greater danger of addiction, and for these reasons it is not used in medicine.

Poisoning by sedatives

Barbituric acid derivatives. These are among the most wide-spread medications, and due to their sedative and hypnotic effects, their accessibility, and their widespread use. Barbiturate intoxication is one of the most common forms of suicide.

From its first synthesis – 1903 Veronal – numerous derivatives have come into use, 1912 Luminal, then in the '20s and '30s one after another Amobarbital, Pentobarbital, and Hexobarbital.

Barbituric acid is a whitish, bitter crystalline substance which dissolves poorly in water, but their salts are better soluble.

They are classed into four groups according to their effects, *long-acting* (barbiturate, phenobarbiturate), medium-acting (butobarbital), *short-acting* (pentobarbital, secobarbital), and *ultra-short-acting* (thiopental, hexobarbital).

After oral ingestion they are absorbed from the stomach and small intestine relatively quickly. Some of the barbiturates are absorbed more quickly and effectively through the rectum than from the stomach. It is distributed in the tissues and body fluids, and also crosses the placental barrier and can be detected in the tissues of the fetus. Its metabolism occurs by oxidation at the C–5 position, the ethyl group being resistant to oxidation, with the longer acetyl group oxidized to secondary alcohols, and the carboxyl derivatives undergoing beta oxidation. Among the derivatives the phenol or alcohol metabolites are conjugated with glucuronic acid. Metabolization occurs in the liver, primarily in the microsomal fraction. The barbiturates and their metabolites are eliminated primarily in the urine and only a small part can be found in the stool. Elimination is quite a long process and traces of the medication can be found in the urine even 12 days after ingestion.

The usual therapeutic dosage – providing there is no hypersensitivity reaction – causes no harm. Acute intoxication occurs with the ingestion of an amount 5–10 times the therapeutic dosage which results in a plasma level of about 0,8–19 mg/l. The diagnosis of poisoning is based on the anamnestic data and the clinical signs as well as on the results of the toxicological examination. General signs are depression, a fall in body temperature, hypoxia, cyanosis, urine retention, then stupor, coma and depressed respiration. In more serious cases circulatory insufficiency develops. Later, due to circulatory and respiratory insufficiency, bronchopneumonia develops in the hypostatic areas. For therapy the first thing recommended is to remove the unabsorbed drug from the stomach. (In our own practice we have several times noticed at the autopsy of barbiturate poisoning victims who had died days after ingestion of the drug, that a large quantity of tablet remnants could be found in the stomach, the continuous slow absorption of which resulted in a high barbiturate blood level.)

The autopsy of victims of sedative poisoning is usually characteristic. Red, bullous dermal alterations can be found on the skin of 6% of the poisoning victims, which are the result of local vessel spasms due to hypersensitivity. With histological examination of some of the areas of the bullae, a histological picture similar to the Leyel syndrome is portrayed, so the formation of bullae on barbiturate poisoning victims reflects the toxic effect of the material. The blood is fluid, the urinary bladder full, and hypostatic pneumonia develops.

Sending urine and blood samples from the intoxicated patient for toxicological examination is imperative.

Chronic barbiturate intoxication can be easily mistaken for neuropsychiatric illness or chronic alcoholism. The chronic ingestion of sedatives usually involves pentobarbital, secobarbital, or amobarbital. When beginning administration the sleep time is lengthened, and then depending on development of tolerance, the period returns to its previous length. Withdrawal causes varying complaints, with sometimes convulsions, other times hallucinations developing. The clinical presentation resembles alcohol intoxication or acute barbiturate poisoning. It can be differentiated from alcohol intoxication in that the physical deterioration of the chronic alcoholic is not found. With chronic administration mental alterations develop: decrease in emotional control, paranoia, antagonistic behavior, and suicide attempts, but the true toxic hallucinations and psychosis are rare. Neurological signs are dysarthria, ataxia, nystagmus, tremor and a positive Babinsky.

Tranquilizers

Benzodiazepine derivates

Three forms are recognized in medical practice: chlordiazepoxide, diazepam and oxazepam (oxazepam is the metabolite of diazepam!). They have sedative, anticonvulsive, and muscle relaxant effects. In elderly patients even small doses can depress the central nervous system. They have an accumulative effect, the half life in large doses being 48 hours in the organism. The highest blood level is achieved 40–60 minutes after ingestion. The effect of chlordiazepoxide is the longest while that of oxazepam is the shortest. They are rapidly absorbed through the small intestine within 30–180 minutes after ingestion with a portion being secreted into the stomach from where it is reabsorbed or eventually eliminated in the stool. They are quickly and practically totally metabolized and the metabolites are eliminated in the urine. During their metabolization active substances are produced. Their properties are rather common, but do not cause a serious toxic harm, so that even after ingestion of 500–1500 mg serious signs do not appear. (With this amount the blood level is 18 micrograms/ml.) The literature of 1979 reports 1239 cases of poisoning by benzodiazepine derivatives with two of them fatal. Damage to the respiratory center may accompany intravenous dosing. It may appear rather symptomless, with sleepiness or coma. At the beginning of the poisoning extrapyramidal signs may appear with dryness of the mouth, dilated pupils and tachycardia. Among the side effects are sleepiness, ataxia, lethargy, changes in libido, ovulatory and menstrual complaints, and a decrease in tolerance to alcohol may play a role in syncope with elderly patients. With a continual high dosing (chlordiazepoxide 300 mg, diazepam 80 mg/day) a physical dependency may develop with withdrawal symptoms appearing upon cessation.

The autopsy findings are not characteristic.

Meprobamate

This is a tranquillizer with muscle relaxant effects. The therapeutic blood level is 1 mg% and lethal dose is 15 mg%. The half life is 10–11 hours. It is 4–5 times less toxic than barbiturates, with a lethal poisoning occurring with the ingestion of 10–40 g. With intoxication insomnia, pin-point pupils, stupor, coma, areflexia, fall in blood pressure, decrease in pulse rate, and respiratory and cardiovascular collapse develop. The highest blood level is reached 1–2 hours after ingestion and remains for hours. The significant portion is metabolized and 90% of the metabolized forms are eliminated in the urine. In the break down process hydroxymeprobamate is formed and then conjugated with glucuronic acid, but this has no pharmacological significance. The remaining 10% is eliminated in the urine unchanged.

Hemodialysis and hemoperfusion is used in treatment, but peritoneal dialysis has not yielded good results. It, and especially its metabolites, can be demonstrated in the urine. The autopsy findings are not characteristic.

Phenothiazide derivates

The phenothiazides belong to the class of major tranquillizers, and are used mainly in the treatment of psychiatric disorders. Tricyclic compounds with substitutions at the number 10 and 2 positions yield the three major groups: 1. aliphatic, 2. piperidine, 3. piperazine derivatives.

The common property of all three groups is that they block both peripheral and central dopamine receptors. They are administered both orally and parenterally. The highest blood level is reached 2–4 hours after ingestion of a therapeutic dosage. The level remains for 3–4 hours and then decreases. The drug is bound almost 100% to plasma albumin. With oral ingestion an enterohepatic circulation can be expected. The greater portion of the absorbed phenothiazide is secreted with the bile into the intestine and reabsorbed. (Even with parenteral administration an enterohepatic circulation can be observed.) The main form of biotransformation in the liver is by demethylation and hydroxylation. The metabolites have less effect than the original form has, but their side effects are significant. The next step in biotransformation of the newly formed compounds is binding to glucuronic acid. The conjugated metabolites are eliminated in the urine. About nine metabolites are eliminated in the urine of humans following administration of chlorpromazine. Due to retention in the tissues the phenothiazide derivatives can be detected in the urine six months after administration. They have a broad application due to their antiemetic, potentiation (narcotics), and antipsychotic effects. Due to their potentiation effect they should be used with care, or avoided, when morphine or morphine-like substances, barbiturates, antihistamines or alcohol are also used. With preoperative use a hypotonic crisis may develop during the course of anesthesia.

With acute intoxication the central nervous system is depressed with the development of insomnia, ataxia, apathy, vomiting, dilated pupils, visual disturbances, dryness of the mouth, tachycardia, chills, constipation, hypotonia and coma. Parkinson-like symptoms can be expected.

Among the side effects accompanying chronic use agranulocytosis is mentioned, hypotonia, hepatitis and photosensitive dermatitis. The lethal blood level is between 1,0–5,0 mg/l and the therapeutic blood level is 0.5mg/l. The autopsy findings are not characteristic. For the toxicological examination of the corpse a large amount must be taken from the liver.

Alcohol intoxication

The alcohols are hydroxyl derivatives of longer or shorter chain aliphatic carbohydrates. Their toxicity increases with the length of the carbon chain, with the exception of methanol, which is a great deal more toxic than ethanol. The divalent alcohols, or glycols with their sweet taste are conspicuous in this group and their wide-spread use accounts for their frequent appearance in poisoning cases. Their clinical signs, their metabolization by the same enzymes and the characteristics of the therapy justify the classification of these members into one group.

Ethylene glycol

Ethylene glycol is a colorless, odorless, sweet liquid which mixes well with water and alcohol. Its boiling point is 197.5 °C. It is widely used in industry, laboratories, automobile cooling and brake fluid and these latter few account for the bulk of the cases of poisoning (due to its sweetening property it played a prominent role in the production of fake Austrian wines which caused numerous poisonings when ethylene glycol was used to improve the wines, but in 1987 in Pécs (Hungary) ethylene glycol also got into the water pipe system and also caused mass intoxication).

The lethal dose of ethylene glycol is 100 g, but some have survived the ingestion of 240 ml. The lethal blood level is 200 mg%. The signs of intoxication appear a short time after ingestion – 1–2 hours. The victim appears drunk, but there is no odor of alcohol on the breath. There is nausea, vomiting, abdominal pains, diarrhea, a burning warm feeling in the mouth and throat, irritability, babbling, ataxia, increase in pulse rate, depression, and dyspnoe. Deep depression, coma, increases in pulse and breathing rate, convulsions, serious acidosis, oliguria, capillary damage and hematuria develop 3–12 hours later.

The autopsy findings include subpleural and subendocardial hemorrhages, bleeding in the tissue of the lungs, heart, kidneys and brain, edema of the brain, damage to the pyramidal cells, the appearance of calcium oxalate crystals, then pulmonary edema and bronchopneumonia.

In the later stages of intoxication 3–4 days following ingestion kidney damage dominates the pathological picture. The epithelial cells of the proximal tubules show damage, with calcium oxalate crystals and lipoid deposits accumulating. The epithelial cells of the convoluted tubules necrotize, the glomeruli swell with the basal membrane becoming thicker and containing granular deposits. The clinical picture reflects acidosis from the effect of the metabolic by-products.

Alcohol dehydrogenase (ADH) plays a significant role in the metabolisation of ethylene glycol. In the course of metabolization glycol aldehyde, then glycolic acid, glyoxylic acid, formic acid and oxalic acid are formed. The significant portion of the metabolites is eliminated in the urine (the deposition of calcium oxalate crystals from the urine has pathological significance!), but the unmetabolized ethylene glycol is also eliminated. About 0.25–2.5% of the ethylene glycol forms oxalic acid.

The competitive effect of ethanol is used in the treatment. In the presence of alcohol ADH does not break down ethylene glycol and thus the metabolization of ethylene glycol – which would yield numerous toxic metabolites – is delayed. Alcohol therapy – 10 g/hour – must begin within eight hours of intoxication and continue for five days. Among the metabolites glycolic acid level in the serum and urine reflect the seriousness of the intoxication and the effectiveness of the treatment. With children the alcohol treatment does not always yield good results and hemodialysis should be preferred for a better effect.

Methyl alcohol poisoning

The physical characteristics are similar to those of ethyl alcohol. I has a boiling point is 64 °C, is inflammable and dissolves well in water. The lethal dose, depending upon sensitivity, is 75 ml. It has an industrial use – as an organic solvent and in the production of paints and plastics – and laboratory use. Imperfectly distilled drinks sometimes contain as much as 5%. It is absorbed through the skin and airways, which may be the main mode of effect in accidents, while oral ingestion happens by mistaking it for ethanol.

- In our practice we have examined massive methanol intoxication. 103 poisoning victims were admitted to the institute in 1965 when several liters of methanol were stolen from a railroad storage car and consumed. Three died and several suffered damage to the optic nerves.

Six to 24 hours after intoxication headache, nausea, vomiting, fatigue, dizziness, and diplopia develop, then abdominal pains, visual disturbances and shallow breathing begin with delirium, unconsciousness, coma and death. A pronounced acidosis is characteristic the manifestation of which is due to the role played by the methanol metabolites. Methanol metabolism, ingested by the organism resembles ethanol except that it is oxidized nine times slower by ADH. Besides this other mechanisms are involved in the elimination of methanol, the most probable part being taken by catalase system which breaks down the alcoholic hydroxyl radicals of other compounds besides methanol. (In animal experiments the role of catalase has been unambiguously shown to break down methanol.) During metabolization ADH generates formaldehyde from methanol which is then oxidized to formic acid.

$$\underset{\text{methanol}}{CH_3OH} \xrightarrow{\text{ADH}} \underset{\text{formaldehyde}}{CH-COH} \xrightarrow{\text{ALDH}} \underset{\text{formic acid}}{HCOOH} + CO_2 + H_2O.$$

The latter is responsible for the development of acidosis in the victim. Those examinations in which after ingestion of methanol the direct inhibition of ADH by administration of pyrazole results in delayed or significantly decreased metabolization and no acidosis illustrate the role of ADH. The above break down process of methanol is slow, taking days to be eliminated under experimental circumstances.

Four ml of methanol can cause visual damage, partly from the formaldehyde and partly from the formic acid. In animal experiments a high level of formic acid has been described while the formaldehyde concentration was not significant. The inhibitory effect of formic acid on the activity of cytochrome oxidase lies behind the damage. The morphological basis of the visual damage is degeneration of the retina and optic nerve, and the process is slow, sometimes developing over a period of months.

The autopsy findings are not characteristic. The organs are engorged with blood, and have an odor of alcohol if a large amount was ingested. Sometimes small subarachnoidal or subpleural hemorrhages can be found which can be demonstrated 2–3 days after poisoning with methanol in the body fluids.

In the treatment the competitive effect of ethanol as described in the treatment of ethylene glycol poisoning is employed. Otherwise symptomatic treatment – management of acidosis – and later removal of the metabolites by hemodialysis can be used.

Ethyl alcohol

It has been used not only as a flavoring substance, but as an important medication before the damaging effects were known. In the textbook of pharmacology written 35 years ago we can find such descriptions of alcohol by the author of the excellent roborant effect upon dosing with alcohol and carbohydrate group. Similarly pregnant women were offered a daily infusion of alcohol to ensure a 1.00‰ blood level against threatened abortion. Today, due to the damaging effect of alcohol these treatment modalities are no longer used.

Ethyl alcohol is a colorless liquid with a characteristic odor, in greater concentrations causes a burning sensation in the mouth and pharynx, and completely dissolves in water. The alcohol content of different drinks varies, in beer 3–6, in wines 9–16, in vermouth 15–20, in liqueurs 20–25, in concentrated distilled spirits 35–50 volume percent. Spirits also contain a small amount of *fuel oils* which share the greatest homology with ethanol, especially amyl alcohol and capronic acid. The quantities of these can significantly influence the intoxicating effect of these drinks and create later complaints, the so-called "hang-over".

Ethanol primarily affects the central nervous system, easily crossing the biological membranes due to its excellent water solubility and small molecular size, and influences membrane transport. Experiments have verified that ethanol inhibits the activity of the Na^+K^+–ATPase. The effect of ethanol follows the changes in the blood alcohol concentration, the effect on the central nervous system being dependent on the alcohol concentration in the organism which also influences the development of the clinical signs.

Even a small amount can dilate the vessels of the skin resulting in a feeling of warmth, which "protects" the vasoconstriction effect of the cold. It is primarily the result of central vasomotor depression because there is no direct vasodilation among the peripheral effects. Alcohol following the consumption is absorbed from the gastrointestinal tract, firstly from the intestines, the stomach and lastly from the large intestine. Absorption depends on the fullness and content of the stomach. A concentration above 15% inhibits gastric motility and secretion, and irritates the mucous membranes. Resorption may take 35–120 minutes. In this individuality may play a role, since alterations disturbing absorption may prolong the resorption of the alcohol. The character of the drink also carries influence. Drinks with a high CO_2 content and concentrated drinks are absorbed more rapidly. Absorption from a full stomach is prolonged. The content of the gastrointestinal tract may otherwise influence the amount of alcohol absorbed. Food proteins may bind alcohol and fatty acids from the digestion of fats in the small intestine may form esters. Some investigations have been reported in which the general detoxification process has been shown to be responsible for the resorption loss in that alcohol bound to glucuronic acid in the liver is eliminated. Thus in an extreme case about 20% of the ingested alcohol may not be absorbed by the organism. The absorbed alcohol crosses the cell membrane by diffusion and is distributed in the organism's water compartments. This means the greater alcohol concentration in the higher water content organism. Widmark especially noted that alcohol diffusion into the fat tissue is quite low. The distribution forms quickly, the organs well-supplied with blood, reaching a concentration equal to that of the blood first. For example, within 10 minutes of oral ingestion of alcohol the alcohol concentration ratio in the brain to that of the cerebral arteries is 1 : 1.18. In early stages the alcohol content of the cubital venous blood significantly varies from that of the arterial blood. The average calculated 60 minute absorption maximum cannot be considered as an equal distribution (numerous investigations have confirmed that the even distribution develops at different times and over time the organs and body fluids vary significantly in their alcohol concentrations.) In this stadium the distribution is more dependent upon the blood supply of the organ and not its water content. An equal distribution can only be reached after achieving a balance in diffusion. The alcohol concentration in expired air follows relatively regularly after establishment of diffusion balance so that the alcohol content of 2100 ml of air equals that of 1 ml of blood. This provides the basis for the determination of blood alcohol level from the alcohol in the expired air. WIDMARK could also deduce the previous alcohol intake of the organism from the current alcohol level, or the measured alcohol concentration at the time the blood sample was taken reflects the amount of alcohol in the organism.

$$A = ct \times p \times r,$$

A = the alcohol content of the organism in grams,

p = body weight,

r = Widmark factor (for men 0.68–0.85, for women 0.55, on the average 0.7 is used),

ct = blood alcohol level in ‰.

$$r = \frac{\text{alcohol concentration in the organism}}{\text{alcohol concentration in the blood}}.$$

The difference in the values of r in men and women reflects the alcohol distribution in the fat and muscle tissues.

Of the absorbed alcohol, 90% is metabolized and 10% is eliminated unchanged in the expired air and urine. Only a small amount is removed via the saliva, sweat and bile. Metabolization takes place primarily in the liver tissue, although there is an ADH which "specifically" breaks down alcohol outside the liver which can be detected in the lungs, the gastric mucosa and in the kidneys, and which has no small amount and activity in the life of the fetus. Three systems participate in the metabolization of alcohol. The first place is occupied by the *ADH metabolic pathway,* but in especially high alcohol concentrations a significant role is played by the *microsomal ethanol oxidation system* (MEOS), and the role of *catalase* cannot be neglected.

ADH is a NAD^+ dependent enzyme, and the role of NAD is in electron transport. In the first step acetaldehyde is formed, and then later acetyl S CoA is formed which enters the tricarboxylic acid cycle and is oxidized to CO_2 and H_2O. The oxidation of acetaldehyde is rapid, so that after ingestion of alcohol only a small amount of acetaldehyde can be detected even after ingestion of a significant amount of alcohol. Certain drugs are capable of inhibiting the activity of aldehyde dehydrogenase, so that acetaldehyde increases and provides the biochemical basis for the disulfiram treatment.

The metabolism of alcohol brings with it changes in NAD^+–NADH ratios, and because of the number of NAD^+ dependent enzymes is significant, this can explain the practical effect alcohol intoxication can have on metabolism. After alcohol ingestion a NAD depletion develops which primarily affects gluconeogenesis, and this can explain the post-alcoholic hypoglycemia. The amino acids entering the citric acid cycle also are directed into metabolic pathway, and the amount of oxaloacetate pyruvate offer decreases, but the lactate and keto acid levels increase and ketoacidosis develops. The process finally results in fatty degeneration of the liver cells.

Since the 1932 publication by Widmark, it has been accepted that there is a linear decrease with the metabolism of alcohol. Thus the metabolization follows the so-called "zero-order kinetics" and this means that the breakdown rate is independent of substrate concentration. According to this the K_m value of ADH is 9.7 mg% and the V_{max} is 23.3 mg%. If the blood alcohol concentration is given to be 100 mg% (1.00‰), this is ten times the K_m value and according to zero-order kinetics the elimination rate is 100 mg/kg/hour. For a 70 kg individual this amounts to about 7 g of alcohol eliminated per hour. This blood alcohol level of 0.15‰ or 15 mg%/hour, which is also the Widmark beta value. In later years the opinion became divided on the linear state of alcohol elimination and several articles appeared which used the Widmark beta value as a standard, while others pointed out the changeability of the Widmark factor. According to the conditions, the metabolism of alcohol does not occur as a zero-order kinetic reaction, but rather obeys the Michaelis-Menten equation. A faster break down of alcohol occurs at higher alcohol concentrations with the adaptation of ADH and this can be expected not only with high alcohol levels, but with repeated consumption of alcohol. In investigations of alcohol metabolism following a previous chronic ingestion of alcohol, the usual beta value was not measured, but rather a decay rate two or three times higher was found.

From the previous mentioned data the ideal blood-alcohol curve can be derived in which the first 90 minutes represents the absorption phase and this section changes not only with absorption by the individual but also with the occasion, or a distribution time must be expected. In this period the blood-alcohol values are not regular and in this time it is not possible to calculate a real value! This section is followed by such a dynamic state of balance in which there is a balance between alcohol absorption and elimination, and which lasts only a short while and in which follows the development of a balance in diffusion. This is already the elimination section in which the previously described blood-alcohol curve becomes regular and the level decreases evenly hour by hour. In this stadium the blood alcohol concentration can be derived from the blood-alcohol curve by measuring a portion being eliminated *(Fig. 173)*.

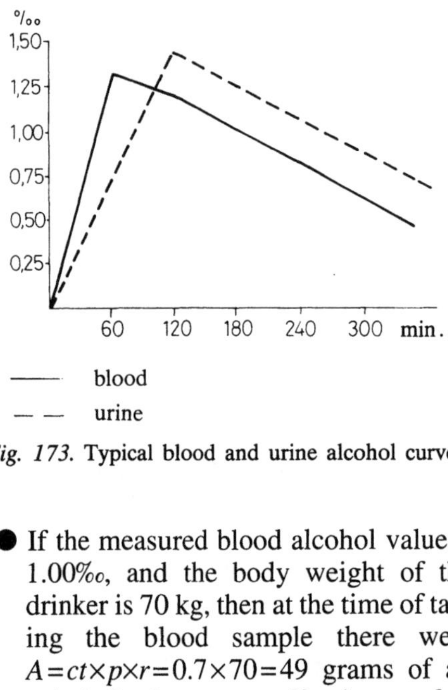

Fig. 173. Typical blood and urine alcohol curves

- If the measured blood alcohol value is 1.00‰, and the body weight of the drinker is 70 kg, then at the time of taking the blood sample there were $A = ct \times p \times r = 0.7 \times 70 = 49$ grams of alcohol. On the average 60 minutes after drinking we can expect the beginning of the elimination. In this stadium we can only calculate backwards to derive the alcohol level of the previous sample. The hourly per mil value is 0.15‰, which expressed in grams is an alcohol level of 7 grams.

The blood-alcohol curve regularity permits the monitoring of changes in urine alcohol values. In the absorption stage, the urinary alcohol remains under the blood alcohol values, and after achievement of a state of balance the urinary alcohol concentration exceeds that of the blood alcohol concentration by a relationship of 1:1.20–1.30. We can use this in deciding whether the blood sample was taken during the absorption stage or the elimination stage. Thus we can avoid the discomfort of a duplicate blood sample giving less information. (The duplicate blood sample is of value if alcohol ingestion had taken place within 10–20 minutes of taking the first sample, and the second sample should be taken 30 minutes later. If one hour lapses between the taking of the two samples, is isn't certain that the second sample might not have been taken when the elimination stage had already begun and from the decreasing value we cannot determine in which stage the intervention took place.) Alcohol in the cerebrospinal fluid also behaves similarly to the concentration of alcohol in the urine.

The urinary alcohol values sometimes significantly exceed the described urinary-blood alcohol ratio. After injury, prolonged unconsciousness, sedative poisoning or cooling an extremely high urinary alcohol value may provide a clue to the previous condition. In such instances the urinary-blood alcohol ratio may reach 1.6–2.2.

Establishing the presence of an alcoholic state by the so-called back calculation brings with it several difficulties. The first is that the blood alcohol curve behaves regularly only under ideal conditions, after ingestion of a simple measured drink. With repeated ingestion a new absorption section starts with each drink, which is followed by the development of a repeated equilibrium state, and if zero order kinetics are involved 7 g of alcohol are evenly broken down and we should derive this value by back calculation.

In elimination of small concentrations of alcohol ADH plays the leading role in which a significant rate of break down by a linear Widmark type elimination is shown and in this case zero-order kinetics are obeyed. With the increase in alcohol tolerance the reaction process speeds up and accelerated elimination of smaller alcohol levels below 1.50‰ can be expected. Besides the adaptation of ADH, the appearance of an atypical isoenzyme whose K_m value is higher plays a part. With higher concentrations of alcohol not only these factors are responsible for the accelerated elimination, but the role of the MEOS must be taken into account as well, which is effective at higher alcohol levels due to its higher K_m value. Genetic factors should also be mentioned in the development of alcohol tolerance, which are characteristic not only of individual populations, but of groups within populations.

In the organism alcohol is distributed in the water compartments. The water content of the living organism is significant, composing 70% of the body weight. Thus it is understandable that after intake of fluids – infusion, transfusion – if it were a significant amount, it can cause a serious change in the blood alcohol level. Thus if a sample was not taken before the medication, it can and must be done either during or after the fluid support, since in any case it is informative. If negative, its influence can be excluded, and if a we get a value indicating its influence, it is the duty of the forensic pathologist to determine what the value was.

The alcohol content of expired air provides the possibility for the so-called *"breathalizer"* test. In expired air 2100 ml contains as much alcohol as 1 ml of blood does. Alcohol disappears from the oral cavity only 30–40 minutes after the ingestion and this depends on the concentration of the drink. Beyond that period the alcohol given off by the lungs is all that is determined. The so-called "breathalizer" is an orientation procedure, and only signifies that the ingestion of alcoholic beverage was possible. It is not possible to measure its influence, because, as already mentioned, a measurement of the flowing air is also required, but even in that case significant errors can be expected. The orientation character of the breathalizer is also shown in that any material that can reduce the probe's reagent will cause a false positive indication of alcohol ingestion. In practice this has happened in many cases, and there is not a single procedure that without exception one can base the demonstration of alcohol in expired air. For this reason it is necessary to follow the regulations scrupulously, since smoking or eating can give a false positive for a little while. If a false positive is suspected, or if the person being tested protests the positivity of the probe, according to the regulations a blood sample must be taken to determine the alcohol level. Many times taking the alcohol level of expired air the possibility was raised that there might have been alcohol vapors in the environmental air, and thus the alcohol content of the inspired air could have had some influence.

● A 40-year-old chemist was driving while intoxicated, the level of intoxication being shown at 1.6‰ blood alcohol level. The physical examination demonstrated being under the influence. Later he stated that in the car a half hour prior to the test a bottle of industrial alcohol was broken and the vapors of the industrial alcohol had caused the influence.

If the alcohol concentration in the air of the work place is 20 mg/l, the consequence is an irritating effect, coughing, burning feeling, and irritation of the conjunctiva and nasal mucosa, but one can get used to it in 10 minutes. With 30 mg/l concentration there is a continuous watering of the eyes and feeling of discomfort. Although the alcohol in the air can get into the airways, such a small amount is resorbed that it does not cause a measurable alcohol concentration in the blood.

In the organism a small amount of ethanol is formed from the food. The origin is fermentation in the intestine, the amount is small and is given as the so-called *endogenous alcohol* level of 0.15 mg% which corresponds to 0.0015%. Among the healthy a higher level will not be expected. Lately Japanese researchers have published results showing that a significant "endogenous" alcohol production can be expected, pointing out that it is primarily found in the Far East. In a 24-hour blood sample of diabetic patients various alcohols can be demonstrated including ethanol. It has similarly been demonstrated in alcohol testing of infected urine. It is nevertheless surprising that today it has been the observation of a significant number of representative cases a high blood alcohol level has been demonstrated in subjects who had not previously ingested alcohol, in such diseases in which there had been a previous high carbohydrate diet and moniliasis. This caused a massive intragastric production of alcohol in which a member of the Candida group – colonizing the intestinal tract – caused the fermentation of alcohol. Such disease cases have also been published in which symptoms of alcohol intoxication developed with the 75% carbohydrate diet of the hospital, with a 2.54‰ blood alcohol concentration and examination of the gastrointestinal tract verified a massive Candida infection. The process has been named the *intragastrointestinal alcohol fermentation syndrome,* and calls to attention the diagnostic possibility and significance. A significant part of the published cases include previous surgical intervention (gastrectomy, cholecystectomy).

The clinical signs of *acute alcohol intoxication* can be characteristic. The autopsy findings in lethal poisoning, however, are weak. The organs smell of alcohol, the esophagus and gastric mucosa show pin-point hemorrhages, and besides pulmonary edema, only the laboratory tests can give the final diagnosis. In cases of suspected alcohol poisoning a blood sample must be taken for testing from the corpse as soon as possible after finding the body. The sample must purposely be taken from such a location where postmortal decay would not be expected to have occurred. The postmortal processes, especially if we examine only the urine sample, can yield misleading results. Widmark had already mentioned how problematic the examination of only the urine sample can be. Since we know that infected urine *in vitro* and if left standing, and in the bladder of the corpse we can count on fermentation processes producing alcohol, and caution is called for. The change in the postmortal ethanol level in the blood sample or the production of alcohol can result in a misleading opinion. Some take into consideration the alcohol fermentation in the corpse of carbohydrate containing infusions. After the examination of a large number of cases, we have not been able to confirm this. For this is necessary not only the consumption of carbohydrates, but the proliferation of such pathogens which are capable of fermenting alcohol. The occasionally formed ethanol does not distribute itself by regular diffusion, but rather a high concentration can be found locally at the site of production. For this reason in the case of suspected postmortal alcohol fermentation it is necessary to take blood from several areas – from the femoral veins on both sides, the cubital veins, the urine, the cerebrospinal fluid, the vitreous humor – and examine the alcohol content. Postmortal alcohol production can be easily verified by specific – gas chromatography, perhaps mass spectrophotometry – examinations, since in this case other products of fermentation besides ethanol can also be detected: acetaldehyde, acetic acid, ketones, furans, pyroles, and alcohols with a molecular weight between 40–160.

Mushroom poisoning

In Europe, where the gathering of wild mushrooms is popular, every year several hundred cases of mushroom poisoning occur. The most common is the amanita type poisoning.

Amanita phalloides, accounts for about 90% of the cases, and the poisoning follows two phases: after a latent period of 8–12 hours the patient develops abdominal pain, nausea, vomiting and profuse diarrhea with an severe lost of fluid and electrolytes, occasionally with fever, tachycardia and hypotonia, then the patient may be symptom-free for a few days, but then the symptoms of liver damage appear with high enzyme values, jaundice, circulatory insufficiency, kidney damage, and hemorrhage. Serious liver damage and hepatocellular necrosis lies behind this, and hepatic coma precedes death. Rarely the renal changes dominate the pathological picture. Death occur 2–4 days later *(Fig. 174).*

Autopsy findings: pin-point hemorrhages in the skin, under the serous membranes and periaortally, fatty degeneration develops in the viscera being most pronounced in the liver and kidneys. The liver is shrunken, yellowish-red and colored by hemorrhages. Histologically, a serious fatty degeneration can be seen in the liver cells, and in the area of the destroyed lobules among the remnants of the necrotic cells hemorrhages and leukocyte infiltration can be found. In the kidneys the epithelia of the proximal tubules are damaged, with fatty degeneration and infiltrated by monocytes. The ingestion of 20 g of mushrooms is lethal, the LD_{50} of amatoxin being 0.1 mg/kg. The toxins of the mushroom, *phallotoxin* and *amatoxin,* are cyclic heptapeptides. Amatoxin is responsible for the hepatorenal damage, its toxicity being 10–20 times that of phallotoxin. It has a significant affinity to hepatocytes and the epithelial cells of the convoluted tubules of the kidney. The effect of the toxin is increased by the enterohepatic circulation and after being eliminated in the bile it is reabsorbed, but the part eliminated by the kidney is also reabsorbed from the glomerular filtrate. Biochemically, amanitin binds to RNA polymerase inhibiting the production of mRNA. As a result, due to the inhibition of protein synthesis, the affected cells are destroyed. The damage to protein synthesis also affects the clotting factors, so that disturbances in factors V–VII–VIII. can account for the hemorrhages found at autopsy, since phallotoxin is membrane-specific and damages the hepatocytes, binding to the protein microfilaments in the plasma of the hepatocytes. In isolated hepatocytes phallotoxin can cause damage within 5–10 minutes. The cells swell up, the calcium level decreases markedly, and lysosomal enzymes are activated. The damage primarily affects the cells with a high protein synthesis. The treatment de-

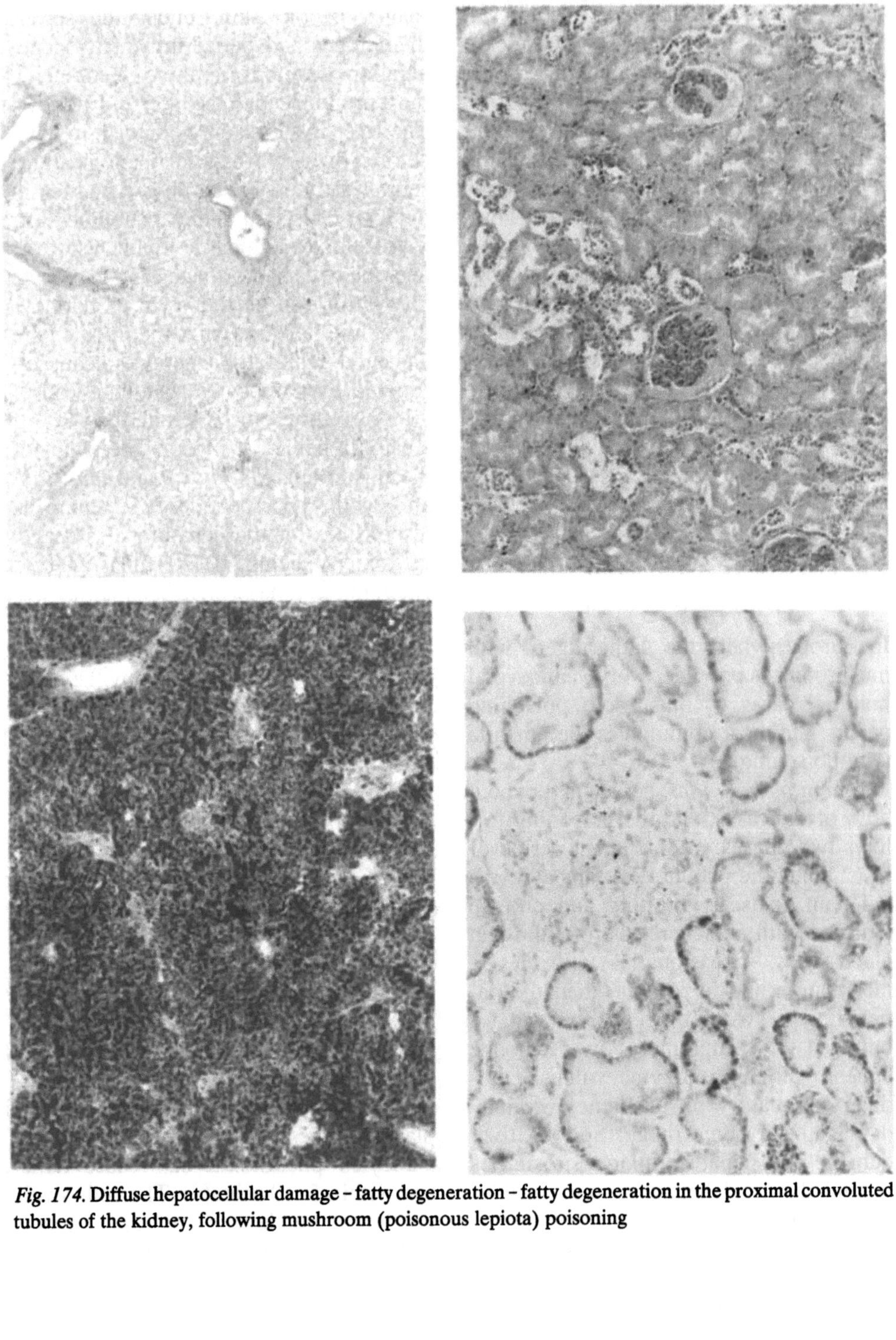

Fig. 174. Diffuse hepatocellular damage – fatty degeneration – fatty degeneration in the proximal convoluted tubules of the kidney, following mushroom (poisonous lepiota) poisoning

pends on early diagnosis. In the spring and summer seasons, when there is the possibility of mushroom poisoning, with the appearance of acute gastrointestinal complaints, one must consider mushroom poisoning. Diagnosis is by demonstration of amatoxin (RIA) in the gastric contents, the blood or the urine. Pumping of the duodenal contents is not only of value in the establishment of the diagnosis, but interrupts the enterohepatic circulation and decreases the effect of the toxin. The toxin can be easily dialyzed, and within 24 hours of discovery of the intoxication, with appropriate treatment, a 70% survival can be achieved.

Amanita muscaria

The mushrooms contains atropine and scopolamine-like substances. The toxin has a peripheral cholinergic effect and does not cross the blood brain barrier. The mushroom toxin consists of isoxasol and amino acids, ibotenic acid and its decarboxylated products, muscimol. Besides the amanita muscaria, these substances can also be found in the false blusher *(Amanita pantherina).* Ibotenic acid and muscimol appear in the urine one hour after ingestion of the mushroom. The signs of poisoning develop within 20–90 minutes, starting with gastroenteritis, midriasis, racing pulse, flushed face, and an hour later drowsiness, fatigue and sleep. The clinical signs depend on the effect of atropine or muscimol. Euphoria follows with a pronounced motor activity, tremor, visual hallucinations, and manic episodes. This state may alternate with other stages of the poisoning. The delirium of the subject and the EEG signs differentiate it from hallucinations induced by psilocybin (species of psilocybe), the alterations being more similar to those produced by belladonna. The most characteristic picture appears in children. After poisoning the symptoms spontaneously subside after 6–9 hours, and with adults it is rarely a serious poisoning, and intervention is required only with the development of serious mania.

The necropsy findings are not specific. In the cases, death occurs within 1–3 hours, following intoxication, the remaining parts of the mushroom can be found in the stomach content.

Helvella esculenta

While not wide-spread in Western and Central Europe, this accounts for 23% of all mushroom poisoning in Poland. It is pleasant-smelling and very toxic with numerous active substances including helvellic acid, which has a powerful hemolytic effect. Besides this several hydrazones, which can be easily hydrolyzed in the organism to toxic monomethylhydrazine. The toxin can be easily extracted with hot water removing 99% of it, but the hydrazine thus extracted remains potent in the cooking water, so if mushroom soup is made, it is the same as consuming fresh mushrooms. The symptoms of mushroom ingestion develop within a short time, 6–8 hours, with stomach pain, diarrhea and vomiting which is not prolonged, but frequent. Twenty-four hours later jaundice, hemolysis, albuminuria, hematuria, oliguria and then anuria develop.

In treatment the property of hydrazine interfering with pyridoxine is employed, so that treatment is initiated with intravenous pyridoxine administration.

Expectations and capabilities of toxicological tests

The *diagnosis of poisoning* is dependent upon numerous factors. Significant roles are played by the anamnestic data, the clinical signs and symptoms and, if the victim dies, the autopsy findings and finally the toxicological examination.

The *anamnestic data,* as has been previously mentioned, provides very relevant clinical, and therefore toxicological, information. For this careful, basic work must be carried out at the scene, which in a significant number of cases falls to the relatives or the ambulance personnel who brought the patient in to the emergency department. The number of cases where a specialist – a forensic medical examiner or police surgeon – whose responsibility it would be to search the premises for the poisoning substance, is on the scene is rather few. If this information does not reach us at our department, during the taking of the history we must consider the occupation of the patient and what kind of poisons he may have had access to, and if the clinical signs indicate a certain poisoning group, we should specifically search out that area in the asking about preceding information.

The *clinical signs* in drug group may be more or less characteristic. It rarely happens that we can discover the poisoning substance on the basis of the clinical picture, but there are many possibilities which should not be missed. Perhaps the odor of the toxin is characteristic, such as in alcohol poisoning, cyanide poisoning, parathion poisoning and benzene intoxication. At other time the *odor of the vomit* may be indicative. Following corrosive poisoning there is a coffee-ground vomit. With arsenic and mercury poisoning the stool is indicative. Further examination of the skin may reveal alterations pointing to some toxin groups. The *color of the skin* and lips with cyanide and carbon monoxide poisoning is cherry red, with methemoglobin poisoning greyish-brown, with corrosive poisoning the oral mucosa and the mucous membranes and skin around the lips are corroded and, depending on the nature of the caustic material, coagulated or colliquated. With chronic lead and mercury poisoning the *discoloration* and *hyperplasia of the gingiva* are characteristic. The formation of bullae on the skin call our attention to barbiturate poisoning.

The *autopsy findings* likewise reflect the characteristic alterations of poisoning groups. Although numerous chemicals can cause specific macro-, micro-, and electron microscopic alterations (parathion, mushrooms poisoning etc.), even so many times the so-called *"negative autopsy"* may raise the possibility of poisoning.

- A 23-year-old man was autopsied in a case of sudden death following uncertain preceding circumstances. At autopsy we found no characteristic alterations of the internal organs and therefore could not explain a death by natural causes. The toxicological examination of an unknown substance, which lately had been used in veterinary medicine, which is metabolized in the organism quite rapidly, raised the possibility of poisoning. In possession of the results of the toxicological examination, the investigator determined that a crime had occurred, in a local drink bar an acquaintance had poured Tetramizol into the drink of the victim as a joke.

Upon opening the body cavities at autopsy, a *characteristic odor* typical of certain types of poisonings, such as was mentioned concerning the clinical data, may be noticed. One must be careful, however, since the decay of the body may hide the smell. Gastric contents found in the abdominal cavity may indicate poisoning by alkali or acid, but the signs of death have already been discussed in that after death the autodigestion of the stomach resembles acid poisoning and can may cause a misleading postmortal malacia, and thus the gastric contents can enter the abdominal cavity. Among the alterations of the internal organs, the notable characteristics of paraquate poisoning include the already mentioned lung alterations, in which the histological presentation with great probability indicated poisoning. The organs are engorged with blood and the perivascular hemorrhages and petechias under the serous membranes accompany such poisonings with which liver damage may also be expected, since the blood clotting factors are also damaged or toxic substances brought about by hypoxia have something to do with the alterations. The characteristic of benzene poisoning is the spotty, hemorrhagic lung tissue, which is not only obvious to the eye, but has a typical odor as well. (Lately specific submicroscopic alterations in the myocardial tissue have been described with carbon monoxide and digitalis poisoning.) Corrosions, erosions and hemorrhages of the gastric mucosa are due not only to toxic causes, but to local circulatory disturbances or congestion. Even so after certain poisonings, such as poisoning with corrosives, arsenic, cyanide and nicotine, the gastric contents and mucosa may be characteristically altered. With cyanide poisoning the odor of the gastric contents and the alkalinity of the gastric contents in nicotine poisoning and the characteristic behavior of the mucosa may occasionally be diagnostic.

As alluded to previously, drugs and toxic substance are detoxified in the liver. Thus the primary target of attack of many toxic substances is the liver tissue. This brings macroscopic and microscopic hepatic alterations. The liver is characteristically altered in arsenic poisoning, mushroom poisoning and with chronic alcohol intoxication.

Toxic substances are also eliminated in the urine, so the kidney tissue may also be a site of damage. The renal alterations with mercuric chloride poisoning unambiguously indicate the fact of intoxication, but the renal tissue also responds characteristically to poisoning by ethylene glycol, too.

In the majority of poisoning cases we can find pathological changes unrelated to the intoxication, thus the evaluation of toxicological cases may cause significant difficulties for the unexperienced physician. In numerous cases the poisoning came to light only later, and in these instances, especially if the xenobiotic is rapidly metabolized or if it is broken down postmortally, verification becomes impossible.

If the possibility of poisoning arises either from the anamnestic data or during the course of autopsy, only the *toxicological examination* can confirm the evidence.

The relationship between the clinician, the forensic pathologist and the toxicologist has grown closer with the rising instances of poisoning, and the role of the toxicologist in the diagnosis of diseases of unknown etiology has become more prominent, since behind so many of these may lie intoxication. Even so if an experienced specialist requests an examination in a poisoning case and sends inappropriate material such inadequacies can result that they not only create unrequired work for the toxicologist, but may jeopardize the results of the examination. For this reason experience is required to recognize the cases in which the determination of poisoning can not be carried out.

In the clinician feels that a toxicological examination is necessary, if possible he should personally contact the toxicologist, and orient him with all such data which would facilitate a fruitful examination. He should come personally to collect the specimen and not entrust it to an incompetent or inexperienced person. The sample should be immediately send for testing, and if not, the appropriate storage is necessary . The material should be sent only to a properly equipped toxicological laboratory since the normal clinical laboratory is not set up for performing exact determinations.

● A 30-year-old male was taken to a department of internal medicine with a clinical picture indicating hepatitis, and for that reason he was transferred to the contagious disease department of the hospital. Here the possibility of paraquate poisoning was raised and a blood sample was taken to the laboratory of the hospital for examination. Here the orientation probe was negative, and therefore for days the patient was treated for hepatitis. Days later after the development of the characteristic pulmonary alterations, he was placed in the intensive care unit. The treatment by both the hospital and intensive care unit proved fruitless, and the patient developed progressive pulmonary fibrosis due to paraquate poisoning two weeks later and died of it.

What kind of material should we send for examination? First of all, blood and urine samples are mandatory. In the urine the remnants of even rapidly metabolized drugs may be found, even if they can't be found in the blood. The fluid of gastric lavage or vomit is regularly sent, and in a large number of cases (especially after the ingestion of a substance that decreases gastric motility), a significant quantity of the substance may be found in the gastric contents. If we consider poisoning with several substances, we also have to take into consideration obtaining a sufficient amount of sample-material for the examinations. Generally the following amounts are enough for toxicological tests:

blood 10–20 ml,
urine 300–400 ml,
all of the vomit,
gastric lavage fluid, the first 500 ml.

Naturally, for each xenobiotic for which there is suspicion, the appropriate material must be collected to cover each examination (with chronic arsenic poisoning, hair; with sedative poisoning, a large amount of urine; with alcohol poisoning, blood, urine etc.). The samples should be kept only in such containers that are clean and free from chemicals, and that can be sealed. We should not add to the sample any preservatives or clotting inhibitors (except citrate) if possible. With the material we should include the patient data, the clinical signs, and occasionally the suspected toxin type. The remnants of the poison brought in with the patient should also be sent along. Finally the name of the requesting physician, his phone number and how urgent the test is.

The method of determination depends not only on the type of toxin, but on the available equipment, too. The toxicological laboratory rarely has every instruments appropriate for determining every rare type of substance. More commonly the determination of each unknown substance is the work of several laboratories. The above mentioned description of packaging and transporting ensures that the least change will occur from improper handling after the sample has been taken. Internal Ministry Regulation 1887 has prescribed the transportation and marking of samples taken for toxicological examination. Since then the number of toxic substances has significantly increased, but the basic principles remain unchanged. Regarding substances taken from a corpse in poisoning the following must be kept in mind:

1. The sample for toxicological examination must be taken as soon as possible after discovery of the corpse.
2. The sample should be transported under refrigeration in order to decrease the postmortal decay or further damage of metabolic products.
3. The substance must be transported to the appropriate toxicological laboratory as quickly as possible.

Public health and toxicological regulations must also be kept in mind regarding the *packaging of the sample.* According to these, organs from a corpse can only be transported in appropriate containers. To serve this purpose the metal covered toxin box must be soldered down. In the toxin box a sealed glass or plastic container should contain the organs. On the container the name and personal data of the deceased, a description of the organs inside, instructions for toxin determination, the time of autopsy, the name of the sending physician and signature should appear on the container. Regarding the containers in the box which are to be dealt with in order, we prepare a list of the container numbers, contents, include a copy of the autopsy record, and especially mention the directions for the toxicological examination.

We may send for examination:

I. Stomach and its contents,
II. Small and large intestine, with contents (in approximately 50 cm sections),
III. Organs (liver 500 g, kidney, brain, lung about 1000 g in their entirety),
IV. Blood (100–200 ml),
V. Urine (200–500 ml), if no urine, then the bladder,
VI. Vomit (all) or gastric lavage fluid,
VII. Toxic substances found in around the corpse.

In addition to the above, with *exhumation* the following should be packaged:

I. Parts of the coffin, clothing of the deceased, shroud,
II. Soil from above or below the coffin, approximately 1 kg each, packaged separately (a significant amount of toxin may be removed from the body with leaching fluids, and the toxic material may be washed out of the soil of the grave),
III. We package separately the paired

organs to exclude postmortal diffusion of the toxin,

IV. Samples of cornified tissue or bone.

If the autopsy or the anamnestic data unambiguously point to the effect of a poison, we must prepare the package accordingly (we send in those organs and body fluids for examination in which the toxic substance is deposited in the greatest amount). Thus with sedative poisoning, the liver, urine and blood samples; with arsenic poisoning, the cornified tissue or with exhumation, the bony tissue; with mercury poisoning, the large intestine and its contents; with mushroom poisoning, the gastrointestinal contents.

The special packaging, however, does not mean that the physician conducting the autopsy who finds in the stomach the remnants of tablets should send them for examination and based on the results received back establish a false diagnosis of poisoning. The remnants of tablets found in the stomach only indicates previous ingestion of a medication, the active substance of which may have been absorbed. Without the determination of the level in the blood or metabolites in the urine the declaration of intoxication is in error and inexcusable.

The toxicologist who receives material for examination works from the given supposition, or performs a general toxin determination, or performs the appropriate procedure to demonstrate the requested toxin type. Numerous methods are known for determination, a brief familiarization with which is necessary for the specialist requiring the toxicological examination.

The first step is the extraction of the toxic substance from the biological material. For this, if we know the nature of the toxic agent, the appropriate solvent and pH value can offer a great help. Some substances can be extracted better near their isoelectric points, since with a deviation from the pH value a significant loss can be expected. Certain solvents are excellent for the extraction of certain drugs, such as the antidepressants with hexane since a mixture of alcohol and chloroform will carry with it, besides the sedatives, numerous other substances. The choice the extracting solution is not only influenced by the amount of the substance to be extracted, but an improper extraction may render the determination impossible. If, for example, the solute chemically affects the extracted material, it may make it difficult to regain the original agent. Although many methods are available for the extraction of toxins from biological materials, generally the following procedures are recommended:

1. Distillation (Tompsett)

Drugs can be extracted from biological material by distillation. The usual extraction by steam distillation of urine can ensure a significant final concentration of the toxic substance. In the first phase of the procedure – 25 ml urine, 25 ml H_2O. 1 g $NaHCO_3$ – we boil it down to 30 ml of distillate, then add 10 ml of nHCl and read it photometrically at 200–350 nm UV against a blank. This is distillate A. After the distillate – now in an acid milieu – we dilute it back to the original level with distilled water and redistill it, and this distillate B we examine in the UV spectrum.

We can examine the extracted substance by gas chromatography or thin layer chromatography methods as well. The procedure are appropriate for those substances which may be found in high concentration in the urine. It isn't a suitable procedure for extraction from blood samples.

2. Extraction by solvent (Kern)

Chemically neutral or acidic or basic materials can be well extracted at the appropriate pH. A significant amount of loss can be expected from using an acidic or basic milieu that deviates significantly, or such hydrolysates may be formed which later disturb the exact determination.

3. Extraction by solvent, salting out (Bastos)

Basic drugs and their metabolites can be extracted with ethanol from the urine, if previously saturated with K_2CO_3. The saturation of the urine decreases the effect of the water as a solute and causes such a physical-chemical response in which the toxic substance appears in the alcohol in greater concentration than with the usual extraction methods. Thus ammonium sulfate is used for the extraction of acidic substances, while K_2CO_3 is used for basic or neutral substances. The significant salt concentration requires such a pH value which facilitates the extraction. With these procedures, for example, 94% of chlordiazepoxide, 100% of diazepam and 91% of morphine can be extracted from the urine.

4. Cation exchange chromatographic procedure (Dole)

Cation exchange thin layer slides can be used to extract narcotics, tranquillizers, amphetamines, and barbiturates from the urine and the substances adsorbed to the ion exchange slide can be well eluted with chloroform citrate buffer, pH 2.2 (1:1) – acidic drugs or barbiturates – or chloroform, isopropanol (3:1), borate buffer, pH 9.3 (1:1) – mainly basic substances –, or chloroform – carbonate buffer, pH 11 (1:1) – amphetamines and primary or secondary amino acids. The procedure can be made simple. We place the strips of 5–6 cm length in the urine – 50–100 ml of urine, diluted with an equal amount of water – and adjust to a pH of 5–6, then, after removing them, we rinse the paper strips twice with distilled water. When dry we can store them or send them for testing.

5. Active charcoal adsorption (Meola)

This is a simple and effective extraction procedure for barbiturates, amphetamines, phenothiazines, quinine, morphine, cocaine, and their metabolites. The toxic substance adsorbs to the surface of the charcoal, and then is eluted with either ethyl ether or chloroform – isopropanol 50:10. Authors report a very good dissolution in thin layer chromatography with interfering groups not being formed.

After extraction the toxicologist must choose between numerous procedures for demonstration. The nature of the substance to be demonstrated to a certain extent determines which procedure to use, but the modern toxicological methods for the identification of each substance promise procedures with many and varied sensitivities, and one should choose a simple demonstration which gives an exact quantitative determination.

The *clinical examination* for toxicological substance should be started with samples taken from the corpse expressly for *thin layer chromatography.* The procedure is quick, inexpensive, and with a little experience it can orient one to the direction of which toxin group to target for further tests. With toxicological examinations the usual Rh values should be used with a great reservation due to the unwanted effects of the biological materials. The presence of conjugated metabolites may be especially disturbing, so therefore the biological material should be purposely hydrolyzed although this also damages the original structure as well. The less damaging enzymatic hydrolysis on the other hand is slow and costly. In spite of these the thin layer chromatography is the usual drug orientation procedure in toxicological laboratories. The property it has that it does not damage the substance emphasizes its significance, and after removal of the spot spectrophotometry, gas chromatography or mass spectroscopy can be used.

Determinations by gas chromatography make for much more accurate examinations than previously possible in that the retention time (Rt) value obtained in this way is much more reliable, and the method is more sensitive than the Rf. data obtained from thin layer chromatography examinations. The problem with gas chromatography procedures is that the presence of small molecular weight substances – metabolites – cannot be identified. For this reason gas chromatography procedures are not the best for the identification of damaging toxic substances through demonstrating a significant metabolisation due to possible decay of the corpse. For this the most appropriate method is gas chromatographic mass spectroscopy. It can with very good resolution verify the capillary gas chromatography procedure when the appropriate temperature program is selected.

With measurement by *mass spectroscopy* in a coupled procedure the components of the toxic substance are separated by gas chromatography equipment, and then the mass spectrum of the separated substances are examined. The mass spectrum for each substance is characteristic and provides the possibility to identify the metabolites or fragments of metabolites. The method can also be used for several possibilities – pyrolysis technique, HPLC – MS, chemical ionization mass spectroscopic procedures – which are today the most modern procedures in forensic toxicology. The drawback to the method is the very high price of the equipment.

UV spectrophotometry has been in use as a method for toxicological determinations for about two decades, but it is one of the most often used procedures in the clinical laboratory. It is used for the quantitative and qualitative determinations of pharmaceuticals from biological material and fluids. It bears special significance for the institution dealing with the care of toxicological patients. With the examination the absorption minimum-maximum values for each drug are characteristic, however besides the numerous advantages in determinations, several drawbacks are also included. Among the advantages are the very easy use and nature of the instrument and analysis, and the procedure itself is not expensive. The material can be analyzed quickly by it and not only qualitative, but quantitative measurements can be performed. Damage to the examined substance occurs very rarely, and therefore further analyses can be performed later with thin layer chromatography and gas chromatography methods. The drawbacks include: certain drugs which have no UV spectrum cannot be analyzed with this procedure, its sensitivity is restricted, and thus, for example, the therapeutic level of numerous drugs cannot be measured. It is not suitable for measuring and differentiating drug mixtures, and thus cannot be compared to gas chromatography even though thin layer chromatography is comparable in accuracy and resolution.

The introduction of *immunological methods* into toxicological examinations sped up analysis, increased sensitivity, and from a certain standpoint increased the specificity and simplicity. With the use of these analytical methods preparation of the material is not necessary. Not only could the extraction losses be dispensed with, the analysis could be made easier by automation.

	CAS	Library Index	Match Quality
1: Phenobarbital (VAN)	000050-06-6	387	9946
2: Moperone	001050-79-9	735	5305
3: Ethotoin	000086-35-1	316	4700
4: Levomenol	023089-26-1	362	2982
5: Primaclone	000125-33-7	351	2249
6: 2,6-Piperidinedione, 3-(4-aminophenyl)-3	000125-84-8	389	1903
7: 1H-Indole	000120-72-9	73	1857
8: Uridine, 2'-deoxy-5-iodo-	000054-42-2	732	1656
9: Methsuximide	000077-41-8	313	1637
10: Floxuridine (USAN)	000050-91-9	422	1499

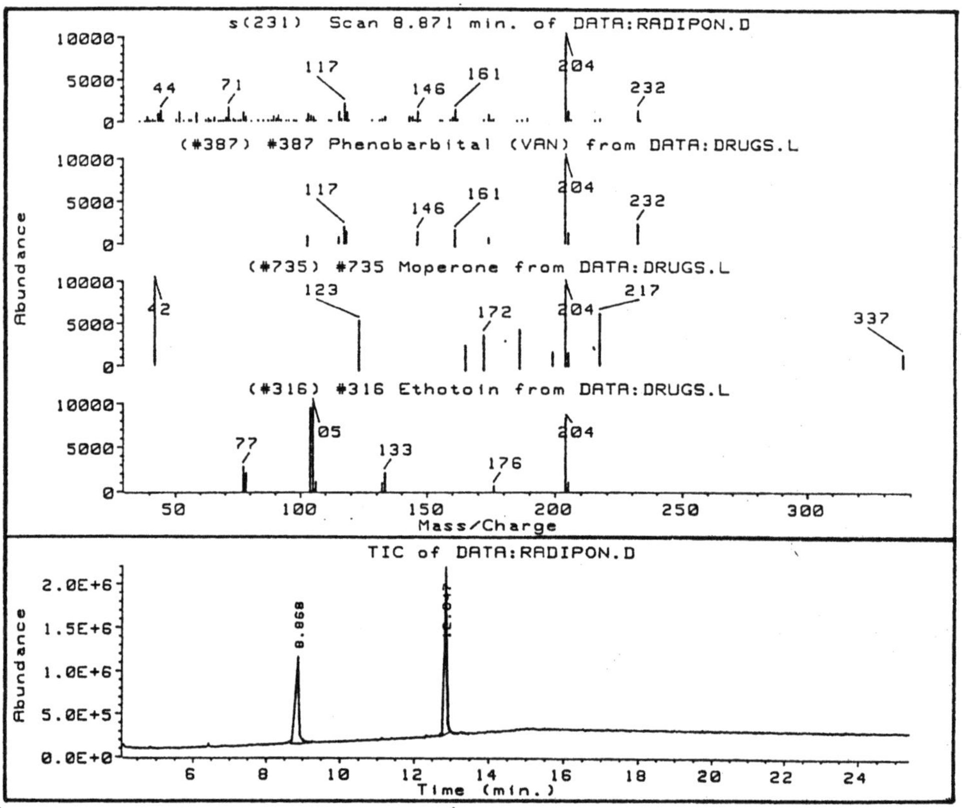

Fig. 175. Modern methods of demonstrating drugs and metabolites. MS–MC determination by computer evaluation

Correlation search of Library file: DATA: DRUGS. L

Scan 8.871 min. of DATA: RADIPON. D
RADIPON, BIOGAL, ETOH EXTRACTED

	CAS	Library Index	Match Quality
1: Codeine	000076-57-3	580	9339
2: 11-Hydroxy-. DELTA.9-tetrahydrocannabinol	036557-05-8	683	8091
3: Hydrocodone	000125-29-1	581	7203
4: 3-Heptanone, 6-(4-morpholinyl)-4,4-diphe	000467-84-5	721	3499
5: 1,3-Benzoidoxole, 5-(2-propenyl)-	000094-59-7	188	3163
6: Diampromide	000552-25-0	668	2928
7: D-2-Bromolysergic acid diethylamide	000478-84-2	799	2697
8: Nicocodine	003688-66-2	804	2632
9: .DELTA.9-Tetrahydrocannabinol (VAN)	001972-08-3	634	2583
10: Chlordiazepoxide (VAN)	000058-25-3	579	2348

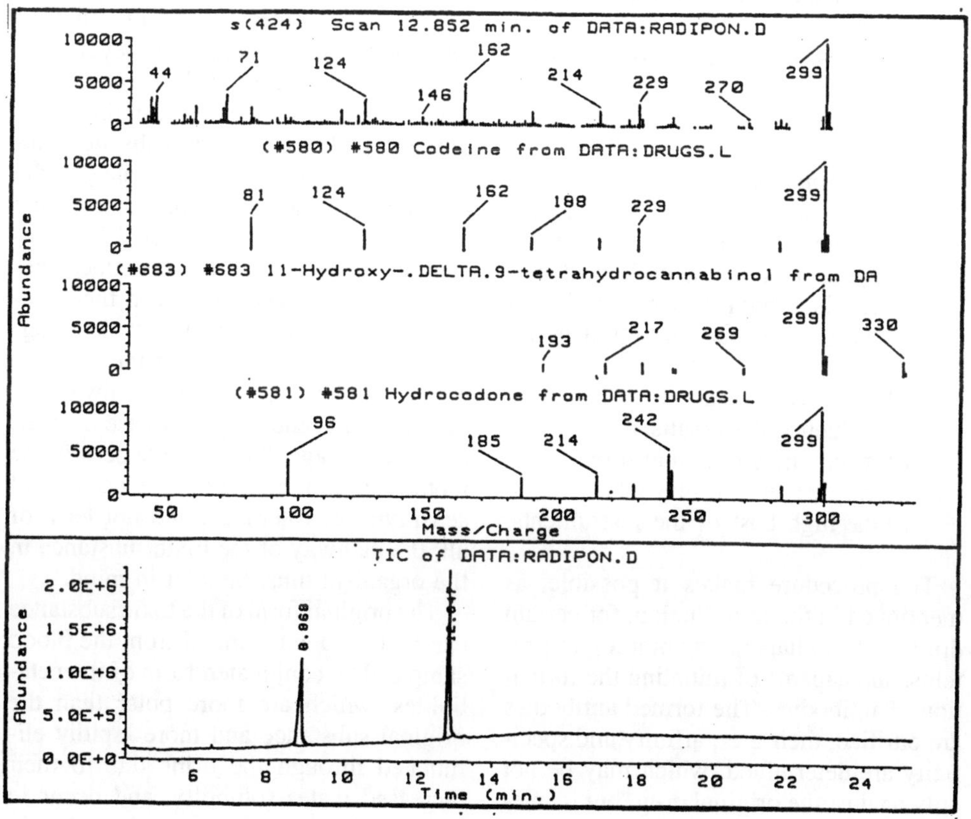

Currently used methods: RIA, hemagglutination inhibition (HI), FRAT (Free Radical Assay Technique), EMIT (Enzyme Multiplication Immunoassay Technique).

Among the numerous *advantages of the methods:*

a) rapid demonstration,
b) low toxic substance (0.5–5.0 μg/ml),
c) beyond morphine they broaden the examination to the demonstration of barbiturates, amphetamines, methadone, cocaine, etc.,
d) requires minimal technical experience.

Its *disadvantages:*

a) false positive results (for example, due to endogenous lysozymal activity in biological materials, which may be so high in the corpse that correction is not possible),
b) the age of the sample, pH changes influence the results,
c) metabolites may interfere,
d) very expensive reagents,
e) the high cost of the instruments.

The procedure makes it possible, as mentioned in the introduction, for certain drugs to form haptens by binding to proteins, and capable of initiating the formation of antibodies. The formed antibodies are purified, their titer, affinity and specificity are determined, which may be not only against the original drug, but its metabolites as well. In EMIT procedure, the enzyme markers lysozyme, glucose-6-phosphate dehydrogenase and malate dehydrogenase are used. The conjugation of the drug and enzyme to the antibody changes the activity of the enzyme, which can be measured as a change in the turbidity of a bacteria suspension (lysozyme), or changes in NAD–NADH (glucose-6-phosphate dehydrogenase, malate dehydrogenase).

Although the methods are primarily used for analysis of the urine, not only body fluids – blood, cerebrospinal fluid, tears – but organs, even formalin-fixed material, can be fruitfully analyzed if the appropriate antibodies are available. The procedure can also be used for further examination of the spot of thin layer chromatography. Because of the possibility of automation, it is especially suited to the monitoring of therapeutic levels.

The *interpretation of the results* of examination results is the responsibility of the forensic pathologist. From the determination procedures of the toxicologist, the presence of xenobiotic types, or concrete toxic substances can be verified, the concentrations present in the examined material given, occasionally with their metabolization products and in their recognition the medical specialist must decide about intoxication. This is not always an easy task. In rendering a precise answer, the toxic dosage, the effective period, the method of administration, the occasional sensitivity or tolerance, and not least of all, the pathway of the toxic substance in the organism must be kept in mind.

The original form of the toxic substance can be best demonstrated from the blood sample. The conjugated form of its metabolites, which are more polar than the original substance and more rapidly eliminated through the urine due to their increased water solubility, and occur in the urine in higher concentrations than in the blood. This is especially relevant regarding the compounds which are rapidly and to a significant degree metabolized. They tend to yield misleading blood levels, if we omit the examination of the urine sample. Among the metabolites, the methylated form of the toxic substances remain in the blood in relatively high concentrations. With certain drugs, such as the tricyclic antidepressants, there is a significant variation between their dosage and blood level, and the blood level does not reflect the amount ingested, nor does it reflect the clinical signs. The blood level is also dependent upon the method of administration. With certain substances the maximal blood level is reached the fastest by intravenous administration. Toxic substances may reach a higher blood level by the inhalation route than by being administered orally, intramuscularly or subcutaneously. The latter ones carry a prolonged blood level elevation. The concentration of the toxic substance depends on several factors. The absorption possibility and speed can be influenced, the route of administration (cyanide per os, or via the airway). The amount of the ingested substance not only influences the concentration, but a large amount also prolongs the effect due to a continuous absorption (a high blood level can be expected for days with barbiturates due to the decrease in gastric mobility, if the toxic substance is not removed.) The rate of metabolism also influences the drug level as does the rate of elimination (some drugs or chemicals, due to their rapid metabolism, if the metabolites are neutral with respect to the organism, do not even carry out a significant toxic effect). The so-called half life, which is dependent upon the metabolization and elimination, influences the level of the original substance. This can develop from the individuality of certain substances, since the half life of an ingested substance in many cases is very short, and after the half life the remaining drug is eliminated only slowly.

Acute or chronic ingestion plays a significant role in the effect of certain toxic substances. While with acute poisoning a smaller amount of the toxic substance is ingested and there is a lower blood and urine level as well as the measured concentration in the organism, with chronic ingestion a much higher level can be measured since it is accumulated gradually and a gradual tolerance develops. (Due to their slow elimination, barbiturates may accumulate, and the with the addiction developed to morphine or its derivatives a tolerance level of several times the toxic dose may appear.) The concentration of the toxic substance in the blood, and in many cases the urine, may not reflect the degree of intoxication, or even the fact of it. In these cases with negative blood and urine tests a significant level may still be measured in the liver. This is why examination of the liver tissue from the corpse for toxicological examination must be pointed out. The toxicologist and the advising medical specialist are in a more fortunate position with the poison determination of the corpse than the clinical toxicology specialist. Such specific samples can be taken from the corpse which can be decisive for the examination of either the original material or its metabolites. Naturally, with the examination of material taken from a dead body, one must count on postmortal alterations, too. Certain substances may be changed, and completely destroyed during the decay or storage of biological material. (Cyanide, CO–Hb, ethanol, chloroform, cocaine, diazepins.) Thus a positive or negative result in these cases may not exclude or sometimes does not support the fact of poisoning.

In the consideration of test results, the question must also be answered how the poisoning occurred, and whether it is an acute or chronic form. The fact of poisoning is shown by the clinical signs and the autopsy results of finding a concentration of poison in the organism. As we have al-

Table 6

SUBSTANCE ADMINISTERED	SUBSTANCE ANALYZED	AVE. BlOOD, PLASMA OR SERUM CONC. (RANGE) (mg/l)	AVE. LIVER CONC. (RANGE) (mg/kg)
Acetaminophen	Same	249B (160–387)	385 (385)
Acetylsalicylic acid	Salicylic acid	661B (61–7320)	420 (2.5–1000)
Aldrin	Same	0.036P	–
	Dieldrin	0.279P	–
Amitriptyline	Same	1.6P (1.1–2.2)	–
	Nortriptyline	1.1B (0.5–1.7)	25 (7.5–64)
Amobarbital	Same	47B (29–68)	219 (106–580)
Amphetamine	Same	8.6B (0.5–41)	30 (4.3–74)
Arsenic	Same	3.3B (0.6–9.3)	29 (2–120)
Barbital	Same	113B (90–225)	509 (108–932)
Benzene	Same	8B (0.9–20)	9 (2.6–16)
Butabarbital	Same	58B (30–88)	112 (51–250)
Caffeine	Same	115B (79–159)	190 (92–329)
Carbon tetrachloride	Same	260B	–
Chlordiazepoxide	Same	32S (3–66)	–
Chlorophorm	Same	32B (10–48)	58 (6–130)
Cocaine	Same	5.2B	–
Codeine	Same	3.6B (1.4–5.6)	–
Diazepam	Same	6.6B (3.2–14.0)	–
Dieldrin	Same	0.27S	–
Digoxin	Same	0.025B (0.004–0.200)	–
Ethylene glycol	Same	2400B (300–4300)	6700 (200–15 100)
Flurazepam	Same	1.8B	–
Halothane	Same	33B	295
Heroin	Morphine	0.43B (0.05–3.00)	–
Lidocaine	Same	54B (11–92)	61 (20–96)
Malathion	Same	815B (100–1880)	1215 (200–1700)
Meprobamate	Same	95B (35–240)	148 (58–360)
Mercury (organic)	Same	2.6B (0.6–6.0)	30 (4.2–78)
Methadone	Same	1.B (0.4–1.8)	3.4 (1.8–7.5)
Morphine	Same	0.7B (0.2–2.3)	3.0 (04–18)
Nicotine	Same	29B (11–63)	–
Nitrazepam	Same	9B	4
Nitrous oxide	Same	18 vol% B	–
Oxazepam	Same	0.5S	–
Paraquat	Same	15B (0–63)	73 (8.8–326)
Parathion	Same	9.0B (0.5–34)	11 (0.1–120)
Pentobarbital	Same	30B (5–169)	130 (23–550)
Phenobarbital	Same	96B (78–116)	185 (89–266)
Procainamide	Same	114B	283
Procaine	Same	49P (21–86)	–
Propranolol	Same	13B (4–29)	198 (60–451)
Quinidine	Same	45B	220
Secobarbital	Same	21B (5–52)	115 (15–330)
Strichnine	Same	26B (0.5–61)	144 (5–257)

TOXIC LEVELS OF DRUGS AND CHEMICALS
R. C. Baselt and R. H. Cravey

ready alluded to, the blood level does not always correspond to the seriousness of the poisoning or the amount ingested. The tables are only collections of data for orientation from which variations may occur in any direction. The tabulated collection is much like the LD_{50} in some poisonings, or for understanding the toxic dose in acute intoxication. Chronic intoxication may vary, since the fact of prolonged subacute or chronic dosing is verifiable only in some cases of poisoning (arsenic, mercury, morphine). Again it must be emphasized that the case of rapidly metabolized substances bring significant difficulties in the confirmation of poisoning. At other times the demonstration of rapidly acting substances (nicotine, cyanide etc.) do not allow the possibility of subacute or chronic dosing.

Occasionally the recognition of a toxicological case is quite simple, at other times it can pose serious difficulties even for the experienced expert. In the case of suspected poisoning the expected tasks are specified. Significant cooperation is called for in the toxicological examination between the treating physician or the physician conducting the autopsy and the toxicologist. Any carelessness can jeopardize the results of the examination for this reason it is necessary to stick to the appropriate instructions. This only means that the toxicologist can only perform his determinations under optimal circumstances. In these results the doctor or the specialist must establish that poisoning has occurred and formulate the opinion *(Table 6).*

References

[1] Aschcraft K. W., R. T. Padulal: The effect of dilute corrosives on the stomach. Pediatrics 53 (1974) 226–232

[2] Bakir F., S. F. Damluji, L. Amin-Zaki, M. Murt A. Khalidim N. Y. Al-Ravi, S. Tikriti, H. I. Dhair, T. W. Clarkson, J. C. Smith, R. A. Doherty: Methylmercury poisoning in Iraq. Science 18 (1973) 230–240

[3] Balogh I.: A szénmonoxidmérgezett szívizom. Kandidátusi Értekezés, 1984

[4] Basett, R. C., R. H. Cravey: A compendium of therapeutic and toxic concentrations of toxicologically significant drugs in human biofluids. J. Anal. Toxicol. 1 (1977) 81–103

[5] Bastianini, R. J., R. C. Phillips, R. S. Schneide, E. F. Ullmann: Homogenous immunochemical drug assays. Am. J. Med. Technol. 39 (1973) 211–216

[6] Bastos, M. L., G. E. Kananen, R. M. Young, J. R. Monforte, I.: Detection of basic organic-drugs and their metabolites in urine. Clin. Chem. 16 (1970) 931–940

[7] Beveridge G. W., A. A. H. Lawson: Occurance of bullous lesions in acute barbiturate intoxication. Br. Med. J. 1 (1965) 835–837

[8] Bidenset, J. H.: Druganalysis by immunoassays. J. Chromatographic Sci. 12 (1974) 293–296

[9] Brandt, M. K.: Thin layer as a method of screening for narcotics usage. Am. J. Med. Technol. 39 (1973) 217–222

[10] Brattin, J. W., J. Sunshine: Immunological assays for drugs in biological samples. Am. J. Med. Technol. 39 (1973) 223–230

[11] Buris, L.: Über den Quotienten Alkoholgehalt im Harn zu Alkoholgehalt im Blut bei verschiedenen Verletzungen und Vergiftungen. Dtsch. Z. ges. gerichtl. Med. 62 (1968) 221–231

[12] Buris, L., Gy. Csabai, M. Fodor, M. Varga: Increase of alcohol dehydrogenase and protein content of liver following chronic ethanol administration. FEBS Letters 183 (1985) 143–144

[13] Brookes, V. J., Poisons, R. E.: Krieger Publ. Co. Huntington N. Y. 1975

[14] McChesney, L., Goldberg, C. K., Pareki, J. C., Russel, G. H. Min: Reappraisal of the toxicology of ethylenglycol II. Food Cosmet. Toxicol. 9 (1971) 21–38

[15] Chhabra, R. S.: Intestinal absorbtion and metabolism of xenobiotics Env. Health Persp. 33 (1979) 61–69

[16] Chiarotti, M., A. Cornevale, N. De Govanni: Capillary gaschromatographic analysis of inicit diamorphine preparations. Forensic Sci. Int. 21 (1983) 245–251

[17] Coburn R. F.: Endogenous carbon monoxide production. N. Engl. J. Med. 282 (1970) 207–209

[18] Copland, G. M., A. Colin, H. S. Shulman: Fatal intraalveolar fibrosis after paraquat ingestion. N. Engl. J. Med. 291 (1974) 290–292

[19] Crabb, D. W., W. F. Bosron, T.–K. Li: Ethanol metabolism. Pharmac. Ther. 34 (1987) 59–73

[20] Cravey, R. H., R. C. Baselt: Introduction to Forensic Toxicology. Biomedical Publ. Davis California (1981)

[21] Cross I. D., I. M. Dale, L. Goolvard, J. M. Lenikon, H. Smith: Methylmercury in blood of dentist. Lancet (1979) 312-313

[22] Curry, A. S.: Advances in Forensic and Clinical Toxicology. CRC Press Cleveland (1972)

[23] Curry, A. S.: Chromatography and forensic chemistry. J. Chromatographic Sci. 12 (1974) 529–534

[24] Dean J. H., M. I. Luster, A. E. Munson, H. Amos: Immunotoxicology and Immunopharmacology. Raven, Pr. N. Y. (1985)

[25] Dillman, R. O., C. K. Gramb, M. J. Lindsky: Lead poisoning from a gunshot wound Am. J. Med. 66 (1979) 509–514

[26] Di Palma J. R.: Drill's Pharmacology in Medicine. Mc.Graw Hill Co. N. Y. (1971) pp. 1089–1097

[27] Dole, V. P., Wan Kyun Kim, I. Eglitis: Detection of narcotic drugs, tranquillisers, amphematines and barbiturates in urine. JAMA, 198 (1966) 349–352

[28] Doull, J., C. D. Klaasen, M. O. Ambdur: Toxicology. McMillen Publ. Co. Inc. N. Y. (1980) pp. 359–408

[29] Dzau, V. J., S. Szabo, Y. C. Chang: Aspiration of metallic mercury, JAMA 238 (1977) 1531–1532

[30] Editorial: Mushroom posoning. Lancet (1980) 351-352

[31] Evans, C. L.: Cobalt compounts as antidotes for hydrocyanic acid. Br. J. Pharmacol. 23 (1964) 455–475

[32] Faulstich H.: Mushroom poisoning. Lancet (1980) 794–795

[33] Finkle, B. S., K. L. McCloskey: The forensic toxicology of cocaine. J. Forensic Sci. 23 (1978) 173–188

[34] Finkle, B. S., K. L. McCloskey, L. S. Goodman: Diasepam and drug associated death. JAMA 242 (1979) 429–434

[35] Forrest, A.: Non-linear kinetics of ethyl alcohol metabolism. Forensic Sci. Soc. 26 (1986) 121–123

[36] Forrest, A.: The estimation of Widmark's factor. Forensic Sci. Soc. 26 (1986) 249–252

[37] Franke, S., U. Freimuth, P. H. List: Über die Giftigkeit der Frühjahrslochel Gyromitra (Helvella) esculenta Fr. Arch. Toxicol. 22 (1967) 293–332

[38] Frankenberg, L., B. Sorbo: Effects of cyanide antidotes on the metabolic conversion of cyanide to thyocyanate. Arch. Toxicol. 33 (1975) 81–89

[39] Franklin, M., W. Bean, P. Hardin: Fowler's solution as an etiological agent in cirrhosis. Am. J. Med. Sci. 219 (1950) 589–596

[40] Fysh, R. R., N. C. H. Oon, K. N. Robinson, R. N. Smith, P. C. White, M. J. Whitehouse: A fatal poisoning with LSD. Forensic Sci. Int. 28 (1985) 109–113

[41] Glaister, J., E. Rentoul: Medical Jurisprudence and Toxicology. Livingstone Ltd. Edinburg (1966)

[42] Goldfrank, L. R.: Goldfrank's Toxicologic Emergencies. ACC/NORWALK Connecticut (1986) 640–650

[43] Gorrod, J. W.: Testing for Toxicity. Taylor-Francis Ltd. London (1981) 11

[44] Green, V. A., G. W. Wise, J. Callenbach: Lead poisoning. Clin. Toxicol. 9 (1976) 33–51

[45] Greenblatt, D. J., M. D. Allen, B. J. Noel, R. I. Shader: Acute overdosage with benzodiasepine derivates. Clinical Pharmacol. Ther. 21 (1977) 497–514

[46] Guerit, J. M., M. M. Meulders, G. Amand: Lead neurotoxicity in clinical asymptomatic children living in the vicinity of an ore smelter. Clin. Toxicol. 18 (1981) 1257–1267

[47] Harada, M.: Congenital Minamata disease. Teratology 18 (1978) 285–288

[48] Harrison, K. L., A. G. Robinson: The effect of maternal smoking on carboxihemoglobin levels and acid-base balance on the fetus. Clin. Toxicol. 18 (1981) 165–168

[49] Hewlett, T. P., K. E. McMart: Ethylene glycol poisoning. Clin. Toxicol. 24 (1986) 389–402

[50] Hoensch, H. P., R. Hut, F. Hartmann: Biotransformation of xenobiotics in human intes-

tinal mucosa. Env. Health. Perspectives 33 (1979) 71–78

[51] Hunt, W. A.: Alcohol and Biological Membranes. Guilford Press N. Y. (1985) 81–88

[52] Iyer, K., J. Goodgold, A. Eberstein, P. Berg: Mercury poisoning in a dentist. Arch. Neurol. 33 (1976) 788–790

[53] Jatlow, P.: Ultraviolet spectrophotometric analysis of drugs in biological fluids. Am. J. Med. Technol. 39 (1973) 231–236

[54] Kaji, H., Y. Asauuma, O. Yahora, H. Shibuea, M. Hisamura, N. Saito, Y. Kavakami, M. Murao: Intragastrointestinal alcohol fermentation syndrome. J. Forensic Sci. Soc. 24 (1984) 461–471

[55] Kerr, H. D., L. A. Sargan: Arsenic content of homeopatic medicins. Clin. Toxicol. 24 (1986) 451–459

[56] Kojima, T., M. Yashiki, T. Une: Experimental study on postmortem formation of carbon monoxide. J. Forensic Sci. Int. 22 (1983) 131–135

[57] Kojima, T., I. Okamoto, M. Yashiti, T. Miyazaki, F. Chikasue, K. Degawa, S. Oshida, K. Sagisaka: Production of carbonmonoxide in cadavers. J. Forensic Sci. Int. 32 (1986) 67–77

[58] Koves, E. M., J. Wells: An evolution of fused silica capillary columns for the screening of basic drugs in postmortem blood qualitative and quantitative analysis. J. Forensic Sci. 30 (1985) 692–707

[59] Laitinen, M. L., K., Hu Hunen: Ethylene glycol intoxication. Clin. Toxicol. 24 (1986) 161–174

[60] Lampe, K. F.: Toxic fungi. Ann. Rev. Pharmacol. Toxicol. 19 (1979) 85–104

[61] Law, N. C.: A modern approach for drug identification. Am. J. Med. Technol. 39 (1973) 237–243

[62] Lester, D., L. Greenberg: The inhalation of ethylalcohol by man. Quatern. J. Stud. Alc. 12 (1951) 167–178

[63] Lewis, M. J.: Inhalation of ethanol vapour. J. Forensic Sci. Soc. 25 (1985) 511

[64] Lewis, M. J.: Blood alcohol: The concentration-time curve and retrospective estimation of level. Forensic Sci. Soc. 26 (1986) 95–113

[65] Lieber, Ch. S.: Metabolism and metabolic effects of alcohol. Medical Clinics N. Am. 68 (1984) 3–31

[66] Lisella, F. S., K. R. Long, H. G. Scott: Toxicology of rodenticides and their relation to human health. J. Environ. Health 33 (1971) 231–237

[67] Lundquist, F., H. Wolthers: The kinetics of alcohol elimination in man. Acta pharmacol. et toxicol. 14 (1958) 265–289

[68] Manicu, P., J. P. Buchet, H. A. Roels, R. Lanwerys: The metabolism of arsen in human. Clin. Toxicol. 18 (1981) 1067–1075

[69] Mannering, G. J., D. R. Van Harken, A. B. Makar, T. R. Tephly, W. D. Watkins, J. I. Goodman: Role of the intracellular distribution of hepatic catalase in the peroxidative oxidation of methanol. Ann. N. Y. Acad. Sci. 168 (1969) 265–280

[70] Martin, W. R., H. F. Fraser: A comparative study of physiological and subjective effects of heroine and morphine administered intravenously in addicts. J.Pharmacol. Exp. Therap. 133 (1961) 388–399

[71] Martin-Amat G., K. E. McMartin, S. S. Hayreh, T. R. Tephly: Methanol poisoning. Ocular toxicity produced by formate. Toxicol. Appl. Pharmacol. 45 (1978) 201–208

[72] McMartin, K. E., A. B. Makar, G. Martin, M. Palese, T. R. Tephly: Methanol poisoning I. Biochem. Med. 13 (1975) 319–333

[73] Mason, J. K., D. J. Blackmore: Experimental inhalation of ethanol vapour. Med. Sci. Law. 12 (1972) 205–208

[74] Matthew, H.: Barbiturates. Clin. Toxicol. 8 (1975) 495–513

[75] Meola, J. M., M. Vanko: Use of charcoal to concentrate drugs from urine before drug analysis. Clin. Chem. 20 (1977) 184–187

[76] Meyer, M. C., A. B. Straughn: Meprobamate. J. Am. Pharmaceutical Assoc. 17 (1977) 173–176

[77] Miller, M. W., T. W. Clarkson: Mercury-mercurials and mercaptons. Plenum Press N. Y. (1973) 233–243

[78] Moriarty, R. W.: Corrosive chemicals acids and alkalis. Drug Therapy 9 (1979) 143–155

[79] Nagy L.: Az alkoholos italok mellékanyagai és azok káros hatásai. Kandidátusi disszertáció (1977)

[80] Nagy L.: A toxicomania helyzete és felszámolásának lehetőségei hazánkban. IM kiadvány (1986)

[81] Nakamura, G. R., T. T. Noguchi: Fatalities from cocaine over doses in Los Angeles county. Clin. Toxicol. 18 (1981) 895–905

[82] Palese, M., T. R. Tephly: Metabolism of formate in the rat. J. Toxicol. Environ. Health 1 (1975) 13–24

[83] Pickett, R. D.: Acute toxicity of heroine alone and in combination with cocaine and quinine. Br. J. Pharmacol. 40 (1970) 145–146

[84] Pounds, C. A., E. F. Pearson, T. D. Turner:

Arsenic in fingernails. J. Forensic Sci. Soc. 19 (1979) 165–173

[85] Powell, L. W., G. T. Mann, S. Kaye: Acute meprobamate poisoning. N. Engl. J. Med. 259 (1958) 716–718

[86] Robinson, A. E., A. I. Coffer, R. D. McDowall: Toxicology of some autopsy cases involving tricyclic antidepressant drugs. Zschr. Rechtsmed. 74 (1974) 261–268

[87] Rubin, M.: Requirements and problems in urinanalysis for abuse drugs: the role of gas-chromatography. Am. J. Med. Technol. 39 (1973) 205–211

[88] Russel, L. A., B. E. Stone, P. A. Rooney: Paraquat poisoning. Clin. Toxicol. 18 (1981) 915–928

[89] Spector, D., D. Whorton, J. Lachary, R. Slavin: Fatal paraquat poisoning, time, concentrations and implications for treatment. John Hopkins Med. J. 142 (1978) 110–113

[90] Sunshine, I., P. I. Jatlow: Methodology for Analytical Toxicology. CRC Press Inc. Florida (1982) 189–214

[91] Thelander, G., J. Jonsson, J. Schuberth: Is urine a suitable material for the preliminary screeaing of drugs in autopsy cases. Forensic Sci. Int. 22 (1983) 189–194

[92] Timbrell, J. A.: Pinciples of biochemical toxicology. Taylor and Francis Ltd. London (1985)

[93] Tollefson, L., F. Cordle: Methylmercury in fish. Env. Health Persp. 68 (1986) 203–208

[94] Tompsett, S. L.: The detection of basic and other drugs in urine by destillation and UV spectrophotometry. Clin. Chem. 15 (1969) 592–599

[95] Vogel, S. N., T. R. Sultan: Cyanide poisoning. Clin. Toxicol. 18 (1981) 367–383

[96] Wauters, J. P., C. Rossel, J. J. Farket: Amanita phalloides poisoning treated by early charcoal hemoperfusion. Br. Med. J. 2 (1978) 1465

[97] Weisdorf, D., J. Kramer, A. Goldberg, H. L. Klawans: Physostigmine for cardiac and neurologic manifestations of phenothiasine poisoning. Clin. Pharm. Ther. 24 (1978) 663–667

[98] WHO Expert Commitee on Drug Dependence. WHO Techn. Rep. Ser. No. 407 (1969)

[99] Widmark, E. M. P.: Die theoretischen Grundlagen und die praktische Verwendbarkeit der gerichtsmedizinischen Alkoholbestimmung. Urban und Schwarzenberg Berlin (1932)

[100] Wills, E.: Biochemical Basis of Medicine. Wright and Bristol (1985)

[101] Winek, C. L., D. P. Singleton, S. P. Shanov: Ethylene and diethylene glycol toxicity. Clin. Toxicol. 13 (1978) 297–324

[102] Yeh, S. H., R. L. McQuinn: GLC determination of heroin and its metabolites in human urine. J. Pharmacol. Sci. 64 (1975) 1237–1239

Chapter 12
Identification

The establishment of identity has an important statistical, judicial and criminal significance. Sometimes the identity even of living persons must be established, such as in psychiatric diseases or unconscious conditions. The identity of an unknown corpse also must be established. It is likewise necessary to clarify the identity of organ or bone remains by examination, too. Mass accidents deserve a special importance in the establishment of identity, with the examination of the victims of traffic accidents. For this appropriate practice and experience in identification as well as the collection of the available appropriate data concerning the victims is indispensable. For this reason in each mass disaster the participation of several well-experienced and specially trained experts is necessary for the examination.

(BARSLEY and co-workers describe in their publication an airline accident in which there were 154 bodies and 117 identifications had to be performed. For this the previous dental records of 123 persons had to be collected and among those working on the identification besides the forensic medical specialist and the radiologist were three forensic dental specialists. On the basis of the dental findings, 75% of the identities could be established.)

Identification may happen:
a) by recognition,
b) on the basis of fingerprints,
c) by dental description,
d) by special identifying markings,
e) by skeletal examination,
f) process of elimination.

Practically all of the listed procedures require such knowledge which can be obtained either from the acquaintances or from the preliminaries. In as much as the information may be in part uncertain, identification is some cases may be difficult or impossible. At other times it may be carried out with utmost certainty, if the appropriate data is available. Thus for example special identification markings, especially if we feel compelled to base each decision on one, may be misleading since they may occur by chance in the population. At the same time fingerprints or dental characteristics can provide an unambiguous identification in most of the cases.

a) Identification by recognition is one of the most commonly used methods. The suitability is indisputable if some previous information already points to the identification of the unknown corpse. It is not, however, suitable for the identification of a large number of unknown corpses. Especially not in the case of disfiguring injuries to the face of the corpse or if decay processes make it difficult or impossible. (In these cases certain procedures can be of help in the reconstruction of the facial lines, so that with fine closure of the injuries and soaking of the decayed and swollen facial soft tissues of the corpse in cold water, after washing the identification may be more fruitful.) In some countries the value of visual recognition is not well trusted.

Even under favorable conditions identification must be given great care. Due to the circumstances the next of kin or acquaintances may be reluctant or even loath to identify the body, and after hardly glancing at it, only later the true identity turns up. The changes in the facial features after death are known. Rigor mortis and after it the relaxation of the muscles can bring such alterations which give occasion for mistakes. The clothing or jewelry of the corpse can give valuable aid in identification. It is relevant that the identification should be performed not on an unclothed body, since each piece of associated clothing or jewelry helps in the immediate identification. The examination of the clothing at the same time can give other relevant indications and sometimes surprising results. In more than one case writing found in the pocket of the corpse brought into the morgue made possible the identification of an unidentified body. Even more surprising was the examination of a body, unidentified for several days which was brought in for identification and his personal identity card was found in the lining of his coat. Similar help may be given from the examination of the surroundings in which the body was found.

- A specialist was called to identity an unidentified body from the skeletal remains. The cause of death was also to be clarified. A hanging had occurred from the limb of a tree about five meters above the ground. Due to the processes of decay the skull was found several meters away from the fallen body while the bones of the trunk and the extremities were lying together covered with forest litter. After removing the layer covering the remains among the pieces of clothing in a plastic envelop a tram pass was found on which was excellently readable the personal data of a university student who had disappeared a year before *(Fig. 176).*

Ökrös identified several of the 62 victims found in the Apafa mass grave, following the II. World War, on the basis of letters and writing found in the clothing.

At other times objects found on or near the corpse can give an indication.

- In the case of the disappearance of a postman, homicide was considered. In the forest in an out of the way place months later the remains of a corpse was found with a postal bag next to it and the great sum of money found in it made the identification possible and excluded the likelihood of a crime.

b) Fingerprints give the possibility for definite identification, however their value is small. Identification can only be performed if the appropriate fingerprint records are available for comparison. For this in our country the department of criminal records must play a role. If fingerprint records are provided for comparison even in a mass accident identification can be performed from one fingerprint. Even mild decay or prolonged submersion in water do not make it impossible to take a print. In these cases the injection of 10% formalin solution injected into the fingertips by a fine gauge needle, or in an urgent

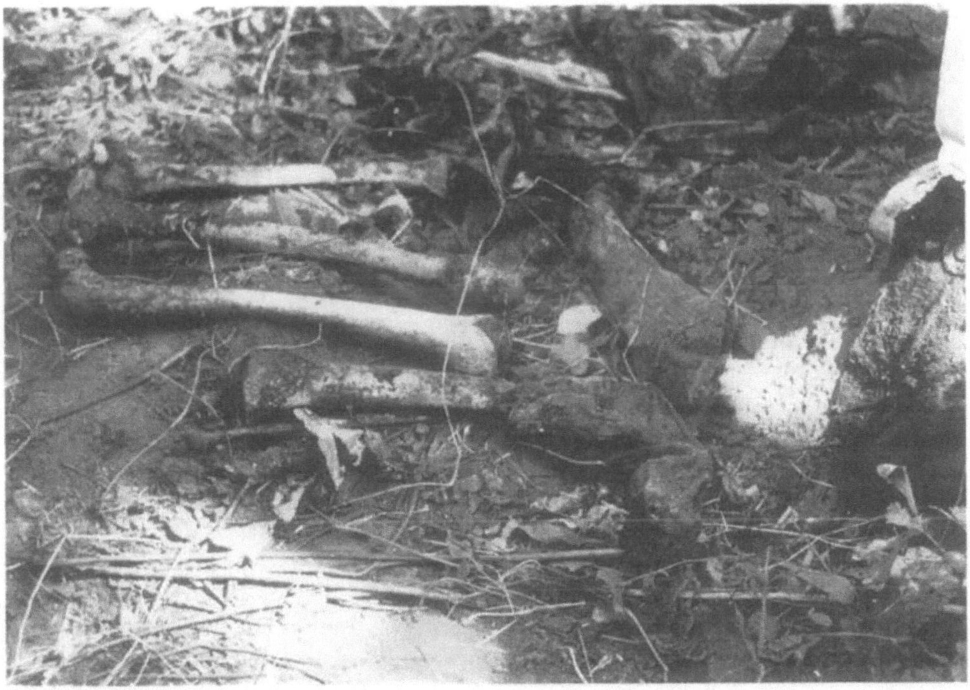

Fig. 176. Skeletal remains of an unidentified body

case water, can stretch out the skin and make it possible to take the fingerprints. (There are a some materials for experimentation for taking the so-called latent fingerprints in cases of identification.) In rigor mortis straightening out the fingers can make taking the fingerprints difficult. Cutting the flexor tendons can solve that problem. In other cases when due to an accident the body may so damaged, for example by fire or corrosives, that the finger print examination cannot be carried out. In these cases examination of the palm prints should be pointed out. In those countries in which a significant portion of the population is routinely fingerprinted and palmprinted for records, these may not only be used in the identification of mass accident victims, but can be used for the identification of prints in hidden places.

c) Identification on the basis of teeth requires appropriate dental records. The possibility of the identification is given by the fact, the teeth and crown keep their structure and characteristics during decay, chemical processes or burning, since neither they nor their repair preparations are much affected by these processes. The precision and possibility is not shown better than in the fact that in some countries where the risk of accidents is high for certain personnel – soldiers and airmen – regular dental records are kept. In the examination of an unknown person for identification a description must be written in a similar manner to the dental record and recorded so that a comparison can be made *(Fig. 177, 178).*

For this the found must not only be described, but their condition, their abnormal al displacement, the location of dental repairs, – post, crown etc. – their type and markings (sometimes the mark of the manufacturer can be found on pros-

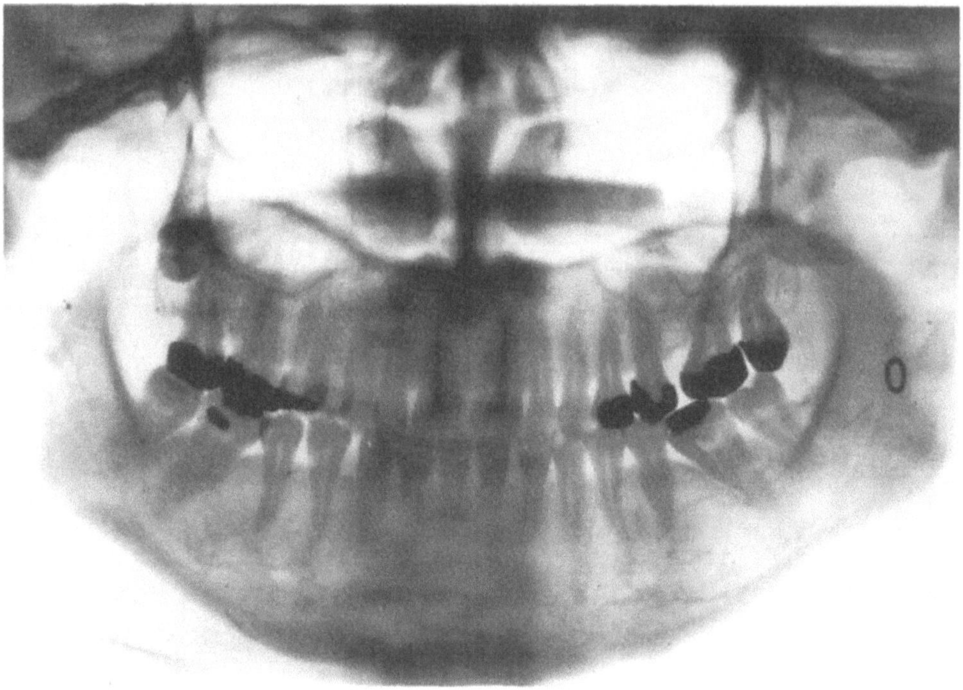

Fig. 177. Panorama X-rays make identification possible

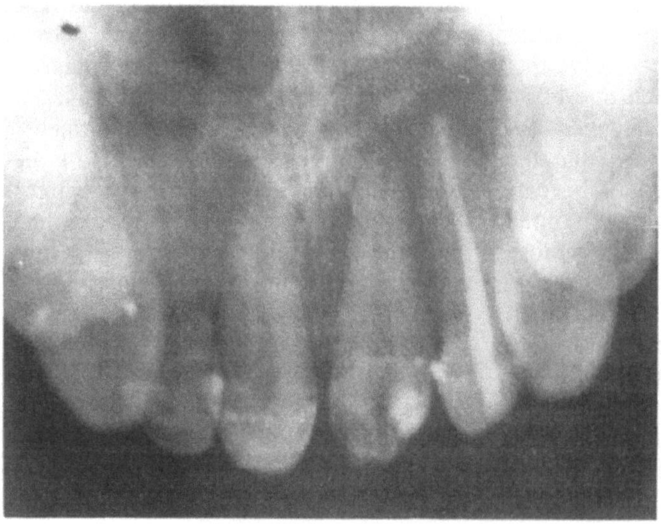

Fig. 178. X-ray of teeth in a cadaver

theses), the traces of visible dental work on the teeth, X-ray a the occasional root fillings, retained teeth fragments etc. must be described. For this an appropriate schematic diagram can be prepared which if properly done can allow for later comparison as well. (Examination of the teeth in a corpse is not easy, and the examination of the molars is especially difficult. They should be examined using a mirror, which makes their description easier.)

In such cases where later importance may be ascribed to the identification and it may be questionable, the possibility should be considered beforehand and an especially careful description of the dental work be carried out. For such an examination a stomatologist is required who can not only provide an expert description, but who can help in matching the dental records with the teeth of the person in question. Likewise it may allow those possibilities in which special filling material or prostheses had been used characteristically during certain periods. Thus metacrylate prostheses and fillings characterize the work between 1930–1956. Furthermore, some work is characteristic of certain countries, and the preservation work may help in identification. The presence of conspicuous orthodontic alterations may also provide useful information.

d) The special identification markings make sometimes possible exact identification. For this reason we must look for them and not only describe them, but in the interests of the hope of later identification, record them photographically. Among the special identification markings are healed *scars* including those that result from common interventions – hernia operations, appendectomies – their localization and occurrence being so common that their value in identification is slight. Those in a conspicuous place, caused by unusual injuries or *amputations* are of more value. The recognition of scars is easy even for inexperienced examiners, although in other cases the stretch marks of pregnancy may look misleadingly like healed scars, or those on the skin of decaying, sodden corpses can cause doubt in differentiation. (The histological examination identifies the scarification alterations unambiguously since in the area of the scar compared with microscopical picture of the neighboring intact area, hair follicles, sebaceous and sweat glands are missing.) Fine scars in the facial area my be a sign of plastic surgery intervention.

Tattoo markings are also considered special identification markings. They are of special value if of an unusual form or in an unusual place *(Fig. 179)*. Tattoos are common among prisoners of penal institutions and primitive people. They often comprise such data – initials of a name, a professional symbol or the symbols of certain institutions – which is important. The most common locations are the skin of the forearm or chest, but they may sometimes be found in unusual places *(Fig. 180)*.

● On one occasion we found a tattoo on the penis of an unidentified body of the words "CHARGE", which helped in identification.

Occupational alterations can also be useful. Hard calluses on the palms of the hands are a sign of heavy physical labor, coal dust in the cracks of the face and hands are characteristic of miners, while the so-called lead lines may be seen in the gums of those who work with lead. Silicosis following the inhalation of quartz dust by miners is described more commonly in the older literature, but may be found rarely today.

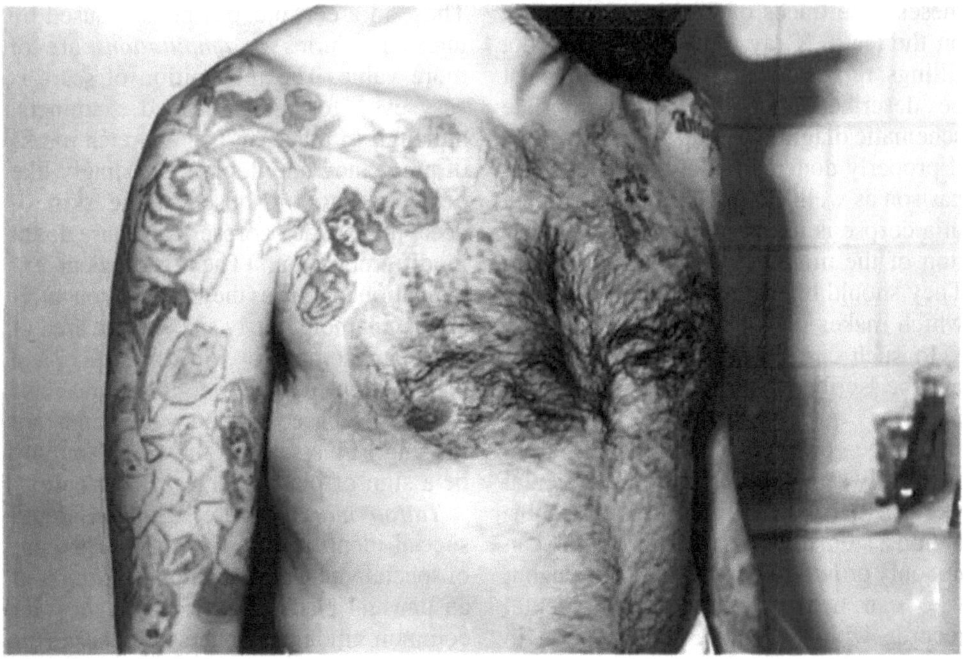

Fig. 179. Tattoos make identification possible

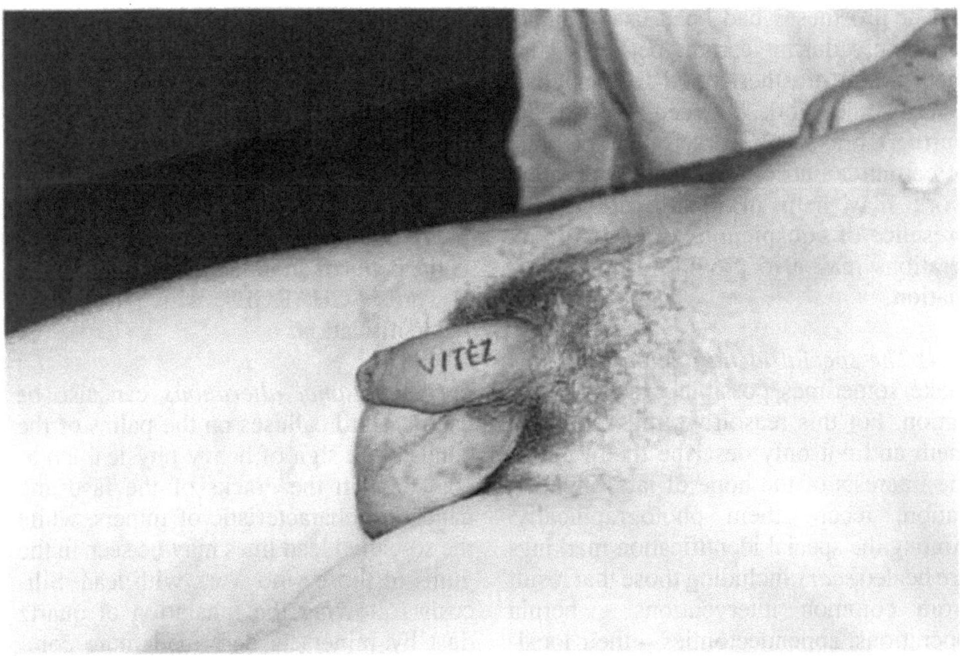

Fig. 180. Tattoo on unusual region ("Hero")

e) The most important thing in identification on the basis of *skeletal remains* is the determination of the age. The forensic pathologist does not deal with skeletal remains more than 50 years old because, due to the statute of limitations, they have no criminal significance. But the determination of how much time has elapsed between death and discovery cannot be neglected. We have already discussed the processes of decay, but in numerous instances recognition through several years of decomposition is important. The establishment of the time lapse since death in these cases starts with the inspection of the remains. Besides the alterations from decay, we examine the clothing, the damage to the soft tissues caused by insects or animals, and turning special attention to the environmental temperature of the place of discovery. Bodies lying in the open after a year become a skeleton with a greasy substance stuck to it, with the remains of a little skin, ligaments and cartilage. Another year later the soft tissues disappear and the bone become dry. The bone marrow dries out and forms a rancid-smelling mass. Corpses buried in dry soil take 5–10 years to be reduced to a skeleton.

Many procedures are used to establish the age of skeletal remains. The consistency and weight of the bone may indicate whether or not the skeletal findings have forensic significance. A sample of the thigh bone at 15 °C usually shows a specific gravity of 1.7–2.2 if fresh or 1.2 if fossilized. The value of 1.7 is the borderline value of specialist examination. If we see cortical corrosion, then the sample is at least 30–40 years old, the alterations primarily appearing on the surface of the joints. In damp soil decomposition of the spongy bone takes place within 20–30 years.

Under UV light a cross-section of bone shows a strong blue-violet light effect, the intensity of which decreases over passage of time following death. (This is useful only in old remains of a hundred years or more.)

With serological reactions we can demonstrate proteins drawn from the bones by anti-human serum. We can get a quick positive Uhlenhut reaction if the death occurred within 20 years, while a drawn-out, sluggish reaction can be expected with samples over 50 years old.

Numerous other methods can also be used and are available for establishment of skeleton age, thus the examination of the lamellar system using polarized optic methods can reveal the formation of adipocere in the Haversian canals. If they are completely filled, death occurred more than 30 years before. In the experience of Berg, the results of optical morphological examinations are much more useful in practice than those obtained by chemistry methods. Thus the fatty impregnation of bone occurs over 0–10 years, the soft tissue remains disappear over 10–20 years, the formation of adipocere is between 30–50 years, while according to his opinion determinations using UV fluorescence and specific gravity have only anthropological interest covering the 500–1000 year interval.

If we have estimated the time of death, the next step may be to determine whether the *remains we are examining are human or animal.* The determination is unambiguous since, as previously indicated, we can use the Uhlenhut method using antihuman serum to determine the origin of skeletal remains. If we are examining an entire skeleton, the recognition is easier.

Determination of the sex of bodily remains may sometimes be problematic. With histological examination of soft tissues, in about 75% of the cells taken from

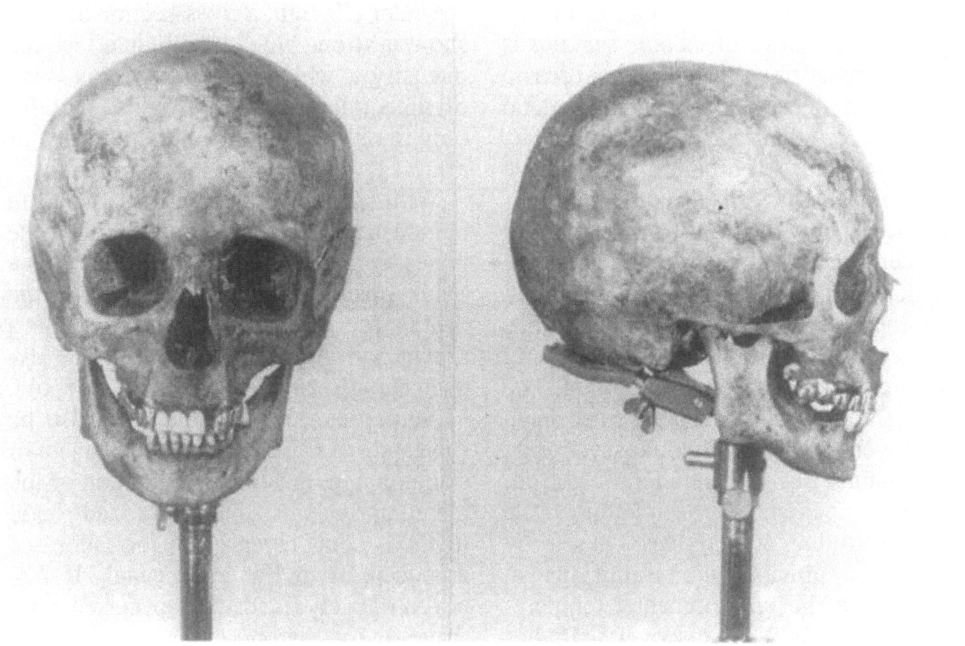

Fig. 181. Female skull

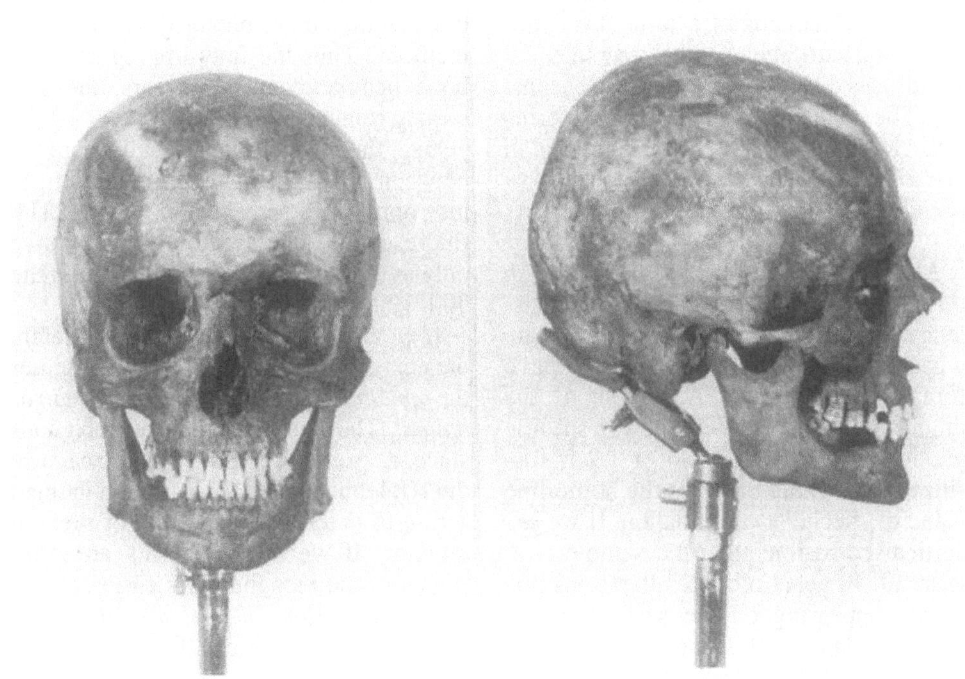

Fig. 182. Male skull (from the collection of Dr. Árpád Szabó)

organ remains of female origin the sex chromatin (Barr body) can be demonstrated, which is a condensed DNA-rich formation which can be well identified using the Feulgen reaction. In soft tissues or remains of male origin the Y chromosome may be detectable, although decay processes and tissue fixation significantly decreases the demonstration of the Y chromosome. Sex determination can be carried out unambiguously from the skeleton only after puberty, and this significantly depends upon the bone found. Examination of the adult skull can determine the sex in 90% of the cases. A similar ratio applies to the pelvis. From the long bones we are successful in only 80% of the cases.

In examination of the skull we take notice of the size, the male skull being larger than that of the female, the points of muscular attachment being more developed, the surface rougher, the mandible thicker and its ascending ramus wide. The frontal eminence and the parietal eminence are not pronounced; the occipital protuberance is thick. The supraorbital area in men is more pronounced, while in women it can hardly be made out. The mastoid process in men is stronger and bigger. On the whole, the female skull is more delicately built. Craniometric measurements can help in a precise examination in which fixed anatomical points are measured and compared *(Fig. 181, 182)*. (These are: the longest dimension of the skull, the shortest distance of its points, the capacity of the cranial vault, the size of the foramen magnum etc.) In examination of the skeleton the pelvis provides the most valuable information. Sexual dimorphism is apparent even from birth, so determination in the young isn't a problem. The differences in adults are even more apparent.

Besides the morphological alterations, numerous morphometric calculations are described which vary within populations, but show significant differences between male and female pelvises. These are mentioned among the objective methods of sex determination. One of the oldest measurement methods is the ratio of the length of the os pubis to that of the os ischii, which is 15% higher in women than in men.

Besides the above, the sexual differences in the thigh bone, the ribs and scapulae can be demonstrated by morphological and statistical calculations. These examinations require such familiarity with anthropology that it exceeds the responsibility of the specialist. The height of the body can be calculated from the length of the tubular bones, – according to Walcher the height of the body is 3.84 times the length of the femur or 5 times that of the humerus.

In examination of the skeleton, the next step is *establishment of age*. The possibilities depend on the condition of the skeletal remains, and the age determination is performed by:

a) dental examination,

b) examination of the ossification centers,

c) description of the ossification of the epiphyseal plates and cranial sutures.

a) The dental description is one of the most broadly used procedures in identification. As previously described, with the presence of the appropriate records, perfect identification can be achieved. The determination of the age can be made almost as perfectly. The appearance of the deciduous teeth, within the limits of individual variation, determine the age at between 5–6 years. At this age the appearance of ossification centers verifies the exact determination. The change of teeth with the appearance of the various permanent teeth allow for more exact data between the ages of 6–14 *(Table 7)*.

Table 7. ***Determination of age based on appearance of teeth according to Krogman***

Tooth	Age
Maxilla	
Anterior incisor	6,5–8,2
Posterior incisor	7,6–9,6
Canine teeth	10,3–13,0
First premolar	8,9–11,8
Second premolar	9,6–12,7
First molar	5,5–7,2
Second molar	11,3–14,0
Mandible	
Anterior incisor	5,7–7,3
Posterior incisor	6,8–8,5
Canine teeth	9,5–12,8
First premolar	9,3–12,2
Second premolar	5,4–13,1
First molar	5,4–7,0
Second molar	10,7–13,5

After age 14 an exact determination of age based on dental characteristics is more difficult. The appearance of the third molar is so individual that there is a variability of two decades. For this reason those examinations which consider age-dependent changes are preferred. Although one must expect many individual variations here as well, by keeping in mind several factors, the possibility of error is greatly diminished. One possibility is based on the Bodecker test in which the wear and abrasions of the teeth, the deposition of secondary dentin in the pulp chamber, apposition of cementum at the roots and gingival atrophy are considered. GUSTAVSON developed this further when in 1947 he suggested the determination of age by dental examination based on six parameters. Although the method applies to the practice of forensic medicine and dentistry, due to its great usefulness, it should be made known. The basis of the *Gustafson* procedure is the age-dependent alterations of the teeth and the assigning of a numerical value to the alterations. The examination takes into consideration:

1. the wear of the chewing surfaces,
2. the degree of paradontosis,
3. secondary dentin, which replaces the soft tissue in the tooth chamber,
4. cementum deposition around the root,
5. root resorption,
6. root transparency.

The above alterations in the teeth are categorized into four stages. The probable age can be read from a nomogram derived from numerical calculations of them *(Fig. 183, 184).*

Although the deviations in individual forms depend on numerous factors, within a population individual characteristics can be demonstrated. The Gustafson procedure is very useable in practice. It is especially important, if the recommendations of the author and those performing later tests are followed, to examine and evaluate several teeth. The test should be carried out by an experienced specialist. After age 50 a significant deviation must be expected.

JONGE puts the limit of enamel wear on the chewing surface at 30 years. The wear reaches the dentin by 40 years of age, and by 50 the dentin is completely exposed. At 60 the chewing surface is worn smooth, while in the 70's the wear extends to the neck of the teeth. The author suggests the process is dependent on the hardness of the enamel and dentin.

Examination of the *ossification centers* in the early years can yield very valuable information in the establishment of the age. In KROGMAN's examinations the appearance of ossification centers in the bones between the periods of birth to five years can be followed not only radiologically but macromorphologically as

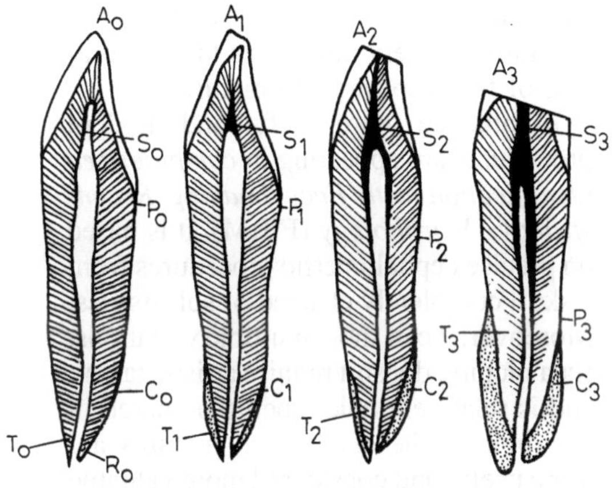

Fig. 183. Age-related changes in the teeth. A: enamel; S: secondary dentin; P: paradentin alterations; C: cementum apposition; T: transparency; R: resorption (according to Gustavson)

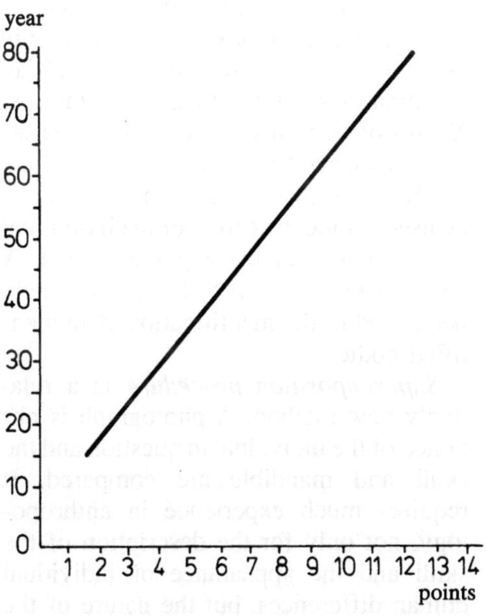

Fig. 184. Age determination based on alterations in the teeth (according to Gustavson)

well. Significant differences between boys and girls were not found, so the data can be applied to both sexes *(Table 8)*.

The ossification of the epiphyseal plates and the cranial sutures offer the third pos-

Table 8. Appearance of ossification centers in certain bones according to Krogman

Age	Ossification center location
Birth	dital epiphysis of femur
	proximal epiphysis of tibia
3 months	head of humerus
	head of femur
	distal epiphysis of tibia
6 months	distal epiphysis of fibula
1 year	II-IV fingers, 1st digit
2 years	V finger, 2nd digit
	lunate bone
3 years	major trochanter of femur
	patella
3 years 10 months	proximal epiphysis of radius
5 years	medial epicondyl of humerus
6 years	distal epiphysis of ulna
8 years	talus
	trochlea of humerus
10 years	lateral epicondyl of humerus

sibility to estimate the age *(Fig. 185)*. The synostosis of the epiphysis and diaphysis means the ossification of the epiphyseal cartilage, which finally becomes continuous with the trabecular bone. Ossification above the center turns peripherally and becomes complete. Thus the radius

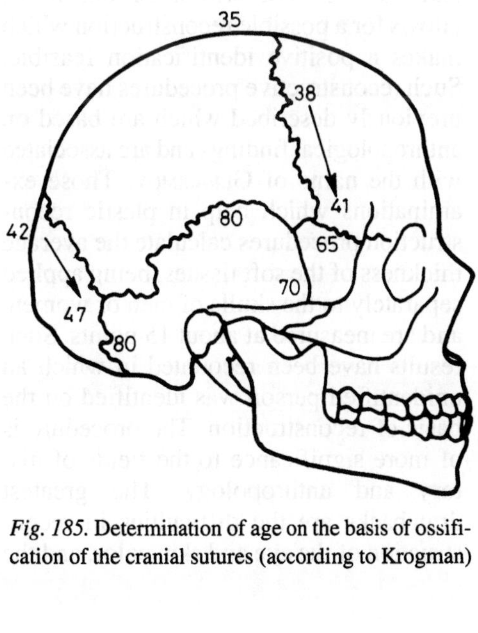

Fig. 185. Determination of age on the basis of ossification of the cranial sutures (according to Krogman)

becomes ossified between 14–15 years of age in the proximal section, between the ages of 18–19 in the distal, the distal epiphysis of the humerus between age 14–15, and its head at age 19–20. The ossification processes of the femur finish by age 17.5–18.5. The ossification processes continue beyond age 20 at the symphysis and cranial bones. Thus the sagittal suture on the skull becomes ossified the earliest. It starts at age 22 and finishes at age 35, while the latest one to ossify is the temporo-sphenoidal suture which starts around age 35–40 and finishes at age 80. In recent years such observations have been published in which the precise determination of age can be performed through measuring the degree of racemization of the protein content in the teeth. This, however, is not only dependent upon the age but on the environmental temperature, too.

With the examination of the bones we must mention the possibility of *reconstruction.* The skull not only helps considerably in the determination of the age and the sex, but within certain limits allows for a possible reconstruction which makes a positive identification feasible. Such reconstructive procedures have been previously described which are based on anthropological findings and are associated with the name of GERASIMOV. Those examinations which help in plastic reconstruction procedures calculate the average thickness of the soft tissues, being applied separately to the skulls of men or women, and are measured at about 15 points. Such results have been recounted in which an unidentified person was identified on the basis of reconstruction. The procedure is of more significance to the fields of history and anthropology. The greatest drawbacks are the difficulties in reconstruction of the eye and skin color, and the hair, and because of this, "artistic interpretation" largely influences the preparation of the reconstructed picture.

In practice more useful and modern procedures are appearing in *computerized identification with Face Imaging Reconstructive Morphology* (FIRM). It is based on precise cephalometric procedures from a skull completely cleaned of soft tissues. Moreover, it can show multiple variations, fix a picture, doesn't require artistic talent, and is relatively quick, being prepared in 4–6 hours. The results and pictures are more useful and considered more valuable than the previously described procedures. The disadvantage is the high set-up cost. With multiple possibilities it provides, it can also be used for exclusion.

Many have considered the possibilities of *radiological examination* and used it in positive identification. Previous X-ray examinations – skull films, chest films and X-rays of fractures – have in many cases made a successful identification possible. An X-ray picture of the frontal sinus can be used for identification or the individual characteristics of the zygomatic arch. A comparison of screening films has already been used in the identification of unidentified bodies.

Superimposition procedure is a relatively new method. A photograph is obtained of the individual in question and the skull and mandible are compared. It requires much experience in anthropology, not only for the description of the skull and the appearance of individual human differences, but the nature of the method demands finding photographs and skull films with identification points which are suitable for comparison and deciding whether the photograph and the skull film are of the same person. The technical description suggests that in the absence of the mandible or significant numbers of teeth, identification cannot be performed. This procedure does not approach the capability of the previously described FIRM. Identification by video camera has recently appeared in the literature. Identification by comparison of the skull with the face picture is more convincing than in the case of the superimposition procedure. Shortly after the appearance of the original publication we successfully performed identification on two skeletons which, having been executed following the revolution of 1956, were exhumed in 1989.

In the last year was published the case, in which a murder victim was identify by typing DNA, receiving the nuclear microsatellite markers from 8 year old skeletal remains.

Determination of the cause of death on the basis of skeletal findings is not easy. Certain injuries and poisonings exist which can be traced back decades or longer. The recognition of the injuries, naturally, is relatively easy if careful exhumation is performed and no damage is inflicted over the course of it. Among the alterations due to rough mechanical effects, on the basis of the characteristic impressions, hacking injuries can be easily identified. In other cases, imprints left on the ribs, sternum or skull by stabbing-incising instruments can be recognized. The recognition of bullet wounds appears easy, but it has happened that worm holes in the corpse have been mistaken for bullet wounds. With wounds caused by soft lead shot, on the edge of the hole a relatively significant amount may be left which can be demonstrated by the proper procedures. With wounds caused by jacketed rounds, the accompanying metal traces have to try to be identified. In any case the evaluation is made significantly more difficult if any group of injuries occurred postmortally, whether during or after burial, and the vital reaction in

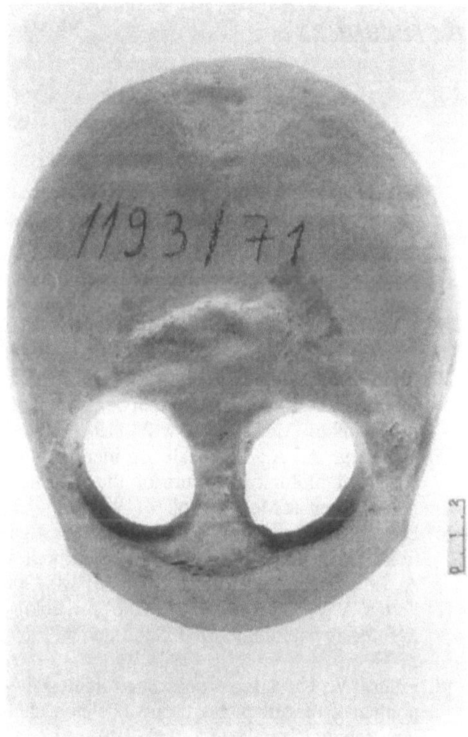

Fig. 186. Healed ritual trepanation injuries to the skull (from the collection of Prof. Arensburg - Tel-Aviv)

these cases offers no help. Interesting findings were published by Arensburg, who in the course of anthropological examinations in Israeli territory, found skeletal remains on which ritual trepanation (cranial "operations") had been performed and which, under the circumstances, were suspected to be injuries *(Fig. 186)*.

Among poisonings, *metal poisoning can be verified centuries later* from the skeletal remains. On this basis arsenic determination was successfully used on skeletal remains so that the sedative-poisoning of Harsányi was demonstrated from the results obtained from bone tissue.

References

[1] Arensburg, B.: Personal communication.

[2] Barsley, R. E., R. F. Carr, J. A. Cottone, J. A. Cuminale: Identification via dental remains. Pan American Flight 759. J. Forensic Sci. 30 (1985) 128–136

[3] Berg, S.: The determination of bone age. In Lundquist F. Methods of Forensic Medicine Vol. II. pp. 231–253, N. Y. Willey and Sons (1963)

[4] Churton, M. C.: Disaster victims identification. The transmission of antemortem dental records by telephoto. Med. Sci. Law 22 (1982) 79–90

[5] Dahlberg, A. A.: Rationale of identification based on biological factors of the dentition. Am. J. Forensic Med. Pathol. 6, (1985) 125–131

[6] Eckert, W. G., S. James, J. Katchis: Investigation of cremation and severely burned bodies. A. J. Forensic Med. Pathol. 9 (1988) 188–200

[7] Fatteh, A. V., G. T. Mann: The role of radiology in forensic pathology. Med. Sci. Law. 9 (1969) 27–30

[8] Földes, V., Kósa, F.: A holttest elföldelési időpontjának megállapítása csontvázleletek alapján. Belügyi Szemle 18 (1980) 108–110

[9] Friedman R. B., K. A. Cornwell, L. Lorton: Dental characteristics of a large military population useful for identification J. Forensic Sci. 34 (1989) 1357–1364

[10] Gatliff, B. P.: Facial sculpture on the skull for identification. Am. J. Forensic Med. Pathol. 5 (1984) 327–332

[11] Gerasimov, M. M.: The Face Finder. J. B. Lippincott, Philadelphia (1971)

[12] Gustafson, G.: Forensic Odontology. Elsevier Publ. Co. N. Y. (1966)

[13] Haertig A., A. Bonnin, L. Lehoux: Role of dental panorama in identification procedures J. Radiol. 72 (1991) 489–490

[14] Hagelberg E., I. C. Gray, A. J. Jeffreys: Identification of the skeletal remains of a murder victim by DNA analysis. Nature 3552, (1991) 427–429

[15] Harsányi, L., Nemeskéri, J., Földes, V.: Személyazonosítás csontvázlelet vizsgálata alapján. Belügyi Szemle 11 (1963) 36–43

[16] Harsányi, L., Leiszner, L.: Csontvázlelet származási idejének és emissiós lumineszcens spektrumának összefüggése. Morfológiai és Ig. Orv. Szemle 9 (1969) 182–186

[17] Harsányi, L., A. Láng, Gy. Farkas: Schlafmittelnachweis im Knochengewebe. A. f. Kriminol. 169 (1982) 149–156

[18] Harsányi, L., Láng, A.: Litium kimutatása csontszövetből. Morfológiai és Ig. Orv. Szemle 24 (1984) 309–311

[19] Harvey, W.: Dental Identification and Forensic Odontology. H. Kimpton Publ. London, (1976)

[20] Helmer, R., J. Schimmler, J. Rieger: Zum Beweiswert der Schadelidentifizierung mit Hilfe der Videobildmischtechnik unter Berücksichtigung der kraniometrischen Individualitat menschlicher Schadel. Z. Rechtsmed. 102 (1989) 451–459

[21] Hershkovitz I., B. Levi, Y. Hiss, B. Arensburg: Medicoritual trephinations in modern Israel Am. J. Forensic Med. Pathol. 12 (1991) 194–199

[22] Hilgendorf, E. L., B. L. Irving: Falsepositivie identification. Medicin Sci. Law. 18 (1978) 255–262

[23] Hill, I. R.: Dental identification in a light aircraft accident. Med. Sci. Law. 19 (1979) 82–85

[24] Hill, I. R.: Mass disaster identification. J. Forensic Sci. 28 (1988) 210–211

[25] Howarth J. H.: Post mortem identification of a body by use of dental evidence. Br. Dent. J. 172 (1992) 158

[26] Imobersteg, C.: The classification of an odontogram. Forensic Sci. Int. 20 (1982) 77–79

[27] Jonge, Th. E.: Des Alterns des Gewisses. Parodontologie 4 (1950) 83–98

[28] Katz, J. D., J. A. Cottone: The present direction of research in forensic odontology. J. Forensic Sci. 33 (1988) 1319–1327

[29] Krogman, W. M.: The human skeleton in forensic medicine I. Postgraduate Medicine 17 (1955) A 48–A 62

[30] Marlin D. C., M. A. Clark, S. M. Standish: Identification of humain remains by comparison of frontal sinus radiographs. J. Forensic Sci. 36 (1991) 1765–1772

[31] Mulhare P., E. McQuillen, C. Collins, F. Howard: An unusual case using DNA polymorphism to determine parentage of human remains. Am. J. Forensic Med. Pathol. 12 (1991) 157–160

[32] Nanko, S.: Decrease of Y chromatin frequency with time after fixation of blood smear. Forensic Sci. Int. 15 (1980) 1–2

[33] Norton, L. E., J. A. Cottone, I. M. Sopher, V. J. M. Dimato: The exhumation and identification of Lee Harvey Oswald J. Forensic Sci. 29 (1984) 19–38

[34] Ohtani S., K. Yamamoto: Racemization velocity of aspartic acid in dentine. Nippon-Hoigaku-Zasshi 44 (1990) 346–351

[35] Perper, J. A., G. A. Patterson, J. S. Backner: Face imaging reconstructive morphology. A new method for physiognomic reconstruction. Am. J. Forensic Med. Pathol. 9 (1988) 126–138

[36] Ritchie, J. G.: An update on estimation of age from teeth J. Forensic Sci. Soc. 28 (1988) 209

[37] Sajantila A., B. Budowle: Identification of induviduals with DNA testing. Ann. Med. 23 (1991) 637–642

[38] Sopher, I. M.: Forensic Dentistry. Ch. C. Thomas Publ. Springfield Ill. (1976)

[39] Washburn, S. L.: Sex differences in the pubic bone. Am. J. Phys. Anthrop. 6 (1948) 199–208

Chapter 13
Legal aspects of medical practice

The 1972 Law (Health Code of Hungary) deals with the requirements related to public health and the authorized stipulations, the most important of which include:

Medical, dental and pharmaceutical activity may be practiced only by those who have received the appropriate diploma from an approved medical university, or from a foreign university with the recognition of a domestic medical university.

The physician or dentist (henceforth physician), except in cases of emergency, is allowed to practice medical or dental (henceforth medical) activity only with a medical diploma, furthermore with the armed services, in a military unit under the existing service requirements, as well as a private medical practice.

If the police, the public attorney or the court orders a medical examination, the physician is obligated to comply. Under this only legally established cases may be exempted.

The National Medical Registry – on request – must accept the Hungarian citizen who has completed medical education at a domestic medical university or foreign university with a diploma recognized by a domestic medical university and whoever does not provide proof of such a diploma must be deleted from the National Medical Registry.

The National Medical Registry must delete that physician who:

a) has died,

b) has been prohibited from practicing medicine by decision of a court of criminal law,

c) has been proscribed from medical activity by the department of public health or under legal disciplinary action,

d) has officially resigned from medical practice.

The physician who had been deleted from the roles of the National Medical Registry for the above *(b-d)* reasons may request reinstatement following the expiration of the reason for deletion.

A physician undergoing treatment in the psychiatry department of the hospital, or the neurology and psychiatry department, upon discharge from the psychiatry department must inform the head of the department of his permanent residence who must in turn inform the appropriate higher level health authority should the necessity arise of restricting the physician's practice of medicine.

If the physician, likewise the pharmacist, according to the opinion of the overseeing health organization, becomes incapable of performing the activities of his profession, he must be restricted for the length of time of the incapacity. The health organization must reexamine this physician or pharmacist who is restricted in practice within two years and render an opinion of his incapacity to practice.

The medical student who, through the opinion of the overseeing health organization for the above mentioned reasons, will not be competent to practice medicine or pharmacy upon receipt of his diploma must be suspended from the continuation of his studies for the period that the reason for the incompetence is in existence.

The physician must also be suspended from professional activity in that case where the physician becomes incapable of carrying on a medical practice due to mental deficiency or some drug dependency (drug or alcohol abuse etc.).

According to the decree of the Minister of Health, barring the physician from practice for the above reasons is brought into force by the chief of psychiatry of the County Hospital to determine that due to mental disturbances, or drug dependency he is incapable of performing the duties of his practice. It is the duty of the overseeing chief physician in the case of a doctor, and of the rector of the medical university in the case of a medical student, to request the examination. Inasmuch as it becomes necessary for the above reasons to bar the physician from practice or to suspend the medical student from studies, the expert medical opinion of the chief medical specialist or the medical records of the patient must be enclosed with the examination which is forwarded by the leadership of the requesting body to the Minister of Health and requests a supervisory opinion. The Forensic Medical Committee of the Health Sciences Council is responsible for requesting the supervisory examination. Before the committee renders its opinion they examine the patient while in possession of the preliminary data and in the opinion after indicating the illness express their judgement of whether it is suitable to recommend treatment and must declare at what time in the future a reexamination will be necessary. The suspended physician, pharmacist or university student may request a supervisory examination of his mental state after two years.

The aim of medical treatment is to protect the health of the population by the prevention and elimination of diseases and by improving the condition of the patient, that is, to effect a cure. By the preamble the WHO Constitution; "the enjoyment of the highest attainable standard of health is one the fundamental rights of every human being...". The *physician has the right and duty* to apply healing and preventative treatment. Among the physician's rights are the freedom of treatment, to refuse to treat, to refuse guidance, to obtain qualifications, the right to private practice and protection from criminal prosecution.

The right of the physician

The physician may choose the methods and possibilities of the patient's treatment. The general view which every treating physician must bear in mind is that the treatment of the patient must be up to date and be administered according to standards of medical science. In the interests of healing, the most specific curative method, intervention and treatment must be employed. This treatment may extend to home treatment, but if necessary the patient must be sent to the special clinic or hospital for examination. The physician must choose the treatment method observing proper consideration for saving the life and restoring the health of the patient in the shortest time. In the preventative and curative procedures, only those may be used which are scientifically based, in accordance with modern medical knowledge, and are accepted methods used in day to day medical practice. The law unequivocally ordains that the physician in the practice of healing and prevention may not use any procedure, treatment method or instrument:

a) which is not at that time accepted by medical science,

b) with which the risk is greater than the postponement of (active) treatment, and for which there is no justifiable reason for the risk,

c) which is legally prohibited or which would involve an act contrary to law.

The physician must *inform the patient* or next of kin of the essentials of the nature of the disease, the condition of the patient, and the treatment method when necessary and when the physician realizes it. In some cases, if the physician has justification, and informing the patient of his condition would result in a deterioration of his psychical status, he may omit informing the patient.

If the patient does not follow the orders or directions of the physician, and this prolongs or obstructs the healing, if the patient by word or deed injures the physician, he *has the right to refuse to treat,* although approval by higher authority is required. However, in emergency cases all that is possible must be done to save the life of the patient, and in that case medical treatment may not be denied.

Among the rights of the physician is included the acquiring of *specialization.*

The physician has the right to *private practice.* That physician or dentist (henceforth physician) has the right to private practice who:

a) is listed in the National Medical Registry,

b) is not legally prohibited by the court, by the health organizations, or under disciplinary action from practicing medicine, or prohibited from engaging in a private practice for disciplinary reasons,

c) maintains a private clinic, or rents and at the place in question maintains facilities, equipment and installations appropriate to public health and specialist requirements,

d) has arranged for the specialty training required by the special area, except when at the time of request is also working in the special area or three years have not elapsed since leaving the specialty.

Every effort is to be made in the interests of supporting the practice of the physician, pharmacist and various workers associated with health.

The responsibilities of the practicing physician

According to the intention of the Health Codes the responsibilities of the physician are also stipulated. Among the most important responsibilities regarding treatment:

In the *activity of treatment and prevention,* every complaint of the patient and pathological sign of disease which the physician encounters must be explored. Among the options extended to the patient is the benefiting from the appropriate therapeutics according to the medical state of the art, the individuality of the patient and extent of the disease. The physician and dentist (henceforth physician) must use the most precise diagnostic procedures, therapeutic methods and equipment available.

The physician must do everything which is in the interest of prevention, life saving, healing and restoring of the ability to work for the patient, with the greatest care and circumspection. The physician must also treat the patient considered incurable with the utmost care.

The responsibilities of medical treatment also involve the methods of *acceptance and care of the patient* as well. The patient may come to the physician during a specified time. The physician or the local authorities stipulate the office hours, and during this time the physician is required to treat the patient who comes to him according to the best of his ability with the appropriate treatment. The physician carries out his treatment of hospitalized patients in order and here the same principles apply as above. In emergency cases the physician is required to treat immediately, or if called to the patient for an emergency, must come immediately. In these cases the physician must interrupt his planned schedule, since an emergency situation takes priority. An emergency case arises when the lack of medical treatment would result in loss of the patient's life, serious danger to physical health, or if over the patient's lifetime would cause such physical damage which would endanger the patient's life or result in permanent injury. An unconscious patient or an accident also constitute an emergency. The law also stipulates that in that case emergency treatment is also appropriate even if the statement from that person calling the physician is not clear. If a physician cannot be found to care for the patient in an emergency case, a certified dentist can be required to render care, naturally within the limits of his alternatives and abilities. In an emergency the physician cannot refuse to treat a patient who comes to him even if the patient does not belong to his district.

The law frees the physician from the responsibilities connected with emergency care when:

a) the physician also is seriously ill,

b) the physician cannot call upon the patient due to immobility for any reason,

c) going to the patient would endanger the physician's life,

d) he is caring for another serious patient, or if an immediate call would endanger a live birth,

e) another physician – duty physician, National Ambulance Service – on the way can ensure immediate care of the patient.

The *responsibilities of medical treatment* are likewise described in the Health Codes. Among other things, the law states that the patient who comes to the physician must be examined and treated according to the appropriate current medical standards. An individual examination means the exploration of the patient's signs and symptoms in light of a detailed case history and familiarization with the previous examination findings. If the patient cannot disclose the facts of the previous illnesses, previous examinations, or the current complaints, the next of kin or those accompanying the patient must be questioned. The examination must explore in detail the general condition of the patient and if the physician considers it necessary, he must perform further investigations which may require examination by specialists or in a medical institution, and if necessary, admitting the patient for hospitalization. The physician may only prescribe medication for the patient after performing the appropriate examinations and may not prescribe medications for a patient without examination.

The physician's responsibilities for record keeping

The physician must keep records of the patients he treats. Besides the personal data on the patient, the physician must record the complaints of the patient, the diagnosis, fact, time and methods of the treatment, and the medications used. With patients under hospital or institutional care, the data of the special investigations, the patient charts and operation records must be maintained daily so that the essentials of the interventions, examinations and medication of the patient can be followed. The daily maintenance of the patient records is the responsibility of the treating physician and may serve as future evidence in a court of law.

Responsibilities of information

The physician must inform the patient or the next of kin of the status of the illness, course and prognosis, and providing the information should be ethical and the patient's confidence should be maintained. It is not allowed to exaggerate the patient's condition and one must endeavor to make the information understandable and unbiased. One may not inform the patient in such a way as to criticize the previous medical treatment and by this undermine the patient's confidence in his previous treatment. The information must extend to the nature of the illness, nursing procedures, the frequency of medical care when relevant and the necessary times, the application of medications, instructions as to diet, and especially with infectious diseases, the mode of transmission, the need for isolation and how to carry it out.

Denial of medical treatment

The physician must deny to the patient any medical treatment or activity, regardless of whether it is requested by the patient or relatives, which conflicts with the law. To this belongs the performing of all interventions which can only be performed properly in an appropriate medical institution and the prescribing of prohibited or restricted medications. It is forbidden to persuade the patient to perform any act contrary to the law (abortion, euthanasia).

Obligation of official confidentiality

The obligation of official confidentiality applies to all information of the status of health (diagnosis, symptoms, prognosis etc.) of the patient, of the individual examined (in a health institution). It further applies to the patient being treated (in a health institution) based on the necessary examinations, the nature of the medical treatment, the circumstances of falling ill, and the known information connected with the examination and treatment.

The physician's obligation to confidentiality also applies to other health care workers. No one is allowed access to the records of the patient other than the physician or the workers involved unless directly for the purpose of necessary procedures or interventions in the interest of the patient, or for consultation with other physicians, or referral of the patient to a special department or for hospitalization. Information concerning his illness may not be disclosed to the relatives without his permission except to obtain information necessary for his treatment. If the patient is a youth, or mentally ill, the patient's guardians or immediate family may be informed of the particulars of the illness without prior permission. All of this must be done in the interest of the patient's treatment and healing. The obligation of confidentiality binds the physician over the course of the treatment of the patient to keep all data pertaining to the patient's treatment confidential, and following that may not supply information even to his relatives without permission of the patient.

The physician's breach of confidentiality is not only a violation of ethics, but may be prosecuted as a violation of personal privacy and for this reason may come under the criminal law codes.

Under certain circumstances the interests of the patient demand that the examination information be brought to the knowledge of the physician or institution continuing the patient's treatment. In this case the physician requesting the examination or prescribing the treatment may request the examination findings from the physician or institution treating him previously.

Every physician and health institution leader is obligated under criminal and civil law to provide, upon the police's, attorney's department's, court's or forensic medical specialist's written request, photocopies signed by the physician or leader of the health institution of the records of the patient's examination or treatment (hospital chart, fever chart, laboratory findings, X-ray findings and pictures etc.) and even the autopsy records if appropriate.

If a physician performs an intervention – for example, an operation – and the treating physician, or any other people besides an assistant also take part, whether doctors or medical assistants or medical students, it is the responsibility of the physician performing the intervention to inform them of the obligation of confidentiality. (If they are to listen to the physician over the course of courtroom proceedings, according to criminal code 65 & (1) under the obligation of medical confidentiality must request the consent of the patient or authorized next of kin regarding the status of the patient, evidence of his treatment and previous saving of his life.)

The obligation of obtaining permission to operate

Obtaining permission to operate is the obligation of the physician of the institution performing the operation. An operation may be performed only with the permission of the patient, or in the case of a minor or mentally incompetent patient, of the next of kin or guardian. While being asked permission, they must also be informed of the nature, consequences and dangers of the operation.

It is not necessary to seek permission in the case when the operation is for the purpose of the immediate saving of a life, nor is it necessary when, during the course of the operation it becomes necessary to expand the operative intervention. Neither is it necessary to obtain permission to operate in the case when the patient is incapable of expressing his will, a minor, incapacitated or mental invalid without next of kin.

Responsibilities of the specialist

The physician, if appointed by the public attorney or the court as expert medical advisor, must fulfill his appointment. Request to be excused may only be made on legal grounds, on the physician's request.

Provisions pertaining to health specialists

The health workers are considered authoritative in such matters which are related to his field of medical care. The authority pertains to such activity for which the health workers have been previously trained, and following the training have undergone the appropriate evaluation of their knowledge to confirm their ability to carry out their duties. The assignment of the commissioned activity must be made in writing and at the same time communicate the criminal and punitive consequences that accompany failure to comply. The permission may at any time be withdrawn.

Responsibilities of the physician

A physician must work within the regulations of his profession. The responsibilities of the physician are also determined by the Health Codes in which is written, "The physician is responsible for the examination and medical treatment of the patient, doing everything in the interests of protecting the patient's health, and withholding nothing essential to it." *The physicians responsibilities may be:*

1. moral or ethical,
2. legal
   a) disciplinary,
   b) breach of regulations,
   c) criminal,
   d) civil.

The physician may become guilty of violation of ethical responsibilities of behavior, since the physician outside the normal ethical practice has to maintain the ethical customs affecting the physicians. Lately the earlier restrictive moral standards, due to their growing importance, have evolved into legal standards inasmuch as they affect other areas of law. (Thus the principle of gratuitousness was a behavioral rule, while now legal drafting outlining the physician's legal responsibilities have come to the fore.)

The physician is guilty of a breach of discipline if he breaks the regulations of the law pertaining to health, either intentionally or unintentionally.

If the physician is guilty of breach, the following disciplinary penalty may be imposed on him/her.

- monetary fine,
- suspension from private medical practice for a period of 3 months to 1 year,
- suspension from all medical activity for a period of 3 months to 1 year.

The monetary fine and the suspension of medical practice may be applied together.

The regulation stipulates that the institution employing the physician or the ethics committee of the Medical Chamber may start the disciplinary procedure.

The responsibilities of the physician with respect to regulations

It may be established:

if he provides narcotics to an unauthorized individual, or to any person above the allowed amount,

if he breaks the responsibilities of registering or storing narcotics,

(This breach of regulations may not necessarily be a physician, although the potential for it is greatest in the medical profession.)

– if he maintains an illegal private practice (only a physician may maintain one).

Malpractice

The practice of medicine is classified as one of the so-called dangerous professions which, even when practiced according to the rules, may involve various dangers. The regulations of the so-called dangerous professions are so written as to forbid certain forms of behavior which if ignored may increase the dangers of the profession. The rules of the medical profession serve the purpose of making the practice of medicine as free from danger as possible.

The Criminal Codes hold the practitioners of the dangerous professions responsible if they break the rules and increase the danger. According to Section 171 (1) of the Criminal Codes: "Whoever by the violation of the regulations of his profession endangers another person or the life of another person, his physical well-being, or health, or causes physical injury is guilty and is punished by one year's imprisonment, social service or monetary fine. The punishment is up to five years imprisonment if the crime results in death."

The Criminal Codes specifically emphasize that individuals falling under the limitations of the professional regulations are not limited to those who are engaged in activities associated with preparation for a specialty, are bound by general acceptance of the written or unwritten regulations and engage in other activities.

The professional regulations of medicine are not inflexible regulations and cannot be applied with validity in the same form in every instance. This is especially true of the factors of medical treatment in which for every patient the appropriate specialist and medical treatment must be applied. In every case, if there is no definitive special rule in the medical treatment, we also find general guidelines and this means that the patient must always be treated with the most modern appropriate medical means and up-to-date information available.

The specialty regulations must take into consideration both the information on which the whole of medical science is based and which is to be found in the medical textbooks, university lectures or notebooks, professional reference books, professional journals, methodology letters and instructions accompanying pharmaceuticals for their use. On the other hand, no physician can be expected to be familiar with the whole body of information related to medicine. Today medical science is divided into numerous specialties, and these special areas educate their members in the appropriate up-to-date level of patient care. This does not mean, however, that the physician operates only within the confines of a narrow specialty area. It is expected of him that he should be familiar enough with medical science outside his area of specialization to apply the appropriate care for a patient in emergency cases.

According to SZUCHOVSZKY, the rules of medicine can be summarized into three broad categories:

> "the first part consists of legal requirements which delineate the form and content of practice,
> the second part consists of regulations of the specialties,
> the third part consists of sui generis regulations, or those from the body of medical knowledge which govern practice. Together these factors provide the regulation of medical practice guaranteeing adequate care for the citizens by the state."

The Criminal Law Codes emphasize carelessness as endangerment in the sphere of the practice of medicine. "A crime is committed by carelessness when one sees the possible consequences of one's behavior, but despite this proceeds recklessly:... it likewise occurs when one does not foresee the consequences due to failure to pay proper attention or take proper precautions" (Section 14).

Two forms of carelessness are recognized, which are knowledgeable *carelessnes (luxuria)* and *negligence (negligently).*

Knowledgeable carelessness means that the perpetrator recklessly ignores the consequences of his behavior. The judgement of this is not the duty of the medical examiner, but of the court.

In determining negligence, it is emphasized that one doesn't see the consequences of his behavior because of failure to render the properly due attention or precautions.

Foresight and foreseeability are the result of numerous subjective factors. According to some, these subjective factors can likewise influence the choice of a particular activity, determine the possibilities of foresight, and thus decide the question of medical crimes of carelessness. Among these can be listed the fatigue and state of health of the physician, which can significantly influence the expectation values. According to SZUCHOVSZKY the responsibility of the physician for foresight is an integral part of the professional regulations of medicine, and as such can be rightfully expected of every physician.

The perpetrator of malpractice can only be such a person who falls under the regulations of that profession. The Supreme Court declared that a person who has not undergone the special medical training does not fall under the regulations of the medical professions, and therefore cannot break the rules of medical practice if he engages in medical activity. Neither does a medical student fall under the regulations of the medical profession. Neither a medical student nor an intern are considered as medical doctors. Medical activity may be performed by them with an outside exclusive supervision and in connection with such activity the responsibility of specialty supervision lies with the treating physician. It must be emphasized, however, that if the medical student or intern does not follow the instructions of the treating physician, then it is not a matter of the appropriate professional regulations, but of general regulations of Criminal Code.

In the *establishment of malpractice, the following conditions should be considered:*

a) the professional regulation broken,

b) culpability in breaking the professional regulation,

c) an immediate danger developed or resulted in physical injury,

d) culpability in the creation of an immediate danger or physical injury,

e) there is a connection between the breaking of the professional regulation and the creation of an immediate danger or physical injury.

If whichever condition from the above mentioned is missing, there are no grounds for establishing criminal responsibility, and the result lies within the realm of medical risk or diagnostic error.

According to the accepted viewpoint, all injurious consequences which come about as a result of medical intervention belong to the category of *medical risk* if the complication:

- was unnecessary,
- was unavoidable,
- could happen even when the physician observes the professional regulations, during the procedures.

In the area of risk we must distinguish between objective and subjective factors. Objective factors originate from the equipment systems and production flaws in the instruments, while subjective factors include the experience of the physician, experience in each procedure, the special and human abilities of those taking part in the treatment of the patient, the assessment of the status of the patient, evaluation of the signs and symptoms, etc. Formulation of the risk incurred naturally does not only involve the surgical specialty, and not only the so-called operational risk by itself, but extends to every area of medical science and those branches must be especially considered which carry particularly high risk factors. Thus, besides the surgical procedures, we include anesthesiology and intensive therapy procedures as well. Dezső expressed the risks of therapy best when he said that therapy itself risks the patients life and health; physical injury is an objective possibility, whether a foreseeable or unforeseeable danger, whether avoidable or unavoidable, which may accompany the therapeutic intervention even when the professional regulations are observed. The medical activity also in essence determines the risk since in practice the medical intervention cannot involve greater risk than the risk if the intervention would not be performed. The physician then oversteps the allowed risk when he puts the patient in greater danger by employing such a procedure which does not correspond to the position of medical science for that particular time, the intervention being performed without the necessary training or practice or prerequisites for the intervention. Likewise the allowed risk is exceeded when such a medication is used which is contraindicated in the given case, or the physician isn't aware of the effects or contraindications.

The objective and subjective factors in *diagnostic error* are practically the same as the above-mentioned objective and subjective factors in the area of the medical risk. Diagnostic error comes under the heading of errors made in good faith which are based on Penal Code, Section 27 (1): "The perpetrator is not liable for such factors of which he could not be aware at the time of committing." Diagnostic error is not considered a breach of professional regulations if the physician took all possible measures to establish the nature of the disease and the diagnosis. If the diagnostic error cannot be verified by these criteria, the physician is excused from legal responsibility.

In summary: the professional regulations are broken and the physician liable if:

- he recognized the behavior required by the regulation but did not act appropriately, exceeding the limits prescribed,
- although recognizing the appropriate regulation, but due to lack of due attention or circumspection did not recognize that the behavior applied to the given situation,
- he did not recognize the professional regulation which applied to the given situation.

Judgement of malpractice is the responsibility of the court, but the answer to special questions is expected from medical examiners. The specialist weighs whether in the given situation the physician behaved in accordance to current medical standards, whether in light of average experience he did everything he could in connection with what the situation demanded. Did he observe foresight and care? According to Dezső "The causal connection – likewise the presence of immediate danger – is a question requiring the opinion of a specialist so that its judgement cannot be made without it. Since the breach of professional regulations and the presence of immediate danger can only be established by a medical examiner, likewise the demonstration of causality can only be made on the basis of expert medical opinion. The judge hasn't the knowledge necessary to make a judgement – and thus cannot be relied on – in the special areas of the ambiguities and uncertainties of the human organism, thus in the determination of causality the part of the medical specialist in very many cases is crucial in deciding whether there is a connection in doubtful cases."

Medical work in numerous cases is a group effort, the result of *teamwork.* It is inevitable that in some cases a judgement may involve group responsibility, or sharing of the responsibility. In general it can be declared that group responsibility in such cases cannot be established. The responsibility must be divided for persons and on the basis of expert medical opinion assigned to the roles of the individual members on the basis of the situation. In the evaluation of a team effort, three tendencies must be differentiated:

One is the acceptance that the leader of the group himself bears responsibility for the errors of the members. This viewpoint is unacceptable as it requires such circumspection and continuous oversight and intimate knowledge of each individual area as cannot be reasonably expected of the leader.

The other concept is the opposite of the previous one. Every member of the group has such unlimited dominion over his area that the leader must be entirely excused in every instance from seeing that the members of the group abide by the rules. Thus the dangerous situation falls to a minimum. The theoretical possibility can be raised in opposition to the idea of absolute autonomy that one member of a group may make an error which is obvious to other members of the group and can not be stopped or corrected by them, and the persons making this error alone could carry the consequences.

The third trend materializes in the theory of so-called limited liability. With this the team leader monitors the appropriate work of the team, and later if someone or some people show uncertainty in the performance of their jobs, or lack of proper experience to perform their tasks, then he takes the appropriate steps to monitor the pertinent individual more closely, and if necessary, dismisses him from the team. If any member of the group notices that someone is not performing his job properly, then he is obliged to report it to the team's leader.

If several groups work together, the given team leaders are likewise obligated to observe the above-mentioned guidelines. This applies especially to the surgery where surgical teams work together with anesthesiology teams.

Health care workers who work in the medical field also come under the professional regulations. In the case of workers, it must be first determined whether they are capable of carrying out their entrusted responsibilities. They can only be entrusted with such responsibilities which have been described in their regulations and their practical skills determined by testing. The tasks of a health worker must be given in writing. At the same time the person must be informed of the legal and criminal responsibilities as well.

The health worker is held responsible for:

breaking any professional regulations applying to his area of work,
properly performing interventions within the area of his responsibility,
voluntarily overstepping the boundaries and performing such interventions which are not his responsibility.

The supervisor – chief physician, department chief – is responsible for the errors of the health worker if:

he assigns to the worker tasks which are prohibited by law,

he assigns tasks to the worker for which he has not been properly trained or tested,
he notices that the worker is incompetent in the fulfillment of his duties and does not remove him from them,
he does not regularly monitor the capabilities of the worker.

Responsibilities of the physician under civil law

The physicians liability under civil law is established where it states, "whoever causes unlawful harm to another is liable for compensation."

The conditions of compensation under civil law are:

- the origin of the damage must be verifiable,
- the damage must be the result of illegal behavior,
- the illegal behavior must be attributable,
- (intentional or due to carelessness),
- there must be connection between the culpability and
- the damage.

There are no grounds for compensation if:

- the damage was not caused illegally,
- damage occurred, but was not of medical origin (no causal connection),
- the physician verifies that it occurred in the
- interests of faultless performance of his duties,
- which under the given circumstances was unavoidable,
- and must be certified (appropriate documentation).

(Faulty performance also means not performing the intervention in the appropriate manner. In an abortion case an obstetrician interrupted an approximately 6 week pregnancy using a so-called abortion forceps. With this he perforated the uterine wall several times causing multiple injuries to the intestines. In the expert medical opinion he was faulted for not using the instrument properly and was convicted of breach of professional regulations. Upon weighing the expert medical opinion the court accepted it inasmuch as it cited improper use of an instrument, and established criminal behavior in the physician as well as a connection with the later consequences.)

The plaintiff (the patient) is most commonly awarded pecuniary damages (a decrease in ability to earn an income, lost profit or use, various expenses or expenditures may be established).

Such an injury may, however, originate in which pecuniary damage cannot be assessed although financial compensation may be appropriate to ease the suffering.

General legal principles (criminality, culpability) may be applied in the establishment of non-pecuniary damage the same way that pecuniary damage is established on legal principles described above.

Non-pecuniary damage applies to damage that permanently or seriously impairs one's participation in social life (cultural, sports, entertainment, finding a mate, choosing a profession, performance of biological functions etc.).

The physician who is employed or associated with a job is not immediately liable for damages caused in connection with the job. The place of work accepts this since the physician himself bears the consequences of ignoring the given civil laws which apply to the private physician.

References

[1] ÁDÁM, GY.: Egészségügyi jogi kézikönyv. Közgazdasági és Jogi Könyvkiadó, Bp. (1990)

[2] Az egészségügyi törvény és végrehajtási utasításai. Eü. Min. kiadványa

[3] BÉKÉS, I.: A gondatlanság a büntetőjogban. Közgazdasági és Jogi Könyvkiadó, Bp. (1974)

[4] BODROGI, GY.: A diagnosztikai iatrogén ártalmak. Orvosi Hetilap 45 (1967) 2129–2132

[5] BRAHAMS, D.: Death in the dentinst's chair. Lancet 2 (1989) 991–992

[6] BUDAVÁRI, R.: Az anaesthesiologia kockázatáról. Morf. és Ig. Orv. Szemle 3 (1963) 229–232

[7] CARMI, A.: Priorities in the delivery of health care. 9th World Congress on Medical Law. Proceedings (1991) 89–126

[8] CHARFOOS, S. L.: Medical malpractice liability. 9th World Congress on Medical Law. Proceedings (1991) 135–142

[9] DEZSŐ, L.: A foglalkozás körében elkövetett veszélyeztetés és a hibás orvosi tevékenység. Magyar jog 4 1971) 228–230

[10] DEZSŐ, L.: Az orvos büntetőjogi felelőssége. BM Könyvkiadó (1979)

[11] DRIPPS, R. D., J. E. ECKENHOFF, L. D. VANDAM: Introduction to anesthesia. The Principles of Safe Practice. W. B. Saunders Co. Philadelphia (1988) 3 pp. 389–416

[12] ECKERT, W. G.: Medicolegal investigations in hospital enviroments. Am. J. Forensic Med. Pathol. 10 (1989) 187–189

[13] FLUSS, S. S.: 25 years of health law: a retrospective from WHO. 9th World Congress on Medical Law. Ghent 1991

[14] FÖLDES, V.: A felelősség megítélése az orvosi tevékenység vitás eseteiben. Rendőrségi Szemle 1 (1962) 65–?

[15] HARSÁNYI, L., SZUCHOVSZKY, GY.: A kórtörténet, mint okirat. Orvosi Hetilap 104 (1963) 1846–1849

[16] HARSÁNYI, L., SZUCHOVSZKY, GY.: Az egészségügyi középkáderek szakmai felelőssége. Orvosi Hetilap 106 (1965) 2424–24264

[17] HARSÁNYI, L., FÖLDES, V., SZUCHOVSZKY, GY.: Vitás műtéti halálesetek szakértői véleményezése. Orvosi Hetilap 107 (1966) 1461–1464

[18] PETERS, J. D., K. S. FINEBERG, D. A. KROLL, V. COLLINS: Anesthesiology and the Law. Health Administration Press (1983) Washington, pp. 7–60

[19] PETERS, J. D., J. C. PERAINO: Malpractice in Hospitals. Ten theories for direct liability. Law Med. and Health Care. 12 (1984) 254–259

[20] ROSENTHAL, M. M.: Dealing with Medical Malpractice. Duke Univ. Press Durham (1988) 1–70

[21] SAMUELS A.: Medical negligence, today, an apraisal. Med. Sci. Law. 23 (1983) 31–36

[22] SCHIFRIN, B. S., H. WEISSMAN, J. WILEY: Electronic fetal monitoring and obstretrical malpractice. Law Med. and Health Care 13 (1985) 100–105

[23] SCHWARTZ, W. B., D. N. MENDELSON: The role of physicianowned insurance companies in the detection and deterrence of negligence. JAMA 262 (1989) 1342–1346

[24] SCHWARTZ, W. B., D. N. MENDELSON: Physicians who have lost their malpractice insurance. JAMA 262 (1989) 1335–1341

[25] SOMOGYI, E.: Új irányok és eredmények az igazságügyi orvostanban. Orvosi Hetilap 114 (1973) 2763–2769

[26] SOMOGYI, E.: Akut appendicitis: gondok és gondolatok. Orvosi Hetilap 113 (1972) 1639–1645

[27] SOMOGYI, E.: Orvosi segítséggel az igazság nyomában. Medicina, Bp. (1977)

[28] SOMOGYI, E., SZUCHOVSZKY, GY.: A műtéti beleegyezési nyilatkozattal kapcsolatos egyes kérdésekről. Orvosi Hetilap 107 (1966) 75–78

[29] SZABÓ, A.: Az aneszteziológia és intenzív terápia művelőinek felelősségéről. Rendőrorvosi Tudományos Ülések (1972) 16–21

[30] SZUCHOVSZKY, GY.: Az orvos büntetőjogi felelősségének egyes kérdéseiről. Orvosi Hetilap 102 (1961) 1633–1639

[31] SZUCHOVSZKY, GY., HARSÁNYI, L.: A műtéti kockázat kérdései az orvosszakértői gyakorlatban. Magyar Sebészet 18 (1965) 1–6

[32] SZUCHOVSZKY, GY., HARSÁNYI, L.: A rendkívüli műtéti halálesetek orvosszakértői vizsgálata. A felróható műtéti hibákról. Magyar Sebészet 27 (1974) 106–112

[33] SZUCHOVSZKY, GY.: Az orvosi működés jogi szabályozása. Szülészet, Nőgyógyászat és Igazságügyi Orvostan. DOTE Női Klinika kiadványa (1984) 5–45

[34] TINKER, J. H.: Anesthetic risk. In: M. C. ROGERS: Current Practice in Anesthesiology. B. C. Decker Inc Toronto (1988) pp. 1–5

[35] TÖRŐ, K.: Az orvos polgári jogi viszony. Közgazd. és Jogi Könyvkiadó Bp. (1965)

[36] TÖRŐ, K.: Az orvos polgári jogi felelőssége. Szülészet, Nőgyógyászat és Igazságügyi Orvostan. DOTE Női Klinika kiadványa (1984) 45–63

Index

A

Abdominal hemorrhage 93, 214
- diagnosis 94
- injury 93, 294

AB0 blood group system 172, 173, 174, 283
- saliva stains 174
- seminal stains 174

Abortion 261–176
- chemical substances 273
- complications 273
- consequences 274
- by instrumental 273
- intervention 272
- recognition of pregnancy 261
- spontaneous 271
- by violence to abdominal wall 95

Abrasion injury 49, 54, 61, 64, 67, 126
- impression 66

Absorption blood group determination 172
Acceleration, contusion 85
Accident involving the lower extremity 303
Accidental injury 299
- disability 299

Acetaldehyde, metabolism of alcohol 349
Acetic acid poisoning 330
Acetylation 317
Acid phosphatase activity demonstration 181
Activity of treatment and prevention 391
Acute airway obstruction 208
Additive effect 314
Adipocere components 25
- formation 25
- – in damp environment 26

Adsorption by active charcoal 362
Age determination 381–384
Age differences, skeletal 381
- by ossification centers 384
- from teeth 382–383

ADH 346, 347, 349, 351
Agglutinin determination 173
Agonal signs 13
Air embolism 52, 275
Air guns 123
Alcohol 347
- absorption 348
- biological membrane 347
- breath examinations 348, 351
- cause of accidents 95–98
- endogene 352
- elimination 348, 350, 351
- hypothermia 147
- metabolism 349
- – diabetic patients 352
- – kinetic reaction 349
- – proteins 348

Alcohol
- – fatty acids 348
- poisoning 352
- – acute 352
- postmortal production 353
- urinary-blood ratio 350

alcoholic state 350
- hypoglycemia 349

Aldrich–Mees lines 324
Aldrin 335
Alkali poisoning 330
Alterations caused by scissors 51
Alternating current 167
Amanita muscaria 355
- phalloides 353

Amatoxin 353

Amniotic fluid aspiration 242–243
Amputation
- lower and upper extremity 304, 306
- - damage assessment 305
Amussat's sign 41, 222, 225
Anatomical healing 163
Aneurysm, 203
- cerebral arteries 194
- dissecting 204
- rupture, sudden death 204
Anoxia 219, 225
Ant bites 27, 29
Antemortem and postmortem injuries 155–159
Antagonist effect 315
Anthropological examinations 288
Aorta, aneurysm 204
- - rupture, sudden death 204
- developmental aberrations 192
AP activity 181
Apoplectiform hemorrhage 87
Aquaplaning 97
Area of compensation 307
Arm, permanent injury 302, 304
Arsenic poisoning 322–324
- - acute 323
- - chronic 324
- autopsy findings 324
- elimination 323
- melanosis 324
Arteriosclerosis 203
Artificial abortion
- irradiation 118–119
- respiration of newborn 242–243
Aspecific granulation tissue 80
Aspiration
- gastric contents 156, 209
- vomit 234
Asthenospermia 279
Atrial defect, sudden death 192
Autoantibody, individual specific 175
Autolytic processes 23
Automatic weapons 122
Automobile accident 103
- autopsy 105
- frontal impact 104
- seat belt 104
Autopsy 34
- cooling death 148
- drowning 41, 232–233
- external examination 35
Autopsy record 35
- - examination of clothing 32
- sudden death 191–192
- suffocation 40, 221, 228
- technique 38
- - hanging 225
- - burned body 18,141
- newborn 239
- - rape 258
- traffic accident 39
- protocol 35
- special 38
- - gunshot 41,129
- - manual strangling 41, 221, 228
- - newborn 38
- - poisoning 357
- - stabbing injuries 60
Azoospermia 279

B

Background radiation 115
Ballistics 124
Barbiturates 342
- and alcohol 315, 343
- metabolism 442
- poisoning 343
Barrel, weapon 124
Benzidine reaction 70
Benzodiazepins 343
Bicycle accident 93, 101
- fall from 101
Biological death 11
Bisexuality 265
Bite marks 184–187
- human tissue 186, 187
- identification 187
- rape 207
- - examination 185
- in sexual offences 185
Black powder 121
Blade edge, 51
- hacking injury 61
- incision injury 50
Blast injury 139
Blister formation 22, 92
- blister injuries 140
Blood
- abscess 69

Blood drop stains 169–177
– – age 175
– – characteristics of 175
– – identification 171
– – rivulets 176
– – specificity 171
– paternity examination 281
– – group heritability 280
– – systems 282
– sample, poisoning 359
– – alcohol 349
– – – alcohol curve 350
– – – dinamic state 350
– – carbon monoxide 225
– – traffic accident 106
– trace demonstration procedures 170–172
Blunt force to the abdomen 92–95
Body
– lying on the road 100
– weight, in relation to alcohol concentration 348
Bone, burned
– age determination 279
– ossification centre 38
– pearls' 107
– penetrating stab injuries 58
Brain
– death 11, 12
– – certain 11
– – determination 12
– – diagnosis 12
– edema 88
– electric shock 108
– embolism, sudden death 192
– emoliation, sudden death 212
– function, irreversible cessation 11
– injury 84–89
– – types 84–89
– temperature 17
– vessel aneurysm 194, 211
– – thrombosis 212
Breathalyser 351
Breath alcohol 351
Braking radiation 114
"Bridge signs" 306
Brown fat 148
Bruising injury 64, 67
– traffic accident 101
Bullet
– effect on target 124–125
Bullet identification of 136–137
– types 121
Burial, decomposition of body 24
Burn degrees 140–141
– hair 141
– injury 140
– – caused by molten metal 143
– – electric shock 108–109
– percentage of surface area 141
– plastic 143
– – PVC 1423

C

Cadaver
– changes over time 16
– – infant 16
– color changes 14
– – in water 16
– soft tissue damage 21
– – by living things 27–30
– – decay 21
temperature 16–17
Calibre 122
Calomel, mercury poisoning 319
Carbon monoxide 325–327
– hemoglobin in blood 325
– – as vital sign 156
– poisoning 325–326
– clinical signs 327
– – oxigen deprivation 325
Cardiac arrest, cuses of
– thoracic injury 90
– reflex mechanism 274
Cardiomyopathy 200
Cardiovascular alterations, sudden death 196–197
– in youth 215
Care, physician's duty of 392
Carelessnes (luxuria) 397
Carp bites 221
Cartridges 121
– identification 138
– – smooth-bore 123
Cataleptic rigor mortis 18
Cataract due to lightnight 113
Cation exchange chromatography procedure 362
Central nervous system tumors, sudden death 213
Cephalhematoma 38
Cerebral hemorrhage 85–88
– coup-contrecoup injuries 85

Cerebral stroke 211
– traumatic 87
– – Courville classification 87
– – secondary 88
Cerebrospinal fluid, brain death 12
Chamber of firearm 124
Characteristic, radiation 114
– desiccation 18
Chelate formation 318
Chemical, antagonism 315
– material causing abortion 273
Chemiluminescence effect 170
Childbed women, mental state 250
Chlorinated hydrocarbons 335
Choke, definition 123
Choking on a swallowed piece (bolus), sudden death 208
– aspirated material, sudden death 208
Chromosomal banding 290
– examinations 289
– – paternity 290
Chronic, subdural hematoma 80
Circulation cessation 14
Circulatory organs, sudden death 192–199
Civil law in medical practice 400
Clinical death 12
Clothing, examination 32
– coroner's report 32
– effect on cooling the body 16
Cocaine 339
Coffin birth 13, 22
Cold effect
– death due to 147
– rigor mortis 18
– survival time in environment 147
Collision 98, 105
– from behind 101, 104
Commotio cerebri 84
Competitive antagonism 346–347
Completely jacketed projectiles 121
Concussion
– cerebral 84
– cardiac 90, 203
Conduction system of the heart 195, 201–203
Congestive cardiomyopathy 201
Congestion, suffocation 220
Conjunctival petechiae 220
– suffocation 220
Connected gene 283
Contact imprint 185
Contaminated zone 125
Contre-coup injury 85
Contusion 64, 67, 69
– cerebral 79, 85
– index 85
Convulsive perpetrator 264
Cooling of body 16, 146, 148
– CK activity 148
– paradox reaction 147
– poisoning 147
Copper poisoning 318–319
Coronary disease, sudden death 193
– atheroclerosis 195
– occlusion 196, 197
Coroner's examination 32
– at scene 44, 225, 227
– certification 162–163
– report 35
Corpuscular radiation 114
Corrosive metal salts 331–332
Corrosives 33, 328
– poisoning 328–332
Cosmic radiation 115
Cranial autopsy 37
– newborn 38
Cranial hemorrhage 112
– vault fracture 75
Criminal abortion 273–274
Criminal responsibility, physician 395
Criminological photography 50
– examinations 169
Crossing over 281
"Crow's feet" type burn injury 141–142
Crude opium cocktail 338
Cyanide poisoning 327–328
– and hypostasis 16
Cytotoxic cerebral edema 89

D

Damage assessment
– in civil law 400
Damage caused by radiating heat 140–141
Damp heat 143
Dashboard injuries 104
Davies–Wilson scheme 183
DDT 335
Death accepted when 11
Death by cooling 146

Death 11–14
- biological 11
- certificate 34
- changes after 14–30
- clinical 12
- determination 11
- drowning 231
- following electrocution 108, 112
- following rape 258
- hanging 225
- natural 31
- sudden 191
- unexpected 31
Decollement bruise 69, 100
Decreased participation in social life 308
Defense injury 51, 59, 72
- types 51
- - incision 51
- - stab 59
- - hacking 63
Degrees of activity following injuries 52, 79, 83
Delayed traumatic apoplexy 87
Demonstration of poisoning 357–372
- immunological methods 368
Dermal alterations 108
- burn injuries 140
- electric shock 109–111
- putrefaction 22
Desiccation 18
- infant 19
Deterioration of health 294
- causes 294
Determination,
- age in identification 381–384
- - from skeletal remains 381
- - bone age 279
- instruments 53, 54, 58, 137
- weapon-calibre 122
Diabetic patient in traffic accident 97
Diagnostic error 398
Diagnostic X-ray examination 115
Diaphragmatic injury 94
Diathermy equipment 120
Diatoms 233
Diazepam 343
Diffuse axonal injury (DAI) 84
Dilatation of circle of Willis, sudden death
Denial of medical treatment 393
Direct
- current 107
Direct rib fracture 89
Disability 293–311
- accidental in character 296
- assessment of degree 296–297
- compensation 295
- disease, causing of 300–301
- decrease 295
- evaluation 299
- herniation of intervertebral disc 306
- theoretical basis 295
- withdrawn 295
Discontinuity, stab injury 54, 55
Diseases of the abdominal organs, sudden death 209
Dissecting aneurysm, sudden death 204
Distillation in toxicology 361
DNA fingerprint 174–175
- postmortal examination 175
- seminal stains 174
Dominant inheritance form 281, 288
Drog dependence 224
Drugs 338
- abuse 339, 340, 341
- blood level 368
- metabolism 339, 341, 342
Drowning 232–234
- autopsy technique 223, 232,
- - stage of 231
Dry
- drowning 231
- heat 140
Duffy blood group system 284
Duodenal injury 94
- ulcers, following burn injury 144, 145

E

Effect of radiation 114–115
Ejaculate examination 180
- demonstration from the vagina 181, 183
- - following rape 181
- paternity 278
- staining of 183
Electric current 107
- burn injuries 108
- power 107
- shock 108
- - death following 108
- - dermal alterations 110

Electric current shock dermal alterations
microscopical findings 110
– – individual sensitivity 107
– – – children 107
– signature 33
– trace 107
Electric stimulability of skeletal muscle 13
Electricity, direct effect 107
– entrance location 107, 110
– immediate effect 107–108
– mechanical injuries 108
– types 107
– voltage 108
Electromagnetic waves 119
Elution blood group determination 173–174
Embolism 204
– cerebral 212
– coronary 196
– fat 70
– pulmonary 204
– sudden death 212
– vital sign 156
Endogenous CO 325
Entry wound 122
Environmental hypothermia 146
Enzyme histochemical alterations
– necrotic myocardial tissue 197, 198
– vital injuries
Epidural hematoma 78
Epileptic patient, sudden death 212
– traffic accident 97
Equivalent dose 114
Erythrophagocytosis 156, 225
Essen–Möller calculation 286
Establishing identity 373
Estimated conception time 280
Ethical responsibility 395
Ethyl alcohol 347–353
Ethylene glycol 348
– competive effect 342
– metabolisation 346
Evidence of rape 137
Examination of bullet 138
– cartridge 138
Examination
– hanging ligature 221
– ossification centers 38
– rape 259
– vaginal secretions 181, 183
Exhibitionism 268
Exhumation 24–25
Exit wound 128
Exitus dilatus 108
– interruptus 108
– momentaneus 108
– retardatus 108
Explosion 138
– boyler 140
– gas appliences 139
Explosive tipped projectiles 121
External
– ballistics 124
– examination, autopsy 35
Eye, hanging 224
– desiccation 19

F

Face imaging reconstructive morphology 384
Facial feature, reconstruction 374
Family law 277
Fat embolism 69–70, 118
– tissue decay 25–26
Fatty infiltration, sudden death 202
Fertility examination 278
Fetal damage, radiation load 116–118
Fetishism 267
Fibrin formation 156
Findings report, filling out 161, 162
Fingernail imprints 221, 228
Fingerprint identification 374
Firearm
– cycle of fire 123–124
– examination of 136–137
– identification 137
– classification 121
– wounds 124–129
Flash
– back 341
– effect 141
– over effect 112
Float test
– infanticide 242
Florance test 181
Fluid release in decay 23
Fly species development 27
Foam 232
Food bolus, sudden death 208
Foot fracture 98, 99
– percentage disability 305

Forensic toxicologist 313
Formaldehyde 346
Fracture 72–75
- healing 74
- hole type 76
- skull base 76
- - newborn 249
- - diagnosis of 76
- traffic accident 98–99
Free radicals 337
Frotteurism 265
Fuel oil 347
Functional
- antagonism 315
- healing 164
Furnace explosion 140

G

Galvanization sign 107
Gammaradiation 113
Gas chromatography 363
- equipment explosion 140
- formation in decomposition 22
Gastric lavage fluid 359
- content examination 36, 359
- mucosa, autodigestion 23
- poisoning 359
Gastrointestinal tract
- air test 39–40, 244
- injury 94
- newborn 39–40
Gc–MS system 363, 364, 365
Gestational age
- calculation on the basis of fetal measure 280
Gingival discoloration, poisoning 319, 157
Gladiator posture 144
Glottic edema 206, 208
Glycosilation 317
Gm system 285
Grave wax 25, 28
Gray hepatization, pneumonia 207
Green-stick fracture 72
Guaiac test 170
Gunpowder 121
- burns-residue 124
- residue 134
- - on hands 129
Gunshot injuries 120
- autopsy technique 41, 129
Gunshot injuries characteristics 125
- direction 133
- identification of the weapon 137
- range 133
- residue 134
Gynecological illnesses, disability 300

H

Hacking injuries 61–64
Heamangioma 211
Hair 177–180
- animal-human 179
- - determination of type 179–180
- burnt 141
- characteristics 177
- core structure-examination 179
- cortical structure 177
- cut 179
- electron microscopic picture 178–179
- examination 178
- formation 177
- growth 177
- injuries 179
- layers 177
- light microscopic picture 177–178
- papilla 177
- structure 177–178
Half-life, poisoning 220
Hand, permanent injury 304
- functional damage 302
- gun 122
Hanging 223–227
- and vessels of the neck 223
- instrument 225
- - padded 224
- mark 223
- - atypical 223
Haptoglobin system 285
Hard drugs 338
Hashish 340
Head injuries 75
- on collision 104, 105
Healing 161–167
- anatomical 163
- establishment of 52, 59, 74
- functional 164
Heart
- decay 23, 25
- injuries 91–92, 104, 110

Heart rupture alterations 91
- stab injury 59
Heat
- conductance capacity 140
- effect, blood 41
- electrocution 109, 111
- stroke 146
Helvella esculenta 355
Hemorrhage
- abdominal 93, 214
- area of the injury 155
- arrosion 209
- amount 177
- bruising 69, 71
- incision injury 53
- intracranial 78, 80, 82, 83, 178
- menstrual 176
- nose 176
- subarachnoideal 82, 212
- traumatic cranial 78, 82, 85, 87
Hemosiderin, formation 157
Herbicides 336
Heritable biochemical characteristics in paternity 284–285
Heroin 342
High voltage 107
Hip joint acetabular fracture, damage assessment 305
Histamine release 158
Histological examination in autopsy 42
Hit-and-run accident 100
HLA system 285
Hole fracture 76
Homemade firearms 123
Homicide,
- gunshot wound 120–139
- hanging 223
- hacking injury 61–64
- incision wound 50–53
- stab wound 53, 60
- strangling 227
Homosexuality 265
Homozygoticity 285
Hot surface 141
- contact 143
- gas inhalation 143
- scald injury 143
Human and animal hair 178
- blood 172
Hummel type gene statistics 286–287
Hunting firearms 123
Hydrochloric acid poisoning 330
Hydrogen peroxide, demonstration of blood stains 170
Hydrolysis 316
Hymen-individual 254, 260
- characteristics 250
- physiological variations 253–254
Hyoid bone fracture 223, 224
Hyperextension 302
Hypospermia 219
Hypostasis
- color 16
- imbibition 16
- poisoning 16
- wandering 14
Hypothermia 146
- early clinical signs 147
- relationship to alcohol 147
Hypoxic condition 219, 325
- acute 219
- chronic 219
- sudden death 202

I

Identification 373–387
- determination of age 381
- - skeletal 379
- - dental 375, 382
Idiopathic hypertrophic subaortic stenosis 201
Imbibition hypostasis 16
Immediate danger
Impact incision injury 51
- abrasion injury 64
- bruising injury 69
- contusion 67
- depth 56
- direction 51
- hatchet injury 62
- laceration 70
- number 51
- size 54
- stab injury 53
Impression fracture 75
- of hacking instruments 62
Impulsive murderer 264
Inability to earn a living 294
- judgement 294–298
- time frame 297

Incised injuries 50
- forms 51
- skid mark 51
- suicidal 51
Increased intracranial pressure 210
Individual effects of toxic materials 313
Induction of drug metabolism 317, 318
Industrial accident 296, 327, 330, 345
Industrially acquired irradiation 115
Infanticide 38, 237–252
- causes of death 242
- questions applying to the mother 252
Infarct, sudden death 197
- myocardial 199
- - papillary muscle rupture 199
Influenza, sudden death 206
Inform the patient 391
Injuries 49
- according to anatomical region 75–95
- burn 340–341
- caused by seat belts 104
- - by steering wheel 104
- contre-coup 85
- definition 49
- determination of age based on histochemical 158
- diaphragm 94
- differentiation
- - antemortem, postmortem 157
- due to heat effect 341
- electric 106–113
- fracture 72–75, 76, 77
- head 75–89, 98, 101, 104
- - newborn 249
- healing 158
- hymen 253–254
- judgement 164–165
- to the pregnant uterus 95
- types 50
Insecticides 333–336
Intermediate
- form of heredity 281
- life 155
Intestinal injury 94
Intracranial hemorrhage 78, 213
- aneurysm 83
- chronic 80
- epidural 178
- lucid intervall 79
- minortrauma 80
Intracranial traumatic 82
Intragastrointestinal alcohol fermentation syndrome 352
Intrauterine oxygen deprivation 240–241
Intussusception in infancy, sudden death 13, 214
Ionizing radiation 113
Irradiation 115
Ischemic heart disease, sudden death 193, 195

J

J-wave 147
Joule's temperature 109
Judgement
- cosmetic injury 308
- malpractice 395
- self defense incapacity 258
- traffic injuries

K

Kell–Cellano system 284
Keratin in hair 178
Kind, elution system of blood grouping 173–174

L

Laceration injuries 64, 70
Lanugo hair 177
Larcher spot 19
Laryngeal
- cartilage, injuries at hanging 222, 223, 225
- - injuries at manual strangulation 229
- - injuries at strangulation 237
- edema, sudden death 208
Latent fingerprints 375
Layered dissection, suffocation 222
LD_{50} expression 313
Lead "lines" 322
- poisoning 321–322
Left heart blood dilution 232
Legal
- aspects of sex life 253, 276
- - libido decrease 263
- - increase 263
- - perversion types 264
- - rape of children 255, 263
- possibilities of mortal danger 165–166
- responsibility 395
Legalities of retirement 295

Lesbian love 265
Lewis group system examination 174
Liability 307–311
Liability judgement 306
Ligamentous injury, damage percentage 303, 305
Ligature mark in hanging 221
Light physical injuries 164
Lightning figure 112
- stroke 112
Linear impression fracture 75
Linked genes 281
Lipids in alcohol resorption 384
Lithopaedion 21
Live birth 240–242
Liver decay 25
Liver rupture 93
Lobular laceration injury 71
Location of tentorial injury 39
Long tract degeneration 84
Loss of virginity 255
Low voltage 107
LSD 339
Lucid interval 79
Luminol test 71
Lung
- fetal 241
- - artificial respiration 243
- injuries 92
- not respirated 240, 241–242
- respirated 241
- suffocation 242
Luxury 397
Lysergic acid diethylamide 339

M

Maceratio 20
Magazine, weapon 122, 138
Maggots 27
Malpractice 395–400
Marijuana 340
Masochism 264
Mass spectroscopy 363
Mature newborn 245
May–Grünwald–Giemsa staining 183
Meconium inhalation 242
Medical certificate 161
- dental and pharmaceutical activity 389
- disability, permanent 164
- findings, with opinion 162, 167–168
Medicolegal
- certificate 161, 167
- endangerment in the professional realm 395
- examination of the body 33–37
- judgement of negligence 397
- legalities of private practice 391
- prohibition from the profession 390
- regulation of function 397
- requirements medical group responsibility 399
- - of informing 393
- responsibility 392–395
- responsibilities toward civil law 400
- risk 397
- tasks at scene 45–46
Medicines
- accidents caused by 342
- causing abortion 273
- metabolization 315–318
Meningeal inflammation, sudden death 212
Meniscus injury, disability 303
Menstrual bleeding 176
Meprobamate 368
Mercury poisoning 319–321
Metabolization of xenobiotics 315–318
Metal complex formation effect 318
Metal compounds 318–324
Methanol 346–347
Methemoglobin 18
Methods in toxicology 361–365
Methylation 319
Microscopy in identification of weapons 138
Microvoltage 107
Microwawe 120
Minor traumas 80
Mixed cell agglutination 173
MN system 173, 283
Morphine 340–342
Motorcyclist injuries 103
- ring fracture 103
Mucus aspiration, newborn 243
Mummification 27
Muscarine type poisoning 335
Muscle, decay 25
Mushroom poisoning 353–355
Myocarditis, sudden death 199–200

N

Narcotic poisoning 338–343
- withdrawal signs 339

Narcotics 338
Neck alterations,
- hanging 291, 224–225
- suffocation 228
- strangulation 229
Neck vessel, hanging 223
- incision injuries 52
- strangling 229
Necrophilia 365
Necrozoospermia 278
Negative autopsy findings, poisoning 357
Negative effect of weather front 98
Negligence,
- forms 397
Nervous system alterations, sudden death in youth 215
Neurological illnesses, disability 300, 305
Neutral position 302
Newborn death
- autopsy 239
- blockage of airway 247
- criminal death 247
- float test 39, 243
- injury 246, 249
- - following death 249
- maternal neglect 246
- mature 243
- natural causes 246
- sudden death 214
- time elapsed from birth 244
Nicotine 33
- type poisoning 335
Nitric acid poisoning 329
Normospermia 278
Nose bleed 176

O

Obligation of official confidentiality 393
Obliterative cardiomyopathy, sudden death 201
Occupational illnesses 296
Oesophageal varix, sudden death 209
Oligospermia 278
Opening the thoracic cavity 37
Opium 340
Organ removal 36
- legal regulation 37
Organophosphate compounds 334
Organs, molecular biological death 12–13
Oxalate cristals 245
Oxidative metabolization 317

P

Pachymeningitis haemorrhagica interna 80
Pancreatic injury 94
Pancreatitis, acute hemorrhage, sudden death 210
Paradoxical reaction, cooling 147
Paraquat 33, 336–337
Paraquat poisoning 369
Paternity
- anthropological investigations 288
- determination 286
- examinations 278–279
- exclusion 287
- fertility 278
- hereditary characteristics 280
- index 287
Pedestrian injuries 99
- lying person 100
Pedophilia 268
Penetrating cranial injury 76
Penetrating fracture 99
Percentage in amputation cases 304–305
Periarteritis nodosa, sudden death 204
Pericardial rupture 90
Peripheral vascular disease, sudden death 203
Permanent disability 165, 301
Permanent injury of upper extremity 302–304
Permanent injury to the lower extremity 303–305
Permanent spinal injury 303
Persistent Botallo duct, sudden death 193
Pesticides 332–333
Phallotoxin 353
Phenol metabolization 316
Phenophthalin test 70
Phenothiazine derivatives 344–345
Photoepilepsy 97
Plant insecticides 333–336
Plastic surgical alterations in identification 375, 377
Pneumonia, sudden death 206–207
Pneumothorax, sudden death 208
Poisoning
- alcohols 345–353
- autopsy 357
- carbon monoxide 325–327

Poisoning clinical signs 357
- corrosives 328–332
- cyanide 327–328
- demonstration procedures 357–369
- diagnosis 357
- herbicides 336–338
- insecticides 333–336
- interpretation of results 366–368
- metal 318–324
- mushroom 353–355
- narcotics 338–342
- pesticides 332–333
- preliminary data 357
- rodenticides 338
- sedatives 242–243
- toxic levels drugs and chemicals 318
- tranquilizers 343–345
Poisonous substances 313
Police medical autopsy 31
Post-alcoholic state 98
Postmortal electric stimulability 18
Potassium hydroxide 330
Potassium permanganate poisoning 331
Potentiating effect 315
Pregnancy 269
- probable signs 269
- reactions 270
- certain signs 270
- following rape 259
- recognition in the cadaver 270–271
- age 271
- ultrasound findings 270
Premature newborn 245
Projectile diameter 137
- construction 122
- searching 130
- surface alterations 137
- visual examination 137
Projectiles 121–122
Pseudoaneurysm 83
Psychiatric
- illnesses for disability 300
- – causing accidents 98
- significance of crimes of perversion 263
Public Health 389
- legal compliance 395
- main areas 389
- regulations 380–395
- responsibilities 391, 393, 394, 395
- workers 399
Pulmonary
- bloody edema 227, 230
- embolism, sudden death 204
Putrefaction 20

R

Radiation
- caused damage 113–119
- consequences 115
- biological effect 114
- dermatitis 117
- direct 116
- dosage 114–115
- fetal damage 116, 118
- ulcer, chronic 117
Radiological examination in identification 384
Rail vehicles 100–101
Rape 253–261
- examination of the suspect 261
- examination of victim 259
- verification 256
Rat bite 28
Recessive inheritance form 281
Recognition 373–374
Recoil effect, weapons 122
Reconstructive possibilities based on skeleton 379–381, 383
Rectal temperature in the cadaver 16
Red blood cell, enzymes 384–385
Reduction 316
Reflex death
- abortion 374
- hanging 235
- manual strangulation 228
Regulation of burial 34
Rehabilitation 299
Renal injury 95
Reparation procedure 158
Reproductive cell death 114
Respiratory organ alterations
- burn injuries 143–144
- sudden death 206–209
Responsibilities of specialists 395
Responsibilities
- information 393
- medical treatment 390, 395
- practicing physician 391
- record keeping 393

Responsibilities specialist 394
- team 399
- under civil law 400
Retraction balls 84
Revolver 122
Rh group system 283
Rib fracture 89
- complication 90
- direct 89
- indirect 90
Right of the physician 390
Rigor mortis 17
- ATP level 17
- cataleptic form 18
- electrical excitability 18
- imitation signs 18
Ring fracture 103
Risus sardonicus (sardonic smile) 17
Rodenticides 338
Rupture of dilated vessel, sudden death 203

S

Saddle thrombus 204
Sadism 264
Sadistic crime in catathymic crisis 264
Salting out in toxicology 362
Scene of the crime 43
- coroner's report at the scene 45, 226
- - searching for biological traces 46
- phaseses 44
- traffic accident 46
Search for the projectile 130
Secondary
- drowning 232
- injury projectiles 132
- shot channel 127
Sedative
- poisoning 342–343
- sedatives 342
Self
- assisted birth 249
- defense injuries 51, 58, 63, 130
- rescue, hanging 225
Separation of fractures 72
Septal defect, sudden death 192
Serious deterioration of health-physical damage 164
Settling hypostasis 14–15
Sexual drive 263
Sexual decrease 263
- increase 264
Sex-determination in identification 379
Shock wave 139
Short-barrelled weapons 122
Shot
- chanel 127
- - direction 133
- - flat bones 128
- - - establishment 133
- - layered dissection 129
- - primary 127
- - temporary 127
- description 129
- distance 133
- range 134
- spread 132
Shotgun cartridge construction 121
- gunshot injuries 132
SIDS 213–214
Sigma unit 181
Significant dose (GNS) 144
Signs of death 14
- early 14
- late 20
Silencer 126
Silver nitrate poisoning 331
Sino-atrial node 195, 203
Skeletal remains 379–381, 383, 384
Skid mark 51
Skull fracture 75–76
- newborn 75
Small intestinal necrosis, sudden death 210
Smoke poisoning 143
Smokeless powder 121
Smooth-bore firearm 123
Sociopaths 98
Sodium hydroxide 330
Soft point projectiles 121
Soft tissue injuries 67
- traffic accident 98
Solvent extraction 362
Somatic death 12
Special identification marks 377
Specialist responsibilities 395
Spectroscopic characteristics of oxyhemoglobin 171
Speedball 339
Sperm cell
- alterations 182, 256
- fragments 182, 183

Sperm recognizability 183
– motility 184, 255
– trace demonstration 180
– examination 181
– number in establishment of paternity 278
Spider web fracture 75
Spinal cord, autopsy 37
– injury in hanging 235
Spine, accidents involving 303
– permanent injury 306
– permanent damage 301
Spiral fracture 72
Splenic injury 93, 210
Spondylosis 301
Spontaneous abortion 271
Stab injury 53, 54
Stabbing incision injury 55
– formation 54
Stain examination
– ejaculate 180
– blood 169
Static electricity effect 112
Steering wheel impact 104
Stenosis of artery supplying the impulse generating center 202
Stool, poisoning 316
Strangulation
– deaths, autopsy technique 41, 229
– by ligature 237
– manual 237
– – injuries 221, 228, 229
– mark 227
Subarachnoideal hemorrhage 82, 212
Subdural hematoma 79
Sublimate poisoning 319
Subpleural suffusion 92
Subtentorial epidural hematoma 79
Sudden death 191–219
– esophageal ulcer 209
– – varicosities 209
– infant 213
– ostium barrier 194
– (SIDS) 213–214
– suffocation 229
Suffocation
– blocking of external air 225, 234
– constriction of thorax 234
– deaths, types 219
– drowning 222, 231
– "dry" 233
Suffocation in muddy water 233
– secondary 222
– signs 221
– sudden death 229
Suicide
– gunshot 131
– hacking 63
– hanging 223
– incision 52
– stab 59
– strangling 227
Sulfuric acid poisoning 329
Superimposition procedure, identification 384
Surgical illnesses, disability 301
Swelling due to decay 22
– temperature dependency 22
Synergistic effect 315
Syphilitic aortic alterations, sudden death 196

T

Takayama reaction, hemochromogenic crystals 171
Team responsibility 399
Teeth
– identification 282–283
– description 281
Teichmann, hemin crystals 171
Temperature induced muscle contraction 144
Temporary deterioration in health 294
Test firing 138
Tentative marks 51
Testicular biopsy material 279
Therapeutic radiation treatment 115
Thermal capacity 141
Thin layer chromatography 362
Thoracic compression 234
Thoracic injury 89
– lung 92
– sudden death 91
Time of
– conception 281
– death 33–36
Tire profile 33, 68
Torpedo projectiles 121
Torsion fracture 103
Toxic effect 313
– side effects 315
Toxicological examinations 359
– immunological methods 363

Toxicological interpretation of examination 365–369
- packaging of samples 359, 360
- possibilities 361–365
Traces of human origin 169–188
- searching the scene of the crime 172
Traffic accident 39, 95
- factors, external 95
- - internal 97
- primary injuries 98
- secondary injuries 98
Transposition of the great vessels, sudden death 192
Traumatic
- cerebral hemorrhage 87
- subarachnoid bleeding 82
Transvestism 267
Tumor induction 116
- radiation load 117

U

Ultrasound equipment 120
- irradiation 120
Ultraviolet irradiation 119
Unexpected death 31, 191
- in hospital 32
- unexplained 31
Upper extremity accident 303
- disability 304
Urate infarction, newborn 244, 245
Urethral injury 95
Urinary alcohol determination 350
Urine sample, poisoning 359
Use of radiopharmacologicals 115
UV spectrophotometry 363

V

Vaginal douche 256
Vaginal SF activity 181
Vascular disease, sudden death 203–205
Vasogenic cerebral edema 88
Vehicle specialist at the scene 106
Venous system thrombosis, sudden death 204
Ventricular fibrillation, electrocution 107
Verification of birth 2551–252
- determination of time elapsed since 251
Vertebral fracture 306
Vessel, arrosion, sudden death 209
Viability of the newborn 249
Vital sign 155
- injuries 155–159
- reaction 157, 225
Vitriol 329
Volatile oils 347
Volvolus 214
Voyeurism 265

W

Waller degeneration 84
Warfarin 338
Washmaid's skin 222
Whiplash fractures 99
Widmark factor 348
Wischnewsky ulcer 148
Work capacity
- accidental in character 296
- assessment of degree 296–297
- decrease 295
- - causing of 300–301
- evaluation 299
- theoretical basis 295
Wound
- hacking 61
- incision
- laceration 64, 70
- measurement 62
- parts 50
- - area 50
- - base 50
- - border 50
- - deepth 65
- - edges 51
- - sides 51
- - surroundings 50
- stab 54
- - forms 54
Wound healing with scars in identification 377

X

Xenobiochemical examination 315
Xg blood group system 284

Z

Zinc chloride poisoning 332
Zoophilia 265

MIX
Papier aus verantwortungsvollen Quellen
Paper from responsible sources
FSC® C105338

If you have any concerns about our products,
you can contact us on
ProductSafety@springernature.com

In case Publisher is established outside the EU,
the EU authorized representative is:
Springer Nature Customer Service Center GmbH
Europaplatz 3, 69115 Heidelberg, Germany

Printed by Libri Plureos GmbH
in Hamburg, Germany

Optimal Control of Nonlinear Processes

Dieter Grass • Jonathan P. Caulkins
Gustav Feichtinger • Gernot Tragler
Doris A. Behrens

Optimal Control of Nonlinear Processes

With Applications in Drugs, Corruption, and Terror

Springer

Dieter Grass
Vienna University of Technology
Institute for Mathematical Methods
in Economics
Argentinierstraße 8
A-1040 Vienna
Austria
dieter.grass@tuwien.ac.at

Jonathan P. Caulkins
RAND Research Center
201 N Craig St Ste 102
Pittsburgh PA 15213-1516
USA
caulkins@andrew.cmu.edu

Gustav Feichtinger
Vienna University of Technology
Institute for Mathematical Methods
in Economics
Argentinierstraße 8
A-1040 Vienna
Austria
gustav@server.eos.tuwien.ac.at

Gernot Tragler
Vienna University of Technology
Institute for Mathematical Methods
in Economics
Argentinierstraße 8
A-1040 Vienna
Austria
tragler@eos.tuwien.ac.at

Doris A. Behrens
University of Klagenfurt
Department of Economics
Universitätsstr. 65-67
9020 Klagenfurt
Austria
doris.behrens@uni-klu.ac.at

ISBN 978-3-540-77646-8 ISBN 978-3-540-77647-5 (eBook)

Library of Congress Control Number: 2008929913

Cover design: WMXDesign GmbH, Heidelberg

Printed on acid-free paper

9 8 7 6 5 4 3 2 1

springer.com

The authors dedicate this book:
to Daniela, Michael, Ilse, and Engelbert;
to Ellen, Jay, Joseph, and Jackie;
to Ingrid, Susanne, Evelyn, Katja, and Basti;
to Elisabeth, Katharina, Helen, and Ayana;
to Lukas, Heinrich, and Marianne.

Preface

The goal of this book is to prepare readers to apply the optimal control theory to nonlinear processes beyond the standard applications. The examples investigated in depth are drawn from drug policy, corruption, and counter-terror, so this book will be of particular interest to economists, epidemiologists, and other scholars interested in the economics of crime, health, and violence. However, the book is designed to simultaneously appeal to an even larger audience of students in mathematics, economics, biosciences, and operations research for whom it fills a gap in the literature between "cookbooks," that give recipes but not deeper understanding, and more formal mathematical textbooks that do not explain how to apply the theory to practical problems.

This innovative balance is inspired by what we and our students have discovered to be essential to productively harnessing optimal control to address novel application areas. In our experience, new models are rarely just minor variants of others whose solution already appears in the literature. So searching through a typical applications-oriented textbook for the right recipe is fruitless; the new model usually has some twist or idiosyncrasy that requires modifying the cookbook recipes, not just applying them. Such modifications require understanding grounded in a more mathematical presentation than cookbooks usually provide. On the other hand, students who read only the more mathematical presentations often have little clue how to go about solving applied problems, either in terms of writing down the original model or in terms of carrying out the numerical computations. For the curious reader, we provide references to formal proofs of key theorems, but do not always reproduce them here, preferring to focus on intuition and applications.

Indeed, even standard applications-oriented textbooks do not always prepare students for studying novel domains. Some authors focus on a specific application; their books are wonderful for students who know they will devote their careers to problems within that one application area, but students' interests and future career trajectories are rarely so well defined. Other authors sprinkle their texts with examples drawn from across the spectrum of application areas. This opens students' minds to the power and flexibility of these methods, so we do some of that ourselves in suggestions for further reading and end of chapter exercises drawn from optimal growth, marketing, production/inventory management, and environmental planning, among other applications. The risk of a broad but shallow approach, however, is that none of the examples is developed in depth, and careers cannot be made by working textbook-like toy problems.

So a second principal innovation of this text is developing in detail examples from three exciting and topical areas: drug, corruption, and counter-terror control. This treatment in depth allows students to learn by example some of the art and craft of good modeling, including the idea of developing layered models starting with highly stylized depictions and then building in greater and greater realism. Compared to most texts, we spend more time discussing why certain functional forms might or might not capture well the underlying system dynamics and how to think about the limitations of modeling approximations, rather than writing down the complete model all at once and simply asserting that it is an accurate reflection of the problem at hand.

We do not expect the majority of students to work professionally in these areas, although the fields of health economics and the economics of crime are growing rapidly. From classroom experience, however, we know students enjoy seeing how mathematics can be used to address these serious and intrinsically fascinating problems. Thinking about how to fight terror, corruption, or illegal drugs is simply more fun for most students than thinking about problems in firms (e.g., inventory management) or mechanics (e.g., balancing an inverted pendulum). Furthermore, the case studies are not just cartoons; the model development in this text mirrors the trajectory of the actual research. This allows the reader to experience some of the same excitement we felt when discovering new results or briefing interpretations that resonated with actual policy-makers with whom we have worked on these problems.

A third innovation is extensive treatment of models with multiple equilibria separated by DNSS points, which are a sort of tipping point. We have found that nonlinear models often have such features, at least for certain parameter constellations, and misleading results can be obtained if the analyst is not sensitized to this possibility.

From a pedagogical perspective, the fourth and perhaps most important innovation is that we have developed a toolbox (`OCMat`)[1] using the MATLAB language to analyze optimal control problems specifically for discounted infinite time horizon models. This toolbox allows (in general) an immediate analysis of the models after the problem formulation, since the necessary files for computation are generated (semi)-automatically. The core framework is the formulation of a boundary value problem, where the infinite time horizon is truncated to a finite horizon and the usual transversality conditions are replaced by so-called asymptotic transversality conditions. This approach is very flexible. It allows consideration of mixed and pure state constraints

[1] `OCMat` is available via `http://www.eos.tuwien.ac.at/OR/OCMat`.

and multi-stage problems, as well as the computation and continuation of DNSS points, junction points between boundary and interior arcs, and heteroclinic connections. Multiple examples are offered for both one and higher-dimensional models.

We are aware that not all readers come to optimal control with the same mathematical background. Hence, after a brief introduction (Chap. 1), Part I of this book continues by summarizing prerequisite material on continuous dynamical systems (Chap. 2). We stress the term "summarizes." A student who has never taken a course in differential equations cannot learn differential equations just by reading Chap. 2. However, for a student who studied differential equations a few years ago or who merely passed the course without attaining a deep understanding of all the material, Chap. 2 offers a valuable review focused specifically on the topics needed to understand optimal control. Appendix A does the same for material from linear algebra, topology, and calculus. That appendix also defines notational conventions, most of which are standard and should be familiar, but are included nonetheless for completeness.

Part II begins with material specifically on nonlinear optimal control. Chapter 3 is in some sense the heart of the book, introducing, explaining, and applying Pontryagin's Maximum Principle. Truly understanding how to apply the theory requires computing numerical solutions, not just proving propositions, so the text refers the student forward to Chap. 7 (Numerical Methods) at appropriate places for tutorials on how to perform the computations. Chapter 4 takes an innovative approach to deepening students' intuition concerning Pontryagin's principle, "deriving" it from standard discrete optimization by viewing continuous optimization as the limit of better and better discrete approximations to the continuous system, where we put "deriving" in quotes because the focus is on building intuition, not mathematical rigor. For a more mathematical class, particularly one for operations research students with a strong background in discrete optimization, Chap. 4 provides some basic ideas for the theory presented in Chap. 3. For others, Chap. 4 may be better appreciated later in the course, after the students have seen and worked on more applied problems.

In either case, the discussion in Chap. 5 of multiple equilibria should be read before proceeding to Part III and, as with Chap. 3, it includes pointers forward to Chap. 7 (Numerical Methods).

Real applications often involve more than just one-dimensional models, so we view the discussion in Chap. 6 of higher-dimensional as another core chapter. What makes higher-dimensional models so much harder is not primarily more advanced theory, but rather practical problems encountered when trying to analyze higher-dimensional systems. Hence, Chap. 6 comprises three detailed case studies, one each from drugs, corruption, and counter-terror. Each case study offers not just a solution, but also a description of the thought processes – including even some of the dead ends we encountered – that went into solving the problem, again with forward references to the parts of Chap. 7 needed for the numerical computations. We believe a complete course on optimal control ought to cover at least one or two of these case studies, but they are not cumulative, so the instructor can pick any subset of them in any order. Chapter 8 discusses advanced topics which is not required material for a basic course in optimal control. Rather, we include just brief discussions of three areas (multi-stage problems, differential games, and distributed parameter models) to give students a sense of the possibilities that exist beyond the standard ordinary differential equation or "compartmental" models.

Acknowledgments

We gratefully acknowledge three groups without whom this book could never have been written. The first are the funding agencies who have supported this project: The Austrian National Bank, the Austrian Science Fund, the Qatar Foundation for Education, Science, and Community Development, and the Robert Wood Johnson Foundation Investigator Awards in Health Policy Research. The views expressed imply no endorsement by any of these funders. Part of the work on drug modeling was written while the fifth author was with the DPMP team at NDARC (University of New South Wales) funded by Colonial Foundation Trust, Drug Policy Modelling Program.

The second are colleagues who collaborated with us on the original research projects that provided the foundation for this text and/or read and commented carefully on earlier drafts of the manuscript. We thank in particular Christian Almeder, Tamer Başar, Raouf Boucekkine, Roswitha Bultmann, Herbert Dawid, Engelbert Dockner, Harri Ehtamo, Jacob Engwerda, Caius Gavrila, Alessandra Gragnani, Lars Grüne, Hendrik Halbach, Richard Hartl, Josef Haunschmied, Franz Hof, Philipp Hungerländer, Steffen Jørgensen, Yalcin Kaya, Michael Kopel, Mark Kleiman, Daniela Knie, Peter Kort, Jacek Krawczyk, Alexander Kurzhanski, George Leitmann, Guiomar Martín-Herrán, Helmut Maurer, Lukas Mayr, Andreas Novak, Geert Olsder, Rosalie Pacula, Harold Pollack, Marion Rauner, Peter Reuter, Markus Riegler, Alison Ritter, Cagri Saglam, Andrea Seidl, Suresh Sethi, Gerhard Sorger, Cornelia Spreitzer, Mathias Staudigl, Alois Steindl, Maria Toda, Vladimir Veliov, Florian Wagener, Dagmar Wallner, Sandra Ward, Franz Wirl, Stefan Wrzaczek, Georges Zaccour, Irmgard Zeiler, and many colleagues at RAND's Drug Policy Research Center. We give special thanks as well to our editor, Werner Müller, for his vision and support throughout the project.

The third are our families, who have tolerated our obsession with this project over the past years and all the travel and extra hours of work it has entailed.

The first author also wants to thank Kornelia Hauser, Robert Peroni, and the people of East-Greenland, who played an important role for his return to the field of mathematics.

Contents

Preface VII

Acknowledgments XI

Part I Background

1 Introduction 3
- 1.1 Taking Rocket Science Beyond the Frontiers of Space 3
- 1.2 Why Drugs, Corruption, and Terror? 5
- 1.3 Questions Optimal Control Can Answer 7

2 Continuous-Time Dynamical Systems 9
- 2.1 Nonlinear Dynamical Modeling 9
- 2.2 One-Dimensional Systems 10
- 2.3 A One-Dimensional Corruption Model 14
- 2.4 Dynamical Systems as ODEs 17
  - 2.4.1 Concepts and Definitions 19
  - 2.4.2 Invariant Sets and Stability 21
  - 2.4.3 Structural Stability 25
  - 2.4.4 Linearization and the Variational Equation 26
- 2.5 Stability Analysis of a One-Dimensional Terror Model 27
- 2.6 ODEs in Higher Dimensions 30
  - 2.6.1 Autonomous Linear ODEs 31
  - 2.6.2 Autonomous Nonlinear ODEs 42
- 2.7 Stability Behavior in a Descriptive Model of Drug Demand ... 51
- 2.8 Introduction to Bifurcation Theory 55
  - 2.8.1 Terminology and Key Ideas of Bifurcation Theory 56
  - 2.8.2 Normal Forms and the Center Manifold: The Tools of Bifurcation Theory 57
  - 2.8.3 Local Bifurcations in One Dimension 63

2.9 Bifurcation Analysis of a One-Dimensional Drug Model 68
2.10 The Poincaré–Andronov–Hopf Bifurcation 71
2.11 Higher-Dimensional Bifurcation Analysis of a Drug Model 74
2.12 Advanced Topics 78
2.12.1 Stability of Limit Cycles 78
2.12.2 Boundary Value Problems 85
Exercises 89
Notes and Further Reading 96

Part II Applied Optimal Control

3 Tour d'Horizon: Optimal Control 101
3.1 Historical Remarks 101
3.2 A Standard Optimal Control Problem 104
3.3 The Maximum Principle of Optimal Control Theory 108
3.3.1 Pontryagin's Maximum Principle 108
3.3.2 Some General Results 113
3.3.3 The Maximum Principle for Variable Terminal Time ... 115
3.3.4 Economic Interpretation of the Maximum Principle 117
3.3.5 Sufficiency Conditions 119
3.3.6 Existence of an Optimal Solution 122
3.3.7 How to Solve an Optimal Control Problem: A Simple Consumption vs. Investment Model 124
3.4 The Principle of Optimality 127
3.4.1 The Hamilton–Jacobi–Bellman Equation 127
3.4.2 A Proof of the Maximum Principle 130
3.5 Singular Optimal Control 131
3.5.1 The Most Rapid Approach Path (MRAP) 134
3.5.2 An Example From Drug Control that Excludes Singular Arcs 137
3.5.3 An Example From Terror Control with an MRAP Solution 139
3.6 The Maximum Principle With Inequality Constraints 142
3.6.1 Mixed Path Constraints 144
3.6.2 General Path Constraints 147
3.6.3 Sufficiency Conditions 154
3.7 Infinite Time Horizon 155
3.7.1 Definitions of Optimality for Infinite Horizon Problems 155
3.7.2 Maximum Principle for Infinite Time Horizon Problems 156
3.7.3 Sufficiency Conditions 159
3.8 Discounted Autonomous Infinite Horizon Models 159
3.8.1 The Michel Theorem 160
3.8.2 The Ramsey Model for an Infinite Time Horizon 165

3.8.3 Structural Results on One-State Discounted, Autonomous Systems 167
3.9 An Optimal Control Model of a Drug Epidemic 168
3.9.1 Model Formulation 168
3.9.2 Stability Analysis 170
3.9.3 Phase Portrait Analysis 176
Exercises 177
Notes and Further Reading 183

4 The Path to Deeper Insight: From Lagrange to Pontryagin 189
4.1 Introductory Remarks on Optimization 189
4.1.1 Notational Remarks 190
4.1.2 Motivation and Insights 190
4.1.3 A Simple Maximization Problem 192
4.1.4 Finite-Dimensional Approximation of an Infinite-Dimensional Problem 195
4.2 Static Maximization 197
4.2.1 Basic Theorems and Definitions 198
4.2.2 Theory and Geometric Interpretation of Lagrange and Karush–Kuhn–Tucker 202
4.2.3 The Envelope Theorem and the Lagrange Multiplier 208
4.2.4 The Discrete-Time Maximum Principle as a Static Maximization Problem 210
4.3 The Calculus of Variations 214
4.3.1 A Simple Variational Example 214
4.3.2 The First Variation 216
4.3.3 Deriving the Euler Equation and Weierstrass–Erdmann Conditions 218
4.4 Proving the Continuous-Time Maximum Principle 223
4.4.1 The Continuous-Time Maximum Principle Revisited 223
4.4.2 Necessary Conditions at Junction Points 227
Exercises 231
Notes and Further Reading 234

5 Multiple Equilibria, Points of Indifference, and Thresholds 237
5.1 Occurrence of Multiple Equilibria 238
5.2 The Optimal Vector Field 239
5.2.1 Finite vs. Infinite Time Horizon Models 239
5.2.2 Discounted Autonomous Models for an Infinite Time Horizon 243
5.3 A Typical Example 244
5.3.1 Existence and Stability of the Equilibria 245

5.3.2 Determining the Optimal Vector Field and the Optimal Costate Rule 247
5.4 Defining Indifference and DNSS Points 252
5.4.1 Multiplicity and Separability 253
5.4.2 Definitions 254
5.4.3 Conclusions from the Definitions 256
5.5 Revisiting the Typical Example 260
5.6 Eradication vs. Accommodation in an Optimal Control Model of a Drug Epidemic 266
Exercises 269
Notes and Further Reading 272

Part III Advanced Topics

6 Higher-Dimensional Models 279
6.1 Controlling Drug Consumption 280
6.1.1 Model of Controlled Drug Demand 280
6.1.2 Deriving the Canonical System 283
6.1.3 The Endemic Level of Drug Demand 286
6.1.4 Optimal Dynamic Policy away from the Endemic State 287
6.1.5 Optimal Policies for Different Phases of a Drug Epidemic 292
6.2 Corruption in Governments Subject to Popularity Constraints 296
6.2.1 The Modeled Incentive for Being Corrupt 297
6.2.2 Optimality Conditions 299
6.2.3 Insights About the Incentive to Be Corrupt 300
6.2.4 Is Periodic Behavior Caused by Rational Optimization? 302
6.3 Is It Important to Manage Public Opinion While Fighting Terrorism? 308
6.3.1 What One Should Know when Fighting Terrorism 309
6.3.2 Derivation of the Canonical System 310
6.3.3 Numerical Calculations 311
6.3.4 Optimal Strategy for a Small Terror Organization 314
Exercises 316
Notes and Further Reading 323

7 Numerical Methods for Discounted Systems of Infinite Horizon 327
7.1 General Remarks 327
7.1.1 Problem Formulation and Assumptions 328
7.1.2 Notation 329

7.1.3 Numerical Methods for Solving Optimal Control Problems . . . 330
7.1.4 Boundary Value Problems from Optimal Control . . . 330
7.2 Numerical Continuation . . . 332
7.2.1 Continuation Algorithms . . . 333
7.2.2 Continuing the Solution of a BVP . . . 338
7.3 The Canonical System Without Active Constraints . . . 342
7.4 Calculating Long-Run Optimal Solutions . . . 343
7.4.1 Equilibria . . . 344
7.4.2 Limit Cycles . . . 346
7.5 Continuing the Optimal Solution: Calculating the Stable Manifold . . . 349
7.5.1 Stable Manifold of an Equilibrium . . . 350
7.5.2 Stable Manifold of Limit Cycles . . . 354
7.6 Optimal Control Problems with Active Constraints . . . 359
7.6.1 The Form of the Canonical System for Mixed Path Constraints . . . 360
7.6.2 The Form of the Canonical System for Pure State Constraints . . . 360
7.6.3 Solutions Exhibiting Junction Points . . . 362
7.7 Retrieving DNSS Sets . . . 366
7.7.1 Locating a DNSS Point . . . 366
7.7.2 Continuing a DNSS Point . . . 368
7.8 Retrieving Heteroclinic Connections . . . 368
7.8.1 Locating a Heteroclinic Connection . . . 368
7.8.2 Continuing a Heteroclinic Connection in Parameter Space . . . 369
7.9 Numerical Example from Drug Control . . . 370
7.9.1 Stating the Necessary Conditions . . . 370
7.9.2 Equilibria of the Canonical System . . . 372
7.9.3 Numerical Analysis . . . 372
7.9.4 Optimal Vector Field for $\nu = 4{,}000$ . . . 373
7.9.5 Optimal Vector Field for $\nu = 12{,}000$ . . . 377
Exercises . . . 380
Notes and Further Reading . . . 382

8 Extensions of the Maximum Principle . . . 385
8.1 Multi-Stage Optimal Control Problems . . . 386
8.1.1 Necessary Optimality Conditions for Two-Stage Control Problems . . . 386
8.1.2 Two-Stage Models of Drug Control . . . 387
8.1.3 Counter-Terror Measures in a Multi-Stage Scenario . . . 388
8.2 Differential Games . . . 391
8.2.1 Terminology . . . 392
8.2.2 Nash Equilibria . . . 394

8.2.3 Tractable Game Structures ... 397
8.2.4 A Corrupt Politician vs. the Tabloid Press ... 397
8.2.5 Leader–Follower Games ... 404
8.2.6 A Post September 11th Game on Terrorism ... 407
8.3 Age-Structured Models ... 417
8.3.1 A Maximum Principle for Distributed Parameter Systems ... 419
8.3.2 Age-Structured Drug Initiation ... 420
8.4 Further Optimal Control Issues ... 422
8.4.1 Delayed Systems ... 422
8.4.2 Stochastic Optimal Control ... 424
8.4.3 Impulse Control and Jumps in the State Variables ... 425
8.4.4 Nonsmooth Systems ... 426
Exercises ... 426
Notes and Further Reading ... 436

Part IV Appendices

A Mathematical Background ... 443
A.1 General Notation and Functions ... 443
A.2 Finite-Dimensional Vector Spaces ... 447
A.2.1 Vector Spaces, Linear Dependence, and Basis ... 447
A.2.2 Linear Transformations and Matrices ... 450
A.2.3 Inverse Matrices and Linear Equations ... 453
A.2.4 Determinants ... 455
A.2.5 Linear Form and Dual Space ... 457
A.2.6 Eigenvalues and Eigenvectors ... 459
A.2.7 Euclidean Vector Space $\mathbb{R}^n$ ... 461
A.3 Topology and Calculus ... 463
A.3.1 Open Set, Neighborhood, and Convergence ... 463
A.3.2 Continuity and Differentiability ... 464
A.3.3 Maximization of Real-Valued Functions in $\mathbb{R}^n$ ... 471
A.3.4 Convex Analysis ... 473
A.3.5 Taylor Theorem and Implicit Function Theorem ... 475
A.3.6 Integration Theory ... 477
A.3.7 Distributions ... 481

B Derivations and Proofs of Technical Results ... 483
B.1 Separation Theorems, Farkas Lemma and Supergradient ... 483
B.2 Proof of the Michel Theorem ... 486
B.2.1 Augmented and Truncated Problem ... 487
B.2.2 Optimal Solution of Problem (B.8) ... 487
B.2.3 Necessary Conditions for Problem (B.8) ... 488
B.2.4 Limit of Solutions for Increasing Time Sequence ... 489

B.3 Proof of the Transversality Condition in Proposition 3.74 491
B.4 The Infinite Horizon Transversality Condition Revisited 492
B.5 Monotonicity of the Solution Path 494
B.6 Admissible and Quasi-Admissible Directions 496
B.7 Proof of the Envelope Theorem 498
B.8 The Dimension of the Stable Manifold 499
B.9 Asymptotic Boundary Condition 502
B.9.1 Equilibrium 502
B.9.2 Limit Cycle 503

References 505

Glossary 531

Index 535

Author Index 545

Part I

Background

1

Introduction

> *"Our universe is the most perfect system, designed by the most wise Creator. Nothing in it will happen without emerging, to some extent, from a* **maximum or minimum principle**.*"*
> *Leonhard EULER* *(1707–1783)*

1.1 Taking Rocket Science Beyond the Frontiers of Space

The methods of dynamic optimization are rocket science – and more. Quite literally when NASA or the European Space Agency plan space missions, they use the methods described in this book to determine when to launch, how much fuel to carry, and how fast and how long to fire thrusters. That's exciting, but it's old news. Engineers have appreciated the power of this branch of mathematics for decades. What is news is the extent to which these methods are now contributing to business, economics, public health, and public safety.

The common attribute across these diverse domains, from medicine to robotics, is the need to control or modify the behavior of dynamical systems to achieve desired goals, typically maximizing (or minimizing) a performance index. The mathematics of *optimal control theory* make this possible. In particular, the discovery of the *Maximum Principle* for optimal paths of a system is what led the way to successful designs of trajectories for space missions like Sputnik and the Apollo program and myriad applications here on earth.

What is also new is that theoretical and numerical advances coupled with improved computing technology now allow exploration of much richer models than could be addressed in the past. An example of a recent theoretical development discussed here are new Maximum Principles for distributed parameter control problems. An example of an advance in numerical methods is the ability to locate thresholds separating competing basins of attraction in optimal control problems.

Distributed parameter methods greatly expand the range of applications for optimal control theory. Lumped parameter systems sufficed in many traditional applications. One state of an aeronautical system was the rocket's velocity. Unless something was going badly wrong, every part of the rocket moved together as a single body, so it was a very good approximation to imagine that all of the rocket had one velocity. Heterogeneity in populations can make the parallel approximations less compelling in demographics or economics. Hence age-structured "cohort" or "vintage" models of aging, migration, and technological and economic progress are increasingly popular, but until recently they were primarily descriptive. Now, however, various maximum principles for distributed parameter control problems provide a powerful tool to analyze such vintage problems.

Likewise, the world is full of nonlinearities, not all of which can be modeled well by the handful of functional forms that permit closed-form analysis, so using dynamic optimization requires an investment in creating numerical solution procedures. That investment has often been a barrier to both true understanding and practical application of these methods, but this volume devotes a chapter to explaining what numerical methods we have found to be vital over our collective 100 years of experience applying dynamic optimization to important problems. A companion website makes our computer code freely available to the reader to download.

The goal of this volume is to teach how the modern theory of dynamic optimization can be harnessed to gain insight into practical problems, including those in emerging areas. Typical texts draw examples from a wide range of applications, e.g., growth theory, dynamics of the firm (e.g., marketing), resource management and environmental planing. This demonstrates the flexibility of the methods, but the examples are inevitably a bit superficial, since the reader can't be presumed to have much domain knowledge in each of the many diverse applications.

Here in addition we develop a focused collection of interrelated examples drawn from three specific domains: counter-terror, corruption, and, most notably, illicit drug markets and their control. Focusing attention on three domains lets each be explored in depth with nested models of increasing complexity and with multiple complementary models, preserving the genuine excitement of nontrivial discoveries that characterizes professional use of these mathematical methods – excitement which is too often obscured in traditional treatments.

For example, we begin discussion with a simple one-state one-control model of treating drug users, and then expand it to two controls to show the dynamic interaction among two contrasting policies, one carrot (drug treatment) and one stick (drug enforcement). That model also illustrates the idea that where it is optimal to end up can depend on where one starts (so-called Dechert–Nishimura–Sethi–Skiba or DNSS separating thresholds), and that whichever direction one heads, the mix of interventions ought to vary dynamically over the course of an epidemic. That one-state model does not allow a very prominent role for drug prevention. Adding a second state to differentiate between new/light users and long-time/heavier users does a better job of elucidating how the relative roles of the two principal demand side interventions (drug prevention and treatment) vary over an epidemic. It also helps explain observed oscillations in the magnitude and character of drug epidemics. For other purposes it is useful to add a different second state, one that represents people who are "susceptible" to drug use, but who have not yet started.

On the other hand, to refine understanding of drug treatment, it is useful to add a third state elaborating the effects of accumulating "careers" of heavy drug use, particularly with regard to how they affect the "reputation" a drug has for being dangerous or benign and how that reputation then feeds back to influence initiation. Initiation into some drug epidemics seems to be cyclic with two different periods, one short and the other longer. Explaining that requires adding a fourth state to differentiate those who have tried and quit recently from other nonusers. To explore how prevention interacts with recurrent long-wave cycles of drug use, it is even useful to expand to an infinite number (a continuum) of states in an age-distributed structure.

This evolution of related drug models powerfully makes a number of important meta-points about modeling, such as the idea that a single system may usefully be addressed by multiple models of varying complexity depending on what particular question is of interest and the notion of exploring the sensitivity of results to the structure of the underlying model used to describe the system. It likewise supports discussion of a range of mathematical topics, including optimal dynamic control, multiple equilibria and DNSS points, limit cycles, bifurcation analysis, path constraints, McKendrick systems, dynamic games, and more.

1.2 Why Drugs, Corruption, and Terror?

This book does *not* draw its examples from drugs, corruption, and terror in the belief that most readers will work professionally on those topics. On the contrary; they are innovative – even unusual – applications for dynamic optimization. However, the range of potential applications is so broad that no one of them is likely to be the professional focus of more than a very small proportion of readers of any book on dynamic optimization.

Rather, we believe drugs, corruption, and terror are good exemplars for other reasons. First, they push the boundaries of optimal control beyond such early economic applications as macroeconomic growth models and exploitation of natural resources.

Second, they are topical. Since September 11th, terrible acts of terror have been visited on Madrid, London, Moscow, Bali and Beslan. Terrorists strike with even greater frequency in Colombia, South and Central Asia, and the Middle East. Terror control has scored noteworthy successes, such as dismantling the November 17th organization in Greece, but there is great need for more and better ideas.

Corruption is not a new problem and lacks a catalyzing event akin to the destruction of New York's Twin Towers, but it is important nonetheless, smothering economic development across vast stretches of the globe, notably in Africa and the former Soviet Union. The World Bank estimates the annual cost of corruption at over US $80 billion worldwide – more than the total of all economic assistance for development. Experts estimate that corruption adds some 25% to the costs of large government contracts. Thus, corruption can substantially reduce a country's growth rate. Corruption also undermines economic development in more insidious ways. Bribes harm a country's economy if civil servants pursue personal enrichment rather than the public good. Pervasive corruption can discourage investment and even erode political stability.

The production and distribution of illegal drugs intersects terrorism and corruption, as well as the spread of infectious diseases such as HIV/AIDS and Hepatitis, and it is a first-order problem in its own right. Drug production is thought to have accounted for as much as 30% of Afghanistan's GDP (Byrd & Ward, 2004) and fuels South America's longest-running civil war. Cost of illness studies find that drug abuse poses enormous costs on traditional consuming nations such as the US, Australia, and parts of Europe. Disturbingly, the United Nations finds that use of many drugs, particularly cocaine and stimulants, is spreading rapidly in parts of the world that heretofore have not had such severe problems. Globalization spreads inexpensive consumer goods around the world – including addictive drugs.

That drugs, corruption, and terror are important problems is not their only appeal for present purposes. They also have a certain morbid or salacious appeal that can hold the reader's interest when the math gets challenging. More substantively, corruption, counter-terror, and drug control are all usefully thought about in terms of populations, incentives, and interventions, concepts which map well into the framework of optimal dynamic control.

The hallmark of dynamic control is the notion that there is such a thing as a "state" of the system that evolves over time, in part subject to its own underlying dynamics and in part in response to nudging from some "social planner" who has an interest in the system. In rocket science the state of the system could be the rocket's position (in three dimensions) as well as its attitude (yaw, pitch, and role), associated derivatives (velocity, acceleration, etc.), and "inventories" (e.g., amount of fuel remaining). The internal dynamics are those set down by Isaac Newton, and the nudging is quite literal and is accomplished by thrusters.

In our applications the state of the system typically includes the numbers of people in each of various categories or activities. In a corruption model there might be two states, one each for the number of honest and dishonest actors. The two states in a drug model be the number of "light" (recreational, casual) users and the number of "heavy" (frequent or dependent) users. A state in a terror model might be the number of terrorists in a given organization. Most but not all states are counts; a terror model might also encode as a dynamic variable the state of world opinion toward terrorists or terror control.

The dynamics of bicycles and space shuttles evolve according to Newton's laws, but people's movements back and forth between different states of activity are driven by far more complex influences. One might think it is impossible to model systems in which humans are key moving parts, but that misunderstands the very definition of modeling. A model is a simplified representation of reality, not a perfect representation. Models of human systems simplify by omitting many factors, but so does any model. There may be more judgment involved in determining what constitutes a requisite model when analyzing human systems, but that makes systems like corruption, drugs, and terror better not worse topics for a book such as this. There is little value in learning all the mathematics if one still lacks skill in the art of judging what aspects of the complicated real world can and be excluded from a model in order to improve its tractability – and also what cannot be excluded.

Still, the inherent complexity of human systems ironically implies that there is particular wisdom in keeping the models simple, simple enough that one can understand intuitively "what makes the model work." Often we will model people's exit from a state as occurring at a constant per capita rate or in proportion to the number of random contacts between two states, perhaps modulated by external factor (such as price). Controls will sometimes be defined directly in terms of how they affect flows, although we will also consider models in which the control represents spending on some program, and the model structure explicitly reflects the "production function" that translates such spending into tangible effects.

1.3 Questions Optimal Control Can Answer

We close by describing at a conceptual level the kinds of questions that dynamic optimization can address. The most basic is *"Where should we go?"* The state space is comprised of an uncountably infinite number of points, each representing a potential destination. Which is best? Sometimes several satisfy all the necessary conditions for optimality, and yet one must determine which better achieves the true objectives. Sometimes no point is best, and the best target in the long run is a limit cycle around which one should cycle forever, rather than settling on any one point.

Static analytic models compare state levels at just two discrete points, e.g., the equilibrium before and after some change. Such "comparative statics" analysis can be informative, but all too often what's important is not only what the new equilibrium is, but also how one gets there (the "transient" path). As John Maynard Keynes observed, "In the long run we all are dead," but most people still have preferences about how their life evolves between now and the time of their death.

Hence, after figuring out where to go, there remains the crucial question: *"What's the best way to get from here to there?"* There are various definitions of "best." When driving to the store, it might be the quickest way. When flying to the moon it might be the way that consumes the least fuel. When driving an epidemic of corruption or drug use down to near zero ("de minimus") levels, the best path might minimize a weighted sum of the amount spent on control and the amount of corruption or drug dependence.

A related question is, *"How should we drive down that path?"* Such questions are trivial in a car with just one directional control (the steering wheel) and narrow lanes that constrain one's options. There are more ways to fight terror, so even if one knows what path to follow, there remain difficult questions about what mix of controls to use and how that mix should vary over time.

When answering these questions, one must understand how the answers would be amended if some of the assumptions underlying the model changed, particularly assumptions embodied in the values of model parameters. With static models, sensitivity analysis with respect to parameters often boil down to a single number, such as a derivative giving the "shadow price" of a marginal increment in some right-hand value. In dynamic optimization the shadow prices themselves vary over time (as "costate variables"). Furthermore, with nonlinear dynamics one must confront (often via "bifurcation diagrams") more fundamental questions of how the very structure of the solution does or does not vary when parameters change. For example, in our four-state drug epidemic model, modest changes in one parameter can flip the system through regimes of stability, instability, oscillation, and chaos.

Questions such as *"Where should we go?"*, *"What paths should we take?"*, and *"How should we drive down that path?"* can be asked about all sorts of systems, and the framework of dynamically evolving states is quite flexible. Besides the drug, corruption and terror control applications mentioned in this book, we have applied it to such diverse areas as fashion design, endangered species protection, dieting, growth economics, and HIV/AIDS control. Others have applied it to chemotherapy (Swan, 1988), nuclear magnetic resonance (Frueh et al., 2005), and even eating cake (Ozdenoren, Salant, & Silverman, 2006).

Before proceeding to the mathematics underpinning optimal control theory, we encourage the reader to identify a few interesting applications and sketch "stocks and flows" diagrams for each. Identify at least qualitatively the relevant states, flows in and out of those states, and controls that can influence those states and/or flows. In the course of reading the book, it may be instructive to reflect on how the various concepts introduced and illustrated for our drugs, corruption, and terror models might be applicable in these domains of interest to the reader.

2

Continuous-Time Dynamical Systems

The importance of continuous dynamical systems for optimal control theory is twofold. First, dynamical systems already occur in the problem formulation, in which the evolution of the states to be controlled is formulated as a differential equation. Second, and more important, the techniques for calculating and analyzing the solutions of optimal control problems, in the form in which we introduce them, profoundly rely on results provided by the theory of continuous dynamical systems. Therefore in this chapter we elaborate the theory in some detail.

To help the reader, not acquainted with dynamical systems, we first provide a historical introduction, and then present the simple case of a one-dimensional dynamical system, introducing important concepts in an informal manner. Subsequently we restate these concepts and the required theory in a rigorous way.

2.1 Nonlinear Dynamical Modeling

Since the seventeenth century dynamical modeling has been of particular importance for explaining a long list of phenomena. Sir Isaac Newton (1643–1727) invented differential and integral calculus, published afterwards in his book *Method of Fluxions*, to describe universal gravitation and the laws of motion. Gottfried Wilhelm Leibniz (1646–1716) independently developed his calculus around 1673. The notation we use today is mostly that of Leibniz, with the well-known exception of Newton's "dot-notation" representing the derivative with respect to time.

Nowadays dynamical systems theory is a flourishing interdisciplinary subject, which is applied not only in many traditional sciences such as physics, aeronautics, astronomy, chemistry, biology, medicine, and engineering, but also in economics, sociology, and psychology. But this was not always the case. Only reluctantly did the social sciences and the humanities adopt dynamical modeling. For instance, the famous economist Joseph Schumpeter

(1883–1950), felt compelled sought to convey his argument for a dynamic approach by coining the phrase that *neglecting dynamic aspects in economic modeling was like performing Shakespeare's Hamlet without the prince of Denmark.* (Additional information about the role and development of dynamics in various disciplines can be found in the Notes p. 96.)

The core attributes of most dynamical systems are nonlinearities that arise from many different sources. In the social sciences, for example, interaction between agents and their mutual interdependencies generate inherent nonlinearities. Linear systems are much simpler to analyze and thus more thoroughly explored. Nonetheless, when it comes to modeling real-world phenomena, linear systems are the exception rather than the rule. The Polish mathematician Stanislav Ulam (1909–1984) remarked that dividing systems into "linear" and "nonlinear ones" makes as much sense as dividing fauna into "elephants" and "non-elephants." Once again, "elephant problems" are often amenable to analytical solution, whereas this is not the case for most "non-elephant problems." However, there exist powerful tools for tackling nonlinear dynamical systems at least numerically. By the way, it has to be admitted that in general a most important part of the dynamics can be described by a linear approximation, indicating the importance of studying linear systems. The purpose of this section is to give an introduction to the general theory and techniques we need in the following chapters.

2.2 One-Dimensional Systems

Real world problems such as those pertaining to drugs, corruption, and terror are inherently nonlinear and inherently dynamic. The nonlinearities stem among other things from the complex interactions between the constituent states of the systems, e.g., social interactions, and they are obviously dynamical since they evolve over time. Some knowledge of the theory of nonlinear dynamical systems is therefore essential to understand what is going on in the modeled real world representations we aim to set up here. We launch this process by discussing one-dimensional continuous dynamical systems to give a first intuition of what dynamics are, how they behave, and what insights we can obtain from their analysis.

We start by considering one-dimensional autonomous[1] systems, given by the following ordinary differential equation (ODE):[2]

$$\dot{x}(t) = f\left(x(t)\right), \quad t \in [0, T] \tag{2.1a}$$

subject to (s.t.)

---

[1] Differential equations in which the independent variable t does not occur explicitly in the function f are called *autonomous.*

[2] For exact definition see Sect. 2.4.

$$x(0) = x_0 \in \mathbb{R}, \tag{2.1b}$$

where $\dot{x}(t)$ is the time derivative of the function $x(\cdot)$ at time t. Solving (2.1) means finding a differentiable function $x(\cdot)$ satisfying (2.1a) and the *initial condition* (2.1b). To ease the notation (if there is no ambiguity) the time argument t is often omitted and (2.1a) becomes

$$\dot{x} = f(x).$$

One-dimensional systems can exhibit only a very limited range of behaviors so that their analysis is quite simple[3] and can be done graphically. In the following sections the crucial concepts are defined rigorously, but examining one-dimensional systems graphically allows us to introduce these concepts – notably ideas related to stability, linearization, and the graphical tool known as a *phase portrait* – in an informal way that carries over to higher-dimensional systems.

To give an example, consider the following ODE:

$$\dot{x}(t) = x(t)\left(1 - x(t)^2\right), \quad t \in [0, \infty) \tag{2.2a}$$

$$\text{s.t.} \quad x(0) = x_0 \in \mathbb{R}. \tag{2.2b}$$

As the reader may verify (by simple differentiation of (2.3)), the explicit solution of (2.2) is given by

$$x(t) = \begin{cases} \left(1 - \mathrm{e}^{-2t}\left(1 - \frac{1}{x_0^2}\right)\right)^{-1/2} & x_0 > 0 \\ 0 & x_0 = 0 \\ -\left(1 - \mathrm{e}^{-2t}\left(1 - \frac{1}{x_0^2}\right)\right)^{-1/2} & x_0 < 0. \end{cases} \tag{2.3}$$

There are basically two ways to analyze the solution of an ODE like (2.2a) or the general case of (2.1). First, the time path of the solution can be (analytically or numerically) calculated (see (2.3)) and depicted in the (t, x)-plane (see Fig. 2.1b). This allows directly reading off the level of the variable at any instant of time depending, of course, on the variable's initial level. The second way is to plot a *phase portrait* in the $(x, \dot{x})$-plane (see Fig. 2.1a). To grasp the meaning of such an analysis, it is helpful to imagine that a phase portrait of a one-dimensional system depicts a particle that is starting its movement at x_0 and is traveling along the x-axis with a certain velocity (direction and speed) as given by $\dot{x}$ that in turn depends on the position of x on the axis as given by the right-hand side of equation (2.2). The particle's path represents then the solution of the ODE starting from the initial condition x_0. Since direction and

[3] Even in the one-dimensional (nonlinear) case finding explicit solutions is rather the exception than the rule. Thus the use of the term "simplicity" refers only to the limited range of system behavior, but does not refer to simplicity with respect to analytical tractability.

speed play an important role it is convenient to augment the graph of $\dot{x}$ vs. x with arrows on the x-axis to indicate the direction of movement, where the flow is to the right when $\dot{x} > 0$ and to the left when $\dot{x} < 0$ (as is illustrated for (2.2) in Fig. 2.1a). The associated concepts of a phase portrait analysis described so far carry over to higher-dimensional systems, where important elements are the system's equilibria. An equilibrium $\hat{x}$ is defined by

$$f(\hat{x}) = 0.$$

In our example (2.2) these are the roots of $x(1 - x^2) = 0$, yielding the three equilibria $\hat{x} = 0, \ \pm 1$.

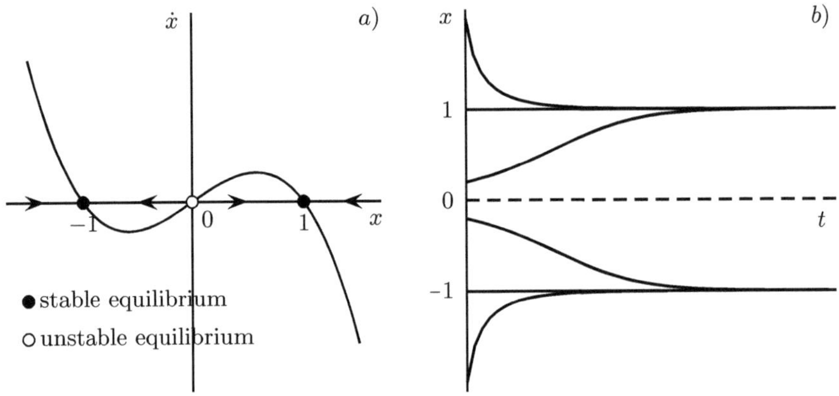

Fig. 2.1. A portrait of (2.2) is depicted in panel (**a**). Panel (**b**) shows several solution paths converging toward the equilibria together with equilibrium solutions

These equilibria represent *equilibrium solutions* (also called fixed points, stationary points, steady states, or critical values) in which the flow induced by the system $f(x(\cdot))$ stagnates. If one starts the system exactly in $x_0 = \hat{x}$, then $x(t) = \hat{x}$ for all time. It is now of interest what happens if we start the system *almost* in $\hat{x}$. We say that $\hat{x}$ is "stable" if the system remains near $\hat{x}$. I.e., trajectories beginning with small perturbations of the equilibrium remain close to the equilibrium. If those perturbed trajectories do not only remain close but eventually return to the equilibrium (even if that takes an infinite amount of time to *exactly* reach the equilibrium), then another form of stability called "asymptotic stability" pertains.

To put it more precisely, an equilibrium $\hat{x}$ is called *stable* if any solution of (2.1a) with initial condition $x(0) = x_0$ "close" to $\hat{x}$ remains in a small neighborhood of $\hat{x}$ for all $t \geq 0$. It is called *asymptotically stable* if it is stable and if there exists a small neighborhood of $\hat{x}$ such that for any solution that starts within that neighborhood it holds that $\lim_{t\to\infty} x(t) = \hat{x}$. If the "small neighborhood" in the definition of asymptotic stability can be expanded to embrace the whole domain (of definition) of $f(x(\cdot))$, then the equilibrium $\hat{x}$ is said to be *globally asymptotically stable* because all trajectories, no matter where in the phase space they start, will eventually approach $\hat{x}$.

The qualitative behavior of a one-dimensional *autonomous* system is limited, since the motion happens along a line. A solution path either approaches an equilibrium, if $f_x(\hat{x}) < 0$, or it goes away from it, where such an unstable equilibrium is characterized by $f_x(\hat{x}) > 0$; see Fig. 2.1a, where the stable equilibria are depicted by a black dot and the unstable equilibrium by an open circle. Note that asymptotically stable equilibria are called *sinks* or *attractors*, and unstable ones are called *sources* or *repellers*.

In the case of our illustrative example we find for the equilibria $0, \pm 1$ with $f_x = -3x^2 + 1$

$$f_x(\hat{x}) = \begin{cases} -2 & \hat{x} = \pm 1 \\ 1 & \hat{x} = 0. \end{cases}$$

Thus the two equilibria ± 1 are attractors, whereas the equilibrium at the origin is a repeller.

As mentioned, nonlinearities are ubiquitous, and it is the linearity (rather than nonlinearity) assumption that has to be justified. Hence, we need to justify the time we are about to spend studying linear systems. There are two primary justifications. First, since linear models are mathematically much simpler to deal with, it is easier to learn first about linear systems and then about nonlinear systems than it is to jump directly into nonlinear systems. Second, many nonlinear models can be linearized, and solutions of linearized systems are reasonable approximations of the solutions of the nonlinear systems in a neighborhood about the point where the linearization was done. In general the most interesting part of the dynamical behavior is covered by its linearization.

If the function $f(x)$ in (2.1a) is not linear in x, one can linearize it by approximating it by its first derivative about an equilibrium $\hat{x}$ as follows. Let $y = x - \hat{x}$ be a small perturbation of $\hat{x}$. By expanding $f(\hat{x} + y)$ about $\hat{x}$, one obtains

$$\dot{y} = \dot{x} = f(\hat{x} + y) = f(\hat{x}) + f_x(\hat{x})y + o(y),$$

where $o(y)$ represents quadratic and higher-order terms. Since $f(\hat{x}) = 0$, we get

$$\dot{y} = f_x(\hat{x})y \tag{2.4}$$

by neglecting higher-order terms. The linear differential equation (2.4) for y is called the *linearization* of f about $\hat{x}$. It says that the deviation y increases exponentially if $f_x(\hat{x}) > 0$ and decreases if $f_x(\hat{x}) < 0$. In the hairline case $f_x(\hat{x}) = 0$ the higher-order terms must be included in a stability analysis. Note further that $|f_x(\hat{x})|$ measures the rate of exponential growth or decay of a solution near the equilibrium $\hat{x}$.

This finishes our short introduction to one-dimensional dynamical systems. We shall now illustrate them with an example from the field of corruption.

Subsequently we shall present a thorough survey of dynamical systems in which the concepts only loosely introduced here are rigorously defined.

2.3 A One-Dimensional Corruption Model

A simple one-dimensional model of corruption suggests that there are two kinds of people, honest and corrupt. We denote them by the subscripts h and c, respectively. Let the state variable $x(t)$ be the proportion of people who are corrupt at time t, i.e., $0 \leq x(t) \leq 1$. The temptation to become corrupt is usually financial, and so the incomes of corrupt people are assumed to be higher than those who are honest, by some constant amount per unit of time: $w_c > w_h$. The primary practical (as opposed to moral) disadvantage of being corrupt is exposure to the risk of capture. The total amount of sanctions that the police can impose is spread across all corrupt people, so-called "enforcement swamping" (Kleiman, 1993). That is, the more people who are corrupt, the less likely it is that any given corrupt person will get caught.

One component of the sanctioning stems from the formal corruption control program, denoted by u, but there can also be a certain fixed amount u_0 of sanctioning even when there is no active control. That constant can represent sanction risk from general policing, as opposed to dedicated anti-corruption efforts. It might also represent social approbation that is subject to "stigma swamping" (the informal social-controls analogous to enforcement swamping).

It is common in economic models to assume that individuals respond to incentives. In these models, that often means that people move back and forth between states in response to differences in the reward or payoff offered by the various states. By this logic people would move back and forth between behaving honestly and dishonestly in response to the difference in "utility" each state offers, where utility is simply the income minus the expected sanction

$$U_c(t) - U_h(t) = w - \frac{u_0 + u(t)}{x(t)}, \tag{2.5}$$

where the constant w is the "premium" or "reward" for dishonesty, i.e., $w = w_c - w_h > 0$, and u is a "control" variable allowing the decision-maker to influence the system. At this stage the control u is assumed to be fixed; but in the following chapters the theory is introduced allowing one to choose this control optimally, relative to some cost or utility functional.

The model assumes that if being honest offers a higher utility, then corrupt people will flow back into the honest state at a per capita rate that is proportional to the difference in utility. However, if being corrupt offers a higher utility, then corrupt people will "recruit" honest people into corruption at a rate that is proportional to $U_c - U_h$, so that the aggregate rate is proportional to the product of the number of corrupt people and the utility difference. This recruitment could be unconscious, as in sociological models of the diffusion of deviance. It could also be conscious. Corrupt people have an incentive to corrupt others because the more corrupt people there are, the lower is the risk of sanction for any given corrupt person.[4] (The reader is invited to explore what that argument would imply for the model equations and solution.) An assumption underlying the model dynamics is that honest people cannot become corrupt without some contact with a corrupt person, perhaps because they do not know the difference in utility between being corrupt and being honest without such contact.[5]

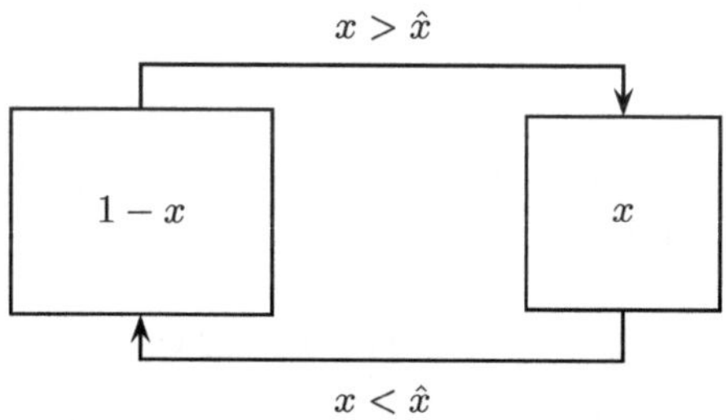

Fig. 2.2. Flow diagram for the corruption model (2.6). Here x denotes the corrupt proportion of society, whereas $1 - x$ represents the honest part. $\hat{x} = (u_0 + u)/w$ is the equilibrium

In the symmetric case, where the proportionality constants for transitions from corrupt behavior to being honest, and vice versa, are the same, $k > 0$ (see Fig. 2.2), one gets the linear state dynamics

$$\dot{x}(t) = f(x(t), u(t)) = kx(t)(U_c(t) - U_h(t)) = k\left(wx(t) - (u_0 + u(t))\right). \quad (2.6)$$

It is instructive to first identify the equilibria. In (2.6) there is only one, given by

$$\hat{x} = \frac{u_0 + u}{w}.$$

Since $w > 0$, $\hat{x} \geq 0$, and is only zero in the unsanctioned case, where $u = u_0 = 0$.

Next, one could ask what happens in the neighborhood of $\hat{x}$. We might argue intuitively that if there were more corrupt people (larger x), that would

4 One might also argue, to the contrary, that the more corrupt agents there are, the more competitive is the market for providing corruption "services" (compare Andvig, 1991).

5 If we disregard this assumption, the flow from the honest to the corrupt people will be proportional to $1 - x$ (see Exercise 2.3).

reduce the sanction risk for corrupt people while having no effect on the income of corrupt or honest people; and so it would make being corrupt more appealing, spurring a further flow of people into corruption. Conversely, a small reduction in the number of corrupt people would make corruption less appealing, leading to a further flow out of corruption. Hence the system will tend to move away from $\hat{x}$, so that the equilibrium can be characterized as unstable.

If the model were more complex, and such intuitive arguments were not sufficient, we could still find the same answer mathematically by noting that the derivative of f evaluated at $\hat{x} = \hat{x}(u)$ is

$$f_x(\hat{x}(u), u) = kw > 0.$$

Thus the gap between the actual state x and the equilibrium $\hat{x}$ will always tend to increase when the state is near $\hat{x}$

$$\frac{\mathrm{d}}{\mathrm{d}t}(\hat{x} - x) = f_x(\hat{x}(u), u)(\hat{x} - x).$$

Hence it is shown that $\hat{x}$ is an *unstable* equilibrium, where small perturbations lead to divergence from this state. As the movement in this simple model takes place along the x-axis, this means that left of $\hat{x}$ the proportion of corrupt people decreases, while right of it the number of corrupt people increases. We therefore have to consider different scenarios, depending on the actual value of $\hat{x}$, given by the total sanction $u_0 + u$, and the difference in the income w. If w is fixed, three scenarios are possible:

No sanctions: $u_0 + u = 0$. Only a society that is totally non-corrupt will remain honest, and even that is an unstable situation. Whenever corruption appears, $x(t) > 0$, corruption will increase exponentially until everyone is corrupt (see Fig. 2.3a).

Medium sanctions: $0 < u_0 + u < w$. Depending on the actual proportion of corrupt people, corruption will increase for $x(t) > \hat{x}$ or decrease for $x(t) < \hat{x}$. This outcome is plausible, given that the risk of sanctions decreases with the proportion leading to corruption (see (2.5) and Fig. 2.3b).

High sanctions: $u_0 + u = w$. The risk of sanctions exceeds the expected profit for any given proportion x and corrupt people become honest. We end up with a totally honest population regardless of the initial state. If $\hat{x} = 1$ the totally corrupt society is an unstable situation. A small fraction of honest people suffices to convert the whole population into one that is entirely free of corruption (see Fig. 2.3c).

With the same argumentation we get analogous results for a fixed amount of sanctions and a varying wage w, "high," "medium," and "low." Note that if sanctions are positive then with increasing wage w, we can still hope that society becomes totally honest.

In a nutshell only if sanctioning makes being corrupt sufficiently unattractive (Fig. 2.3b, c) does society have a chance to approach a state of honesty.

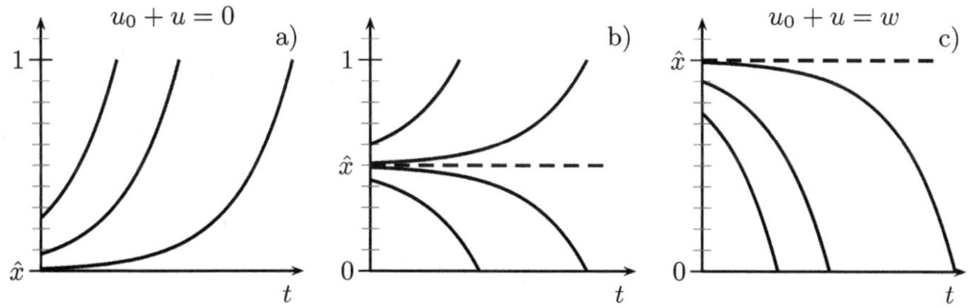

Fig. 2.3. The three cases of zero, medium, and high sanctions. Note that 0 and 1 are model inherent boundaries; thus the solutions are considered only within this range and the dynamics are set to zero otherwise

What we have already introduced informally for the one-dimensional case will now be established in a general and formal way.

2.4 Dynamical Systems as ODEs

In dynamic models usually time is an independent variable.[6] The dependent (state) variables are then functions of time. Changes in these variables over time involve the derivatives of functions with respect to time.

We let t denote the real-valued time argument, and $x(t)$ denotes the value of some variable x at time t. The derivative of $x(\cdot)$ at any moment of time t is denoted by

$$\frac{\mathrm{d}x(t)}{\mathrm{d}t}, \quad \text{or} \quad \dot{x}(t).$$

To describe the process of change we must link the rate of change in $x(\cdot)$ at t to the values of $x(t)$ and t. Hence we consider equations of the form:

$$\dot{x}(t) = f\left(x(t), t\right), \quad t \in [t_0, t_1] \subset \mathbb{R} \tag{2.7a}$$

$$x(t_0) = x_0 \in \mathbb{R}^n, \tag{2.7b}$$

where $x(t)$ is the *state* of the system at time t and $f : \mathbb{R}^n \times \mathbb{R} \to \mathbb{R}^n$ is a function continuous in t and continuously differentiable in x, called the *(state) dynamics* of x. Hence the rate of change, $\dot{x}(t)$, depends on the current state $x(t)$ and the time t. A solution of (2.7) is defined as:

Definition 2.1 (ODE, IVP, and Solution). *The equation (2.7a) is called an* ordinary differential equation (ODE) *and the system (2.7) is called an* initial value problem (IVP) *for the* initial condition *(2.7b).*

The function $x : [t_0, t_1] \to \mathbb{R}^n$ is called a solution *to the IVP (2.7) if $\dot{x}(t)$ satisfies (2.7a) for all $t \in [t_0, t_1]$ and $x(t_0) = x_0$.*

[6] Here we assume that time is the only independent variable.

Remark 2.2. It is common practice to assume that the dynamics f is only considered on a set $D \times \mathbb{R} \subset \mathbb{R}^n \times \mathbb{R}$ with D open in $\mathbb{R}^n$. To simplify notation we omit the reference to the set D. In case that f is only defined on a set with D closed the solution at the boundary ∂D has to be analyzed carefully. As an example reconsider the model of Sect. 2.3, where the set $D = [0, 1]$ was a closed set.

An important existence and uniqueness result is stated by:

Theorem 2.3 (Picard–Lindelöf). *Let the dynamics $f(x, t)$ of the ODE (2.7a) be continuous and Lipschitz continuous in x for all $t \in [0, T]$; then the IVP (2.7) has a unique solution on $[0, T]$.*

Remark 2.4. For further questions of existence the reader is referred to any of the numerous textbooks on ODEs, e.g., Hartman (1982).

Remark 2.5. The term *ordinary* in ODE is used to indicate that there is only a single independent variable. Otherwise, partial derivatives would appear and we would have a partial differential equation; such equations are briefly outlined in Sect. 8.3.

Remark 2.6. Opposite to an IVP we may consider a so-called *boundary value problem (BVP)*. For IVPs we know exactly where we start, i.e. $x(t_0) = x_0 \in \mathbb{R}^n$ at a time t_0 is given, whereas in the latter case we only have partial information about both the initial state and the final state, i.e.,

$$b\left(x(t_0), x(t_1)\right) = 0,$$

where b is a vector-valued function $b : \mathbb{R}^n \to \mathbb{R}^n$. In the following sections we exclusively consider IVPs and return to the BVPs in Sect. 2.12.2.

An equivalent formulation for a solution of (2.7) is then the following:

Proposition 2.7 (Integral Equation). *The function $x : [t_0, t_1] \to \mathbb{R}^n$ is a solution of the IVP (2.7) iff $x(\cdot)$ is continuous and satisfies*

$$x(t) = x_0 + \int_{t_0}^{t} f\left(x(s), s\right) \mathrm{d}s, \quad \textit{for all } t \in [t_0, t_1]. \tag{2.8}$$

The equation (2.8) is called an integral equation.

When the time variable is integer-valued, i.e., the change in time is only considered at discrete steps, we speak of *difference equations*

$$x(t+1) = f\left(x(t), t\right), \quad t \in \mathbb{Z}, \tag{2.9}$$

where the variable t is often replaced by the variable n, indicating that only integers are considered.

In this book we focus on continuous-time problems largely leaving aside discrete-time systems. The only reason why we mention them at all is that some results based on the stability of discrete systems play an important role in characterizing the stability behavior of periodic solutions of continuous systems (Sect. 2.6.2).[7]

Another differentiating criterion for ODEs is:

Definition 2.8 (Autonomous and Nonautonomous ODE). *The ODE (2.7a) is called an* autonomous *ODE if the dynamics does not explicitly depend on the time variable t, i.e.,*

$$\dot{x}(t) = f\left(x(t)\right), \quad x \in \mathbb{R}^n, \ \ t \in [t_0, t_1], \tag{2.10}$$

Remark 2.9. Note that in case of an autonomous ODE the dynamics f is only a function of the state variable x, i.e., $f : \mathbb{R}^n \to \mathbb{R}^n$.

otherwise it is called a nonautonomous *ODE.*

From the definition of an autonomous ODE we find:

Lemma 2.10 (Time-Shift Invariant Solution). *Let the ODE (2.10) be autonomous and $x(\cdot)$ be a solution of (2.10) with initial condition $x(t_0) = x_0$ then the time-shifted function*

$$y(t) := x(t + t_0), \quad \textit{with} \quad t \in [0, t_1 - t_0]$$

is a solution of the ODE (2.10) with initial condition $y(0) = x_0$.

Due to Lemma 2.10 we may restrict our considerations, without loss of generality, to the ODE (2.10) on the time interval $[0, T]$ and initial condition $x(0) = x_0$.

In this book we are almost solely confronted with autonomous and thus time-shift invariant problems. In the rare cases where we consider a nonautonomous problem, we shall explicitly refer the reader to this point.

2.4.1 Concepts and Definitions

Next we consider the autonomous problem (2.10) and give the following definitions:

Definition 2.11 (Trajectory, Orbit, and Phase Space). *Let $x(\cdot)$ be a solution of the autonomous ODE (2.10); then $x(\cdot)$ is called the* trajectory *or* solution path*) through x_0.*

The ordered subset[8]

[7] Much of what we present for differential equations has a close analogy for difference equations. Albeit we have to admit that difference equations can exhibit complex, like chaotic, behavior even in the one-dimensional case.

[8] The ordering $\preccurlyeq$ is given by the time argument, i.e.,

$$x(t_1) \preccurlyeq x(t_2) \quad \text{iff} \quad t_1 \le t_2.$$

$$\mathrm{Or}(x_0) := \{x(t) \in \mathbb{R}^n : x(0) = x_0,\ t \in \mathbb{R}\} \subset \mathbb{R}^n,$$

is called the orbit *through* x_0. *The graphical representation of all orbits is called the* phase space.

Remark 2.12. Note that the orbit is the projection of a trajectory $x(\cdot)$ into the phase space while retaining its time orientation.

For an autonomous ODE we can attach to every point $x \in \mathbb{R}^n$ a vector $f(x) \in \mathbb{R}^n$ giving rise to the following definition

Definition 2.13 (Vector Field, Flow, and Dynamical System). *Given the autonomous ODE (2.10) the image of the function* $f : \mathbb{R}^n \to \mathbb{R}^n$ *is called the* vector field *of (2.10). It is said that the vector field* $f(x)$ *generates a* flow $\varphi^t : \mathbb{R}^n \to \mathbb{R}^n$, *which transforms an* initial state x_0 *into some state* $x(t) \in \mathbb{R}^n$ *at time* $t \in \mathbb{R}$

$$\varphi^t(x_0) := x(t).$$

The triple

$$(f, \mathbb{R}^n, \varphi^t(\cdot))$$

is called a dynamical system *derived from the ODE (2.10).*

For a comprehensive introduction into the field of dynamical systems the reader is referred to Arrowsmith and Place (1990).

Remark 2.14. Note that the trajectories of the ODE (2.10) are continuously differentiable functions following the vectors tangentially (see Fig. 2.4). Due to its definition the $\varphi^t(\cdot)$ satisfies (2.10), i.e.,

$$\frac{\mathrm{d}\varphi^t(x_0)}{\mathrm{d}t} = f\left(\varphi^t(x_0)\right), \quad \text{and} \quad \varphi^0(x_0) = x_0.$$

From the definition of a flow two properties immediately follow:

- $\varphi^0 = \mathbb{I}^{(n)}$, which implies that the system does not change its state "spontaneously." This assures that the flow at time zero starts at the initial position x_0.
- $\varphi^{s+t} = \varphi^s \circ \varphi^t$, which implies that the state dynamics does not change in time. Thus the state at time $s + t$ is the same as if we first consider the state $x(s)$ at time s and then consider the state after time t when starting from $x(s)$.

The three objects "trajectory," "orbit," and "flow" are similar, but they emphasize different aspects of the same phenomenon (see Fig. 2.5).

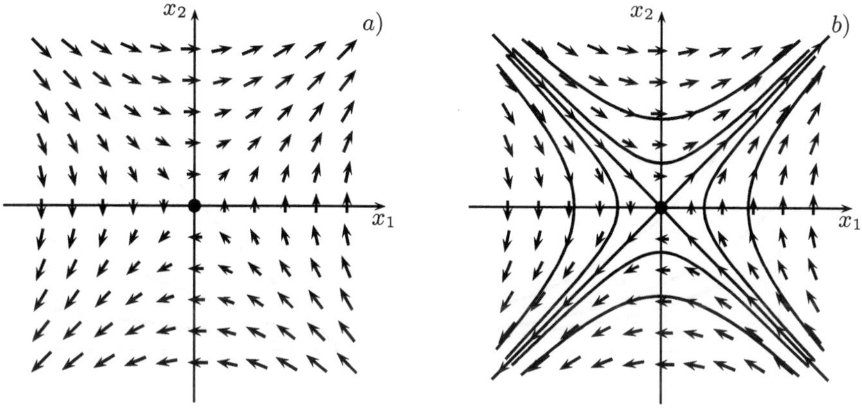

Fig. 2.4. In (**a**) the two-dimensional vector field for $\dot{x}_1 = x_2$ and $\dot{x}_2 = x_1$ is depicted, where at each point x, the corresponding directional vector $f(x) = (x_2, x_1)$ is attached. Panel (**b**) depicts some solution curves within this vector field

2.4.2 Invariant Sets and Stability

The simplest object of a dynamical system is an equilibrium:

Definition 2.15 (Equilibrium). *Let* $(f, \mathbb{R}^n, \varphi^t(\cdot))$ *be a dynamical system derived from the ODE (2.10) then a point* $\hat{x} \in \mathbb{R}^n$ *is called an* equilibrium (steady state, fixed point, critical state) *if* $\varphi^t(\hat{x}) = \hat{x}$ *for all* $t \in \mathbb{R}$. *The solution* $\hat{x}(\cdot) \equiv \hat{x}$ *of the ODE (2.10) is called an* equilibrium solution.

Definition 2.16 (Isocline). *Let*

$$\dot{x} = f(x),\ x \in \mathbb{R}^2,$$

with $f = (f_1, f_2)'$ *and* $x = (x_1, x_2)'$ *be an ODE; then the contour lines*

$$N_{f_1}(c) = \{(x_1, x_2) : f_1(x_1, x_2) = c\}, \quad \textit{and} \quad N_{f_2}(c) = \{(x_1, x_2) : f_2(x_1, x_2) = c\}$$

are called the $\dot{x}_1$-isocline *and* $\dot{x}_2$-isocline *for value c, respectively. For* $c = 0$ *they are simple called the* $\dot{x}_1$*-isocline and* $\dot{x}_2$*-isocline.*

Remark 2.17. From (2.10) it follows that an equilibrium $\hat{x}$ is characterized by the equation

$$f(\hat{x}) = 0.$$

For a two-dimensional system an equilibrium is therefore given by the crossing of its zero isoclines.

Another important object of a dynamical system is a trajectory which loops forever with a certain fixed time period between successive passages through a given point:

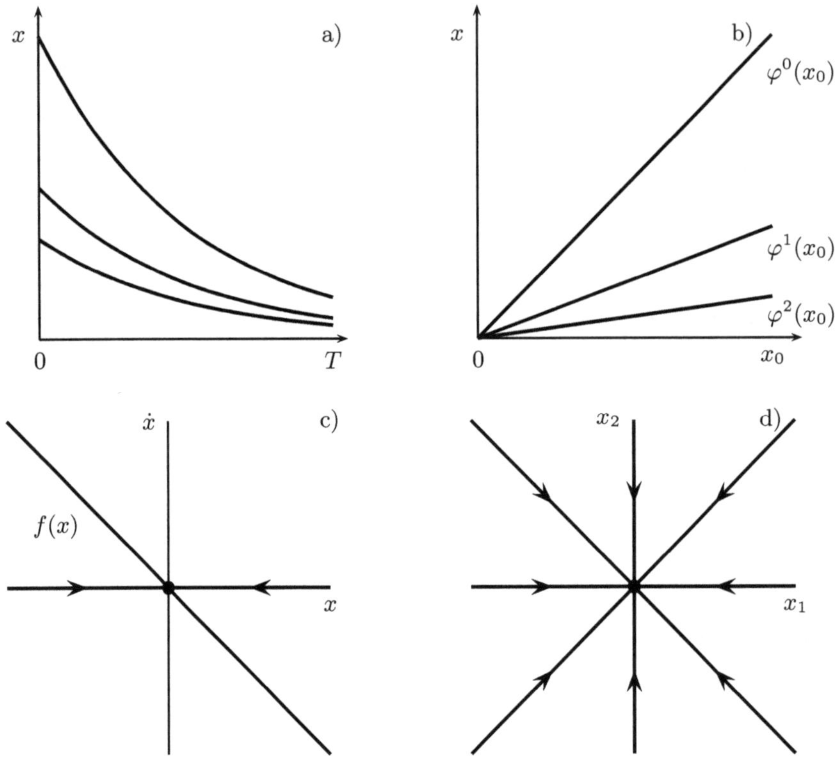

Fig. 2.5. For the linear ODE $\dot{x} = -x$ depicts (**a**) three different trajectories, (**b**) the corresponding flow $\varphi^t(x_0)$ drawn for different times t and (**c**) the corresponding phase portrait. Additionally in panel (**d**) some orbits for the two-dimensional ODE $\dot{x}_1 = -x_1$ and $\dot{x}_2 = -x_2$ are depicted

Definition 2.18 (Cycle and Periodic Solution). *Let* $(f, \mathbb{R}^n, \varphi^t(\cdot))$ *be a dynamical system derived from the ODE (2.10) then* $\Gamma \subset \mathbb{R}^n$ *is called a* cycle *if there exists a* $\Theta > 0$ *such that for every* $x_0 \in \Gamma$, $\varphi^{t+\Theta}(x_0) = \varphi^t(x_0)$ *for all* t*. The minimal* Θ *satisfying this property is called the* period *of the cycle. A solution* $\Gamma(\cdot)$ *of the ODE (2.10) with* $\Gamma(0) \in \Gamma$ *is called a* periodic solution *with* period Θ.

Remark 2.19. Note that there exist infinitely many trajectories representing a cycle Γ, since every solution $x(\cdot)$ with initial condition $x(0) \in \Gamma$ describes the orbit Γ. If we do not refer to one specific trajectory we sometimes write (if there is no ambiguity) Γ instead of $\Gamma(\cdot)$ for a trajectory representing the cycle. But the reader should be aware that Γ and $\Gamma(\cdot)$ are different objects.

Definition 2.20 (Limit Cycle). *An isolated cycle Γ is called a* limit cycle.[9]

An equilibrium and a limit cycle are each particular objects within a general class called a *limit set*:

Definition 2.21 (Limit Set). *Let φ^t be a flow of (2.10) on $\mathbb{R}^n$. Then the set*

$$\omega(x_0) = \left\{x \in \mathbb{R}^n : \lim_{k\to\infty} \varphi^{t_k}(x_0) = x, \text{ and } \lim_{k\to\infty} t_k = \infty \text{ with } t_k < t_{k+1}\right\}$$

is called the (positive) limit set (ω-limit set) *for x_0 and*

$$\alpha(x_0) = \left\{x \in \mathbb{R}^n : \lim_{k\to\infty} \varphi^{t_k}(x_0) = x, \text{ and } \lim_{k\to\infty} t_k = -\infty \text{ with } t_{k+1} < t_k\right\}$$

is called the negative limit set (α-limit set) *for x_0.*

A limit set describes the states that a trajectory can reach in the "long run."

Remark 2.22. For higher-dimensional systems, $n > 2$, more complex solutions may occur where, e.g., the trajectories exhibit *aperiodic* behavior; which means that although the trajectories are bounded, they do not converge to equilibria or limit cycles. Additionally, in *chaotic* systems the solutions can exhibit sensitive dependence on the initial conditions.

Both, equilibrium and cycle, exhibit another important property, namely that of invariance, i.e., starting at an equilibrium or cycle, the trajectory remains at the equilibrium or cycle forever. This property can generally be defined as follows:

Definition 2.23. *An* invariant set *of a dynamical system is a subset* $\mathrm{S} \subset \mathbb{R}^n$ *such that $x_0 \in \mathrm{S}$ implies*

$$\varphi^t(x_0) \in \mathrm{S}, \quad \text{for all} \quad t.$$

Thus Definition 2.23 formalizes the property of "remaining somewhere forever."

Remark 2.24. Other invariant sets are like the stable and unstable manifold of an equilibrium or a heteroclinic/homoclinic connection and will subsequently be defined.

For an invariant set S the concept of stability can be introduced:

Definition 2.25. *An invariant set* S *of a dynamical system is called*

1. Stable *if for every neighborhood U of* S*, which is sufficiently small, there exists a neighborhood V of* S*, such that $x_0 \in V$ implies $\varphi^t(x_0) \in U$ for all $t \in \mathbb{R}$.*

9 *Isolated* denotes that there is no other cycle in its neighborhood; for a counter example see Fig. 2.6a, where through any point $x \in \mathbb{R}^2$ there passes a cycle.

2. Attracting *if there exists a neighborhood* V *of* S *such that* $x_0 \in V$ *implies*

$$\lim_{t \to \infty} \varphi^t(x_0) \in \mathrm{S}\,.$$

The set $\bigcup_{t \leq 0} \varphi^t(V)$ *is called the* basin of attraction

3. Repelling *if it is attracting for the reversed time* $t \to -t$.

4. Unstable *if it is not stable.*

5. Asymptotically stable *if it is both stable and attracting.*

6. Globally (asymptotically) stable *if the neighborhood* V *of attraction for* S *can be chosen as* $\mathbb{R}^n$.

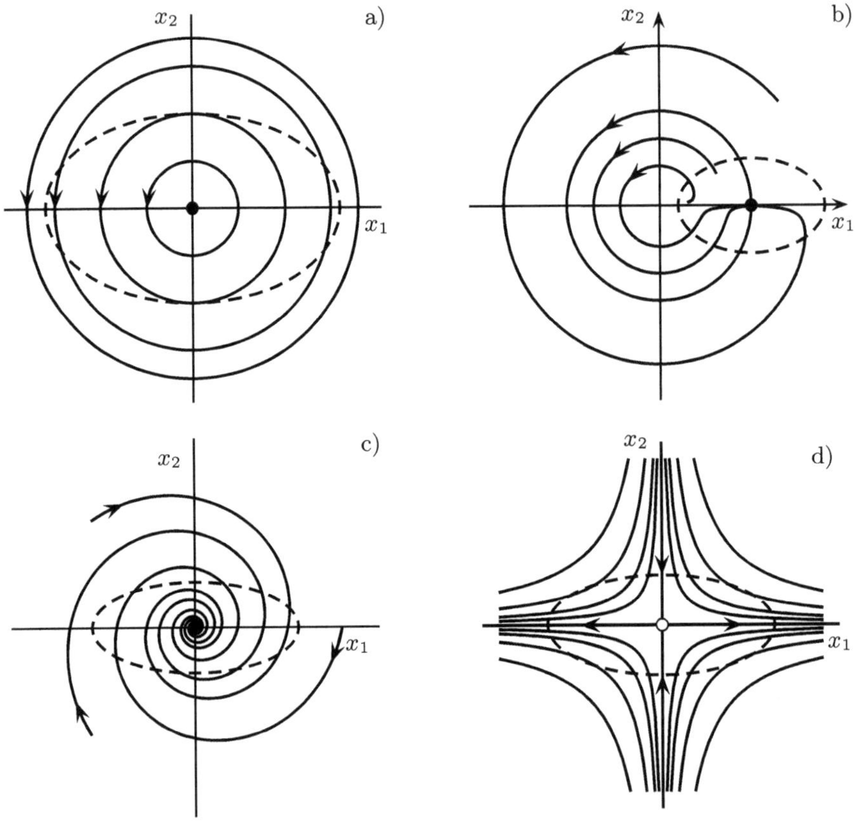

Fig. 2.6. In (**a**) the orbits around the equilibrium at the origin are cycles; thus it is a stable but not attracting equilibrium also called a *center*. In (**b**) every orbit converges to the equilibrium at $(1, 0)$ and is therefore attracting, but not stable since for every neighborhood V of $(1, 0)$ there exist orbits leaving V. In (**c**) an asymptotically stable equilibrium is depicted, and (**d**) shows an example of an unstable equilibrium

Remark 2.26 (Semistability). An equilibrium $\hat{x}$ of a one-dimensional system is called a *semistable* equilibrium if there exist $x' < \hat{x} < x''$ such that

$$\hat{x} = \omega(x') = \alpha(x'') \quad \text{or} \quad \hat{x} = \omega(x'') = \alpha(x').$$

Such an equilibrium may occur if a stable and an unstable equilibrium collide (see, e.g., p. 64).

A limit cycle Γ of a two-dimensional system is called a *semistable* limit cycle if there exist x' and x'' such that

$$\Gamma = \omega(x') = \alpha(x'') \quad \text{or} \quad \Gamma = \omega(x'') = \alpha(x').$$

Such a limit cycle may occur if a stable and an unstable limit cycle collide.

Remark 2.27. In particular, an attracting equilibrium $\hat{x}$ is called an *attractor* and a repelling equilibrium is called a *repeller*.

Remark 2.28. Note that stability and attraction are distinct concepts. A center in the linear case (discussed below on p. 39) is stable but not attracting. On the other hand, there are examples of autonomous ODEs exhibiting attracting but not stable limit sets (see Fig. 2.6).

2.4.3 Structural Stability

In the last section we introduced the concept of stability for invariant sets. This subsection answers the question of how sensitive the solution is in the long run to small disturbances of the initial states near an invariant set. But especially from an applied point of view another kind of stability is interesting. Namely to consider changes not only for the initial states but for the whole vector field. It is the idea of finding how robust the solution of a model is when facing *small perturbations* of its describing functions.

We therefore define:

Definition 2.29 (Topological Equivalence). *Let $f_1, f_2 : \mathbb{R}^n \to \mathbb{R}^n$ be continuously differentiable functions defining the flows φ_1^t and φ_2^t. Then f_1 and f_2 are called* topologically equivalent *if there exists a C^0-homeomorphism h mapping φ_1^t onto φ_2^t, i.e.,*

$$h(\varphi_1^t(x)) = \varphi_2^t(h(x)).$$

This is a very strong definition of equivalence since it requires that systems with, e.g., different time parameterization are *not* topological equivalent. Thus to get a more coarse classification of systems we introduce a less strict definition of equivalence:

Definition 2.30 (Topological Orbital Equivalence). *Let $f_1, f_2 : \mathbb{R}^n \to \mathbb{R}^n$ be continuously differentiable functions defining the flows φ_1^t and φ_2^t. Then*

f_1 and f_2 are called topologically orbitally equivalent *if there exists a C^0-homeomorphism h mapping the orbits of φ_1^t onto the orbits of φ_2^t, preserving the direction of time, i.e.,*

$$h(\varphi_1^t(x)) = \varphi_2^{\tau_y(t)}(y), \quad \text{with} \quad y = h(x)$$

and $\tau_y(t)$ increasing in t.

We are now able to give an exact definition for the term structural stability:

Definition 2.31 (Structural Stability). *Let*

$$\dot{x} = f_1(x), \quad x \in \mathbb{R}^n, \quad f_1 \in C^1 \tag{2.11}$$

define a dynamical system. Then system (2.11) is called structurally stable *in the region $U \subset \mathbb{R}^n$ if any system*

$$\dot{x} = f_2(x), \quad x \in \mathbb{R}^n, \quad f_2 \in C^1$$

which is close to f_1 relative to the C^1 norm is topologically orbitally equivalent in U to the system (2.11).

In a local form this definition can be rewritten as:

Definition 2.32. *A dynamical system $(f^1, \mathbb{R}^n, \varphi_1^t)$ is called* locally topologically *equivalent* near an equilibrium $\hat{x}_1$ *to a dynamical system $(f^2, \mathbb{R}^n, \varphi_2^t)$* near an equilibrium $\hat{x}_2$ *if there exists a homeomorphism $h : \mathbb{R}^n \to \mathbb{R}^n$ that*

1. *Is defined in a small neighborhood $U \subset \mathbb{R}^n$ of $\hat{x}_1$*
2. *Satisfies $\hat{x}_2 = h(\hat{x}_1)$*
3. *Maps orbits of the first system in U onto orbits of the second system in $V = f_1(U) \subset \mathbb{R}^n$, preserving the direction of time*

For a detailed presentation of structural stability and interrelated questions the reader is referred to Arrowsmith and Place (1990) and Arnold (1983).

2.4.4 Linearization and the Variational Equation

Having found some specific solution $x(\cdot)$ of (2.10), e.g., an equilibrium or limit cycle, we are interested in the behavior of solutions starting near this solution. Therefore the following differential equation can be considered:

$$\dot{y}(t) = f\left(x(t) + y(t)\right) - f\left(x(t)\right), \tag{2.12}$$

where $y(t)$ "measures" the deviation from $x(t)$ at time t and (2.12) describes how the perturbation evolves over time. Equation (2.12) exhibits the special solution $y \equiv 0$ characterizing the undisturbed case. Drawing conclusions about the nearby trajectories from the solutions of (2.12) is straightforward.

An obvious simplification of (2.12) is its linear approximation by the Taylor theorem, according to which (2.12) is rewritten as

$$\dot{y}(t) = f_x\left(x(t)\right)y(t) + o\left(y(t)\right). \tag{2.13}$$

Neglecting the higher-order terms in (2.13) yields the so-called *variational equation of solution* $x(\cdot)$:

$$\dot{y}(t) = f_x\left(x(t)\right)y(t),$$

which in general is a linear nonautonomous system with $J(t) = f_x(x(t))$, where the Jacobian matrix $J(\cdot)$ of $f(\cdot)$ is evaluated along the trajectory $x(\cdot)$.

2.5 Stability Analysis of a One-Dimensional Terror Model

We introduce a simple, one-state model that aims to shed light on the question of how best to prosecute the "war on terror." Counter-terror measures may range from homeland security operations to invading certain territories to targeted assassinations of terrorists, or freezing assets of organizations with links to potential terrorists. Some types of counter-terror operations have more, and others have fewer, unwanted "side-effects." As a proxy for the heterogeneity of counter-terror activities, the model here distinguishes between two abstract categories:

"Fire strategies" include killing terrorists via aerial bombing of residential neighborhoods, aggressively searching all people passing through a checkpoint or roadblock, or other tactics that involve significant collateral damage or inconvenience to innocent third parties (generating resentment among the populations from which terrorist organizations seek recruits). Thus "fire," denoted by v, may have the direct benefit of eliminating current terrorists but the undesirable indirect effect of stimulating recruitment rates (see Keohane & Zeckhauser, 2003).

"Water strategies," on the other hand, are intelligence-driven arrests or "surgical" operations against individuals who are known with very high confidence to be guilty and which do not harm innocent parties. Thus "water," denoted by u, "plays by the rules" in the eyes of the general population and does not fuel (additional) recruitment, but u is more expensive and more difficult to be applied than v. So both controls have their advantages, and both have their drawbacks. We cannot generally claim that one control measure is "better than the other one." The best mix of these two strategies to employ depends on the current state of the problem and the current strength of the terrorist organization.

The strength of the terrorist organization at time t is reflected by a state variable, $S(t)$. Most simply, $S(t)$ may be thought of as the number of active terrorists, but more generally it could also reflect the organization's total resources including financial capital, weapons, and technological know-how, as in Keohane and Zeckhauser (2003).

The strength (or size) of terrorist organizations changes over time. What makes the organization stronger (or weaker)? In modeling criminal enterprises a small part of recruitment (initiation) is usually scripted, represented by a constant term τ, but most is treated as an increasing function of the current state (Caulkins, 2005). Following the lead of other authors (e.g., Castillo-Chavez & Song, 2003) who have applied this reasoning to the recruitment of terrorists, we also adopt this approach. This means that new terrorists are recruited by existing terrorists. Accordingly, when an organization is small, the growth rate ought to be increasing approximately in proportion to the current number of terrorists, say kS with $k > 0$. Yet, growth is not exponential and unbounded. At some point, growth per current member should slow down because of limits on the number of potential recruits, limits on the capacity of the organization to train and absorb new recruits, etc. The degree of slowing down is modeled by the parameter $\alpha \leq 1$. Moreover, the aggressive use of "fire," v, also increases recruitment. A functional form modeling this behavior is

$$I(S, v) = \tau + (1 + \rho v)kS^{\alpha},$$

with $\tau, \rho \geq 0, k > 0$ and $0 \leq \alpha \leq 1$. See also (2.14) below.

We distinguish between three types of outflows from the stock of terrorists. The first represents people who leave the organization, die in suicide attacks, or fall victim to routine or background enforcement efforts that are in addition to those the decision-maker in this problem is actively managing. This outflow, $O_1(S)$, is a function of only S and is represented by μS, with $\mu > 0$. Two additional outflows, $O_2(S, u)$ and $O_3(S, v)$, reflect the consequences of water-type and fire-type operations, respectively. The more aggressive the terror control, the greater the number of terrorists eliminated. The outflow due to water-type strategies is presumed to be concave in S because actionable intelligence is limited and heterogeneous, $O_2(S, u) = \beta(u)f_1(S)$. There may also be diminishing returns if more specialized skills are needed, and so there is a limited number of units that conduct water operations. In particular, concavity is modeled by a power function, $f_1(S) = S^{\theta}$ with $\theta \leq 1$. In contrast, the outflow due to fire strategies, $O_3(S, v) = \gamma(v)f_2(S)$, is modeled as being linear in S because the methods are perceived to be "shotgun" or "undirected" methods and hence $f_2(S) = S$. The more targets there are (i.e., the larger S is), the greater the number of terrorists that will be hit.

We use the same concave functional form for both $\beta(u) = \beta \ln(1 + u)$ and $\gamma(v) = \gamma \ln(1+v)$ so that any differences in the way water and fire type operations are employed stem from differences in their character, not from arbitrary decisions concerning functional forms. It turns out that a logarithmic function constitutes a convenient choice for the purpose of our analysis. Both functions include a leading constant, representing the efficiency of the operations. Since water-type operations are more expensive in the sense that for any given level of spending z, $\beta(z) < \gamma(z)$, the constant for water-type interventions $\beta > 0$ is smaller than the corresponding constant $\gamma > 0$ for fire-type operations.

Combining the above features, the "terror dynamics" in this model can be written as

$$\dot{S} = \tau + (1 + \rho v)kS^{\alpha} - \mu\, S - \beta\, \ln(1 + u)\, S^{\theta} - \gamma\, \ln(1 + v)\, S, \tag{2.14}$$

with τ, ρ, k, α as before and μ, β, $\gamma > 0$, $\beta < \gamma$, $0 \le \theta \le 1$.

For convenience we normalize the units used to measure the size of the terrorist organization to one. Specifically, the normalization is such that in the absence of baseline recruitment ($\tau = 0$) and counter-terror measures ($u = v = 0$) the long-run size of a terrorist organization equals one. Thus

$$\dot{S} = kS^{\alpha} - \mu S,$$

yields $k = \mu$ for $\dot{S} = 0$ at $S = 1$.

We formulate the model presented so far bearing in mind the optimal control framework, which is the main issue of this book. Thus the two operations of fire and water are assumed to be dependent on time, i.e., $u(t)$, $v(t)$, allowing a situational reaction in the form of anti-terror measures that depends on the actual state. Then $u(t)$ and $v(t)$ should be feedbacks $u(t, S)$ and $v(t, S)$, respectively (see Exercise 7.2).

As a preliminary step and to obtain a first insight into the model's complexity, one may consider the model where the controls are fixed, i.e., $u(\cdot) \equiv u$, $v(\cdot) \equiv v$. Reformulating (2.14) in that way, one can try to determine its dynamical behavior, including the computation of the equilibria of the system. Unfortunately it is not possible to find closed-form solutions of the equilibria for arbitrary parameter values of α and θ. Hence we shall specify these values as $\alpha = 1$ and $\theta = 1/2$. Together with the assumption $k = \mu$, this finally yields

$$\dot{S} = \tau + \mu\rho v S - \beta\, \ln(1 + u)\, \sqrt{S} - \gamma\, \ln(1 + v)\, S. \tag{2.15}$$

To find the equilibria of (2.15) we therefore have to solve the equation

$$(\mu\rho v - \gamma\, \ln(1 + v))\, S - \beta\, \ln(1 + u)\, \sqrt{S} + \tau = 0,$$

which for $\mu\rho v - \gamma\, \ln(1 + v) \neq 0$ becomes a quadratic equation in $\sqrt{S}$ with the following solutions

$$\begin{aligned}\sqrt{\hat{S}_{1,2}} &= \frac{\beta\, \ln(1 + u) \pm \sqrt{\beta^2 \ln^2(1 + u) - 4\tau\, (\mu\rho v - \gamma\, \ln(1 + v))}}{2\, (\mu\rho v - \gamma\, \ln(1 + v))} \\ &= \frac{\beta\, \ln(1 + u)}{2\, (\mu\rho v - \gamma\, \ln(1 + v))} \left(1 \pm \sqrt{1 - \Omega}\right),\end{aligned}$$

where

$$\Omega := \frac{4\tau\left(\mu\rho v - \gamma\ \ln(1+v)\right)}{\beta^2 \ln^2(1+u)}.$$

If $\mu\rho v - \gamma\ \ln(1+v) = 0$ the equilibrium is given by

$$\hat{S}_1 = \left(\frac{\tau}{\beta\ \ln(1+u)}\right)^2.$$

To determine the stability of the equilibria we have to consider the Jacobian J of the state dynamics, evaluated at the equilibrium, given by

$$J(\hat{S}) = \frac{\mathrm{d}\dot{S}(\hat{S})}{\mathrm{d}S} = \mu\rho v - \gamma\ \ln(1+v) - \frac{\beta\ \ln(1+u)}{2\sqrt{\hat{S}}},$$

therefore yielding

$$J(\hat{S}) = \begin{cases} -\dfrac{\beta^2 \ln^2(1+u)}{2\tau} & \mu\rho v - \gamma\ \ln(1+v) = 0 \\ (\mu\rho v - \gamma\ \ln(1+v))\dfrac{\pm\sqrt{1-\Omega}}{1 \pm \sqrt{1-\Omega}} & \mu\rho v - \gamma\ \ln(1+v) \neq 0. \end{cases}$$

This provides the following stability properties of the equilibria, depending on the size and sign of Ω.

Region	$\hat{S}_1$	$\hat{S}_2$
$\Omega \leq 0$	Asymptotically stable	–
$0 < \Omega < 1$	Repelling	Asymptotically stable
$\Omega = 1$	Semistable	Semistable
$\Omega > 1$	–	–

In the region $\Omega \in (0,\ 1)$, where both equilibria exist $\hat{S}_1 > \hat{S}_2$, whereas for $\Omega = 1$ both equilibria coincide to a semistable equilibrium. For an interpretation of the equilibria in terms of the counter-terror measures see Exercise 2.2.

For the above cases, $\Omega < 0$ and $0 < \Omega < 1$, the equilibria and their first derivatives depend continuously on the parameter values. Thus it can easily be argued that the signs of the derivatives do not change for slight parameter changes, a property that will later be called *hyperbolic* (see Definition 2.42). Therefore these stability and existence results will also hold true for parameter values α and θ near 1 and 1/2 (see also Fig. 2.7, where the solution is depicted for the set of parameter values specified in Table 2.1).

2.6 ODEs in Higher Dimensions

We now proceed to examine the special cases of linear and nonlinear autonomous ODEs in more detail.

Table 2.1. Parameter values specified for the numerical calculation of the ODE (2.15)

β	μ	γ	ρ	τ	u	v
1.00	3.00	1.00	0.10	0.12	1.00	10.00

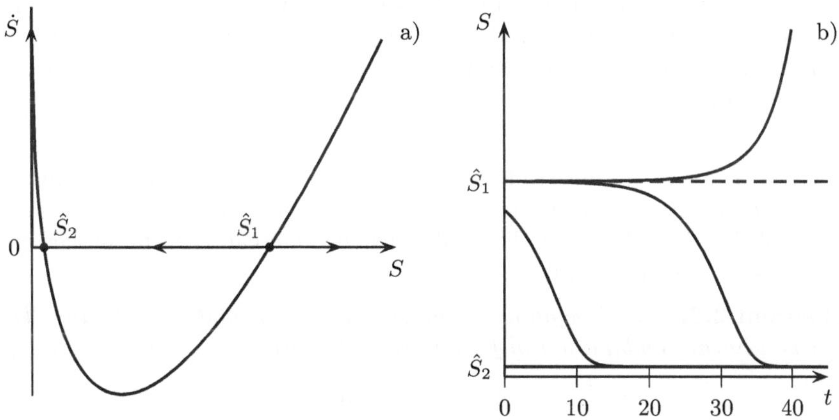

Fig. 2.7. In (**a**) the phase portrait of the ODE (2.15) is depicted and in (**b**) some solution trajectories are shown

2.6.1 Autonomous Linear ODEs

In the simplest case, the dynamics $f(x)$ is given by a linear function in $x \in \mathbb{R}^n$, i.e.,

$$\dot{x} = Jx, \quad x(0) = x_0 \in \mathbb{R}^n, \tag{2.16}$$

where J is an $n \times n$ matrix. From vector space theory we know that in the nonsingular case, i.e., where J is invertible, $\hat{x} = 0$ is the only equilibrium.

In the one-dimensional case, where $J \in \mathbb{R}$ is a scalar, one can see by inspection that the solution of (2.16) is

$$x(t) = \mathrm{e}^{Jt} x_0, \quad t \in \mathbb{R}.$$

Thus $x(\cdot)$ is an exponential function exhibiting one of three possible structural behaviors, depending on the sign of the scalar J:

$J > 0$: The origin is a globally repelling equilibrium.
$J < 0$: The origin is a globally attracting equilibrium.
$J = 0$: The degenerate case, in which every point x_0 is a (stable) equilibrium.

In analogy to the one-dimensional case, the explicit solution of (2.16) for the higher-dimensional case in which J is an $n \times n$ matrix can be written as

$$x(t) = e^{Jt} x_0, \quad t \in \mathbb{R}, \tag{2.17}$$

where the exponential function of a matrix e^{Jt} is defined as the infinite sum

$$e^{Jt} := \mathbb{I}^{(n)} + Jt + \frac{J^2}{2!}t^2 + \frac{J^3}{3!}t^3 + \cdots . \tag{2.18}$$

In Exercise 2.7 the reader is invited to prove that (2.18) satisfies (2.16). Note that (2.17) gives an explicit formula for the flow φ^t of (2.16) as a linear mapping. Although (2.17) is the exact and explicit solution, however, it is not more than a formality if we cannot explicitly calculate the power functions J^n. Using the identity

$$e^{Q^{-1}JQ} = Q^{-1} e^J Q,$$

where $Q \in \mathbb{R}^{n\times n}$ is invertible, creates the possibility of transforming the matrix J into its Jordan normal form (see Theorem A.56) for which (2.17) can explicitly be calculated. The following theorem can then be proved (see, e.g., Hirsch & Smale, 1974):

Theorem 2.33. *Let J be an $n \times n$ matrix and $x(\cdot)$ a solution of (2.16). Then $x(\cdot)$ is a linear combination of functions of the form*

$$at^k e^{\alpha t}\cos(\beta t),\ bt^l e^{\alpha t}\sin(\beta t), \quad a, b \in \mathbb{R},$$

where $\xi = \alpha + i\beta$ runs through all eigenvalues of J, with $\beta \geq 0$ and

$$k, l \leq m(\xi) - 1.$$

Here $m(\xi)$ denotes the algebraic multiplicity of the eigenvalue ξ.

Remark 2.34. Note that Theorem 2.33 delivers the possibility of calculating the solution of the linear ODE (2.16) without having to resort to the matrix Q and therefore to the Jordan normal form. Thus the eigenvalues and their properties have to be determined and the actual solution is then calculated by comparison of coefficients.

Remark 2.35 (Inhomogeneous ODE). The ODE

$$\dot{x} = Jx + C, \quad x(0) = x_0 \in \mathbb{R}^n, \tag{2.19}$$

with $J, C \in \mathbb{R}^{n\times n}$ and $C \neq 0$, is called an *autonomous*[10] *inhomogeneous linear ODE* in contrast to (2.16), which is then called an autonomous *homogeneous* linear ODE. Provided J is invertible the inhomogeneous ODE (2.19) can uniquely[11] be transformed to the homogenous ODE (2.16) by setting

$$y := x + J^{-1}C,$$

which corresponds to a shift of the (unique) equilibrium at the origin to $-J^{-1}C$. Thus all results for the homogeneous problem have an immediate counterpart for the inhomogeneous problem.

---

[10] In the nonautonomous case, i.e., $C = C(t)$, a solution of the ODE (2.19) can be found by the so-called *variation of constants method*, see Exercise 2.20.

[11] Otherwise, if J is not invertible, the uniqueness of the transformation gets lost.

The main purpose of the following parenthesis is to help the reader better understand the analogous considerations for the linear nonautonomous case in Sect. 2.12.1.

The Superposition Principle, Fundamental Matrix, and Wronski Determinant

The *principle of superposition* states that for linear systems the linear combination of solutions $x_i(t) \in \mathbb{R}^n$ of (2.16), i.e.,

$$x(t) = \sum_{i=1}^{n} \gamma_i x_i(t) = X(t)\gamma$$

with

$$X(t) = (x_1(t), \cdots, x_n(t)), \quad \text{and} \quad \gamma = (\gamma_1, \ldots, \gamma_n)', \tag{2.20}$$

is a solution of (2.16) satisfying the initial condition

$$x_0 = X(0)\gamma = \sum_{i=1}^{n} \gamma_i x_i(0).$$

The reader is invited to prove the superposition principle in Exercise 2.8.

Let us restate these considerations with a slightly different perception. Assuming that we know n solutions $x_i(t)$ of (2.16); the matrix $X(t)$ defined in (2.20) satisfies the matrix ODE:[12]

$$\begin{aligned} \dot{X}(t) &= JX(t) \\ \text{s.t.} \quad X(0) &= (x_1(0), \ldots, x_n(0)). \end{aligned} \tag{2.21}$$

If $X(0)$ has full rank, i.e., $(x_1(0), \ldots, x_n(0))$ are linearly independent, then the following proposition is true:

Proposition 2.36 (Full Rank Condition). *Let $X(t)$ satisfy the matrix ODE (2.21). If $X(0)$ has full rank, then $X(t)$ has full rank for all t.*

In Exercise 2.9 the reader is invited to prove this proposition. Proposition 2.36 justifies the notation of a linearly independent solution matrix $X(t)$, since this property is verified either at every time point t or at none. We call such a linearly independent matrix solution $X(t)$ a *fundamental solution* of (2.21). Especially distinguished is the fundamental matrix satisfying $X(0) = \mathbb{I}^{(n)}$, called the *principal matrix solution* of (2.21). Every fundamental matrix solution $Y(t)$ can be transformed into a principal matrix solution defining

$$X(t) = Y(t)Y^{-1}(0),$$

[12] The matrix ODE is understood in a coordinatewise sense. Thus every column of the matrix $X(t)$ is a solution of (2.16).

where the inverse matrix exists due to the full-rank condition.

Finally, we can specify the explicit solution form of a principal matrix solution $X(t)$ by using (2.17) as

$$X(t) = \mathrm{e}^{Jt} X(0) = \mathrm{e}^{Jt} \tag{2.22}$$

since $X(0) = \mathbb{I}^{(n)}$.

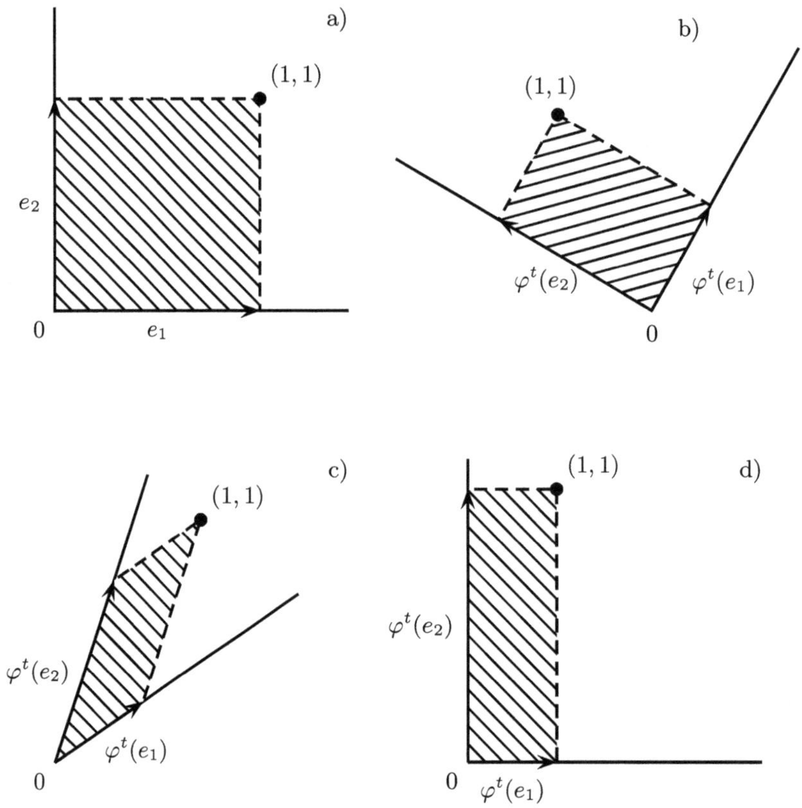

Fig. 2.8. The time evolution of a fundamental matrix starting at the generic basis e_1 and e_2 of $\mathbb{R}^2$, is depicted for a linear system – for time zero in (**a**), and at time t for a stable focus (rotation and shrinking of the axis) in (**b**), for a stable node (squeezing and shrinking of the axis) in (**c**), and for a saddle (stretching and shrinking of the axis) at the origin in (**d**)

Remark 2.37. What is the geometric meaning of fundamental matrix solutions? Imagine the columns of the matrix $X(0)$ as basis vectors of $\mathbb{R}^n$ attached to the origin. The evolution of $X(t)$ characterizes the deformation of the coordinate system under the dynamics (2.16). Hence a point represented by the coordinates x_0 at time $t = 0$ moves in space according to the coordinate systems change. If, e.g., the origin is a stable equilibrium then the time-varying coordinate system shrinks continuously and a point described by the coordinates $x_0 \neq 0$ approaches the origin when following the dynamics (see Fig. 2.8).

Remark 2.38. Pushing this geometric approach further we consider the time-varying volume of the parallelepiped given by the column vectors of the fundamental matrix $X(t)$ (see the shadowed area in Fig. 2.8)

$$\operatorname{vol} X(t) = \det X(t) = \det\left(\mathrm{e}^{Jt} X(0)\right). \tag{2.23}$$

Using (A.5), we can restate (2.23) as

$$\det X(t) = \det X(0)\, \mathrm{e}^{\operatorname{tr} Jt}.$$

Defining, for every fundamental solution matrix $X(t)$, the *Wronski determinant*

$$W(t) := \det X(t),$$

therefore yields

$$W(t) = W(0)\mathrm{e}^{\operatorname{tr} Jt}. \tag{2.24}$$

Now we turn to the important case of a *two-dimensional* or *planar* system.

Planar Linear Systems

In the two-dimensional case, the Jacobian J is a 2×2 matrix

$$J = \begin{pmatrix} a & b \\ c & d \end{pmatrix}$$

and the differential equation can be written in coordinate form as

$$\begin{pmatrix} \dot{x}_1 \\ \dot{x}_2 \end{pmatrix} = \begin{pmatrix} ax_1 + bx_2 \\ cx_1 + dx_2 \end{pmatrix}. \tag{2.25}$$

To apply Theorem 2.33, one has to determine the eigenvalues of matrix J, which are given by

$$\xi_{1,2} = \frac{\operatorname{tr} J \pm \sqrt{(\operatorname{tr} J)^2 - 4 \det J}}{2}, \tag{2.26}$$

where

$$\operatorname{tr} J = a + d, \quad \text{and} \quad \det J = ad - bc.$$

Note that the eigenvalues, as the solution of the quadratic characteristic equation, can have two real or a pair of conjugate complex solutions. If the roots of the characteristic equation

$$\xi^2 - \xi \operatorname{tr} J + \det J = 0$$

are distinct, the corresponding eigenvectors ν_1 and ν_2 are linearly independent. Any initial condition x_0 can then be written as a linear combination of ν_1 and ν_2, say

$$x_0 = \gamma_1\nu_1 + \gamma_2\nu_2,$$

and the general solution of (2.26) is

$$x(t) = \gamma_1 e^{\xi_1 t}\nu_1 + \gamma_2 e^{\xi_2 t}\nu_2.$$

Let us first assume that neither eigenvalue is zero. This implies that J is nonsingular and that the origin is the unique equilibrium. To simplify the analysis, note that for any 2×2 real matrix J, a real matrix Q exists such that $Q^{-1}JQ = A$, where A can take only one of the following four types of Jordan normal forms:

$$A = \begin{pmatrix} \xi_1 & 0 \\ 0 & \xi_2 \end{pmatrix}, \qquad A = \begin{pmatrix} \xi & 0 \\ 0 & \xi \end{pmatrix},$$

$$A = \begin{pmatrix} \xi & 0 \\ 1 & \xi \end{pmatrix}, \qquad A = \begin{pmatrix} \alpha & \beta \\ -\beta & \alpha \end{pmatrix},$$

where ξ_1 and ξ_2 are distinct real roots, ξ is a double root, with corresponding one- or two-dimensional eigenspace, respectively, and $\alpha \pm \mathrm{i}\beta$ are conjugate complex roots of the characteristic equation for J and A. The linear transformation Q^{-1} defines a new variable $y = Q^{-1}x$. Thus $\dot{x} = Q\dot{y}$, and (2.25) becomes

$$\dot{y} = Ay. \tag{2.27}$$

The solutions of (2.27) and (2.16) are qualitatively the same, and so we describe the qualitative properties of (2.27). The key observation is that there are, in a sense, only six types of possible solutions to system (2.27) and therefore also to (2.25). Furthermore, the names and intuition of those *six types* carry over to higher-dimensional systems.

Phase Diagram Representation of the Solution

Recall that the origin is the only equilibrium point of (2.27) under our assumption that $\det J \neq 0$ (i.e., there are no zero roots). Throughout, we denote the initial point by (y_1^0, y_2^0) at $t = 0$ and assume that it is not the origin. (Since the origin is an equilibrium, if the initial point is at the origin the system will always remain at the origin.) In the following we briefly present the different types of solutions arranged by the importance for the solution of optimal control models, especially for models we analyze in this book.

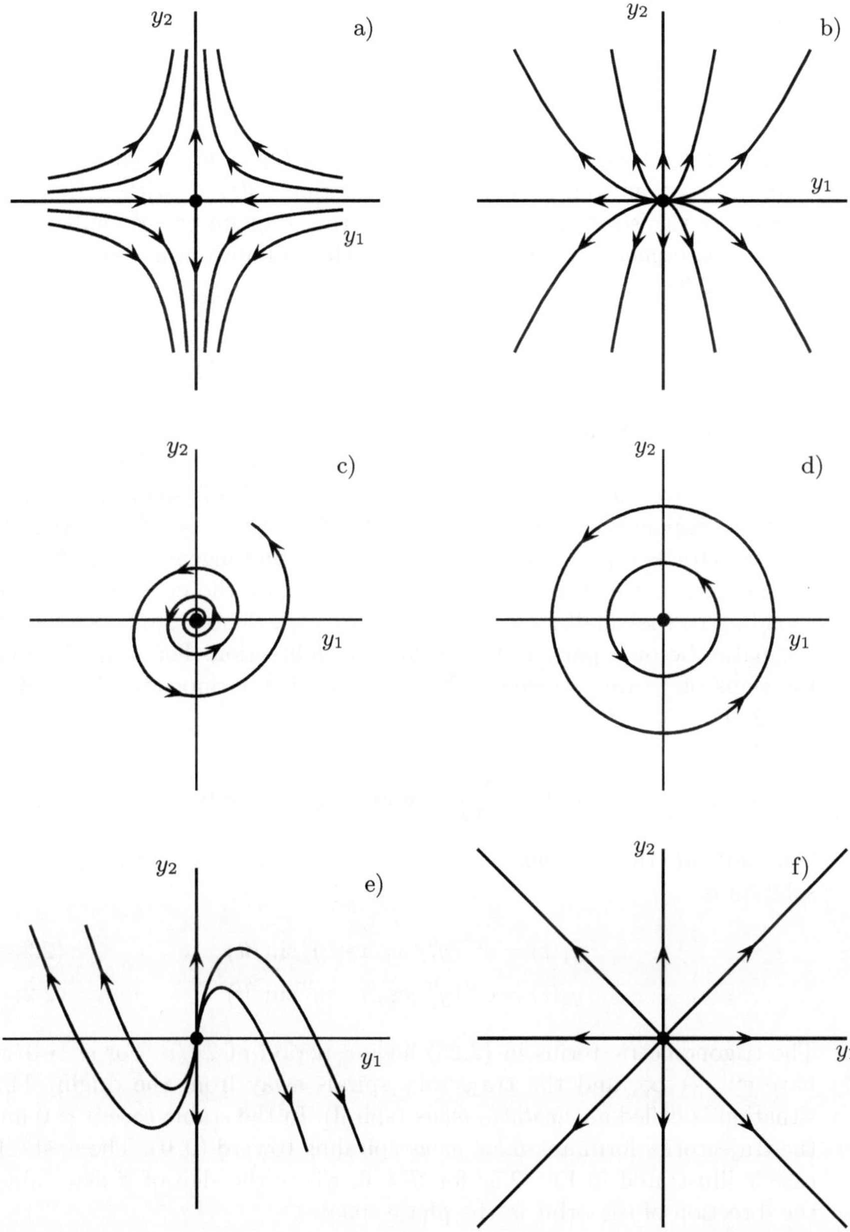

Fig. 2.9. Phase portraits for planar (linear) systems of ODEs, with (**a**) $\xi_1 < 0 < \xi_2$; (**b**) $\xi_1 > \xi_2 > 0$; (**c**) $\alpha > 0$, $\beta > 0$; (**d**) $\alpha = 0$, $\beta > 0$; (**e**) $\xi > 0$, $\mathrm{rk}(A - \xi\mathbb{I}^{(2)}) = 1$; (**f**) $\xi > 0$, $\mathrm{rk}(A - \xi\mathbb{I}^{(2)}) = 0$

a) *Saddle point*:

$$A = \begin{pmatrix} \xi_1 & 0 \\ 0 & \xi_2 \end{pmatrix}, \quad \text{and} \quad \operatorname{sgn} \xi_1 \neq \operatorname{sgn} \xi_2.$$

Thus the roots of the characteristic equation are real, and distinct. Assume $\xi_1 < 0 < \xi_2$, then there exists a solution $y_1(t) = y_1^0 e^{\xi_1 t}$ converging to 0 for $t \to \infty$ as well as a diverging solution $y_2(t) = y_2^0 e^{\xi_2 t}$. Here the abscissa is the *stable manifold*, whereas the ordinate corresponds to the *unstable manifold* (see Definition 2.45). The equilibrium is a *saddle point* (see Fig. 2.9a).

b) *Node*:

$$A = \begin{pmatrix} \xi_1 & 0 \\ 0 & \xi_2 \end{pmatrix}, \quad \text{and} \quad \operatorname{sgn} \xi_1 = \operatorname{sgn} \xi_2.$$

The characteristic roots are real and distinct. The solution is $y_1(t) = y_1^0 e^{\xi_1 t}, y_2(t) = y_2^0 e^{\xi_2 t}$. The trajectories will be unstable if the eigenvalues ξ_i are positive, and stable if they are negative. Both solutions explode or decay exponentially (see Fig. 2.9b for $0 < \xi_1 < \xi_2$). Geometrically, the trajectories typically emanate from the origin tangentially to the slow eigendirection, which is the direction spanned by the eigenvector corresponding to the smaller eigenvalue ξ_1 (see, e.g., Shub, 1987). For $t \to \infty$ the paths become parallel to the fast eigendirection. For a stable node the signs of ξ_i are reversed and arrows are in the opposite direction in Fig. 2.9b.

c) *Focus*:

$$A = \begin{pmatrix} \alpha & \beta \\ -\beta & \alpha \end{pmatrix}, \quad \text{and} \quad \alpha \neq 0,\ \beta \neq 0.$$

The roots are the complex conjugates $\alpha + i\beta$ and $\alpha - i\beta$ with $\alpha \neq 0$. The solution is

$$y_1(t) = e^{\alpha t}(y_1^0 \cos \beta t + y_2^0 \sin \beta t), \tag{2.28a}$$
$$y_2(t) = e^{\alpha t}(y_2^0 \cos \beta t - y_1^0 \sin \beta t). \tag{2.28b}$$

The trigonometric terms in (2.28) have a period of $2\pi/\beta$. For $\alpha > 0$ we have $e^{\alpha t} \to \infty$, and the trajectory spirals away from the origin. This situation is called an *unstable focus* (spiral). In the stable case $\alpha < 0$ and the trajectories form an *stable focus* spiraling toward $(0, 0)$. The unstable case is illustrated in Fig. 2.9c for $\beta < 0$, where the sign of β determines the direction of the orbit in the phase space.

The equilibria considered so far are structurally stable in the sense that small perturbations of the defining matrix A do not change the qualitative behavior of the system. Contrary to that, the subsequent equilibria are hairline cases, i.e., they are sensitive to small perturbations of A. The theory analyzing the occurrence of such sensitive equilibria is called *bifurcation theory* and will be introduced in Sect. 2.8.

d) *Center*:

$$A = \begin{pmatrix} 0 & \beta \\ -\beta & 0 \end{pmatrix}, \quad \text{and} \quad \beta \neq 0.$$

In the case of pure imaginary eigenvalues, i.e., for $\alpha = 0$, all solutions are closed circles with period $\Theta = 2\pi/\beta$. The oscillations have fixed amplitude and the equilibrium is called a *center*. As we shall see in Sect. 2.10, this case becomes important when analyzing the Poincaré–Andronov–Hopf bifurcation. The counterclockwise movement, i.e., $\beta < 0$, is illustrated in Fig. 2.9d. Note that for a center the origin is stable but not asymptotically stable.

e) *Degenerate node*:

$$A = \begin{pmatrix} \xi & 0 \\ 1 & \xi \end{pmatrix}.$$

There is a single real root, but no real matrix Q can transform J into a diagonal matrix (the eigenspace is of dimension one). The solution has the form:

$$y_1(t) = y_1^0 \mathrm{e}^{\xi t}, \quad y_2(t) = (y_2^0 + y_1^0 t)\mathrm{e}^{\xi t}.$$

For $\xi > 0$, both $y_1(t)$ and $y_2(t)$ diverge from the origin for $t \to \infty$. The flow is illustrated in Fig. 2.9e. The equilibrium is called a *degenerate* or *improper node* and is unstable since $\xi > 0$. When $\xi < 0$, the trajectories follow the same lines in the opposite direction and the origin is therefore stable. There is only one eigendirection (the y_2-axis). As $t \to \pm\infty$ all trajectories become parallel to it.

f) *Star node*:

$$A = \begin{pmatrix} \xi & 0 \\ 0 & \xi \end{pmatrix}.$$

There is a single real eigenvalue ξ (the eigenspace is of dimension two). The solution is $y_1(t) = y_1^0 \mathrm{e}^{\xi t}, y_2(t) = y_2^0 \mathrm{e}^{\xi t}$. Since $y_2(t)/y_1(t)$ is constant, the trajectories are rays through the origin. If $\xi < 0$, it is globally asymptotically stable; if $\xi > 0$, the node is unstable (see Fig. 2.9f illustrating the unstable case).

In the following we shall give a summary of the classification of the equilibrium at the origin with respect to the characteristic roots.

Classification of Equilibria

For a planar linear system with constant coefficients, the type and stability of all equilibria can be characterized in a single diagram (see Fig. 2.10).

Let the abscissa measure the trace $\tau = \operatorname{tr} A$ and the ordinate measure the determinant $\Delta = \det A$ of the matrix of the planar system. Then the solution of the characteristic equation may be written, using (2.26),

$$\xi_{1,2} = \frac{1}{2}\left(\tau \pm \sqrt{\tau^2 - 4\Delta}\right).$$

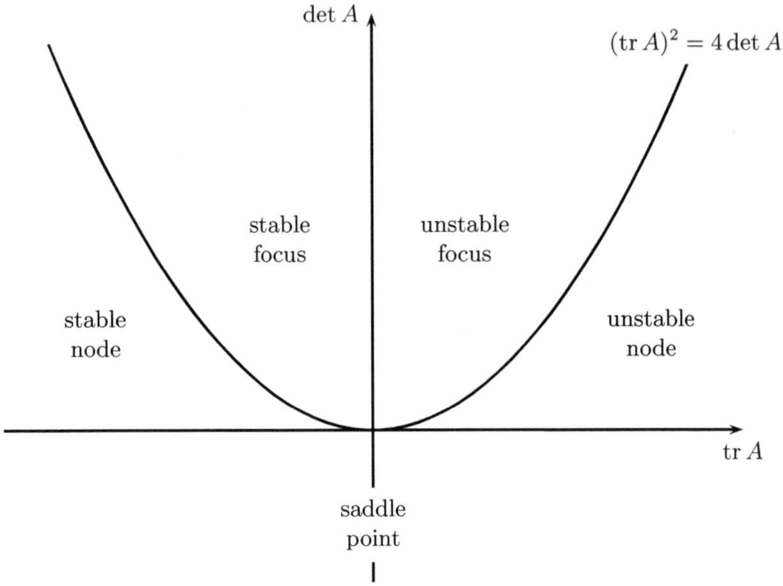

Fig. 2.10. Classification of equilibria in planar systems $\dot{x} = Ax$

By observing that (2.26) may be written as $(\xi - \xi_1)(\xi - \xi_2) = 0$, we also get

$$\tau = \xi_1 + \xi_2, \quad \Delta = \xi_1 \xi_2.$$

Considering the six cases above and Fig. 2.10 leads to the following conclusions:

1. For $\Delta < 0$, the eigenvalues are real and have opposite signs. Hence the origin is a *saddle point.*
2. For $\Delta > 0$, the eigenvalues are either real with the same sign (*nodes*), or complex conjugate (*foci* and *centers*), where the sign of the discriminant $D = \tau^2 - 4\Delta$ determines which case arises. For $D > 0$, nodes occur, and foci are obtained for $D < 0$.
   a) The origin is a repelling node (focus) if $\tau > 0$.
   b) The origin is an asymptotic stable node (focus) if $\tau < 0$.
3. In Fig. 2.10 it is easy to recognize the other cases as hairline cases. Since for $\tau = 0$, centers occur, whereas $D = 0$ corresponds to the star and degenerate node. Finally, $\Delta = 0$ characterizes the case of equilibria, where the matrix A is singular and hence the origin may not be the unique equilibrium.

Higher-Dimensional Linear Systems

Since the world is largely nonlinear, we are not interested in linear systems per se. We have discussed planar linear systems in such detail because the categorization of the six broad types of equilibria provides useful intuition that carries over to higher-dimensional systems, including nonlinear systems, where an important strategy is to examine the linearization about an equilibrium. In what follows, therefore, we shall need to generalize to higher dimensions the idea of keeping track of which eigenvalues $\xi_i, i = 1, \dots, n$ have positive, negative, or zero real parts, since those counts play a crucial role in determining the stability of linear systems of all dimensions, not just planar systems. Thus we define the following (generalized) eigenspaces:

$$\mathrm{E}^s = \operatorname{span}\{\nu_j \in \mathbb{R}^n : \operatorname{Re}(\xi_j) < 0\}, \quad \dim \mathrm{E}^s = n_- \tag{2.29a}$$

$$\mathrm{E}^u = \operatorname{span}\{\nu_j \in \mathbb{R}^n : \operatorname{Re}(\xi_j) > 0\}, \quad \dim \mathrm{E}^u = n_+ \tag{2.29b}$$

$$\mathrm{E}^c = \operatorname{span}\{\nu_j \in \mathbb{R}^n : \operatorname{Re}(\xi_j) = 0\}, \quad \dim \mathrm{E}^c = n_0, \tag{2.29c}$$

where $n_- + n_+ + n_0 = n$ is the number of state variables (dimension of the system). Then E^s is called the *stable*, E^u is called the *unstable* and E^c is called the *center* eigenspace.

Considering that $J^i\nu_j = \xi_j^i\nu_j$ and using the infinite sum (2.18), we see that the eigenspaces $\mathrm{E}^s, \mathrm{E}^u$, and E^c are invariant under the linear flow $\varphi^t(\cdot) = \mathrm{e}^{Jt}(\cdot)$, i.e., $\varphi^t(\mathrm{E}^s) \subset \mathrm{E}^s$, etc. Using Theorem 2.33 one can furthermore show that

$$\lim_{t\to\infty} \varphi^t(\mathrm{E}^s) = 0, \quad \text{and} \quad \lim_{t\to-\infty} \varphi^t(\mathrm{E}^u) = 0,$$

justifying the notation of E^s as the stable and E^u as the unstable subspace. Contrary to that, one cannot designate the long-run behavior of the trajectories in the center subspace E^c without knowing further details of the algebraic multiplicity of the eigenvalues. This exceptional position of the center subspace plays a crucial role in bifurcation theory and will be further explained in Sect. 2.8.3. The equilibrium at the origin satisfying $n_0 = 0$ is called *hyperbolic* (see Definition 2.42).

Remark 2.39. Note that the difference between the (un)stable and the center subspace is also one of persistence by slight changes of the defining (linear) dynamics J. Since the eigenvalues continuously depend on the matrix J, it easily follows that if J is changed to $J_\varepsilon = J + \Delta J$, with ΔJ small, the eigenvalues with a positive/negative real part will not change their sign. This is unlike the case for the zero eigenvalues, where the slightest change of J will move it to the positive or negative side. Thus a system in which $n_0 = 0$, i.e., $\mathrm{E}^c = \emptyset$, is "structurally stable" for small (linear) disturbances of the matrix J, whereas in the case of $n_0 > 0$ the system's behavior may change considerably.

Summing up, we find the following classification of a hyperbolic equilibrium at the origin, i.e., $n_0 = 0$:

$n_- > 0, n_+ = 0$ the origin is an attractor.
$n_- = 0, n_+ > 0$ the origin is a repeller.
$n_- > 0, n_+ > 0$ the origin is unstable, exhibiting trajectories converging to and diverging from it, and is therefore a saddle (point).

This classification (in a local form) can also be transformed to the nonlinear case (see Sect. 2.6.2).

Remark 2.40. For the sink (and reversing time also for the source) we can give a geometric intuition for its asymptotic stability using (2.24), which describes the volume change of the fundamental matrix solution (coordinate system); and we see that

$$\tau = \operatorname{tr} J = \sum_{i=1}^{n} \xi_i < 0.$$

Hence

$$\det X(t) = \det X(0) \mathrm{e}^{t\tau},$$

is contracting, a condition that provides the geometric intuition for a shrinking coordinate system and therefore an asymptotic convergence of all paths to the origin.

Next, the theory of autonomous systems is continued for the nonlinear case.

2.6.2 Autonomous Nonlinear ODEs

In the majority of models presented in this book the system dynamics is given by a nonlinear function $f : \mathbb{R} \to \mathbb{R}^n$:

$$\dot{x}(t) = f(x(t)) \tag{2.30a}$$
$$\text{s.t.} \quad x(0) = x_0 \in \mathbb{R}^n,$$

where f is continuously differentiable.

Remark 2.41. In general it is not possible to state a closed-form solution of (2.30), therefore we have to rely on numerical methods, when solving an explicit ODE.

Equilibria and Their Stability

Next we describe the dynamic behavior of trajectories in the neighborhood of an equilibrium $\hat{x}$. Therefore we define:

Definition 2.42 (Hyperbolic Equilibrium). *An equilibrium $\hat{x}$ is called* hyperbolic *if the corresponding Jacobian $J(\hat{x})$ has no zero or purely imaginary eigenvalues, i.e., $n_0 = 0$, otherwise it is called a* nonhyperbolic *equilibrium.*

Using the properties of a hyperbolic equilibrium in Hartman (1982) the following theorem is proved:

Theorem 2.43 (Hartman–Grobman Theorem). *Let $\hat{x}$ be a hyperbolic equilibrium of the ODE (2.30a). Then there exists a neighborhood $U \subset \mathbb{R}^n$ of $\hat{x}$ and a neighborhood $U' \subset \mathbb{R}^n$ of the origin such that the ODE (2.30a) restricted to U is topological equivalent to the variational equation of $\hat{x}$*

$$\dot{x}(t) = f_x(\hat{x})x(t) = J(\hat{x})x(t), \quad x(0) \in U'.$$

This theorem formally states that the dynamical behavior of a nonlinear system near a hyperbolic equilibrium can be fully described by its linearization. Thus the stability behavior of an equilibrium for an ODE is characterized by the eigenvalues ξ of the Jacobian matrix $J(\hat{x}) = f_x(\hat{x})$:

Theorem 2.44. *Let $\hat{x}$ be an equilibrium of the ODE (2.30a). If for every eigenvalue ξ of the Jacobian matrix $J(\hat{x}) = f_x(\hat{x})$*

$$\operatorname{Re}\xi < 0$$

holds, then $\hat{x}$ is asymptotic stable. If there exists an ξ with

$$\operatorname{Re}\xi > 0,$$

then $\hat{x}$ is unstable.

This result is analogous to the linear case (see p. 41), and a proof can be found in Hartman (1982).

An important concept is that of a *local stable and unstable manifold* of an equilibrium $\hat{x}$. These are defined by:

Definition 2.45 (Local Manifolds). *Let $\hat{x}$ be an equilibrium of the ODE (2.30a) and U be a neighborhood of $\hat{x}$; then the set*

$$\mathrm{W}^s_{loc}(\hat{x}) = \{x \in U : \lim_{t\to\infty} \varphi^t(x) = \hat{x}, \text{ and } \varphi^t(x) \in U, t \geq 0\}$$

is called the stable local manifold *of $\hat{x}$ and the set*

$$\mathrm{W}^u_{loc}(\hat{x}) = \{x \in U : \lim_{t\to\infty} \varphi^{-t}(x) = \hat{x}, \text{ and } \varphi^{-t}(x) \in U, t \geq 0\},$$

is called the unstable local manifold *of $\hat{x}$.*

Now the following theorem can be proved (see Carr, 1981; Marsden & McCracken, 1976; and Kelley, 1967):

Theorem 2.46 (Manifold Theorem for Flows). *Suppose that $\hat{x}$ is an equilibrium of (2.30a), where $f \in C^k(\mathbb{R}^n)$, and $\hat{J} = f_x(\hat{x})$. Let n_+, n_- and n_0 be the corresponding dimensions of the stable, unstable, and center subspaces E^s, E^u, and E^c. Then there locally exist the local stable and unstable C^k manifolds $\mathrm{W}^s_{loc}(\hat{x}), \mathrm{W}^u_{loc}(\hat{x})$, and a* local center manifold *$\mathrm{W}^c_{loc}(\hat{x})$ of the dimensions n_+, n_- and n_0 and being tangent to $\mathrm{E}^s, \mathrm{E}^u$, and E^c (see (2.29)). The manifolds $\mathrm{W}^s_{loc}(\hat{x}), \mathrm{W}^u_{loc}(\hat{x})$, and $\mathrm{W}^c_{loc}(\hat{x})$ are under the flow of f. The stable and unstable manifolds are unique, whereas the center manifold need not be unique.*

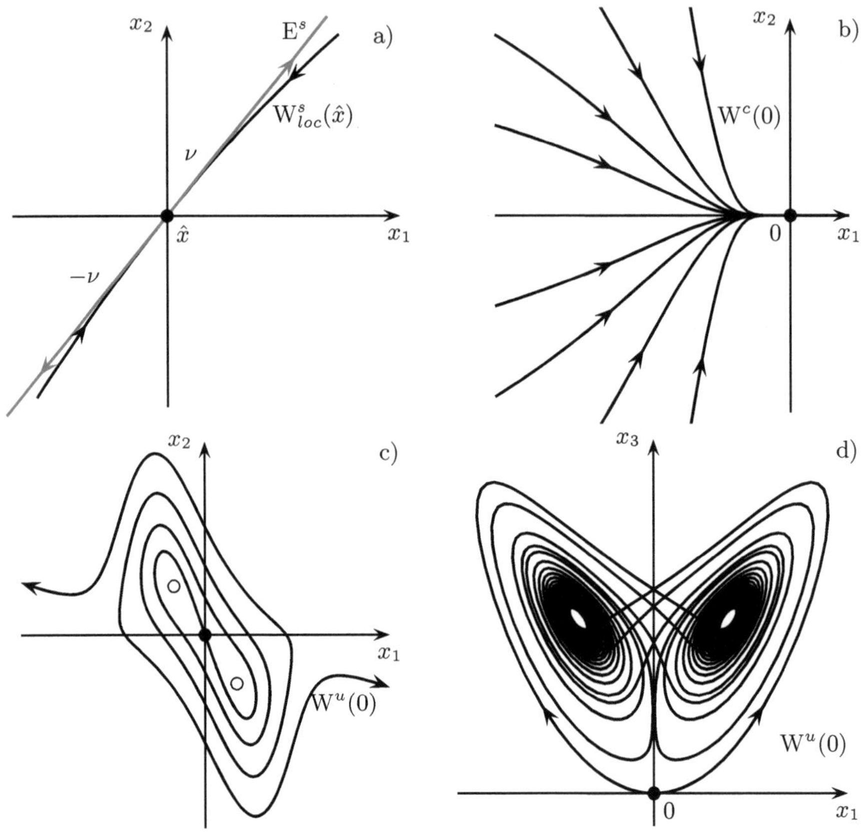

Fig. 2.11. In (**a**) the local stable manifold $W^s_{loc}(\hat{x})$ is depicted together with the stable eigenspace E^s spanned by the eigenvector ν. In (**b**) the existence of infinitely many center manifolds $W^c(0)$ is illustrated for the system (2.31). In (**c**) the stable (*solid*) as well as the unstable (*dashed*) global manifold is depicted for an equilibrium at the origin. The last panel (**d**) shows the Lorenz attractor projected into the (x_1, x_3)-plane as an example for complex global behavior of a one-dimensional unstable manifold

Furthermore, the local manifolds $W^s_{loc}(\hat{x}), W^u_{loc}(\hat{x})$ have global extensions $W^s(\hat{x}), W^u(\hat{x})$ by letting points in $W^s_{loc}(\hat{x})$ flow backward in time and those in $W^u_{loc}(\hat{x})$ flow forward:

Definition 2.47 (Global Manifolds of an Equilibrium). *Let $\hat{x}$ be an equilibrium of (2.30a); then the set*

$$W^s(\hat{x}) = \bigcup_{t \geq 0} \varphi^{-t}(W^s_{loc})(\hat{x})$$

is called the global stable manifold *of $\hat{x}$ and*

$$W^u(\hat{x}) = \bigcup_{t\geq 0} \varphi^t(W^u_{loc})(\hat{x})$$

is called the global unstable manifold *of* $\hat{x}$ *(see Fig. 2.11b,d).*

A trajectory $x(\cdot)$ *of the ODE (2.30) is called a* stable path *of* $\hat{x}$ *if the corresponding orbit* $\mathrm{Or}(x_0)$ *satisfies* $\mathrm{Or}(x_0) \subset W^s\,\hat{x}$ *and* $\lim_{t\to\infty}\varphi^t(x_0) = \hat{x}$.

A trajectory $x(\cdot)$ *of the ODE (2.30) is called an* unstable path *of* $\hat{x}$ *if the corresponding orbit* $\mathrm{Or}(x_0)$ *satisfies* $\mathrm{Or}(x_0) \subset W^u\,\hat{x}$ *and* $\lim_{t\to\infty}\varphi^{-t}(x_0) = \hat{x}$.

For $n_+ = 1$ the situation is depicted in Fig. 2.11a.

Definition 2.48 (Saddle Point). *An equilibrium* $\hat{x}$ *satisfying* $n_+ > 0$ *and* $n_- > 0$ *is called a* saddle point *or shortly* saddle.

Remark 2.49 (Saddle Point Stability). In economic dynamics a saddle $\hat{x}$ is often referred to as an equilibrium exhibiting *saddle point stability.* Here the term "stability" only refers to the fact, that converging paths exist, and must not be confused with a stable equilibrium (see, e.g., Sect. 5.1).

Remark 2.50. Note that this special construction of the global stable manifold becomes immediately clear when one considers that the points reached by letting the time flow backward are exactly those from where the forward trajectories will end up in the stable local manifold when moving forward in time. This idea constitutes the basis for a simple method to numerically compute the stable manifold (see Sect. 7.4.1).

Remark 2.51. Some few results exist guaranteeing the existence of the global manifolds (see, e.g., Hartman, 1982, Chap. VIII). These results rely on geometric considerations, which, for the planar case, are depicted in Fig. 2.12. Since these results are, in our context, only of minor practical importance we refrain from presenting their explicit formulation.

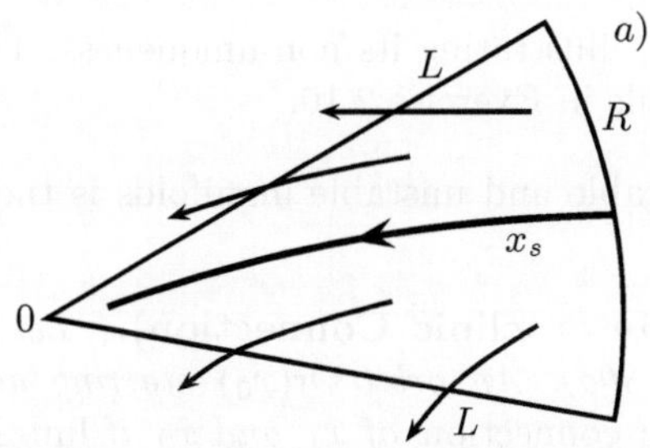

Fig. 2.12. The situation assuring the existence of a global saddle path. From geometric intuition it is evident that under the given assumptions a trajectory moving to the origin has to exist

Example 2.52 (Non-Unique Center Manifold). A typical example illustrating the non-uniqueness of the center manifold is given by the following ODE:

$$\dot{x}_1 = x_1^2 \tag{2.31a}$$

$$\dot{x}_2 = -x_2. \tag{2.31b}$$

Linearizing the system (2.31) around the equilibrium at the origin yielding

$$\begin{pmatrix} \dot{x}_1 \\ \dot{x}_2 \end{pmatrix} = \begin{pmatrix} 0 & 0 \\ 0 & -1 \end{pmatrix} \begin{pmatrix} x_1 \\ x_2 \end{pmatrix}$$

reveals that 0 is an eigenvalue of the Jacobian and therefore the equilibrium is nonhyperbolic. The manifold theorem for flows assures the existence of a local center manifold $\mathrm{W}^c_{loc}(0)$ tangential to the corresponding eigenspace $\mathrm{E}^c(0)$. This eigenspace is given by the x_1-axis as the reader may verify. Moreover the x_1-axis is such a center manifold since $x_2 \equiv 0$ implies $\dot{x}_2 = 0$ and is therefore tangential to $\mathrm{E}^c(0)$ (in fact it coincides).

But additionally there exist further center manifolds (see Fig. 2.11b). For $x_1 \neq 0$ we divide both dynamics of (2.31) yielding the one-dimensional nonautonomous ODE

$$\dot{x}_2 = -\frac{x_2}{x_1^2}.$$

The solution of this ODE is explicitly given by

$$x_2(x_1) = x_2(0)\mathrm{e}^{-\frac{1}{x_1(0)}}\mathrm{e}^{\frac{1}{x_1}},$$

which corresponds to the orbits of the system (2.31) and reveals that for $x_1(0) < 0$ the solution converges tangentially to the origin. Thus every orbit given by

$$x_2(x_1) = \begin{cases} x_2(0)\mathrm{e}^{-\frac{1}{x_1(0)}}\mathrm{e}^{\frac{1}{x_1}} & x_1 < 0 \\ 0 & x_1 \geq 0 \end{cases}$$

is a center manifold, illustrating its non-uniqueness. The reader is invited to accomplish the details in Exercise 2.10.

Connected to the stable and unstable manifolds is the so-called heteroclinic connection:

Definition 2.53 (Heteroclinic Connection). *Let $\hat{x}_1$ and $\hat{x}_2$ be equilibria of the ODE (2.30a). An orbit* $\mathrm{Or}(x_0)$ *starting at a point $x_0 \in \mathbb{R}^n$ is called a* heteroclinic connection *of $\hat{x}_1$ and $\hat{x}_2$ if $\lim_{t\to-\infty}\varphi^t(x_0) = \hat{x}_1$ and $\lim_{t\to\infty}\varphi^t(x) = \hat{x}_2$.*

Remark 2.54. From Definition 2.53 it immediately follows that the heteroclinic connection is part of the unstable manifold of $\hat{x}_1$ as well as of the stable manifold for $\hat{x}_2$ (see Fig. 2.13).

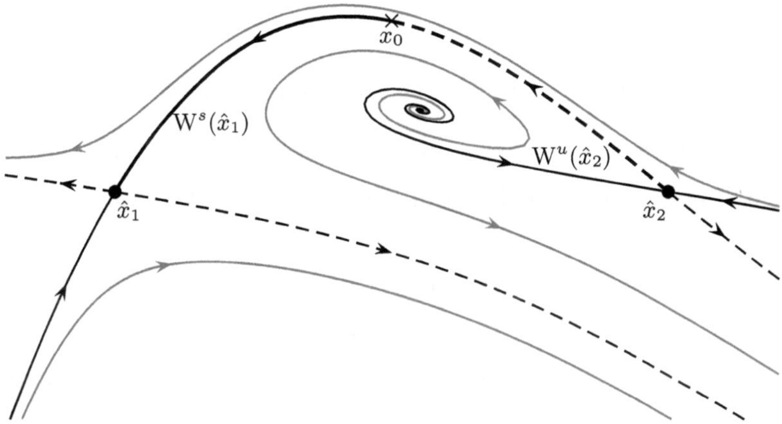

Fig. 2.13. A heteroclinic connection between the equilibria $\hat{x}_1$ and $\hat{x}_2$ is depicted, where the stable manifold of $\hat{x}_1$ coincides with the unstable manifold of $\hat{x}_2$. For illustration a point x_0 lying on the heteroclinic connection is shown, where the corresponding trajectory converges to $\hat{x}_1$ in positive time and to $\hat{x}_2$ in negative time

Remark 2.55. The introduction of heteroclinic connections is not an end in itself but becomes important in the analysis of the occurrence of multiple optimal solutions (see Chap. 5).

Definition 2.56 (Homoclinic Connection). *Let $\hat{x}$ be an equilibrium of the ODE (2.30a). Then an orbit* $\mathrm{Or}(x_0)$ *starting at a point $x_0 \in \mathbb{R}^n$ is called a* homoclinic connection *of $\hat{x}$ if* $\lim_{t\to\pm\infty} \varphi^t(x_0) = \hat{x}$.

Next we turn our attention to the nonhyperbolic case, which becomes important for the analysis of structural changes of dynamical systems (see Sect. 2.8).

Example 2.57 (Calculation of the Center Manifold). In this subsection we present a planar system with a nonhyperbolic equilibrium at the origin. By means of this planar system we exemplify the calculation of the corresponding center manifold to determine the stability of the equilibrium. For a generalization of the here presented transformation the reader is referred to Guckenheimer and Holmes (1983) and Kuznetsov (1998).

Given the two-dimensional system:

$$\dot{x}_1 = x_1 x_2 + x_1^3 \tag{2.32a}$$

$$\dot{x}_2 = -x_2 - 2x_1^2, \tag{2.32b}$$

we determine the stability of the equilibrium at the origin. The corresponding Jacobian

$$J = \begin{pmatrix} 0 & 0 \\ 0 & -1 \end{pmatrix}$$

reveals that $n_0 = n_- = 1$, yielding the corresponding eigenspaces

$$\mathrm{E}^s = \{(x_1, x_2) : x_1 = 0\}, \quad \mathrm{E}^c = \{(x_1, x_2) : x_2 = 0\}.$$

First, it is obvious that the linear approximation $\dot{x} = Jx$, explicitly written as

$$\dot{x}_1 = 0$$
$$\dot{x}_2 = -x_2,$$

is insufficient for determining the behavior of the system in a neighborhood of the origin.

Therefore, we use a quadratic approximation of the center manifold $\mathrm{W}^c_{loc}(0)$ in a neighborhood of the origin and analyze the dynamics restricted to this approximation.

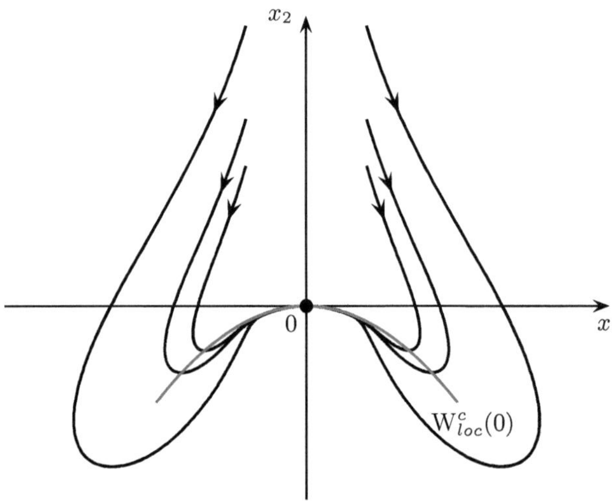

Fig. 2.14. The phase portrait for the dynamics (2.32) is depicted confirming the (asymptotic) stability of the nonhyperbolic equilibrium at the origin. The *gray line* shows the quadratic approximation of the local center manifold $\mathrm{W}^c_{loc}(0)$

The manifold theorem for flows assures the existence of the center manifold near the origin, which can be written as $x_2 = C(x_1)$ and is tangential to the center eigenspace E^c. This yields

$$C(0) = 0, \quad \text{and} \quad C_{x_1}(0) = 0.$$

Using the Taylor theorem $C(x_1)$ can quadratically be approximated

$$x_2 = C(x_1) = \frac{c}{2}x_1^2 + o(x_1^2). \tag{2.33}$$

To calculate the constant c we consider the total time derivative of (2.33)

$$\dot{x}_2 = \frac{\mathrm{d}C(x_1)}{\mathrm{d}t}$$

which becomes

$$\begin{aligned}\dot{x}_2 &= \frac{\partial C(x_1)}{\partial x_1}\dot{x}_1 = cx_1(x_1x_2 + x_1^3) + o(x_1)(x_1x_2 + x_1^3) \\ &= c\left(\frac{c}{2}+1\right)x_1^4 + o(x_1^4). \end{aligned} \tag{2.34}$$

Substituting (2.33) into (2.32b) yields

$$\dot{x}_2 = -x_2 - 2x_1^2 = -\left(\frac{c}{2}+2\right)x_1^2 + o(x_1^2). \tag{2.35}$$

When comparing the leading coefficients of x_1^2 for both representations (2.34) and (2.35) of $\dot{x}_2$, we find

$$\frac{c}{2} + 2 = 0 \quad \text{implying} \quad c = -4.$$

Thus the quadratic approximation of the center manifold is given by

$$x_2 = -2x_1^2$$

and the dynamics for x_1 restricted to the local center manifold becomes

$$\dot{x}_1 = x_1C(x_1) + x_1^3 = -2x_1^3 + x_1^3 + o(x_1^3) = -x_1^3 + o(x_1^3).$$

This proves that the equilibrium at the origin is stable (see Fig. 2.14).

The Occurrence of Limit Cycles

As has already been mentioned limit cycles are, beside equilibria, other important limit sets often occurring in higher-dimensional (nonlinear) systems.

The reader may already be familiar with periodic system behavior. The well-known *predator–prey model*, for instance, can exhibit recurrence of population numbers. When there are lots of rabbits (the *prey population*), the birth rate of foxes (the *predator population*) will increase in response to the bountiful food supply. This increases the fox population, but these additional foxes also eat more rabbits. As the number of rabbits shrinks, food for foxes becomes scarce, and their birth rate declines. Eventually the smaller predator population allows the prey population to recover and the whole cycle starts again.

Thus the descriptive two-state predator–prey model and various models addressed in this chapter's Exercises can exhibit an attracting limit cycle.

But in general it is much harder to detect such a limit cycle than finding an equilibrium. However, for planar systems it is at least possible to formulate conditions under which such cyclical solutions exist, known as the Poincaré–Bendixson theorem:

Theorem 2.58 (Poincaré–Bendixson). *If a nonempty compact ω- or α-limit set of a planar flow does not contain an equilibrium then it is a limit cycle.*

For a proof see Hirsch and Smale (1974) or Hartman (1982).

The Poincaré–Bendixson theorem is very intuitive. Basically it says that if a trajectory of a continuous dynamical system stays in a bounded region of the $\mathbb{R}^2$ forever, it has to approach "something." This "something" is either a point or a cycle. So if it is not a point, then it must be the other. If you enter a room and remain there forever without being allowed to stand still, sooner or later you will retrace your steps. Just because you would eventually have to walk over a spot you had already visited does not mean you would then have to walk in circles forever, but that is because you retain the capacity to make choices. For a trajectory whose motion depends entirely and only on its current position, once the trajectory returns to a place in the plane it has already visited, that trajectory is trapped and must then cycle forever.

The condition in the Poincaré–Bendixson theorem that no equilibrium is contained in the limit set is important as Fig. 2.15 illustrates, where in the long-run the solutions converge to a *heteroclinic cycle*, which is constituted by equilibria and heteroclinic connections, and not a limit cycle.

The Poincaré–Bendixson theorem is intuitive, but often not terribly helpful. How do you know what region to consider? And how would you know that any trajectory that entered the region could not ever leave? But most important, the Poincaré–Bendixson theorem is valid only for planar systems. As soon as one has to add a third-state variable, it will not be able to break the phase space into an interior and an exterior of a closed orbit and the theorem becomes completely worthless. Fortunately bifurcation theory provides tools to find periodic orbits by the important *Poincaré–Andronov–Hopf theorem*, as will be presented in Sect. 2.10.

Analogous to equilibria, the stability of limit cycles are of great importance for the long-run behavior of the dynamical system. But since the necessary theory is more involved than in the case of equilibria, we postponed this part in Sect. 2.12.1.

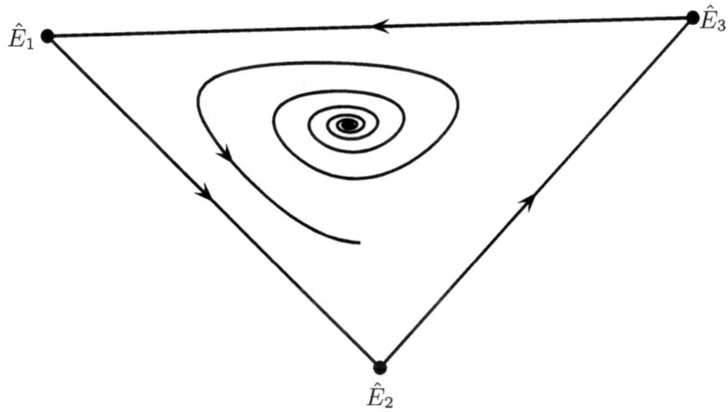

Fig. 2.15. The limit set, given by the equilibria $\hat{E}_1$, $\hat{E}_2$, $\hat{E}_3$ and their heteroclinic connections, is a compact set but is *not* a limit cycle. It is a so-called heteroclinic cycle (see, e.g., Arrowsmith & Place, 1990, Chap. 5)

2.7 Stability Behavior in a Descriptive Model of Drug Demand

Patterns of drug use vary over time not only owing to external factors such as sanctions and prices, but also as a result of the progression of users through various types or "states" of drug use (Kandel, 2002). Modeling the various drug use states and associated transitions at the aggregate or population level can improve projections about future trends and assist with policy analysis. "System dynamics" models of this sort have been developed for tobacco (Levy, Chaloupka, Gitchell, Mendez, & Warner, 2002; Mendez & Warner, 2000; Mendez, Warner, & Courant, 1998; Tengs, Ahmad, Moore, & Gage, 2004; Tengs, Osgood, & Chen, 2001), heroin (Annemans et al., 2000; Caulkins et al., 2006; Levin, Roberts, & Hirsch, 1975; Rossi, 2001), cocaine (Caulkins, Behrens, Knoll, Tragler, & Zuba, 2004; Everingham & Rydell, 1994; Everingham, Rydell, & Caulkins, 1995; Homer, 1993a,b), and injection drug use generally (Caulkins, Dietze, & Ritter, 2007).

In this section we present a model from the field of drug control, where we take care about the enormous heterogeneity across users in rates of consumption. Heavy cocaine users may consume 100+ grams per year, whereas weekly users may consume more like 10 grams per year. Indeed, someone who used cocaine just once in the past 12 months (≈0.1 grams) would still be recorded as a "past-year" user. Furthermore, the relative numbers of less- and more-frequent users can change dramatically over time (Everingham and Rydell, 1994). Hence, distinguishing the numbers of users at different intensities of drug use can help track trends in total drug consumption more accurately.

As a first approach to reflecting this heterogeneity Everingham and Rydell (1994) and Behrens, Caulkins, Tragler, Haunschmied, and Feichtinger (1999) use two states to distinguish people who use cocaine "at least weekly" (defined to be "heavy users," $H(t)$), from those who used cocaine "at least once within the last year but who used less than weekly" (defined as "light users," $L(t)$). Both studies assume there are so many more nonusers than users that the number of nonusers is essentially a constant and does not need to be modeled explicitly.[13]

The biggest difference between the Behrens et al. (1999) and Everingham and Rydell (1994) models (besides the latter being a discrete-time model) is the approach taken to modeling initiation. Everingham and Rydell (1994) were primarily interested in describing past trends, so initiation over time was simply set equal to historical trends in initiation. Behrens et al. (1999) sought to model initiation as an endogenous function of the current state of the drug epidemic, to enable projections of future trends and model the effects of various drug-control interventions.

Figure 2.16 gives a schematic representation of the resulting model, whose equations can be summarized as in the following figure.

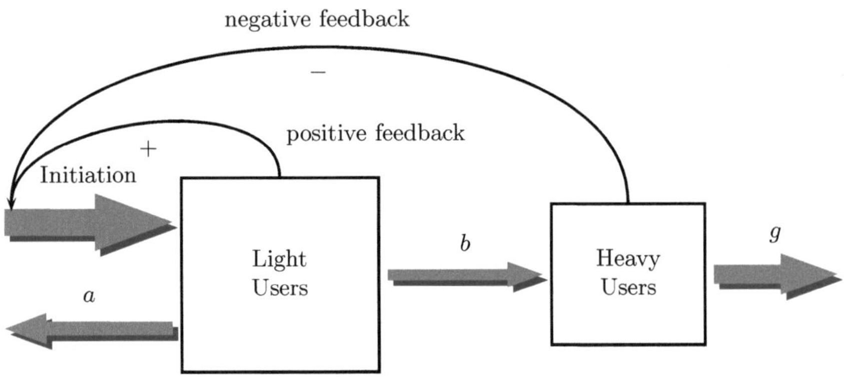

Fig. 2.16. Flow diagram for the *LH*-model (2.36)

$$\dot{L} = I(L,H) - (a+b)L, \qquad L(0) = L_0, \qquad (2.36a)$$
$$\dot{H} = bL - gH, \qquad H(0) = H_0, \qquad (2.36b)$$

[13] Other studies explicitly model the number of nonusers who are "susceptible" to initiation via an additional time-varying state variable, $S(t)$. This recognizes that as drug use spreads, the pool of potential initiates shrinks, helping to limit the drug epidemic from growing forever. We shall explore such models below, but they lump all drug users together into a single state. Merging the ideas of tracking susceptibles and distinguishing different types of users within a single model of illicit drug use is an active area of current research.

$L > 0$	...	number of light users,
$H > 0$	...	number of heavy users,
$I(L, H)$	...	initiation into light use,
a	...	average rate at which light users quit,
b	...	average rate at which light users escalate to heavy use,
g	...	average rate at which heavy users quit.

In Behrens et al. (1999) it is assumed that the number of current users influences initiation in two distinct ways. First, most people who start using drugs do so through contact with a friend or sibling who is already using and is happy with that use. The metaphor of a drug "epidemic" is commonly used precisely because of this tendency for current users to "infect" new users. Hence Behrens et al. (1999) model initiation as increasing in the number of light users.

Initiation is modeled as being promoted by light users because light users are rarely dependent, so their continued use indicates that they enjoy drug use. In contrast many, if not most, heavy users manifest obvious adverse effects of drug use, notably drug dependence but also various ill effects on work, social relationships, and health. So Behrens et al. (1999) believe heavy users are not effective recruiters of new initiates. (Note: This is not a universally held position. Some epidemiologists believe that heavy users also recruit new initiates, and the reader may enjoy thinking about how that alternative perspective could be built into a drug-prevalence model and what implications that would have on the results derived below.)

Musto (1987) argues that, in addition, knowledge of adverse effects of drug use can deter initiation. He hypothesizes that drug epidemics die out when a new generation of potential users becomes aware of the risks of drug abuse and, as a result, does not try drugs. One might expect the perception or reputation of a drug to be influenced by the relative number of light and heavy users. If most drug users are heavy users, the drug would be perceived as dangerous or harmful. Thus a model of drug initiation might have the following properties.

1. Initiation is proportional to the number of light users $L(t)$.
2. The rate at which light users "recruit" initiates is moderated by the drug's reputation for harmfulness, which in turn is governed by the relative number of heavy and light users.
3. Although most new users are "recruited," some enter the using population for other reasons (intrinsic interest, immigration, etc.). In the jargon of diffusion models, these individuals are "innovators" as opposed to "imitators."

Behrens et al. (1999) used the following initiation function to capture these three ideas.

$$I(L, H) = \tau + sLe^{-q\frac{H}{L}}, \tag{2.37}$$

$L > 0$ ... number of light users,
$H > 0$ ... number of heavy users,
s ... average rate at which light users attract nonusers,
q ... constant measuring the deterrent effect of heavy drug abuse,
τ ... number of innovators.

This initiation model implies that large numbers of heavy users are "bad" (for the drug's reputation), because they consume at high rates and impose costs on society, but also "good" because they discourage initiation. Heavy users impose costs in the near term, but generate a perverse sort of "benefit" for the future by reducing initiation and thus future use. The impact of a heavy user on initiation depends on the number of other heavy and light users, so that the magnitude of the "benefit" of a heavy user depends on the stage of the drug epidemic. Thus one would expect the effectiveness of various drug-control interventions, particularly treatment, to vary over the course of the epidemic. We explore that assumption in Sect. 6.1, where we introduce optimal control to the model.

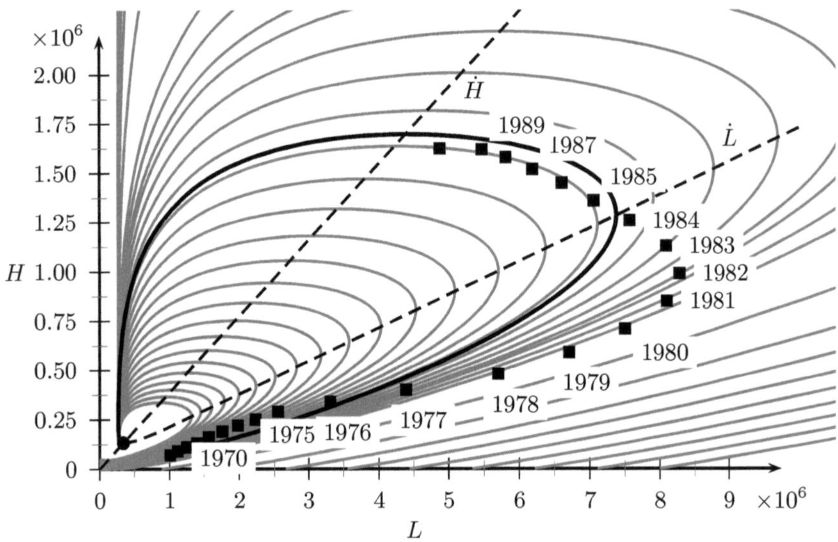

Fig. 2.17. Phase portrait, including smoothed historical trajectory of the current US cocaine epidemic (annual data are represented by *squares*)

For now it suffices to note that this rather simple model can do a surprisingly good job of reproducing trends in certain drug epidemics. Figure 2.17 shows this by mapping the outcome of this two-state model (2.36) in the phase portrait with parameter values estimated for the US cocaine epidemic as $a = 0.163$, $b = 0.024$, $\tau = 50{,}000$, $g = 0.062$, $s = 0.61$, $q = 7$ (Behrens et al., 1999).

Next we analyze the model in respect to occurring equilibria. The reader is invited to check that as L approaches zero, $\dot{L}$ is always positive, and as H goes to zero, $\dot{H}$ is always positive if L is positive. Hence we restrict our analysis to the (invariant) positive quadrant of the (L,H)-plane. The equilibrium, $\hat{X} = (\hat{L},\hat{H}) = \{(L,H) | \dot{L} = 0, \dot{H} = 0\}$, of the planar system (2.36) can be determined as a function of the system parameters:

$$\hat{X} = \begin{pmatrix} \hat{L} \\ \hat{H} \end{pmatrix} = \frac{\tau}{\Omega} \begin{pmatrix} 1 \\ \frac{b}{g} \end{pmatrix}, \tag{2.38}$$

where

$$\Omega := a + b - sR$$

with

$$R = R(q,b,g) := \mathrm{e}^{-\frac{qb}{g}}$$

denoting the equilibrium reputation of cocaine. Equilibrium prevalence (determined by (2.38)) is positive as long as $\Omega > 0$. The associated Jacobian matrix evaluated at (2.38) is calculated as

$$\hat{J} = \begin{pmatrix} I_L(\hat{L},\hat{H}) - (a+b) & I_H(\hat{L},\hat{H}) \\ b & -g \end{pmatrix} = \begin{pmatrix} s\frac{qb}{g}R - \Omega & -sqR \\ b & -g \end{pmatrix}.$$

By (2.26) the corresponding eigenvalues of the Jacobian are calculated as follows

$$\xi_{1,2} = \frac{1}{2}\left(\operatorname{tr}\hat{J} \pm \sqrt{(\operatorname{tr}\hat{J})^2 - 4\det\hat{J}}\right), \tag{2.39}$$

where $\operatorname{tr}\hat{J} = -g - \Omega + sRqb/g$ and $\det\hat{J} = g\Omega > 0$.

Using the results of Sect. 2.6.2 on the linearized system, we find that the equilibrium (2.38) is a stable focus for the parameter values given by Behrens et al. (1999). Thus drug use approaches a relatively high long-rum level, and the trajectory converging to the equilibrium $(\hat{L},\hat{H})$ happens to follow the pattern of damped oscillations (see also Sect. 2.11).

2.8 Introduction to Bifurcation Theory

Bifurcation theory is in itself a huge field encompassing a broad range of applications. Thus this introductory section cannot provide more than a glimpse to the subject, and the reader interested in theoretical as well as numerical details is referred to good textbooks on that subject, e.g., Guckenheimer and Holmes (1983) and Kuznetsov (1998). Nonetheless, the analysis of optimal control problems involves to a large extent the study of dynamical systems; and as the problems considered here have a variety of parameters, which are at best known to lie in some interval, bifurcation theory is necessary to analyze the possible changes in the dynamical behavior of the models. The next subsections introduce the reader to selected problems analyzed by bifurcation theory and should facilitate the first steps for anyone who wants to undertake a more detailed study by presenting its terminology and underlying ideas.

2.8.1 Terminology and Key Ideas of Bifurcation Theory

The basic object under investigation by means of bifurcation theory is

$$\dot{x}(t) = f(x(t), \mu), \quad \text{with} \quad x(t) \in \mathbb{R}^n,\ \mu \in \mathbb{R}^p,\ t \in [0, \inf) \tag{2.40}$$

a parameter-dependent ODE, whereby bifurcation theory tries to explain disruptions in the dynamical behavior of (2.40), while changing the parameter(s) μ. Thus we define:

Definition 2.59 (Bifurcation). *The appearance of a topologically nonequivalent, in the sense of Definition 2.30, phase portrait of (2.40) under variation of parameters μ is called a* bifurcation.

A parameter value, where such a change takes place, is called a bifurcation value *or* critical value *of the parameter and will be denoted by μ_c.*

Generally we distinguish between two types of structural changes, namely those changes that occur via *local bifurcations* and those induced by *global bifurcations.*[14] While the latter has to consider, e.g., the global stable or/and unstable manifolds, local bifurcations can be sufficiently characterized by the local stability analysis of equilibria, limit cycles, or other types of limit sets. Since global bifurcations need rather more advanced techniques, we shall not present any general results on this topic but instead refer the interested reader to Guckenheimer and Holmes (1983) or Kuznetsov (1998).

Remark 2.60. In optimal control theory global bifurcations, especially the heteroclinic bifurcation,[15] play a crucial role in connection with multiple optimal solutions (see Chap. 5).

Since there exists an unmanageably large number of possible dynamics, the problem of classification is reminiscent of Sisyphus's challenge to finish this task, and it is obvious that bifurcation theory will always be a work in progress. But fortunately phase portraits are not totally arbitrary, and recurring patterns can be identified and transformed to "simple" ODEs. The important tools of bifurcation theory are therefore the representation of ODEs in their

[14] Global bifurcations involve the entire phase space rather than just the neighborhood of an equilibrium or limit cycle and are therefore harder to deal with and harder to be detected.

[15] At a *heteroclinic bifurcation* a heteroclinic connection between two equilibria emerge at the critical value of the parameter.

normal form and the projection into the subspace, where the bifurcation occurs, i.e., the center manifold.

To introduce these tools in a concise way is beyond the scope of this book and even is not necessary for its application to the models of optimal control theory presented here. Therefore we introduce the necessary terms by means of a simple example to facilitate comprehension without becoming too technical. The following derivation and its generalizations can be found in Kuznetsov (1998).

2.8.2 Normal Forms and the Center Manifold: The Tools of Bifurcation Theory

To analyze local bifurcations of equilibria, it is useful to consider the dynamics restricted to the center manifold, since a qualitative change by varying a parameter can only occur for this part of the dynamics. The dynamics along the (un)stable manifolds are robust against small disturbances. But the restriction to the center manifold is only the first step in the analysis. Moreover, we shall find further coordinate transformations that simplify the analytic expressions of the vector field on the center manifold. This simplified dynamics is then called *normal form*. The analysis of the normal forms yields a qualitative picture of the flows of each bifurcation type, and we shall subsequently present only the most common ones.

For a more general theory of normal forms the reader is, e.g., referred to Guckenheimer and Holmes (1983). We settle for the presentation of the coordinate transformation of a concrete example, yielding the normal form of the so-called fold bifurcation, where two equilibria emerge by varying the bifurcation parameter.

Let us therefore consider the following two ODEs:

$$\dot{x} = g(x, \beta) = \beta(1 + x) + x^3 + \frac{x^2 - 1}{x^2 + 1} + 1, \quad x, \beta \in \mathbb{R}, \tag{2.41}$$

and

$$\dot{x} = f(x, \mu) = \mu + x^2 \quad x, \mu \in \mathbb{R}. \tag{2.42}$$

Considering the functional forms of (2.41) and (2.42), it is not immediately reasonable that both equations exhibit, at least locally, the "same" dynamical structure. But for $\mu_c = \beta_c = 0$ both systems exhibit a nonhyperbolic equilibrium at the origin, i.e., $f_x(0, 0) = g_x(0, 0) = 0$. Moreover, the phase portraits of both systems at $\mu_c = \beta_c = 0$ suggest an equivalent dynamical behavior near the origin; see Fig. 2.18a. Clearly, this only concerns the local behavior, as Fig. 2.18b illustrates. Equation (2.42) is obviously easier to analyze, therefore it is of general interest to identify conditions under which an ODE of the complexity of (2.41) can locally be transformed to (2.42).

Remark 2.61. Note that in our example the restriction to the center manifold is trivially satisfied, since the dynamics is one-dimensional and therefore already represents its critical part.

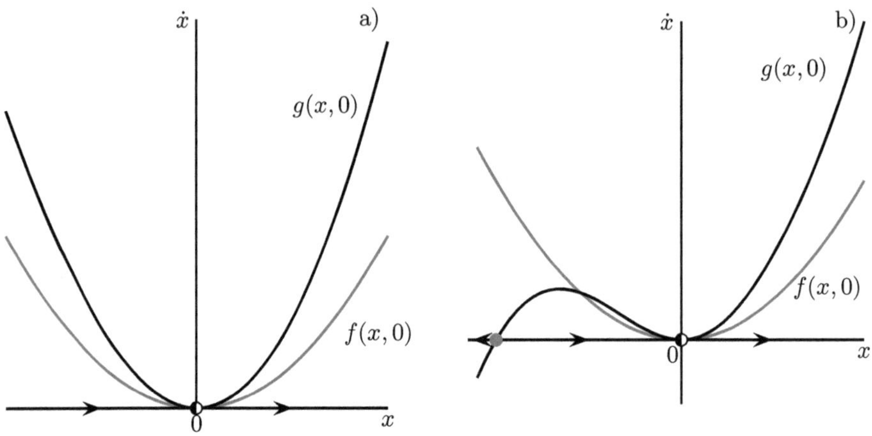

Fig. 2.18. Panel (**a**) depicts the phase portraits of (2.41) and (2.42) for the critical parameter value $\beta = \mu = 0$ illustrating the local equivalence of both systems. In panel (**b**) the global difference of both systems is portrayed

Coordinate Transformation

In a first step we show that (2.41) can be transformed into a system

$$\dot{x} = \mu + x^2 + o(x^2), \tag{2.43}$$

which approximates (2.42) up to terms of order two. Subsequently we prove that these higher-order terms can be neglected for describing the local dynamical behavior. In other words we show that both systems are locally topologically equivalent.

To carry out the transformation process we use the Taylor theorem to consider a cubic approximation of (2.41) about the equilibrium $\hat{x} = 0$ and small β. Thus we find

$$g(x,\beta) = g(0,\beta) + g_x(0,\beta)x + \frac{1}{2}g_{xx}(0,\beta)x^2 + \frac{1}{6}g_{xxx}(0,\beta)x^3 + o(x^3).$$

Utilizing

$$g(0,\beta) = \beta, \quad g_x(0,\beta) = \beta, \quad g_{xx}(0,\beta) = 4, \quad g_{xxx}(0,\beta) = 6 \tag{2.44}$$

yields

$$g(x,\beta) = \beta + \beta x + 2x^2 + x^3 + o(x^3). \tag{2.45}$$

Next we remove the linear term in (2.45) by applying the linear transformation $z = x + \delta$, where $\delta(\beta)$ is some parameter, depending on β and satisfying $\delta(0) = 0$. Now (2.45) becomes

$$\begin{aligned} g(z,\delta,\beta) &= \beta + \beta(z-\delta) + 2(z-\delta)^2 + (z-\delta)^3 + o\left((z-\delta)^3\right) \\ &= \beta - \beta\delta + 2\delta^2 + \left(\beta - 4\delta - 3\delta^2\right)z + (2+3\delta)\,z^2 + o(z^2) + o(\delta^2). \end{aligned}$$

To remove the linear coefficient $C(\beta,\delta) = \beta - 4\delta - 3\delta^2$ of z, we use the implicit function theorem. Since the nondegeneracy condition

$$C_\delta(0,0) = -g_{xx}(0,0) = -4 \neq 0 \tag{2.46}$$

is satisfied the implicit function theorem (see Theorem A.125) assures the local existence of a function $\delta(\beta)$ satisfying $C(\beta,\delta(\beta)) = 0$. This function is given by

$$\delta(\beta) = \frac{\beta}{4} + o(\beta). \tag{2.47}$$

Substituting (2.47) into $g(z,\delta,\beta)$ yields

$$\dot{z} = \beta + o(\beta) + \left(2 + \frac{3\beta}{4} + o\left(\beta\right)\right) z^2 + o(z^2). \tag{2.48}$$

Remark 2.62. What can be inferred if condition (2.46) is not satisfied? Either the dynamics is substantially different from (2.43), e.g.,

$$\dot{x} = \mu + x^3,$$

or higher-order terms have to be considered, e.g.,

$$\dot{x} = \mu + x^4.$$

Parameter Transformation

In a next step we introduce the new parameter $\bar{\mu}$ for the constant term of (2.48), i.e.,

$$\bar{\mu} = \beta + o(\beta).$$

To replace β in the coefficient of z^2, we have to assure that β can be expressed as a function of $\bar{\mu}$. Using the inverse function theorem (see Theorem A.126) this is guaranteed if the derivative $\bar{\mu}'(0)$ does not vanish. By virtue of (2.48) this condition can be restated as

$$\bar{\mu}'(0) = g_\beta(0,0) = 1 \neq 0. \tag{2.49}$$

Thus we find

$$\beta = \bar{\mu} + o(\bar{\mu}). \tag{2.50}$$

Substituting (2.50) into (2.48) yields

$$\dot{z} = \bar{\mu} + \left(2 + \frac{3\bar{\mu}}{4} + o(\bar{\mu})\right) z^2 + o(z^2). \tag{2.51}$$

Remark 2.63. What can be inferred if condition (2.49) is not satisfied? The following examples

$$\dot{x} = \mu^2 + x^2$$

and

$$\dot{x} = \mu^3 + x^2,$$

violate (2.49). But whereas in the first case the system exhibits different dynamical behavior for varying μ compared to (2.42), the latter is topological equivalent to (2.42).

Scaling the Coordinate

In a last step we scale (2.51), using $y = |2 + \frac{3\bar{\mu}}{4} + o(\bar{\mu})|z$, which yields

$$\dot{y} = \mu + y^2 + o(y^2), \tag{2.52}$$

with $\mu = \bar{\mu}|2 + \frac{3\bar{\mu}}{4} + o(\bar{\mu})|$.

Remark 2.64. Inspecting the scaling carefully reveals that in general we derive a system satisfying

$$\dot{y} = \mu \pm y^2 + o(y^2),$$

where the actual sign of y^2 depends on the sign of the coefficient of z^2 evaluated at $\bar{\mu} = 0$.

What remains is to show that the term $o(y^2)$ does not change the local behavior of the dynamics and therefore the systems are locally topologically equivalent.

Topological Equivalence

To prove the local topological equivalence of the local system's dynamics (2.43) and (2.42), we have to show that for $|\mu|$ small:

1. Both systems exhibit locally the same number of equilibria.
2. A homeomorphism exists transforming the orbits of (2.51) into orbits of (2.52) and preserving the direction of time.

For the first part we consider the manifold of equilibria for (2.51), i.e.,

$$F(y,\mu) = \mu + y^2 + o(y^2) = 0. \tag{2.53}$$

Since

$$\frac{\partial F(0,0)}{\partial \mu} = 1$$

the implicit function theorem implies the existence of a function $\mu = b(y)$, satisfying $F(y, b(y)) = 0$, whereby

$$b(y) = g(0) + b_y(0)y + \frac{1}{2}b_{yy}(0)y^2 + o(y^2).$$

Using $b(0) = 0$, together with the formulas for implicit first and second derivatives, yields

$$b_y(0) = 0, \quad b_{yy}(0) = -2,$$

implying

$$b(y) = -y^2 + o(y^2).$$

Proving that for $|y|$ small enough $b(y)$ is negative and therefore (2.53) exhibits two equilibria, $\hat{y}_{1,2}(\mu)$, for $\mu < 0$. These equilibria are near $\hat{x}_{1,2}(\mu) = \pm\sqrt{-\mu}$, proving the first part.

For the proof of the second part we consider the homeomorphism $y = h(x)$

$$h(x) = \begin{cases} \mathrm{Id}(x) & \mu \geq 0 \\ a(\mu) + b(\mu)x & \mu < 0, \end{cases}$$

where $a(\mu)$ and $b(\mu)$ are determined such that $\hat{y}_{1,2} = h(\hat{x}_{1,2})$. Thus h maps the equilibria of (2.52) onto equilibria of the perturbed system (2.51). That h is really a homeomorphism follows from the fact that for one-dimensional systems an orbit is an interval on the real line and that for $\lim_{t\to\infty} x(t) = \hat{x}_{1,2}$ we have $\lim_{t\to\infty} h(x(t)) = \hat{y}_{1,2}$; if necessary we have to consider $t \to -\infty$. This ends our proof for the topological equivalence of (2.41) and (2.42).

Remark 2.65. In general the normal form is a polynomial system with mostly integer coefficients, exhibiting a special kind of bifurcation. It is important to consider under which conditions the simplification of an ODE to a normal form is possible (see, e.g., Guckenheimer & Holmes, 1983).

Remark 2.66. Finally, let us return to the conditions that have been identified along the previous proof as sufficient to guarantee the existence of a transformation into the normal form, namely (2.46) and (2.49). The first condition assures that the function is not "too" degenerate (and is therefore called the *nondegeneracy condition*, whereas the second condition is the so-called *transversality condition* on the parameter(s). Here the term transversality is derived from the geometric property of a transversal crossing. Consider, e.g., the already presented system

$$\dot{x} = \mu^2 + x^2.$$

Then the transversality condition is violated since $f_\mu(0,0) = 0$. Obviously this system exhibits a different behavior, since no equilibria exist for $\mu \neq 0$. Portrayed graphically, the graph of the dynamics at $x = 0$ for $\mu \to 0$ touches the x-axis tangentially, contrary to the original system, in which the graph of μ crosses the x-axis transversally (see Fig. 2.19).

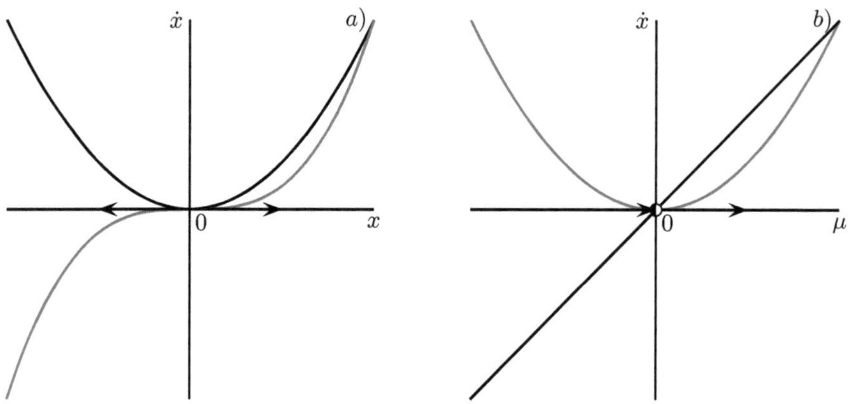

Fig. 2.19. In (**a**) the system dynamics, for $\mu = 0$, $\dot{x} = x^3$ (*gray line*) violates the nondegeneracy condition and exhibits a different local behavior at $x = 0$ as compared with (2.52). Panel (**b**) depicts the case in which the dynamics at $x = 0$ is given by $\dot{x} = \mu^2$ and therefore violates the transversality condition

Another very important and prominent example of using a normal form representation of an ODE is that of the Poincaré–Andronov–Hopf bifurcation presented in Sect. 2.10. Even though the same idea underlies the derivation of the corresponding normal form, the actual calculations are more involved and we therefore refer the reader to Kuznetsov (1998).

Last, we want to touch on the importance of the manifold theorem for flows for bifurcation theory, especially the part on the center manifold.

Center Manifold

The center manifold and its local representation is of crucial importance for the numerical computation of bifurcations and the reduction to normal forms. The manifold theorem for flows assures that the stable, unstable and center manifolds are invariant under the given dynamics. This allows the reduction of the dynamics to its bifurcation-relevant part, i.e., to the center manifold also called the *reduced equation*. In the simplest cases the determination of the bifurcation type can be done, by searching for equilibria exhibiting eigenvalues with zero real part. Then the center manifold and the reduced dynamics have to be computed. Checking the nondegeneracy and transversality conditions lets us determine the type of bifurcation.

As an elementary example, let us consider the system:

$$\dot{x}_1 = \mu + x_1^2 + x_2 \tag{2.54a}$$

$$\dot{x}_2 = -x_2. \tag{2.54b}$$

Then, using calculations analogous to the computation of the center manifold in Example (2.57), we find that the center manifold is given by

$$x_2 = o(x_1^2).$$

Thus the dynamics projected onto the center manifold is locally given by

$$\dot{x}_1 = \mu + x_1^2 + o(x_1^2).$$

Since for the reduced equation the properties of nondegeneracy (2.42) and transversality (2.43) are satisfied, we proved that the system (2.54) exhibits a fold bifurcation already analyzed in the section before, when discussing the prototypical example

$$\dot{x} = \mu + x^2.$$

For an in-depth treatment of a computation algorithm of the center manifold, the reader is referred to Kuznetsov (1998).

2.8.3 Local Bifurcations in One Dimension

In this section we focus on local bifurcations along the real line and analyze the asymptotic, or long-run, stability behavior of a dynamical system if the value of a single parameter is varied far enough to reach a *bifurcation value* μ_c.

In what follows we give a brief introduction to local bifurcation theory, dealing only with changes in stability properties of equilibria. We start by presenting the three simplest types (in normal form) of bifurcations in a one-dimensional setting, where only one parameter, μ, is varied. These bifurcations are not confined to $\mathbb{R}$ and can occur in higher-dimensional systems as well, as we have already mentioned in the previous section. Once these basic tools have been mastered, discussions of more advanced bifurcations may be of interest.

One useful way to depict the change in the dynamics of the system is to plot the phase-portrait at the ordinate-axis vs. the parameter, μ, at the abscissa, which is called a *bifurcation diagram* and will be used to present the following bifurcations.

Saddle-Node Bifurcation

Saddle-node bifurcation is the most fundamental type of bifurcation in which equilibria are created or destroyed. It is also called a *fold* (or *tangent*) bifurcation or *blue sky bifurcation.* The latter denotation refers to the sudden appearance of a pair of equilibria "out of the blue sky" as Abraham and Shaw (1982) describe it. We have already met this bifurcation type in the previous section, where we introduced normal forms by means of a prototypical example.

Consider the following flow on the real axis:

$$\dot{x} = \mu + x^2, \tag{2.55}$$

where $x \in \mathbb{R}$ and $\mu \in \mathbb{R}$ is a parameter. When $\mu < 0$ there are two equilibria, one stable and one unstable (see Figs. 2.20 and 2.21).

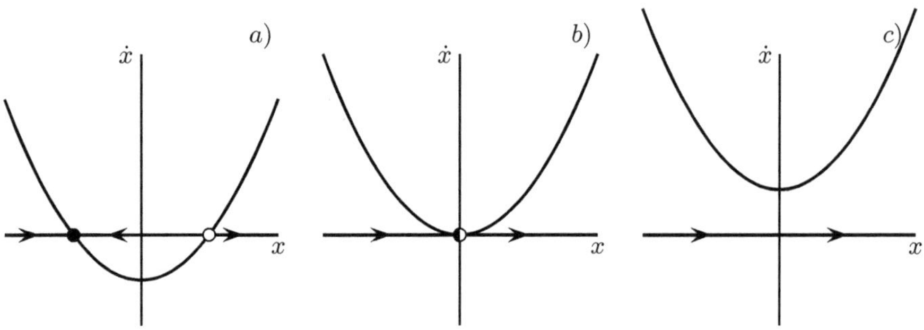

Fig. 2.20. The phase portrait of the dynamics (2.55) is depicted for (**a**) $\mu < 0$, (**b**) $\mu = 0$, and (**c**) $\mu > 0$

For $\mu > 0$ there is no equilibrium. If μ moves downward, an equilibrium arises "out of the blue sky" that is semistable. The bifurcation value $\mu = 0$ separates two qualitatively different vector fields.

The dynamics (2.55) is in a specific sense prototypical for *all* saddle-node bifurcations as we have explained in the last section on normal forms. Hence the following theorem can be formulated:

Theorem 2.67 (Fold Bifurcation). *Any one-dimensional system*

$$\dot{x} = f(x, \mu), \quad x, \mu \in \mathbb{R},$$

with $f \in C^2(\mathbb{R})$ exhibiting an equilibrium at $x = 0$ for $\mu = 0$ with $f_x(0,0) = 0$, and satisfying

A.1: $f_{xx}(0,0) \neq 0$,
A.2: $f_\mu(0,0) \neq 0$,

is locally topologically equivalent to the system

$$\dot{x} = \mu \pm x^2.$$

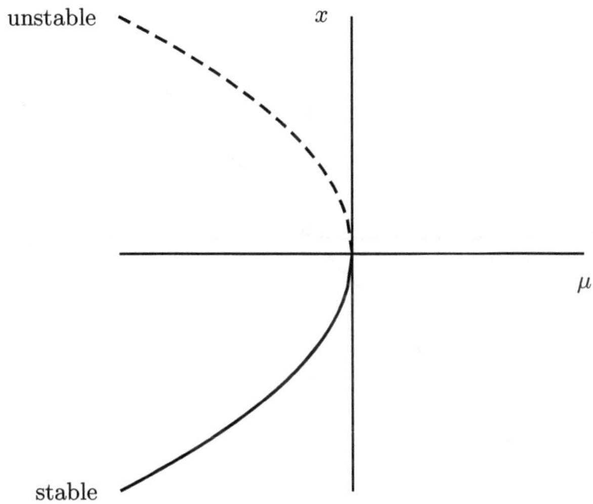

Fig. 2.21. Bifurcation diagram for a saddle-node or "blue sky" bifurcation

Transcritical Bifurcation

Transcritical bifurcation provides a mechanism for an exchange of stability of persisting equilibria.

The normal form for the transcritical bifurcation is

$$\dot{x} = \mu x - x^2, \quad x, \mu \in \mathbb{R}. \tag{2.56}$$

The three parts of Fig. 2.22 sketch the dynamics of the vector field depending on the parameter μ.

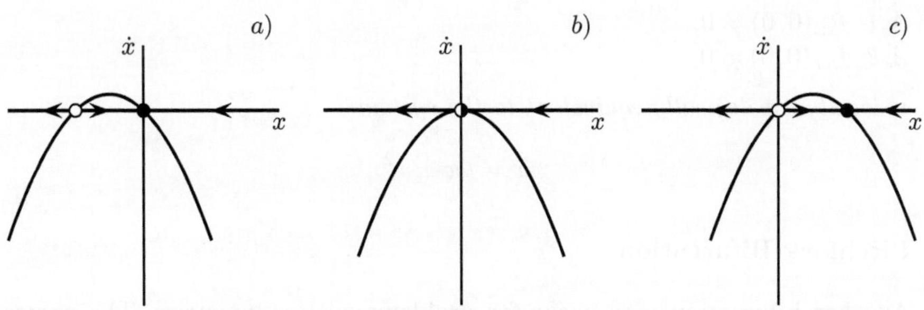

Fig. 2.22. The phaseportrait of the dynamics (2.56) is depicted for (**a**) $\mu < 0$, (**b**) $\mu = 0$, (**c**) $\mu > 0$

For $\mu < 0$ there is an unstable equilibrium at $\hat{x} = \mu$ and a stable one in the origin. For increasing μ, these two equilibria collide for $\mu = 0$, and

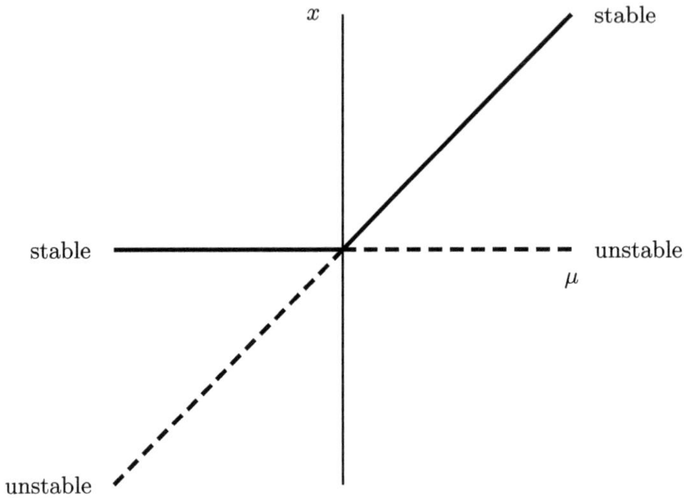

Fig. 2.23. Bifurcation diagram for a transcritical bifurcation

the resulting equilibrium is semistable. For $\mu > 0$, $x = 0$ becomes unstable, whereas $\hat{x} = \mu$ is now stable. The exchange of stabilities is marked in the bifurcation diagram shown in Fig. 2.23.

Generally we find:

Theorem 2.68 (Transcritical Bifurcation). *Any one-dimensional system*

$$\dot{x} = f(x, \mu), \quad x, \mu \in \mathbb{R},$$

with $f \in C^2(\mathbb{R})$ exhibiting an equilibrium at $x = 0$ for $\mu = 0$ with $f_x(0,0) = 0$, and satisfying

A.1: $f_{xx}(0,0) \neq 0$,
A.2: $f_{\mu x}(0,0) \neq 0$,

is locally topologically equivalent to the system

$$\dot{x} = \mu x \pm x^2.$$

Pitchfork Bifurcation

Another bifurcation may occur for problems with symmetries. The normal form of the so-called *supercritical pitchfork bifurcation* is given as

$$\dot{x} = \mu x - x^3, \quad x, \mu \in \mathbb{R}. \tag{2.57}$$

A transformation $x \to -x$ leads to an equivalent flow on the line, i.e., to left–right symmetry. This is illustrated in Fig. 2.24.

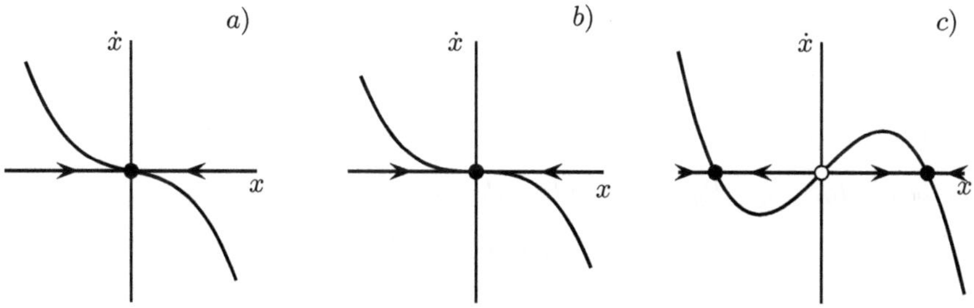

Fig. 2.24. The phaseportrait of the dynamics (2.57) is depicted for (**a**) $\mu < 0$, (**b**) $\mu = 0$, (**c**) $\mu > 0$

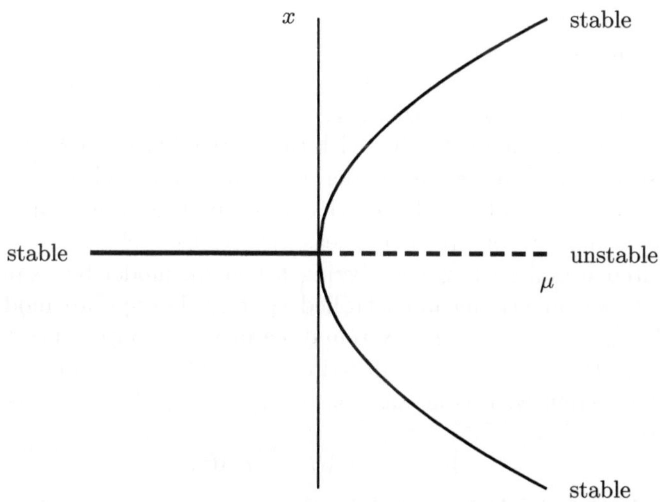

Fig. 2.25. Bifurcation diagram for a (supercritical) pitchfork bifurcation

For $\mu < 0$ there is only one equilibrium, i.e., the origin, and it is stable. $x = 0$ remains stable[16] for $\mu = 0$. For $\mu > 0$, the origin becomes unstable, and two additional stable equilibria arise symmetrically to $x = 0$, where $\hat{x} = \pm\sqrt{\mu}$.

Figure 2.25 reveals the denotation "pitchfork."

For the subcritical bifurcation, $\dot{x} = \mu x + x^3$, the bifurcation diagram is inverted. Note that the cubic term now destabilizes the system, whereas it acts to stabilize it for the supercritical bifurcation.

Generally we find:

Theorem 2.69 (Pitchfork Bifurcation). *Any one-dimensional system*

$$\dot{x} = f(x, \mu), \quad x, \mu \in \mathbb{R},$$

[16] This case provides an example of a vanishing linearization.

with $f \in C^2(\mathbb{R})$ *exhibiting an equilibrium at* $x = 0$ *for* $\mu = 0$ *with* $f_x(0,0) = f_{xx}(0,0) = 0$, *and satisfying*

A.1: $f_{xxx}(0,0) \neq 0$,
A.2: $f_{\mu x}(0,0) \neq 0$,

is locally topologically equivalent to the system

$$\dot{x} = \mu x \pm x^3.$$

2.9 Bifurcation Analysis of a One-Dimensional Drug Model

Here we present in some sense the simplest of all possible drug prevalence models, because it has just one state variable, $A(t)$, which counts the total number of drug users at time t. Finding the optimal demand side policy subject to some epidemic dynamics is challenging, and so it makes sense to start with a one-state model instead of starting with the more advanced LH-model (2.36). This one-state model, based on Tragler, Caulkins, and Feichtinger (2001), has two control variables, $u(t)$ and $v(t)$, that describe the expenditures at time t for treatment and law enforcement measures, respectively.

It is often useful to begin analyzing a control model by examining the behavior of the underlying uncontrolled (purely descriptive) model. Hence, we consider first Tragler et al.'s system dynamics with both controls set equal to zero, i.e., $u(t) = v(t) = 0$ for all t (in Exercise 2.4 the reader is invited to analyze the system with constant control $u(\cdot) \equiv u$). This reduces the state equation to

$$\dot{A}(t) = kf(A(t)) - \mu A(t), \tag{2.58}$$

where $kf(A(t))$ and $\mu A(t)$ denote initiation into and desistance from drug use at time t, respectively. Note that for ease of exposition, in what follows we shall mostly omit the time argument t.

Equation (2.58) states that users quit at a constant rate μ and initiation is a function of the current number of users. This reflects the fact that most initiates are introduced to drug use by an existing user, often a friend or family member, and so $f(A)$ should be an increasing function, at least initially.[17] However, once use is widespread, the ill effects of drug consumption become visible and suppress initiation (cf. Musto, 1987); this suggests that $f(A)$ should become a decreasing function for high enough values of A. The reader may enjoy comparing the modeling approach (2.36) with (2.58) as the latter model describes the same facts, but by means of a single variable. We use here what is perhaps the simplest function covering these two aspects, the logistic function

$$f(A) = kA\left(\bar{A} - A\right). \tag{2.59}$$

[17] This assumption is identical to one modeled transmission mechanism of the LH-model (2.36).

Remark 2.70. The original analysis published in Tragler (1998) and Tragler et al. (2001) used the monotonously increasing power function $f(A) = kA^\alpha$, and so in this respect we depart from the original studies. The power function is in some ways slightly more realistic, but the logistic function is better for present purposes.

While we first wrote the state equation (2.58) with separate inflow and outflow terms describing initiation and quitting, respectively, with $f(A)$ from (2.59), the system dynamics may be rewritten as an equivalent, purely logistic model

$$\dot{A} = \left(k\bar{A} - \mu\right) A \left(1 - \frac{k}{k\bar{A} - \mu} A\right) =: r_0 A \left(1 - \frac{A}{K}\right), \tag{2.60}$$

where $r_0 := k\bar{A} - \mu$ is the maximal growth rate at $A = 0$ and $K := \frac{k\bar{A}-\mu}{k}$ is the so-called carrying capacity (maximum number of users there could ever be).

This model has two equilibria, $\hat{A}_1 = 0$ and $\hat{A}_2 = K$, which we obtain by solving the equation $\dot{A} = 0$. The stability properties of these equilibria can be determined by using the first-order derivative of $\dot{A}$ with respect to A, i.e.,

$$\frac{\partial}{\partial A}\dot{A} = r_0 \left(1 - \frac{2A}{K}\right) = k\bar{A} - \mu - 2kA. \tag{2.61}$$

More formally, (2.61) gives the 1×1 Jacobian matrix of our one-state descriptive drug model. Evaluation of (2.61) at the equilibria gives

$$\left.\frac{\partial}{\partial A}\dot{A}\right|_{\hat{A}_i} = \begin{cases} r_0 & i = 1 \\ -r_0 & i = 2. \end{cases}$$

These results for the equilibria allow us to illustrate a transcritical bifurcation occurring in this model when allowing r_0 to change continuously from a negative to a positive value (follow Fig. 2.26). Note first that $\hat{A}_1 = 0$ and $\hat{A}_2 = \frac{r_0}{k}$ exist for any value of r_0 with the first being constant and the second being linear in r_0, where the sign of $\hat{A}_2$ is the same as that of r_0. For any negative value of r_0, the eigenvalue of the Jacobian at $\hat{A}_1 = 0$ is negative, implying that $\hat{A}_1 = 0$ is locally stable. Vice versa, the eigenvalue at $\hat{A}_2$ is positive for $r_0 < 0$, which implies that $\hat{A}_2$ is locally unstable. At the critical value $r_0 = 0$, the two equilibria coincide at $\hat{A}_1 = \hat{A}_2 = 0$ with the eigenvalue being 0, too. This is where the transcritical bifurcation occurs. That means, continuing with positive values of r_0, $\hat{A}_1 = 0$ becomes locally unstable, while $\hat{A}_2 = \frac{r_0}{k}$ becomes both positive and locally stable.

For our modeling purposes, r_0 and K should clearly have positive values, so that we shall assume later that

$$k\bar{A} > \mu. \tag{2.62}$$

Under this assumption, $\hat{A}_1 = 0$ is locally unstable, while $\hat{A}_2 = \frac{r_0}{k}$ is strictly positive and locally stable.

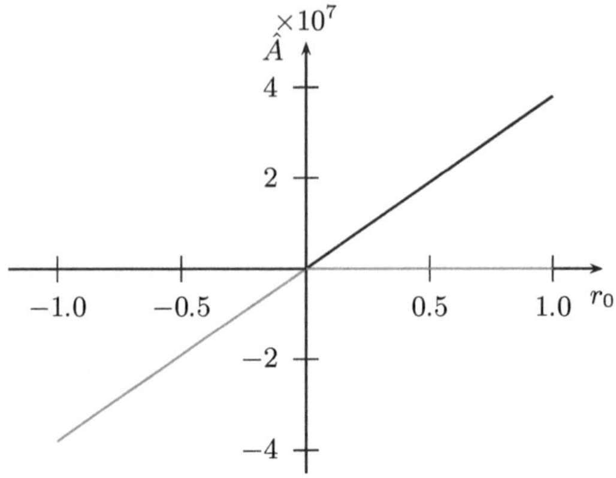

Fig. 2.26. Illustration of a transcritical bifurcation occurring at $r_0 = 0$

From a more dynamic point of view, the solution of the logistic equation (2.60) is well known to be

$$A(t) = \frac{A_0 K}{A_0 + (K - A_0)\,\mathrm{e}^{-r_0 t}},$$

where $A_0 := A(0)$ is the initial number of cocaine users.

From a global perspective, for any positive initial number of users A_0 we have

$$\begin{aligned}\lim_{t\to\infty} A(t) &= \lim_{t\to\infty} \frac{A_0 K}{A_0 + (K - A_0)\,\mathrm{e}^{-r_0 t}} \\ &= \frac{A_0 K}{A_0 + (K - A_0)\lim_{t\to\infty}\mathrm{e}^{-r_0 t}} = K = \hat{A}_2.\end{aligned}$$

That means that, unless $A_0 = 0 = \hat{A}_1$ (in which case the epidemic never starts), any positive initial number of users produces a time path converging monotonously to the carrying capacity $K = \hat{A}_2$, which turns out to be globally attracting. If A_0 is less/greater than K, the number of users increases/decreases monotonously while approaching the level K. This is illustrated in Fig. 2.27, where we see four time paths starting at $A_0 = 1, \frac{K}{2}, \frac{3K}{2}, 2K$, respectively. The parameter values used ($r_0 = 0.324854$, $K = 12,204,200$) were derived with the purpose of fitting the model to data for the current US cocaine epidemic (cf. Bultmann, Caulkins, Feichtinger, & Tragler, 2007).

In the rest of this chapter we deal with local bifurcations in the plane and beyond.

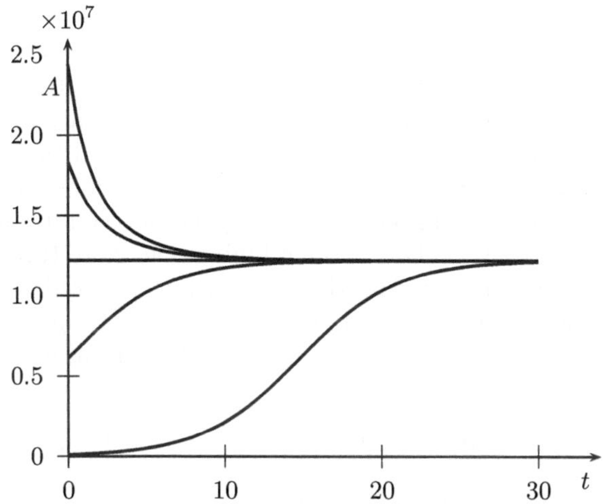

Fig. 2.27. Time paths $A(t)$ for $t \in [0, 30]$ and different initial numbers of users A_0

2.10 The Poincaré–Andronov–Hopf Bifurcation

Section 2.8.3 showed that in *fold* (or *blue-sky*), *transcritical*, and *pitchfork bifurcations* the equilibria of one-dimensional continuous dynamical systems were created or destroyed, had their stability behavior exchanged, or had their numbers doubled, respectively. As we have already mentioned, evidence of these types of bifurcations can be generalized from the $\mathbb{R}$ to the $\mathbb{R}^n, n \geq 2$ in a straightforward way, by projection into the center manifold.

Planar systems:

$$\begin{pmatrix} \dot{x}_1 \\ \dot{x}_2 \end{pmatrix} = \dot{x} = f(x) = \begin{pmatrix} f_1(x_1, x_2) \\ f_2(x_1, x_2) \end{pmatrix}$$

as a special case of the general nonlinear case (cf. Sect. 2.6.2), potentially exhibit richer system behavior, e.g., limit cycles or heteroclinic cycles, than one-dimensional systems do. While one-state ODEs have only a single eigenvalue that must be a real number (because complex eigenvalues occur only in pairs), planar systems have two eigenvalues (of the linearized system evaluated at an equilibrium if the system dynamics is nonlinear). Therefore an additional type of structural change can occur where the eigenvalues are purely imaginary. This bifurcation type is a so-called *Poincaré–Andronov–Hopf bifurcation (PAH-bifurcation)* usually denoted as *Hopf bifurcation*, where an equilibrium bifurcates into an equilibrium and a limit cycle.

Having in mind the normal form as the "simplest" possible representation of a system exhibiting some special type of bifurcation, one can ask about the normal form of a PAH-bifurcation. Since in this case a pair of eigenvalues becomes purely imaginary, two eigenvalues are affected, namely ξ and its complex conjugate $\bar{\xi}$. Thus the generic system exhibiting a PAH-bifurcation is at least of dimension two. Subsequently we shall state sufficient conditions (Poincaré–Andronov–Hopf theorem) to guarantee the existence of a transformation to its normal form, analogous to the fold bifurcation Theorem 2.67. During the proof of Theorem 2.71 a function $l_1(\mu)$, called the *Lyapunov coefficient*, occurs; an explicit formula is given in the remark below. This function plays a crucial role as it provides a nondegeneracy condition and its sign constitutes the stability of the emerging limit cycle. Note that for reasons of simplicity the theorem is stated for the case in which the equilibrium is already shifted to the origin and the critical bifurcation parameter μ_c is shifted to zero too. A full proof for arbitrary dimension $n \geq 2$ is given, e.g., in Kuznetsov (1998):

Theorem 2.71 (Poincaré–Andronov–Hopf in $\mathbb{R}^2$). *Suppose the ODE*

$$\dot{x} = f(x, \mu), \quad \textit{with} \quad x \in \mathbb{R}^2, \ \mu \in \mathbb{R},$$

has for small $|\mu|$ an equilibrium at the origin with eigenvalues

$$\xi_{1,2}(\mu) = \eta(\mu) \pm \mathrm{i}\omega(\mu),$$

satisfying $\eta(0) = 0$, $\omega(0) > 0$.

If the following conditions are satisfied,

1. *$l_1(0) \neq 0$, (for an explicit formula of l_1 see (2.64)),*
2. *$\eta'(0) \neq 0$,*

then the system is locally topologically equivalent near the origin $k = 0$, $\mu = 0$ to one of the following normal forms:

$$\begin{pmatrix} \dot{y}_1 \\ \dot{y}_2 \end{pmatrix} = \begin{pmatrix} \beta & -1 \\ 1 & \beta \end{pmatrix} \begin{pmatrix} y_1 \\ y_2 \end{pmatrix} \pm (y_1^2 + y_2^2) \begin{pmatrix} y_1 \\ y_2 \end{pmatrix}, \tag{2.63}$$

where $\beta(\mu) = \eta(\mu)/\omega(\mu)$ and the sign of the cubic term is determined by $\operatorname{sgn} l_1(0)$.

Remark 2.72. That the system described by the normal form (2.63) exhibits a limit cycle can easily be seen by transforming it into polar coordinates, where it becomes

$$\begin{aligned} \dot{R} &= \pm R(\beta - R^2) \\ \dot{\theta} &= 1, \end{aligned}$$

with $x_1 = R\cos\theta$ and $x_2 = R\sin\theta$ and $R \geq 0$. In Fig. 2.28 the case is depicted for a positive R dynamic.

Contrary to the fold bifurcation, it is not possible to eliminate, during the transformation into the normal form, all terms of greater order than two. One of the occurring cubic terms remains and is called *resonant term*, where $l_1(\mu)$ is

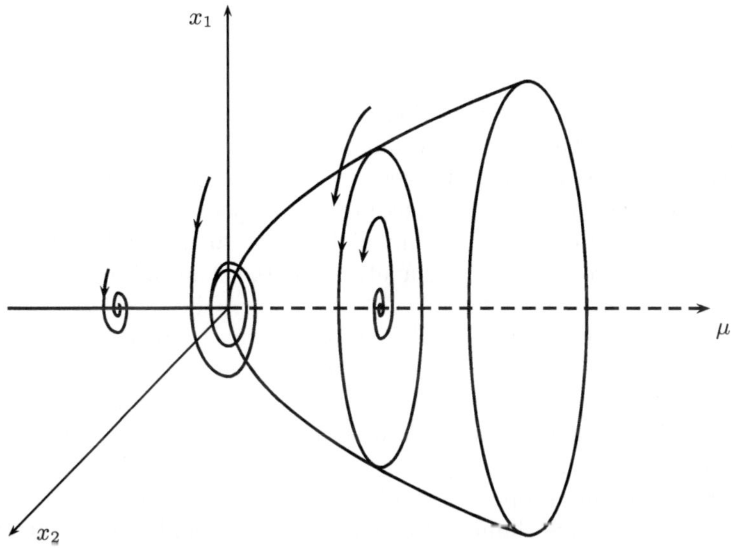

Fig. 2.28. Poincaré–Andronov–Hopf bifurcation

its coefficient. In particular its sign for $\mu = 0$ determines the stability behavior of the limit cycle and is therefore of great importance in the numerical analysis. A lengthy calculation (see, e.g., Guckenheimer & Holmes, 1983; Kuznetsov, 1998) shows that the Lyapunov coefficient $l_1(\mu)$ can explicitly be written as

$$\begin{aligned} l_1 &= \frac{1}{16}\left[\frac{\partial^3 g_1}{\partial x_1^3} + \frac{\partial^3 g_1}{\partial x_1 \partial x_2^2} + \frac{\partial^3 g_2}{\partial x_1^2 \partial x_2} + \frac{\partial^3 g_2}{\partial x_1^3}\right] \\ &+ \frac{1}{16\omega(0)}\left[\frac{\partial^2 g_1}{\partial x_1 \partial x_2}\left(\frac{\partial^2 g_1}{\partial x_1^2} + \frac{\partial^2 g_1}{\partial x_2^2}\right) - \frac{\partial^2 g_2}{\partial x_1 \partial x_2}\left(\frac{\partial^2 g_2}{\partial x_1^2} + \frac{\partial^2 g_2}{\partial x_2^2}\right)\right] \\ &- \frac{1}{16\omega(0)}\left[\frac{\partial^2 g_1}{\partial x_1^2}\frac{\partial^2 g_2}{\partial x_1^2} - \frac{\partial^2 g_1}{\partial x_2^2}\frac{\partial^2 g_2}{\partial x_2^2}\right], \end{aligned} \tag{2.64}$$

where $g = (g_1, g_2)'$ is the nonlinear part of the dynamics $f = (f_1, f_2)'$ evaluated at the equilibrium, i.e.,

$$\dot{x} = f(x, \mu) = \hat{J}(\mu)x + g(x, \mu),$$

and ω the imaginary part of the eigenvalue. Thus the following characterization holds:

1. For $l_1(0) < 0$ closed orbits emerge in a *supercritical* PAH-bifurcation and correspond to *stable* limit cycles.
2. For $l_1(0) > 0$ closed orbits emerge in a *subcritical* PAH-bifurcation and correspond to *unstable/repelling* cycles.

Thus the Poincaré–Andronov–Hopf theorem allows us to establish the existence of a limit cycle as well as its stability behavior, which is very useful for locating limit cycles as used in Sect. 7.4.2.

Obviously a PAH-bifurcation can also occur for higher-dimensional systems. This implies that a two-dimensional center manifold exists in the n-dimensional space that is tangent to the eigenspace spanned by the corresponding eigenvectors $\nu, \bar{\nu}$. Thus projecting (locally) the dynamics near the equilibrium onto this center manifold leads to a two-dimensional system, wherein the projection can be analyzed by the Poincaré–Andronov–Hopf theorem.

To illustrate a *supercritical PAH-bifurcation* ($l_1(0) < 0$), we imagine that – without loss of generality – the orbits emerge for $\mu > 0$. (The orbits could also emerge for $\mu < 0$, but this would not alter anything about the validity of this illustration.) Thus as long as $\mu < 0$ holds, the equilibrium $\hat{x}(\mu)$ is stable. As the bifurcation parameter attains its critical value, $\mu = 0$, $\hat{x}(\mu)$ alters its stability properties and becomes repelling, and closed orbits emerge. The union of these limit cycles forms a paraboloid that is tangent to the set expanded by the eigenvectors belonging to the eigenvalues with purely imaginary parts, $\xi_{1,2}(0) = \pm \mathrm{i}\omega(0)$, the center manifold.

These ideas will be made concrete by giving an intuitive example of a supercritical PAH-bifurcation taken from the field of drug research.

2.11 Higher-Dimensional Bifurcation Analysis of a Drug Model

Let us reconsider the two-state model of US cocaine consumption given by the planar system (2.36) – but this time from a bifurcation perspective. In Sect. 2.7 we already established the existence of a unique equilibrium

$$\hat{X} = \begin{pmatrix} \hat{L} \\ \hat{H} \end{pmatrix} = \frac{\tau}{\Omega} \begin{pmatrix} 1 \\ \frac{b}{g} \end{pmatrix}, \tag{2.65}$$

where

$$\Omega := a + b - sR > 0, \text{ by assumption}$$

with

$$R = R(q, b, g) := \mathrm{e}^{-\frac{qb}{g}}.$$

The associated Jacobian matrix is given by

$$\hat{J} = \begin{pmatrix} I_L(\hat{L}, \hat{H}) - (a+b) & I_H(\hat{L}, \hat{H}) \\ b & -g \end{pmatrix} = \begin{pmatrix} s\frac{qb}{g}R - \Omega & -sqR \\ b & -g \end{pmatrix}.$$

Since $\det \hat{J} > 0$ always holds for the equilibrium as determined by (2.38), $\hat{J}$ exhibits a pair of purely imaginary eigenvalues iff the trace of the Jacobian matrix disappears, i.e., $\operatorname{tr}\hat{J} = 0$. Thus the nondegeneracy condition in the Poincaré–Andronov–Hopf theorem is satisfied if

$$\operatorname{tr}\hat{J} = -g - \Omega + \frac{sRqb}{g} = 0. \tag{2.66}$$

Therefore the equation $sqbR = g(\Omega + g)$ defines a surface in the five-dimensional parameter space along which system (2.36) possesses two purely imaginary eigenvalues, $\xi_{1,2} = \pm i\sqrt{g\Omega}$. As one crosses this surface by variation of a single parameter, while all other parameter values remain unchanged (what economists call a ceteris paribus condition), the real part of the pair of complex conjugate eigenvalues, $\nu_{1,2}$, changes its sign, while the imaginary part remains nonzero, i.e., the system exhibits a PAH-bifurcation. The associated conditions for the entire set of system parameters, $\{a, b, g, s, q\}$, are given by Behrens et al. (1999); but here we focus on a particular one, namely the parameter g. This parameter describes the outflow from the state of heavy use, $H(t)$, and can, for instance, be increased or decreased by funding more or fewer drug treatment programs.

The reason why we analyze g is that when the exit rate from the heavy-use state is low, the heavy-use state has considerable inertia that can prevent a drug epidemic from repeating. A low g does not protect society from a first epidemic. Regardless of g's value, if initially there are enough light users to make the ratio H/L small and hence give the drug a benign reputation, then a positive feedback loop can be created by the sL part of the initiation term that feeds the L state. The resulting explosion in light users implies that, over time, many people will escalate to the heavy-use state. Eventually that alters the drug's reputation, undercutting initiation and short-circuiting the positive feedback loop. In short, the drug moves from an epidemic to an endemic problem, with numbers of both light and heavy users gradually declining.

Whether there is a second explosive epidemic, however, depends on what the ratio of H/L is as the number of drug users decays and hence on the relative rates at which light and heavy users quit. The exit rate from light use ($a = 0.163$ for US cocaine) is a function of the drug and societal parameters generally, but the exit rate from heavy use (g) is more amenable to manipulation by policy interventions, so that it is the key parameter to examine via bifurcation analysis.

When the rate at which heavy users quit obtains its *PAH-bifurcation critical value*, $g_c = \{g : \ a + b + g - sR(1 + qb/g) = 0\}$; then the change in the real part of the pair of conjugate complex eigenvalues (as given by 2.39) as the bifurcation parameter g varies is different from zero as long as

$$sqbR(g_c) \neq \frac{g_c^3}{qb}$$

holds. Thus a PAH-bifurcation occurs at $(\hat{X}(g_c), g_c)$ as one crosses the surface defined by (2.66), i.e.,

$$\left.\frac{\partial \operatorname{Re}\xi_{1,2}(g)}{\partial g}\right|_{g=g_c(a,q,s,b)} = \frac{1}{2}\left(\frac{sR(g_c)q^2b^2}{g_c^3} - 1\right) \neq 0.$$

We already know that on the center manifold the motion tends neither toward the equilibrium nor away from it, but remains in a certain region of the phase space forever. Thus the center manifold is determined by the following transformation of system (2.36) into a linear and nonlinear part

$$\begin{pmatrix} \dot{L} \\ \dot{H} \end{pmatrix} = \begin{pmatrix} 0 & -\sqrt{g_c\Omega(g_c)} \\ \sqrt{g_c\Omega(g_c)} & 0 \end{pmatrix} \begin{pmatrix} L - \hat{L}(g_c) \\ H - \hat{H}(g_c) \end{pmatrix} + \begin{pmatrix} \phi(L,H) \\ \psi(L,H) \end{pmatrix},$$

where

$$\begin{pmatrix} \phi(L,H) \\ \psi(L,H) \end{pmatrix} = \begin{pmatrix} I(L,H) - (a+b)L + \sqrt{g_c\Omega(g_c)}(H - \hat{H}(g_c)) \\ bL - gH - \sqrt{g_c\Omega(g_c)}(L - \hat{L}(g_c)) \end{pmatrix}.$$

As long as

$$sqR(g_c) \geq \sqrt{g_c\Omega(g_c)} =: \omega \tag{2.67}$$

holds at the *PAH-bifurcation critical value*, ceteris paribus, the normal-form calculation yields a negative coefficient

$$\begin{aligned} l_1(0) &= \frac{1}{16}\left(\phi_{LLL} + \phi_{LHH} + \psi_{LLH} + \psi_{HHH}\right) \\ &\quad + \frac{1}{16\omega}\left(\phi_{LH}\left(\phi_{LL} + \phi_{HH}\right) - \psi_{LH}\left(\psi_{LL} + \psi_{HH}\right) - \phi_{LL}\psi_{LL} + \phi_{HH}\psi_{HH}\right) \\ &= \frac{1}{16\omega}\left(\omega\left(I_{LLL} + I_{LHH}\right) + I_{LH}\left(I_{LL} + I_{HH}\right)\right) \\ &= \frac{-I_{HH}}{16L\omega}\left(\underbrace{\omega\left(3\frac{H^2}{L^2} + 1\right)}_{>0} + \underbrace{q\frac{H}{L}\left(\frac{H^2}{L^2} + 1\right)}_{>0}\underbrace{(sRq - \omega)}_{\text{Eq. 2.66}\geq 0}\right) < 0. \end{aligned}$$

Hence there exist periodic solutions that correspond to stable limit cycles for $g > g_c$. In other words when $g > g_c$, the unique equilibrium, (2.65), changes its stability because the real parts of the characteristic roots, (2.39), become positive such that the eigenvalues cross the imaginary axis of the complex plain with positive velocity (the transversality condition of Poincaré–Andronov–Hopf theorem). Since additionally condition (2.67) holds, we obtain a supercritical PAH-bifurcation. The equilibria have the local property of unstable foci, and the periodic orbits are attracting (for $g > g_c$).

On the one hand, if the exit rate from the heavy-use state is low ($g < g_c = 9.405\%$), the ratio of H/L will remain large enough to keep the drug from again getting a benign reputation. That is, the deterrent effect of heavy drug use is sufficient to suppress initiation into light use so that the epidemic declines and does not recur, at least with comparable force. On the other hand, if a high percentage of heavy users receives treatment or otherwise exits heavy use ($g > 13.8\%$), there is almost no deterrence and light users recruit nonusers with rate $s = 0.61$, so that prevalence can again grow exponentially. Between these values of g ($g_c < g < 13.8\%$) the deterrent force of heavy users is not strong enough to prevent further initiation, but is strong enough to prevent nearly proportional initiation. This interplay causes cycles (see Fig. 2.29).

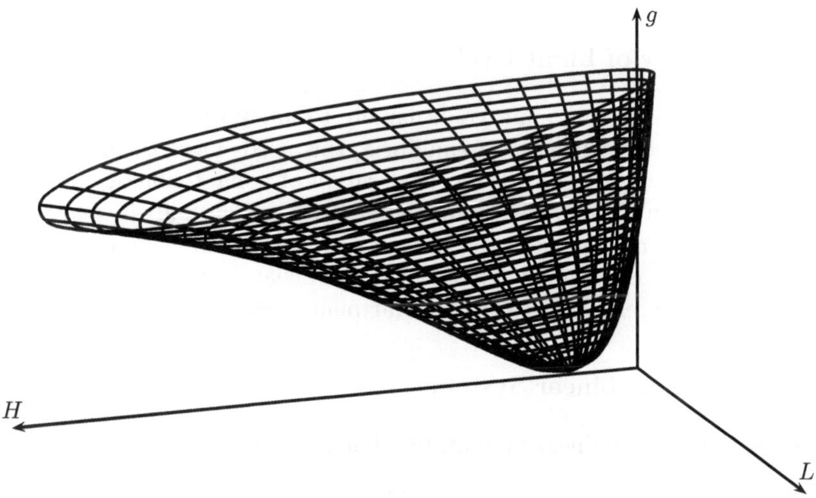

Fig. 2.29. Cyclical prevalence for parameter set $a = 0.163$, $b = 0.024$, $s = 0.61$, $q = 7.0$, $\tau = 50{,}000$ and for different values of the rate at which heavy users quit, $g_c \approx 0.0925 \leq g \leq 0.099$

Close to the PAH-bifurcation equilibrium $\hat{X}(g_c) = (576000, 149000)'$ the approximate radius of the cycles (as well as their period) may be estimated as a function of the parameter values (see, e.g., Hassard, Kazarinoff, and Wan (1981, p. 90); Strogatz (1994, p. 251) and Sect. 7.4.2). One realizes that the cycles "grow" – close to the bifurcation point with the size proportional to $\sqrt{g - 0.09405}$ and the periods estimated by $2\pi/\omega(g)$ – until g reaches 0.138, which corresponds to the hypothetical case of 89.5% of heavy users receiving treatment each year.

Thus, as Fig. 2.29 depicts, for a flow rate only infinitesimally larger than 0.09405, the numbers of light and heavy users would cycle counterclockwise forever with a period of approximately 70 years. Since such cycling in a social system is usually undesirable, this suggests that treating a constant, large proportion of heavy users throughout an epidemic, regardless of its course, may not always be the best policy. This leads directly to the idea explored in Behrens, Caulkins, Tragler, and Feichtinger (2000b), namely how treatment and other drug-control interventions should vary over the course of a drug epidemic. A brief summary is given in Sect. 6.1.

2.12 Advanced Topics

In this section we subsumed parts of the theory of dynamical systems not necessarily to be considered by the reader, who is not interested in the basic fundamentals for numerical calculations. Nonetheless, the following theory will play a crucial role in Chap. 7 where the numerical methods for computing optimal solutions are presented and can therefore not be neglected.

2.12.1 Stability of Limit Cycles

This subsection has one main goal, namely to analyze the stability of limit cycles. Compared to the case of equilibria, this needs more theoretical background and heavily relies on the consideration of nonautonomous linear systems. Thus even though nonautonomous systems play only a marginal, if any, role in the models presented here, we provide a brief summary of some principal results concerning nonautonomous linear systems. For a detailed presentation the reader is referred to Hartman (1982).

Nonautonomous Linear Systems

In a nonautonomous linear system, the dynamics becomes

$$\dot{x}(t) = J(t)x(t), \quad t \in \mathbb{R} \tag{2.68a}$$

$$\text{s.t.} \quad x(t_0) = x_0, \quad x_0 \in \mathbb{R}^n, \tag{2.68b}$$

where $J(t)$ is an $n \times n$ matrix explicitly depending on time t.

Remark 2.73. Note that we cannot restrain the initial condition to the time point $t_0 = 0$, since the function $J(t)$ describing the dynamics explicitly depends on t and therefore a time shift of the form $t \to t - t_0$ leads for the same initial condition x_0 to a different solution of (2.68) (see Fig. 2.30). Thus if we want to point to this initial time dependence, the solution of (2.68) will be written in the form $x(t, t_0)$.

We shall now present the concept of a fundamental (principal) matrix in a way analogous to autonomous systems (see p. 33), in which the former considerations may help the reader to understand the underlying idea. The only, but important, difference is the dependence on the initially chosen time point t_0, which can always be assumed to be 0 for autonomous problems.

As the reader may directly verify, the superposition principle also holds in the nonautonomous case (see Exercise 2.8).

Now, assume that we know n solutions $x_i(t)$ of (2.68a) with initial conditions $x_i(t_0) = x_i^0$. Then the matrix $X(t, t_0)$ composed of the columns $x_i(t)$

$$X(t, t_0) = (x_1(t), \dots, x_n(t))$$

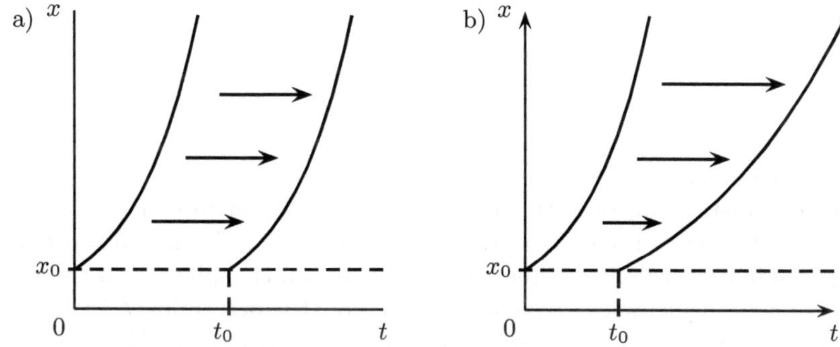

Fig. 2.30. In (**a**) the time-shifted solution of an *autonomous* ODE is depicted, exhibiting the invariance of the solution to such a transformation. In (**b**) we see the time-shifted solution of a *nonautonomous* ODE, revealing the dependence on the initial state x_0 as well on the initial time point t_0

satisfies the matrix differential equation

$$\dot{X}(t, t_0) = J(t)X(t, t_0) \tag{2.69}$$

with the initial condition $X(t_0, t_0) = \left(x_1^0, \dots, x_n^0\right)$. Note that, contrary to the analogue definition for autonomous systems, the initial time point t_0 is an argument of $X(t, t_0)$. Given the uniqueness of the solution of (2.68) and the superposition principle, the analogue proposition to Proposition 2.36 immediately follows:

Proposition 2.74. *The columns of a matrix solution $X(t, t_0)$ of (2.69) are linearly independent for all t iff they are linearly independent for some $t_1 \in \mathbb{R}$, especially $t = t_0$.*

The proof is analogous to that of Proposition 2.36 and is left to the reader (Exercise 2.16).

Now we can define:

Definition 2.75 (Fundamental Matrix Solution). *The time-dependent matrix $X(t, t_0)$ is called a* fundamental matrix solution *of (2.69) if it satisfies*

$$\dot{X}(t, t_0) = J(t)X(t, t_0)$$

with $\det X(t_0, t_0) \neq 0$, *i.e., $X(t_0, t_0)$ is invertible.*

Every fundamental matrix solution $X(t, t_0)$ can be transformed into a so-called *principal matrix solution* $Y(t, t_0)$ satisfying $Y(t_0, t_0) = \mathbb{I}^{(n)}$, by defining

$$Y(t, t_0) = X(t, t_0)X^{-1}(t_0, t_0).$$

Principal matrix solutions exhibit the following properties:

1. $Y(t,t_0) = Y(t,s)Y(s,t_0)$.
2. $Y(t,t_0)^{-1} = Y(t_0,t)$.
3. Given $Y(t,t_0)$, any solution $x(t)$ of (2.68) can be written in the form

$$x(t) = Y(t,t_0)x_0.$$

as the reader may verify.

The geometric interpretation presented for the autonomous case (see p. 33) clearly holds true for the nonautonomous problem, wherein the transformation of the original coordinate system $X(t_0)$ now depends explicitly on the initial time point t_0. Nonetheless, we can also ask how the determinant (volume) of the fundamental matrix (coordinate system) varies over time. By considering the Wronski determinant, the so-called *Liouville Formula* (2.70) can be proved (see, e.g., Hartman, 1982):

Proposition 2.76. *Let $X(t,t_0)$ be a fundamental matrix solution of the ODE (2.69), then the Wronski determinant $W(t,t_0)\det X(t,t_0)$ satisfies*

$$W(t,t_0) = W(t_0)\mathrm{e}^{\int_{t_0}^{t} \operatorname{tr} J(s)\,\mathrm{d}s}. \tag{2.70}$$

Remark 2.77. Note that (2.70) is exactly (2.24) for a time-varying $J(t)$.

However, the fundamental matrix solutions are more of theoretical than practical interest, since in general it is not possible to find an explicit solution matrix of (2.68). Nonetheless, further important properties can be derived if the dynamics $J(t)$ is periodic, a case that will subsequently be presented.

Floquet Theory

For the following considerations we analyze the ODE

$$\dot{x} = J(t)x, \tag{2.71}$$

where the corresponding dynamics $J(t)$ is periodic, i.e.,

$$J(t+\Theta) = J(t), \quad \text{for some} \quad \Theta > 0.$$

Owing to this functional form of the dynamics, the solutions exhibit a special structure, which is subsequently analyzed. In that case the solution of (2.68) is analogous to that of the linear autonomous case. This is stated in the following theorem (see, e.g., Hartman, 1982).

Theorem 2.78. *Let the system (2.68) have a periodic matrix function $J(t)$ with $t \in \mathbb{R}$ of period Θ. Then any fundamental matrix $X(t,t_0)$ of (2.68) has a representation of the form*

$$X(t,t_0) = \mathrm{e}^{Rt}C(t), \quad \textit{where} \quad C(t+\Theta) = C(t), \tag{2.72}$$

and $R \in \mathbb{C}^{n\times n}$ is a constant matrix.

Remark 2.79. Note that (2.72) is similar to the formula (2.22) for the autonomous system, with $C(t) \equiv X_0$ and $R = J$.

Adjoint Systems

In this book we are often confronted with so-called adjoint problems, which naturally occur in optimization problems. In some sense the adjoint problem describes the solutions orthogonal to the original space (see remark below). Thus associated to (2.68a) is the nonautonomous linear system

$$\dot{x}(t) = -J'(t)x(t), \tag{2.73}$$

which is called the *adjoint system*. This system plays an important role, e.g., in the numerical calculation of the (un)stable manifolds of a limit cycle (see Sect. 7.5.2).

Remark 2.80. Let us once more return to the geometric interpretation of a fundamental matrix solution as a coordinate system at the origin. Since the fundamental matrices $Y(t,t_0)$ of the adjoint equation (2.73) are the transposed inverse fundamental matrices $(X'(t,t_0))^{-1}$ of the original system (2.68a), the rows of $Y(t,t_0)$ are orthogonal to the columns of $X(t,t_0)$. This property makes it easy to describe solutions being orthogonal to solutions of the original system as solutions of the adjoint system.

The previous remark is proved by the following proposition:

Proposition 2.81. $X(t,t_0)$ *is a fundamental matrix solution of (2.68a) iff* $(X'(t,t_0))^{-1} = \left(X^{-1}(t,t_0)\right)'$ *is a fundamental matrix solution of (2.73).*

Where the proof is left as an exercise for the reader (Exercise 2.21).

Applying the Floquet Theory

Finally, we are ready to reap the fruit of this preliminary work and can tackle the question of stability for limit cycles. Thus let us consider a periodic solution $\Gamma(\cdot)$ with period Θ of the autonomous ODE

$$\dot{x}(t) = f(x(t)), \quad x(t) \in \mathbb{R}^n, \quad t \in [0, \Theta]. \tag{2.74}$$

Then the corresponding variational equation is given by

$$\dot{y}(t) = f_x(\Gamma(t))y(t), \tag{2.75}$$

where the matrix $J(t) = f_x(\Gamma(t))$ is periodic with period Θ. The ODE (2.75) expresses the evolution of the deviation $y(\cdot) = \Gamma(\cdot) - x(\cdot)$, where $x(\cdot)$ is a solution of (2.74) for an initial condition $x(0) = \Gamma(0) + \delta x$. Similar to the case of an equilibrium, one would like to characterize the stability of the limit cycle $\Gamma(\cdot)$ by analyzing the associated variational equation (2.75).

Utilizing the results of the previous Sect. 2.12.1, we define:

Definition 2.82 (Monodromy Matrix). *Let $\Gamma(\cdot)$ be a periodic solution of the ODE (2.74), with period Θ, and let $X(\cdot)$ be a principal matrix solution of the variational equation (2.75) then the matrix*

$$\mathrm{M} = X(\Theta),$$

is called the monodromy matrix M *of the periodic solution $\Gamma(\cdot)$.*

Let ξ_i, $i = 1, \dots, n$ be the eigenvalues of the monodromy matrix M *then*

$$n_+ := \{i : |\mathrm{Re}\,\xi_i| < 1\}, \; n_- := \{i : |\mathrm{Re}\,\xi_i| > 1\}, \; \textit{and}\; n_0 := \{i : |\mathrm{Re}\,\xi_i| = 1\}.$$

It can be proved that the eigenvalues of the monodromy matrix M do not depend on the specifically chosen periodic solution $\Gamma(\cdot)$ ascribing the orbit, denoted by Γ, of the periodic solution. Using this property the following definition can be given:

Definition 2.83 (Hyperbolic Limit Cycle). *Let Γ be a limit cycle of the ODE (2.74); then the limit cycle Γ is called* hyperbolic *if a monodromy matrix* M *of Γ exhibits only one eigenvalue ξ with $\xi = 1$.*

If $n_+ n_- > 0$, then the limit cycle $\Gamma(\cdot)$ is called of hyperbolic saddle-type.

Remark 2.84. When considering a limit cycle $\Gamma(\cdot)$ we have to distinguish between its representation as a periodic solution and the corresponding limit set, denoted by Γ. Since the stability of the limit cycle (as a limit set) only depends on the eigenvalues of a corresponding monodromy matrix, which itself is independent of the actually chosen representation $\Gamma(\cdot)$, we will use the term limit cycle as a periodic solution and limit set synonymously.

Definition 2.85 (Manifolds of a Limit Cycle). *Let Γ be a limit cycle of the ODE (2.74) then the set*

$$\mathrm{W}^s(\Gamma) = \{x : \lim_{t\to\infty} \varphi^t(x) \in \Gamma\}$$

is called the stable manifold *of the limit cycle Γ and the set*

$$\mathrm{W}^u(\Gamma) = \{x : \lim_{t\to-\infty} \varphi^t(x) \in \Gamma\}.$$

is called the unstable manifold *of the limit cycle Γ*

The eigenvalues of a monodromy matrix M characterize the stability of a limit cycle Γ:

Theorem 2.86 (Stability of a Limit Cycle). *Let Γ be a limit cycle of the ODE (2.74) and let* M *be a monodromy matrix of the limit cycle. If $n_+ = n-1$ then the limit cycle is unstable, while if $n_- = n - 1$ the limit cycle is stable.*

The Liouville formula in Proposition 2.76 applied to the monodromy matrix yields

$$\det \mathrm{M} = \mathrm{e}^{\int_0^{\Theta} \operatorname{tr} f_x(\Gamma(t))\,\mathrm{d}t}.$$

This provides another criterion to check whether a limit cycle is unstable or not because utilizing Theorem 2.90, one can rewrite this identity as

$$\xi_1 \xi_2 \cdots \xi_{n-1} = \mathrm{e}^{\int_0^{\Theta} \operatorname{tr} f_x(\Gamma(t))\,\mathrm{d}t},$$

since $\det \mathrm{M} = \xi_1 \xi_2 \cdots \xi_{n-1}$. Thus the following corollary holds:

Corollary 2.87. *Let $\Gamma(\cdot)$ be a limit cycle of (2.74) with period Θ. If*

$$\mathrm{e}^{\int_0^{\Theta} \operatorname{tr} f_x(\Gamma(t))\,\mathrm{d}t} > 1$$

holds, then the cycle Γ is unstable.

Proof. This easily follows from the consideration that at least one of the eigenvalues has to satisfy $|\xi_i| > 1$; otherwise the product cannot be greater than one.

Similar to the case of an equilibrium the stability properties of limit cycles are now determined by the eigenvalues of the monodromy matrix. I.e., the monodromy matrix plays a similar role for cycles, than the Jacobian matrix does for the analysis of equilibria. What is the reason for such a characterization? In the following we give a short motivation for this interrelation.

Motivation for the Stability Results of a Limit Cycle

To motivate Theorem 2.86, we make a short detour by introducing the so-called Poincaré map, describing the dynamic behavior of points near an arbitrarily chosen point $x_\Gamma \in \Gamma$ of a limit cycle Γ.

Considering such a point x_Γ, we take the $n-1$-dimensional hyperplane

$$\Sigma = \{x : \ f(x_\Gamma)\,(x - x_\Gamma) = 0\}, \tag{2.76}$$

which is the plane crossing the limit cycle orthogonally at x_Γ (see Fig. 2.31).

Hence, in a neighborhood $U \subset \Sigma$ of x_Γ, we can define a (unique) function $\mathrm{P} : U \to \Sigma$, which is called the *Poincaré map*, by

$$\mathrm{P}(x) = \varphi^{\tau}(x),$$

where τ is the *first time* such that the trajectory starting at x crosses the plane Σ in a local neighborhood U of x_Γ, i.e., $\varphi^{\tau}(x) \cap \Sigma \cap U \neq \emptyset$ (see, e.g., Hartman, 1982).

Owing to this construction x_Γ is a critical value[18] of the Poincaré map, since $\mathrm{P}(x_\Gamma) = \varphi^{\Theta}(x_\Gamma) = x_\Gamma$. Moreover, the Poincaré map can (locally) be

[18] The critical value of a difference equation is the analogon to the equilibrium of a differential equation, i.e., the corresponding dynamics is zero.

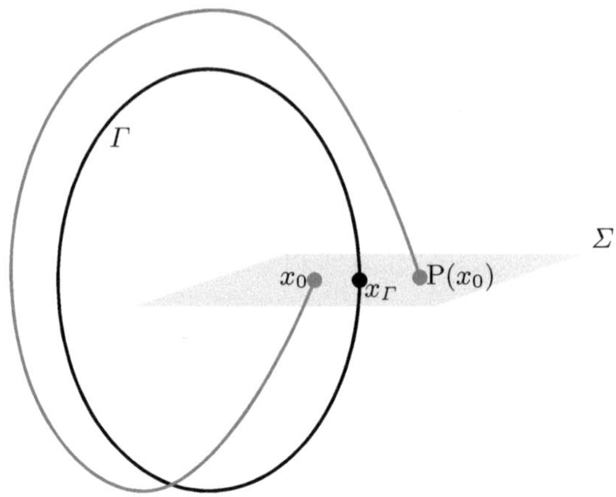

Fig. 2.31. Here the Poincaré map P of $\Gamma(\cdot)$ is illustrated

written as a discrete dynamical system in $\mathbb{R}^{n-1}$, since P is a map from $U \subset \Sigma$ into the $n-1$-dimensional hyperplane Σ. Hence the stability of x_Γ is described by the eigenvalues $\xi_i, i = 1, \dots, n-1$ of the Jacobian

$$\frac{\mathrm{d}\,\mathrm{P}}{\mathrm{d}x}(x_\Gamma)$$

of the Poincaré map P at x_Γ.

Remark 2.88. It is important to note that whereas the Poincaré map P depends on the arbitrarily chosen point $x_\Gamma \in \Gamma$, the eigenvalues $\xi_i, i = 1, \dots, n-1$ are independent from the point x_Γ. Thus it is geometrically evident that the stability of x_Γ in respect to the Poincaré map also describes the stability of the limit cycle Γ. In any case this has to be proved where a proof can be found, e.g., in Hartman (1982).

But for a discrete dynamical system an analogues theorem to Theorem 2.44 holds:

Theorem 2.89. *Let $\hat{x}$ be a critical state of the dynamical system (2.9), i.e., $f(\hat{x}) = 0$. If for every eigenvalue ξ of the Jacobian matrix $J(\hat{x}) = f_x(\hat{x})$*

$$|\mathrm{Re}\,\xi| < 1$$

holds, then $\hat{x}$ is stable. If there exist some eigenvalues ξ with

$$|\mathrm{Re}\,\xi| > 1,$$

then $\hat{x}$ is unstable.

The following theorem states the intimate connection between the Poincaré map and the solution of the variational equation:

Theorem 2.90 (Monodromy Matrix and Floquet Multipliers). *The monodromy matrix* M *exhibits the eigenvalues*

$$1, \xi_1, \ldots, \xi_{n-1},$$

where ξ_i correspond to the eigenvalues (characteristic Floquet multipliers*) of the Poincaré map associated with the cycle Γ.*

Here n_- denotes the number of eigenvalues ξ satisfying $|\mathrm{Re}\,\xi| < 1$ and n_+ denotes the number of eigenvalues ξ satisfying $|\mathrm{Re}\,\xi| > 1$.

Remark 2.91. The reason for 1 to be an eigenvalue relies on the geometric fact that the tangent vector on the limit cycle at x_0 is an eigenvector with corresponding eigenvalue 1.

2.12.2 Boundary Value Problems

So far we have concentrated our considerations on ODEs formulated as an IVP, i.e., a differential equation

$$\dot{x}(t) = f(x(t), t), \quad x \in \mathbb{R}^n, \quad t \in [0, T] \tag{2.77}$$

$$\text{s.t.} \quad x(0) = x_0. \tag{2.78}$$

The usual association with this kind of problem is the Newton paradigm, which states that once we know the exact data of a body and any forces affecting it, we can describe its movement forever. But the situation changes if we have only partial information about its initial states. If no further information is available, we obtain a whole set of possible solutions. Providing further conditions for the end time T, we have to chose among the trajectories of this set of solutions, satisfying simultaneously the end constraint. It is obvious that this kind of problem may become more involved, since, depending on the further constraints at time T, one solution, many solutions, or no solution exists. In any case these problems naturally occur in optimal control problems since there we have to determine trajectories satisfying specific optimality conditions (see Chap. 3).

We now consider the general problem of finding a solution $x(t)$, where information is given for the two points $x(0)$ and $x(T)$, i.e.,

$$b\,(x(0), x(T)) = 0, \tag{2.79}$$

where b is a vector-valued function $b : \mathbb{R}^n \to \mathbb{R}^n$ called the *boundary condition*. Problems of the type (2.77) and (2.79) are therefore called *two-point boundary value problems (BVP)*.

Remark 2.92. Note that the IVP can be seen as a special form of the BVP, where the boundary condition (2.79) is given by

$$b\,(x(0), x(T)) = x(0) - x_0 = 0.$$

Naturally one can extend this problem by introducing *multi-point conditions*:

$$b\left(x(0), x(t_1), \dots, x(T)\right) = 0, \quad 0 < t_1 < \dots < t_N = T,$$

which is called a *multi-point boundary value problem.* Nonetheless, this is equivalent to a two-point BVP if one considers the following transformation

$$t \to \frac{t - t_i}{t_{i+1} - t_i}, \quad i = 0, \dots, N-1,$$

normalizing each interval $[t_i,\ t_{i+1}]$ to $[0,\ 1]$. Thus we find an augmented system

$$\dot{\bar{x}} = \bar{f}(\bar{x}, t), \quad \bar{x} \in \mathbb{R}^{Nn}, \quad t \in [0,\ 1], \tag{2.80a}$$

with

$$\bar{x}(0) = \left(x(0), x(t_1), \dots, x(t_{N-1})\right)' \quad \bar{x}(1) = \left(x(t_1), x(t_2), \dots, x(T)\right)',$$

and

$$\bar{f} = \left(t_1 f, \dots, (T - t_{N-1})\, f\right)'.$$

Furthermore the multi-point condition can be rewritten as

$$\bar{b}\left(\bar{x}(0), \bar{x}(1)\right) = 0, \tag{2.80b}$$

with $\bar{b}$ appropriately defined. To guarantee the continuity of the solution $x(\cdot)$ additionally $(N-1)n$ continuity conditions have to be considered, given by

$$\bar{x}(0) - \bar{x}(1) = 0. \tag{2.80c}$$

Thus we have transformed the multi-point BVP into a two-point BVP. This transformation is not without cost, since the system (2.80) is larger in dimension compared to the original system.

The question of existence and uniqueness of a solution for a BVP, even in the linear case, is more difficult to answer than for an IVP. As an example we consider the following simple example:

Example 2.93.

$$\dot{x} = \begin{pmatrix} 0 & -1 \\ 1 & 0 \end{pmatrix} x, \quad 0 \le t \le \pi,$$

under the condition

$$x_1(0) = 0, \quad x_2(\frac{\pi}{2}) = \beta.$$

Under the condition $x_1(0) = 0$ it immediately follows that $x_1(t) = \tau \sin t$ for τ arbitrary, whereas $x_2(t) = \tau \cos t$. Thus, if $\beta = 0$, there exist infinitely many solutions, whereas for $\beta \neq 0$ no solution exists at all. This is contrary to the situation of an IVP, where the problem with initial condition $x_2(0) = \beta$ exhibits a unique solution.

For the nonlinear case the situation can become much more involved, and the reader should be warned to inspect the results of BVPs carefully.

However, a simple consideration associates an IVP with the BVP (2.77) (2.79) and provides a necessary condition for the existence of the solution. If one assumes that the BVP (2.77) and (2.79) has a solution $x(\cdot)$, then the corresponding flow $\varphi^t(x_0)$, with $x(0) = x_0 \in \mathbb{R}^n$, satisfies $b\left(\varphi^0(x_0), \varphi^T(x_0)\right) = 0$. Since for every $y \in \mathbb{R}^n$

$$\begin{aligned} &\dot{x} = f(x,t), \quad t \in [0, T] \\ \text{s.t.} \quad &x(0) = y, \end{aligned}$$

and f continuous and continuously differentiable in x, exhibits a unique solution (see Picard–Lindelöf theorem (Theorem 2.3)). Then the existence of a solution of the BVP is equivalent to the existence of a y_0, satisfying the generally nonlinear equation

$$b\left(\varphi^0(y_0), \varphi^T(y_0)\right) = 0. \tag{2.81}$$

Thus we can formulate:

Theorem 2.94. *Suppose that $f : \mathbb{R}^n \times \mathbb{R} \to \mathbb{R}^n$ is continuous and continuously differentiable in x. Then the BVP (2.77) and (2.79) has as many solutions as there are distinct roots y_0 of (2.81). For each of these y_0 a solution $x(\cdot)$ of the BVP is given by*

$$x(t) = \varphi^t(y_0).$$

Since nonlinear equations may have no solution, a finite number of solutions, or an infinite number of solutions, one can at best hope to prove that if a solution $x(\cdot)$ exists at all, that this solution is at least locally unique. It is possible, however, to prove that a solution $x(\cdot)$ is locally unique if the corresponding variational equation (see Sect. 2.6.2) given by:

$$\begin{aligned} &\dot{y} = f_x\left(x(t), t\right) y \\ \text{s.t} \quad &\frac{\partial b\left(x(0), x(T)\right)}{\partial x(0)} y(0) + \frac{\partial b\left(x(0), x(T)\right)}{\partial x(T)} y(T) = 0 \end{aligned}$$

has the unique solution $y \equiv 0$.

Remark 2.95. Numerical algorithms for solving BVPs mostly use iterative strategies to find a solution, whereby the user has to provide some initial function $\tilde{x}(\cdot) : [0, T] \to \mathbb{R}^n$. On the one hand, this seems different from an IVP, where for a numerical calculation no such function has to be made available; but, on the other hand, the initial condition $x(0) = x_0$ is already a solution function embracing its total future behavior.

Let us stop at this point and refer the reader to textbooks on BVPs, such as Ascher, Mattheij, and Russell (1995).

Examples for BVP Problems Occurring in Applied Optimal Control Theory

The reason why we introduce BVPs at all lies in its importance as an instrument for solving optimal control problems, since the corresponding necessary optimality conditions are given as a BVP of the form (see Sect. 3.3.1):

$$\dot{x} = \mathcal{H}^*_\lambda(x, \lambda) \tag{2.82a}$$

$$\dot{\lambda} = r\lambda - \mathcal{H}^*_x(x, \lambda) \tag{2.82b}$$

$$\text{s.t.} \quad x(0) = x_0 \in \mathbb{R}^n \tag{2.82c}$$

$$\lambda(T) = S_x\left(x(T)\right) \in \mathbb{R}^n, \tag{2.82d}$$

where $\mathcal{H}^* : \mathbb{R}^n \times \mathbb{R}^n \to \mathbb{R}^n$, $S \in \mathbb{R}^n \to \mathbb{R}$. Thus (2.82) is a BVP with linear boundary conditions (2.82c) and (2.82d).

A possible algorithm for solving such a problem is presented in Chap. 7. When solving an optimal control problem one also has to compute of limit cycles. a problem which can be formulated:

$$\begin{aligned}
&\dot{x} = \Theta f(x), \quad t \in [0, 1] \\
&x(0) = x(1) \\
&\psi(x) = 0,
\end{aligned}$$

where Θ is the (unknown) period of the searched for limit cycle and $\psi : \mathbb{R}^n \to \mathbb{R}$ a scalar function characterizing a specific representation of the limit cycle.

Another problem is the calculation of the stable manifold of a saddle $\hat{x}$, which can be stated as:

$$\begin{aligned}
&\dot{x} = f(x), \quad t \in [0, \infty) \\
\text{s.t.} \quad &x(0) \in \mathrm{W}^s \\
&\lim_{t\to\infty} x(t) = \hat{x}.
\end{aligned}$$

Or as a last example we may be interested in an optimal solutions satisfying some constraints, so that at some time point $t_s \in [0, T]$ the dynamics switches between the solution path being in the interior and at the boundary of the constraint region. Then the problem becomes finding a solution $x(\cdot) \in \mathbb{R}^{2n}$ that satisfies

$$\begin{aligned}
&\dot{x}^1 = f^1(x^1), \quad t \in [0, t_s] \\
&\dot{x}^2 = f^2(x^2), \quad t \in [t_s, T] \\
&x^1(0) = x_0 \\
&x^1(t_s) = x^2(t_s) \\
&x^2(T) = 0,
\end{aligned}$$

with $f^i : \mathbb{R}^n \to \mathbb{R}^n$, $i = 1, 2$, which is a typical multi-point BVP.

With all these problems the reader may be confronted when he/she tries to find a numerical solution of an optimal control problem, where algorithms are provided in the numerical part of the book Chap. 7.

This final section on BVPs concludes the preliminary work, and we now turn to the actual topic of this book, namely optimal control theory. In conclusion, the theory of dynamical systems is an indispensable part of optimal control theory, both in its usual formulation and in its numerical computation, justifying their lengthy discussion.

Exercises

2.1 (A Dynamic Model of Terrorism). Recently Udwadia, Leitmann, and Lambertini (2006) divided the population in a given region into three components: terrorists, those susceptible to both terrorist and pacifist propaganda, and nonsusceptibles. The flows between three classes incorporate the effects of both military or police and persuasive interventions.

Denote the number of terrorists in a certain area at time t as $x(t)$. The nonterrorist population in the region is made up of the population of susceptibles, $y(t)$, and nonsusceptibles, $z(t)$.

The number of terrorists in a given period of time can change for several reasons:

1. Recruitment by the terrorists of individuals from the susceptibles; the effectiveness of this is taken to be proportional to the product of the number of terrorists and the number of susceptibles.
2. The effect of antiterrorist measures that are directed at reducing the terrorist population, such as military and police action, which we assume increases rapidly, i.e., quadratically with the number of terrorists.
3. The number of terrorists who are killed in action, including those killed by suicide bombings, a number that we assume to be proportional to the terrorist population itself.
4. The increase in the terrorist population primarily through appeals by terrorists to other terrorist groups.

These four effects are captured in the differential equation

$$\dot{x} = axy - bx^2 + (c-1)x.$$

The change in the number of the susceptibles is likewise caused by several factors:

1. Depletion of their population caused by their direct contact with terrorists whose point of view they adopt.
2. Depletion of the population of susceptibles caused by nonviolent propaganda; this effect assumes that the propaganda intensifies rapidly as the number of terrorists increases, and we assume that the change this causes is proportional to the product x^2y.
3. An increase in the population of susceptibles caused by the propaganda that is created through the publicity of terrorist acts.

4. An increase in the susceptible population when individuals from outside the area are incited to move into the area; we assume that the changes in the y population attributable to this cause and the previous one are proportional to the number of terrorists in the region of concern.
5. The increase in the susceptible population proportional to its own size.

The evolution of the susceptible population adduced from these effects can be expressed as

$$\dot{y} = axy - ex^2y + fx + gy.$$

Last, the change in the number of nonsusceptibles, z, in a given interval of time is described by:

1. Those members of the susceptible population who become nonsusceptibles by virtue of having altered their persuasions because of the nonviolent actions or propaganda.
2. Those who become susceptibles owing to the effects of global propaganda spread by terrorists.
3. The increase in the z-population, which is proportional to its population numbers. This, then, may be described by the equation

$$\dot{z} = ex^2y - \bar{f}x + hz.$$

Udwadia, Leitmann, and Lambertini (2006) claimed that this three-dimensional nonlinear model captures some important features of the dynamics of tensional activity.

To study the long-term dynamical evolution, it is necessary to determine the equilibria. Then a phase-portrait analysis should be carried out. What do the projections in the two-dimensional subspaces look like? Can limit cycles occur?

A critical parameter is c, the ratio of the rate of increase of the terrorists. Can you identify other key parameters of the system?

2.2 (The One-Dimensional Terror Model Revisited). Show the existence and analyze the properties of the equilibria for the one-dimensional terror model (2.14) in Sect. 2.5; prove the following statements and interpret them in terms of the counter-terror measures u and v:

1. Consider $u > 0$ and $\mu\rho < \gamma$:
   a) For $v > 0$, $\mu\rho v - \gamma \ln(1 + v) > 0$.
   b) For $v \ll 1$ only $\hat{S}_1$ exists.
   c) If $v \to 0$, then $\sqrt{\hat{S}_1} \to \frac{\tau}{\beta \ln(1+u)}$.
2. Consider $u > 0$ and $\mu\rho > \gamma$:
   a) There exists $v_0 > 0$, $\mu\rho v_0 - \gamma \ln(1 + v_0) = 0$.
   b) For $v \ll 1$ $\hat{S}_1$ and $\hat{S}_2$ exist.
   c) If $v \to 0$, then $\hat{S}_2 \to \infty$.
3. There exists $v_0 > 0$ such that for $v > v_0$, $\dot{S} > 0$ for every S_0 and every time t.
4. There exists $u_0 > 0$ such that for $u > u_0$ at least one asymptotically stable equilibrium exists.

Hint. For questions (1a) and (2a) consider the first derivative

$$(\mu\rho v - \gamma \ln(1 + v))'.$$

For questions (1b) and (2b) consider the Taylor expansion

$$\ln(1+v) = v - \frac{1}{2}v^2 + o(v^3).$$

For questions (2c) and (2c) consider the Taylor expansion

$$\sqrt{1-\Omega} = 1 - \frac{1}{2}\Omega + o(\Omega).$$

2.3 (A Push–Pull Corruption Model). Formulate and solve the corruption model described in Sect. 2.3, in which the flow from honest state to corrupt state is proportional to corruption $1-x$. Analyze the push–pull case

$$\dot{x} = kx(1-x)(U_c - U_h).$$

2.4 (The One-Dimensional Drug Model with Constant Treatment and Zero Enforcement). Analyze an extended version of the one-dimensional drug model of Sect. 2.9, with the system dynamics given by

$$\dot{A} = kA\left(\bar{A} - A\right) - \mu A - c\sqrt{u}\sqrt{A},$$

where the constant "control" u denotes treatment (see Sect. 3.9). Then

1. Find the equilibria of the system and determine their stability properties.
2. Consider u as a bifurcation parameter.

2.5 (The Rosenzweig & MacArthur Predator–Prey Model). Rosenzweig and MacArthur (1963) described the intertemporal interaction between a *predator population* and its *prey*. The variables $x(t)$ and $y(t)$ denote the population size of the prey and the predator populations, respectively, both at time t. The function $g(x)$ denotes the specific growth rate of the prey population and $h(x,y)$ is the so-called *predator response function*. We can describe the entire ecosystem's dynamics as follows:

$$\begin{pmatrix} \dot{x} \\ \dot{y} \end{pmatrix} = \begin{pmatrix} g(x)x - h(x,y)y \\ eh(x,y)y - my \end{pmatrix}.$$

We assume that the natural habitat of the prey species is confined so that in the absence of the predator species the prey only grows exponentially if the population size is very small. Then the prey population's growth slows down and approaches a maximum level, the so-called *carrying capacity* K. This yields the *logistic growth function*,

$$g(x) = r\left(1 + \frac{x}{K}\right).$$

Thus the prey population x is increased by natural processes and is reduced by intraspecific competition and by the predator y. The predator response function h can be regarded as the per capita prey consumed by every individual of the predator population and measures, therefore, y's difficulty in finding suitable food. This is modeled by a *Holling-type* II (see Holling, 1959) function, i.e.

$$h(x,y) = h(x) = \frac{ax}{b+x},$$

where parameter a denotes an upper limit on daily consumption of the predator and b is the so-called *half-saturation constant*. Parameter e accounts for the metabolic efficiency loss that translates the food of the predator into offspring. Thus the net change in y is determined by subtracting the (exogenous) death rate m from the fertility rate of the predator, defined by $eh(x)$, as by assumption h does not depend on y.

To study the ecological evolution of the two types of species, it is helpful to carry out a bifurcation analysis with respect to e. Thus, when answering these questions it is useful to distinguish between three different efficiency ranges, i.e., intervals for the efficiency e to convert prey into offspring,

$$\left[\frac{m}{a}, \frac{m}{a} + \frac{mb-K}{a}\right), \left[\frac{m}{a} + \frac{mb-K}{a}, \frac{m}{a} + \frac{K+b}{K-b}\right), \left[\frac{m}{a} + \frac{K+b}{K-b}, \infty\right),$$

and draw the corresponding phase plots.

Hint. Utilizing the Poincaré–Bendixson theorem might be useful.

2.6 (Dynamic Fishery Model). Let x denote the size of a population of fish that is harvested at a certain rate $h(x)$. Assume that the growth of this population is bounded by intraspecies competition. Then x grows toward a known carrying capacity K, as embodied in a *logistic growth function.* Together this leads to the following model of the exploitation of a renewable resource (Gordon–Schäfer model Gordon (1954))

$$\dot{x} = rx\left(1 + \frac{x}{K}\right) - h(x). \tag{2.83}$$

Determine the system behavior (including the equilibria) for the following types of harvest functions $h(x)$.

$$h(x) = h, \tag{T1}$$
$$h(x) = Ex, \quad E > 0. \tag{T2}$$

What types of bifurcations can be identified for the bifurcation parameters $h > 0$ and $E > 0$, respectively? What are the consequences for the modeled harvesting strategies?

2.7. Prove by formally differentiating the sum

$$\mathrm{e}^{Jt} := \mathbb{I}^{(n)} + Jt + \frac{J^2}{2!}t^2 + \frac{J^3}{3!}t^3 + \cdots$$

that the exponential function satisfies the linear ODE

$$\dot{x} = Jx.$$

2.8. Prove the principle of superposition for the linear autonomous and nonautonomous problem.

2.9. Prove Proposition 2.36.

Hint. Prove by contradiction that there exists some t_1 such that $X(t_1)$ is singular. Now use the uniqueness of the solution and demonstrate that the zero function is a specific solution.

2.10 (Non-Unique Center Manifold). Consider the ODE (2.31) then:

- Determine the eigenspaces for the Jacobian at the origin
- Approve the equation for the orbits
- Prove that the center manifolds are infinitely often differentiable at 0

2.11. Prove Proposition 2.74, i.e., the columns of a fundamental matrix solution are linearly independent for all t iff they are linearly independent for some $t_1 \geq 0$.

2.12 (An Advertising Diffusion Model). Consider the following marketing model

$$\dot{x} = a(1-x) - \delta x \tag{2.84a}$$

$$\dot{a} = \alpha(x, a), \tag{2.84b}$$

where x denotes the market share of a firm and a its advertising rate. Customers change to another firm (or product) with rate $\delta \geq 0$. The advertising intensity changes according to a feedback rule $\alpha(x, a)$, whereby it makes some sense to assume

$$\alpha_x > 0, \alpha_{xx} \geq 0; \qquad \alpha_a > 0, \alpha_{aa} \leq 0; \qquad \alpha_{xa} \geq 0.$$

Note that the conditions of the first diffusion model of Gould (1970) deliver

$$\alpha(x, a) = \left(r + \frac{\delta}{1-x}\right) a$$

provided that the advertising costs are quadratic ($c(a) = 1/2a^2$) and the return of sales is linear ($\pi(x) = x$); compare Gould (1970) and Feichtinger and Hartl (1986, p. 325), as well as Exercise 3.5.

Carry out a phase-portrait analysis of the system (2.84). Show that the stable manifold has a negative slope and interpret the result.

2.13 (Price Dynamics). Consider the following continuous-time version of the famous Cobweb model. Let the demand for a good at time t be a linearly decreasing function of its price and the supply s a linearly increasing function, i.e.,

$$d = ap + b, \qquad a < 0,\ b > 0$$

$$s = cp + d, \qquad c > 0,\ d < 0.$$

The price dynamics assumes that it adapts according to the excess demand, i.e.,

$$\dot{p} = \gamma\,(d - s)\,,$$

where γ measures the speed of approaching the equilibrium price.

Determine the equilibrium price and describe the adjustment dynamics. Which sign of γ implies the stability of the long-run equilibrium? Find a *discrete* version of the model and illustrate the "cobweb" in a (p_t, p_{t+1})-diagram.

2.14 (Environmental Pollution and Capital Accumulation). Denote by $P(t)$ the stock of pollution at time t and by $K(t)$ the capital stock of an economy. Let $F(K)$ be the produced output by the (single) production factor K ($F' > 0$, $F'' < 0$). Assume that the output can be used for abatement A, being consumed or invested for capital accumulation, I, i.e.,

$$F(K) = A + C + I.$$

To simplify, let us suppose that constant consumption $C = 0$. It is plausible to consider a state-dependent (linear) feedback rule for abatement

$$A = \varphi P, \quad \varphi > 0.$$

Then the interaction of the state variables K and P is described as follows

$$\dot{K} = F(K) - \varphi P - \delta K$$
$$\dot{P} = \varepsilon F(K) - G(\varphi P) - \alpha P,$$

where $\delta \geq 0$ denotes the depreciation rate of the capital, $\varepsilon > 0$ is the emission rate of the production, and α is the natural cleaning rate of the level of pollution. The function $G(A)$ measures the impact of abatement A on the reduction of the pollution ($G' > 0$, $G'' \leq 0$).

Find the isoclines and the equilibrium $(\hat{K}, \hat{P})$. What are the local stability properties of this equilibrium? Carry out a sensitivity analysis of $(\hat{K}, \hat{P})$ with respect to the parameters and interpret the results. Discuss other intuitively appealing feedback mechanisms of P on $\dot{K}$.

2.15 (A Growth Model). Consider the following "variant" of Solow's growth model (Solow, 1956)

$$\dot{K} = sF(K, L) - \delta K,$$

where $s \in (0, 1)$ is the saving rate, δ is the depreciation rate of capital, K is an economy's capital stock, L denotes the economy's labor force, and $F(K, L)$ is the neoclassical production function, assumed, e.g., to be of Cobb–Douglas type

$$F(K, L) = K^{\alpha} L^{\beta}, \qquad \alpha, \beta \in (0, 1).$$

Suppose that the stock of labor force develops according to the difference between the marginal product of labor, F_L and a constant wage rate w (comment on this assumption), i.e.,

$$\dot{L} = L\left(F_L(K, L) - w\right).$$

Carry out a phase-portrait analysis in the (K, L)-plane. Does there exist an equilibrium, and what might be its stability properties?

2.16. Prove Proposition 2.74

2.17 (PAH_Bifurcation in an Advertising Model). In Feichtinger (1992) the following descriptive marketing model is motivated:

$$\dot{x} = k - axy + \beta y \tag{2.85}$$
$$\dot{y} = axy - \delta y,$$

where x denotes the number of potential buyers of a good and y the customers of this brand. The parameter $\delta = \beta + \varepsilon$, where β measures the brand-switching rate and ε measures the dropout rate of the market. The term axy is the usual diffusion term where word-of-mouth is supported by the advertising rate a. According to the so-called Dorfman-Steiner rule, a constant percentage of sales revenue should be allocated to advertising (see, e.g., Feichtinger & Hartl, 1986, p. 314). Thus, by substituting $a = \alpha y$ into (2.85), we get a two-dimensional nonlinear system (which has similarities to the so-called Brusselator[19]).

Carry out a bifurcation analysis. Show that there exists a unique equilibrium. For $\gamma = \alpha k^2/\delta\varepsilon^2$, there exists γ_i, $i = 1,2$ with $0 < \gamma_1 < 1 < \gamma_2$ such that the equilibrium is

$$\begin{array}{lll} \text{an unstable node} & \text{iff} & \gamma \in [0, \gamma_1) \\ \text{an unstable focus} & \text{iff} & \gamma \in (\gamma_1, 1) \\ \text{a stable focus} & \text{iff} & \gamma \in (1, \gamma_2) \\ \text{a stable node} & \text{iff} & \gamma \in (1, \gamma_2). \end{array}$$

Furthermore, show that there exists γ_3 with $\gamma_1 < \gamma_3 < 1$ such that for all $\gamma \in (\gamma_3, 1)$ there is a *stable* limit cycle. Give an economic interpretation of this persistent oscillation by dividing it into four regimes.

2.18 (Easterlin Cycles). In Easterlin (1961) an explanation for the US baby boom and its reversal was offered. The following two-dimensional system connects the per capita capital stock k and the aspiration level measured as an expected income

$$z(t) = \gamma \int_{-\infty}^{t} \mathrm{e}^{-\gamma(t-s)} g(k(s))\, \mathrm{d}s. \tag{2.86}$$

Here $g(k) = f(k) - \delta k$ is the actual net income, where $f(k)$ denotes the per capita production function and δ the depreciation rate of the capital stock. The parameter γ measures the speed of adjustment. Somewhat surprisingly, (2.86) is equivalent to

$$\dot{z} = \gamma\,(g(k) - z)\,.$$

The dynamics of the capital stock is given as

$$\dot{k} = f(k) - \delta k - c - (b-d)k,$$

where $n = b - d$ is the natural growth rate of a (closed) population written as the difference between the crude birth rate, b, and crude death rate, d. While the latter is assumed to be constant, the former is assumed to depend positively on the difference between the actual and the expected income

$$b = b(g(k) - z) \quad \text{with} \quad b > 0,\ b' \geq 0.$$

Finally, suppose consumption per person depends positively on z, i.e.,

$$c = c(z) \quad \text{with} \quad c > 0,\ c' \geq 0.$$

Using the Poincaré–Bendixson theorem derive sufficient conditions for the existence of a stable limit cycle. Try to give a demo-economic interpretation of the cycle's orientation.

2.19 (The Lorenz Attractor). The Lorenz attractor is a well-known example of a *chaotic flow*, noted for its butterfly shape. The equations

---

[19] The Brusselator is an example for an autocatalytic, oscillating chemical reaction.

$$\dot{x} = \sigma(y - x)$$
$$\dot{y} = x(\rho - z) - y$$
$$\dot{z} = xy - \beta z$$

were introduced by Lorenz (1963), who considered an atmospheric model, by simplifying *Navier–Stokes* equations occurring in fluid dynamics. Roughly speaking, the state x measures the rate of convective overturning, the state y denotes the horizontal temperature variation, and the variable z is the vertical temperature variation. The three parameters σ, ρ, and β are proportional to the *Prandtl* number, the *Rayleigh* number, and some physical proportions (see Sparrow, 1982). For the parameter values $\sigma = 10$, $\rho = 28$, and $\beta = 8/3$ calculate the equilibria and paths of the two-dimensional stable manifold at the origin.

2.20 (Inhomogeneous Linear Differential Equation). Consider the ODE

$$\dot{x}(t) = kx(t) + u(t), \quad k, x, u \in \mathbb{R},$$
$$\text{s.t.} \quad x(0) = x_0$$

which is called a *linear inhomogeneous* differential equation. Show that the solution is given by

$$x(t) = \mathrm{e}^{kt}\left(x_0 + \int_0^t \mathrm{e}^{-ks} u(s)\,\mathrm{d}s\right),$$

and that for $k > 0$ the inequality

$$|x(t)| \leq \mathrm{e}^{kt}\left(|x_0| + \int_0^t |u(s)|\,\mathrm{d}s\right)$$

Hint. Use the so-called variation of constants method *by setting* $x(t) = c(t)\mathrm{e}^{kt}$ *and determine* $c(t)$. *To derive the inequality note that for* $k > 0$ $\mathrm{e}^{-ks} \leq 1$ *for all* $s \geq 0$.

2.21 (Adjoint Solution). Prove Proposition 2.81.

Hint. Consider the time derivative $\frac{\mathrm{d}}{\mathrm{d}t}\left(X^{-1}(t, t_0)\right)$, *which follows by differentiating the identity* $X^{-1}(t, t_0)X(t, t_0) = \mathbb{I}^{(n)}$.

Notes and Further Reading

The theory of dynamical systems and ODEs is one of the central areas of mathematical research. It develops techniques required for the analysis of intertemporal decision problems arising in dynamic economics and management sciences. This chapter may be seen as a compact reference (and toolkit) for solving dynamic optimization problems. In addition and among other references, we recommend the following three well-written, application-oriented books: Léonard and Long (1992), on dynamic modeling in the various fields of optimal control theory; Strogatz (1994), on physics and engineering; and Hofbauer and Sigmund (1988), on biomathematics.

A fine introduction to economic applications of nonlinear dynamical systems theory is given by Hommes (1991); compare also Lorenz (1993).

Compared with Léonard and Long (1992), we treat parts of the theory of dynamical systems in more depth, not least because one of our intentions is to present concrete algorithms for solving optimal control problems. An excellent introductory book on the theory of dynamical systems for readers starting from a background of only calculus and elementary linear algebra is Hirsch, Smale, and Devaney (2002) which is a revised edition of the classical textbook Hirsch and Smale (1974).

Our approach has made it necessary to refer to more theoretically oriented books, such as Hartman (1982), in which the theory of linear nonautonomous systems, together with the Floquet theory, are presented. The Floquet theory is helpful for stating and deriving some of the results used in the computation of limit cycles and the corresponding manifolds in Chap. 7.

The presentation of dynamical systems as nonlinear ODEs can be found mainly in the books of Arrowsmith and Place (1990); Strogatz (1994); Wiggins (1990), and Arnold (1983), where the unfamiliar reader is referred to Strogatz (1994).

The introduction of an ODE in the sense of Definition 2.1 is given under very restrictive assumptions. To capture more general problems, extensions in various directions can be considered. One of these extensions is the concept of a Carathéodory solution, where the integral equation (2.8) is understood in the Lebesgue sense. Other extensions allow the dynamics f to be multivalued, yielding a so-called *differential inclusion* (see, e.g, Aubin & Cellina, 1984). Especially useful in the context of PDEs are so-called *viscosity solutions* introduced by Crandall and Lions (1983), which extend the classical solution concept of PDEs.

A good introduction to bifurcation and stability analysis (from equilibrium to chaos) is provided by Seydel (1994), see also the excellent book by Troger and Steindl (1991).

Kuznetsov (1998) and Guckenheimer and Holmes (1983) are highly recommended as advanced books on bifurcation theory. Many of our examples in the text, in particular those of a normal form and nonhyperbolic equilibrium, are taken from Kuznetsov (1998). We also refer the reader to the MATLAB toolbox "MatCont" provided by the group Kuznetsov, which can be used to do numerical bifurcation analysis. This toolbox allows the numerical computation not only of bifurcations concerning equilibria but also of the limit cycles. Moreover bifurcations of higher codimension[20] (codim > 1) can be analyzed.

The section on BVP is taken mainly from Ascher et al. (1995), which includes a comprehensive overview of the numerical methods in the field of BVPs. It also contains a well-written overview of the important results from ODEs.

The Poincaré–Andronov–Hopf bifurcation, where an equilibrium gives rise to a limit cycle, was first studied by the French mathematician Henri Poincaré in 1892 while he was investigating the planetary three-body problem. Poincaré did many things and can be said to have been the originator of both algebraic topology and the theory of analytic functions of several complex variables. Paying tribute to his pioneering work, the theorem (discussed in Sect. 2.10) bears his name, together with the names of A.A. Andronov and H. Hopf. The latter two mathematicians independently discovered periodic behavior to be a result of a local bifurcation – Andronov in the late 1920s (Andronov, 1929) and Hopf in the early 1940s (Hopf, 1943).

[20] The *codimension* of a bifurcation is the number of independent conditions determining the bifurcation.

The corruption model presented in Sect. 2.3 has been selected mainly because of its simplicity. There is a small, but important, literature on dynamic economic modeling of corruption. A good introductory survey is Andvig (1991).

Rinaldi, Feichtinger, and Wirl (1998) studied the dynamics of corruption at the top, i.e., corruption by politicians. Their framework relates actions (positive actions of the politicians, bribery, consumption, and the unveiling of corruption) to the state variables – popularity (as a proxy for power), assets accumulated from bribes, and investigation. The authors differentiate corrupted and uncorrupted systems, and in the class of corrupted systems distinguish between strongly controlled (steady behavior), weakly controlled (cyclic behavior), and uncontrolled (wild behavior). For example, increasing the persistence of investigators can control the system but cannot eliminate corruption, whereas institutional changes that lower the practice of giving and taking bribes can.

Caulkins, Gragnani, Feichtinger, and Tragler (2006) extended the LH-model presented in Sect. 2.11 by considering two additional states that represent in more detail newly initiated ("light") users' response to the drug experience. Those who dislike the drug quickly "quit" and briefly suppress initiation by others. Those who like the drug progress to ongoing ("moderate") use, from which they may or may not escalate to "heavy" or dependent use. Initiation is spread contagiously by light and moderate users, but is moderated by the drug's reputation, which is a function of the number of unhappy users (recent quitters and heavy users). The proposed model generates complex behavior of the solution paths including cycles, quasi-periodic solutions, and chaos. The model has the disquieting property of endogenously generating peaks followed by a crash to low levels and a dramatic resurgence of use. Thus, even if the current drug epidemic ebbs and we enjoy a long period of low rates of use, that does not guarantee that drug epidemics will not return with equal ferocity.

Behrens, Caulkins, Tragler, and Feichtinger (2000a) augmented the LH-model (see Sect. 2.11) by an awareness variable or a "memory of the adverse consequences of heavy-use years" (compare also Sect. 6.1 and Exercise 6.5). If past bad experiences fade away quickly, drug incidence increases. The resulting increase in the number of occasional drug users leads to a future increase in the number of heavy users who contribute to the accumulation of a higher level of awareness or memory that in turn suppresses incidence. This interaction is capable of production cycles.

Heterogeneity in intensity of activity is of course not restricted to the modeling of drug epidemics. It is just as relevant in modeling economic activity (high- and low-wage earners), the transmission of infectious diseases such as HIV/AIDS (people who frequently or less frequently interact with others in ways that can transit the virus), environmental problems (high- vs. low-rate consumers of a natural resource), and a host of other domains.

The logistic model occurring in Exercises 2.5 and 2.6, developed quite early by the Belgian mathematician Verhulst (1838), is often used to describe the growth of populations.

Before refining them along several lines (see, e.g., Exercise 2.5), the "classical" predator–prey model was independently invented in the mid 1920's by and named after A. Lotka and V. Volterra. Hofbauer and Sigmund (1988) provide a good introduction as well as some ramifications.

An extended analysis of the cobweb phenomenon dealt within Exercise 2.13 may lead to instability and even chaos (see Chiarella, 1988).

Part II

Applied Optimal Control

3

Tour d'Horizon: Optimal Control

This chapter presents the fundamentals of optimal control theory. In the first section we give a short historical survey, introducing the reader to the main ideas and notions. Subsequently we introduce the standard problem of optimal control theory.

We state Pontryagin's Maximum Principle, distinguishing between the cases without and with mixed path or pure state inequality constraints. The Hamilton–Jacobi–Bellman equation is used to give an informal proof of the Maximum Principle. Then the Maximum Principle is extended to the case of an infinite planning horizon. This is followed by the presentation of a one-dimensional optimal control model, and we give an economic interpretation of the Maximum Principle.

3.1 Historical Remarks

Control theory is a fruitful and interdisciplinary area of research that combines several mathematical traditions to address a rich array of applications spanning many fields. Our topic, *optimal control*, is only one of many branches of control theory, but it is an important one. Before proceeding to explain Pontryagin's Maximum Principle, which underpins optimal control theory, we give a short history of the origins of control theory generally, and its marriage with optimization to form optimal control theory. For more complete accounts of the history of optimal control theory, see Dreyfus (1965); Fernández and Zuazua (2003); Fleming (1988); Neustadt (1976), and Pesch and Bulirsch (1994).

As is quite often the case, necessity was the mother of invention, and the methods explored in this book are founded not just on basic mathematics, but also on efforts to solve practical engineering problems. Maxwell's analysis of the stability of steam engines (ca 1868), the feedback concept developed by control engineers in the 1920s, and Wiener's "cybernetics" contributions in the 1940s are usually mentioned as milestones in the development of what has been called systems, or control, engineering. However, Fernández and Zuazua

(2003) traced these roots much further back, referring to the Romans, Greeks, and even ancient Mesopotamia, where the control of irrigation systems was well-known.

Around the middle of the twentieth century progress in *automatic* control, coupled with a number of noteworthy mathematical achievements including Wald's sequential analysis, Bellman's dynamic programming, and Pontryagin's Maximum Principle, led to the emergence of control theory as a recognized new field. Positioned as it is at the interaction of control (or systems) engineering and mathematics, control theory may be seen as one of the most interdisciplinary areas of science today.

Another important intellectual thread is *optimization.* This branch of mathematics deals with the improvement of a decision variable in order to minimize a cost or to maximize a utility. After the Second World War, linear and nonlinear programming showed a remarkable development in both theory and applications from which optimal control draws heavily.

The mathematics of control theory has its roots in the calculus of variations. This important part of mathematical analysis was created in the second half of the seventeenth century. In 1662 Fermat derived the *law of refraction* as the solution to a minimum time problem. Almost one-quarter of a century later, Newton determined the optimal shape of a ship's bow as a trade-off between a low *resistance* in the water and a high cargo load of the ship (cf. Goldstine, 1980). Usually the famous brachistochrone problem of Johann Bernoulli is seen as a starting point of the calculus of variations. Bernoulli asked the "most ingenious mathematicians of the whole globe" to find the time-minimal path of a mass point between two points in the gravitational field of the earth.[1] Bernoulli and, later Euler and Lagrange, contributed substantially to the development of the calculus of variations. In the nineteenth century, Hamilton, Weierstrass, and Jacobi developed the theory further. The resulting methods have been (and still are) of great value in analytical mechanics. (Hence we speak of "Hamiltonian systems.") A century later, related ideas played a role in dynamic economics (compare, e.g., Magill, 1970).

The rise of the calculus of variations was closely connected with problems arising in physics. It took about 250 years until the first economic applications were made. Evans (1924) studied the dynamic pricing problem for a monopolist, whereas Ramsey (1928) analyzed neoclassical capital accumulation by using Euler's equation.[2] Other early highlights include an analysis of the optimal exploitation of exhaustible resources, see Hotelling (1931).

[1] In a fine survey on the development of optimal control, Sussmann and Willems (1997) stated that optimal control was born in 1696 with Bernoulli's solution of the brachistochrone problem.

[2] Ramsey's model is the fundamental optimal growth model. Based on it, a series of substantial extensions has been proposed. It may be interpreted not only as a macroeconomic model for nationwide capital accumulation, but also in a microeconomic framework for a firm that determines its optimal capital accumulation program over time.

Pontryagin's Maximum Principle likewise had its roots in engineering problems. In the 1950s, engineers in the Soviet Union were wrestling with problems arising in steering aircraft. They discussed their problems with mathematicians at the Steklov Institute in Moscow. Pontryagin and his group became interested in this field, and their research resulted in the famous *Maximum Principle*, the technique that underpins much of the present book and others on optimal control theory (see Boltyanski, Gamkrelidze, & Pontryagin, 1956).

It is not surprising that such a momentous result drew on the work of several individuals or that controversy should emerge over who should get how much credit for which ideas. This is not the place to delve into the melodrama of geniuses' egos. The priority questions have been discussed by others; see, e.g., Boltyanski (1994); Gamkrelidze (1978) and Pesch and Bulirsch (1994). What is clear now is that there have been important precursors of Pontryagin, Boltyanski, Gamkrelidze, and Mishchenko (1962), e.g., Bushaw (1952); Hestenes (1950, 1965); McShane (1939) and Valentine (1937) in the US, as well as Feldbaum (1965), and others in Russia. Likewise, it seems clear that there are several independent roots of optimal control theory. There is, however, no doubt that optimal control is an extension of the calculus of variations and that one essential contribution of the Russian school was the introduction of an explicit control variable. Even today the control variable is often denoted by the letter u, taken from the Russian word *upravlenije* meaning *control* (compare Boltyanski, 1994, p. 9).

Another independent intellectual thread in the development of intertemporal optimization is Bellman's approach, known as *dynamic programming*. Note that this method was also invented by Isaacs (1965) (see Breitner, 2005, for a comprehensive discussion). Remarkably enough, Pesch and Bulirsch (1994) recently discovered that precursors of both the Maximum Principle and the Bellman equation can already be found in Carathéodory's work (Carathéodory, 1926, 1935). Using the so-called *royal road in the calculus of variations*, it turned out that the optimal control conditions are consequences of Carathéodory's results.

After the publication of Pontryagin's *Mathematical Theory of Optimal Processes* in English (1962), Pontryagin's Maximum Principle started its triumphal journey, transforming thinking in many fields, including applications in economics and management.[3] Among the first important publications were Arrow and Kurz (1970); Cass (1965, 1966); Hadley and Kemp (1971); Intriligator (1971) and Shell (1967, 1969) in *economics*, as well as

[3] The first book on applications of Pontryagin's Maximum Principle to economic problems was Arrow and Kurz (1970), in which an analysis of optimal growth was given. The applications explored the question of whether or not fiscal instruments (taxation, expenditures, and debt management) led to an optimal intertemporal allocation of resources in the presence of constraints imposed by private-sector behavior. It took another four years for the publication of a monograph on Operations Research applications. Bensoussan, Hurst Jr., and Näslund (1974) dealt with production, inventory, marketing, and other management issues.

Bensoussan et al. (1974); Näslund (1966, 1969); Sethi (1978) and Thompson (1968) in *management problems* and *Operations Research.*

The recent history of optimal control theory has been characterized by three types of development that have a prominent place in this book:

1. The Maximum Principle is extended to new types of problems, e.g., distributed parameter problems such as those discussed in Sect. 8.3.
2. Advances in computational power and numerical methods allow larger and more complicated problem formulations to be addressed, cf. Chap. 7.
3. Novel application areas are explored outside of physics and engineering and the classic applications in growth economics and firm management, notably in health, natural resources, pollution, environment, epidemiology, demography, and the economics of crime.

An interesting survey on developments of optimal control theory has been collected by Fleming (1988). This booklet, a *Panel on Future Directions in Control Theory,* surveyed a variety of emerging directions in optimal control theory and its applications.

The *European Journal of Control* (vol. 13/1, 2007) provides a readable collection on the development of control from its beginnings to the present (and even to the "day after tomorrow"). Particularly interesting are the papers by Willems (2007), Mayne (2007) and Kurzhanski (2007). That issue gives a comprehensive survey on the development of control theory and its various (mostly engineering) applications,[4] it contains also interesting details on the origins of optimal control in the fifties and sixties.

The spectrum of control techniques and applications is much too wide to be reviewed in this book. Our intention is to develop some decidedly non-traditional applications (drug control, crime, and counter-terror) to open the reader's mind to the variety of possibilities and to inspire a new generation to carry these wonderful mathematical tools into new application areas.

3.2 A Standard Optimal Control Problem

One main purpose of this book is to introduce the reader to the process of modeling and solving optimal control problems in economics, management, environmental planning, resource extraction, health planning, and other fields. Our aim is to present a mathematical description that is general enough to apply to many intertemporal decision situations and simple enough to assure tractability.

[4] One reason for this collection of papers was the 50th anniversary of The International Federation of Automatic Control (IFAC), founded in 1957. The dawn of modern control theory was the appearance of the papers of Pontryagin and his associates on the Maximum Principle, by Bellman on dynamic programming and Kalman on the general theory of control systems at the first IFAC World Congress (1960) in Moscow.

We consider a class of optimal control problems that frequently occurs in the modeling of dynamic processes, starting with a standard problem that can serve as a basis for extensions.

Suppose that the state of a system at time t can be described by an n-dimensional real column vector[5]

$$x(t) = (x_1(t), x_2(t), \dots, x_n(t))' \in \mathbb{R}^n, \quad t \in [0, T].$$

Here $T > 0$ denotes the *terminal time* or *horizon date* of the process. In many economic applications the terminal time is infinity. In that case the time interval $[0, T]$ is replaced by $[0, \infty)$. These are referred to as *infinite time horizon* problems and will be considered in Sect. 3.7.

Suppose that there is a decision-maker who is able to influence the development of the state variable over time by choosing an m-dimensional *control value* $u(t)$ at time t

$$u(t) = (u_1(t), u_2(t), \dots, u_m(t))' \in \Omega\,(x(t), t)\,, \quad t \in [0, T],$$

where the control (function) $u(\cdot)$ is piecewise continuous. One of the flavors of optimal control theory is the inclusion of constraints on the control variables; that means that a *control region* $\Omega(x(t), t)$ is given with $u(t) \in \Omega\,(x(t), t)$. In the denotation of the control region we omit the arguments and shortly write Ω, if there is no ambiguity.

We assume that the evolution of the state can be described by an ODE

$$\dot{x}(t) = f(x(t), u(t), t) \quad \text{for} \quad t \in [0, T] \tag{3.1a}$$

$$\text{s.t.} \quad x(0) = x_0, \tag{3.1b}$$

and *terminal* or *end constraints*:

$$x_i(T) = x_i^T, \quad i = 1, \dots, n' \tag{3.1c}$$

$$x_i(T) \geq x_i^T, \quad i = n' + 1, \dots, n'' \tag{3.1d}$$

$$x_i(T)\,\text{free}, \quad i = n'' + 1, \dots, n, \tag{3.1e}$$

where $n' \geq 0$, $n'' \geq 0$, $n' + n'' \leq n$, $f : \mathbb{R}^n \times \mathbb{R}^m \times \mathbb{R} \to \mathbb{R}^n$ is a vector-valued function $f = (f_1, f_2, \dots, f_n)'$, where for all $i = 1, \dots, n$, $f_i(x, u, t)$ and $\partial f_i(x, u, t)/\partial x$ are continuous with respect to their arguments. Equation (3.1a) is called the *system dynamics* or the *state dynamics*. It describes how the current state $x(t)$ and the decision-maker's action $u(t)$ at time t influence the rate of change of the state at time t.

Definition 3.1 (Admissible Pair and Control). *The pair of functions* $(x(\cdot), u(\cdot)) : [0, T] \to \mathbb{R}^n \times \mathbb{R}^m$ *is called an* admissible pair *of (3.1) if* $u(\cdot)$ *is piecewise continuous, for which the left- and right-hand limit exist and* $x(\cdot)$

[5] Note that $(\dots)'$ denotes the transposition of a row vector to a column vector.

is continuous and piecewise continuously differentiable, which satisfies for all points t where $u(\cdot)$ is continuous:

$$\begin{aligned} \dot{x}(t) &= f(x(t), u(t), t) \\ \text{s.t.} \quad x(0) &= x_0, \end{aligned}$$

and at the terminal time T

$$\begin{aligned} x_i(T) &= x_i^T, \quad i = 1, \dots, n' \\ x_i(T) &\geq x_i^T, \quad i = n'+1, \dots, n'' \\ x_i(T) &\textit{ free}, \quad i = n''+1, \dots, n \end{aligned}$$

and

$$u(t) \in \Omega\,(x(t), t)\,, \quad \textit{for all} \quad t \in [0,\, T].$$

The function $x(\cdot)$ is called a state trajectory *or simply a* trajectory *with* initial condition x_0 *and* terminal conditions *(3.1c)–(3.1e), the function $u(\cdot)$ is called an* admissible control. *For conventional reasons we decide that at a point of discontinuity t of the control $u(\cdot)$*

$$u(t) := u(t^-),$$

and the control is defined to be continuous at time zero and the terminal time T.

The goal of the decision-maker is to choose an admissible control $u(\cdot)$ in an optimal way. For this purpose, we suppose that the decision-maker has the *objective functional*

$$V(u(\cdot)) = \int_0^T \mathrm{e}^{-rt} g(x(t), u(t), t)\,\mathrm{d}t + \mathrm{e}^{-rT} S(x(T), T). \tag{3.2}$$

The expression $g(x(t), u(t), t)$, where $g : \mathbb{R}^n \times \mathbb{R}^m \times \mathbb{R} \to \mathbb{R}$, measures the instantaneous *profit* (*utility, cost*) derived by applying the control $u(t)$ at time t when the current state is $x(t)$ and r is nonnegative and called *discount rate*. The term $S(x(T), T)$ denotes the *salvage* or *scrap value* associated with the *terminal state* $x(T)$. The salvage value can be thought of as the payoff or reward for being in state $x(T)$ at the end of the planning horizon. The functions $g(x, u, t)$ and $\partial g(x, u, t)/\partial x$ are assumed continuous with respect to their arguments and the salvage value $S : \mathbb{R}^n \times \mathbb{R} \to \mathbb{R}$ is assumed to be continuously differentiable with respect to x and T.

The basic optimal control problem consists of maximizing[6] the functional $V(\cdot)$ defined in (3.2) over all admissible controls $u(\cdot)$, while taking into account that the evolution of the state is determined by the system dynamics (3.1a), the initial condition (3.1b), and the terminal constraints (3.1c)–(3.1e).

The role of the state variable x has already been mentioned. It is the concept of the state that distinguishes static optimization from intertemporal optimization (dynamic programming). It should be stressed that the current state $x(t)$ cannot be influenced *directly* by the decision-maker. The state variable summarizes the result of *past* decisions.[7]

The instrument by which the evolution of the system can be steered is the control variable $u(t)$. Capital accumulation by investment is an example that makes this distinction clear. The capital stock, $x(t)$, is a state whose future value can be influenced (indirectly) by the current investment rate, $u(t)$, but the decision-maker cannot simply decide to have an arbitrary amount of capital at this instant. Capital can be accumulated only over time.

Let us summarize the optimal control problem in the standard form denoted as (OC):[8]

$$\max_{u(\cdot)} \left\{ \int_0^T \mathrm{e}^{-rt} g(x(t), u(t), t)\, \mathrm{d}t + \mathrm{e}^{-rT} S(x(T), T) \right\} \tag{3.3a}$$

$$\text{s.t.} \quad \dot{x}(t) = f(x(t), u(t), t), \quad t \in [0, T] \tag{3.3b}$$

$$x(0) = x_0 \tag{3.3c}$$

$$x_i(T) = x_i^T, \quad i = 1, \ldots, n' \tag{3.3d}$$

$$x_i(T) \geq x_i^T, \quad i = n' + 1, \ldots, n'' \tag{3.3e}$$

$$x_i(T)\ \text{free}, \quad i = n'' + 1, \ldots, n \tag{3.3f}$$

$$u(t) \in \Omega\left(x(t), t\right), \quad \text{for all} \quad t \in [0, T], \tag{3.3g}$$

where the problem is to find an admissible pair $(x(\cdot), u(\cdot))$ maximizing the objective functional (3.3a). The optimal control problem OC is called a problem of *free end value* if $x_i(T)$ is free for all $i = 1, \ldots, n$, otherwise it is called a problem with *terminal constraints*.

---

6 Throughout this book the problems are formulated as maximization problems. Note that any minimization problem can be transformed into a maximization problem via multiplication by -1, i.e.,

$$x_0 = \operatorname{argmin}\{g(x)\} \quad \text{iff} \quad x_0 = \operatorname{argmax}\{-g(x)\}.$$

7 The state $x(t)$ contains the *information* required to decide optimally. The assumption is that the state history from $s = 0$ to $s = t$ is *summarized* in $x(t)$. In a sense this feature may be compared to the *Markov property* of stochastic processes.

8 Note that here and in the following time arguments are omitted if there is no ambiguity.

Definition 3.2 (Optimal Solution and Control). *Let* $(x^*(\cdot), u^*(\cdot))$ *be an admissible pair for* OC *(3.3). If*

$$V(u^*(\cdot)) \geq V(u(\cdot)), \quad \textit{for all admissible controls} \quad u(\cdot);$$

then $(x^*(\cdot), u^*(\cdot))$ *is called an* optimal solution (path) *for* OC *(3.3),* $u^*(\cdot)$ *is called an* optimal control *and* $x^*(\cdot)$ *is called an* optimal state trajectory. *A part of the optimal solution* $(x^*(\cdot), u^*(\cdot))$ *is called an* (optimal) arc.

The value function *for* OC *(3.3) with respect to the initial state* x_0 *is denoted by*

$$V^*(x_0) := V(u^*(\cdot)).$$

Remark 3.3. In a general setting and especially to derive existence conclusions for an optimal solution of the problem OC (3.3) the control is assumed to be measurable (instead of piecewise continuous), then the state function is absolute continuous (instead of piecewise continuously differentiable) (see, e.g., Vinter, 2000).

An optimal control problem can have zero, one, or multiple optimal solutions. In what follows we present conditions allowing us to determine optimal solutions, starting with the necessary optimality conditions that are provided by Pontryagin's Maximum Principle.

3.3 The Maximum Principle of Optimal Control Theory

Generally speaking there exist two different approaches to considering dynamic optimization problems. The first approach can be seen as a generalization of the usual maximization problem from calculus (see Chap. 4) and is inseparably connected with the work of Pontryagin et al. (1962). In the second approach the dynamical structure is utilized. In that case the theory of dynamic programming (introduced by Bellman) provides the theory to solve the optimization problem.

In the following sections we present the central result of Pontryagin's approach to optimal control theory, known as Pontryagin's Maximum Principle and also the Hamilton–Jacobi–Bellman (HJB) equations, proved by Bellman (1957). The theorems are stated without rigorous proofs and should be seen as a summary of results needed to tackle optimal control problems.

3.3.1 Pontryagin's Maximum Principle

In this subsection the core theorem of Pontryagin's seminal work is stated. As already noted this approach can be seen as a generalization of the necessary conditions provided by the calculus for maximizing functions or the calculus of variations for maximization of functionals. Pontryagin's Maximum Principle provides necessary conditions that an optimal solution has to satisfy, i.e., given that an optimal solution exists, it has to satisfy the conditions of the Maximum Principle. The necessary conditions will be formulated as an ODE, extending the already given state dynamics into an ODE of dimension $2n$, finally justifying our detailed consideration of ODEs in the previous chapter. Let us state the theorem in one of its simplest forms:

Theorem 3.4 (Pontryagin's Maximum Principle). *Let* $(x^*(\cdot), u^*(\cdot))$ *be an optimal solution of* OC *(3.3) with free terminal state. Then there exists a continuous and piecewise continuously differentiable function* $\lambda(\cdot)$*, with* $\lambda(t) \in \mathbb{R}^n$ *satisfying for all* $t \in [0, T]$*:*

$$\mathcal{H}(x^*(t), u^*(t), \lambda(t), t) = \max_{u \in \Omega(x^*(t),t)} \mathcal{H}(x^*(t), u, \lambda(t), t), \tag{3.4a}$$

and at every point t *where* $u(\cdot)$ *is continuous*

$$\dot{\lambda}(t) = r\lambda(t) - \mathcal{H}_x\left(x^*(t), u^*(t), \lambda(t), t\right). \tag{3.4b}$$

Furthermore the transversality condition

$$\lambda(T) = S_x(x^*(T), T) \tag{3.4c}$$

holds, where

$$\mathcal{H}\left(x, u, \lambda, t\right) := g\left(x, u, t\right) + \lambda f\left(x, u, t\right) \tag{3.4d}$$

is called the Hamiltonian *of the problem* OC *(3.3).*

Equation (3.4b) is called the adjoint equation and the variable λ is called the *costate* or *adjoint variable.* By definition the costate is a row vector $\lambda = (\lambda_1, \dots, \lambda_n)$.

The usual proof of Pontryagin's Maximum Principle via the HJB equation is postponed until Sect. 3.4.1, where the dynamic programming approach is presented. In Chap. 4 two other proofs are presented, where the first proof parallels the theory of mathematical programming and the theory of optimal control and a second proof is given by the calculus of variations.

If the reader is eager to see an example, on how to apply Pontryagin's Maximum Principle we refer him/she to Sect. 3.3.7, where the Ramsey model is presented as an introductory example. Many other examples will follow in the subsequent chapters and many problems are formulated in the exercises at the end of each chapter.

Remark 3.5. In case that the optimal control $u^*(\cdot)$ is discontinuous at $t \in [0, T]$ (3.4a) holds for the left as well as the right-hand limit of $u^*(\cdot)$ at t.

Definition 3.6 (Canonical System and Extremal Solution). *Let* $\hat{u}(\cdot)$ *be an admissible control of* OC *(3.3) satisfying the* Hamiltonian maximizing condition

$$\hat{u}(t) \in \underset{u\in\Omega(x(t),t)}{\operatorname{argmax}} \mathcal{H}(x(t),u,\lambda(t),t);$$

then the ODE

$$\dot{x}(t) = \mathcal{H}_\lambda\left(x(t),\hat{u}(t),\lambda(t),\lambda_0,t\right) = f\left(x(t),\hat{u}(t),t\right) \tag{3.5a}$$

$$\dot{\lambda}(t) = r\lambda(t) - \mathcal{H}_x\left(x(t),\hat{u}(t),\lambda(t),\lambda_0,t\right), \tag{3.5b}$$

is called the canonical system *of* OC *(3.3).*[9]

Let $(\hat{x}(\cdot),\hat{\lambda}(\cdot))$ be a solution of the canonical system (3.5), which satisfies the initial condition (3.3c), the transversality condition (3.4c) and the terminal constraints (3.1c)–(3.1e); then $\hat{x}(\cdot)$ is called an extremal state (trajectory) *and the pair $(\hat{x}(\cdot),\hat{u}(\cdot))$ is called an* extremal solution *of the problem* OC *(3.3).*

Remark 3.7. The canonical system (3.5) together with the initial condition (3.3c) and the transversality condition (3.4c) determines a $2n$ boundary value problem (BVP, see Sect. 2.12.2). Algorithms for solving such problems are presented in Chap. 7.

Remark 3.8. Throughout this book the term *equilibrium* (see Definition 2.15) is used to describe the long-run (asymptotic) behavior of a dynamical system, when it converges to a fixed point. Synonymously, we use the denotation "fixed point" or "steady state" of a differential equation. This concept must not be confounded with an *economic equilibrium*. The latter refers to the equality of supply and demand, i.e., a clearance of the markets or, more generally, to a situation in which the decisions of economic agents (producers, consumers, government, etc.) are made in a consistent manner. An equilibrium in economic sense is inherently different from equilibrium in the sense of dynamical systems, i.e., from a long-run steady state. Whether an optimal path of a control problem or its asymptotic value is an economic equilibrium depends on the economic interpretation of the intertemporal decision problem (e.g., whether the markets are cleared, or the budget restrictions are satisfied). Equilibria in the sense of fixed points of the underlying dynamical systems may or may not be economic equilibria. In an economic equilibriun no one of the agents can gain by a unilateral deviation from the equilibrium solution; compare the concept of a Nash equilibrium given in Definition 8.4.

An important function is the:

Definition 3.9 (Maximized Hamiltonian). *Let $\mathcal{H}(x,u,\lambda,t)$ be the Hamiltonian (3.4d), then the function*

$$\mathcal{H}^*\left(x,\lambda,t\right) = \max_{u\in\Omega(x,t)} \mathcal{H}(x,u,\lambda,t)$$

is called the maximized Hamiltonian.

[9] Note that we define the derivative of a real-valued function with respect to a row vector as a column vector. In particular this convention allows us to omit the transposition sign in (3.5a).

Remark 3.10. At this place we have to note a potential notational confusion between two different fields. The Hamiltonian of classical mechanics corresponds to the maximized Hamiltonian of Pontryagin. One has to take care to distinguish between the Hamiltonian and the maximized Hamiltonian when crossing into the literature on classical mechanics.

Remark 3.11. The Hamiltonian $\mathcal{H}$ defined in (3.4d) is also called the *current-value Hamiltonian* contrary to the *present-value Hamiltonian* defined as

$$\tilde{\mathcal{H}}(x, u, \lambda, t) = \mathrm{e}^{-rt} g\left(x, u, t\right) + \tilde{\lambda}(t) f\left(x, u, t\right).$$

The current-value notation is widely used in optimal control literature, especially in economic fields. For the present-value notation the reader can prove in Exercise 3.1 that the conditions:

$$\tilde{\mathcal{H}}(x^*(t), u^*(t), \tilde{\lambda}(t), t) = \max_{u \in \Omega(x(t),t)} \tilde{\mathcal{H}}(x^*(t), u, \tilde{\lambda}(t), t) \tag{3.6a}$$

$$\dot{\tilde{\lambda}}(t) = \tilde{\mathcal{H}}_x(x^*(t), u^*(t), \tilde{\lambda}(t), t) \tag{3.6b}$$

$$\tilde{\lambda}(T) = \mathrm{e}^{-rT} S_x(x^*(T), T), \tag{3.6c}$$

are equivalent to the necessary conditions (3.4) stated in Pontryagin's Maximum Principle, by the transformation

$$\tilde{\mathcal{H}}(x, u, \lambda, t) := \mathrm{e}^{-rt} \mathcal{H}(x, u, \lambda, t), \quad \text{and} \quad \tilde{\lambda}(t) := \mathrm{e}^{-rt} \lambda(t).$$

Due to the previous remark we define:

Definition 3.12 (Autonomous Optimal Control Problem). *An optimal control problem* OC *(3.3) is called an* autonomous optimal control problem *if the functions $g : \mathbb{R}^n \times \mathbb{R}^m \to \mathbb{R}$, $f : \mathbb{R}^n \times \mathbb{R}^m \to \mathbb{R}^n$ and the control region $\Omega(x)$ do not explicitly depend on the time argument t.*

Remark 3.13. For autonomous optimal control problems the current-value notation has the advantage that the corresponding canonical system becomes an autonomous ODE.

Next we formulate the Maximum Principle for an optimal control problem *OC* (3.3) with terminal constraints:

Theorem 3.14 (Maximum Principle With Terminal Constraints). *Let $(x^*(\cdot), u^*(\cdot))$ be an optimal solution of* OC *(3.3) with terminal constraints (3.1c)–(3.1e). Then there exist a continuous and piecewise continuously differentiable function $\lambda(\cdot)$, with $\lambda(t) \in \mathbb{R}^n$ and a constant $\lambda_0 \geq 0$ such that for all $t \in [0, T]$:*

$$(\lambda_0, \lambda(t)) \neq 0$$

$$\mathcal{H}(x^*(t), u^*(t), \lambda(t), \lambda_0, t) = \max_{u \in \Omega(x(t),t)} \mathcal{H}(x^*(t), u, \lambda(t), \lambda_0, t) \tag{3.7a}$$

and at every point t where u(·) is continuous

$$\dot{\lambda}(t) = r\lambda(t) - \mathcal{H}_x\left(x^*(t), u^*(t), \lambda(t), \lambda_0, t\right),$$

and the transversality conditions

$$\begin{aligned}
&\lambda_i(T) \text{ no conditions} \quad i = 1, \dots, n' \\
&\lambda_i(T) \geq \lambda_0 S_{x_i}(x^*(T), T), \quad \text{and} \\
&\qquad \left(\lambda_i(T) - \lambda_0 S_{x_i}(x^*(T), T)\right)\left(x_i^* - x_i^T)\right) = 0, \quad i = n'+1, \dots, n'' \\
&\lambda_i(T) = \lambda_0 S_{x_i}(x^*(T), T), \quad i = n''+1, \dots, n
\end{aligned}$$

hold, where

$$\mathcal{H}(x, u, \lambda, \lambda_0, t) := \lambda_0 g(x, u, t) + \lambda f(x, u, t). \tag{3.7b}$$

Note that the Hamiltonian (3.7b) explicitly depends on the constant λ_0. In the majority of economic applications λ_0 can be assumed to be greater than zero. However, in general this condition is not satisfied; see, e.g., Example (3.79). Thus we define:

Definition 3.15 (Normal and Abnormal Problems). *If for an optimal solution of an optimal control problem the necessary conditions only hold if* $\lambda_0 = 0$ *the problem is called an* abnormal problem.[10] *Otherwise it is called a* normal problem.

Nevertheless, for a certain class of problems the assumption is satisfied, which we already used in the formulation of Pontryagin's Maximum Principle (Theorem 3.4):

Proposition 3.16. *For an optimal control problem* OC *(3.3) without terminal constraints the problem is normal and* λ_0 *can be set to one.*

Proof. Note that if $\lambda_0 > 0$, the Hamiltonian $\mathcal{H}$ can be divided by λ_0 and taking λ/λ_0 instead of λ satisfies the conclusions of Pontryagin's Maximum Principle, with $\lambda_0 = 1$. Hence we only have to prove that the case $\lambda_0 = 0$ can be excluded. Let us assume that $\lambda_0 = 0$; thus $\mathcal{H} = \lambda f$, which together with the transversality condition (3.4c) yields $\lambda(T) = 0$. Owing to the linearity of equation (3.4b) in λ, we find $\lambda(t) = 0$ for all $t \in [0, T]$, contradicting the necessary condition $(\lambda_0, \lambda(t)) \neq 0$. □

Remark 3.17. In the light of Proposition 3.16 it was therefore justified to formulate the Hamiltonian in Theorem 3.4 without λ_0.

---

[10] The term *abnormal* is used, since in that case the conditions of Pontryagin's Maximum Principle do not change if g is replaced by any other function.

If the functions $f(x,u,t)$ and $g(x,u,t)$ are considered as two times continuously differentiable with respect to u a further necessary condition can be stated:

Theorem 3.18 (Legendre–Clebsch Condition). *Let the Hamiltonian $\mathcal{H}(x,u,\lambda,\lambda_0,t)$ be two times continuously differentiable with respect to u and $(x^*(\cdot), u^*(\cdot))$ be an optimal solution. Then for every $t \in [0, T]$ where $u^*(t)$ lies in the interior of the control region $\Omega(x^*(t),t)$ the Hessian matrix*

$$\mathcal{H}_{uu}(x^*(t),u^*(t),\lambda(t),\lambda_0,t) \quad \textit{is negative semidefinite.} \tag{3.8}$$

This condition is called the Legendre–Clebsch condition. *If the matrix (3.8) is negative definite it is said that a* strict Legendre–Clebsch condition *holds.*

Proof. Since $\mathcal{H}$ is twice continuously differentiable in u, we know from calculus (see Theorem A.104) that, if u^* lies in the interior of the control region Ω, the maximum condition (3.4a) implies $\mathcal{H}_u = 0$ at $(x^*,\ u^*)$. Furthermore for a maximum the Hessian matrix with respect to u has to be negative semidefinite, concluding the proof. □

3.3.2 Some General Results

In the following we summarize some general results concerning the properties of the maximized Hamiltonian and the controls. These results will prove useful in the subsequent chapters:

Definition 3.19 (Regular Hamiltonian). *The Hamiltonian $\mathcal{H}$ is said to be* regular *if for any pair of values $(x,\ \lambda)$ and time $t \in [0,\ T]$ the set*

$$\underset{u\in\Omega(x,t)}{\operatorname{argmax}}\, \mathcal{H}\,(x,u,\lambda,\lambda_0,t)$$

is a singleton.

Lemma 3.20. *For given x, λ and t let the Hamiltonian be strictly concave with respect to u and the control region $\Omega(x,t)$ be convex. Then the Hamiltonian is regular.*

Proof. To the contrary assume there exist x, λ and t such that $u_1 \neq u_2$ are both maximizers of the Hamiltonian, i.e., with $\mathcal{H}(u) := \mathcal{H}(x,u,\lambda,\lambda_0,t)$ we find

$$\mathcal{H}(u_1) = \mathcal{H}(u_2).$$

Then by the strict concavity of $\mathcal{H}$ with respect to u we find for $0 < \kappa < 1$

$$\begin{aligned}\mathcal{H}(\kappa u_1 + (1-\kappa)u_2) &> \kappa\mathcal{H}(u_1) + (1-\kappa)\mathcal{H}(u_2)\\ &= \mathcal{H}(u_2).\end{aligned}$$

By the convexity of $\Omega(x,t)$ the control value $\kappa u_1 + (1-\kappa)u_2 \in \Omega$, contradicting that u_2 is a maximizer of the Hamiltonian. □

An immediate consequence of this lemma is:

Corollary 3.21. *Let the Hamiltonian be two times continuously differentiable with respect to* u *and the Hessian matrix* $\mathcal{H}_{uu}(x, u, \lambda, \lambda_0, t)$ *be negative definite for given* x, λ *and* t *and* $\Omega(x, t)$ *be convex; then the Hamiltonian is regular.*

For a regular Hamiltonian we find:

Proposition 3.22. *Let* $u^*(\cdot)$ *be an optimal control of* OC *(3.3) and let the Hamiltonian be regular; then* $u^*(\cdot)$ *is continuous on* $[0, T]$.

Proof. If $u^*(\cdot)$ is discontinuous at some $t \in [0, T]$ then the left- and right-hand limit at t are different, contradicting the uniqueness of the control value. □

The next proposition taken from Feichtinger and Hartl (1986) proves important to show the existence of points exhibiting multiple optimal solutions (see Chap. 5):

Proposition 3.23. *Let us consider an autonomous and normal problem* OC *(3.3), with* $m \geq n$, $\Omega = \mathbb{R}^m$. *Suppose the Hamiltonian* $\mathcal{H}$ *be two times continuously differentiable in* u, *strictly concave in* u *and* f_u *have full rank for all values of an admissible solution* $(x(\cdot), u(\cdot))$. *Then the maximized Hamiltonian* $\mathcal{H}^*(x, \lambda)$ *with maximizer* $u^*(x, \lambda)$ *is strictly convex in* λ *for any fixed* x, *achieving its minimum for* λ^* *satisfying* $f(x, u^*(x, \lambda^*)) = 0$.

Proof. First, we show the strict convexity of $\mathcal{H}^*$ with respect to λ, which is equivalent to

$$\mathcal{H}^*(x, \kappa\lambda_1 + (1-\kappa)\lambda_2) < \kappa\mathcal{H}^*(x, \lambda_1) + (1-\kappa)\mathcal{H}^*(x, \lambda_2).$$

Therefore let $\lambda_1, \lambda_2 \in \mathbb{R}^n$, and $0 < \kappa < 1$ be arbitrarily chosen, yielding

$$\begin{aligned}\mathcal{H}^*(x, \kappa\lambda_1 + (1-\kappa)\lambda_2) &= \mathcal{H}\left(x, u^*, \kappa\lambda_1 + (1-\kappa)\lambda_2\right)\\ &= \kappa\mathcal{H}\left(x, u^*, \lambda_1\right) + (1-\kappa)\mathcal{H}\left(x, u^*, \lambda_2\right)\\ &\leq \kappa\mathcal{H}^*\left(x, \lambda_1\right) + (1-\kappa)\mathcal{H}^*\left(x, \lambda_2\right),\end{aligned}$$

where $u^* = u^*(x, \kappa\lambda_1 + (1-\kappa)\lambda_2)$.

Next we show that for $\lambda_1 \neq \lambda_2$ equality does not hold. Otherwise assume that for $\lambda_1 \neq \lambda_2$ a κ_0 exists, where equality holds, i.e., there exists a (single!) u^* satisfying

$$\mathcal{H}(x, u^*, \kappa_0\lambda_1 + (1-\kappa_0)\lambda_2) = \kappa_0\mathcal{H}\left(x, u^*, \lambda_1\right) + (1-\kappa_0)\mathcal{H}\left(x, u^*, \lambda_2\right).$$

Thus u^* maximizes the Hamiltonian for each of the costate values λ_1, λ_2.

Owing to the strict concavity of the Hamiltonian with respect to u, its maximum is achieved for $\mathcal{H}_u = 0$ yielding

$$g_u(x, u^*) + \lambda f_u(x, u^*) = 0, \tag{3.9}$$

for $\lambda = \lambda_1, \lambda_2$.

Using the rank condition for f_u and $m \geq n$ we can chose n control coordinates (for simplicity these are the first n coordinates) such that the matrix

$$F := (f_{u_1}(x, u^*), \cdots, f_{u_n}(x, u^*))$$

is invertible and from (3.9), evaluated for λ_1, and λ_2, we find

$$(\lambda_1 - \lambda_2) f_{u_i}(x, u^*)' = 0, \quad i = 1, \ldots, n,$$

and therefore

$$(\lambda_1 - \lambda_2) F = 0.$$

But due to the nonsingularity of F this last equation is only satisfied for $\lambda_1 = \lambda_2$ contradicting the assumption $\lambda_1 \neq \lambda_2$ and proving the strict convexity of $\mathcal{H}^*$ with respect to λ.

To prove the last part of the proposition we use the strict concavity $\mathcal{H}_{uu} < 0$ and the implicit function theorem, yielding the differentiability of u with respect to λ and therefore

$$\mathcal{H}^*_\lambda = f + \mathcal{H}_u \frac{\partial u}{\partial \lambda} = f,$$

since $\mathcal{H}_u = 0$.

A strictly convex and continuously differentiable function achieves its minimum where its derivative equals zero (see Theorem A.104) and therefore

$$\mathcal{H}^*_\lambda = 0 = f(x, u^*),$$

which completes the proof. □

3.3.3 The Maximum Principle for Variable Terminal Time

Extending the problem OC (3.3), we may be interested in choosing the terminal time T optimally. Thus we not only have to find the optimal solution over $[0, T]$, but also to consider T as a controlled variable, such that the objective function is maximized on an optimally chosen time interval $[0, T^*]$, i.e., we replace the objective function (3.3a) of OC (3.3) by

$$\max_{u(\cdot), T} \left\{ \int_0^T \mathrm{e}^{-rt} g(x(t), u(t), t) \, \mathrm{d}t + \mathrm{e}^{-rT} S(x(T), T) \right\},$$

with $T > 0$.

Remark 3.24. Note that the explicit dependence of the salvage value on the terminal time T is now of importance.

For these problems the following theorem provides a further necessary condition:

Theorem 3.25 (Maximum Principle for Variable (Free) Terminal Time). *Given the optimal control problem* OC *(3.3) with variable terminal time T and without terminal constraints, let $(x^*(\cdot),\, u^*(\cdot))$ be an optimal solution on the optimal time interval $[0,\, T^*]$, with $T^* \in (0,\, \infty)$. Then the conditions of Theorem 3.4 are satisfied together with*

$$\mathcal{H}\left(x^*(T^*), u^*(T^*), \lambda(T^*), T^*\right) = rS\left(x^*(T^*), T^*\right) - S_T\left(x^*(T^*), T^*\right). \quad (3.10)$$

Given the results of Pontryagin's Maximum Principle the condition (3.10) can be deduced by simple calculus.

Proof. Consider the function

$$V(t) = \int_0^t \mathrm{e}^{-rs} g\left(\tilde{x}(s), \tilde{u}(s), s\right)\, \mathrm{d}s + \mathrm{e}^{-rt} S\left(\tilde{x}(t), t\right),$$

on a slightly increased time interval $[0, T^* + \varepsilon)$ with $\varepsilon > 0$, where

$$\tilde{u}(s) := \begin{cases} u^*(s) & s \in [0,\, T^*] \\ u^*(T^*) & s \in (T^*, T^* + \varepsilon), \end{cases}$$

and let $\tilde{x}(\cdot)$ be the corresponding solution of the state dynamics. The extended control $\tilde{u}(\cdot)$ is admissible and can be assumed continuous on $(T^* - \varepsilon, T^* + \varepsilon)$ for ε small enough. Therefore the state trajectory $\tilde{x}(\cdot)$ and hence $V(\cdot)$ are continuously differentiable on $(T^* - \varepsilon, T^* + \varepsilon)$. Denoting the time variable as T, a necessary condition (see Theorem A.103) for $V(\cdot)$ to achieve its maximum at T^* yields

$$\frac{\mathrm{d}V(T^*)}{\mathrm{d}T} = 0.$$

Using the transversality condition (3.4c) this equation can therefore explicitly be written as

$$\begin{aligned}\frac{\mathrm{d}V(T^*)}{\mathrm{d}T} &= \mathrm{e}^{-rT^*}\left(g(T^*) + S_x \dot{x}(T^*) + S_T\left(T^*\right) - rS\left(T^*\right)\right) \\ &= \mathrm{e}^{-rT^*}\left(g(T^*) + \lambda(T^*) f(T^*) + S_T\left(T^*\right) - rS\left(T^*\right)\right) \\ &= \mathrm{e}^{-rT^*}\left(\mathcal{H}(T^*) + S_T\left(T^*\right) - rS\left(T^*\right)\right) = 0.\end{aligned}$$

Dividing the last equation by e^{-rT^*} finally proves condition (3.10). □

The problem of variable terminal time can further be extended to the case in which the optimal terminal time T^* can only be chosen from a time interval $T^* \in [\underline{T},\, \bar{T}]$. In that case the following theorem holds:

Theorem 3.26 (Maximum Principle for Constrained Variable Time). *Given the optimal control problem* OC *(3.3) with variable terminal time T restricted to the interval $[\underline{T}, \bar{T}]$ and without terminal constraints, let $(x^*(\cdot), u^*(\cdot))$ be an optimal solution on the optimal time interval $[0, T^*]$. Then the conditions of Theorem 3.4 are satisfied together with*

$$\begin{array}{c}\mathcal{H}\left(x^*(T^*), u^*(T^*), \lambda(T^*), T^*\right) - \\ rS\left(x^*(T^*), T^*\right)\end{array} \begin{cases} \leq -S_T\left(x^*(T^*), T^*\right) & \text{for } T^* = \underline{T} \\ = -S_T\left(x^*(T^*), T^*\right) & \text{for } \underline{T} < T^* < \bar{T} \\ \geq -S_T\left(x^*(T^*), T^*\right) & \text{for } T^* = \bar{T}. \end{cases}$$

Remark 3.27. Theorem 3.26 also embraces the problem of an unconstrained terminal time with $\underline{T} = 0$ and $\bar{T} = \infty$.

If the optimal control problem with terminal constraints is considered we find:

Corollary 3.28. *Given the optimal control problem* OC *(3.3) with variable terminal time T restricted to the interval $[\underline{T}, \bar{T}]$ and with terminal constraints, let $(x^*(\cdot), u^*(\cdot))$ be an optimal solution on the optimal time interval $[0, T^*]$. Then the conditions of Theorem 3.14 are satisfied together with*

$$\begin{array}{c}\mathcal{H}\left(x^*(T^*), u^*(T^*), \lambda(T^*), \lambda_0, T^*\right) - \\ r\lambda_0 S\left(x^*(T^*), T^*\right)\end{array} \begin{cases} \leq -\lambda_0 S_T\left(x^*(T^*), T^*\right) & \text{for } T^* = \underline{T} \\ = -\lambda_0 S_T\left(x^*(T^*), T^*\right) & \text{for } \underline{T} < T^* < \bar{T} \\ \geq -\lambda_0 S_T\left(x^*(T^*), T^*\right) & \text{for } T^* = \bar{T}. \end{cases}$$

3.3.4 Economic Interpretation of the Maximum Principle

We now turn to one of the most important considerations in the economic application of optimal control theory, the reliance of dynamic cost-benefit analysis on the concept of a shadow price and the Hamiltonian. Many optimal control problems in economic applications can be written as (OCE):

$$\max_{u(\cdot)} \left\{ \int_0^T \mathrm{e}^{-rt} g(x(t), u(t))\, \mathrm{d}t + \mathrm{e}^{-rT} S(x(T), T) \right\}$$
$$\text{s.t.} \quad \dot{x}(t) = f(x(t), u(t)), \quad t \in [0, T]$$
$$x(0) = x_0,$$

where T is often assumed to be infinite (see Sect. 3.7).

The widespread application of the Maximum Principle to economic problems has at least two explanations:

- The first is that it provides a system of $2n$ differential equations for the state and the costate vectors. The *qualitative* analysis of these (generally) nonlinear differential equations provides valuable structural insight into the shape of the optimal paths. This will be discussed in detail in most of the control models to follow.

- The second explanation is the usefulness of the interpretation of the adjoint variable as a shadow price (or imputed value):

$$\lambda(t) = V_x^*(x(t)), \tag{3.11}$$

where $V^* : \mathbb{R}^n \to \mathbb{R}$ is the value function of the optimal control problem (see Definition 3.2). Therefore $\lambda(t)$ measures the marginal worth of an increment in the state at time t when moving along the optimal trajectory. In other words, $\lambda(t)$ is the highest (hypothetical) price that a rational decision-maker would be willing to pay for an additional unit of the state variable at time t when the problem is solved optimally.

Note that

$$\lambda f = \sum_{j=1}^{n} \lambda^j f^j = \sum_{j=1}^{n} \frac{\partial V^*}{\partial x^j} \frac{\mathrm{d}x^j}{\mathrm{d}t}$$

measures the total marginal change in the objective functional value for an infinitesimal change of all state variables.

Let us now interpret the Hamiltonian in economic terms. Assume that a decision-maker is facing a standard optimal control problem. At any instant of time t, he or she considers the state of the system $x(t)$ and has to choose the control value $u(t)$ optimally. The selection of the control value has *two* effects:

- A *direct* one, namely to generate an instantaneous profit $g(x(t), u(t))$
- An *indirect* effect, namely to change the state through $f(x(t), u(t))$

It is possible to maximize the direct utility without taking into consideration the future development of the dynamical system. Such myopic behavior is clearly suboptimal in a genuine intertemporal decision problem. In the context of the capital accumulation problem such a policy would mean consuming everything and investing nothing. (*Devil may care.*) The other extreme is the *Stalinist policy* of minimal consumption. The decision-maker consumes virtually nothing and invests the whole product to increase the capital stock as fast as possible.

It is intuitively clear that a rational decision-maker avoids such extreme solutions. He or she solves the dynamic decision problem by maximizing a "weighted" sum of both goals, namely by maximizing the instantaneous profit and the rate of change of the state variable. Or, to put it in other words: Since we cannot compare apples to pears, it is necessary to "weight" the rate of change of the state, i.e., $\mathrm{d}x/\mathrm{d}t$, by its value $\partial V^*/\partial x$. Thus we get

$$\mathcal{H}(x, u, \lambda) = g(x, u) + \lambda f(x, u) = g(x, u) + V_x^*(x)\dot{x}.$$

Note that the dimensions of the given quantities, denoted by square brackets $[\cdot]$, are compatible since:

$$[\mathcal{H}] = [g] = \text{value/time unit},$$
$$[V_x^*] = \text{value/state unit, and}$$
$$[\dot{x}] = \text{state/time unit.}$$

The economic interpretation of the Hamiltonian maximizing condition is that the Maximum Principle decouples the *dynamic* optimization problem in $[0, T]$ to create an infinite set of *static optimization* problems at any $t \in [0, T]$. The Hamiltonian can be interpreted as a *generalized* profit rate, including direct and indirect profits, to be maximized at each instant of time t.

It remains for us to interpret the adjoint equation that describes the evolution of the dynamic shadow prices. Rewritten as

$$-\dot{\lambda} + r\lambda = g_x + \lambda f_x, \tag{3.12}$$

the adjoint equation admits an economic equilibrium interpretation of the type *marginal cost equals marginal revenue.* The left side of (3.12) denotes the rate of decrease or increase of the shadow price $-\dot{\lambda}$, plus the (bank) interest rate $r\lambda$, i.e., the marginal cost of holding the capital. The total marginal value $\mathcal{H}_x$ of investing the capital equals the sum of the direct marginal contribution, g_x, and the indirect marginal contribution, λf_x. This gives the marginal revenue of investing the capital. The shadow price is determined by equalizing marginal cost and marginal revenue.

The economic interpretation of the transversality (terminal) condition (3.4c) is obvious, since at the horizon date T only the marginal revenue has to be considered and therefore $\lambda(T) = S_x(x(T), T) = V_x^*(x(T))$.

To interpret the optimality conditions for the optimal terminal time T^*, we consider (3.10). Here S_T denotes the change of the salvage value per unit shift of the terminal time T. The term rS gives the opportunity cost if the process is not stopped at time T. Equation (3.10) provides a trade-off between termination of the process at time T on the one hand, and the continuation during a small time unit on the other.

To give the concrete interpretation for an investment production problem, by selling a machine at time T one gets $S(x, T)$ Euros and interests rS during the next time unit. Or the machine runs for this additional time unit generating a direct profit g, as well as a changing the selling price for $S_x f + S_T$.

If T^* is the optimal selling time, both decisions, i.e., to sell at T^* or to keep it for another time unit, lead to the same utility. This can be seen indirectly: if the internal marginal utility exceeds (is smaller than) the interest on the salvage value it is better to keep the machine (to sell it earlier). In both cases T^* is not optimal.

3.3.5 Sufficiency Conditions

In general Pontryagin's Maximum Principle only provides necessary conditions that an optimal solution has to satisfy. Under specific concavity or convexity, respectively, assumptions on the involved functions these conditions are also sufficient:

Theorem 3.29 (The Mangasarian Sufficiency Conditions). *Let the pair $(x^*(\cdot), u^*(\cdot))$, and function $\lambda(\cdot)$ satisfy Pontryagin's Maximum Principle with $\lambda_0 = 1$. Suppose that $\Omega(x,t)$ is convex for every $x \in \mathbb{R}^n$, $t \in [0, T]$, the partial derivatives of $g(x,u,t)$ and $f(x,u,t)$ are continuous with respect to their arguments and the Hamiltonian $\mathcal{H}$ is jointly concave in (x,u) for all t and additionally the salvage function $S(x,t)$ is concave in x; then $(x^*(\cdot), u^*(\cdot))$ is an optimal solution.*

If the Hamiltonian $\mathcal{H}$ is strictly concave in (x,u), then $(x^*(\cdot), u^*(\cdot))$ is the unique solution.

The following proof can also be found in Seierstad and Sydsaeter (1986).

Proof. We have to prove that for any admissible pair $(x^*(\cdot), u^*(\cdot))$

$$V(u^*) - V(u) = \int_0^T \mathrm{e}^{-rt} \left(g(x^*, u^*, t) - g(x,u,t)\right) \mathrm{d}t \\ + \mathrm{e}^{-rT} \left(S(x^*(T), T) - S(x(T),T)\right) \geq 0. \quad (3.13)$$

For the following derivation we use the abbreviations

$$\mathcal{H} := \mathcal{H}(x,u,\lambda,t), \ \mathcal{H}^* := \mathcal{H}(x^*, u^*, \lambda, t), \ S^* = S(x^*(T),T), \ S = S(x(T),T).$$

Then from the concavity of the $\mathcal{H}$ and S the inequalities (see Proposition A.112)

$$\mathcal{H}^* - \mathcal{H} \geq \mathcal{H}^*_x(x^* - x) + \mathcal{H}^*_u(u^* - u), \quad S^* - S \geq S^*_x(x^* - x)$$

follow, together with (see Proposition A.113)

$$\mathcal{H}^*_u(u^* - u) \geq 0 \quad \text{iff} \quad u^* \text{ satisfies the maximizing condition (3.7a).}$$

Combining these inequalities yields

$$\mathcal{H}^* - \mathcal{H} \geq \mathcal{H}^*_x(x^* - x) = \dot{\lambda}(x - x^*). \quad (3.14)$$

Therefore rewriting (3.13) as

$$V(u^*) - V(u) = \int_0^T \mathcal{H}^* - \mathcal{H} \,\mathrm{d}t + \int_0^T \lambda(\dot{x} - \dot{x}^*) \,\mathrm{d}t + \mathrm{e}^{-rT}(S - S^*),$$

we find by means of (3.14)

$$\begin{aligned} V(u^*) - V(u) &\geq \int_0^T \dot{\lambda}(x - x^*) \,\mathrm{d}t + \int_0^T \lambda(\dot{x} - \dot{x}^*) \,\mathrm{d}t + \mathrm{e}^{-rT} S^*_x(x^* - x) \\ &= \int_0^T \frac{\mathrm{d}}{\mathrm{d}t} \left(\lambda(x - x^*)\right) \mathrm{d}t + \mathrm{e}^{-rT} S^*_x(x^* - x) \\ &= \lambda(T)(x(T) - x^*(T)) - \mathrm{e}^{-rT} S^*_x(x - x^*) = 0, \end{aligned}$$

where for the last step we used the transversality condition.

In case of strict concavity the inequality is strict if either $x \neq x^*$ or $u \neq u^*$, concluding the proof. □

A further sufficiency condition can be stated known as:

Theorem 3.30 (The Arrow Sufficiency Conditions). *Let $(x^*(\cdot), u^*(\cdot))$, and function $\lambda(\cdot)$ satisfy Pontryagin's Maximum Principle with $\lambda_0 = 1$. If the maximized Hamiltonian $\mathcal{H}^*$ exists for all x and is concave in x for all t, and the salvage function $S(x, T)$ is concave in x, then $(x^*(\cdot), u^*(\cdot))$ is an optimal solution.*

If $\mathcal{H}^*$ is strictly concave in x, then $x^*(\cdot)$ (but not necessarily $u^*(\cdot)$) is unique.

The following proof uses a result of the theory of convex analysis (see Appendix A.3.4), specifically the existence of a supergradient.

Proof. Considering the proof of Theorem 3.29 we see that the crucial step was the derivation of the inequality (3.14). Thus if we can prove the inequality

$$\mathcal{H}(x^*, u^*, \lambda, t) - \mathcal{H}(x, u, \lambda, t) \geq \dot{\lambda}(x - x^*)$$

we are finished. From the definition of the maximized Hamiltonian we find

$$\mathcal{H}(x^*, u^*, \lambda, t) - \mathcal{H}(x, u, \lambda, t) \geq \mathcal{H}^*(x^*, \lambda, t) - \mathcal{H}^*(x, \lambda, t),$$

where $u \in \Omega(x, t)$ is arbitrary.

Since $\mathcal{H}^*$ is concave there exists a supergradient a (see Proposition A.121) satisfying

$$\mathcal{H}^*(x^*, \lambda, t) - \mathcal{H}^*(x, \lambda, t) \geq a(x^* - x).$$

Thus combining the last two inequalities the function

$$k(x) := \mathcal{H}(x^*, u^*, \lambda, t) - \mathcal{H}(x, u^*, \lambda, t) - a(x^* - x)$$

has the following properties

$$k(x) \geq 0, \quad \text{and} \quad k(x^*) = 0.$$

Since $k(x)$ is continuously differentiable and x^* is a minimizer $k_x(x^*) = 0$ has to hold. This yields

$$k_x(x^*) = -\mathcal{H}_x(x, u^*, \lambda, t) + a = 0,$$

showing that the supergradient is given by

$$a = -\dot{\lambda}$$

proving (3.14).

If $\mathcal{H}^*$ is strictly concave in x the strict inequality holds for $x \neq x^*$, whereas nothing can be said for the case $u \neq u^*$, which concludes the proof. □

Remark 3.31. Notice that the assumptions of the Mangasarian sufficiency conditions Theorem 3.29 imply the concavity of the maximized Hamiltonian $\mathcal{H}^*$ in x (see Exercise 3.13). Thus the sufficiency conditions of Arrow type are weaker than those of Mangasarian type.

Remark 3.32. Inspecting the proof of the previous theorem carefully shows that we do not need concavity of the maximized Hamiltonian for all state values x. If the set of admissible states $A(t) \subset \mathbb{R}^n$ at time t is convex, and the extremal state $x(t)$ is an interior point of $A(t)$, then Theorem 3.30 holds provided the maximized Hamiltonian is concave for $x(t) \in A(t)$ for all $t \in [0, T]$.

3.3.6 Existence of an Optimal Solution

We have to admit that the question of existence of an optimal solution for an optimal control problem is an important question in its own right. Searching among the solutions satisfying the necessary conditions overlooks the fact that there need not exist a solution at all. Early in the last century Tonelli (1915) recognized this important fact and formulated the *direct method of optimization*. It consists of the following steps for finding an optimal solution:

1. Show the existence of an optimal solution
2. Search among the paths satisfying the necessary conditions for those exhibiting the highest objective value

Only if both steps are carried out is it guaranteed that an optimal solution can be found. To clarify this point we take an example from Vinter (2000), where the unique path satisfying the necessary conditions is not an optimal solution. Let us consider the optimal control problem:

$$\max_{u(\cdot)} \left\{ - \int_0^1 x(t)u(t)^2 \, dt \right\} \tag{3.15a}$$

$$\text{s.t.} \quad \dot{x}(t) = u(t), \quad t \in [0, 1] \tag{3.15b}$$

$$x(0) = 0, \quad x(1) = 0. \tag{3.15c}$$

Remark 3.33. Omitting the first step of Tonelli's direct optimization method, we shall subsequently identify a unique path satisfying the necessary optimality conditions. But a simple calculation proves that, e.g., the pair

$$(u(t), x(t)) = (a(1 - 2t), at(1 - t)), \quad a \in \mathbb{R}$$

is an admissible solution, exhibiting an objective value of

$$a^3 \int_0^1 t(1 - t)((1 - 2t))^2 \, dt = \frac{a^3}{30}.$$

Thus for $a \in \mathbb{R}$ the absolute objective value can be made arbitrarily large, proving that in the set of admissible paths neither a maximizer nor a minimizer exist. At this point we are finished. In more complex situations it is not so easy to see, if either an optimal solution exists or not. Therefore the question of existence is often ignored and it is assumed that the optimal solution is among those satisfying the necessary conditions. At best one can give heuristic arguments for the existence of an optimal solution. For this problem the pathology is produced by the objective function (3.15a), which "rewards" an increase in the state as well as an increase in the control. Thus there is no mechanism for making it optimal to restrict either the state or the control.

The misleading result of a naive approach, in which the question of existence is omitted, is now analyzed in detail for the given problem. Using Theorem 3.14 we find the following necessary conditions, where the Hamiltonian

$$\mathcal{H}(x, u, \lambda, \lambda_0) = -\lambda_0 x u^2 + \lambda u$$

is continuously differentiable in u with $u \in \mathbb{R}$. Then the Hamiltonian maximizing condition yields

$$\mathcal{H}_u(x(t), u(t), \lambda(t), \lambda_0) = -2\lambda_0 x(t) u(t) + \lambda(t) = 0. \tag{3.16}$$

The problem is normal since otherwise, if $\lambda_0 = 0$, (3.16) becomes $\lambda(t) = 0$ contradicting $(\lambda_0, \lambda(t))$ for all t. Using (3.16) the costate can be expressed as

$$\lambda(t) = 2x(t)u(t) = 2x(t)\dot{x}(t)$$

yielding the adjoint equation

$$\begin{aligned} \dot{\lambda}(t) &= -\mathcal{H}_x(x(t), u(t), \lambda(t)) = u(t)^2 \\ \lambda(t) &= \lambda(0) + \int_0^t u(s)^2 \, \mathrm{d}s. \end{aligned}$$

Since (3.16) has to hold for every t it has to hold especially for $t = 0$, which implies $\lambda(0) = 0$ and therefore

$$\lambda(t) = \int_0^t u(s)^2 \, \mathrm{d}s.$$

But this last equation can be restated as

$$\begin{aligned} 2x(t)\dot{x}(t) &= \int_0^t u(s)^2 \, \mathrm{d}s \\ \frac{\mathrm{d}}{\mathrm{d}t}\left(x(t)^2\right) &= \int_0^t u(s)^2 \, \mathrm{d}s \\ x(1)^2 &= \int_0^1 \int_0^t u(s)^2 \, \mathrm{d}s \, \mathrm{d}t. \end{aligned} \tag{3.17}$$

Obviously $u \equiv 0$ satisfies the necessary conditions, but owing to (3.17) this is also the only admissible control. Since for any admissible control $u \not\equiv 0$, which satisfies the necessary conditions, the integral $\int_0^1 \int_0^t u(s)^2 \, ds \, dt > 0$, and therefore the terminal constraint $x(1) = 0$ is violated. On the other hand $u \equiv 0$ is not a maximizer, since, e.g., $\varepsilon t(1-t)$ with $\varepsilon > 0$, exhibits a larger objective value and is arbitrarily close to $u \equiv 0$.

This example clarifies the importance of existence theorems. But these theorems are generally of only limited practical use and are outside the scope of this book, especially for solving problems involving infinite time horizons. Therefore we do not state any of these theorems and instead refer the interested reader to Seierstad and Sydsaeter (1986) and Vinter (2000).

Remark 3.34. The optimal control problem (3.15) is analogous to the static optimization problem $\max_x x^3$. For the static problem zero is the unique point which satisfies the first order necessary conditions, but no maximizer or minimizer exist.

Another approach to finding a maximizer could be called the *indirect optimization method* in contrast to Tonelli's *direct optimization method.* This leads to the sufficiency conditions, in which the class of considered problems is restricted in such a way that one can show that a solution satisfying the necessary conditions is already an optimal solution. Some of these theorems are stated throughout the book. But these theorems are also of only limited use, since in many practical problems these restricted conditions are not satisfied.

Summing up, we have to admit that we cannot provide an easy tool for enabling the reader to decide whether the computed trajectory is an optimal solution or not. We can only refer to this delicate topic and caution the reader to argue carefully when denoting a solution of the canonical system as the optimal solution.

Next, we consider the neoclassical growth model of Ramsey (1928), which was one of the first applications of the Maximum Principle in economics.

3.3.7 How to Solve an Optimal Control Problem: A Simple Consumption vs. Investment Model

A core question in economics is how much of a given output (or income) should be used for consumption and how much should be invested. To focus on this optimal allocation problem, let us consider an economy with a single production factor K, i.e., capital. Denote by $F(K)$ the output produced by this capital stock. That output can either be consumed or invested. Let C be the amount of output allocated for consumption, so $I = F(K) - C$ is the corresponding investment rate. The capital stock develops according to the equation

$$\dot{K} = I - \delta K = F(K) - C - \delta K, \quad K(0) = K_0,$$

where δ denotes the rate of depreciation of capital, which is assumed to be a constant.

The Optimal Control Model

Let $U(C)$ be the utility society derives from consuming at rate C and r be the social discount rate. Then a central planner may consider the following problem:

$$\max_{C(\cdot)} \left\{ \int_0^T \mathrm{e}^{-rt} U(C)\,\mathrm{d}t + \mathrm{e}^{-rT} S\left(K(T)\right) \right\} \tag{3.18a}$$

$$\text{s.t.} \quad \dot{K} = F(K) - \delta K - C \tag{3.18b}$$

$$K(0) = K_0 > 0. \tag{3.18c}$$

Furthermore the following assumptions on the functions U and F are assumed to hold:

$$U'(C) > 0, \ \ U'(0) = \infty, \ \ U''(C) < 0, \quad \text{for all} \quad C \geq 0 \tag{3.19a}$$

$$F'(K) > 0, \ \ F''(K) < 0, \quad \text{for all} \quad K > 0 \tag{3.19b}$$

$$F(0) = 0, \ \ F'(0) > r + \delta, \ \ F'(\infty) < \delta. \tag{3.19c}$$

$$S''(K) \leq 0. \tag{3.19d}$$

The properties summarized in (3.19c), i.e., that the (production) function is "steep enough" at zero and "flat enough" for large arguments, are known as *Inada-conditions*.

The steps accomplished in the next paragraphs provide the starting point for all the models presented in this book. There is not one recipe for all optimal control problems: solving optimal control problems often takes ingenuity. However, it is usually sensible to try these steps, and for certain well-behaved standard problems, they are all that is required.

Maximizing the Hamiltonian

To use Pontryagin's Maximum Principle we have to consider the corresponding current-value Hamiltonian

$$\mathcal{H} = U(C) + \lambda \left(F(K) - \delta K - C\right). \tag{3.20}$$

Note that in absence of terminal constraints the problem is normal. From the assumption (3.19a) it follows that the Hamiltonian satisfies $\mathcal{H}_{CC} = U'' < 0$ and is therefore strictly concave in C. Thus the maximizer C^* of $\mathcal{H}(K, C, \lambda)$ for fixed K and λ lies in the interior of $\Omega = [0, \infty)$ and therefore satisfies

$$\mathcal{H}_C(K, C^*, \lambda) = U'(C^*) - \lambda = 0.$$

Therefore the Maximum Principle (3.4a) yields

$$\lambda = U'(C^*). \tag{3.21}$$

Since the function U is strictly concave, the inverse function U'^{-1} exists and C^* considered as a function of the costate λ is given by

$$C^*(\lambda) = U'^{-1}(\lambda). \tag{3.22}$$

Moreover the Hamiltonian is strictly concave in (K, C). To see that we use the positivity of λ, which can be deduced from (3.21) and (3.19a), implying the negative definiteness of the matrix

$$\begin{pmatrix} \mathcal{H}_{KK} & \mathcal{H}_{KC} \\ \mathcal{H}_{KC} & \mathcal{H}_{CC} \end{pmatrix} = \begin{pmatrix} \lambda F''(K) & 0 \\ 0 & U'' \end{pmatrix},$$

and therefore the concavity of the Hamiltonian. Since the salvage function is assumed concave in K (see (3.19d)) we can apply Theorem 3.29 assuring that any solution satisfying the necessary conditions is already optimal.

Deriving the Canonical System

Next we derive the adjoint equation using (3.4b). For the Hamiltonian (3.20) this yields

$$\dot{\lambda} = r\lambda - \mathcal{H}_K = r\lambda + \lambda(\delta - F'(K)) = (r + \delta - F'(K))\lambda. \tag{3.23}$$

Substituting (3.22) into the state equation (3.18b) establishes

$$\dot{K} = F(K) - \delta K - U'^{-1}(\lambda). \tag{3.24}$$

These equations (3.23) and (3.24) constitute the canonical system. Finally the transversality condition (3.4c) reads as

$$\lambda(T) = S_K(K(T)) \tag{3.25}$$

establishing, together with the initial condition (3.18c), a boundary value problem (BVP).

Transformation into the State–Control Space

From an application oriented point of view it is often more convenient to transform the canonical system into the state–control space. This representation allows an immediate interpretation of the results in the problem constituting terms. By means of the implicit function theorem, it follows that the optimal control given by (3.22) is differentiable with respect to time. Therefore we consider the total time derivative of $\mathcal{H}_C(K, C, \lambda) = 0$ yielding

$$\frac{\mathrm{d}}{\mathrm{d}t}\mathcal{H}_C = U''(C)\dot{C} - \dot{\lambda}.$$

Using the adjoint equation (3.23) and (3.21) we find

$$\dot{C} = \frac{U'(C)}{U''(C)}(\delta + r) - \frac{F'(K)}{U''(C)}$$

yielding, together with the state dynamics (3.18b), an ODE in K and C. Using (3.25) and (3.22) the boundary value for C at the terminal time T is given by

$$C(T) = {U'}^{-1}\left(S_K\left(K(T)\right)\right).$$

The analysis of this system, over an infinite time horizon, is postponed to Sect. 3.7.2, but can also be found in Arrow and Kurz (1970) and Intriligator (1971).

3.4 The Principle of Optimality

In the following subsections we first derive the Hamilton–Jacobi–Bellman (HJB) equation utilizing the principle of optimality and subsequently use the results to give a proof of the Maximum Principle, at least under a strong differentiability assumption of the value function. For notational simplicity we set, in this section, the discount rate r equal to zero.

3.4.1 The Hamilton–Jacobi–Bellman Equation

Besides the Maximum Principle another approach to solving optimal control problems is that of dynamic programming. Dynamic programming relies on a general principle in mathematics of embedding the original problem in a larger class of problems which are then solved.[11]

The optimal control problem OC (3.3) is therefore embedded in a family of problems (OCF), that are stated as follows:

$$\max_{u(\cdot)} \left\{ \int_t^T g(x(s), u(s), s)\, \mathrm{d}s + S(x(T), T) \right\} \tag{3.26a}$$

$$\text{s.t.} \quad \dot{x}(s) = f(x(s), u(s), s), \quad s \in [t, T] \qquad x(t) = \xi. \tag{3.26b}$$

For any pair (ξ, t) it is assumed that the corresponding optimal control problem exhibits an optimal solution. Then the value function (3.26a) is a function in (ξ, t) and is called the Bellman function $W(\xi, t)$. It is defined as

$$W(\xi, t) = \max_{u(\cdot)} \left\{ \int_t^T g(x(s), u(s), s)\, \mathrm{d}s + S(x(T), T) \right\}. \tag{3.27}$$

[11] A well-known example is the derivation of roots of a cubic equation, where the clue is the embedding of the real line into the complex plane.

Remark 3.35. In general the Bellman function $W(\xi, t)$ has to be defined as a supremum instead of a maximum, since in general the existence of an optimal solution cannot be assured. Nevertheless, the definition in (3.27) suffices for our needs. Moreover note that the Bellman function $W(\xi, t)$ and the value function $V^*(\xi)$ coincide at time $t = 0$, i.e., $W(\xi, 0) = V^*(\xi)$.

The derivation of the HJB equation uses the *principle of optimality*, which is formulated verbally in Bellman (1957) as:

Principle of Optimality. *An optimal policy has the property that whatever the initial state and initial decision are, the remaining decisions must constitute an optimal policy with regard to the state resulting from the first decision.*

In a mathematical formulation it becomes:

Theorem 3.36 (Principle of Optimality). *Assume that for each (ξ, t) with $t \in [0, T]$, $\xi \in \mathbb{R}^n$ there exists an admissible solution $(x^*(\cdot), u^*(\cdot))$ of problem* OCF *(3.26). Then $(x^*(\cdot), u^*(\cdot))$ is an optimal solution for the problem of class* OCF *(3.26) with $x(t) = \xi$ iff*

$$W(\xi, t) = \int_t^s g(x^*(\tau), u^*(\tau), \tau)\, \mathrm{d}\tau + W(x^*(s), s) \tag{3.28a}$$

$$\text{and} \quad W(x^*(T), T) = S(x^*(T), T). \tag{3.28b}$$

Relation (3.28a) is of major importance since it allows us to extract information about the relative change of $W(\xi, t)$ with respect to ξ when s tends to t, which results in the HJB equation:

Theorem 3.37 (Hamilton–Jacobi–Bellman Equation). *Let the Bellman function $W(\xi, t)$ be continuously differentiable with respect to ξ and t. Furthermore, for every initial point ξ and time t there exists an admissible control $u^*(\cdot)$ with a corresponding state trajectory $x^*(\cdot)$. Then $(x^*(\cdot), u^*(\cdot))$ is an optimal solution of* OCF *(3.26) iff the Bellman function $W(\xi, t)$ satisfies the* Hamilton–Jacobi–Bellman equation (HJB)*:*

$$-W_t(\xi, t) = \max_u \left\{ g(\xi, u, t) + W_x(\xi, t) f(\xi, u, t) \right\}, \tag{3.29a}$$

$$\text{and} \quad W(\xi, T) = S(\xi, T), \tag{3.29b}$$

for all $(\xi, t) \in \mathbb{R}^n \times [0, T]$ for which $u^*(\cdot)$ is continuous.

Remark 3.38. The derivation below relies on the continuous differentiability of the Bellman function $W(\xi, t)$ with respect to the state[12] ξ and time t. In general this assumption is not satisfied, even if the defining functions $g(x, u, t)$ and $f(x, u, t)$ are arbitrarily often differentiable in x and u (see, e.g., Example (3.81)). But also in this case analogous results can be proved. For this purpose a generalized concept of derivatives is introduced as in nonsmooth optimization (see, e.g., Clarke, 1983).

[12] Note that the derivative with respect to the state is denoted by W_x.

Proof. To prove the necessary part of the theorem we use (3.28) yielding

$$W(x^*(s), s) - W(\xi, t) = -\int_t^s g(x^*, u^*, \tau)\,\mathrm{d}\tau. \tag{3.30}$$

Owing to the assumed continuity of u^* at t, elementary calculus provides

$$\lim_{s \to t} \frac{-\int_t^s g(x^*, u^*, \tau)\,\mathrm{d}\tau}{s - t} = -g(x^*(t), u^*(t), t) = -g(\xi, u^*(t), t).$$

Under the given assumption of differentiability, the left-hand side of (3.30) can be written as

$$W(x^*(s), s) - W(\xi, t) = (W_x(\xi, t) f(\xi, u, t) + W_t(\xi, t))\,(s - t) + o\,(|s - t|)$$

yielding the identity

$$W_x(\xi, t) f(\xi, u^*(t), t) + W_t(\xi, t) + g(\xi, u^*(t), t) = 0$$

along an optimal solution $(x^*(\cdot), u^*(\cdot))$ with $\dot{x} = f(x, u, t)$. Thus to prove (3.29a) we only have to assure that the inequality

$$W_x(\xi, t) f(\xi, u, t) + W_t(\xi, t) + g(\xi, u, t) \leq 0$$

holds for any admissible (ξ, t) and control value u. Consider an arbitrary control value u and fix a state ξ and time t. For a small interval $[t,\ t + \varepsilon]$, where u is kept constant, the principle of optimality yields

$$W(\xi, t) \geq \int_t^{t+\varepsilon} g(\xi, u, t)\,\mathrm{d}t + W\left(x(t + \varepsilon), t + \varepsilon\right),$$

which can also be written as

$$h(\varepsilon) = W\left(x(t + \varepsilon), t + \varepsilon\right) - W(\xi, t) + \int_t^{t+\varepsilon} g(\xi, u, t) \leq 0.$$

Using $h(0) = 0$, we obtain

$$0 \geq \lim_{\varepsilon \to 0} \frac{h(\varepsilon) - h(0)}{\varepsilon} = W_x(\xi, t) f(\xi, u, t) + W_t(\xi, t) + g(\xi, u, t),$$

proving the HJB (3.29a).

To prove the sufficient part of the theorem let $u(\cdot)$ be an admissible control on the time interval $[t, T]$ with a corresponding state trajectory $x(\cdot)$ satisfying $x(t) = \xi$. From the HJB equation we find for all t

$$\begin{aligned} 0 &\geq g(x, u, t) + W_x f(x, u, t) + W_t(x, t) \\ &= g(x, u, t) + \frac{\mathrm{d}}{\mathrm{d}t} W(x, t) \end{aligned}$$

and therefore

$$0 \geq \int_t^T g(x,u,t)\,\mathrm{d}t + W(x(T),T) - W(x(t),t)$$

$$W(x(t),t) \geq \int_t^T g(x,u,t)\,\mathrm{d}t + S(x(T),T).$$

Using the same derivation for $(x^*(\cdot), u^*(\cdot))$ yields

$$W(\xi,t) = \int_t^T g(u^*,x^*,t)\,\mathrm{d}t + S(x^*(T),T).$$

This proves that $u^*(\cdot)$ maximizes the objective functional (3.26a) and therefore $(x^*(\cdot), u^*(\cdot))$ is an optimal solution. □

3.4.2 A Proof of the Maximum Principle

We now use the HJB equation to derive Pontryagin's Maximum Principle. The proof relies on the strong assumption that the Bellman function $W(\xi,t)$ is twice continuously differentiable with respect to ξ, which in general is not satisfied (see Example (3.81)). However, under this assumption the proof is exact.

Proof. From Theorem 3.37 we know that the HJB equation

$$-W_t(\xi,t) = \max_u \{g(\xi,u,t) + W_x(\xi,t)f(\xi,u,t)\} \tag{3.31}$$

$$\text{and} \quad W(\xi,T) = S(\xi,T)$$

are satisfied for an optimal solution $(x^*(\cdot), u^*(\cdot))$. If we formally define

$$\lambda(t) := W_x(x^*(t),t), \tag{3.32}$$

we may identify the right-hand side of the HJB equation as the Maximum Principle (3.4a)

$$\mathcal{H}(x^*,u^*,\lambda,t) = \max_u \mathcal{H}(x^*,u,\lambda,t).$$

Restating (3.31) in the form

$$\max_u \{g(\xi,u,t) + W_x(\xi,t)f(\xi,u,t) + W_t(\xi,t)\} = 0,$$

we see that for $u^*(t)$ the function

$$\Xi(\xi,t) := g(\xi,u^*(t),t) + W_x(\xi,t)f(\xi,u^*(t),t) + W_t(\xi,t)$$

achieves its maximum value of zero at $x^*(t)$. Since $W(\xi,t)$ is assumed to be two times continuously differentiable, $\Xi(\xi,t)$ is continuously differentiable in ξ, yielding

$$\Xi_x(x^*(t),t) = 0, \quad \text{for all } t$$

and therefore

$$g_x(x^*(t),u^*(t),t)+W_{xx}(x^*(t),t)f+W_x(x^*(t),t)f_x(x^*(t),u^*(t),t)+W_{tx}(x^*(t),t) = 0.$$

Using the identity

$$\begin{aligned}\frac{\mathrm{d}}{\mathrm{d}t}W_x(x^*(t),t) &= W_{xx}(x^*(t),t)\dot{x}^*(t) + W_{xt}(x^*(t),t)\\ &= W_{xx}(x^*(t),t)f(x^*(t),u^*(t),t) + W_{tx}(x^*(t),t)\end{aligned}$$

yields the adjoint equation

$$\dot{\lambda}(t) = -\mathcal{H}_x^*(x^*(t),u^*(t),\lambda(t),t).$$

And the transversality condition follows from the definition of $\lambda(t)$

$$\lambda(T) = W_x(x,T) = S_x(x,T),$$

which concludes the proof. □

The identity (3.32) provides an interpretation of the costate λ as a shadow price (see also Sect. 3.3.4).

3.5 Singular Optimal Control

The term *singular optimal control* applies to an important class of problems, for which the Legendre–Clebsch condition, that the Hamiltonian is negative semidefinite is trivially satisfied because $\det \mathcal{H}_{uu} = 0$.

Consider the optimal control problem OC (3.3) with the Hamiltonian

$$\mathcal{H}(x,u,\lambda,\lambda_0,t) = \lambda_0 g(x,u,t) + \lambda f(x,u,t), \tag{3.33}$$

and the occurring functions being two-times continuously differentiable with respect to u. Then a control value u^* lying in the interior of the control region Ω and satisfying the Maximum Principle will necessarily meet the condition

$$\mathcal{H}_u(x,u^*,\lambda,\lambda_0,t) = 0.$$

If, moreover, the strict Legendre–Clebsch condition holds, then u^* is a (local) maximizer of the Hamiltonian. Yet the Legendre–Clebsch condition is only of restricted use when it is trivially satisfied, i.e.,

$$\det \mathcal{H}_{uu}(x,u^*,\lambda,\lambda_0,t) = 0. \tag{3.34}$$

In a one-control model (3.34) reduces to $\mathcal{H}_{uu}(x,u^*,\lambda,\lambda_0,t) = 0$.

Remark 3.39. Depending on the rank k of the Hessian $\mathcal{H}_{uu}$, the Legendre–Clebsch condition provides only necessary conditions for k control coordinates and further conditions are necessary to characterize the remaining optimal control coordinates.

An important class of models exhibiting this kind of singularity are those problems in which the control variable u only appears linearly in the Hamiltonian $\mathcal{H}$. Therefore we define:

Definition 3.40. *Let the Hamiltonian $\mathcal{H}$ of (3.33) be linear in the control variable u. Then the optimal control $u^*(\cdot)$ is called a* singular control *on $[\underline{t}, \bar{t}]$ if*

$$\mathcal{H}_u\left(x^*(t), u^*(t), \lambda(t), \lambda_0, t\right) = 0,$$

for all $t \in [\underline{t}, \bar{t}]$. The corresponding optimal solution $(x^*(\cdot), u^*(\cdot))$ is called a singular path *or* singular arc.

To simplify the exposition we restrict ourselves to the case of a scalar control u and the linear problem (LP):

$$\max_{u(\cdot)} \int_0^T \mathrm{e}^{-rt} \left(g_1(x(t),t) + g_2(x(t),t)u(t)\right) \mathrm{d}t + \mathrm{e}^{-rT} S(x(T),T) \tag{3.35a}$$

$$\text{s.t.} \quad \dot{x}(t) = f_1(x(t),t) + f_2(x(t),t)u(t), \quad t \in [0, T] \tag{3.35b}$$

$$x(0) = x_0 \tag{3.35c}$$

$$u \in [a, b]. \tag{3.35d}$$

Another basic class for this kind of model comprise the so-called *linear–quadratic problems* (LQ):

$$\begin{aligned} &\max_{u(\cdot)} \int_0^T \mathrm{e}^{-rt} \left(x'(t)Qx(t) + u'(t)Pu(t)\right) \mathrm{d}t + \mathrm{e}^{-rT} S(x(T),T) \\ \text{s.t.} \quad &\dot{x}(t) = f_1(t)x(t) + f_2(t)u(t) + f_3(t), \quad t \in [0, T] \\ &x(0) = x_0 \\ &\Omega = \{u : \ u_i \in [a_i, b_i], \ i = 1, \dots, m, \quad \text{and} \quad a_i \le b_i \in \mathbb{R}\}. \end{aligned}$$

The values a_i and b_i may also depend on time t.

These linear and linear–quadratic problems are not the only models exhibiting singular arcs, since the defining property in Definition 3.40 may also hold for models in which not all control variables appear linearly. Moreover, examples of singular arcs exist in which the singular control is given by a nonlinear function. A classical example from orbit-transfer can be found in Breakwell (1964).

Considering (3.35), we define the so-called *switching function* as

$$\sigma(t) = \mathcal{H}_u(x(t), u(t), \lambda(t), \lambda_0, t). \tag{3.36}$$

The sign of the switching function $\sigma(\cdot)$ determines the optimal control value at time t, i.e., $u(t)$, by the Hamiltonian maximizing condition (3.4a)

$$u(t) = \begin{pmatrix} a \\ \text{singular} \\ b \end{pmatrix} \quad \text{if} \quad \sigma(t) \begin{pmatrix} < \\ = \\ > \end{pmatrix} 0.$$

To see this, remember that a bounded linear function achieves its maximum at the upper bound if it is strictly increasing, whereas for a strictly decreasing function the lower bound yields its maximum. Models of this type often exhibit a *bang-bang* solution. A *bang-bang control* denotes a control jumping from one boundary to another, i.e., jumping discontinuously from one extreme, say, a, to the other extreme b.[13]

Research in singular optimal control includes the analysis of the junction points between nonsingular and singular arcs and the formulation of necessary conditions characterizing those junction points and optimal singular arcs. For this, the concept of the *order of a problem* is of great importance:

Definition 3.41. *Let $u^*(\cdot)$ be a singular control; then the* (problem) order *is the smallest number q such that the $2q$th time derivative*

$$\frac{\mathrm{d}^{2q}}{\mathrm{d}t^{2q}} \mathcal{H}_u(x^*(t), u^*(t), \lambda(t), \lambda_0, t)$$

explicitly contains the control variable u. If no derivative satisfies this condition we define $q := \infty$.

Remark 3.42. Note that the odd time derivatives of $\mathcal{H}_u$ are always zero and therefore the order q is an integer. This is a consequence of the linearity of the functions in the control variable u and has first been proved in Robbins (1967). This concept of order can also be extended to the nonlinear case.

Remark 3.43. This definition of order can be extended to the case of a vector valued control. In that case one has to distinguish between singular and nonsingular coordinates of the control.

Remark 3.44. Strictly speaking, one has to distinguish between the *problem order* q and the *arc order* p, where the latter is defined as the non-vanishing of the $2p$th total time-derivative of $\mathcal{H}_u$ along the optimal solution $(x^*(\cdot), u^*(\cdot))$ (see Lewis, 1980). The arc order p may exceed the problem order q but not *vice versa.* However, since this distinction plays no role in subsequent material in this book, we simply assume that $p = q$ holds.

Now, the *generalized Legendre–Clebsch condition* can be formulated as a further necessary condition. The classical proof can be found in Robbins (1967).

[13] They have been called "bang-bang" controls because of the noise they made in mechanical implementations of such systems.

Theorem 3.45 (Generalized Legendre–Clebsch Condition). *Let the pair $(x^*(\cdot), u^*(\cdot))$ be an optimal solution of* LP *(3.35) with (problem) order $q < \infty$. Then the following property holds*

$$(-1)^q \frac{\partial}{\partial u} \frac{\mathrm{d}^{2q}}{\mathrm{d}t^{2q}} \mathcal{H}_u(x^*(t), u^*(t), \lambda(t), \lambda_0, t) \leq 0, \quad \textit{for every} \quad t \in (\underline{t}, \bar{t}). \quad (3.37)$$

This condition can also be derived for a vector-valued control. For further results the reader is referred to the survey article Michel (1996).

Another important approach, dating to Miele (1962), for solving a special class of singular optimal control models is presented in the following section. note that at this place we had to accept a compromise, since in the problem formulation of the following subsection the time horizon is assumed as infinite, which is an anticipation of Sect. 3.7. Anyhow, the infinite time horizon does not impose some new conditions, therefore we decided to present the theory in this form.

3.5.1 The Most Rapid Approach Path (MRAP)

An important class of optimal control models has the property that a singular arc should be approached as fast as possible. If one starts out on the singular arc, it is optimal to stay there. Otherwise the optimal solution is such that the singular arc is reached in the fastest possible manner.

This most rapid approach path (MRAP) relies on Green's integral theorem. It provides a useful tool for classifying the solution structure for one-state optimal control models. The specific technique used in the proof does not allow an immediate generalization to the higher-dimensional case and is therefore restricted to one-dimensional models.

We now consider the following class of one-dimensional autonomous optimal control models over an infinite time horizon:

$$\max_{u(\cdot)} \int_0^\infty \mathrm{e}^{-rt} g(x(t), u(t))\, \mathrm{d}t \quad (3.38a)$$

$$\text{s.t.} \quad \dot{x} = f(x(t), u(t)), \quad x(0) = x_0 \quad (3.38b)$$

$$u \in [u_1(x),\, u_2(x)] \quad (3.38c)$$

$$x \in [\underline{x},\, \bar{x}] \subset \mathbb{R}, \quad (3.38d)$$

with

$$g(x, u) = A(x) + B(x)\Phi(x, u) \quad (3.38e)$$

$$f(x, u) = a(x) + b(x)\Phi(x, u), \quad (3.38f)$$

where all functions occurring in (3.38e) and (3.38f) are assumed to be continuously differentiable with respect to x and u and $b(x) \neq 0$.

The following definition describes an MRAP:

Definition 3.46 (Most Rapid Approach Path (MRAP)). *A* most rapid approach path (MRAP) $x^*(\cdot)$ *to a given path* $\tilde{x}(\cdot)$ *has the property*

$$|x^*(t) - \tilde{x}(t)| \leq |x(t) - \tilde{x}(t)|, \quad \textit{for all} \quad t \in [0, \infty)$$

for all admissible state trajectories $x(\cdot)$, *i.e., trajectories satisfying (3.38b) and (3.38d).*

The following result transforms the problem into a more suitable form:

Proposition 3.47. *The model class (3.38) may be written in the following equivalent form:*

$$\max_{x(\cdot)} \int_0^\infty \mathrm{e}^{-rt} \left(M(x(t)) + N(x(t))\dot{x}(t) \right) \mathrm{d}t \tag{3.39a}$$

$$s.t. \quad x(0) = x_0, \quad \dot{x}(t) \in \Omega(x(t)), \quad x \in [\underline{x}, \bar{x}], \tag{3.39b}$$

where $M(x)$ *and* $N(x)$ *are continuously differentiable and the domain* Ω *depends continuously on* x.

Proof. From (3.38f) and $b(x) \neq 0$ it follows that

$$\Phi(x, u) = \frac{1}{b(x)} \left(\dot{x} - a(x) \right).$$

By inserting this into (3.38e), we obtain (3.39a) with

$$M(x) = A(x) - a(x)B(x)/b(x)$$
$$N(x) = B(x)/b(x).$$

Furthermore,

$$\Omega(x) = \{ a(x) + b(x)\Phi(x, u) : u \in [u_1(x), u_2(x)] \}.$$

□

Note that (3.39a) and (3.39b) define a variational problem.

Let us choose

$$v = \dot{x}$$

as a new control variable. According to the definition of the switching function $\sigma(t)$ in (3.36), a singular solution is given by the following relations:

$$\mathcal{H} = M(x) + N(x)v + \lambda v \tag{3.40a}$$
$$\sigma = \mathcal{H}_v(x, v, \lambda) = N(x) + \lambda = 0 \tag{3.40b}$$
$$\dot{\sigma} = N'(x)v + \dot{\lambda} = 0 \tag{3.40c}$$
$$\dot{\lambda} = r\lambda - \mathcal{H}_x = r\lambda - M'(x) - N'(x)v. \tag{3.40d}$$

From (3.40) we obtain the following equation to determine a singular solution $x = \hat{x}$:

$$I(\hat{x}) := rN(\hat{x}) + M'(\hat{x}) = 0. \tag{3.41}$$

The following theorem shows the optimality of the MRAP to the singular solution $\hat{x}$ or the boundaries $\underline{x}$ or $\bar{x}$, respectively:

Theorem 3.48 (MRAP Theorem). *Assume that (3.41) has a unique solution $\hat{x}$, which is admissible, i.e.,*

$$0 \in \Omega(\hat{x}), \quad \textit{and} \quad \underline{x} \leq \hat{x} \leq \bar{x}. \tag{3.42}$$

Assume further that

$$I(x) \begin{Bmatrix} > \\ < \end{Bmatrix} 0 \quad \textit{for} \quad \begin{cases} \underline{x} \leq x < \hat{x} \\ \hat{x} < x \leq \bar{x}, \end{cases} \tag{3.43}$$

and for any admissible trajectory $x(\cdot)$ it holds that

$$\lim_{t\to\infty} \mathrm{e}^{-rt} \int_{x(t)}^{\hat{x}} N(\xi)\mathrm{d}\xi \geq 0. \tag{3.44}$$

If for any $x_0 \in [\underline{x}, \bar{x}]$ an MRAP exists, then it is the optimal solution.

If there exists no admissible solution $\hat{x}$ of (3.41) and if

$$I(x) \begin{Bmatrix} > \\ < \end{Bmatrix} 0, \quad \textit{for all} \quad x \in [\underline{x}, \bar{x}]\,, \textit{ then the MRAP to } \begin{Bmatrix} \underline{x} \\ \bar{x} \end{Bmatrix} \textit{ is optimal.}$$

The core of the proof uses the fact that the integral in (3.39a) may be written as a curve integral. Transforming it by Green's theorem to a two-dimensional area integral allows one to show that any admissible solution gives a smaller integral than the MRAP solution. See Feichtinger and Hartl (1986, Chap. 3) or Kamien and Schwartz (1991, Sect. 13) for a full proof.

The MRAP theorem says that if it is possible to reach the singular arc, it should be done as fast as possible. Any departure from the singular level is suboptimal.

For a finite-time horizon optimal control problem with given terminal state $x(T) = x_T$, the result is carried over in an obvious way. If the planning horizon is large enough, it is optimal to reach the singular level $\hat{x}$ as fast as possible, then to stay on it as long as possible and leave $\hat{x}$ to arrive at the terminal state x_T. If, on the other hand, T is short, then the optimal path has the property that it approaches $\hat{x}$ as fast as possible (without violating the initial condition and terminal constraint). If (3.41) has more than one solution, there are multiple long-run equilibria (see Fig. 3.1):

Theorem 3.49. *Let $\hat{x}_1 < \tilde{x}_1 < \hat{x}_2 < \tilde{x}_2 < \cdots < \hat{x}_n$ be solutions of (3.41) with*

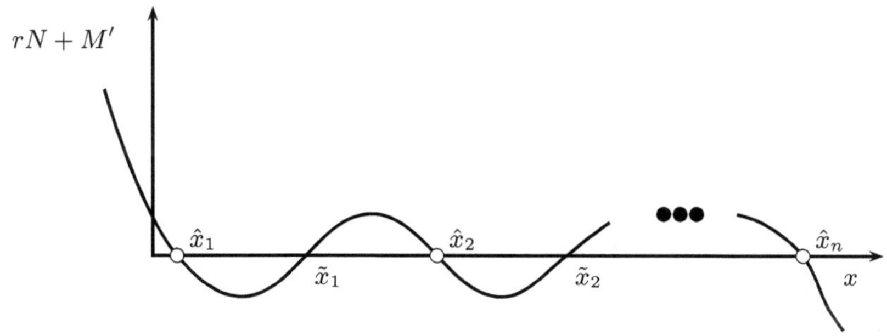

Fig. 3.1. The function $rN + M'$ in the case of multiple equilibria

$$I(x)\begin{Bmatrix} > \\ < \end{Bmatrix} 0 \quad for \quad x \in \begin{cases} (\tilde{x}_{i-1}, \hat{x}_i) & or\ x < \hat{x}_1 \\ (\hat{x}_i, \tilde{x}_i) & or\ x > \hat{x}_n. \end{cases}$$

Then the optimal solution is an MRAP reaching one of the equilibria given by $\hat{x}_1, \hat{x}_2, \ldots, \hat{x}_n$.

3.5.2 An Example From Drug Control that Excludes Singular Arcs

Crackdowns are a popular approach to drug enforcement. Kleiman (1988) defines them as "an intensive local enforcement effort directed at a particular geographic target." Frequently the target is a so-called "open-air" drug market where there is flagrant dealing that causes serious problems for the surrounding community. Caulkins (1993) developed a dynamical systems model of crackdowns, which we convert to an optimal control formulation in a manner similar to that in Baveja, Feichtinger, Hartl, Haunschmied, and Kort (2000). Unlike supply control efforts targeted elsewhere in the distribution chain, street-level enforcement has little impact on the drug price. Rather, its immediate objective is typically to drive markets underground, often to so-called "beeper markets" where transactions are surreptitious and arranged by cellular phone. Driving markets underground may reduce consumption by increasing so-called search-time costs, which are the nonmonetary costs of locating, purchasing, and using drugs (Kleiman, 1988; Moore, 1973). The primary goal, however, is not so much reducing drug use as restoring the civility of local communities by reducing the disorder, fear, and violence associated with flagrant markets. Ironically, street-level enforcement can be expensive precisely because catching dealers operating in flagrant markets is so easy. Aggressive crackdowns can swamp the criminal justice system because there are more dealers than prosecutors and prisons can handle. Hence the objective is to minimize the number of dealers $x(t)$ in the market while using the least possible amount of enforcement (denoted $u(t)$) over time, typically with some upper bound on the amount of enforcement that can be employed at any given time $u(t) \leq \bar{u}$. Thus by letting the constant k denote the social cost per active dealer relative to the monetary cost of enforcement, the objective is to

$$\max_{u(\cdot)} \int_0^T \mathrm{e}^{-rt} \left(-kx - u\right) \mathrm{d}t.$$

As in the one-state corruption model discussed in the previous chapter, Caulkins et al. (2006) suggested that dealers can be modeled as moving back and forth between selling in a particular market and alternative "employment" (whether legitimate work or selling drugs in other places or ways) in response to the difference in net wage. However, in the Caulkins et al. (2006) model the rate of movement is absolute, not per capita; since there are few "barriers to entry" into retail selling, there is no notion that people moving into deviance must be recruited by people who are already deviant. In the special case where dealers are risk-neutral, the state dynamics are written as

$$\dot{x} = c\left(\frac{\pi Q(x)}{x} - \frac{u}{x} - w_0\right),$$

where π is the "net profit" per sale, w_0 is the "reservation wage" available through alternative forms of work, and $Q(x)$ is the number of sales per day in that market. Sales are presumably an increasing but concave function of the number of sellers working in the market. An analytically convenient concave function is

$$Q(x) = \alpha x^\beta, \quad \beta \in (0, 1].$$

Since this model is of the form (3.38) we are inclined to find an MRAP as the optimal solution. Thus we transform the problem into the form (3.39) with

$$\begin{aligned}
M(x) &= x(w_0 - k) - \pi\alpha x^\beta \\
N(x) &= \frac{x}{c} \\
I(x) &= \frac{rx}{c} + w_0 - k - \beta\pi\alpha x^{\beta-1} \\
\Omega(x) &= c\left(\pi\alpha x^{\beta-1} - \frac{u}{x} - w_0\right).
\end{aligned}$$

In the previous section we have seen that a singular solution, in terms of the state, is a zero of $I(x)$, yielding

$$w_0 - k = \beta\pi\alpha x^{\beta-1} - \frac{rx}{c}. \tag{3.45}$$

A closer inspection reveals that condition (3.43) is violated, excluding the MRAP as an optimal solution (see Fig. 3.2). Still, singular arcs may exist unless they can be ruled out by the generalized Legendre–Clebsch condition in Theorem 3.45. Thus we determine the problem order q.

The corresponding calculations are elementary but tedious, finally yielding $q = 1$ since

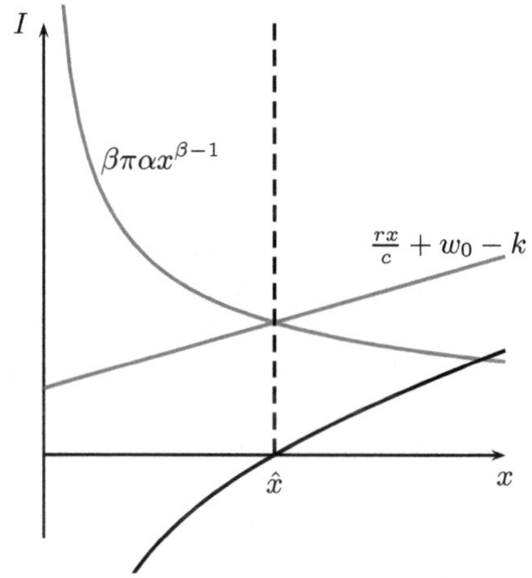

Fig. 3.2. Equation (3.45) is schematically depicted, revealing that $I(x) < 0$ for $x < \hat{x}$ and $I(x) > 0$ for $x > \hat{x}$

$$\begin{aligned}\frac{\partial}{\partial u}\ddot{\mathcal{H}}_u &= \frac{c^2}{x^3}\left((w_0 - k) + \beta\pi\alpha x^{\beta-1}(\beta - 2)\right)\\ &= \frac{c^2}{x^3}\left(-\frac{rx}{c} + \beta\pi\alpha x^{\beta-1}(\beta - 1)\right) < 0,\end{aligned}$$

where we used (3.45).

Therefore

$$-\frac{\partial}{\partial u}\ddot{\mathcal{H}}_u > 0$$

does not satisfy the generalized Legendre–Clebsch condition (3.37), which implies that singular arcs can be excluded.

Thus the optimal control $u^*(\cdot)$ is given by

$$u^*(t) = \begin{cases} 0 & \dot{\sigma} = \mathcal{H}_u < 0 \\ u \in [0, \bar{u}] & \dot{\sigma} = \mathcal{H}_u = 0 \\ \bar{u} & \dot{\sigma} = \mathcal{H}_u > 0. \end{cases}$$

3.5.3 An Example From Terror Control with an MRAP Solution

In this model we both simplify and extend the counter-terror model introduced in Sect. 2.5. Recall that the strength of a terror organization is given by $S(t)$ and that the control v ("fire strategies") both helps by inducing an outflow from the current stock of terrorists and hurts by increasing terrorists' recruitment. We simplify by omitting the other control ("water strategies") and by making the control-induced outflow linear instead of concave in the amount spent on the control. We extend it by allowing this control to vary over time so it is a dynamic, not a static control variable. Hence, the state dynamics taking into account these effects is given by

$$\dot{S}(t) = \tau + (k + \epsilon v(t))S(t)^{\alpha} - \mu S(t) - \eta v(t)S(t), \tag{3.46a}$$

with $k, \epsilon, \alpha, \mu, \eta > 0$ and $k > \mu$. (At this place we kept the time argument to stress the difference to the fire-and-water model in Sect. 2.5.)

In linear models it is important to include explicit bounds on the amount of control employed, so the counter-terror measure $v(\cdot)$ is constrained by $[0, \bar{v}]$.

We also extend the model formulation by introducing an objective functional. The goal is presumed to be minimizing the (discounted) weighted sum over time of the strength of the terrorist organization and the amount spent on terror control, or formulated as a maximization problem

$$\max_{v(\cdot)} \int_0^{\infty} \mathrm{e}^{-rt} \left(-cS(t) - v(t)\right) \mathrm{d}t. \tag{3.46b}$$

The model (3.46) has the form of problem OC (3.3) so we may try to apply the MRAP theorem (3.48).

To keep the analysis simple consider the special case with $\alpha = 1$ and $\tau = 0$. Hence the dynamics (3.46a) reduces to

$$\dot{S} = gS + \theta v S,$$

with $g = k - \mu > 0$ and $\theta = \epsilon - \eta$. Note that for $\theta \geq 0$ the counter-terror intervention is useless. It both costs money and increases the number of terrorists. Obviously it would never be optimal to use such a strategy, so to exclude such a situation we assume $\theta < 0$, together with $g + \theta\bar{v} \leq 0$.

We first have to determine the functions $M(S)$, $N(S)$ and $I(S)$ and the set $\Omega(S)$, which are

$$\begin{aligned}
M(S) &= -cS + \frac{g}{\theta} \\
N(S) &= -\frac{1}{S\theta} \\
I(S) &= -\frac{r}{S\theta} - c \\
\Omega(S) &= gS + \theta v S.
\end{aligned}$$

By the assumptions on the parameter values we find that condition (3.42), i.e., $0 \in \Omega(S)$, is satisfied. Next we have to prove the conditions (3.43) and (3.44). From the functional form of $I(S)$ the following results can be derived

$$\lim_{S\to 0} I(S) = \lim_{S\to 0} -\frac{r}{S\theta} - c = \infty > 0,$$

and

$$\lim_{S\to\infty} I(S) = \lim_{S\to\infty} -\frac{r}{S\theta} - c = -c < 0,$$

with

$$I(\hat{S}) = 0 \quad \text{for} \quad \hat{S} = -\frac{r}{c\theta},$$

proving (3.43). Likewise, from the positivity of $N(S)$, we see that (3.44) is verified. Hence the conditions of Theorem 3.48 are satisfied, and the optimal solution is the MRAP to the singular state $\hat{S}$.

For $S(0) < \hat{S}$ the optimal strategy is "do nothing," i.e., $v = 0$ until the state $\hat{S}$ is reached, then switch to the singular control $v^* = -\frac{g}{\theta}$. Otherwise, if $S(0) > \hat{S}$ one applies full control ($v^* = \bar{v}$) and switches at $S = \hat{S}$ to the singular control $v^* = -\frac{g}{\theta}$ (see Fig. 3.3a,b).

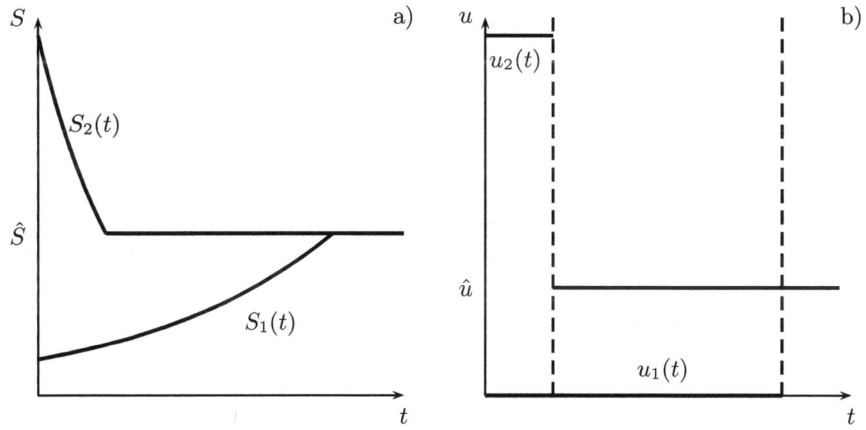

Fig. 3.3. Panel (**a**) depicts two MRAP solutions $S_1(t)$ and $S_2(t)$ of model (3.46), for which the initial states lie either beneath or above the state $\hat{S}$. Additionally panel (**b**) shows the corresponding optimal controls

In terms of the exogenous parameters c and θ the interpretation of the long-run state $\hat{S} = -\frac{r}{c\theta}$ is straight forward; an increase/decrease of the costs per terrorist or the efficiency of the counter-terror measures leads to a decrease/increase in the long-run optimal strength of the terrorists. In terms of the discount parameter r a myopic policy-maker is more willing to tolerate long-run growth in the terrorists strength than is a far sighted decision-maker. The reader is invited to analyze the model for the general case, with $\alpha \neq 1$ and $\tau > 0$, and provide parallel interpretations with respect to those additional parameters.

3.6 The Maximum Principle With Inequality Constraints

In this subsection we extend the standard problem OC (3.3) by allowing inequality constraints on the path. We formulate the following extended optimal control problem with inequality constraints (OCC):

$$\max_{u(\cdot)} \left\{ \int_0^T \mathrm{e}^{-rt} g(x(t), u(t), t)\,\mathrm{d}t + \mathrm{e}^{-rT} S(x(T), T) \right\} \tag{3.47a}$$

$$\text{s.t.} \quad \dot{x}(t) = f(x(t), u(t), t) \tag{3.47b}$$

$$x(0) = x_0, \quad t \in [0, T] \tag{3.47c}$$

$$c(x(t), u(t), t) \geq 0, \quad t \in [0, T] \tag{3.47d}$$

$$h(x(t), t) \geq 0, \quad t \in [0, T] \tag{3.47e}$$

$$a(x(T), T) = 0 \tag{3.47f}$$

$$b(x(T), T) \geq 0, \tag{3.47g}$$

where the functions $f : \mathbb{R}^n \times \mathbb{R}^m \times \mathbb{R} \to \mathbb{R}^n$, $g : \mathbb{R}^n \times \mathbb{R}^m \times \mathbb{R} \to \mathbb{R}$, $S : \mathbb{R}^n \times \mathbb{R} \to \mathbb{R}$, $c : \mathbb{R}^n \times \mathbb{R}^m \times \mathbb{R} \to \mathbb{R}^l$, $h : \mathbb{R}^n \times \mathbb{R} \to \mathbb{R}^k$, $a : \mathbb{R}^n \times \mathbb{R} \to \mathbb{R}^{l'}$, $b : \mathbb{R}^n \times \mathbb{R} \to \mathbb{R}^{l''}$ are continuously differentiable with respect to all their arguments. The problem is to find an admissible control $u^*(\cdot)$ maximizing the objective functional (3.47a) subject to the state dynamics (3.47b) and initial condition (3.47c), path constraints (3.47d–3.47e), and terminal constraints (3.47f–3.47g).

Note that the control region Ω is now explicitly given by

$$\Omega(x, t) = \{u : c(x, u, t) \geq 0\}.$$

Thus further necessary conditions can be stated taking the special form of the control region into account.

The path constraint given by the inequality $c(x, u, t) \geq 0$ is called *mixed path constraint* since it includes control as well as state variables. Whereas the inequality $h(x, t) \geq 0$ only includes state variables and is therefore called *pure state constraint*. This distinction is reasonable from a theoretical point of view since the pure state constraint cannot directly be transformed into a restriction of the control region Ω and can therefore not be formulated as a standard problem OC (3.3).

Mixed path constraints are easier to handle. This fact can intuitively be understood by considering that the control is under the direct influence of the decision-maker. Therefore nothing really dramatic changes if the control constraint becomes active. The optimal policy only has to be kept at this "boundary" value $c(x, u, t) = 0$ for a while. So the change from the inactive to the active constraint is "smooth." In the case of pure state constraints the situation is different. The decision-maker has no possibility of influencing the state directly; hence a considerably change in the control may be necessary to keep the state at its "boundary" value.

In the context of constraints, an important bit of terminology is that of entry and exit time. These denote the time points at which the constraints become active or inactive, respectively. These instants of time are defined as follows:

Definition 3.50. *Let $h(x,t) \geq 0$ be a pure state constraint. The time $\underline{t}$ is called an* entry time *if there exists an $\varepsilon > 0$ such that*

$$\begin{cases} h(x,t) > 0 & \underline{t} - \varepsilon < t < \underline{t} \\ h(x,t) = 0 & \underline{t} \leq t < \underline{t} + \varepsilon, \end{cases}$$

or $\bar{t}$ is called an exit time *if*

$$\begin{cases} h(x,t) = 0 & \bar{t} - \varepsilon < t \leq \bar{t} \\ h(x,t) > 0 & \bar{t} < t < \bar{t} + \varepsilon, \end{cases}$$

or $\underline{\bar{t}}$ is called a contact time *if*

$$\begin{cases} h(x,t) > 0 & \underline{\bar{t}} - \varepsilon < t < \underline{\bar{t}} \\ h(x,t) = 0 & t = \underline{\bar{t}} \\ h(x,t) > 0 & \underline{\bar{t}} < t < \underline{\bar{t}} + \varepsilon. \end{cases}$$

This definition applies in an obvious way to mixed path constraints $c(x,u,t) \geq 0$. The points of entry/exit and contact time are consequently called *entry/exit* and *contact points*, where entry and exit points are summarized as *junction points* and the corresponding times $\tilde{t}$ as *junction times.*

Definition 3.51 (Inactive/Active Constraint and Interior/Boundary Arc). *Let for x, u and t*

$$\mathcal{I}_m(x,u,t) := \{i : c_i(x,u,t) = 0, \ x \in \mathbb{R}^n, u \in \mathbb{R}^m, t \in [0, T], 1 \leq i \leq l\},$$

and

$$\mathcal{I}_s(x,u,t) := \{j : h_j(x,t) = 0, \ x \in \mathbb{R}^n, t \in [0, T], 1 \leq i \leq k\},$$

and let $(x(\cdot), u(\cdot))$ be an admissible pair of OCC *(3.47); then c_i or h_j is called an* active constraint *for $(x(\cdot), u(\cdot))$ at t if $i \in \mathcal{I}_m(x(t), u(t), t)$ or $j \in \mathcal{I}_s(x(t), t)$ otherwise it is called an* inactive constraint.

Let

$$T_I := \{t \in [0, T] : \mathcal{I}_m(x(t), u(t), t) = \emptyset, \ \text{and} \ \mathcal{I}_s(x(t), t) = \emptyset\},$$

and

$$T_B := \{t \in [0, T] : \mathcal{I}_m(x(t), u(t), t) \neq \emptyset, \text{ or } \mathcal{I}_s(x(t), t) \neq \emptyset\},$$

then

$$(x, u) : T_I \to \mathbb{R}^n \times \mathbb{R}^m$$

is called an interior arc *of* $(x(\cdot), u(\cdot))$, *and*

$$(x, u) : T_B \to \mathbb{R}^n \times \mathbb{R}^m$$

is called a boundary arc *of* $(x(\cdot), u(\cdot))$.

3.6.1 Mixed Path Constraints

Mixed path constraints explicitly depend on the control value and possibly also on the state and time. To assure that the necessary conditions formulated in the following theorem hold, the following *constraint qualification* (see also Sect. 4.2.4) has to be satisfied, namely that the $l \times (l+1)$ matrix

$$\begin{pmatrix} c_u^1(x(t), u(t), t) & c^1(x(t), u(t), t) & \cdots & 0 \\ \vdots & \vdots & \ddots & \vdots \\ c_u^l(x(t), u(t), t) & 0 & \cdots & c^l(x(t), u(t), t) \end{pmatrix} \tag{3.48}$$

has, along the optimal solution $(x^*(\cdot), u^*(\cdot))$, full rank for every $t \in [0, T]$. At points of discontinuity of the optimal control (3.48) has to hold for the left- and right-hand limit separately.

The first-order necessary conditions are as follows:

Theorem 3.52 (Maximum Principle for Mixed Path Constraints). *Let $(x^*(\cdot), u^*(\cdot))$ be an optimal solution of* OCC *(3.47a)–(3.47d) satisfying the constraint qualification (3.48). Then there exist a continuous and piecewise continuously differentiable function $\lambda(\cdot)$, with $\lambda(t) \in \mathbb{R}^n$, and a piecewise continuous multiplier function $\mu(\cdot)$, with $\mu(t) \in \mathbb{R}^l$ satisfying the following conditions at every time t where $u^*(\cdot)$ is continuous:*

$$\mathcal{H}(x^*(t), u^*(t), \lambda(t), t) = \max_{u \in \Omega(x,t)} \mathcal{H}(x^*(t), u, \lambda(t), t)$$
$$\mathcal{L}_u(x^*(t), u^*(t), \lambda(t), \mu(t), t) = 0$$
$$\dot{\lambda}(t) = r\lambda(t) - \mathcal{L}_x(x^*(t), u^*(t), \lambda(t), \mu(t), t),$$

with the complementary slackness condition

$$\mu(t) \geq 0, \quad \mu(t)c(x^*(t), u^*(t), t) = 0,$$

and the transversality condition

$$\lambda(T) = S_x(x^*(T), T).$$

The Hamiltonian $\mathcal{H}$ and Lagrangian $\mathcal{L}$ are defined by

$$\mathcal{H}(x, u, \lambda, t) = g(x, u, t) + \lambda(t) f(x, u, t)$$
$$\mathcal{L}(x, u, \lambda, \mu, t) = \mathcal{H}(x, u, \lambda, t) + \mu(t) c(x, u, t).$$

For an informal derivation of Theorem 3.52, see Sect. 4.4.2.

Remark 3.53. For the case that the constraint qualification is not satisfied see the discussion in Seierstad and Sydsaeter (1986, Note 4.2.7).

In Léonard (1981) the following theorem is proved deriving conditions on the sign of the costate $\lambda(\cdot)$:

Theorem 3.54 (Signs of the Costate Variables). *Let $(x^*(\cdot), u^*(\cdot))$ be an optimal solution of the optimal control problem (3.47a)–(3.47d). Assume that there is a partition N^+ and N^- of the set $N = \{1, \dots, n\}$, i.e., $N^+ \cup N^- = N$ and $N^+ \cap N^- = \emptyset$, such that at any point of the optimal path the following conditions are true:*

1. *$i \in N^+$ implies $g_{x_i} \geq 0$ and $c^k_{x_i} \geq 0$ for all $k = 1, \dots, l$,*
   $i \in N^-$ implies $g_{x_i} \leq 0$ and $c^k_{x_i} \leq 0$ for all $k = 1, \dots, l$.
2. *$f^j_{x_i} \geq 0$ if i and j belong to the same group, $i \neq j$,*
   $f^j_{x_i} \leq 0$ if i and j belong to different groups.
3. *There exists a non-empty subset of N, called N_1, such that for all $i \in N_1$ either $g_{x_i} \neq 0$ or $\mu_r c^r_{x_i} \neq 0$ for some r.*
4. *For all $i \in N_1$, $f^j_{x_i} \neq 0$ for some $j \in N_1$.*

Then $i \in N^+$ implies $\lambda_i(t) > 0$, and $i \in N^-$ implies $\lambda_i(t) < 0$ for all $t \in [0, T)$.

Remark 3.55. From the economic interpretation of λ_i as the shadow price of stock x_i we can say that for $g_{x_i} > 0\,(< 0)$ stock i has positive (negative) intrinsic worth and therefore stock i is called a good (bad) stock if $i \in N^+$ (N^-) and the strict inequality holds.

Ramsey's Model With Mixed Path Constraints

Considering again Ramsey's model, formulated in Sect. 3.3.7, and assume that at any time one cannot consume and invest more than the output. Thus the problem is restricted by the following mixed path constraint

$$0 \leq C(t) \leq F(K(t)), \quad \text{for all} \quad t \geq 0.$$

The assumption

$$U'(0) = \infty$$

is dropped, which only served the purpose of excluding the case that it might be optimal to consume nothing.

Then the model is written as:

$$\max_{C(\cdot)} \left\{ \int_0^T e^{-rt} U(C)\, dt + e^{-rT} S(K(T)) \right\}$$

$$\text{s.t.} \quad \dot{K} = F(K) - \delta K - C, \quad K(0) = K_0 > 0$$

$$0 \leq C \leq F(K). \tag{3.49}$$

We use Pontryagin's Maximum Principle Theorem 3.52 to derive the necessary conditions for an optimal solution. Thus we have to consider the Lagrangian (in current-value notation)

$$\mathcal{L}(K, C, \lambda, \mu_1, \mu_2) = U(C) + \lambda\left(F(K) - \delta K - C\right) + \mu_1 C + \mu_2\left(F(K) - C\right).$$

Note that the constraint qualification (3.48) is satisfied since not both control constraints can become active at the same time (as long as $K > 0$). Thus the matrix

$$\begin{pmatrix} 1 & C(t) & 0 \\ -1 & 0 & F\left(K(t)\right) - C(t) \end{pmatrix}$$

has full rank two.

Note that the Hamiltonian is strictly concave in C and the interior region

$$\Omega(K) = \{C : 0 \le C \le F(K)\}$$

is convex in C for given K. Therefore the Hamiltonian is regular implying continuity of the control $C(\cdot)$.

Thus the necessary conditions can be stated for all $t \in [0, T]$ as:

$$\mathcal{L}_C = U'(C) - \lambda + \mu_1 - \mu_2 = 0 \tag{3.50a}$$

$$\dot{\lambda} = r\lambda - \mathcal{L}_K = \lambda\left(r + \delta - F'(K)\right) - \mu_2 F'(K) \tag{3.50b}$$

$$\lambda(T) = S_K\left(K(T)\right) \tag{3.50c}$$

$$\mu_1 \ge 0, \quad \mu_1 C = 0 \tag{3.50d}$$

$$\mu_2 \ge 0, \quad \mu_2\left(F(K) - C\right) = 0. \tag{3.50e}$$

We have to distinguish between the different cases of an interior arc and a boundary arc. We concentrate on the latter, since the first case has already been considered in Sect. 3.3.7.

Boundary Arc I: Zero Consumption $C = 0$

The complementary slackness conditions (3.50e) yield $\mu_2 = 0$ and hence

$$\mathcal{L} = U(C) + \lambda\left(F(K) - \delta K - C\right) + \mu_1 C.$$

To derive an explicit formula for the Lagrange multiplier $\mu_1(\cdot)$ along the boundary arc we can use (3.50a) together with $C = 0$, yielding

$$\mu_1(t) = -U'(0) + \lambda(t).$$

Due to the nonnegativity condition in (3.50d)

$$\lambda(t) \ge U'(0)$$

has to be satisfied.

The adjoint equation (3.50b) for the boundary arc ($C = 0$) reads as

$$\dot{\lambda} = \lambda \left(r + \delta - F'(K) \right),$$

which together with the corresponding state equation

$$\dot{K} = F(K) - \delta K$$

gives the canonical system.

Boundary Arc II: Maximum Consumption $C = F(K)$

For the boundary arc along maximum consumption $C = F(K)$ we find $\mu_1 = 0$, and the corresponding Lagrangian is given by

$$\mathcal{L} = U(C) + \lambda \left(F(K) - \delta K - C \right) + \mu_2 \left(F(K) - C \right).$$

From (3.50a) the Lagrange multiplier μ_2 is given by

$$\mu_2(t) = U' \left(F(K(t)) \right) - \lambda(t),$$

and therefore

$$\lambda(t) \le U' \left(F(K(t)) \right)$$

has to hold along the boundary arc.

For $C = F(K)$ the state equation reduces to

$$\dot{K} = -\delta K$$

and the adjoint equation becomes

$$\dot{\lambda} = \lambda \left(r + \delta \right) - U'(F(K))F'(K).$$

This example is pursued in Sect. 3.6.2, where additionally pure state constraints are considered.

3.6.2 General Path Constraints

Consider the general *OCC* (3.47). The obvious analytical difference between mixed path and pure state constraints is the independence of $h(x,t)$ from the control variable u. We therefore introduce the following definition (see also Hartl, Sethi, & Vickson, 1995):

Definition 3.56 (Order of State Constraint). *Let $h : \mathbb{R}^n \times \mathbb{R} \to \mathbb{R}$ be $q \in \mathbb{N}$ times continuously differentiable and the functions $d^{(i)} : \mathbb{R}^n \times \mathbb{R}^m \times \mathbb{R} \to \mathbb{R}$, $i = 0, \ldots, q$ be recursively defined*

$$\begin{aligned} d^{(0)}(x,u,t) &:= h(x,t) \\ d^{(1)}(x,u,t) &:= \dot{h}(x,t) = h_x(x,t) f(x,u,t) + h_t(x,t) \\ &\vdots \\ d^{(q)}(x,u,t) &:= \dot{d}^{(q-1)}(x,u,t) = d_x^{(q-1)}(x,u,t) f(x,u,t) + d_t^{(q-1)}(x,u,t). \end{aligned}$$

If

$$d_u^{(i)}(x,u,t) = 0,\ 0 \le i < q, \quad \textit{and} \quad d_u^{(q)}(x,u,t) \neq 0,$$

then the pure state constraint $h(x,t)$ *is called of* order q. *For* $h : \mathbb{R}^n \times \mathbb{R} \to \mathbb{R}^k$ *the order is determined for each coordinate function* h_j, $j = 1, \dots, k$, *and the* j*th state constraint is called of* order q_j.

Remark 3.57. Intuitively speaking the order q of the state constraint is given by the number for which a control variable explicitly occurs in $\frac{\mathrm{d}^q h}{\mathrm{d}t^q}$ for the first time.

In many economic applications the state constraint is of order one in each of its coordinates. Therefore we set

$$\begin{aligned} d(x,u,t) := d^{(1)}(x,u,t) &= h_x(x,t)\dot{x} + h_t(x,t) \\ &= h_x(x,t)f(x,u,t) + h_t(x,t) \end{aligned} \tag{3.51}$$

with

$$d(x,u,t) = \left(d^1(x,u,t), \dots, d^k(x,u,t)\right)',$$

and restrict the following formulations to state constraints of order one.

Remark 3.58 (Indirect Approach). Considering the total time derivative of $h(x,t)$ allows the derivation of necessary conditions via the so-called *indirect* approach, which historically preceded the *direct*[14] approach used here. The indirect approach exploits the fact that for active constraints $h(x,t) = 0$ the function (3.51) should satisfy

$$d(x,u,t) \ge 0.$$

Since $d(x,u,t) < 0$, the state constraint decreases, implying $h(x,t) < 0$ and therefore violating the state constraint. Thus for the indirect approach, a modified set, $\tilde{\Omega}(x,t)$, of admissible control values can be used

$$\tilde{\Omega}(x,t) = \{u : c(x,u,t) \ge 0, \text{ and } d(x,u,t) \ge 0 \text{ if } h(x,t) = 0\}.$$

Using this condition the pure state constraints explicitly appear in the set of admissible control values and therefore the corresponding optimal control problem can be formulated as a standard optimal control problem *OC* (3.3).

Before we state the general Maximum Principle for problem *OCC* (3.47), we formulate the following constraint qualification for the pure state constraint. Let the matrix

[14] The terms direct and indirect are caused by the considered Lagrangian. For the direct approach the pure state constraint is directly adjoined, whereas in the indirect approach the derived function $d(x,u)$ is adjoined.

$$\begin{pmatrix} d_u^1(x,u,t) & h^1(x,t) & \cdots & 0 \\ \vdots & \vdots & \ddots & \vdots \\ d_u^k(x,u,t) & 0 & \cdots & h^k(x,t) \end{pmatrix} \tag{3.52}$$

have full rank for every $t \in [0, T]$. If the order of the jth pure state constraint is $q_j > 1$, d_u^j has to be replaced by $(d^j)_u^{(q_j)}$.

Moreover for the terminal constraints (3.47f) and (3.47g) the following constraint qualification has to hold

$$\begin{pmatrix} b_x^1(x,T) & b^1(x,T) & \cdots & 0 \\ \vdots & 0 & \ddots & 0 \\ b_x^{l''}(x,T) & 0 & \cdots & b^{l''}(x,T) \\ a_x^1(x,T) & 0 & \cdots & 0 \\ \vdots & \vdots & \ddots & \vdots \\ a_x^{l'}(x,T) & 0 & \cdots & 0 \end{pmatrix} \tag{3.53}$$

has full rank for all possible values x and T.

In analogy to the Maximum Principle for mixed path constraints Theorem 3.52 we now state a theorem, which is better to be denoted as an informal theorem. Since it has not fully been proved in the literature (see also Hartl et al., 1995).

Remark 3.59. In Seierstad and Sydsaeter (1986) the following necessary conditions are called *almost necessary conditions* since, very rarely, problems are encountered where the optimal solutions require more complicated multipliers and costates.

Theorem 3.60 (Informal Maximum Principle for General Inequality Constraints). *Let $(x^*(\cdot), u^*(\cdot))$ be an optimal solution of* OCC *(3.47), where the constraint qualification (3.48), (3.52) and (3.53) are satisfied. Assume that $x^*(\cdot)$ has only finitly many junction times. Then there exist a piecewise*[15] *absolutely continuous function $\lambda(\cdot)$, with $\lambda(t) \in \mathbb{R}^n$, piecewise continuous multiplier functions $\mu(\cdot)$, $\nu(\cdot)$, with $\mu(t) \in \mathbb{R}^l$, $\nu(t) \in \mathbb{R}^k$, a vector $\eta(\tilde{t}_i)$ for each point $\tilde{t}_i$, $i = 1, \dots, q$ of discontinuity of $\lambda(\cdot)$ and constants $\lambda_0 \geq 0$, $\alpha \in \mathbb{R}^{l'}$, $\beta \in \mathbb{R}^{l''}$, $\gamma \in \mathbb{R}^k$ satisfying for almost all*[16] *$t \in [0, T]$:*

$$\left(\lambda_0, \lambda(t), \mu(t), \nu(t), \alpha, \beta, \gamma, \eta(\tilde{t}_1), \dots \eta(\tilde{t}_q)\right) \neq 0 \tag{3.54a}$$

$$\mathcal{H}(x^*, u^*, \lambda, \lambda_0, t) = \max_{u \in \Omega} \mathcal{H}(x^*, u, \lambda, \lambda_0, t) \tag{3.54b}$$

$$\mathcal{L}_u(x, u, \lambda, \lambda_0, \mu, \nu, t) = 0 \tag{3.54c}$$

$$\dot{\lambda}(t) = r\lambda(t) - \mathcal{L}_x(x^*(t), u^*(t), \lambda(t), \lambda_0, \mu(t), \nu(t), t) \tag{3.54d}$$

---

[15] There exists a partition of the time interval $[0, T]$ such that $\lambda(\cdot)$ is absolutely continuous on each subinterval.

[16] The term *almost all* has its origin in measure theory, where it characterizes properties which hold for all elements except some set of measure zero. In our case it means at every time t except finitely many.

with the complementary slackness conditions

$$\mu(t) \geq 0, \quad \mu(t)c(x^*, u^*, t) = 0 \tag{3.54e}$$
$$\nu(t) \geq 0, \quad \nu(t)h(x^*, t) = 0. \tag{3.54f}$$

At the end point T the following transversality condition has to hold:

$$\lambda(T^-) = \lambda_0 S_x(x^*(T), T) + \gamma h_x(x^*(T), T) + \\ \alpha a_x(x^*(T), T) + \beta b_x(x^*(T), T) \tag{3.54g}$$

with the complementary slackness conditions

$$\beta \geq 0, \quad \beta b(x^*(T), T) = 0 \tag{3.54h}$$
$$\gamma \geq 0, \quad \gamma h(x^*(T), T) = 0. \tag{3.54i}$$

Discontinuities of the costate λ and the Hamiltonian $\mathcal{H}$ at time $\tilde{t}$ are of the form[17]

$$\lambda(\tilde{t}^+) = \lambda(\tilde{t}^-) - \eta(\tilde{t})h_x(\tilde{t}), \tag{3.54j}$$
$$\mathcal{H}(\tilde{t}^+) = \mathcal{H}(\tilde{t}^-) + \eta(\tilde{t})h_t(\tilde{t}), \tag{3.54k}$$

with

$$\eta(t) \geq 0, \quad \textit{and} \quad \eta(t)h(t) = 0. \tag{3.54l}$$

The Hamiltonian $\mathcal{H}$ and Lagrangian $\mathcal{L}$ are defined by

$$\mathcal{H}(x, u, \lambda, \lambda_0, t) = \lambda_0 g(x, u, t) + \lambda(t) f(x, u, t)$$
$$\mathcal{L}(x, u, \lambda, \lambda_0, \mu, \nu, t) = \mathcal{H}(x, u, \lambda, \lambda_0, t) + \mu(t)c(x, u, t) + \nu(t)h(x, t).$$

The reader is also referred to Sect. 4.4.2 where we use a variational approach, to prove that the costate and Hamiltonian, respectively, can be discontinuous at junction points, (see also Hartl et al., 1995, Theorem 4.2).

Remark 3.61. The conditions (3.54j) and (3.54k) are called *corner conditions* and are the analogous of the *Weierstrass–Erdmann conditions* from calculus of variations (see Sect. 4.3.3).

For a regular Hamiltonian (see Definition 3.19) we can prove:

Proposition 3.62. *Let $(x^*(\cdot), u^*(\cdot))$ be an optimal solution of* OCC *(3.47). If the Hamiltonian is regular, then $u^*(\cdot)$ is continuous at junction times.*

The proof is straightforward and can also be found in Feichtinger and Hartl (1986).

[17] For notational simplicity we set $\mathcal{H}(t) := \mathcal{H}(x(t), u(t), \lambda(t), \lambda_0, t)$.

Proof. Considering the left- and right-hand side limits of the control $u^*(\cdot)$ and costate $\lambda(\cdot)$ at $\tilde{t}$, denoted as u^-, λ^-, and u^+, λ^+, respectively we find

$$\begin{aligned}\mathcal{H}(x,u^-,\lambda^-,\lambda_0,\tilde{t}) &= \lambda_0 g(x,u^-,\tilde{t}) + \lambda^- f(x,u^-,\tilde{t}) \\ &= \lambda_0 g(x,u^-,\tilde{t}) + \left(\lambda^+ + \eta h_x\right) f(x,u^-,\tilde{t}) \\ &= \mathcal{H}(x,u^-,\lambda^+,\lambda_0,\tilde{t}) + \eta h_x f(x,u^-,\tilde{t}) \\ &\le \mathcal{H}(x,u^+,\lambda^+,\lambda_0,\tilde{t}) + \eta h_x f(x,u^-,\tilde{t}) \\ &= \mathcal{H}(x,u^-,\lambda^-,\lambda_0,\tilde{t}) + \eta h_x f(x,u^-,\tilde{t}) + \eta h_t,\end{aligned} \tag{3.55}$$

which yields the inequality

$$\mathcal{H}(x,u^-,\lambda^-,\lambda_0,\tilde{t}) \le \mathcal{H}(x,u^-,\lambda^-,\lambda_0,\tilde{t}) + \eta d^-, \tag{3.56}$$

where d is defined in (3.51) and d^- denotes the left-hand side limit. Therefore we get

$$\eta d^- \ge 0.$$

Next we exclude the case $\eta d^- > 0$. Therefore we distinguish the cases of an exit, contact, and entry point. In the latter case we immediately find

$$d^- = \frac{\mathrm{d}h^-}{\mathrm{d}t} = \lim_{s\to 0^-} \frac{h(x^*(\tilde{t}+s),\tilde{t}+s) - h(x^*(\tilde{t}),\tilde{t})}{s} = \lim_{s\to 0^-} \frac{0-0}{s} = 0,$$

whereas for the former cases we derive

$$d^- = \frac{\mathrm{d}h^-}{\mathrm{d}t} = \lim_{s\to 0^-} \frac{h(x^*(\tilde{t}+s),\tilde{t}+s) - h(x^*(\tilde{t}),\tilde{t})}{s} = \lim_{s\to 0^-} \frac{h(\tilde{t}+s)}{s} \le 0,$$

since $s < 0$ and $h(\tilde{t}+s) \ge 0$.

Together with (3.56) this yields $\eta d^- = 0$. Note that this is a general result since the regularity assumption was not used for its derivation.

This identity implies that equality has to hold at (3.55) yielding

$$\mathcal{H}(x,u^-,\lambda^+,\lambda_0,\tilde{t}) = \mathcal{H}(x,u^+,\lambda^+,\lambda_0,\tilde{t}).$$

But this says that u^- as well as u^+ maximize the Hamiltonian

$$\mathcal{H}(x,u,\lambda^+,\lambda_0,\tilde{t}).$$

Thus by the regularity of the Hamiltonian the uniqueness of $u^*(\tilde{t})$ follows and therefore the continuity of the control. □

For the next proposition, characterizing a continuous costate, we assume a strengthened form of the constraint qualifications (3.48) and (3.52). Thus the matrix

$$\begin{pmatrix} c_u^1(x,u,t) & c^1(x,u,t) & \cdots & 0 & 0 & \cdots & 0 \\ \vdots & \vdots & \ddots & \vdots & \vdots & \ddots & \vdots \\ c_u^l(x,u,t) & 0 & \cdots & c^l(x,u,t) & 0 & \cdots & 0 \\ d_u^1(x,u,t) & 0 & \cdots & 0 & h^1(x,t) & \cdots & 0 \\ \vdots & \vdots & \ddots & \vdots & \vdots & \ddots & \vdots \\ d_u^k(x,u,t) & 0 & \cdots & 0 & 0 & \cdots & h^k(x,t) \end{pmatrix} \tag{3.57}$$

has full rank for all $t \in [0, T]$. Then the following, can be proved (Feichtinger & Hartl, 1986):

Proposition 3.63. *Let $h(x,t) \geq 0$ be a state constraint of order one with an extremal state having an interior arc that joins a boundary arc at $\tilde{t}$. Then $\eta(\tilde{t}) = 0$ if one of the following conditions is satisfied:*

1. *The control $u(\cdot)$ is continuous and the constraint qualification (3.57) is satisfied.*
2. *The exit or entry is nontangential, i.e., $d(\tilde{t}^+) > 0$ or $d(\tilde{t}^-) < 0$, respectively (cf. Fig. 3.4).*

The proof is straight forward and can be found, e.g., in Feichtinger and Hartl (1986).

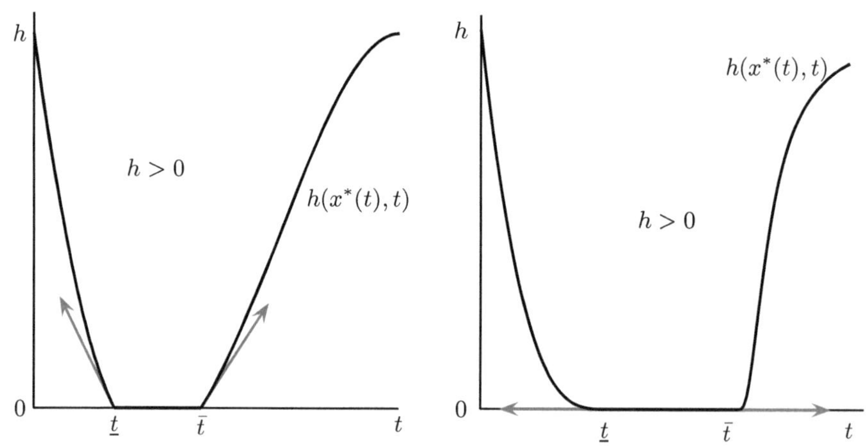

Fig. 3.4. The cases of (**a**) a nontangential entry and exit point and (**b**) a tangential entry and exit point are depicted

For a comprehensive survey of the Maximum Principle under state constraints, the reader is referred to Hartl et al. (1995). An example and economic interpretation of a model with discontinuous costate can be found in Verheyen (1992). In Chap. 4 we give an informal proof explaining the possible discontinuity of the costate and Hamiltonian, respectively.

Ramsey's Model With General Constraints

Next we extend the Ramsey model by introducing the pure state constraint

$$K(t) \geq \underline{K}, \quad \text{for all} \quad t \geq 0, \tag{3.58}$$

where for the initial state $K(0) = K_0 \geq \underline{K}$ is assumed.

To analyze the Ramsey model including the mixed constraints (3.49) as well as the pure state constraint (3.58) we use Pontryagin's Maximum Principle Theorem 3.60. Therefore we have to consider the Lagrangian

$$\mathcal{L}(K, C, \lambda, \mu_1, \mu_2, \nu) = \\ U(C) + \lambda \left(F(K) - \delta K - C\right) + \mu_1 C + \mu_2 \left(F(K) - C\right) + \nu \left(K - \underline{K}\right).$$

Then the necessary conditions become:

$$\mathcal{L}_C = U'(C) - \lambda + \mu_1 - \mu_2 = 0 \tag{3.59a}$$

$$\dot{\lambda} = r\lambda - \mathcal{L}_K = \lambda \left(r + \delta - F'(K)\right) - \mu_2 F'(K) - \nu \tag{3.59b}$$

$$\lambda(T) = S_K\left(K(T)\right)$$

$$\mu_1 \geq 0, \quad \mu_1 C = 0$$

$$\mu_2 \geq 0, \quad \mu_2 \left(F(K) - C\right) = 0 \tag{3.59c}$$

$$\nu \geq 0, \quad \nu \left(K - \underline{K}\right) = 0. \tag{3.59d}$$

First we note that the constraint (3.58) is of order one since the total time derivative of the state constraint $h(K) := K - \underline{K}$

$$\frac{\mathrm{d}}{\mathrm{d}t} h(K) = \dot{K} = F(K) - \delta K - C$$

explicitly contains the control variable C. We restrict our analysis to the case where the state and control constraint do not become active at the same time. Then the constraint qualification (3.57) for matrix

$$\begin{pmatrix} 1 & C(t) & 0 & 0 \\ -1 & 0 & F\left(K(t)\right) - C(t) & 0 \\ -1 & 0 & 0 & K(t) - \underline{K} \end{pmatrix}$$

is trivially satisfied. The regularity of the Hamiltonian implies the continuity of the optimal control(see Proposition 3.62). Thus using the constraint qualification we can apply Proposition 3.63 proving the continuity of the costate at junction points.

Minimum Capital Stock $K = \underline{K}$

After these initial considerations we analyze the case where the state constraint becomes active. Thus for $K_0 > \underline{K}$ there shall exist an interval $(\underline{t}, \bar{t})$ satisfying

$$K(t) = \underline{K} \quad \text{for} \quad t \in (\underline{t}, \bar{t}).$$

Since $K(t)$ is constant on the interval $(\underline{t}, \bar{t})$ its time derivative is zero. Hence to keep the state on the boundary arc the control value is given by

$$\underline{C} = F(\underline{K}) - \delta \underline{K}.$$

To derive the adjoint equation we consider the total time derivative of (3.59a) yielding

$$\frac{\mathrm{d}}{\mathrm{d}t}\mathcal{L}_C = U''\dot{C} - \dot{\lambda} = 0,$$

where we used $\mu_1 = \mu_2 = 0$, since no control constrains are active. At the boundary arc $C = \underline{C}$ is constant implying $\dot{C} = 0$ and thus $\dot{\lambda} = 0$. Transforming (3.59b) and using (3.59a) yields an explicit formula for the multiplier ν

$$\nu = U'(\underline{C})\left(r + \delta - F'(\underline{K})\right).$$

By assumption $U'(C) > 0$; thus a necessary condition for the boundary arc to be optimal is $F'(\underline{K}) < r + \delta$.

In Exercise 3.11 the reader is invited to analyze Ramsey's model for the finite time horizon T, whereas in Sect. 3.8.2 the analysis is done for the infinite time horizon.

3.6.3 Sufficiency Conditions

Next we formulate sufficient conditions for problems *OCC* (3.47):

Theorem 3.64 (The Arrow Sufficiency Conditions). *Let $(x^*(\cdot), u^*(\cdot))$ be an admissible solution for problem* OCC *(3.47). Assume that there exist a piecewise continuously differentiable function $\lambda : [0, T] \to \mathbb{R}^n$, piecewise continuous functions $\mu : [0, T] \to \mathbb{R}^l$, and $\nu : [0, T] \to \mathbb{R}^k$, such that conditions (3.54b)–(3.54f) of Theorem 3.60 hold with $\lambda_0 = 1$. Assume further that there exist a $\alpha \in \mathbb{R}^{l'}$ and $\beta \in \mathbb{R}^{l''}$ such that (3.54g) and (3.54h)–(3.54h) hold and assume that at all points $\tilde{t}_i$, $i = 1, \ldots, q$ of discontinuity of $\lambda(\cdot)$, there exist $\eta(\tilde{t}_i) \in \mathbb{R}^n$, $i = 1, \ldots, q$, such that (3.54j)–(3.54l) hold. If the maximized Hamiltonian $\mathcal{H}^*$ exists for all x and is concave in x for all t, and the salvage function $S(x, T)$ is concave in x, $c(x, u, t)$ is quasiconcave in (x, u), $h(x, t)$ and $b(x, t)$ are quasiconcave in x, and $a(x, t)$ is linear in x then $(x^*(\cdot), u^*(\cdot))$ is an optimal solution.*

If $\mathcal{H}^*$ is strictly concave in x, then $x^*(\cdot)$ (but not necessarily $u^*(\cdot)$) is unique.

An analogous theorem holds for:

Theorem 3.65 (The Mangasarian Sufficiency Conditions). *Let the assumptions of Theorem 3.64 hold and replace the concavity of the maximized Hamiltonian by the concavity of the Hamiltonian in (x, u) for all t, then Theorem 3.64 remains valid.*

3.7 Infinite Time Horizon

So far an optimal control problem OC has been defined up to some finite time T. However, it is often useful to consider an infinite time horizon. A justification for this can be found in Arrow and Kurz (1970, p. xviii):

> The infinite horizon is an idealization of the fundamental point that the consequences of investment are very long-lived; any short horizon requires some methods of evaluating end-of-period capital stocks, and the only proper evaluation is their value in use in the subsequent future.

There are many interesting economic models formulated as optimal control problems over an infinite time horizon (OCI):

$$\max_{u(\cdot)} \int_0^\infty \mathrm{e}^{-rt} g(x(t), u(t), t)\,\mathrm{d}t \tag{3.60a}$$

$$\text{s.t.} \quad \dot{x}(t) = f(x(t), u(t), t) \tag{3.60b}$$

$$x(0) = x_0. \tag{3.60c}$$

This problem entails some theoretical difficulties, however. One is the derivation of a transversality condition. Another problem is that (3.60a) denotes an improper integral, which may not converge. If it does not converge, then it is even not clear what is meant by optimality. Therefore new concepts of optimality have to be introduced. In both cases an answer will be found by approximating the infinite time problem by appropriate finite time problems.

3.7.1 Definitions of Optimality for Infinite Horizon Problems

In our models the objective value is almost always finite, i.e., the integral (3.60a) converges. However the reader may at some point encounter problems for which it diverges. The results presented so far do not provide criteria for comparing the objective value for different admissible solutions, let alone a way to characterize an optimal solution. Different attempts have been made to find optimality criteria covering problems of this kind. We present three main concepts, which can be further refined (see, e.g., Carlson, Haurie, and Leizarowitz, 1991; Stern, 1984).

Define the truncated objective functional V_T with $T > 0$,

$$V_T(u(\cdot)) = \int_0^T \mathrm{e}^{-rt} g(x(t), u(t), t)\,\mathrm{d}t,$$

for the problem OCI (3.60). The subsequent definitions give some optimality criteria using the truncated objective functional:

Definition 3.66 (Optimality Criteria). *The admissible control $u^*(\cdot)$ is called:*

(O) Overtaking optimal *if, for any admissible control* $u(\cdot)$*, there is a* $T(u(\cdot))$ *such that for every* $T \geq T(u(\cdot))$

$$V_T(u(\cdot)) \leq V_T(u^*(\cdot))$$

(C) Catching up optimal *if, for any admissible control* $u(\cdot)$ *and for every* $\varepsilon > 0$*, there is a* $T(u(\cdot), \varepsilon)$ *such that for every* $T \geq T(u(\cdot), \varepsilon)$

$$V_T(u(\cdot)) < V_T(u^*(\cdot)) + \varepsilon$$

(S) Sporadically catching up optimal *if, for any admissible control* $u(\cdot)$ *for every* $\varepsilon > 0$ *and for every* $\bar{T}$*, there exists a* $T = T(u(\cdot), \varepsilon, \bar{T}) \geq \bar{T}$ *such that*

$$V_T(u(\cdot)) < V_T(u^*(\cdot)) + \varepsilon$$

For the above definitions the ordering also denotes an order in strength. That is, (O) implies (C) implies (S) (see also Fig. 3.5).

In light of the above definitions problem *OCI* (3.60) can be reformulated as: find an admissible pair ($x^*(\cdot)$, $u^*(\cdot)$) such that this pair is optimal in the sense of one of the given definitions (O), (C), or (S). In the following we shall state a Maximum Principle for the infinite horizon.

3.7.2 Maximum Principle for Infinite Time Horizon Problems

For the infinite horizon case a Maximum Principle was first formulated by Halkin (1974) as:

Theorem 3.67 (Maximum Principle for an Infinite Time Horizon). *Let the pair* ($x^*(\cdot)$, $u^*(\cdot)$) *be an optimal solution of* OCI *(3.60) according to any definition of optimality in Definition 3.66. Then there exist a continuous and piecewise continuously differentiable function* $\lambda(\cdot)$*, with* $\lambda(t) \in \mathbb{R}^n$ *and a constant* $\lambda_0 \geq 0$ *satisfying for all* $t \geq 0$*:*

$$(\lambda_0, \lambda(t)) \neq 0$$
$$\mathcal{H}(x^*(t), u^*(t), \lambda(t), \lambda_0, t) = \max_u \mathcal{H}(x^*(t), u, \lambda(t), \lambda_0, t),$$

and at every point t *where* $u(\cdot)$ *is continuous*

$$\dot{\lambda}(t) = r\lambda(t) - \mathcal{H}_x \left(x^*(t), u^*(t), \lambda(t), \lambda_0, t\right).$$

Note that there is no transversality condition in the sense of (3.4c), a result that is a consequence of the proof strategy presented in Halkin (1974).

Proof. The main idea of the proof is to consider truncated versions of the infinite rime horizon problem *OCI* (3.60) for an increasing time sequence T_k with $\lim_{k\to\infty} T_k = \infty$. Thus we consider for every T_k the problem defined by (3.60b–3.60c) together with the truncated objective function

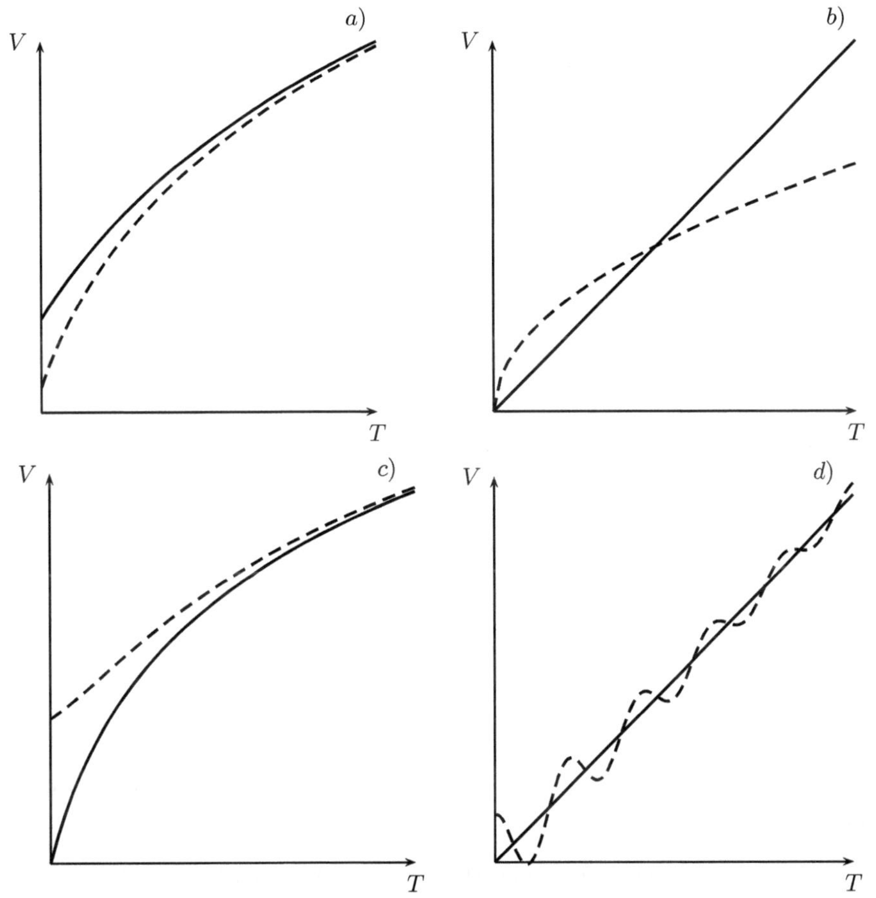

Fig. 3.5. Typical examples for the optimality definitions are depicted. The *solid line* denotes $V_T(u^*(\cdot))$ and the *dashed line* denotes $V_T(u(\cdot))$. In (**a**) $V_T(u(\cdot)) \le V_T(u^*(\cdot))$ for all T whereas in (**b**), the overtaking criterion becomes relevant because $V_T(u^*) \ge V_T(u(\cdot))$ only for sufficiently large T. In (**c**) the catching-up criterion is shown, and (**d**) gives a typical example of the sporadically catching-up criterion. Note that for each case the stronger criterion does not apply

$$\max_{u(\cdot)} \int_0^{T_k} \mathrm{e}^{-rt} g(x, u, t)\, \mathrm{d}t,$$

and the terminal state constraints

$$x(T_k) = x^*(T_k).$$

It can be proved that for these problems the restriction of $(x^*(\cdot), u^*(\cdot))$ to the interval $[0,\ T_k]$ is an optimal solution, for any of the three definitions of optimality.

From Pontryagin's Maximum Principle we know that for every k, there exist $\lambda_0^{(k)} \ge 0$ and a continuous and piecewise continuously differentiable

$\lambda^{(k)}(\cdot)$ satisfying

$$(\lambda_0^{(k)}, \lambda^{(k)}(0)) \neq 0 \tag{3.61a}$$

$$\mathcal{H}(x^*, u^*, \lambda^{(k)}, \lambda_0^{(k)}, t) = \max_u \mathcal{H}(x^*, u, \lambda^{(k)}, \lambda_0^{(k)}, t) \tag{3.61b}$$

$$\dot{\lambda}^{(k)} = r\lambda^{(k)} - \mathcal{H}_x(x^*, u^*, \lambda^{(k)}, \lambda_0^{(k)}, t) \tag{3.61c}$$

for every $t \in [0, T_k]$ where the control $u^*(\cdot)$ is continuous. As $(\lambda_0^{(k)}, \lambda^{(k)}(0))$ appear linearly in $\mathcal{H}$, we can normalize these vectors without changing (3.61) such that $\|\lambda_0^{(k)}, \lambda^{(k)}(0))\| = 1$ holds. Hence we can construct a sequence of bounded vectors, where, by elementary calculus, a converging subsequence exists (see the Bolzano–Weierstrass theorem (Theorem A.71)) satisfying

$$\lim_{i\to\infty} (\lambda_0^{(k_i)}, \lambda^{(k_i)}(0)) = (\lambda_0, \lambda(0)),$$

such that $\|(\lambda_0, \lambda(0))\| = 1$.

Let $\lambda(\cdot)$ be the unique solution[18] of the differential equation

$$\dot{\lambda} = r\lambda - \mathcal{H}_x^*(x^*, \lambda, t) \tag{3.62}$$

with the initial condition $\lambda(0) = \lim_{i\to\infty} \left(\lambda_0^{(k_i)}(0)\right)$; then

$$\lambda(t) = \lim_{i\to\infty} \left(\lambda^{(k_i)}(t)\right)$$

holds due to the uniqueness of the solution (3.62), together with (3.61c). Therefore

$$\mathcal{H}(x^*, u^*, \lambda, t) = \lim_{i\to\infty} \max_u \mathcal{H}(x^*, u, \lambda^{(k_i)}, t) = \max_u \mathcal{H}(x^*, u, \lambda, t)$$

is satisfied as $\mathcal{H}$ is linear in $\lambda_0^{(k_i)}$ as well as $\lambda^{(k_i)}(\cdot)$, which proves the theorem. □

Remark 3.68. Considering the problem *OCI* (3.60), which additionally includes mixed path and pure state constraints of the form (3.47d) and (3.47d). Then the analogous (informal) theorem to Theorem 3.60 can be proved according to any of the optimality conditions of Definition 3.66, but also without a transversality condition.

Theorem 3.67 is significantly weaker than Pontryagin's Maximum Principle since it lacks the formulation of an analogue to the transversality condition. One might expect that a kind of transversality condition, like $\lim_{T\to\infty} \lambda(T) = 0$, but that is not generally true, as counter-examples (see Example (3.78)) confirm. Nevertheless, under some additional conditions we can derive transversality conditions holding at infinity.

[18] The adjoint equation is linear in λ, therefore yielding existence and uniqueness of a solution.

3.7.3 Sufficiency Conditions

The following sufficiency results are direct generalizations of the finite time horizon problem results in Sect. 3.3.5. We restrict attention to the case in which the objective value is finite, but similar results are available in the general case, in which the weaker definitions of optimality have to be considered. For these results the reader is referred to Seierstad and Sydsaeter (1977):

Theorem 3.69 (The Mangasarian Sufficiency Conditions for Infinite Time Horizon). *Let $(x^*(\cdot), u^*(\cdot))$, and $\lambda(\cdot)$ satisfy Pontryagin's Maximum Principle with $\lambda_0 = 1$ and for all admissible $x(\cdot)$ the limiting transversality condition*

$$\lim_{t\to\infty} \lambda(t)\,(x(t) - x^*(t)) \geq 0$$

holds. Suppose that $\Omega(x,t)$ is convex for every $x \in \mathbb{R}^n$, $t \in [0, T]$, the partial derivatives of $g(x,u,t)$ and $f(x,u,t)$ are continuous with respect to their arguments and the Hamiltonian $\mathcal{H}$ is jointly concave in x and u for all t and λ, then $(x^*(\cdot), u^*(\cdot))$ is an optimal solution.

If $\mathcal{H}^*$ is strictly concave in x and u, then $(x^*(\cdot), u^*(\cdot))$ is the unique optimal solution.

The transversality condition (3.63) is in general not a necessary condition.[19]

Proof. Following the argumentation of Theorem 3.29 we find

$$V(u^*) - V(u) \geq \lambda(T)(x(T) - x^*(T)) \geq 0$$

which together with the limiting condition (3.63), finishes the proof. □

Analogously the Arrow Sufficiency conditions can be proved for the infinite case:

Theorem 3.70 (The Arrow Sufficiency Conditions for Infinite Time Horizon). *Suppose $(x^*(\cdot), u^*(\cdot))$, and $\lambda(\cdot)$ satisfy Pontryagin's Maximum Principle with $\lambda_0 = 1$, and for all admissible $x(\cdot)$ the limiting transversality condition*

$$\lim_{t\to\infty} \lambda(t)\,(x(t) - x^*(t)) \geq 0 \tag{3.63}$$

holds. If the maximized Hamiltonian $\mathcal{H}^*$ is concave in x for all t and λ, then $(x^*(\cdot), u^*(\cdot))$ is an optimal solution.

3.8 Discounted Autonomous Infinite Horizon Models

In many economic applications the problems are formulated as autonomous optimal control problems. We shall subsequently refer to these specific problems as (DAM):

[19] For the infinite horizon case different transversality conditions exist, see Seierstad and Sydsaeter (1986).

$$\max_{u(\cdot)} \int_0^\infty \mathrm{e}^{-rt} g(x(t), u(t))\, \mathrm{d}t \tag{3.64a}$$

$$\text{s.t.} \quad \dot{x}(t) = f(x(t), u(t)) \tag{3.64b}$$

$$x(0) = x_0, \tag{3.64c}$$

where f and g are assumed to be continuously differentiable with respect x and u. Moreover it is assumed that the integral (3.64a) converges for every admissible pair $(x(\cdot), u(\cdot))$. Hence the definitions of optimality (O), (C), and (S) coincide.

For this special kind of model, conditions can be stated allowing us to derive the necessity of a transversality condition.

3.8.1 The Michel Theorem

For *DAM* (3.64) the necessary conditions for the infinite time horizon problem can be strengthened by the following theorem:

Theorem 3.71 (Michel Theorem). *Let the pair $(x^*(\cdot), u^*(\cdot))$ be an optimal solution of* DAM *(3.64). Then there exist a continuous and piecewise continuously differentiable function $\lambda(\cdot)$, with $\lambda(t) \in \mathbb{R}^n$ and a constant $\lambda_0 \geq 0$ such that for all $t \geq 0$ the following conditions hold:*

$$(\lambda_0, \lambda(t)) \neq 0 \tag{3.65a}$$

$$\mathcal{H}(x^*(t), u^*(t), \lambda(t), \lambda_0) = \max_u \mathcal{H}(x^*(t), u, \lambda(t), \lambda_0), \tag{3.65b}$$

and for all $t \geq 0$ where $u(\cdot)$ is continuous

$$\dot{\lambda}(t) = r\lambda(t) - \mathcal{H}_x(x^*(t), u^*(t), \lambda(t), \lambda_0) \tag{3.65c}$$

$$\mathcal{H}(x^*(t_0), u^*(t_0), \lambda(t_0), \lambda_0) = r\lambda_0 \int_{t_0}^\infty \mathrm{e}^{-rt} g(x^*(t), u^*(t))\, \mathrm{d}t \tag{3.65d}$$

together with the transversality condition

$$\lim_{t\to\infty} \mathrm{e}^{-rt} \mathcal{H}(x^*(t), u^*(t), \lambda(t), \lambda_0) = 0. \tag{3.65e}$$

Remark 3.72. Even though the theorem is stated for problems without restrictions on the control value u and state x, the result can be adapted to the case of equality and inequality constraints.

Remark 3.73. We present the proof of Theorem 3.71 in Appendix B.2 as its results are of great importance for the models we are analyzing. As does Halkin in his proof, Michel uses a finite-time approximation. But since he presupposes stronger assumptions in the model – i.e., the existence of the improper integral (3.64a) and the autonomous form of the state dynamics (3.64b) – he can use a different proof-strategy by introducing a salvage value and considering a further state and control variable, which in addition allows the derivation of the transversality condition (3.65e).

Under further assumptions on the functions g and f the transversality condition (3.65e) can be strengthened to:

Proposition 3.74 (Transversality Condition). *If $g(x,u) \geq 0$ and the set of possible values of the state dynamics, evaluated along an optimal state trajectory $x^*(\cdot)$ for an arbitrary control value u*

$$\{f(x^*(t),u) : \; u \in \mathbb{R}^m\} \tag{3.66}$$

contains an open neighborhood of zero for all $t \geq T_0 \geq 0$, then the transversality condition

$$\lim_{t\to\infty} \mathrm{e}^{-rt}\lambda(t) = 0 \tag{3.67}$$

holds for problem DAM *(3.64).*

The proof can be found in Appendix B.2.

The following proposition generalizes (3.65d) and is of great practical use, since it provides a formula allowing an explicit computation of the objective functional without carrying out the integration process:

Proposition 3.75 (Objective Value Given by the Hamiltonian). *Let the pair $(\hat{x}(\cdot), \hat{u}(\cdot))$ satisfy the necessary conditions (3.65) of Theorem 3.71 with $\lambda_0 = 1$, then*

$$\int_0^\infty \mathrm{e}^{-rt} g(\hat{x}(t), \hat{u}(t))\,\mathrm{d}t = \frac{1}{r}\mathcal{H}\left(x(0), u(0), \lambda(0)\right). \tag{3.68}$$

Remark 3.76. This result is a consequence of the proof of Theorem 3.71 and is related to (3.65d). However, it is stronger as we do not assume $(\hat{x}(\cdot), \hat{u}(\cdot))$ to be an optimal solution, but only to satisfy the necessary conditions. Thus Proposition 3.75 proves useful when multiple paths (see Sect. 5.4) satisfy the necessary conditions and therefore the corresponding objective values have to be compared.

Proof. The crucial part concerns the identity of the total and partial time derivative of the *present-value* Hamiltonian along a trajectory satisfying the necessary conditions. This identity holds in the general case, but for a better understanding we derive it under the assumption that the Hamiltonian maximizing condition is achieved for $\mathcal{H}_u = 0$. Then the following identity holds:

$$\begin{aligned}\frac{\mathrm{d}}{\mathrm{d}t}\mathcal{H} &= \mathcal{H}_x\dot{x} + \mathcal{H}_\lambda\dot{\lambda} + \mathcal{H}_u\dot{u} + \frac{\partial}{\partial t}\mathcal{H}\\ &= \mathcal{H}_x f - f'\mathcal{H}_x + \frac{\partial}{\partial t}\mathcal{H}\\ &= \frac{\partial}{\partial t}\mathcal{H}.\end{aligned}$$

Hence with

$$\mathcal{H} = \mathrm{e}^{-rt} g(x,u) + \lambda f(x,u)$$

we get

$$\dot{\mathcal{H}} = \frac{\partial}{\partial t}\mathcal{H} = -r\mathrm{e}^{-rt} g(x,u),$$

or in integrated form,

$$\mathcal{H}(t) - \mathcal{H}(0) = -r \int_0^t \mathrm{e}^{-rt} g(x,u)\,\mathrm{d}t.$$

Utilizing (3.65e), $\lim_{t\to\infty} \mathcal{H}(t) = 0$, proves (3.68). □

Remark 3.77. Since at time zero the current and present-value Hamiltonian yield the same value, formula (3.68) also holds for the current-value Hamiltonian.

The formula in (3.68) allows an immediate computation of the objective value of trajectories satisfying the necessary optimality conditions. Hence in the case of multiple candidates for an optimal solution it is easy to compare the corresponding objective values.

The reader should be aware that the assumption (3.68) on the state dynamics in Proposition 3.74 cannot be weakened without violating the transversality condition, and $\lambda_0 > 0$ cannot be guaranteed in general. This can be seen from the following counter-examples, taken from Halkin (1974).

Example 3.78 (Violation of the Transversality Condition). For the problem:

$$\begin{aligned} &\max_{u(\cdot)} \int_0^\infty (1 - x(t))\, u(t)\,\mathrm{d}t \\ \text{s.t.}\quad &\dot{x}(t) = (1 - x(t))\, u(t), \\ &x(0) = 0, \quad u(t) \in [0,\ 1], \quad t \geq 0 \end{aligned}$$

the transversality condition (3.67) is not satisfied. The formal reason for the failing of the transversality condition is that the assumption (3.66) in Proposition 3.74 on the dynamics is violated, since for every $\varepsilon > 0$ there exists a $T > 0$ such that for all $t > T$ and all $u \in [0,\ 1]$

$$|\dot{x}^*(t)| = |\mathrm{e}^{-t} u| < \varepsilon.$$

From the state equation we derive

$$x(t) = 1 - \mathrm{e}^{-\int_0^t u(s)\,\mathrm{d}s},$$

and the objective value function V_T at time T is given by

$$V_T\left(u(\cdot)\right) = \int_0^T \dot{x}(t)\,\mathrm{d}t = x(T).$$

Thus for an arbitrary admissible $u(\cdot)$ the inequality

$$V_T\left(u(\cdot)\right) = 1 - \mathrm{e}^{-\int_0^T u(s)\,\mathrm{d}s} \leq 1 - \mathrm{e}^{-T} = V_T\left(x_0, 1\right)$$

holds, proving that $u^* \equiv 1$ is the optimal control with the corresponding optimal state trajectory

$$x^*(t) = 1 - \mathrm{e}^{-t}.$$

Applying the necessary optimality conditions yields, given the Hamiltonian

$$\begin{aligned}\mathcal{H}(x(t), u(t), \lambda(t), \lambda_0) &= \lambda_0 \left(1 - x(t)\right) u(t) + \lambda \left(1 - x(t)\right) u(t) \\ &= u(t) \left(\lambda_0 + \lambda(t)\right) \mathrm{e}^{-\int_0^t u(s)\,\mathrm{d}s},\end{aligned}$$

the costate equation becomes

$$\dot{\lambda}(t) = \lambda_0 + \lambda(t)$$

which exhibits the solution

$$\lambda(t) = \left(\lambda_0 + \lambda(0)\right) \mathrm{e}^t - \lambda_0.$$

It remains to show that

$$\lim_{t\to\infty} \lambda(t) \neq 0.$$

But from the Maximum Principle we know that

$$\max_{u\in[0,\,1]} u \left(\lambda_0 + \lambda(t)\right) \mathrm{e}^{-\int_0^t u(s)\,\mathrm{d}s}$$

is achieved for $u = 1$ yielding $u^* \equiv 1$. Therefore, as the Hamiltonian is linear in u, this requires $\lambda_0 + \lambda(t) \geq 0$ for all t, especially for $t = 0$. From $(\lambda_0, \lambda(t)) \neq 0$ it follows that either $\lambda_0 = 0$, and hence $\lambda(0) > 0$, or $\lambda_0 > 0$. Thus, in any case the transversality condition is not satisfied.

In the following example, also presented in Halkin (1974), it is shown that for infinite horizon problems $\lambda_0 > 0$ cannot be guaranteed.

Example 3.79 (Abnormal Infinite Horizon Problem). In the problem:

$$\begin{aligned}&\max_{u(\cdot)} \int_0^\infty \left(u(t) - x(t)\right) \mathrm{d}t \\ \text{s.t.}\quad &\dot{x}(t) = u(t)^2 + x, \\ &x(0) = 0, \quad u(t) \in [0,\,1], \quad t \geq 0\end{aligned}$$

it holds that $\lambda_0 = 0$.

Utilizing $u \equiv 0$ yields

$$V_T(0) = 0, \quad \text{for all} \quad T.$$

The state equation has the solution

$$x(t) = \int_0^t u^2(s)\mathrm{e}^{s-t}\,\mathrm{d}s.$$

This implies that

$$V_T(u(\cdot)) = \int_0^T \left(u(t) - \int_0^t u(s)^2(s)\mathrm{e}^{s-t}\,\mathrm{d}s\right)\,\mathrm{d}t < 0.$$

In particular $\lim_{T\to\infty} V_T(u(\cdot)) = -\infty$ for any other (piecewise continuous) choice of $u \not\equiv 0$, as $\int u(t)\,\mathrm{d}t$ grows at most linearly, whereas $\int x(t)\,\mathrm{d}t$ grows exponentially. Thus $u^* \equiv 0$ is the optimal control, with the corresponding state trajectory $x^* \equiv 0$. From the necessary conditions we derive, using the Hamiltonian

$$\mathcal{H}(x(t), u(t), \lambda(t), \lambda_0) = \lambda_0\,(u(t) - x(t)) + \lambda\left(u(t)^2 + x\right)$$

the costate equation

$$\dot{\lambda}(t) = -\lambda(t) + \lambda_0$$

exhibits the solution

$$\lambda(t) = (\lambda(0) - \lambda_0)\,\mathrm{e}^{-t} + \lambda_0.$$

Since the Maximum Principle demands that

$$\max_{u\in[0,\,1]} \lambda_0 u + \lambda u^2$$

be achieved for $u = 0$, $\lambda_0 > 0$ is ruled out. Otherwise, for $\lambda_0 > 0$, the costate equation reveals that we can find a $T > 0$ such that for all $t > T$,

$$\lambda(t) > 0$$

holds. But this yields $u^*(t) = 1$ for $t > T$, which contradicts the result $u^* \equiv 0$.

Remark 3.80. Another argument why the transversality condition may not hold for infinite horizon problems is considered in Appendix B.4.

The next example takes up again the question of differentiability of the value function for an optimal control problem.

Example 3.81 (A Nondifferentiable Value Function). Let us consider the following example:

$$\max_{u(\cdot)} \int_0^\infty \mathrm{e}^{-rt}x(t)u(t)\,\mathrm{d}t \tag{3.69a}$$

$$\text{s.t.}\quad \dot{x}(t) = -x(t) + u(t) \tag{3.69b}$$

$$x(0) = x_0 \in \mathbb{R}$$

$$u(t) \in [-1, 1], \quad t \geq 0. \tag{3.69c}$$

The state equation (3.69b) reveals that for any $x_0 < 0$ the negative control $u \equiv -1$ gives the largest decrease of $x(t)$ and keeps $x(t) < 0$ therefore maximizes the product $x(t)u(t)$, and likewise $u \equiv 1$ does this for the case $x_0 > 0$. By symmetry, if $x = 0$, both $u \equiv -1$ and $u \equiv 1$ yield the same objective function and are hence both optimal. Thus the optimal pair is given by

$$u^* \equiv \begin{cases} -1 & x_0 < 0 \\ -1 \text{ or } 1 & x_0 = 0 \\ 1 & x_0 > 0, \end{cases}$$

and

$$x^*(t) = \begin{cases} -1 + \mathrm{e}^{-t}(x_0 + 1) & x_0 < 0 \\ \pm 1 \mp \mathrm{e}^{-t} & x_0 = 0 \\ 1 + \mathrm{e}^{-t}(x_0 - 1) & x_0 > 0. \end{cases}$$

Note that for $x_0 = 0$ two optimal paths exist, which is analyzed in more detail in Sect. 5.4.1. For the moment we are only interested in the properties of the corresponding value function $V^*(x_0)$.

An elementary calculation yields

$$V^*(x_0) = \begin{cases} \frac{1-rx}{r(r+1)} & x_0 < 0 \\ \frac{1}{r(r+1)} & x_0 = 0 \\ \frac{rx+1}{r(r+1)} & x_0 > 0, \end{cases} \quad \text{and} \quad V_x^*(x_0) = \begin{cases} -\frac{1}{r+1} & x_0 < 0 \\ \text{nondifferentiable} & x_0 = 0 \\ \frac{1}{r+1} & x_0 > 0. \end{cases}$$

This example reveals that even for functions g and f which are arbitrary often differentiable the value function may not be differentiable at all.

3.8.2 The Ramsey Model for an Infinite Time Horizon

We consider the Ramsey model introduced on p. 124 for an infinite time horizon. In that case the salvage function $S(K)$ is omitted yielding the model:

$$\max_{C(\cdot)} \int_0^\infty \mathrm{e}^{-rt} U(C)\, \mathrm{d}t$$

$$\text{s.t.} \quad \dot{K} = F(K) - \delta K - C, \quad K(0) = K_0.$$

$$0 \le C \le F(K) \tag{3.70a}$$

$$K \ge \underline{K}. \tag{3.70b}$$

In Sect. 3.6.2 we already derived the canonical system for the state–control space

$$\dot{K} = F(K) - \delta K - C \tag{3.71a}$$

$$\dot{C} = \frac{U'(C)}{U''(C)} \left(r + \delta - F'(K)\right). \tag{3.71b}$$

It cannot be proved from the Proposition 3.74 that the transversality condition (3.67) is a necessary condition. Since for an open neighborhood of zero $N_\varepsilon(0)$ the inclusion

$$N_\varepsilon(0) \subset F(K) - \delta K - C, \quad C \geq 0$$

can only be assured if $F(K) - \delta K > 0$, which is not necessarily true.

Next we do a phase portrait analysis of the nonlinear dynamical system given by (3.71a) and (3.71b). Therefore we have to consider the $\dot{K}$- and $\dot{C}$-isoclines yielding

$$C = F(K) - \delta K \tag{3.72a}$$

$$F'(K) = r + \delta. \tag{3.72b}$$

Utilizing the assumptions (3.19b) and (3.19c) we see that the $\dot{K}$-isocline (3.72a) is a strictly concave function being zero both at the origin and for some $\tilde{K} > 0$ and exhibiting its maximum at some $0 < K_m < \tilde{K}$ (see Fig. 3.6a). Moreover the $\dot{C}$-isocline is a vertical line, where (3.19c) together with (3.72b) assures the existence of a unique $\hat{K}$ satisfying (3.72b). Thus we finally find a unique equilibrium at $(\hat{K}, \hat{C})$ with $\hat{C} = F(\hat{K}) - \delta\hat{K}$ and the corresponding Jacobian

$$\hat{J}\left(\hat{K}, \hat{C}\right) = \begin{pmatrix} F'(\hat{K}) - \delta & -1 \\ -\dfrac{U'(\hat{C})}{U''(\hat{C})} F''(\hat{K}) & 0 \end{pmatrix}.$$

Since $\det \hat{J} < 0$ the equilibrium is a saddle point, exhibiting a stable path. Thus for initial states in a neighborhood of $\hat{K}$ the stable path is a possible candidate for an optimal solution. In fact by a careful inspection of the phase portrait it can be proved that this solution is the unique optimal solution, see Arrow and Kurz (1970, p. 64).

In presence of mixed path constraints (3.70a) there exist exit points $\bar{K}_1 < \bar{K}_2$, where for initial states between these points the stable path is the unique optimal solution (see Fig. 3.6a). The exit point $\bar{K}_1$ is an intersection point of the stable path with the axis $C = 0$ and the exit point $\bar{K}_2$ is given by the intersection of the stable path with the curve $C = F(K)$. In Sect. 3.6.1 we have already proved that the optimal control is continuous. Thus the optimal solutions depicted in Fig. 3.6a are the unique optimal paths.

In case of an additional pure state constraint (3.70b) the optimal solution for $\hat{K} < \underline{K} < \bar{K}_1$ is depicted in Fig. 3.6b. In that case it is optimal to control the system into the boundary equilibrium $(\underline{K}, \underline{C})$. The optimality of the depicted solution for initial states lying between $\underline{K}$ and $\bar{K}_1$ can explicitly be shown, using Theorem 3.70. Since for these states the maximized Hamiltonian is strictly concave in K (see Sect. 3.3.7). Moreover the limiting transversality condition is satisfied, since $\lambda(t) \geq 0$ for all t and $\lim_{t\to\infty} K(t) \geq \hat{K}$ for any admissible state trajectory. Since the costate and control are continuous (see Sect. 3.6.2) at the exit point $\bar{K}_1$ the depicted solution in Fig. 3.6b is the unique optimal solution.

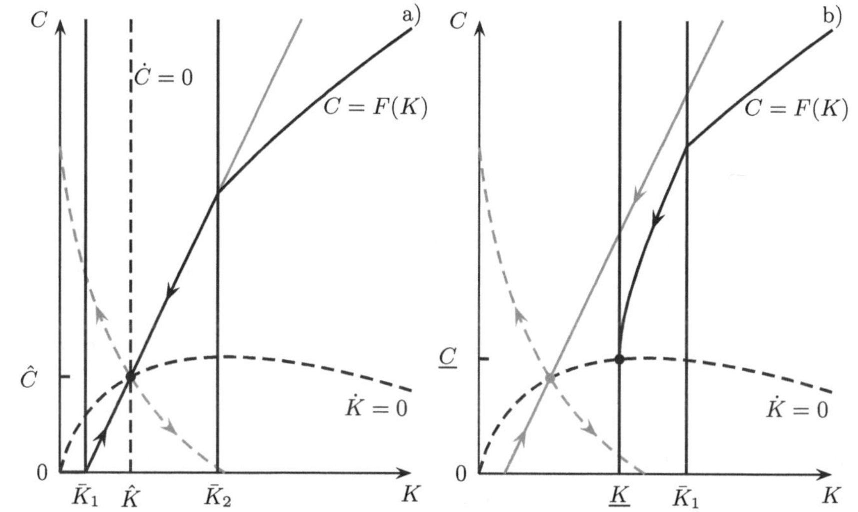

Fig. 3.6. Panel (**a**) depicts the optimal solution path (black solid curve) for the Ramsey model over an infinite time horizon and with mixed path constraints. Starting between the states $\bar{K}_1$ and $\bar{K}_2$ the stable path converging to the saddle $(\hat{K}, \hat{C})$ is the optimal solution. For initial states outside this interval the optimal control lies on its boundary until the exit point $\bar{K}_1$ or $\bar{K}_2$, respectively, is reached. There it is optimal to move along the stable path. In panel (**b**) also the pure state $K \geq \underline{K}$ has to be considered. In that case for states lying between $\underline{K}$ and $\bar{K}_1$ the optimal control value lies in the interior of the control region and the optimal path leads to the boundary equilibrium $(\underline{K}, \underline{C})$. For states $K > \bar{K}_1$ the control values are chosen from the upper boundary of the control region, until the exit point $\bar{K}_1$ is reached, there one switches to the interior of the control region as described before.

Remark 3.82. For Fig. 3.6 we used the functional forms

$$F(K) = \sqrt{K}, \quad \text{and} \quad U(C) = \log C,$$

and the parameter values $r = 0.1$ and $\delta = 0.5$.

3.8.3 Structural Results on One-State Discounted, Autonomous Systems

We summarize some propositions revealing structural properties of the solutions of autonomous, discounted systems over an infinite time horizon. The long-run behavior of the optimal solution is interesting from an economic point of view, first to see whether the optimal trajectory converges to some equilibrium (or in higher dimensions also to a limit cycle).

Under appropriate concavity assumptions one can show that asymptotic paths are the optimal solutions (see, e.g., Carlson et al., 1991, Chap. 6). But in general for nonlinear, nonconcave models these paths are only candidates, and one has to exclude other possible paths explicitly. See, e.g., Arrow and Kurz (1970, p. 64), in which such an argument is given for a simple capital accumulation model.

The main computational effort for solving optimal control models of this type is calculating the stable manifolds of the occurring saddles (see Sect. 7.4).

Equilibria are of significant importance for analyzing autonomous infinite horizon problems, especially for one-state models, and the following proposition summarizes some crucial properties; for a proof see Wagener (2003):

Proposition 3.83. *For one-state models of type* DAM *(3.64) with* $r > 0$*, unstable equilibria are the only possible limit sets of the corresponding canonical system.*

Sketch of Proof. The first part of the proposition uses the fact that the Jacobian $\hat{J}$ of the canonical system at an equilibrium $(\hat{x}, \hat{\lambda})$ is given by

$$\hat{J} = \begin{pmatrix} \mathcal{H}^*_{\lambda x} & \mathcal{H}^*_{\lambda\lambda} \\ -\mathcal{H}^*_{xx} & r - \mathcal{H}^*_{x\lambda} \end{pmatrix},$$

yielding $\operatorname{tr} J = r > 0$. This property also rules out limit cycles.

Thus saddles and their stable paths are identified as the most important candidates for optimal solutions under the assumption that an optimal solution converges to an equilibrium.

Remark 3.84. The instability of optimal equilibria and limit cycles for $r > 0$ is proved for arbitrary dimensions in Sect. 7.4.

For one-state models the monotonicity of the state trajectory can be proved:

Proposition 3.85. *Let* $(x^*(\cdot), u^*(\cdot))$ *be the unique optimal solution of a one-state model of type* DAM *(3.64). Then the state trajectory is monotone for all* $t \geq 0$.

An elementary proof is presented in Appendix B.5, (see also Hartl, 1987).

Remark 3.86. The assumption of uniqueness is crucial for the validity of the proposition and is shown by a counter-example in Hartl (1987). There an optimal state trajectory following a damped oscillation exists, since the optimal control is not unique.

With these arguments in mind, we now analyze an optimal control problem of the US cocaine epidemic.

3.9 An Optimal Control Model of a Drug Epidemic

3.9.1 Model Formulation

As a simple optimal control problem example, we augment the descriptive model of a drug epidemic from Sect. 2.9 with one control that increases the rate of exit from drug use, which we will refer to as *treatment*. More precisely, the control variable $u(t)$ denotes treatment expenditure at time t. As in Tragler, Caulkins, and Feichtinger (2001) we assume that the rate at which users quit in response to treatment may be described by

$$c\left(\frac{u(t)}{A(t)}\right)^z. \tag{3.73}$$

The interpretation is that outflow due to treatment is proportional to treatment spending $u(t)$ per capita $A(t)$ raised to an exponent z $(0 < z < 1)$ that reflects diminishing marginal efficiency of treatment, with c being a positive constant. Such diminishing returns have been included in several related models (e.g., Everingham and Rydell, 1994) and reflect "cream skimming." The idea is that some users are easier to treat than others, and the treatment system has some capacity to focus first on individuals who are more likely to benefit from treatment. As treatment funding and the number of people treated grow, however, the system can afford to be less and less selective.

For ease of exposition, we will mostly omit the time argument t in what follows. Multiplying the rate from (3.73) by the number of users A, we get

$$c\left(\frac{u}{A}\right)^z A = cu^z A^{1-z} \tag{3.74}$$

as the number of users per unit time who quit in response to treatment when treatment spending is at level u. Note that (3.74) also holds for $A = 0$, which can be shown using l'Hospital's rule. Plugging (3.74) into the descriptive dynamics (2.58) and using the logistic function (2.59) for initiation, we get

$$\dot{A} = kA\left(\bar{A} - A\right) - cu^z A^{1-z} - \mu A \tag{3.75a}$$

as the state equation for our control model. Equation (3.75a) states that we consider one inflow term, initiation, and two outflow terms: outflow due to treatment and the "natural" outflow.

For the optimal control model we still have to specify the objective functional, which describes the optimization goal of the decision-maker. We formulate the objective as minimizing the discounted sum of the costs associated with drug use plus the costs of treatment. For simplicity we assume that the societal costs of drug use are proportional to the number of users, with parameter ρ denoting the average annual costs per user. If we assume an infinite planning horizon, we get the formulation

$$\min_{u(\cdot)} \int_0^\infty \mathrm{e}^{-rt}\left(\rho A(t) + u(t)\right) \mathrm{d}t, \tag{3.75b}$$

where r is the time discount rate. The minimization is subject to the system dynamics (3.75a) and the nonnegativity constraint

$$u(t) \geq 0, \quad \text{for all} \quad t \tag{3.75c}$$

as a reasonable condition for the control.

3.9.2 Stability Analysis

For the purpose of applying Pontryagin's Maximum Principle to the autonomous optimal control problem specified by (3.75), we first multiply the objective functional by -1 to obtain a maximization problem. Next, we formulate the current-value Hamiltonian

$$\mathcal{H}(A, u, \lambda) = -\rho A - u + \lambda \left(kA\left(\bar{A} - A\right) - cu^z A^{1-z} - \mu A\right),$$

where λ is the current-value costate variable. Recall that the costate λ may be interpreted as a shadow price of the stock A of users. More precisely, in this problem we expect that λ will be negative with the absolute value describing the incremental costs of having one more drug user.

As a necessary condition for optimality we have the Hamiltonian maximizing condition $\mathcal{H}_u = 0$, which gives

$$u = (-cz\lambda)^{\frac{1}{1-z}} A = u(A, \lambda). \tag{3.76}$$

For negative λ, $\mathcal{H}_{uu} = -cz(z-1)\lambda u^{z-2} A^{1-z}$ is negative in the admissible domain, so the control u from (3.76) indeed maximizes the Hamiltonian. Furthermore, u is nonnegative whenever A is, so we don't have to take into account the nonnegativity constraint on u (3.75c) explicitly. Substituting the expression (3.76) for u in the costate equation

$$\dot{\lambda} = r\lambda - \mathcal{H}_A$$

gives

$$\dot{\lambda} = \lambda\left(r - k\left(\bar{A} - 2A\right) + (1-z)\left(-c^{\frac{1}{z}} z\lambda\right)^{\frac{z}{1-z}} + \mu\right) + \rho \tag{3.77}$$

as the dynamics of the costate. Analogously, we paste u from (3.76) into the state equation (3.75a) to get

$$\dot{A} = kA\left(\bar{A} - A\right) - \left(-c^{\frac{1}{z}} z\lambda\right)^{\frac{z}{1-z}} A - \mu A. \tag{3.78}$$

The canonical system of the two differential equations (3.77–3.78) will now be used to derive the solution of our optimal control problem. We start by computing the equilibria of the canonical system, which we get by solving $\dot{A} = 0$ and $\dot{\lambda} = 0$ simultaneously. Obviously, $\dot{A} = 0$ is quadratic in A and can easily be solved, giving the two solutions

$$\hat{A}_1 = 0 \tag{3.79}$$

and

$$\tilde{A} = \bar{A} - \frac{\mu}{k} - \frac{1}{k}\left(-c^{\frac{1}{z}} z\lambda\right)^{\frac{z}{1-z}} = \tilde{A}(\lambda). \tag{3.80}$$

Pasting either of the two solutions (3.79–3.80) into $\dot{\lambda} = 0$, we get a nonlinear equation in λ, where the nature of the nonlinearity is determined by the value of the exponent $\frac{z}{1-z}$. For $z \in (0,\, 1)$, this exponent is monotonously increasing in z and may take any value in $(0,\, \infty)$. This implies that there is exactly one value of z leading to a quadratic equation in λ, i.e., $z = 0.5$, with the exponent taking the value 1. In past analyses, z has been set to 0.4 (Zeiler, 2004), 0.5 (Wallner, 2005), or 0.6 (Behrens et al., 2000b; Tragler et al., 2001). We shall use the medium-sized value

$$z = 0.5.$$

This has the advantage of allowing for an analytical solution of the equation $\dot{\lambda} = 0$, while any other value of z would require numerical solution methods for the remaining steps of the analysis.

We first compute the equilibria of the canonical system at $\hat{A}_1$ and $\tilde{A}$, respectively. Then we study the stability properties of these equilibria by analyzing the associated eigenvalues of the Jacobian matrix.

Boundary Equilibrium $\hat{A}_1$

Substituting $\hat{A}_1 = 0$ into $\dot{\lambda} = 0$ yields the quadratic equation

$$\lambda^2 - \frac{4\left(r - k\bar{A} + \mu\right)}{c^2}\lambda - \frac{4\rho}{c^2} = 0,$$

the solutions of which are given by

$$\hat{\lambda} = \frac{2\left(r - k\bar{A} + \mu\right)}{c^2} \pm \sqrt{\frac{4\left(r - k\bar{A} + \mu\right)^2}{c^4} + \frac{4\rho}{c^2}}. \tag{3.81}$$

Defining as in Sect. 2.9

$$r_0 := k\bar{A} - \mu,$$

we can rewrite (3.81) more concisely as

$$\hat{\lambda} = \frac{2}{c}\left(\frac{(r - r_0)}{c} \pm \sqrt{\frac{(r - r_0)^2}{c^2} + \rho}\right). \tag{3.82}$$

It makes sense to assume that condition (2.62) holds, i.e., r_0 is positive. Without loss of generality we will further assume that the social cost parameter ρ is strictly positive.[20] We now first observe that the radicand (i.e., the argument of the square root) in (3.82) is strictly positive, implying that the square root

[20] A negative value of ρ does not make sense from an economic point of view. The hairline case $\rho = 0$ reduces the objective to the minimization of treatment spending, which results in the trivial optimal solution $u \equiv 0$, i.e., the uncontrolled problem discussed earlier in Sect. 2.9.

gives a positive real number. Furthermore, the square root dominates the term $\frac{(r-r_0)}{c}$, irrespective of the sign of this term. Hence we conclude that only the solution with the negative square root gives a negative costate, yielding the appropriate equilibrium solution $\hat{\lambda}_1$ given by

$$\hat{\lambda}_1 = \frac{2}{c}\left(\frac{(r-r_0)}{c} - \sqrt{\frac{(r-r_0)^2}{c^2} + \rho}\right). \tag{3.83}$$

Interior Equilibrium $\tilde{A}$

Substituting $\tilde{A} = \bar{A} - \frac{\mu}{k} - \frac{1}{k}\left(-c^{\frac{1}{z}} z\lambda\right)^{\frac{z}{1-z}} = \tilde{A}(\lambda)$ into $\dot{\lambda} = 0$ yields a quadratic equation in λ,

$$\lambda^2 + \frac{4\left(r + k\bar{A} - \mu\right)}{3c^2}\lambda + \frac{4\rho}{3c^2} = 0,$$

the roots of which are given by

$$\hat{\lambda}_{2/3} = \frac{2}{3c^2}\left(-\left(r + r_0\right) \pm \sqrt{\left(r + r_0\right)^2 - 3c^2\rho}\right). \tag{3.84}$$

The associated equilibrium values of A are given by

$$\hat{A}_{2/3} = \frac{1}{3k}\left(2r_0 - r \pm \sqrt{\left(r + r_0\right)^2 - 3c^2\rho}\right), \tag{3.85}$$

where we define $\hat{A}_2$ ($\hat{A}_3$) as the solution in (3.85) with the *negative* (*positive*) square root term.

As we are looking for real roots, we need to demand that the radicand, given by

$$\Delta := \left(r + r_0\right)^2 - 3c^2\rho \tag{3.86}$$

and being the same for $\hat{\lambda}_{2/3}$ and $\hat{A}_{2/3}$, is nonnegative:

$$\Delta \geq 0 \quad \text{iff} \quad \rho \leq \frac{\left(r + r_0\right)^2}{3c^2} =: \rho_{bs}. \tag{3.87}$$

Assuming that (3.87) holds, $\hat{\lambda}_{2/3}$ given by (3.84) are not only real but also negative, implying that in this case we get two more candidates for equilibria making economic sense.

Whether or not condition (3.87) holds obviously depends on the relative sizes of the parameters involved. For a better understanding let us assume that all parameters except for the social cost parameter ρ are kept fixed, while we let ρ vary in $(0, \infty)$. In other words, we will perform a *bifurcation analysis* with respect to the average social costs per user per unit of time, a graphical representation of which we display in Fig. 3.7.

With Δ from (3.86) and

$$\Phi := 2r_0 - r$$

$\hat{A}_{2/3}$ can be presented more clearly as

$$\hat{A}_{2/3} = \frac{1}{3k}\left(\Phi \pm \sqrt{\Delta}\right). \tag{3.88}$$

(3.87) states that the equilibria at $\hat{A}_{2/3}$ exist iff the social cost parameter ρ is less or equal to ρ_{bs}, implying that a *blue sky* bifurcation occurs for $\rho = \rho_{bs}$, where $\Delta = 0$ and $\hat{A}_2 = \hat{A}_3 = \frac{\Phi}{3k}$. Furthermore, observing that Δ is increasing for decreasing values of ρ, we find that $\hat{A}_2$ and $\hat{A}_3$ are decreasing and increasing, respectively, when we move along the ρ-axis from right to left (see Fig. 3.7). Finally, at $\rho = 0$ (i.e., the minimum value for the social costs) we compute $\hat{A}_{2/3} = \frac{1}{3k}\left(\Phi \pm (r + r_0)\right)$, where $\hat{A}_3 = \frac{r_0}{k}$ corresponds to the steady state level of A in the uncontrolled (descriptive) problem (cf. Sect. 2.9).

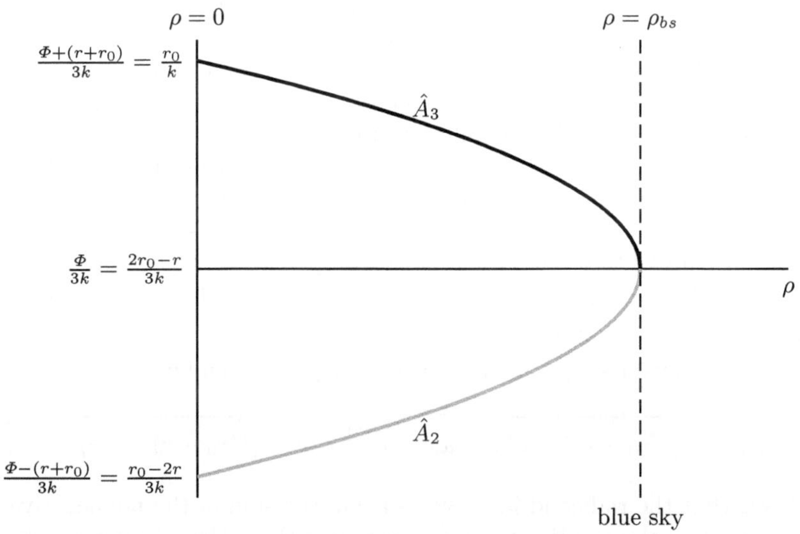

Fig. 3.7. Bifurcation diagram for ρ, keeping all other parameters constant. The equilibria at $\hat{A}_{2/3}$ exist iff $\rho \le \rho_{bs}$, where ρ_{bs} is the location of the blue sky bifurcation

This concludes a basic discussion of the equilibria that may arise in our optimal control model of drug use. We proved that there may be up to three equilibria, the admissibility and stability properties of which we will discuss next.

Admissibility and Stability Properties of the Equilibria

An equilibrium $(\hat{A}_i, \hat{\lambda}_i)$, $i = 1, 2, 3$, is *admissible* if both $\hat{A}_i \geq 0$ and $\hat{\lambda}_i \leq 0$ hold. We concluded above that this is always true for the equilibrium at $\hat{A}_1 = 0$ with $\hat{\lambda}_1$ from (3.83), implying that there is always at least this one equilibrium solution.

Assuming again fixed values for all parameters except for ρ, we find that we need ρ less or equal to $\rho_{bs} = \frac{(r+r_0)^2}{3c^2}$ for $\left(\hat{A}_{2/3}, \hat{\lambda}_{2/3}\right)$ to exist. If they exist, our considerations above concluded that $\hat{\lambda}_{2/3}$ will be nonpositive, so the costates have the right sign. What remains to be checked are the signs of $\hat{A}_2$ and $\hat{A}_3$, respectively.

First recall Fig. 3.7. There, the horizontal axis is at the level $\Phi = 2r_0 - r$, which can have any sign. The main question is where to put the horizontal line representing $\hat{A}_1 = 0$ which separates the admissible solutions (lying above) from the ones which are not admissible (lying below). What we do know is that $\hat{A}_3$ at $\rho = 0$ is $\frac{1}{3k}\left(\Phi + (r + r_0)\right) = \frac{r_0}{k}$, which is always positive due to our basic nonnegativity assumption for r_0 (recall (2.62)). While this observation allows us to conclude that the horizontal axis $\hat{A}_1 = 0$ must be located below $\frac{r_0}{k}$, we cannot say more without knowing the relative sizes of r and r_0. In other words, depending on those sizes of r and r_0, we may imagine to find the axis $\hat{A}_1 = 0$ anywhere below the level $\frac{r_0}{k}$. An immediate conclusion is that it is possible to find all three equilibria in the admissible domain.

For ease of exposition, let us choose one particular scenario as illustrated in Fig. 3.8, where we find the horizontal axis $\hat{A}_1 = 0$ somewhere between the levels $\frac{\Phi}{3k}$ and $\frac{r_0 - 2r}{3k}$. This is the case whenever $r \in \left[\frac{r_0}{2}, 2r_0\right]$. Furthermore, let us in parallel to discuss the stability properties of the equilibria which we do by analyzing the two eigenvalues $\alpha_i^{(1)}$ and $\alpha_i^{(2)}$ of the Jacobian matrix, evaluated at the equilibria $(\hat{A}_i, \hat{\lambda}_i)$, $i = 1, 2, 3$.

The eigenvalues $\alpha_1^{(1)}$ and $\alpha_1^{(2)}$ at $(\hat{A}_1, \hat{\lambda}_1)$ are given by

$$\alpha_1^{(1)} = \sqrt{(r_0 - r)^2 + c^2\rho}, \quad \text{and} \quad \alpha_1^{(2)} = r - \sqrt{(r_0 - r)^2 + c^2\rho}. \tag{3.89}$$

We see that the radicand in (3.89) is again the sum of the nonnegative term $(r_0 - r)^2$ and the positive term $c^2\rho$, implying that these eigenvalues are real. While $\alpha_1^{(1)}$ is (always) positive, $\alpha_1^{(2)}$ can have any sign. What we may say, though, is that for ρ sufficiently high, the radicand will be large enough for $\alpha_1^{(2)}$ becoming negative. In particular, after a few lines of algebraic operations we find that

$$\alpha_1^{(2)} < 0 \quad \text{iff} \quad r_0^2 - 2r_0 r + c^2\rho =: \Omega > 0.$$

In terms of a condition for ρ, $\alpha_1^{(2)}$ is negative and, hence, $(\hat{A}_1, \hat{\lambda}_1)$ is a saddle point iff

$$\Omega > 0 \quad \text{iff} \quad \rho > \frac{r_0\,(2r - r_0)}{c^2} =: \rho_t,$$

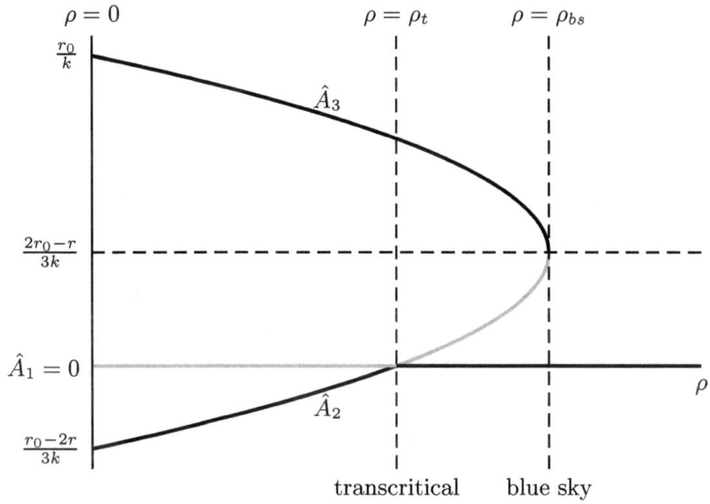

Fig. 3.8. Bifurcation diagram for ρ, keeping all other parameters constant. Starting with high values of ρ, there is only one equilibrium at $\hat{A}_1 = 0$, which is a saddle. With ρ decreased, a blue sky bifurcation occurs, creating a medium-sized unstable equilibrium and a high saddle point. With ρ decreased further, a transcritical bifurcation emerges where the medium-sized equilibrium becomes negative and at the same time the equilibrium changes its stability property, i.e., becoming a saddle, while the equilibrium at $\hat{A}_1 = 0$ becomes unstable

while it is unstable otherwise. Not surprisingly, under parameter values leading to a graphical representation as illustrated in Fig. 3.8, not only we find a change of the stability of $(\hat{A}_1, \hat{\lambda}_1)$ at ρ_t, but also it is exactly this value of ρ where $\hat{A}_2$ changes its sign, because $\hat{A}_2$ is positive exactly if $\rho > \rho_t$. Furthermore, analyzing the eigenvalues $\alpha_2^{(1)}$ and $\alpha_2^{(2)}$ at $(\hat{A}_2, \hat{\lambda}_2)$ given by

$$\alpha_2^{(1)/(2)} = \frac{r}{2} \pm \frac{1}{\sqrt{3}} \sqrt{\Delta + \frac{3}{4} r^2 - \Phi \sqrt{\Delta}}, \tag{3.90}$$

we find that $(\hat{A}_2, \hat{\lambda}_2)$ is a saddle point iff $\rho < \rho_t$, while otherwise it is unstable. We conclude that we just proved the existence of a *transcritical* bifurcation at $\rho = \rho_t$ as illustrated in Fig. 3.8 (cf. Sect. 2.8.3).

Finally, the eigenvalues $\alpha_3^{(1)}$ and $\alpha_3^{(2)}$ at $(\hat{A}_3, \hat{\lambda}_3)$ are given by

$$\alpha_3^{(1)/(2)} = \frac{r}{2} \pm \frac{1}{\sqrt{3}} \sqrt{\Delta + \frac{3}{4} r^2 + \Phi \sqrt{\Delta}}.$$

In a scenario as depicted in Fig. 3.8 with positive $\Phi = 2r_0 - r$, both eigenvalues are real and have opposite sign, so $(\hat{A}_3, \hat{\lambda}_3)$ is a saddle point and $\hat{A}_3$ is positive for all ρ in $[0, \rho_{bs}]$.

This concludes the discussion of existence, admissibility, and stability properties of the equilibria of the canonical system (3.77–3.78). What remains to be done is a phase portrait analysis.

3.9.3 Phase Portrait Analysis

We have shown above that the simple model of a drug epidemic considered here has either one, two, or three admissible equilibria, as is best illustrated by a bifurcation diagram such as the one in Fig. 3.8. Keeping all parameters except for the social cost parameter ρ constant, we find the following three possible regimes determined by the particular value that is chosen for ρ:

$0 \leq \rho < \rho_t$: The equilibria at $\hat{A}_1 = 0$ and $\hat{A}_3 > 0$ are admissible. $(\hat{A}_1, \hat{\lambda}_1)$ is unstable, $(\hat{A}_3, \hat{\lambda}_3)$ is a saddle point. For any positive initial number of users $A(0) =: A_0$, the optimal trajectory is the saddle point path starting at A_0 and converging to the *high* equilibrium at $\hat{A}_3$ as shown in Fig. 3.9a. In this regime, which is characterized by low costs of drug use, optimal treatment spending is moderate, resulting in a high long-run equilibrium. As already discussed earlier, in the special case $\rho = 0$ where no costs of drug use occur irrespective of the number of users, optimal treatment spending is zero for obvious reasons, so the optimal equilibrium corresponds to the highest possible number of users, i.e., the equilibrium level of the uncontrolled system $\frac{r_0}{k}$. However, with increasing costs of drug use ρ, treatment becomes more and more attractive, so the equilibrium level of users to be approached is decreasing (but positive).

$\rho_t < \rho < \rho_{bs}$: All three equilibria are admissible. $(\hat{A}_1, \hat{\lambda}_1)$ and $(\hat{A}_3, \hat{\lambda}_3)$ are saddle points, $(\hat{A}_2, \hat{\lambda}_2)$ is unstable. This case will be discussed later in Sect. 5.6. We will see that both saddle points can be optimal, with their basins of attraction in terms of the initial number of users A_0 being separated by a so-called DNSS point.

$\rho > \rho_{bs}$: The only admissible equilibrium is at the *low* level $\hat{A}_1 = 0$. Hence, for all initial numbers of users A_0 it is optimal to follow the saddle point path leading to the lowest possible number of users $\hat{A}_1 = 0$ as illustrated in Fig. 3.9b. The economic interpretation is that for large enough costs of drug use $(\rho > \rho_{bs})$ optimal treatment spending will be relatively excessive, allowing for an eradication of drug use.

Remark 3.87. The scenario we discussed above assumed $r \in \left[\frac{r_0}{2}, 2r_0\right]$. For $r < \frac{r_0}{2}$ or $r > 2r_0$ the corresponding bifurcation diagrams are different from the one in Fig. 3.8 in that the location of the horizontal axis representing the steady state at $\hat{A}_1$ is lower or higher, respectively. When $r < \frac{r_0}{2}$, $\hat{A}_2$ is positive for all nonnegative values of ρ, so the transcritical bifurcation occurs for a negative value of ρ. When $r > 2r_0$, $\hat{A}_2$ is negative for all nonnegative values of ρ, so there are at most two admissible steady states. More precisely, for $\rho > \rho_t$ the only admissible equilibrium is at $\hat{A}_1$, implying that the eradication

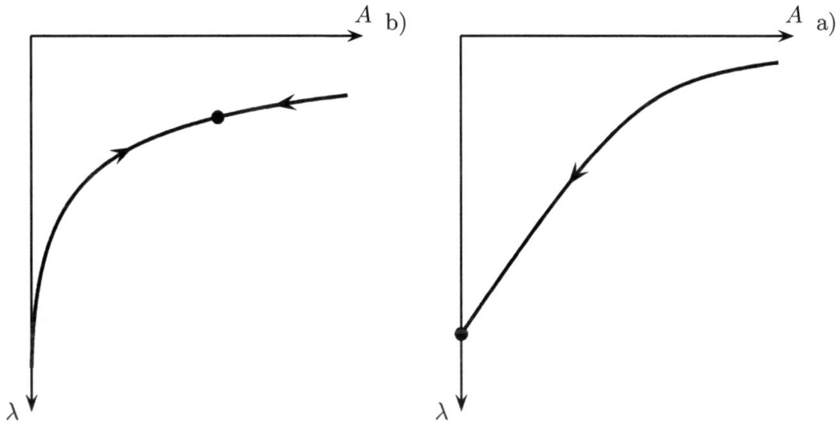

Fig. 3.9. In (**a**) the phase diagram for a case in which only the high equilibrium is optimal is shown. In panel (**b**) the phase diagram for a case in which only the equilibrium at $\hat{A}_1 = 0$ is optimal is depicted

policy is optimal. For $\rho \leq \rho_t$ $(\hat{A}_3, \hat{\lambda}_3)$ is both admissible and a saddle point, while $(\hat{A}_1, \hat{\lambda}_1)$ is unstable, so the optimal policy is to converge to the high equilibrium at $\hat{A}_3$. We will provide more insightful discussions about possible scenarios and their implications for optimal policies in Sect. 5.6.

Exercises

3.1 (Present- and Current-Value Notation). Prove that for the present-value notation (see Remark 3.11) the necessary conditions (3.6) can be derived from the necessary conditions (3.4).

Hint. Consider the transformation $\tilde{\mathcal{H}} = \mathrm{e}^{-rt}\mathcal{H}$, *and* $\tilde{\lambda} = \mathrm{e}^{-rt}\lambda$.

3.2 (Control and Terminal Constraints). Solve the following problem:

$$\min_{u(\cdot)} \int_0^4 x \, \mathrm{d}t$$
$$\text{s.t.} \quad \dot{x} = u, \quad x(0) = 1$$
$$1 + u \geq 0, \quad 1 - u \geq 0$$

for the following alternative terminal constraints
(a) $x(4) = 1$, (b) $x(4) \geq 1$, (c) $x(4) \leq 1$, (d) $x(4)$ free. Show that in case (b) one gets $x(4) = 1$. Note that the complementary slackness condition

$$\lambda(4)\,(x(4) - 1) = 0$$

says that at the end "nothing valuable is left" (i.e., $x(4) > 1$ is suboptimal for $\lambda(4) \neq 0$).

Hint. Use Pontryagin's Maximum Principle Theorem 3.52.

3.3 (Pure State Constraints). Solve Exercise 3.91 for $x(4) - 1 = 0$ and the additional path constraint

$$h(x) = x \geq 0 \quad \text{for} \quad 0 \leq t \leq 4.$$

Hint. Use the optimality conditions of Pontryagin's Maximum Principle Theorem 3.60, particularly the complementary slackness conditions (3.54f). Does the costate jump?

3.4 (The Nerlove-Arrow Model). The following model provides one of the first applications of optimal control in economics. It dates back to 1962 and was then solved by variational calculus.

Nerlove and Arrow (1962) conceived advertising as an investment to accumulate goodwill. Advertising expenditures spent today influence future demand. Goodwill is interpreted as "advertising capital" or, more simply, as the number of customers, who have bought the product so far.

Denoting by a the advertising expenditure rate at time t and by A the goodwill stock by time t, we get

$$\dot{A} = a - \delta A, \quad A(0) = A_0,$$

where the rate $\delta > 0$ measures the rate at which the customers leave the firm or stop using the product. Here it is assumed that one monetary unit spent on advertising causes a (gross) increase of goodwill by one unit.

If we assume a constant selling price, the sales revenue of the firm depends solely on A and we consider a strictly concave return function $\pi(A)$. The objective of the firm is to maximize its discounted profit stream

$$\max_{a(\cdot)\geq 0} \int_0^\infty \mathrm{e}^{-rt} \left(\pi(A) - a\right) \mathrm{d}t.$$

Show the existence of an MRAP solution and interpret the turnpike property of the singular solution. Extend the analysis to a monopolistic firm for which the sales depend not only on A but also on the price.

3.5 (Advertising and Diffusion–Gould's First Diffusion Model). This example refers to another early application of optimal control techniques in marketing (Gould, 1970). We consider a single firm on the supply side, and many consumers on the demand side. Assume a market for a durable good with a constant number of potential buyers, i.e., a market potential $\bar{x}$. Denote by x the number of the firm's customers by time t. Denote also the advertising rate of the firm at time t by $a(t)$ and assume that the advertising costs $c(a)$ are convex, with $c(0) = 0$, $c'(a) > 0$, $c''(a) > 0$. The state dynamics

$$\dot{x} = a\,(\bar{x} - x) - \delta x, \quad x(0) = x_0$$

describes the transition of potential buyers to customers by means of advertising as well as the "obsolescence" of the product (e.g., by brand switching). The firm's objective is to maximize the present value of its net profit:

$$\max_{a(\cdot)\geq 0} \int_0^T \mathrm{e}^{-rt} \left(\pi(x) - c(a)\right) \mathrm{d}t + \mathrm{e}^{-rT} S x(T).$$

Here $\pi(x)$ is the profit obtained by the sales (net of the production costs), while S denotes the salvage value per customer at the end of the planning horizon T.

Usually it makes sense to assume $S = 0$. But one can imagine the case in which at the terminal time the firm sells its clientele.

Carry out a saddle point analysis. Discuss the dependence of the solution on the model parameters.

3.6 (Optimal Maintenance and Replacement). Consider a machine whose resale value $x(\cdot)$ gradually declines over time t. Assume that it is possible to slow the rate of decline of the resale value by preventive maintenance. Denote by T the sale date of the machine and by u the expenditures on preventive maintenance.

The decline of the resale value is determined by two components: a technological obsolesce rate $\gamma(t)$ (aging and technological progress reduces the productivity of the machine) and a rate of successive deterioration $\delta(t)$, both of which are subsequently considered constant. The dynamics of the resale value is given by

$$\dot{x} = -\gamma - \delta x + g(u, t), \tag{3.92}$$

where $g(u, t)$ measures the effectiveness of maintenance.

It seems reasonable to assume $\gamma \geq 0$ and $g_t \leq 0$. It is realistic to assume that preventive maintenance is not so effective as to enhance the resale value over its previous values; i.e.,

$$-\gamma + g(\bar{u}, t) \leq 0 \quad \text{for} \quad t \in [0, T],$$

where $\bar{u}$ denotes the maximum maintenance rate.

The machine produces goods or services. Suppose that the revenue of the production depends on the state of the machine. Assuming for simplicity that the revenue is given by πx, then the firm wants to maximize the discounted stream of production revenue minus maintenance costs during its lifetime, plus the discounted resale value at T

$$\max_{u(\cdot) \in [0, \bar{u}]} \int_0^T \mathrm{e}^{-rt} (\pi x - u) \, \mathrm{d}t + \mathrm{e}^{-rT} x(T)$$

subject to (3.92) and a given initial value $x(0) = x_0 > 0$.

The problem typically consists of simultaneously determining the optimal rate of preventive maintenance and the sale date of the machine.

Assuming that $\pi > r + \delta$ for $t \in [0, T]$, show that there exists a switching point τ such that

$$u(t) = \begin{cases} \bar{u} & \text{for } 0 \leq t \leq \tau \\ 0 & \text{for } \tau \leq t \leq T. \end{cases}$$

Discuss the "corner" solutions $\tau = 0$ and $\tau = T$, respectively.

3.7 (Free Terminal Time; Optimal Replacement). In Exercise 3.6 the planning horizon T was fixed. Assume now that T has to be determined optimally. Use the condition (3.10) to determine the optimal replacement time of a machine. Which assumptions imply the existence of a non-degenerate T^*?

Note that (3.10) admits a nice economic interpretation given in Sect. 3.3.4.

3.8 (A Production–Inventory Model). Assume that a firm has to satisfy the demand for a good by production. If production exceeds demand, the excess is put into inventory. Denote the demand as d, the production rate as v, and the stock of inventory as z. These three quantities are connected by the following accounting equation:

$$\dot{z} = v - d,$$

where the initial inventory $z(0) = z_0 \geq 0$ is given. Demand $d(\cdot)$ is exogenously given. Clearly, the production intensity must be nonnegative, $v \geq 0$.

Assuming that no shortages are allowed, a pure state constraint $z \geq 0$ is imposed.

Assuming convex production costs, $c(v)$, and linear inventory costs, hz, we see that the firm's goal is to minimize the total costs over a fixed and finite planning period:

$$\min_{v(\cdot)} \int_0^T (c(v) + hz)\, dt,$$

where h is the per-unit inventory cost and $c(v)$ is the production cost function.

Characterize the optimal production program by combining interior and boundary solutions, i.e., $z > 0$ and $z = 0$. It turns out that the optimal production policy is a "smoothed" version of the demand trajectory. "Peaks" of demand are pulled down, whereas "dips" are filled up.

If we set $d \equiv 0$ and $z(T) = z_T > 0$, the model deals with the problem of determining an optimal production program to meet a certain demand x_T at a given deliver date T. Prove that in general there is an initial period of no production or inventory. Ascertain the time t^* when production commences in order to meet the final demand.

3.9 (Monopolist Pricing with Dynamic Demand and Production Cost). Formulate and solve the following dynamic price model of a firm faced with carryover effects and learning by doing (Kalish, 1983).

For many durable goods, sales at time t depend not only on the price $p(t)$ but also on past sales, i.e., the cumulated sales until t. Assume that for a given price during the earlier stages of the product's lifecycle the sales at time t increase with the cumulated sales until t, $X(t)$, whereas later the opposite is true. Thus the demand at t is given by $\eta(p(t))\varphi(X(t))$, where $\eta'(p) < 0$ and $\varphi'(X) \gtreqless 0$ for $X \lesseqgtr \bar{X}$, and where $\bar{X}$ is a positive constant.

Suppose further that the cost of producing one unit $c(X)$ depends negatively on X, i.e., $c'(X) < 0$ ("learning by doing"). Formulate an intertemporal decision problem for a profit-maximizing firm that must determine an optimal pricing policy.

3.10 (Consumption–Pollution Trade-Offs). The following model goes back to Forster (1977). It studies the trade-off between consumption and pollution. In order to focus on this basic problem, we assume away problems of natural-resource exhaustion, population growth, technical progress, and capital accumulation. Its purpose is to show how the solution is modified when the equilibrium occurs on the boundary of the state space.

Assume that economic welfare is measured by a strictly concave utility function $U(C, P)$ of current consumption C and a stock of pollution P. The marginal utility of consumption is positive but diminishing. The marginal utility of pollution is negative and decreasing. As the pollution level rises, these effects are aggravated. In particular, we assume that $U_{CP} \leq 0$ (e.g., a rise in the dust-particle level in a picnic area will drive down the enjoyment derived from an additional sandwich).

In each time period a fixed output ψ^0 is produced and is allocated to consumption C or to pollution control E. That is,

$$\psi^0 = C + E.$$

Posing the problem in this way allows us to focus solely on the consumption–pollution abatement trade-off.

Whereas consumption contributes with a convex flow $g(C)$ to pollution, P is cleaned up by a concave function $h(E)$. The net contribution to the flow of pollution is given by

$$Z(C) = g(C) - h(E) = g(C) - h(\psi^0 - C).$$

The accumulation of waste is governed by the ODE

$$\dot{P} = Z(C) - \alpha P, \tag{3.93}$$

where α denotes the natural cleaning rate. Given the above assumptions, Z is a concave function.

Note that there exists a level of consumption, $\bar{C}$, that will sustain a clean environment:

$$Z(C) \lesseqqgtr 0 \quad \text{for} \quad C \lesseqqgtr \bar{C}.$$

The planning problem is

$$\max_{C(\cdot)} \int_0^\infty \mathrm{e}^{-rt} U(C, P)\, \mathrm{d}t$$

subject to (3.93), $P(0) = P_0$, $0 \le C \le \psi_0$ and, the *pure state constraint*

$$P(t) \ge 0, \quad \text{for all} \quad t.$$

Carry out a saddle point analysis, and give an economic interpretation of the long-run equilibrium describing the consumption–pollution trade-off. Discuss the two essential cases, namely:

- An environment that is polluted over the long run (interior equilibrium)
- A clean long-run (boundary) equilibrium

Prove and interpret the condition

$$U_C(\bar{C}) \lesseqqgtr \frac{-U_P(0) Z'(\bar{C})}{r + \alpha},$$

which is crucial to distinguish the two cases.

3.11 (Optimal Capital Accumulation). Consider the Ramsey model over an infinite time horizon defined in Sect. 3.8.2:

1. Prove that the canonical system for the admissible control $C(t) = 0$ admits only the equilibria $(0, 0)$ and $(\tilde{K}, 0)$ with $F'(\tilde{K}) < \delta$.
2. Derive the canonical system for maximum consumption, i.e., $C = F(K)$.
3. Calculate the optimal solution for the functional forms and parameter values defined in Sect. 3.8.2.
4. Solve Ramsey's problem for a finite planning horizon with a fixed end-point condition $K(T) = K_T$. (Note that the inequality $K(T) \ge K_T$ would give the same solution.)

Hint. For question 1 note that $F(K) - \delta K$ exhibits its maximum at some $\hat{K}$ with $F'(\hat{K}) = \delta$.
For question 3 use one of the algorithms to calculate the stable path defined in Sect. 7.4.

Note that for a linear production function $F(K) = gK$ the model admits another interpretation, as follows. A decision-maker inherits a capital stock $K_0 > 0$ and intends to maximize the present value of the stream of consumption utility by allocating the available capital between consumption and an investment that pays an interest rate g.

3.12. Prove that the matrix (3.48) has full rank iff the gradients $c_u^i(x(t), u(t), t)$ are linearly independent, when the ith constraint is active.

Hint. If the ith constraint is active, $c^i = 0$.

3.13. Let $\Omega \subset \mathbb{R}^m$ be convex and let $f(x, u)$ be a real-valued concave function of (x, u), $x \in \mathbb{R}^n$, $u \in \Omega$. Then prove that

$$f^*(x) := \max_{u \in \Omega} f(x, u)$$

is concave in x, provided that the maximum value exists for each $x \in \mathbb{R}^n$.

Hint. Let $x_1, x_2 \in \mathbb{R}^n$, $\theta \in [0, 1]$ *and choose* $u_1, u_2 \in \Omega$ *such that* $f^*(x_i) = f(x_i, u_i)$, $i = 1, 2$.

3.14. The objective functional (3.2) is known as *Bolza* form. If the salvage value vanishes, $S(x(T)) = 0$, we have a so-called *Lagrange problem*. If $g(x, u, t) = 0$, the control problem is called a *Mayer problem*. It is *not* true that a Bolza problem is more general than the other forms.
Prove that the three forms of an optimal control problem are equivalent.

Hint. The salvage value S *can be written as*

$$S(x(T), T) = S(x_0, 0) + \int_0^T S_x(x(t), t)\dot{x}(t) + S_t(x(t), t)\,\mathrm{d}t.$$

Moreover, the integral $\int_0^T g(x, u, t)\,\mathrm{d}t$ *may be written as a salvage value by adding an additional state variable* $y(t)$ *as follows*

$$\int_0^T g(x, u, t)\,\mathrm{d}t = y(t)$$
$$\text{s.t.} \quad g(0) = 0, \quad \dot{y}(t) = g(x, u, t).$$

3.15 (Jorgenson's Investment Model). The following model by Jorgenson (1963, 1967) provides a cornerstone of most models in the area of the "dynamics of the firm" (compare Ludwig, 1978; van Hilten, Kort, & van Loon, 1993; and van Loon, 1985)

$$\max_{I(\cdot), L(\cdot)} \int_0^\infty \mathrm{e}^{-rt}\left(pF(K, L) - cI - wL\right)\mathrm{d}t$$
$$\text{s.t.} \quad \dot{K} = I - \delta K, \quad K(0) = K_0$$
$$\underline{I} \le I \le \bar{I}.$$

Here $K(t)$ denotes the capital stock owned by a firm at time t, $L(t)$ the labor force employed by the firm, and $I(t)$ the gross investment rate. The selling price p, the investment cost c, the wage rate w, and the depreciation rate δ are constant. The production function $F(K, L)$ is assumed to be concave jointly in (K, L). Note that $\underline{I} < 0$ allows for disinvestments.

Since the control variable, L, does not appear in the state equation, it can be determined by static maximization. Denoting this maximum by

$$\pi(K) = \max_{L(\cdot)} (pF(K, L) - cI - wL) \tag{3.94}$$

we get, by means of the envelope theorem, $\pi'(K) = pF_K > 0$. Furthermore, the concavity of F implies $\pi''(K) < 0$. By (3.94) we obtain a function $L = L(K)$, and by substituting this we get a one-control model.

Show that there exists an MRAP and interpret the singular solution $\hat{K}$, $\hat{L} = L(\hat{K})$. What is the economic meaning of the derived optimal investment policy and the optimal employment?

In a more realistic approach, the firm's labor force is dealt with as an additional state variable that can be controlled by hiring and firing. Formulate such a two-state model including hiring/firing costs.

3.16 (Optimal Alcohol Consumption at a Party). Assume that a person derives utility from consuming alcohol but disutility from a level of inebriation that is too high. Too much drinking at earlier stages of a party may cause displeasure in the later stages and a hangover afterward. There is a utility $U(u, x)$ depending not only on the drinking rate u, but also on the accumulated consumption (level of inebriation) x. The dynamics are

$$\dot{x} = u - \delta x, \quad x(0) = x_0.$$

Formulate an optimal control problem including a (negative) salvage value of $x(T)$. Discuss the properties of U for various kinds of drinking behavior. While defensive drinking may be characterized by $U_{ux} < 0$, addiction might mean $U_{ux} > 0$ (see Exercise 6.2). Show that in the first case the optimal consumption path monotonically decreases. Show that a permille limit (i.e., a pure state constraint $x \leq \bar{x}$ limiting inebriation), gives rise to a smaller consumption rate at least during the earlier stages of the party. See Feichtinger (1987) for a detailed analysis of this unusual optimal control model.

Notes and Further Reading

At the end of Sect. 3.1 we briefly mentioned some important references for the application of Pontryagin's Maximum Principle to economics and Operations Research. There are at least four standard references to books on optimal control of economic processes.

Sethi and Thompson (2000), (originally published in 1981, 2nd edition in 2000), provides a valuable introductory textbook to the field. Since the mathematical apparatus is kept simple (without being a collection of recipes), it is well-suited for beginners. The book contains examples from many fields, such as finance, production/inventory, marketing, maintenance/replacement, and resource management.

Another good introductory book is that by Kamien and Schwartz (1991). Fundamental concepts and results are introduced mainly with simple economic examples.

While the first part introduces variational calculus, the second part presents optimal control.

A mathematically more sophisticated approach is provided in the monograph by Seierstad and Sydsaeter (1986). Although it avoids measure theory and functional analysis, problems of the existence of solutions, path constraints, and other delicate issues are carefully discussed. Moreover, it analyzes several interesting economic models.

The book by Léonard and Long (1992) is a remarkable one. It begins with an introduction to nonlinear programming, an approach that is also pursued in this book. Many examples from various economic fields make it a very useful textbook.

Another introduction to optimal control of economic processes is the German-language book by Feichtinger and Hartl (1986). It contains a rich survey of models in production/inventory, maintenance/replacement, marketing, investment, employment, dynamics of the firm, resource management, and environmental planning.

Other texts dealing with economic applications of optimal control are Tu (1991) and Chiang (1992). Caputo (2005) provided a monograph on optimal control theory and its economic applications. A hallmark of this excellent book are the applications of the envelope conditions to a dynamic comparative analysis.

After the formulation of the Maximum Principle by Pontryagin et al. (1962) and the dynamic programming approach by Bellman (1957), the need for tools for nonsmooth (i.e., not differentiable) problems became apparent. Clarke (1983) provided such a tool with his concept of *generalized gradients*, while at the same time Crandall and Lions (1983) introduced their concept of viscosity solutions proving the existence of generalized solutions of the HJB equation. A self-contained presentation of this modern approach to optimal control theory can be found in Vinter (2000).

A nice capital theoretic interpretation of the Maximum Principle has been given by Dorfman (1969). His main thesis is that optimality conditions can be attained by "strictly economic reasoning." While the converse might be true (see Sect. 3.3.4), Dorfman's statement may somewhat be exaggerated.

There exist several proofs of the Maximum Principle. In the work of Pontryagin et al. (1962) *needle variations*, (so called because in the limit the graphs of such variations are "needle shaped"), were considered. Other proofs rely on the HJB equation: Arrow and Kurz (1970) did so, where the objective function is assumed to be twice continuously differentiable. For the general case, which relies on the concept of viscosity solutions, an exact proof can be found in Barron and Jensen (1986) or Cesari (1983). Long and Shimomura (2003) used the envelope theorem to prove the Maximum Principle. A proof under reduced differentiability hypotheses can be found in Arutyunov and Vinter (2004) or Shvartsman (2007).

Pontryagin's Maximum Principle provides only necessary conditions of the first order, i.e., the first derivatives are considered. But if the functions are at least twice continuously differentiable, quadratic approximations can be considered for a theory of second-order conditions (meaning that second derivatives are used). In fact, these conditions are formulated as a (matrix) Riccati differential equation but are in general hard to verify. They provide further conditions for classifying a possible optimal solution and proving at least the local optimality of a calculated extremal. For a detailed presentation of this theory the interested reader is referred to Caroff and Frankowska (1996); Malanowski, Maurer, and Pickenhain (2004); Maurer and Pickenhain (1995); Zeidan (1984) and Zeidan and Zezza (1988).

In many applications (e.g., in engineering sciences and in economics) linear–quadratic control problems play an important role. An LQ control problem is a problem with linear dynamics and a quadratic objective function. In the LQ case the HJB equation leads to a matrix Riccati equation which may be used to synthesize a feedback controller. A good reference is Bryson and Ho (1975); compare also Sethi and Thompson (2000) for a short introduction.

In the basic optimal control problems OC (3.3) no conditions for the terminal state $x(T)$ are imposed. In some cases, however, terminal constraints on the $x(T)$ play a role, either as fixed-end point problems or in the form of inequality constraints (see Sect. 3.6). Sethi and Thompson (2000) provided a complete study of terminal conditions (see their table on p. 75).

An interesting use of the generalized Legendre–Clebsch condition was its application to a problem in space navigation, known as Lawden's spiral. Lawden (1964) showed that a singular arc of this model satisfied Pontryagin's Maximum Principle and was therefore an optimal candidate. But Kelley, Kopp, and Moyer (1967) falsified its optimality, applying the generalized Legendre–Clebsch condition.

The idea of exploiting Green's integral theorem to prove the MRAP property traces back to Miele (1962); see also Bell and Jacobson (1975). Sethi (1977) was the first to apply the MRAP concept in economics and OR. He used the term "nearest feasible path," but the term MRAP became popular. Note that Sethi's study of multiple equilibria also provided an early approach to indifference points (see Chap. 5).

Note also the relation of MRAPs to turnpikes and saddle points occurring in mathematical economics and growth theory; compare McKenzie (1986).

As already mentioned in Remark 3.58 the direct method was earlier used (see Pontryagin et al., 1962). More information on the treatment of pure state constraints are given by Feichtinger and Hartl (1986) and Hartl et al. (1995).

To the knowledge of the authors a comprehensive economic interpretation of the possible jump of the shadow price in problems with pure state constraints is still outstanding. A partial explanation was given by Verheyen (1992). In his illustration of an economy with irreversible investments, it appears that the jump is caused by a sudden change in the cost of capital and, therefore, in the marginal net present value of the capital stock.

The optimal control model of a drug epidemic presented in Sect. 3.9 with one state variable representing the number of users, A, is only one out of several variants of the so-called A-model that was first discussed in Tragler (1998) and Tragler et al. (2001) where in addition to the one control considered here (*drug treatment*) a second control was included (*price-raising law enforcement*). In Moyzisch (2003) Zeiler (2004) and Swaton (2005) *prevention* was included as third control variable. Recognizing that price-raising drug enforcement may increase property crime, Caulkins et al. (2000) used an optimal control model to provide recommendations about whether convicted drug-involved property offenders should be incarcerated or should receive some form of drug treatment. Acknowledging that *harm reduction* is gaining increasing interest as an alternative form of drug policy, Wallner (2005) Rudel (2006) and Caulkins et al. (2007) adopted the A-model appropriately. The impact of *supply shocks* on optimal dynamic drug policies was studied recently in a multi-stage framework (see Sect. 8.1) by Bultmann (2007), Bultmann et al. (2007) and Bultmann et al. (2008). Only recently, Zeiler (2008) coupled two identical A-models for the purpose of studying multiple drug use in two distinct drug user populations. While basically all these variants of the A-model were parameterized with data from the current US cocaine epidemic, there also exist a few studies using data for the Australian heroin epidemic (e.g., Mautner (2002), Großlicht (2003), Morawetz (2003)).

Price-raising drug enforcement suppresses drug use, but it may increase property crime. Using an optimal control model Caulkins, Dworak, Feichtinger, and Tragler (2000) provided recommendations about whether convicted drug-involved property offenders should be incarcerated or should receive some form of drug treatment.

The "optimal maintenance and replacement" model presented in Exercise 3.6 traces back to Thompson (1968) and provides one of the very first applications of optimal control to management science. In addition to his analysis, there are many papers in this field (see Feichtinger & Hartl, 1986, Chap. 10 as well as Sethi & Thompson, 2000, Chap. 9 for an introduction to the field). An interesting extension of the maintenance and replacement problems deals with a chain of machines. By this we mean that a machine will be replaced by a new one; compare Sethi and Thompson (2000, Sect. 9.3) and Feichtinger and Hartl (1986, Sect. 2.8).

For a nice economic interpretation of the terminal condition (3.10) compare Feichtinger and Hartl (1986, p. 46). Note that the proof of Theorem 3.25 is independent of the Maximum Principle and uses only calculus; see Hartl and Sethi (1983).

Exercise 3.8 refers to another important field of application for Pontryagin's Maximum Principle; see Sethi and Thompson (2000, Chap. 6) for a detailed survey of control-theoretic production/inventory models. These models trace back to Arrow, Karlin, and Scarf (1958), and it can be seen as the basis of numerous extensions; (see e.g., Feichtinger & Hartl, 1986, Chap. 9).

The pricing problem sketched in Exercise 3.9 is just one among a vast field of marketing applications for optimal control theory. For pertinent models on pricing, advertising, and product quality, see Feichtinger and Hartl (1986, Chap. 11) and Feichtinger, Hartl, and Sethi (1994).

Exercise 3.10 on consumption–pollution trade-offs exemplifies a growing domain of applications dealing with the efficient control of environmental pollution; see also Feichtinger and Hartl (1986, Chap. 15). There is a striking similarity between crime control and environmental control, where the stock of offenders/pollution is controlled by prevention/abatement as well as treatment/clean-up measures see Feichtinger (2001).

A whole spectrum of optimal control applications can be found for "unorthodox" situations. Feichtinger and Mehlmann (1986) contains a non-exhaustive survey of the field "planning the unusual," covering such areas as literature, theology, ethics, sports, and history. Although some of the models seem to lack seriousness, they often have hidden benefits, (e.g., clarifying principles of optimal control) and in some cases may even offer valuable features for real-life decisions. To illustrate a few points on this unorthodox spectrum, let us briefly mention two models discussed in Feichtinger and Mehlmann (1986). The first is a health care model in which the patients are under the care of a physician with various remuneration patterns. For example, a physician is rewarded for each treatment or is paid for each patient or each successful cure (and maybe punished in case of failure); alternatively, the physician may be remunerated by the healthy part of the population. The second model is a predator–prey model describing the dilemma of a vampire that draws utility from sucking blood but, by biting human beings, creates competitors (other vampires) that also exploit the prey.

In Exercise 3.16 the utility function depends not only on the control (i.e., the consumption rate), but also on the state variable. *State-dependent* utility functions play an important role in dynamic economies, e.g., in habit formation (see, e.g., Ryder and Heal, 1973), environmental pollution (compare Exercise 3.10). Brock circumscribed state dependency nicely as "*money sings.*" Its validity fosters complex behavior of consumption paths, i.e., periodic and aperiodic oscillations, even chaos. A nice example of state-dependent utility functions is status seeking, where the status is determined by relative wealth; see, e.g., Fisher and Hof (2005).

Majumdar, Mitra, and Nishimura (2000) and Nishimura and Sorger (1996) studied cyclical chaotic equilibrium paths in deterministic optimal growth models with infinitely lived agents.

4

The Path to Deeper Insight: From Lagrange to Pontryagin

In the last chapter we presented Pontryagin's Maximum Principle and the Hamilton–Jacobi–Bellman equation to solve optimal control problems. Now we deal with its exposition from a different point of view. In this chapter we first describe an intuitive approach to the Maximum Principle and its results, in which we reformulate the continuous-time problem of optimal control theory as a discrete-time problem. Then we introduce the problem of static optimization under equality and inequality constraints. The Lagrangian approach is used to find first-order necessary optimality conditions for the optimal solution. From this formulation we derive a discrete form of Pontryagin's Maximum Principle. Thereafter it is easy to understand how the discrete principle might be extended to the continuous case. In the course of this informal approach we also introduce the main ideas of the calculus of variations, the forerunner of optimal control theory. This allows us to derive the necessary conditions of the Maximum Principle in a concise way but also to give an explanation for the jump condition for the costate in the case of pure state constraints.

4.1 Introductory Remarks on Optimization

With this goal in mind, we start by making some notational comments and give an introduction to optimization theory. It is intended to present the general questions of optimization and thus to characterize the optimal control problems as one specification of a general problem. From this enhanced point of view it is easier to discern similarities in the formulations of conditions specifying optimal solutions for such apparently distinct areas as maximizing a real function and finding the optimal strategy in an economic model. We shall not present a general theory of optimization but rather provide some insight into the mathematical thinking and reasoning in the field of optimization – a global map, so to speak, to keep the reader from getting lost in the details.

4.1.1 Notational Remarks

Einstein instructed that a model should be as simple as possible but not simpler. Likewise, we try to keep the notation as simple as possible but also as complex as necessary. This is not an easy task, especially as we present results from several mathematical fields, each with its own notational standard. To keep these parts notationally consistent while also depicting the analogy between *static optimization* and *optimal control theory*, we have had to strike some compromises. In the discussion of static optimization we use uppercase letters for functions (e.g., G, F) and occurring variables (e.g., X), whereas in the part dealing with optimal control theory we use lowercase letters for the corresponding functions (e.g., g, f) and variables (e.g., x). Maximizers are denoted by an asterisk, e.g., X^* and the corresponding value function is given by $G^* := G(X^*)$.

4.1.2 Motivation and Insights

An optimal control problem can be considered as a special case of the general maximization problem (*GMP*): Let $(\mathbb{V}, \|\cdot\|)$ be a normed vector space (see Appendix A.2.7), and let G be a real-valued function(al) $G: \mathbb{V} \to \mathbb{R}$ called the *objective functional* or *objective function*, then the constrained maximization problem, written as:

$$\max_X G(X) \tag{4.1a}$$

$$\text{s.t.} \quad X \in \Omega \subset \mathbb{V} \tag{4.1b}$$

is, to find an element X^* with

$$X^* \in \underset{X\in\Omega}{\operatorname{argmax}}\, G(X). \tag{4.2}$$

Explicitly written (4.2) becomes

$$X^* \in \Omega \subset \mathbb{V} \tag{4.3a}$$

such that the following inequality

$$G(X) \le G(X^*) \quad \text{holds for all} \quad X \in \Omega. \tag{4.3b}$$

If such an element X^* exists, it is called a *maximizer* or *maximal (optimal) solution* of problem *GMP* (4.3).

In this context the important questions are:

- Does a maximizer X^* exist? (existence).
- Can conditions be stated distinguishing a maximizer from any other element in Ω? (necessary optimality conditions).

- Do the necessary conditions suffice to identify a maximizer? (sufficient optimality conditions).

All three of these questions are of importance to solve a maximization problem, where in our presentation we concentrate on the second question (see also Appendix A.3.3). Anyhow, without specifying the properties of the function G and the structure of the set Ω, mathematics can do little to answer these questions. And depending on how much information is given, answers vary greatly in character, ranging from abstract theorems of existence to concrete algorithms of how to calculate a maximizer.

Since the set $\mathbb{V}$ is assumed to be a normed vector space, the concept of neighborhood can be applied and therefore the following definition can be given:

Definition 4.1 (Local/Global Maximum). *Let X^* be a maximizer for problem* GMP *(4.3) restricted to the set $N_\varepsilon(X^*) \cap \Omega$, where $N_\varepsilon(X^*)$ is an open ε-neighborhood of X^*; then X^* is called a* local maximizer. *If X^* is the unique local maximizer; then it is called a* strict local maximizer.

If X^* is a (unique) maximizer of GMP *(4.3); then it is called a* (strict) global maximizer.

A coarse classification of the type of maximization problems is given by the dimension of the vector space $\mathbb{V}$, i.e., finite- or infinite-dimensional problems, respectively. Typical examples of the finite-dimensional case are maximizations in $\mathbb{V} := \mathbb{R}^n$, whereas an optimal control problem can be seen as an example for an infinite-dimensional maximization problem, with

$$\mathbb{V} := C_p^{0,1}([0,T],\mathbb{R}^n) \times C_p^0([0,T],\mathbb{R}^m),$$

which is the set of continuous and piecewise continuously differentiable (state) functions and piecewise continuous (control) functions (for its definition see Appendix A.3.2).

A further distinction is the specification of the set $\Omega \subset \mathbb{V}$, which is often given in the form of equality or inequality constraints

$$\Omega := \{X \in \mathbb{V} : \; F(X) = 0, \quad \text{and} \quad H(X) \geq 0\}.$$

The corresponding problem is then called a *maximization problem under equality and/or inequality constraints.*

Another possibility to classify maximization problems is that of specifying properties of the occurring functions G, F, and H. Especially if these are differentiable or nondifferentiable, yielding the distinction between smooth and nonsmooth maximization problems.

We restrict our considerations to smooth problems. This approach is, without doubt a significant restriction to set of admissible solutions, but makes mathematical life much easier and can be justified for a broad range of applications.

Having given a short survey of possible specifications of optimization problems, we shall now present a simple problem introducing the underlying ideas for solving these problems. At this stage technical terms are used in a naive sense but will be defined precisely in the subsequent sections.

4.1.3 A Simple Maximization Problem

Problem Formulation

Let us start by analyzing the simple problem of maximizing the real-valued function $G(X) = X(X^2 - 1/2)$ restricted to the interval $\Omega = [-1, 1]$, i.e., to the problem:

$$\begin{aligned} &\max_X X(X^2 - 1/2) \\ \text{s.t.} \quad &X + 1 \geq 0 \\ &1 - X \geq 0, \end{aligned}$$

where $\mathbb{V} = \mathbb{R}$, $G : \mathbb{R} \to \mathbb{R}$ is continuously differentiable, and

$$\Omega = [-1, 1] = \{X : H(X) \geq 0\}$$

with $H(X) := (X + 1, 1 - X)'$ (see the graph in Fig. 4.1).

In light of our discussion above, this is a smooth, finite-dimensional optimization problem with inequality constraints. Rephrasing the problem formulation, we search for some criterion allowing us to characterize possible *candidates* for the optimal solution.

Local Criterion for Characterizing a Maximizer

In general such a criterion relies on the *local* behavior of the function G, which reduces the complexity of the problem, since locally the behavior of the function G may be "nice," whereas the global behavior can be complicated. It is evident that for every candidate $\hat{X}$ as a maximizer we have to assure the validity of the inequality (4.3b), at least in some *neighborhood*. To validate this inequality for such a point $\hat{X}$ we consider the objective values, while we vary the point along an arbitrary *admissible direction* δS. Admissible means that the varied point has to satisfy the constraints. In other words, we have to prove that at a possible maximizer $\hat{X}$ admissible changes of this point do not increase the value of the objective function. From this formulation we conclude that we can split the problem into two parts. First, we have carefully to examine how to characterize an admissible direction or admissible change and, second, we have to find some concept that allows us to describe the change in the functional values as simple as possible. Our example is simple enough to apply these considerations heuristically.

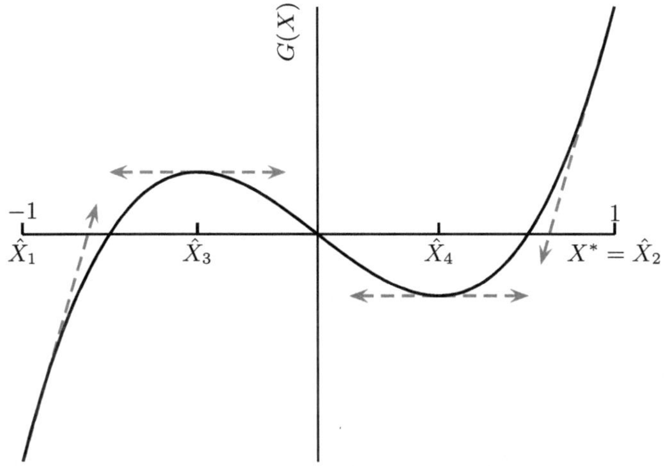

Fig. 4.1. For the simple case of a cubic polynomial the main principles of maximization are depicted. In general the condition that the derivative is zero for points lying in the interior of the admissible region yields only local extremals ($\hat{X}_{3,4}$). On the boundary $\hat{X}_{1,2}$ one has to determine the admissible directions δS and check whether the objective function G increases or decreases along these directions

Admissibility and First-Order Conditions

Let us start with the problem of admissibility. If we consider some point X lying in the interior of the interval, changes in the positive direction as well as in the negative direction satisfy the constraints. If we consider $+1$ and -1 as vectors of the real line, any admissible direction δS can be written as $\varepsilon \cdot (+1)$ or $\varepsilon \cdot (-1)$ with $\varepsilon \geq 0$, where for ε small enough $X \pm \varepsilon$ stay in the interval Ω. At the boundary $\{\pm 1\}$ of the interval the admissible directions are $+1$ for the left boundary point and -1 for the right boundary point.

Given the polynomial form of function G, we find the functional value for a "slightly" varied point $X + \varepsilon\delta S$, and $\delta S \in \{-1, 1\}$ as

$$G(X + \varepsilon\delta S) = G(X) + \underbrace{\left(3X^2 - 1/2\right)}_{G_X(X)} \varepsilon\delta S + o(\varepsilon^2). \tag{4.4}$$

Here (4.4) follows from the polynomial form of G. In general the Taylor theorem provides such a polynomial approximation.

From our previous arguments we know that for any admissible change of X the functional value must not increase; hence $G(X + \varepsilon\delta S) - G(X) \leq 0$. If we consider (4.4) for all $\varepsilon > 0$ (small enough), this reduces to the *necessary optimality condition*

$$G_X(X)\delta S = \lim_{\varepsilon \to 0^+} \frac{G(X + \varepsilon\delta S) - G(X)}{\varepsilon} \leq 0, \tag{4.5}$$

where (4.5) denotes the directional derivative of G along δS. Thus it is claimed that the directional derivative along an admissible direction δS is nonpositive.

If we inspect this condition carefully, we see that at an *interior point* X of the interval, the directions 1 as well as -1 are admissible. Therefore at an interior point (4.5) can be satisfied only if

$$G_X(X) = 0, \tag{4.6}$$

which is the well-known result from unconstrained optimization of differentiable functions (see Appendix A.3.3).

Candidates That Are Not Maximizers

Equations (4.5) and (4.6) just provide a necessary condition, and hence points satisfying these conditions are only candidates for a maximizer. This can already be seen in our introductory example, in which the interior points $\hat{X}_{3,4} = \mp\sqrt{1/6}$ satisfy (4.6) but are not maximizers, although $\hat{X}_3 = -\sqrt{1/6}$ is at least a *local* maximizer. The boundary point $\hat{X}_2 = 1$ satisfies (4.5) and is therefore a (local) maximizer. The second boundary point $\hat{X}_2 = -1$ does not satisfy the necessary conditions and can therefore be excluded. For this simple example we know that a maximizer exists (see Theorem A.102). Moreover we know that $\hat{X}_{2,3,4}$ are the only candidates and therefore in a final step we have to compare the objective values of these points identifying $\hat{X}_2$ as the global maximizer. From this line of argument it already becomes obvious that for more involved problems the justification for a candidate to be a (local) maximizer can get rather complicated. If the occurring functions are twice continuously differentiable, further (second-order) necessary conditions can be stated that a maximizer has to satisfy.

Existence of a Maximizer

One aspect is often ignored or overlooked, namely that of the existence for a maximizer/minimizer. For our previous example the general theorem, that a continuous function exhibits a maximum and minimum on a compact set, assures its existence (see Theorem A.102). In general, however, the question of existence cannot easily be answered. But since the necessary conditions are derived under the assumption that a maximizer exists, its existence is of fundamental importance. Otherwise the detected solutions may not have a meaning anyhow as the *Perron paradoxon* impressively shows:

Perron paradoxon. *One is the largest natural number.*

Proof. Suppose the largest natural number is N, then if $N > 1$ we find $N^2 > N$ contradicting the assumption on N and therefore $N = 1$.

Even though the proof is logical correct, its conclusion fails since its assumption, the existence of a largest natural number, is false. Thus the reader should be aware that the question of existence is not only one of mathematical subtlety, but it is of fundamental relevance for a correct interpretation of the detected solutions satisfying the necessary optimality conditions.

Therefore consider the problem:

$$\max_X X^3$$
$$\text{s.t.} \quad X \in \mathbb{R}.$$

For this problem $X = 0$ is the unique solution satisfying the first order necessary condition (4.6), i.e., $3X^2 = 0$, but obviously it is not a maximizer nor a minimizer. Thus the necessary condition failed to identify an optimal solution since there exists no maximum or minimum in $\mathbb{R}$ (cf. Sect. 3.3.6).

4.1.4 Finite-Dimensional Approximation of an Infinite-Dimensional Problem

To conclude this motivational section let us finally reformulate, in a heuristic manner, the continuous optimal control problem (infinite-dimensional) as a discrete optimal control problem (finite-dimensional). This step, although seemingly straightforward, has difficulties of its own, e.g., the discretization of a continuous problem need not have a solution at all or may not be an approximation of the original problem (see, e.g., Cullum, 1969). For our current goal, however, it suffices to state the possible pitfalls without solving them.

An Infinite-Dimensional Problem

In the previously stated scheme, the optimal control problem:

$$\max_{u(\cdot)} \int_0^T g(x(t), u(t))\,\mathrm{d}t + S(x(T)) \tag{4.7a}$$

$$\text{s.t.} \quad \dot{x} = f(x(t), u(t)), \quad t \in [0, T] \tag{4.7b}$$

$$x(0) = x_0 \tag{4.7c}$$

$$c(x(t), u(t)) \geq 0, \quad \text{for all} \quad t \in [0, T] \tag{4.7d}$$

$$h(x(t)) \geq 0, \quad \text{for all} \quad t \in [0, T] \tag{4.7e}$$

$$a(x(T)) = 0 \tag{4.7f}$$

$$b(x(T)) \geq 0 \tag{4.7g}$$

is an infinite-dimensional maximization problem, where the corresponding objective functional G is given by

$$G(x(\cdot), u(\cdot)) = \int_0^T g(x(t), u(t))\,\mathrm{d}t + S(x(T)),$$

and $(x(\cdot), u(\cdot))$ is an element of the vector space

$$\mathbb{V} := C_p^{0,1}([0, T], \mathbb{R}^n) \times C_p^0([0, T], \mathbb{R}^m).$$

What about the subset $\Omega \subset \mathbb{V}$? Here we find

$$F(x(\cdot), u(\cdot)) = \begin{cases} \dot{x}(t) - f(x(t), u(t)) & t \in [0, T] \\ x(0) - x_0 \\ a(x(T)) \end{cases}$$

$$H(x(\cdot), u(\cdot)) = \begin{cases} c(x(t), u(t)) & t \in [0, T] \\ h(x(t)) & t \in [0, T] \\ b(x(T)). \end{cases}$$

Approximation

In line with our chosen approach we now transform the infinite-dimensional optimization problem *OCC* (4.7) by discretizing the model on a finite time grid. For numerical as well as for theoretical purposes the way of discretizing the continuous-time problem is of great importance. For our informal approach the discretization is of less importance since it should only help the reader to become acquainted with the underlying ideas. But we hope that this approach facilitates the reader doing the step from static to dynamic optimization.

Remark 4.2. This approach can also be found in the book of Léonard and Long (1992) albeit there it is not accomplished to the extent we will present the theory here.

Now the discretization is done in a straightforward manner. Thus the time interval $[0, T]$ is subdivided into $N-1$ equal-sized intervals of length $\tau = T/(N-1)$. Using basic calculus, we replace the integral in (4.7a) by a finite sum of step width τ

$$\max_{(u_1,\dots,u_{N-1})} \sum_{i=1}^{N-1} \tau g(x_i, u_i) + S(x_N),$$

where $x_i = x((i-1)\tau)$, $u_i = u((i-1)\tau)$, for $i = 1, \dots, N$.

Furthermore, the differential equation (4.7b) is replaced by the difference equation

$$\frac{x_{i+1} - x_i}{\tau} = f(x_i, u_i),$$

and hence we find for the initial condition (4.7c)

$$\begin{aligned} & x_{i+1} = x_i + \tau f(x_i, u_i), \quad i = 1, \dots, N-1 \\ \text{s.t.} \quad & x_1 = x(0) = x_0. \end{aligned}$$

The constraints on the paths and at the terminal time become:

$$\begin{aligned}
&c(x_i, u_i) \geq 0, \quad i = 1, \dots, N-1\\
&h(x_i) \geq 0, \quad i = 1, \dots, N\\
&b(x_N) \geq 0\\
&a(x_N) = 0.
\end{aligned}$$

Summing up, this yields a discrete-time optimization problem (DOC), which approximates the continuous-time problem (4.7):

$$\max_{(u_1,\dots,u_{N-1})} \sum_{i=1}^{N-1} \tau g(x_i, u_i) + S(x_N) \tag{4.8a}$$

$$\text{s.t.} \quad x_{i+1} = x_i + \tau f(x_i, u_i), \quad i = 1, \dots N-1$$
$$x_1 = x_0 \tag{4.8b}$$
$$c(x_i, u_i) \geq 0, \quad i = 1, \dots N-1 \tag{4.8c}$$
$$h(x_i) \geq 0, \quad i = 1, \dots N \tag{4.8d}$$
$$b(x_N) \geq 0 \tag{4.8e}$$
$$a(x_N) = 0, \tag{4.8f}$$

where $x_i \in \mathbb{R}^n$ and $u_i \in \mathbb{R}^m$.

Remark 4.3. Note that the factor τ appears because of the discretization process and has no influence on the maximization. Therefore, if exclusively studying the discrete problem, we shall assume $\tau = 1$.

4.2 Static Maximization

In this section we develop the theory of static maximization under equality and inequality constraints insofar as it is needed to derive a special form of the discrete-time Maximum Principle. Our paradigmatic object of investigation in this section is that of a real-valued, finite-dimensional, and smooth maximization problem under equality and inequality constraints. In formal terms, let $G : \mathbb{R}^n \to \mathbb{R}$, $F : \mathbb{R}^n \to \mathbb{R}^m$ and $H : \mathbb{R}^n \to \mathbb{R}^k$ be continuously differentiable functions; then the problem, subsequently referred to as finite-dimensional static maximization (FSM), is written as:

$$\max_{X \in \mathbb{R}^n} G(X) \tag{4.9a}$$
$$\text{s.t.} \quad F(X) = 0 \tag{4.9b}$$
$$H(X) \geq 0, \tag{4.9c}$$

where $F(X) = 0$ is called the *equality constraint* and $H(X) \geq 0$ is called the *inequality constraint.*

4.2.1 Basic Theorems and Definitions

In this subsection the necessary conditions and theorems are presented to develop the Lagrange theory for solving problem *FSM* (4.9). Thus we have to find a maximizer X^* satisfying the equations $F(X^*) = 0$ and lying in a region bounded by the inequalities $H(X^*) \geq 0$. As we have seen for the motivating example in Sect. 4.1.3, it is important to distinguish between points lying in the interior and at the boundary of the region Ω (see Fig. 4.2a). Therefore we specify the set $\mathcal{I}(X)$ of indices with the active inequality constraints at a point X, i.e.,

$$\mathcal{I}(X) := \left\{ j : H^j(X) = 0 \right\},$$

where the argument X is omitted if there is no ambiguity.

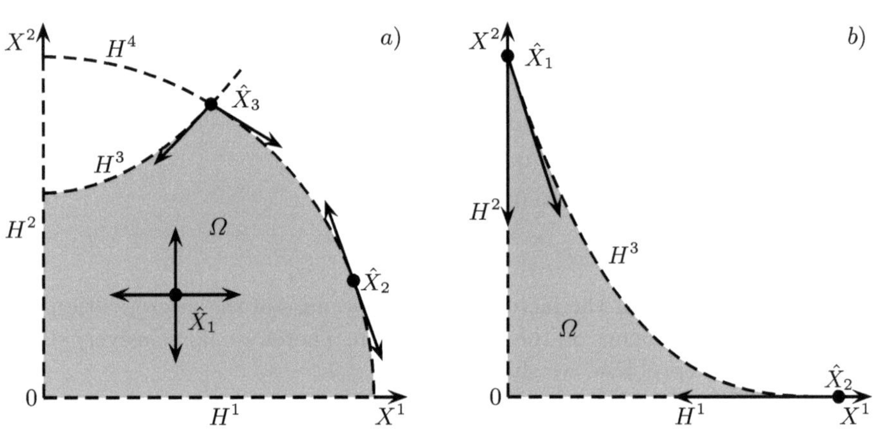

Fig. 4.2. In (**a**) the (*gray*) region Ω, given by the inequality constraints H^1 to H^4, is depicted together with an inner point $\hat{X}_1$ and the two points at the boundary $\hat{X}_2$ and $\hat{X}_3$. The admissible directions are given by the convex hull of the depicted vectors. Thus at the inner point $\hat{X}_1$ every direction is admissible. Panel (**b**) depicts the admissible directions for the points $\hat{X}_1$ and $\hat{X}_2$. In $\hat{X}_2$ the constraints H^1 and H^3 intersect tangentially therefore the admissible directions are lying in the negative half-line at $\hat{X}_2$

The introductory example showed that admissible direction is a central term for stating necessary conditions for a (local) maximizer. Obviously, an admissible point lies in the region restricted by the constraints, and a point given by a possibly infinitesimal change of $\hat{X}$ along an admissible direction should also satisfy the constraints. Formally these concepts are defined by:

Definition 4.4 (Admissibility). *A point $\hat{X} \in \mathbb{R}^n$ is called* admissible *for problem* FSM *(4.9) if it satisfies the conditions (4.9b) and (4.9c).*

A vector $\delta S \in \mathbb{R}^n$ is called an admissible direction (at $\hat{X}$) *if there exists a sequence $X_j \in \mathbb{R}^n$, $j \in \mathbb{N}$ of admissible points with*

$$\lim_{j\to\infty} X_j = \hat{X}$$

and

$$\lim_{j\to\infty} \frac{X_j - \hat{X}}{\|X_j - \hat{X}\|}\|\delta S\| = \delta S. \tag{4.10}$$

A vector δS which is not admissible is called a nonadmissible direction.

Remark 4.5. Note that the zero vector is an admissible direction, since in that case (4.10) is trivially satisfied for any sequence of admissible points converging to $\hat{X}$.

Remark 4.6. Geometrically this definition refers to the fact that a point $\tilde{X}$ given by

$$\tilde{X} = \hat{X} + \varepsilon\delta S,$$

with $\varepsilon \geq 0$ chosen small enough is admissible. The formulation as a limiting process is necessary to include the case, where the admissible direction is tangential to the boundary of the constraint. In Fig. 4.3a the case of a nonadmissible direction δS is shown. Here it is not possible to find a sequence of admissible points satisfying Definition 4.4.

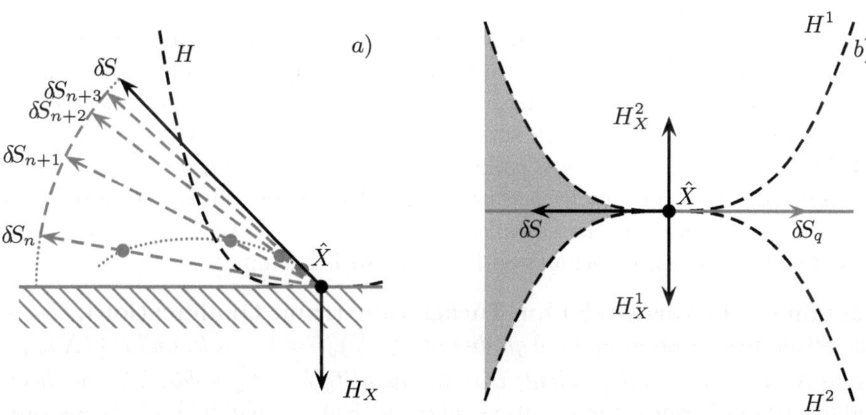

Fig. 4.3. Panel (**a**) shows that any direction δS not satisfying $H_X\delta S \geq 0$ is not admissible, since for any sequence δS_j converging to δS nearly all corresponding points $\hat{X}_j$ (*gray dots*) violate the constraints. In (**b**) the case is shown in which quasi-admissible directions δS_q exist (*gray arrow*), which are not admissible

Remark 4.7. The symbol δS for an admissible direction anticipates already its generalization in the calculus of variations (see Sect. 4.3), where it is convenient to use the symbol δ for variational terms. We employ this terminology here to make it easier for the reader to recognize the similarities of both theories.

Since the definition of an admissible direction at the point $\hat{X}$ is not very amenable to manipulation, it is convenient to consider the related set of *quasi-admissible directions at* $\hat{X}$, denoted as $\mathbb{A}_q$, which is obtained by the linear approximation of the constraints; that is,

$$\mathbb{A}_q = \{\delta S : F^i_X(\hat{X})\delta S = 0, i = 1, \dots, k,\ H^j_X(\hat{X})\delta S \geq 0,\ j \in \mathcal{I}(\hat{X})\}.$$

Unfortunately, the sets of admissible and quasi-admissible directions are, in general, not identical (see Fig. 4.3b). In general only the following conclusion holds:

Proposition 4.8. *Every admissible direction at* $\hat{X}$ *is also a quasi-admissible direction at* $\hat{X}$*; that is*

$$\mathbb{A} \subset \mathbb{A}_q.$$

The geometric argument for Proposition 4.8 in the complementary formulation

$$\mathbb{R}^n \setminus \mathbb{A}_q \subset \mathbb{R}^n \setminus \mathbb{A}$$

is depicted in Fig. 4.3a. Since, if you chose a vector $\delta S \mathbb{R}^n \setminus \mathbb{A}_q$, which is not quasi admissible, in that case $H_X \delta S < 0$, then Definition 4.4 cannot be satisfied and is therefore also not admissible. The formal proof can be found in Appendix B.6.

As already stated the converse inclusion of Proposition 4.8 does not hold in general. Thus deriving necessary optimality conditions, where quasi-admissible directions are utilized rather than admissible directions, one has to assure the identity of both sets by some additional property. Such an additional *regularity property* is called a *constraint qualification.*

One of these properties assuring the identity of admissible and quasi-admissible direction is the so-called *Karush–Kuhn–Tucker (KKT) constraint qualification*, which is formulated in the following lemma:

Lemma 4.9 (Karush–Kuhn–Tucker Constraint Qualification). *Let* $\hat{X}$ *be an admissible point and the gradients* $F^i_X(\hat{X})$, $i = 1, \dots, k$, *and* $H^j_X(\hat{X})$, $j \in \mathcal{I}$ *at* $\hat{X}$ *be linearly independent; then the identity* $\mathbb{A} = \mathbb{A}_q$ *holds. The condition of linearly independent gradients is called the* Karush–Kuhn–Tucker constraint qualification.

The main idea of the proof is depicted in Fig. 4.4, whereas the technical details are presented in Appendix B.6.

Remark 4.10. The KKT constraint qualification assures that admissible directions can be specified by (in)equalities without explicitly referring to the construction process of Definition 4.4.

The KKT constraint qualification can also be stated in the form, that the matrix

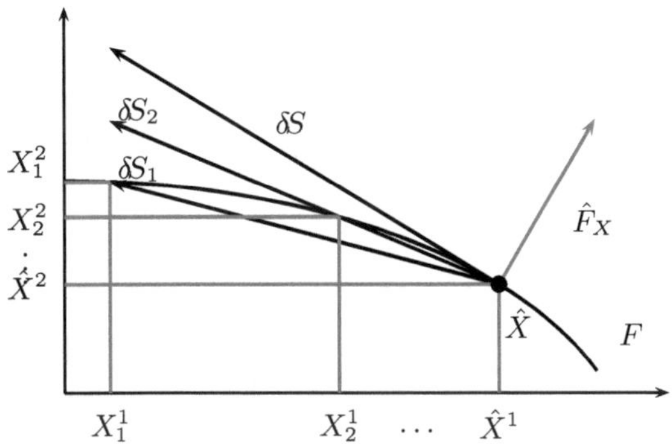

Fig. 4.4. The process of constructing a sequence of vectors δS_i converging to the quasi-admissible direction δS, that is $\hat{F}_X \delta S = 0$, is depicted. The implicit function theorem assures the explicit calculation of a sequence of admissible points $X_i = (X_i^1, X_i^2)$. Since for $X_i^1 = \hat{X}^1 + \theta_i \delta S^1$ we find X_i^2 from satisfying $F(X_i^1, X_i^2) = 0$, where $\theta_i = \|X_i - \hat{X}\|/\|\delta S\|$ and $\lim_{i \to \infty} \theta_i = 0$

$$\begin{pmatrix} F_X^1(X) & 0 & \cdots & 0 \\ \cdots & \cdots & \cdots & \cdots \\ F_X^k(X) & 0 & \cdots & 0 \\ H_X^1(X) & H^1(X) & \cdots & 0 \\ \cdots & \cdots & \cdots & \cdots \\ H_X^l(X) & 0 & \cdots & H^l(X) \end{pmatrix}, \tag{4.11}$$

evaluated at an admissible point $\hat{X}$, exhibits full rank. The reader is invited to prove this reformulation in Exercise 4.6.

Next we state the necessary conditions for a maximizer X^* of problem *FSM* (4.9), which has already been formulated in the simple case of the introductory example in Sect. 4.1.3:

Theorem 4.11 (General Necessary Condition). *Let X^* be a (local) maximizer of* FSM *(4.9); then*

$$G_X(X^*)\delta S \le 0, \tag{4.12}$$

for any admissible direction δS.

Proof. We prove the theorem by contradiction. First observe that for $\delta S = 0$ (4.12) is trivially satisfied. Thus assume the existence of an admissible direction at X^*, $\delta S \neq 0$, satisfying

$$G_X(X^*)\delta S > 0. \tag{4.13}$$

By Definition 4.4 we find a sequence

$$\delta S_i := \theta_i (X_i - X^*), \quad \theta_i = \frac{\|\delta S\|}{\|X_i - X^*\|} > 0, \ \ i \in \mathbb{N},$$

where $X_i \neq X^*$ are admissible points. Next we consider

$$\begin{aligned} G(X_i) &= G\left(X^* + \theta_i^{-1}\delta S\right) \\ &= G(X^*) + \theta_i^{-1} G_X(X^*)\delta S + o(\theta_i^{-1}) \end{aligned}$$

yielding

$$\begin{aligned} 0 \geq G(X_i) - G(X^*) = \theta_i^{-1} G_X(X^*)\delta S + o(\theta_i^{-1}) \\ 0 \geq G_X(X^*)\delta S + \frac{o(\theta_i^{-1})}{\theta_i^{-1}} \\ 0 \geq \lim_{i\to\infty} \left(G_X(X^*)\delta S + \frac{o(\theta_i^{-1})}{\theta_i^{-1}} \right) = G_X(X^*)\delta S. \end{aligned}$$

But this is a contradiction to (4.13), concluding the proof. □

Theorem 4.11 provides a condition that every maximizer of *FSM* (4.9) has to satisfy, but in general (without further restrictions on function G) this condition is not sufficient. Hence points $\hat{X}$ may exist, satisfying (4.12), which are neither local nor global maximizers of *FSM* (4.9). Therefore we define:

Definition 4.12 (Extremal). *Every point $\hat{X}$ satisfying (4.12) is called an* extremal point of *FSM* (4.9).

This completes our general exposition of definitions and elementary theorems. We shall now introduce the Lagrange theory of optimization.

4.2.2 Theory and Geometric Interpretation of Lagrange and Karush–Kuhn–Tucker

Here we analyze the problem *FSM* (4.9) using the theory of Lagrange and Karush–Kuhn–Tucker. Doing so will subsequently allow us to derive the first-order necessary conditions of discrete optimal control problems.

In coordinate notation, problem *FSM* (4.9) becomes:

$$\begin{aligned} &\max_{X\in\mathbb{R}^n} G(X) \\ \text{s.t.} \quad &F^1(X) = 0, \dots, F^k(X) = 0 \\ &H^1(X) \geq 0, \dots, H^l(X) \geq 0. \end{aligned}$$

Necessary Conditions for a Maximizer of *FSM* (4.9)

In the following the Lagrange–Karush–Kuhn–Tucker theorem provides first-order necessary conditions to identify a maximizer of problem *FSM* (4.9). Its proof relies considerably on the analysis of the (local) change of the objective function along admissible directions $\delta S \in \mathbb{A}$. Hence an easy-to-manage characterization of these directions is needed. Since such a characterization is provided by quasi-admissible directions $\delta S \in \mathbb{A}_q$, the identity of both sets $\mathbb{A}_q = \mathbb{A}$ has to be guaranteed.

Using the Karush–Kuhn–Tucker constraint qualification we find the theorem:

Theorem 4.13 (Lagrange–Karush–Kuhn–Tucker). *Let X^* be a local maximizer of problem* FSM *(4.9) and let the matrix (4.11) have full rank. Then there exist unique row vectors $\Lambda = (\Lambda_i)_{i=1}^k$ and $\Pi = (\Pi_j)_{j=1}^l$ such that:*

$$\mathcal{L}_X(X^*) = 0 \tag{4.15a}$$

$$\Pi \geq 0 \tag{4.15b}$$

$$\Pi H(X^*) = 0, \tag{4.15c}$$

where $\mathcal{L} = G + \Lambda F + \Pi H$ is called the Lagrangian *of problem* FSM *(4.9) and the vector (Λ, Π) is called the* Lagrange multiplier. *The condition (4.15c) is called* complementary slackness condition. *The nonnegativity condition (4.15b) together with the complementary slackness condition are also known as the* Karush–Kuhn–Tucker conditions.

Proof. Lemma 4.9 assures that $\mathbb{A} = \mathbb{A}_q$ holds. From the necessary conditions stated in Theorem 4.11 we find $G_X(X^*)\delta S \leq 0$ for every admissible and therefore quasi-admissible direction δS. Furthermore, any equality constraint $F^i = 0$ can be separated into $F^i \geq 0$ and $-F^i \geq 0$. Thus from the definition of quasi-admissible directions we end up with $\pm F^i_X \delta S \geq 0$ and $H^j_X \delta S \geq 0$ with $j \in \mathcal{I}(\hat{X})$.

Now we can apply the Farkas lemma (Theorem A.36), for $-G_X(X^*)$, which assures the existence of vectors $\Lambda_1 \geq 0, \Lambda_2 \geq 0$, and $\Pi^j \geq 0,\ j \in \mathcal{I}(\hat{X})$. If we set $\Pi^k = 0$ for $k \notin \mathcal{I}(\hat{X})$ the Farkas lemma (Theorem A.36) yields

$$G_X + \Lambda_1 F_X - \Lambda_2 F_X + \Pi H_X = 0.$$

Collecting the factors of F_X to $\Lambda = \Lambda_1 - \Lambda_2$, we have proved (4.15a), the nonnegativity condition (4.15b), and the complementary slackness condition (4.15c). □

Remark 4.14. Note that contrary to the inequality constraints, where Π_j has to be nonnegative, the sign of Λ_i is not determined.

Necessary Conditions Without Constraint Qualifications

Let us define the following set $A' = \{\delta S : G^*_X \delta S \leq 0\}$; then Theorem 4.11 yields $\mathbb{A} \subset A'$, but not necessarily $\mathbb{A}_q \subset A'$. The constraint qualification in the Lagrange–Karush–Kuhn–Tucker theorem ensures the inclusion $\mathbb{A} = \mathbb{A}_q \subset A'$ as well as the uniqueness of the multiplier (Λ, Π). If the KKT constraint qualification is dropped, two things can happen. First, $\mathbb{A}_q \subset A'$ can still hold yielding the results of the Lagrange–Karush–Kuhn–Tucker theorem but losing the uniqueness of the Lagrange multiplier. Or second, $\mathbb{A}_q \not\subset A'$, then in the proof of the Lagrange–Karush–Kuhn–Tucker theorem, the assumptions of the Farkas lemma (Theorem A.36) do not hold and no conclusion can be drawn from it. Without constraint qualification, the following weaker form of the Lagrange–Karush–Kuhn–Tucker theorem can be proved:

Theorem 4.15 (Weak Lagrange–Karush–Kuhn–Tucker). *Let X^* be a local maximizer of the problem* FSM *(4.9). Then there exist a real number $\Lambda_0 \geq 0$ and row vectors $\Lambda = (\Lambda_i)_{i=1}^k$ and $\Pi = (\Pi_j)_{j=1}^l$ with $(\Lambda_0, \Lambda, \Pi) \neq 0$ satisfying*

$$\begin{aligned}
&\mathcal{L}_X(X^*) = 0 \\
&\Pi \geq 0 \\
&\Pi H(X^*) = 0,
\end{aligned}$$

where $\mathcal{L} = \Lambda_0 G + \Lambda F + \Pi H$ is called the general *Lagrangian. The vector $(\Lambda_0, \Lambda, \Pi)$ is called a* Fritz John (FJ) multiplier.

In case of $\mathbb{A}_q \not\subset A'$ the linear dependence of the gradients F_X^i is a necessary condition, which is equivalent to $\Lambda_0 = 0$ and $(\Lambda, \Pi) \neq 0$. This was first proved by John (1948) for inequality constraints, whereas the complete proof for equality and inequality constraints can be found in Mangasarian and Fromovitz (1967). In fact only two cases have to be considered, namely $\Lambda_0 = 0$ and $\Lambda_0 = 1$. Since if $\Lambda_0 > 0$ holds, the Lagrangian can be divided by Λ_0 without changing the results.

In the following subsection we present the geometric intuition for the Lagrange–Karush–Kuhn–Tucker theorem. In many of the optimization textbooks the Lagrange–Karush–Kuhn–Tucker theoremis proved by making the subsequent presented geometric steps rigor (see, e.g., Apostol, 1977; Fletcher, 1987).

Geometric Intuition of the Lagrangian Approach

For the underlying geometric idea of the Lagrange–Karush–Kuhn–Tucker theorem let us consider a problem in the plane, where the function $G(X)$ has to be maximized due to the constraint $F : \mathbb{R}^2 \to \mathbb{R}$:

$$\max_{X \in \mathbb{R}^2} G(X) \tag{4.16a}$$

$$\text{s.t.} \quad F(X) = 0. \tag{4.16b}$$

For notational simplicity we write $X = (x, y)'$. Let $X^* = (x^*, y^*)'$ be a solution of this problem and $F_X(x^*, y^*) \neq 0$. Especially we assume $F_y(x^*, y^*) \neq 0$, then by the implicit function theorem there exists an open neighborhood $N_\varepsilon(x^*) =$

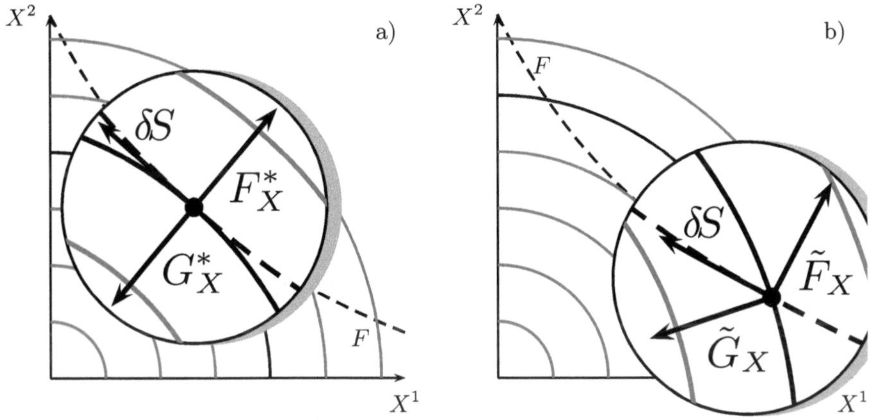

Fig. 4.5. In the optimal case (**a**) an admissible direction δS may not increase the optimal value G^*, where G is shown by its *contour lines*. Hence δS is orthogonal to the contour line at G_X^* as well as to the equality constraint F_X^* (*dashed curve*). This implies the linear dependence of G_X^* and F_X^* and therefore the existence of a Lagrange multiplier Λ with $G_X^* + \Lambda F_X^* = 0$. Case (**b**) visualizes the argument that δS has to be orthogonal to G^*, as otherwise a step in an admissible direction would increase the objective value G

$(x^* - \varepsilon, x^* + \varepsilon)$ and a continuously differentiable function $y(x) : N_\varepsilon(x^*) \to \mathbb{R}$ satisfying

$$F(x, y(x)) = 0, \quad \text{for all} \quad x \in N_\varepsilon(x^*).$$

Next we show that the gradient $F_X(X^*)$ is perpendicular to the tangent vector of $y(x)$ at x^*, which is an admissible direction δS and given by

$$\delta S = \left(1, \frac{\mathrm{d}y(x^*)}{\mathrm{d}x}\right)'.$$

That δS is an admissible direction is a consequence of the implicit differentiation formula applied to $y(x)$

$$(F_x(x^*, y^*), F_y(x^*, y^*)) \left(1, -\frac{F_x(x^*, y^*)}{F_y(x^*, y^*)}\right)' = F_x(x^*, y^*) - F_x(x^*, y^*) = 0.$$

We next show that the gradient $G_X(x^*, y^*)$ is also perpendicular to $y(x)$ at x^* (see Fig. 4.5). Therefore consider the problem

$$\max_x G(x, y(x)), \quad \text{with} \quad x \in N_\varepsilon(x^*),$$

which is a real-valued maximization problem of a continuously differentiable function and therefore

$$\frac{\mathrm{d}}{\mathrm{d}x} G(x^*, y(x^*)) = 0 \tag{4.17}$$

has to hold at X^*. Using the chain rule, the derivative (4.17) becomes

$$0 = (G_x(x^*, y^*), G_y(x^*, y^*)) \left(1, -\frac{F_x(x^*, y^*)}{F_y(x^*, y^*)}\right)',$$

proving that $G_X(X^*)$ is perpendicular to the curve at X^*. Since $G_X(X^*)$ as well as $F_X(X^*)$ are perpendicular to $y(x)$ they are linearly dependent and therefore a $\Lambda \neq 0$ exists satisfying

$$G_X(X^*) + \Lambda F_X(X^*) = 0.$$

An Example Failing the Constraint Qualification

The Lagrangian method may fail if the constraint qualification is not satisfied. To study such a case we analyze the following problem:

$$\max G(x, y) = -y \tag{4.18a}$$

$$\text{s.t.} \quad H(x, y) = y^3 - x^2 \geq 0. \tag{4.18b}$$

Obviously $x = y = 0$ is the (unique) maximizer. But since

$$H_X(0, 0) = \begin{pmatrix} 0 \\ 0 \end{pmatrix},$$

there exists no λ satisfying (4.15a), which for this specific case becomes

$$\begin{pmatrix} 0 \\ 0 \end{pmatrix} = \begin{pmatrix} 0 \\ -1 \end{pmatrix} + \lambda \begin{pmatrix} 0 \\ 0 \end{pmatrix}.$$

In Fig. 4.6 the admissible region of the problem (4.18) is depicted, showing that there is a cusp[1] at the origin. Thus the curve

$$\gamma := \{(x, y) : \; y^3 - x^2\}$$

given by (4.18b), is not differentiable at (0, 0) and therefore the chain of previous reasoning cannot be drawn. Considering the set of admissible directions we see that (4.18b) can be split into the two constraints

$$\tilde{H}^{1,2}(x, y) := \pm y^{\frac{3}{2}} - x \geq 0.$$

We see that the corresponding sets of admissible directions $\mathbb{A} = \{(x, 0) : \; x \geq 0\}$ and quasi-admissible directions $\mathbb{A}_q = \{(x, 0) : \; x \in \mathbb{R}\}$ are not identical and thus the constraint qualification is not satisfied (see Fig. 4.6).

So far we answered the question which necessary conditions a maximizer has to satisfy. In the next subsection we address the question under which conditions these necessary conditions are also sufficient.

[1] A *cusp point* is a point at which two branches of a curve meet such that the tangents of each branch are equal.

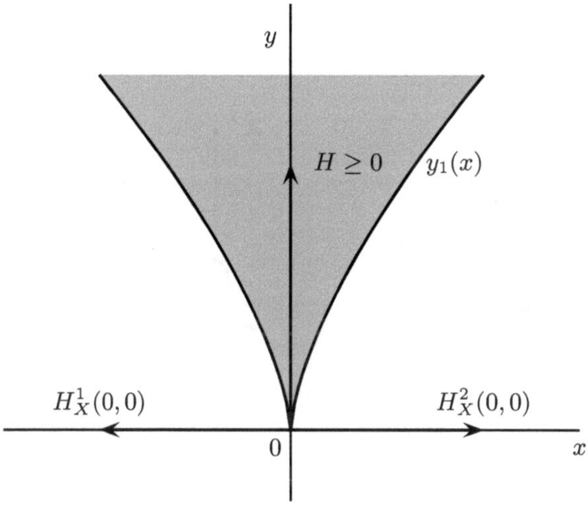

Fig. 4.6. The admissible region $H \geq 0$ of problem (4.18) exhibits a cusp point at the origin. Since the gradients $H_X^{1,2}(0,0)$ are linearly dependent the constraint qualification is violated and the Lagrange–Karush–Kuhn–Tucker theorem cannot be applied

Sufficiency Conditions for a Maximizer of *FSM* (4.9)

Under appropriate concavity assumptions the necessary conditions become also sufficient:

Theorem 4.16 (Global Sufficiency). *Let X^* satisfy the conditions of the Lagrange–Karush–Kuhn–Tucker theorem and let the Lagrangian $\mathcal{L}$ be (strictly) concave in X; then X^* is a (strict) global maximizer of problem* FSM *(4.9).*

Proof. We have to show that $G(X) \leq G(X^*)$ holds for every admissible X. This follows from

$$\begin{aligned} G(X) - G(X^*) &= \mathcal{L}(X) - \mathcal{L}(X^*) \\ &\leq \mathcal{L}_X(X^*)(X - X^*) \\ &= 0. \end{aligned}$$

For a strictly concave function the strict inequality follows, and hence X^* is the unique maximizer, which concludes the proof. □

Under the assumption that the functions G and F are two times continuously differentiable a local form of Theorem 4.16 can be stated:

Theorem 4.17 (Local Sufficiency). *If X^* is an extremal point of* FSM *(4.9) and if the Hessian matrix of the Lagrangian at X^* satisfies*

$$\delta S' \mathcal{L}_{XX} \delta S < 0, \quad \text{for every } \delta S \neq 0 \text{ and } \delta S \in \mathbb{A},$$

then X^* is a strict local maximizer of FSM *(4.9).*

For a geometric interpretation of Theorem 4.17 see Fig. 4.7.

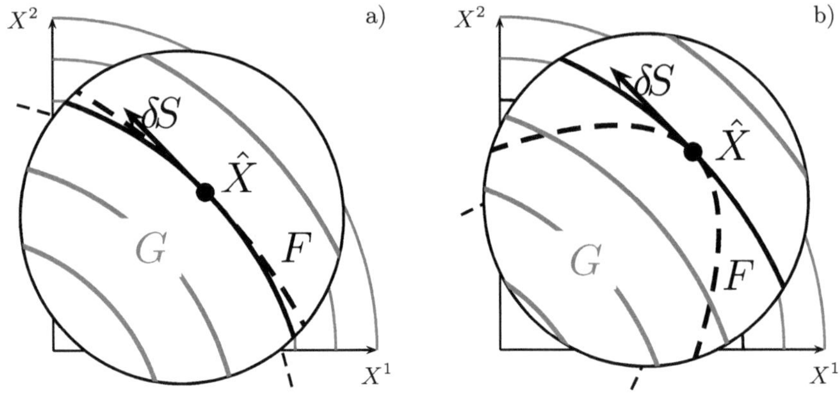

Fig. 4.7. For $G = \|X\|$ the contour lines of G (*solid curves*) and the constraint F (*dashed curve*) are depicted. It is illustrated that for an extremal $\hat{X}$ (a change along an admissible direction δS does not change the objective value), the curvature of G and F in $\hat{X}$ is of importance. In case (**a**) the objective value is not increased in second-order approximation in a neighborhood of $\hat{X}$ and hence is a maximizer, whereas in case (**b**) the curvature of F is that large that the objective value for a point X in the neighborhood of $\hat{X}$ exceeds that of $\hat{X}$

Remark 4.18. The inequality

$$\delta S' \mathcal{L}_{XX} \delta S \leq 0, \quad \text{for all} \quad \delta S \in \mathbb{A},$$

is a necessary condition of second order for a maximizer X^* of *FSM* (4.9). If the constraint qualification hold the set of admissible directions $\mathbb{A}$ can be replaced by the set of quasi-admissible directions $\mathbb{A}_q$. For optimal control problems such second-order conditions can also be stated but are in general difficult to prove.

After this short excursion to sufficient and second-order conditions, we consider an important tool for the sensitivity analysis of solutions of *FSM* (4.9) provided by the envelope theorem.

4.2.3 The Envelope Theorem and the Lagrange Multiplier

The sensitivity of the value function of an optimization problem, which depends on exogenously given parameter values, is an important question to be analyzed. The envelope theorem and its generalizations answer these questions. Let us therefore extend problem *FSM* (4.9) to the case including the exogenous parameter $\mu \in \mathbb{R}^p$ (*FSMP*):

$$\begin{aligned} &\max_{X \in \mathbb{R}^n} G(X, \mu) \\ \text{s.t.} \quad &F^1(X, \mu) = 0, \dots, F^k(X, \mu) = 0, \\ &H^1(X, \mu) \geq 0, \dots, H^l(X, \mu) \geq 0, \end{aligned}$$

where the given functions G, F and H are continuously differentiable with respect to X and μ. Then the corresponding Lagrangian is given by

$$\mathcal{L}(X, \Lambda, \Pi, \mu) = G(X, \mu) + \Lambda F(X, \mu) + \Pi H(X, \mu). \tag{4.19}$$

Defining the value function

$$G^*(\mu) = \begin{cases} G\left(X^*(\mu), \mu\right) & X^*(\mu) \in \operatorname*{argmax}_{X \in \Omega(X,\mu)} G(X, \mu) \\ \infty & \operatorname*{argmax}_{X \in \Omega(X,\mu)} G(X, \mu) = \emptyset \end{cases} \tag{4.20}$$

the following theorem can be proved:

Theorem 4.19 (Envelope Theorem For Constrained Maxima). *Let the value function (4.20) be finite for every $\mu \in \Gamma \subset \mathbb{R}^p$ and Γ be open. For every $\mu \in \Gamma$ there exists a multiplier $(\Lambda^*(\mu), \Pi^*(\mu))$ for the Lagrangian (4.19) satisfying*

$$\mathcal{L}_X\left(X^*(\mu), \Lambda^*(\mu), \Pi^*(\mu), \mu\right) = 0.$$

Assume that $X^* : \Gamma \to \mathbb{R}^n$, $\Lambda^* : \Gamma \to \mathbb{R}^k$ and $\Pi^* : \Gamma \to \mathbb{R}^l$ be continuously differentiable in μ; then the value function (4.20) is continuously differentiable in μ and

$$\frac{\mathrm{d}G^*}{\mathrm{d}\mu}(\mu) = \frac{\partial \mathcal{L}}{\partial \mu}\left(X^*(\mu), \Lambda^*(\mu), \Pi^*(\mu), \mu\right).$$

Remark 4.20. A comprehensive exposition of the envelope theorem in context of optimal control theory and comparative dynamics can be found in Caputo (2005).

For the proof see Appendix B.7.

Remark 4.21. For the consideration of a parametrized maximization problem under weaker assumptions the reader is referred to Clarke, Ledyaev, Stern, and Wolenski (1998).

An important corollary of this result enables us to find an interpretation of the Lagrange multiplier:

Corollary 4.22. *Let X^* be a maximizer of the problem* FSM *(4.9) and let the vector $\varepsilon = (\varepsilon_1, \dots, \varepsilon_{k+l})'$ denote a change in the constraint levels, i.e.,*

$$F(X) + \begin{pmatrix} \varepsilon_1 \\ \vdots \\ \varepsilon_k \end{pmatrix} = 0, \quad \text{and} \quad H(X) + \begin{pmatrix} \varepsilon_{k+1} \\ \vdots \\ \varepsilon_{k+l} \end{pmatrix} = 0.$$

Under the assumptions of Theorem 4.19 we find

$$(\Lambda, \Pi) = \frac{\mathrm{d}G(X^*)}{\mathrm{d}\varepsilon}.$$

Proof. For the given maximization problem the Lagrangian $\mathcal{L}$ is written as

$$\mathcal{L}(X, \Lambda, \varepsilon) = G(X) + \sum_{i=1}^{k} \Lambda_i \left(F^i(X) - \varepsilon_i\right) + \sum_{j=1}^{l} \Pi_j \left(H^j(X) - \varepsilon_{j+k}\right).$$

Thus we find

$$\frac{\mathrm{d}G^*}{\mathrm{d}\varepsilon} = \frac{\mathrm{d}\mathcal{L}}{\mathrm{d}\varepsilon} = (\Lambda, \Pi),$$

which concludes the proof. □

Remark 4.23. From Cor. 4.22 it follows that the entries of the Lagrange multiplier denote the change of the value function G^* if the constraint levels are relaxed. For reasons of simplicity we only consider the case of an equality constraint. Setting

$$\Lambda_j = \frac{\mathrm{d}G^*(0)}{\mathrm{d}\varepsilon} \approx \frac{\Delta G^*(0)}{\Delta\varepsilon}$$

we see that Λ_j can be interpreted as the *shadow price* of the jth constraint. Compare this with the economic interpretation of the costate in optimal control problems in Sect. 3.3.4.

4.2.4 The Discrete-Time Maximum Principle as a Static Maximization Problem

In this subsection we use the results from Lagrange theory to prove a discrete version of the Maximum Principle. We start with reformulating the discrete optimal control problem as stated in Sect. 4.1.4.

Reformulation of the Discrete-Time Optimal Control Problem

First we analyze the maximum condition posed on the objective function (4.8a)

$$\max_{u \in \mathbb{R}^M} \left\{ \sum_{i=1}^{N-1} g(x_i, u_i) \right\} + S(x_N),$$

with $u = (u_1', \dots, u_{N-1}')'$ and $M = (N-1)m$.

Here the maximization is formulated only for the controls u_i at the steps $i = 1, \dots, N-1$. It is now possible to take two different positions. First, the states x_i, $i = 1, \dots, N$, can be considered as an independent variable $x \in \mathbb{R}^K$ satisfying the constraints (4.8b–4.8f), which is equivalent to the maximization

$$\max_{(u,x)\in\mathbb{R}^M\times\mathbb{R}^K}\left\{\sum_{i=1}^{N-1} g(x_i,u_i)+S(x_N)\right\}.$$

Pursuing this line leads to the discrete-time Maximum Principle by using the Lagrange–Karush–Kuhn–Tucker theorem. Second, one can also refer to the recursive structure of the discrete state dynamics given in (4.8b) and keep the original maximum condition (4.8a), which corresponds to the dynamic programming approach.

In this subsection we adopt the Lagrangian point of view and consider the problem *DOC* (4.8) as a maximization problem for the objective function

$$G(X)=\sum_{i=1}^{N-1} g(x_i,u_i)+S(x_N),$$

with

$$X=(u_1',x_1',\dots,u_i',x_i',\dots,x_N')'\in\mathbb{R}^K,\quad K=Nn+(N-1)m.$$

The equality constraint $F(X)=0$ is given as

$$F(X)=\begin{cases} x_1-x_0=F^{(0)}(x_1) \\ -x_i+x_{i+1}-f(x_i,u_i)=F^{(i)}(u_i,x_i,x_{i+1}) & i=1,\dots,N-1 \\ a(x_N)=F^{(N)}(x_N), \end{cases}$$

representing the state dynamics, together with initial and terminal constraints.

Finally, the inequality constraint $H(X)\geq 0$ is combined in

$$H(X)=\begin{cases} c(x_i,u_i) & i=1,\dots,N-1 \\ h(x_i) & i=1,\dots,N-1 \\ b(x_N). \end{cases}$$

Rewriting the discrete-time optimal control problem in this form, we get:

$$\max_{X\in\mathbb{R}^K} G(X) \tag{4.21a}$$

$$\text{s.t.}\quad F(X)=0 \tag{4.21b}$$

$$H(X)\geq 0. \tag{4.21c}$$

After this reformulation of the discrete problem *DOC* (4.8) as a static maximization problem, (4.21) can be analyzed via the Lagrange theory.

The Discrete Maximum Principle

We start with the formulation of the discrete Maximum Principle for *DOC* (4.8):

Theorem 4.24 (Discrete Maximum Principle). *Let the sequence of vectors* (x_i^*, u_i^*), $i = 1, \dots, N-1$, *be an optimal solution of* DOC *(4.8). Then there exist row vectors* $\lambda^i \in \mathbb{R}^n$, $\nu^i \in \mathbb{R}^k$, *and* $\mu^i \in \mathbb{R}^l$ *with* $i = 1, \dots, N-1$ *and constants* $\lambda_0 \geq 0$, $\alpha \in \mathbb{R}^{l'}$ *and* $\beta \in \mathbb{R}_+^{l''}$ *with* $(\lambda_0, \lambda^i, \nu, \mu, \alpha, \beta) \neq 0$ *where* $\nu = (\nu^1, \dots, \nu^{N-1})$, $\mu = (\mu^1, \dots, \mu^{N-1})$ *satisfying the following conditions:*

$$\mathcal{L}_{u_i}(x_i^*, u_i^*, \lambda^i, \mu^i, \nu^i, \lambda_0) = 0 \tag{4.22a}$$

$$\lambda^i = \lambda^{i-1} - \mathcal{L}_{x_i}(x_i^*, u_i^*, \lambda^i, \mu^i, \nu^i, \lambda_0), \quad i = 2, \dots, N-1 \tag{4.22b}$$

together with the complementary slackness conditions

$$\mu^j \geq 0, \quad c^j(x_i^*, u_i^*)\mu^j = 0, \quad j = 1, \dots, l \tag{4.22c}$$

$$\nu^j \geq 0, \quad h^j(x_i^*)\nu^j = 0, \quad j = 1, \dots, k. \tag{4.22d}$$

At the end point the following transversality condition has to hold

$$\lambda^{N-1} = S_x(x_N^*) + \nu^N h_x(x_N^*) + \alpha a_x(x_N^*) + \beta b_x(x_N^*)$$

with the complementary slackness conditions

$$\beta \geq 0, \quad \beta b(x_N^*) = 0.$$

The function

$$\mathcal{L}(x_i, u_i, \lambda^i, \mu^i, \nu^i, \lambda_0) = \mathcal{H}(x_i, u_i, \lambda^i, \lambda_0) + \sum_{i=1}^{N-1} \left(\mu^i c_i + \nu^i h_i\right) \tag{4.22e}$$

is called the Lagrangian *and*

$$\mathcal{H}(x_i, u_i, \lambda^i, \lambda_0) = \lambda_0 g(x_i, u_i) + \lambda^i f(x_i, u_i)$$

the Hamiltonian *of the problem.*

Remark 4.25. For a more general formulation of the problem the reader is referred to Ravn (1999).

Proof. For the proof we apply the results of the weak Lagrange–Karush–Kuhn–Tucker theorem to the problem (4.21).

At first we define the overall Lagrangian[2] $\mathbb{L}$ of the problem as

$$\mathbb{L} = \lambda_0 \left(\sum_{i=1}^{N-1} g(x_i, u_i) + S(x_N) \right) + \sum_{i=1}^{N-1} \lambda^i \left(x_i - x_{i+1} + f(x_i, u_i)\right)$$
$$+ \sum_{i=1}^{N-1} \mu^i c(x_i, u_i) + \sum_{i=1}^{N} \nu^i h(x_i) + \kappa\,(x_1 - x_0) + \alpha a(x_N) + \beta b(x_N),$$

[2] Note that $\mathbb{L}$ denotes the Lagrangian of the problem *DOC* (4.8) considered as a static maximization problem and is different to the Lagrangian $\mathcal{L}$ in (4.22e), where the correspondence is given in (4.23).

or when using (4.22e)

$$\begin{aligned}\mathbb{L} = &\sum_{i=1}^{N-1} \mathcal{L}(x_i, u_i, \lambda^i, \mu^i, \nu^i, \lambda_0) + \sum_{i=1}^{N-1} \lambda^i (x_i - x_{i+1}) \\ &+\nu^N h(x_N) + \alpha a(x_N) + \beta b(x_N). \end{aligned} \tag{4.23}$$

The condition (4.15a) of the Lagrange–Karush–Kuhn–Tucker theorem applied to $\mathbb{L}$ yields

$$\mathbb{L}_{u_i} = \mathcal{L}_{u_i} = 0, \quad i = 1, \dots, N-1 \tag{4.24}$$

$$\mathbb{L}_{x_1} = \mathcal{L}_{x_1} + \lambda^1 + \kappa = 0 \tag{4.25}$$

$$\mathbb{L}_{x_i} = \lambda^i + \mathcal{L}_{x_i} - \lambda^{i-1} = 0, \quad i = 2, \dots, N-1 \tag{4.26}$$

$$\mathbb{L}_{x_N} = \lambda_0 S_{x_N} - \lambda^{N-1} + \nu^N h_{x_N} + \alpha a_{x_N} + \beta b_{x_N} = 0. \tag{4.27}$$

From (4.24) we find

$$\mathcal{L}_{u_i} = 0,$$

identifying the control value at time i as an extremal point of the Lagrangian $\mathcal{L}$. Note that in the absence of inequality constraints $\mathcal{L}_{u_i} = 0$ reduces to $\mathcal{H}_{u_i} = 0$, i.e., u_i is an extremal of the Hamiltonian, which is a local form of the Hamiltonian maximizing condition.

Using (4.25) and (4.26) yield

$$\mathcal{L}_{x_1} = \mathcal{H}_{x_1} + \lambda^1 + \mu^1 c_{x_1} + \nu^1 h_{x_1} = -\kappa \tag{4.28}$$

$$\lambda^i = \lambda^{i-1} - \mathcal{L}_{x_i}(x_i, u_i). \tag{4.29}$$

Thus (4.29) adds an adjoint system of recursive relations to the state system, in which the vectors λ^i are the *adjoint variables* or *costates*. From (4.28) it follows that λ^1 is free. Whereas (4.27) restricts λ^{N-1} to

$$\lambda^{N-1} = \lambda_0 S_{x^N} + \nu^N h_{x_N} + \alpha a_{x_N} + \beta b_{x_N}, \tag{4.30}$$

yielding the *transversality condition.*

Note that in the absence of any terminal constraints on the state, (4.30) reduces to

$$\lambda^{N-1} = \lambda_0 S_{x^N},$$

or if $S \equiv 0$

$$\lambda^{N-1} = 0.$$

□

Remark 4.26. The formal analogy between the discrete-time Maximum Principle and the continuous-time Maximum Principle is obvious and the reader may, e.g., derive the adjoint differential equation from its discrete analog (4.22b) in an informal way by a simple limiting argument. Anyhow, a rigorous derivation of the continuous Maximum Principle from the discrete-time Maximum Principle is formally tricky and beyond the scope of this book.

Remark 4.27. One of the main drawbacks of the Lagrangian approach is that the Hamiltonian maximizing condition

$$u^* = \underset{u}{\operatorname{argmax}} \mathcal{H}(x, u, \lambda)$$

can only be derived in the local form

$$\mathcal{H}_u(x, u^*, \lambda) = 0.$$

Thus the optimal control value u^* is only specified as an extremal point of the Hamiltonian $\mathcal{H}$.

Next we introduce the calculus of variations to present a further proof of Pontryagin's Maximum Principle, which allows us to derive the corner conditions specific only to the continuous-time problem.

4.3 The Calculus of Variations

This is not the place to present the theory of the calculus of variations in depth; for that the reader is referred, e.g., to the textbooks on the calculus of variations by Bliss (1925); Sagan (1969), and Smith (1974). Nonetheless, an introduction to calculus of variations as a direct predecessor of optimal control theory should be given (see the historical remarks in Sect. 3.1). The calculus of variations extends the methods of ordinary calculus to the case of functionals. This allows a generalization of the Lagrange–Karush–Kuhn–Tucker theory and will be explored in some detail in the following section.

4.3.1 A Simple Variational Example

In this subsection we present one of the simplest problems, which can be formulated as a problem of the calculus of variations, namely to determine the (continuously differentiable) path of minimum length connecting two points $a \neq b$ in the plane.

Problem Formulation

From calculus we know that the arc length of a continuously differentiable function $x : [0, T] \to \mathbb{R}^2$ is given by

$$G(x(\cdot)) = \int_0^T \|\dot{x}(t)\| \, dt.$$

Then the problem can be stated as the minimization problem:

$$\min_{x(\cdot)\in C^1([0,T])} \int_0^T \|\dot{x}(t)\| \, \mathrm{d}t \tag{4.31a}$$

$$\text{s.t.} \quad x(0) = a, \quad x(T) = b, \tag{4.31b}$$

where subsequently the integrand of (4.31a) is abbreviated by

$$g(\dot{x}) := \|\dot{x}\| = \sqrt{\dot{x}_1^2 + \dot{x}_2^2}.$$

Thus among all continuously differentiable curves $x(\cdot)$ connecting the points a and b, one has to identify the curve exhibiting the smallest arc length. At this point we assume a naive point of view and forget that we already know the solution given by the connecting line.

As in the previously discussed case of static optimization we next consider small variations of the minimizer $x^*(\cdot)$. These variations together with an analysis of the corresponding objective value will then lead to necessary conditions characterizing a minimizer of problem (4.31). Therefore we first have to identify admissible variations.

Admissible Variations

Suppose that $x^*(\cdot)$ is a solution of problem (4.31). Since $x^*(\cdot)$ is assumed to be continuously differentiable with fixed initial and terminal state, we only consider variations such that the perturbed curve is in the same class of functions. Thus the set

$$\mathbb{A} := \{\delta S(\cdot) \in C^1([0,T]) : \delta S(0) = \delta S(T) = 0\}$$

satisfies these conditions, since for $\varepsilon > 0$ the varied curve

$$x^\varepsilon(\cdot) := x^*(\cdot) + \varepsilon \delta S(\cdot) \in C^1([0,T]), \quad \delta S \in \mathbb{A} \tag{4.32}$$

is continuously differentiable with $x^\varepsilon(0) = a$ and $x^\varepsilon(T) = b$.

Moreover, this thus defined set of admissible variations $\mathbb{A}$ is a vector space exhibiting the important property

$$\delta S(\cdot) \in \mathbb{A} \quad \text{iff} \quad -\delta S(\cdot) \in \mathbb{A}.$$

This property allows us to chose ε in (4.32) not only for $\varepsilon \in \mathbb{R}_+$ but for all $\varepsilon \in \mathbb{R}$. For $\delta S(\cdot) \in \mathbb{A}$ the real-valued function

$$V(\varepsilon) := G(x^\varepsilon(\cdot)) = \int_0^T g\left(\dot{x}^*(t) + \varepsilon \dot{\delta S}(t)\right) \mathrm{d}t$$

is then continuously differentiable with respect to ε and defined in an open neighborhood of zero, which exhibits a (local) minimum at $\varepsilon = 0$ (see Definition 4.28). This approach reduces the "functional" problem to the well known real-valued problem, which will subsequently be exploited.[3]

[3] Note that $\dot{\delta S}(\cdot)$ denotes the time derivative $\frac{\mathrm{d}}{\mathrm{d}t}\delta S(\cdot)$ of the variation $\delta S(\cdot)$ and *must not* be varied independently from $\delta S(\cdot)$.

Local Criterion for a Minimizer

Given the continuous differentiablity of $V(\cdot)$, its derivative has to be zero at $\varepsilon = 0$ (see Appendix A.3.3). Interchanging integration and differentiation and applying the chain rule therefore yields

$$V'(0) = \int_0^T \left\langle g_x\left(\dot{x}^*(t)\right), \dot{\delta S}(t)\right\rangle \,\mathrm{d}t = 0. \tag{4.33}$$

To reformulate (4.33) in a more applicable form we apply the Dubois–Reymond lemma (Lemma A.140), for each of the terms occurring in the scalar product of (4.33). This yields the final condition, that for the minimizer $x^*(\cdot)$ there exists a constant $C \in \mathbb{R}^2$ satisfying

$$g_x\left(\dot{x}^*(t)\right) = C = (C_1, C_2)' \in \mathbb{R}^2, \quad \text{for all} \quad t \in [0, T].$$

Or using the definition of g we find

$$\frac{\dot{x}^*(t)}{\|\dot{x}^*(t)\|} = C, \quad \text{for all} \quad t \in [0, T].$$

Since for $a \neq b$, $\dot{x}(0) \neq 0$ we find $\|C\| = 1$ for all t, which implies that at least one of the coordinates is unequal to zero. Assuming $C_2 \neq 0$ we set $y = x_1$, and $z = x_2$. Thus y can be considered as a function $y(z)$ yielding

$$y'(z) = \frac{\dot{y}}{\dot{z}} = \frac{C_1}{C_2}.$$

This proves that the minimizer $x^*(\cdot)$ is a straight line.

Having considered this specific problem of the calculus of variations let us return to the general case.

4.3.2 The First Variation

Let us reconsider the general problem of maximization (GMP):

$$\max_X G(X) \tag{4.34a}$$

$$\text{s.t.} \quad X \in \Omega \subset \mathbb{V}, \tag{4.34b}$$

where $\mathbb{V}$ is assumed to be a real vector space, e.g., $\mathbb{V} = C_p^{0,1}([0, T])$.

In the previous subsection we considered "small" variations $\varepsilon\delta S$ of X^* to determine necessary conditions a maximizer X^* of problem (4.34) has to satisfy. For these variations the relative changes

$$\frac{G(X^* + \varepsilon\delta S) - G(X^*)}{\varepsilon}, \quad \text{with} \quad \varepsilon > 0$$

in direction of δS are analyzed. We therefore define the first variation of the functional G in direction δS by the following:

Definition 4.28 (First Variation). *Let $G : \mathbb{V} \to \mathbb{R}$ with $\hat{X} \in \mathbb{V}$ and $\delta S \in \mathbb{V}$. If the following limit*

$$\delta G(\hat{X}, \delta S) := \lim_{\varepsilon \to 0^+} \frac{G(\hat{X} + \varepsilon \delta S) - G(\hat{X})}{\varepsilon},$$

exists, then $\delta G(\hat{X}, \delta S)$ is called the first variation *of $G(\hat{X})$ at $\hat{X}$ in direction δS.*

Remark 4.29. The first variation $\delta G(\hat{X}, \delta S)$ is the right side derivative of $G(\hat{X} + \varepsilon \delta S)$ with respect to ε, denoted by

$$\frac{\mathrm{d}}{\mathrm{d}\varepsilon} G(\hat{X} + \varepsilon \delta S)\bigg|_{\varepsilon = 0^+} := \delta G(\hat{X}, \delta S).$$

Remark 4.30. For a differentiable function $G : \mathbb{R}^n \to \mathbb{R}$ the first variation denotes the directional derivative, which is given by

$$\delta G(\hat{X}, \delta S) = G_X(\hat{X}) \delta S = \sum_{i=1}^{n} \frac{\partial G(\hat{X})}{\partial X_i} \delta S_i,$$

where $\delta S = (\delta S_1, \dots, \delta S_n)'$.

Next, we define the set of admissible variations:

Definition 4.31 (Admissible Variation). *A vector $X \in \mathbb{V}$ is called* admissible *for* GMP *(4.34) if $X \in \Omega$. A vector $\delta S \in \mathbb{V}$ is called an* admissible variation *of an admissible vector X if $X + \varepsilon \delta S \in \Omega$ for all $\varepsilon \in [0, 1]$. The set of admissible variations is denoted by $\mathbb{A}$.*

We can now formulate the analog to Theorem 4.11 as:

Theorem 4.32 (Necessary Optimality Condition). *Let $G : \mathbb{V} \to \mathbb{R}$ possess a first variation at $X^* \in \mathbb{V}$ for every $\delta S \in \mathbb{A}$. Suppose G exhibits a relative maximum at X^*, then*

$$\delta G(X^*, \delta S) \le 0.$$

If the set $\mathbb{A}$ is a vector space, then

$$\delta G(X^*, \delta S) = 0.$$

Proof. To prove the first part we only have to consider that if X^* is a local maximizer, we find for $\varepsilon > 0$ small enough

$$\frac{G(X^* + \varepsilon \delta S) - G(X^*)}{\varepsilon} \le 0$$

yielding

$$\delta G(X^*, \delta S) = \lim_{\varepsilon \to 0+} \frac{G(X^* + \varepsilon \delta S) - G(X^*)}{\varepsilon} \le 0. \tag{4.35}$$

For the second part we use the fact that the first variation is homogenous, i.e.,

$$\delta G(X^*, \mu \delta S) = \mu \delta G(X^*, \delta S), \quad \mu \in \mathbb{R},$$

which is an immediate consequence of the definition; the reader is invited to prove this property in Exercise 4.7. Given the homogeneity and using the fact that, since $\mathbb{A}$ is a vector space, with $\delta S \in \mathbb{A}$ also $-\delta S \in \mathbb{A}$, we get

$$\delta G(X^*, -\delta S) = -\delta G(X^*, \delta S) \le 0.$$

This yields, together with (4.35), the equality

$$\delta G(X^*, \delta S) = 0$$

and concludes the proof. □

To derive the necessary optimality conditions of an optimal control problem we first prove the Euler equation and Weierstrass–Erdmann conditions of the calculus of variations.

4.3.3 Deriving the Euler Equation and Weierstrass–Erdmann Conditions

We start analyzing the following optimal control problem:

$$\max_{u(\cdot)} \int_0^T g(x(t), u(t), t)\, \mathrm{d}t \tag{4.36a}$$

$$\text{s.t.} \quad \dot{x}(t) = u(t) \tag{4.36b}$$

$$x(0) = x_0, \quad x(T) = x_T, \tag{4.36c}$$

where $x(\cdot) \in C_p^{0,1}([0, T])$, $u(\cdot) \in C_p^0([0, T])$, and g is two times continuously differentiable in x and u. This problem can equivalently be rewritten as a problem of the calculus of variations:

$$\max_{x(\cdot)} \int_0^T g(x(t), \dot{x}(t), t)\, \mathrm{d}t \tag{4.37a}$$

$$\text{s.t.} \quad x(0) = x_0, \quad x(T) = x_T. \tag{4.37b}$$

Then the following theorem holds:

Theorem 4.33 (Euler Equation and Weierstrass–Erdmann Conditions). *Let $x^*(\cdot)$ be a maximizer of problem (4.37) with a kink at $\tilde{t}$ and satisfying the regularity assumption*

$$\det g_{\dot{x}\dot{x}}(x^*(t), \dot{x}^*(t), t) \neq 0, \quad \textit{for all} \quad t \in [0, T]; \tag{4.38}$$

then the following conditions have to be satisfied:

Euler Equation: On each interval $[0, \tilde{t})$ *and* $(\tilde{t}, T]$

$$\frac{\mathrm{d}}{\mathrm{d}t} g_{\dot{x}}(x^*(t), \dot{x}^*(t), t) = g_x(x^*(t), \dot{x}^*(t), t). \tag{4.39}$$

First Weierstrass–Erdmann condition: at time $\tilde{t}$

$$g_{\dot{x}}(x^*(\tilde{t}), \dot{x}^*(\tilde{t}^-), \tilde{t}) = g_{\dot{x}}(x^*(\tilde{t}), \dot{x}^*(\tilde{t}^+), \tilde{t}). \tag{4.40}$$

Second Weierstrass–Erdmann condition: at time $\tilde{t}$

$$\mathcal{H}(x^*(\tilde{t}), \dot{x}^*(\tilde{t}^-), \tilde{t}) = \mathcal{H}(x^*(\tilde{t}), \dot{x}^*(\tilde{t}^+), \tilde{t}) \tag{4.41}$$

with

$$\mathcal{H}(x, \dot{x}, t) := g(x, \dot{x}, t) - \dot{x} g_{\dot{x}}(x, \dot{x}, t). \tag{4.42}$$

Remark 4.34 (Regularity Assumption). The regularity assumption (4.38) assures that the optimal solution $x^*(\cdot)$ is two times continuously differentiable on each of the intervals $[0, \tilde{t}]$ and $[\tilde{t}, T]$, where at the boundaries the left- and right-hand side derivatives, respectively, are considered (see also Exercise 4.12).

Proof. The solution $x^*(\cdot)$ is a maximizer of (4.37) iff $(x^*(\cdot), u^*(\cdot))$ is an optimal solution of problem (4.36), with $\dot{x}^*(\cdot) = u^*(\cdot)$ and a discontinuity of $u^*(\cdot)$ at $\tilde{t}$.

To derive the necessary optimality conditions we have to determine the set of admissible variations (see Fig. 4.8a). Therefore we consider variations $\delta x(\cdot) \in C_p^{0,1}([0, T])$ with a kink at $\tilde{t}$, and variations $\delta\tilde{t}$ of the junction time $\tilde{t}$. Varying the junction time $\tilde{t}$ causes a shift of the kink. But since the variation $\delta x(\cdot)$ exhibits the kink at $\tilde{t}$ we have to introduce a time transformation assuring that both variations can be considered simultaneously (see Fig. 4.8c). Thus we define the transformation

$$\tau(t, \varepsilon) := \begin{cases} \dfrac{t}{\tilde{t} + \varepsilon\delta\tilde{t}}\tilde{t} & 0 \le t \le \tilde{t} + \varepsilon\delta\tilde{t} \\ \tilde{t} + \dfrac{t - \tilde{t} - \varepsilon\delta\tilde{t}}{T - \tilde{t} - \varepsilon\delta\tilde{t}}(T - \tilde{t}) & \tilde{t} + \varepsilon\delta\tilde{t} \le t \le T, \end{cases} \tag{4.43}$$

which satisfies $\tau(t, 0) = t$. This time transformation is defined such that $\tau(t, \varepsilon)$ maps the intervals $[0, \tilde{t} + \varepsilon\delta\tilde{t}]$ and $[\tilde{t} + \varepsilon\delta\tilde{t}, T]$ onto $[0, \tilde{t}]$ and $[\tilde{t}, T]$.

The derivative of (4.43) with respect to the perturbation variable at $\varepsilon = 0$ is given by

$$\tau_\varepsilon(t, 0) = \begin{cases} -\dfrac{t}{\tilde{t}}\delta\tilde{t} & 0 \le t \le \tilde{t} + \varepsilon\delta\tilde{t} \\ -\dfrac{T - t}{T - \tilde{t}}\delta\tilde{t} & \tilde{t} + \varepsilon\delta\tilde{t} \le t \le T, \end{cases}$$

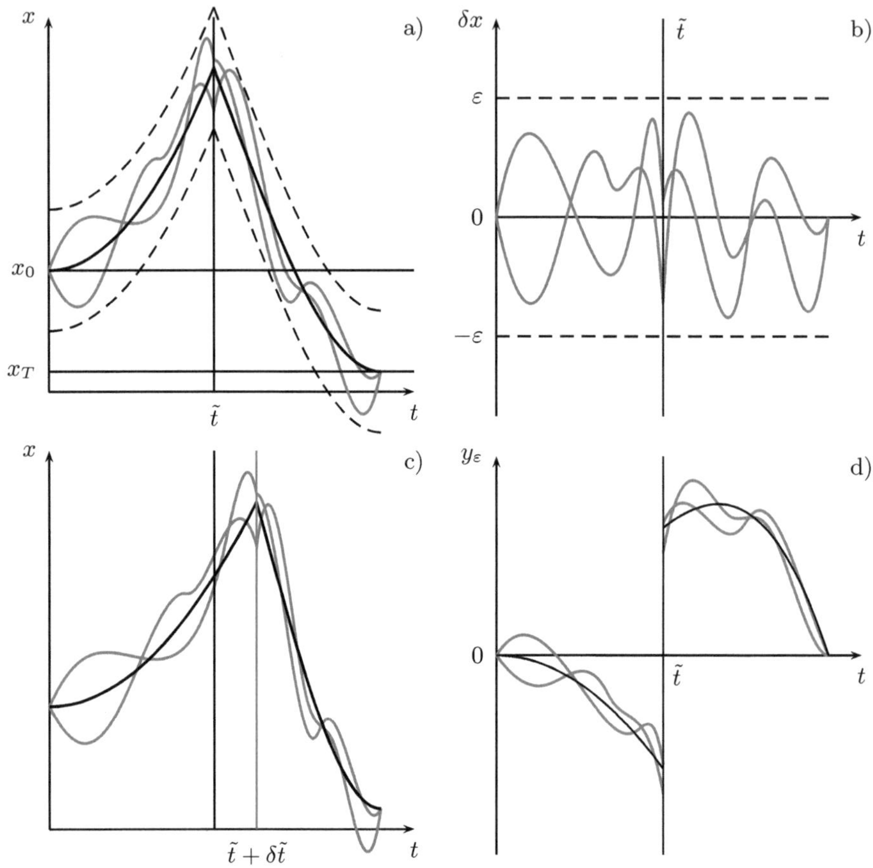

Fig. 4.8. Panel (**a**) depicts the solution path $x^*(\cdot) \in C_p^{0,1}([0, T])$ (*black curve*), with a kink at $\tilde{t}$, and two varied paths (*gray curve*) $x^*(\cdot) + \delta x_i(\cdot)$, $i = 1, 2$ enclosed in a region bounded by the *dashed curves*. Corresponding to these varied paths in (**b**) the variations $\delta x_i(\cdot)$, $i = 1, 2$ are shown. In panel (**c**) additionally the variation $\delta\tilde{t}$ of $\tilde{t}$ is considered. Therefore the time transformation (4.43) is applied to the solution path as well as the variations, yielding the varied paths $y_i(\tau(t, \varepsilon))$, $i = 1, 2$ given by (4.45). The variations $(y_i)_\varepsilon$ of y_i, $i = 1, 2$ (*gray curve*) are shown in (**d**). This change is composed of a part stemming from the time transformation and given by $-\dot{x}^*(\cdot)\delta\tilde{t}$ (*black curve*), therefore the discontinuity at $\tilde{t}$, and the variation $\delta x_i(\cdot)$, $i = 1, 2$

yielding at $t = \tilde{t}$

$$\tau_\varepsilon(\tilde{t}, 0) = -\delta\tilde{t}. \tag{4.44}$$

Using the time transformation (4.43), we can define a path $y(\cdot)$, which denotes the variation of $x^*(\cdot)$ with respect to x as well as t by

$$y(\tau(t,\varepsilon)) := x^*(\tau(t,\varepsilon)) + \varepsilon\delta x(\tau(t,\varepsilon)). \tag{4.45}$$

Then $y(\tau(t,\varepsilon))$ satisfies $y(\tau(t,0)) = y(t) = x^*(t)$ and the derivative of (4.45) with respect to the perturbation variable at $\varepsilon = 0$ is given by

$$\begin{aligned} y_\varepsilon(\tau(t,0)) &= \dot{x}^*(\tau(t,0))\tau_\varepsilon(t,0) + \delta x(\tau(t,0)) \\ &= \dot{x}^*(t)\tau_\varepsilon(t,0) + \delta x(t) = y_\varepsilon(t), \end{aligned} \tag{4.46}$$

yielding for the left- and right-hand side limit at $\tilde{t}$

$$y_\varepsilon(\tilde{t}^-) = -\dot{x}^*(\tilde{t}^-)\delta\tilde{t} + \delta x(\tilde{t}^-), \quad \text{and} \quad y_\varepsilon(\tilde{t}^+) = -\dot{x}^*(\tilde{t}^+)\delta\tilde{t} + \delta x(\tilde{t}^+).$$

Owing to the continuity of $\delta x(\cdot)$ we can define

$$\delta x(\tilde{t}^-) = \delta x(\tilde{t}^+) =: \delta\tilde{x},$$

which denotes the variation of the state at time $\tilde{t}$.

In Remark 4.34 we pointed to the fact that the optimal solution is two times continuously differentiable on each of the intervals $[0, \tilde{t}]$ and $[\tilde{t}, T]$. Therefore the time derivative $\dot{y}_\varepsilon(t)$ is well defined on each of these intervals as can be seen by (4.46). This will be important in the subsequent derivation.

We set

$$g(\tau(t,\varepsilon)) := g(y(\tau(t,\varepsilon)), \dot{y}(\tau(t,\varepsilon)), t)$$

and omit the time arguments if there is no ambiguity. Then applying first the Leibniz rule (Proposition A.139) and afterwards the integration by parts (Proposition A.138) formula the first variation of the objective functional

$$V(x(\cdot)) := \int_0^T g(x(t), \dot{x}(t), t)\,\mathrm{d}t,$$

from (4.37a) is given by

$$
\begin{aligned}
\left.\frac{\mathrm{d}V(\varepsilon)}{\mathrm{d}\varepsilon}\right|_{\varepsilon=0^+} &= \left.\frac{\mathrm{d}}{\mathrm{d}\varepsilon}\left(\int_0^{\tilde{t}+\varepsilon\delta\tilde{t}} g(\tau(t,\varepsilon))\,\mathrm{d}t + \int_{\tilde{t}+\varepsilon\delta\tilde{t}}^{T} g(\tau(t,\varepsilon))\,\mathrm{d}t\right)\right|_{\varepsilon=0^+} \\
&= g(\tilde{t}^-)\delta\tilde{t} - g(\tilde{t}^+)\delta\tilde{t} + \int_0^{\tilde{t}} (g_x y_\varepsilon + g_{\dot{x}}\dot{y}_\varepsilon)\,\mathrm{d}t + \int_{\tilde{t}}^{T} (g_x y_\varepsilon + g_{\dot{x}}\dot{y}_\varepsilon)\,\mathrm{d}t \\
&= \left(g(\tilde{t}^-) - g(\tilde{t}^+)\right)\delta\tilde{t} + g_{\dot{x}}(\tilde{t}^-)y_\varepsilon(\tilde{t}^-) - g_{\dot{x}}(\tilde{t}^+)y_\varepsilon(\tilde{t}^+) \\
&\quad + \int_0^{\tilde{t}} \left(g_x - \frac{\mathrm{d}}{\mathrm{d}t}g_{\dot{x}}\right) y_\varepsilon\,\mathrm{d}t + \int_{\tilde{t}}^{T} \left(g_x - \frac{\mathrm{d}}{\mathrm{d}t}g_{\dot{x}}\right) y_\varepsilon\,\mathrm{d}t \\
&= \left(g(\tilde{t}^-) - g_{\dot{x}}(\tilde{t}^-)\dot{x}^*(\tilde{t}^-) - g(\tilde{t}^+) + g_{\dot{x}}(\tilde{t}^+)\dot{x}^*(\tilde{t}^+)\right)\delta\tilde{t} \\
&\quad + \left(g_{\dot{x}}(\tilde{t}^-) - g_{\dot{x}}(\tilde{t}^+)\right)\delta\tilde{x} \\
&\quad + \int_0^{\tilde{t}} \left(g_x - \frac{\mathrm{d}}{\mathrm{d}t}g_{\dot{x}}\right) y_\varepsilon\,\mathrm{d}t + \int_{\tilde{t}}^{T} \left(g_x - \frac{\mathrm{d}}{\mathrm{d}t}g_{\dot{x}}\right) y_\varepsilon\,\mathrm{d}t.
\end{aligned}
\tag{4.47}
$$

Since with $y_\varepsilon(\cdot)$ admissible also $-y_\varepsilon(\cdot)$ is admissible Theorem 4.32 states that the first variation of the objective functional (4.47) has to be zero. Then

$$\left(g_{\dot{x}}(\tilde{t}^-) - g_{\dot{x}}(\tilde{t}^+)\right)\delta\tilde{x} = 0$$

yields the first Weierstrass–Erdmann condition (4.40) and

$$\left(g(\tilde{t}^-) - g_{\dot{x}}(\tilde{t}^-)\dot{x}^*(\tilde{t}^-) - g(\tilde{t}^+) + g_{\dot{x}}(\tilde{t}^+)\dot{x}^*(\tilde{t}^+)\right)\delta\tilde{t} = 0$$

the second Weierstrass–Erdmann condition (4.41).

Using the Dubois–Reymond lemma (Lemma A.140) on each interval $[0, \tilde{t}]$ and $[\tilde{t}, T]$ we find that the integrals in (4.47) yield the Euler equation (4.39), which concludes the proof. □

Remark 4.35 (Reformulation in Optimal Control Notation). Setting

$$\lambda(t) := -g_{\dot{x}}(x^*, \dot{x}^*, t), \quad \text{and} \quad \mathcal{H}(x, u, \lambda, t) := g(x, u, t) + \lambda(t)u(t),$$

the Euler equation (4.39) becomes

$$\dot{\lambda}(t) = -\mathcal{H}_x(x, u, \lambda, t).$$

The usual costate equation for the optimal control problem (4.36) and the Weierstrass–Erdmann conditions assure the continuity of the costate and the Hamiltonian, respectively at $\tilde{t}$, i.e.,

$$
\begin{aligned}
&\lambda(\tilde{t}^-) = \lambda(\tilde{t}^+) \\
&\mathcal{H}\left(x(\tilde{t}), u(\tilde{t}^-), \lambda(\tilde{t}), (\tilde{t})\right) = \mathcal{H}\left(x(\tilde{t}), u(\tilde{t}^+), \lambda(\tilde{t}), (\tilde{t})\right).
\end{aligned}
$$

Remark 4.36 (Transversality Condition). Consider the problem (4.37) with free terminal time, then the following *transversality conditions* can be derived

$$g_{\dot{x}}(x(T), \dot{x}(T), T) = 0 \tag{4.48a}$$
$$g(x(T), \dot{x}(T), T) - \dot{x}(T) g_{\dot{x}}(x(T), \dot{x}(T), T) = 0. \tag{4.48b}$$

In Exercise 4.13 the reader is invited to prove the transversality conditions repeating the arguments of the previous proof.

These results will now be used to prove Pontryagin's Maximum Principle.

4.4 Proving the Continuous-Time Maximum Principle

The Euler equation and Weierstrass–Erdmann conditions are now used to prove the necessary conditions stated in Pontryagin's Maximum Principle. This approach allows a more detailed analysis of the question of continuity and differentiability of the costate – a question that is omitted from most books that survey this subject on this mathematical level – and is an extension of the problem considered in Sect. 4.3.3.

Using the results of the previous subsections we present a proof of the Maximum Principle in local form. The following presentation is mainly based on the excellently written (in German) lecture note in Oberle (2006). For the *local* Maximum Principle the Hamiltonian maximizing condition

$$\mathcal{H}(x^*(t), u^*(t), \lambda(t), t) = \max_u \mathcal{H}(x^*(t), u, \lambda(t), t)$$

is replaced by the condition

$$\mathcal{H}_u(x^*(t), u^*(t), \lambda(t), t) = 0, \tag{4.49}$$

implying that the control value $u^*(t)$ is an extremal point of the Hamiltonian.

Let us restate the optimal control problem, which we subsequently consider:

$$\max_{u(\cdot)} \left\{ \int_0^T g(x(t), u(t), t)\, dt \right\} \tag{4.50a}$$
$$\text{s.t.} \quad \dot{x}(t) = f(x(t), u(t), t) \tag{4.50b}$$
$$x(0) = x_0, \quad x(T) = x_T, \quad t \in [0, T], \tag{4.50c}$$

where the functions $f : \mathbb{R}^n \times \mathbb{R}^m \times \mathbb{R} \to \mathbb{R}^n$ and $g : \mathbb{R}^n \times \mathbb{R}^m \times \mathbb{R} \to \mathbb{R}$ are continuous and continuously differentiable with respect to x and u.

4.4.1 The Continuous-Time Maximum Principle Revisited

To apply the results of Theorem 4.33 to the optimal control problem (4.50) we have to restate the problem, transforming it into a calculus of variation problem. Therefore we introduce the new variables

$$v(t) := \int_0^t u(s)\,\mathrm{d}s, \quad \text{and} \tag{4.51a}$$

$$\rho(t) := \int_0^t \lambda(s)\,\mathrm{d}s, \tag{4.51b}$$

where $\lambda(\cdot)$ is assumed some piecewise continuous function (see Remark 4.37).
Then we consider the new problem:

$$\max_{v(\cdot),x(\cdot),\rho(\cdot))} \int_0^T \left(g(x(t),\dot{v}(t),t) + \dot{\rho}(t)\left(f(x(t),\dot{v}(t),t) - \dot{x}(t)\right)\right)\,\mathrm{d}t \tag{4.52a}$$

$$\text{s.t.} \quad x(0) = x_0, \quad v(0) = 0, \quad \rho(0) = 0, \tag{4.52b}$$

Setting

$$\tilde{g}(x,\dot{x},\dot{v},\dot{\rho},t) := g(x(t),\dot{v}(t),t) + \dot{\rho}(t)\left(f(x(t),\dot{v}(t),t) - \dot{x}(t)\right),$$

and

$$y := (x, v, \rho)$$

(4.52a) becomes

$$\max_{y(\cdot)} \int_0^T \tilde{g}(y,\dot{y},t)\,\mathrm{d}t$$
$$\text{s.t.} \quad y(0) = (x_0, 0, 0)',$$

and problem (4.50) is therefore stated as a problem of the calculus of variations in the form (4.37) and we can use Theorem 4.33 to derive the necessary optimality conditions. In fact this problem is slightly different, since there are no terminal conditions stated. Thus so-called transversality conditions have to be satisfied (see Remark 4.36).

Proof of the Local Maximum Principle

First we consider the function $\mathbb{H}$ defined in (4.42), yielding

$$\mathbb{H}(y,\dot{y},t) := \tilde{g}(y,\dot{y},t) - \dot{y}\tilde{g}_{\dot{y}}(y,\dot{y},t). \tag{4.53}$$

Subsequently we need the following derivatives

$$\tilde{g}_y = \begin{pmatrix} g_x + \dot{\rho} f_x \\ 0 \\ 0 \end{pmatrix}, \quad \tilde{g}_{\dot{y}} = \begin{pmatrix} -\dot{\rho} \\ g_{\dot{v}} + \dot{\rho} f_{\dot{v}} \\ f - \dot{x} \end{pmatrix},$$

and

$$\tilde{g}_{\dot{y}\dot{y}} = \begin{pmatrix} 0 & 0 & -\mathbb{I}^{(n)} \\ 0 & g_{\dot{v}\dot{v}} + \dot{\rho} f_{\dot{v}\dot{v}} & 0 \\ -\mathbb{I}^{(n)} & 0 & 0 \end{pmatrix}. \tag{4.54}$$

Considering (4.54) we see that the regularity assumption is equivalent to the nonsingularity of $g_{uu} + \dot{\rho} f_{uu}$, which is equivalent to the non singularity of $\mathcal{H}_{uu}$, where

$$\mathcal{H} := g + \lambda f$$

is the usual Hamiltonian.

Under the assumption that $\tilde{g}_{\dot{y}\dot{y}}$ is nonsingular for all $t \in [0, T]$ the necessary optimality conditions of Theorem 4.33 have to be satisfied. In that case the Euler equation yields

$$\frac{\mathrm{d}}{\mathrm{d}t} \tilde{g}_{\dot{y}}(y^*(t), \dot{y}^*(t), t) = \tilde{g}_y(y^*(t), \dot{y}^*(t), t)$$

or explicitly written for each of its components

$$\dot{\lambda} = -(g_x + \lambda f_x) \tag{4.55a}$$

$$\frac{\mathrm{d}}{\mathrm{d}t} \mathcal{H}_u = 0 \tag{4.55b}$$

$$\frac{\mathrm{d}}{\mathrm{d}t} (f - \dot{x}) = 0, \tag{4.55c}$$

where we used the identities $\dot{v}(t) = u(t)$ and $\dot{\rho}(t) = \lambda(t)$. Since these identities hold piecewise, we find, using (4.55b) and (4.55c), that the terms

$$\mathcal{H}_u, \quad \text{and} \quad f - \dot{x}$$

are piecewise constant.

At a point $\tilde{t}$, where the solution exhibits a discontinuous derivative the Weierstrass–Erdmann conditions have to be satisfied. Thus using the first Weierstrass–Erdmann condition we get

$$\tilde{g}_{\dot{y}}(y^*(\tilde{t}), \dot{y}^*(\tilde{t}^-), \tilde{t}) = \tilde{g}_{\dot{y}}(y^*(\tilde{t}), \dot{y}^*(\tilde{t}^+), \tilde{t})$$

or for its coordinates

$$\lambda(\tilde{t}^-) = \lambda(\tilde{t}^+) \tag{4.56a}$$

$$\mathcal{H}_u(\tilde{t}^-) = \mathcal{H}_u(\tilde{t}^+) \tag{4.56b}$$

$$f(\tilde{t}^-) - \dot{x}(\tilde{t}^-) = f(\tilde{t}^+) - \dot{x}(\tilde{t}^+). \tag{4.56c}$$

Thus the first identity (4.56a) proves that the costate $\lambda(\cdot)$ is continuous for every $t \in [0, T]$, which in consequence says, that the solution $y^*(\cdot)$ can only have a discontinuous derivative if the optimal control $u^*(\cdot)$ is discontinuous. Moreover (4.56b) and (4.56c) prove that with $c_1, c_2 \in \mathbb{R}$

$$\mathcal{H}_u \equiv c_1 \tag{4.57a}$$
$$f - \dot{x} \equiv c_2, \tag{4.57b}$$

these terms are constant on the interval $[0, T]$.

Next we consider the transversality condition (4.48a)

$$\tilde{g}_{\dot{y}}(y(T), \dot{y}(T), T) = 0,$$

which becomes in coordinate form

$$\begin{aligned} &\lambda(T) = 0 \\ &\mathcal{H}_u(x(T), u(T), \lambda(T), T) = 0 \\ &f(x(T), u(T), T) - \dot{x}(T) = 0. \end{aligned} \tag{4.58}$$

This finally proves the transversality condition (4.58) of the optimal control problem together with $c_1 = c_2 = 0$. Therefore we find the local Maximum Principle be satisfied as

$$\mathcal{H}_u(x(t), u(t), t) = 0, \quad \text{for all} \quad t \in [0, T],$$

and retrieve the state dynamics

$$\dot{x}(t) = f(x(t), u(t), t), \quad \text{for all} \quad t \in [0, T].$$

In a last step we analyze the function $\mathbb{H}$, yielding

$$\begin{aligned} \mathbb{H} &= g + \lambda(f - \dot{x}) + \dot{x}\lambda - u(g_u + \lambda f_u) - \lambda(f - \dot{x}) \\ &= g + \lambda f = \mathcal{H}. \end{aligned} \tag{4.59}$$

From the second Weierstrass–Erdmann condition we find

$$\mathbb{H}(y^*(\tilde{t}), \dot{y}^*(\tilde{t}^-), \tilde{t}) = \mathbb{H}(y^*(\tilde{t}), \dot{y}^*(\tilde{t}^+), \tilde{t})$$

and using (4.59) this yields

$$\mathcal{H}(\tilde{t}^-) = \mathcal{H}(\tilde{t}^+),$$

and therefore the continuity of the Hamiltonian for every t, which concludes the local Maximum Principle.

Remark 4.37. The critical part of the proof is the assumption on the costate $\lambda(\cdot)$, since in the definition (4.51) we assumed that $\lambda(\cdot)$ is integrable, which cannot a priori be assumed. In a general framework using results from functional analysis it can at least be proved that $\lambda(\cdot)$ is a function of bounded variation and that the corresponding Lagrangian does therefore exist in the Riemann–Stieltjes sense.

Remark 4.38 (Needle Variations). To derive not only the local Maximum Principle but the usual global Maximum Principle a different type of variations has to be considered. For the previous proof we considered variations $\varepsilon\delta u(\cdot)$, which converge to zero in the maximum norm, i.e., $\lim_{\varepsilon\to 0}\max\varepsilon\|\delta u(\cdot)\| = 0$. In Pontryagin, Boltyanski, Gamkrelidze, and Mishchenko (1962) so-called *needle variations* $\delta u_N(\cdot)$ (see Fig. 4.9) were used, which converge to zero in the integral norm, i.e.,

$$\lim_{\varepsilon\to 0}\varepsilon\int_0^T \|\delta u_N(t)\|\,\mathrm{d}t = 0$$

but not necessarily in the maximum norm.

Next we introduce mixed path and pure state constraints for the previously given optimal control problem and derive necessary corner conditions.

4.4.2 Necessary Conditions at Junction Points

For the definition of the terms used in this subsection the reader is referred to Sect. 3.6. In this section we concentrate on the derivation of the necessary conditions at a junction time $\tilde{t}$. In case of mixed path constraints the necessary optimality conditions at the junction time $\tilde{t}$ reduce to:

$$\lambda(\tilde{t}^+) = \lambda(\tilde{t}^-) \tag{4.60a}$$
$$\mathcal{H}(\tilde{t}^+) = \mathcal{H}(\tilde{t}^-), \tag{4.60b}$$

which simply states the continuity of the costate and Hamiltonian, whereas for pure state constraints $h(x,t)$ the following conditions have to be satisfied:

$$\lambda(\tilde{t}^+) = \lambda(\tilde{t}^-) - \eta(\tilde{t})h_x(x(\tilde{t}),\tilde{t}) \tag{4.61a}$$
$$\mathcal{H}(\tilde{t}^+) = \mathcal{H}(\tilde{t}^-) + \eta(\tilde{t})h_t(x(\tilde{t}),\tilde{t}) \tag{4.61b}$$
$$\eta(\tilde{t}) \geq 0. \tag{4.61c}$$

These conditions are called the *corner conditions*, which correspond to the *Weierstrass–Erdmann conditions* from the calculus of variations.

Using variational principles we derive the corner conditions and explain the differences between the case of mixed path constraints (4.60) and that of pure state constraints (4.61). For notational simplicity we consider a system with only one state and one control.

Derivation of the Corner Conditions

To analyze necessary optimality conditions in the case of mixed path or pure state constraints at a junction time $\tilde{t}$ we use the same definitions as in Sect. 4.4.1, where we derived the necessary conditions without any path

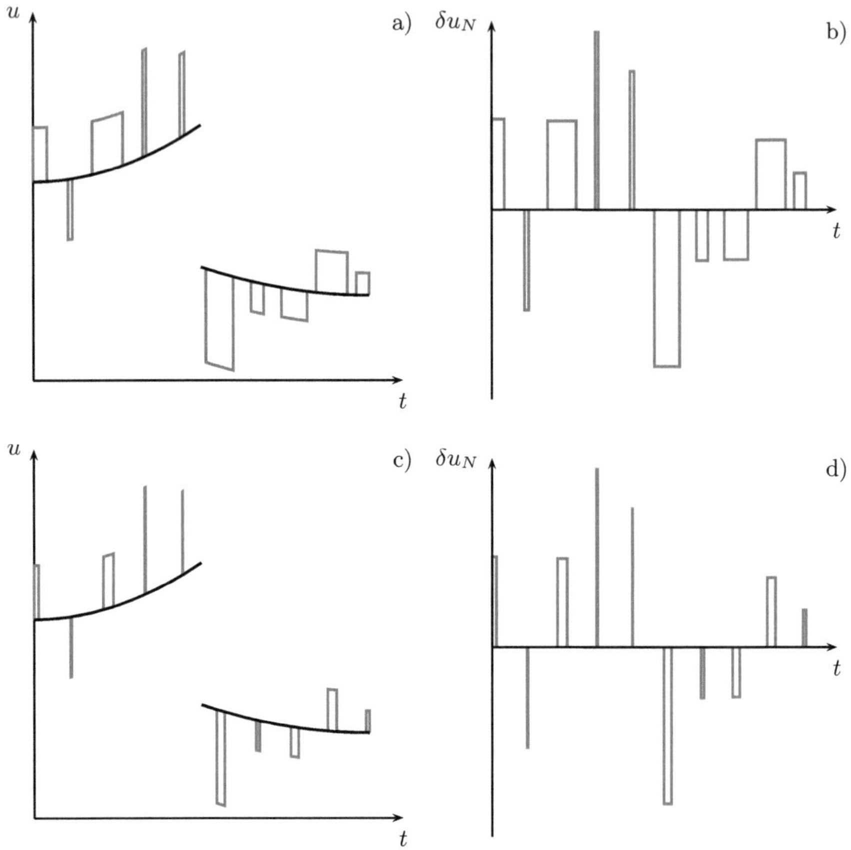

Fig. 4.9. In (**a**) the control path $u(\cdot)$ together with varied control $u(\cdot)+\delta u_N(\cdot,\varepsilon)$ is illustrated, where the needle variation $\delta(\cdot,\varepsilon)$ is shown in (**b**). In the panels (**c**) and (**d**) the situation is captured for a smaller ε, where the change in the control values are the same, but the support of the variation δu_N is smaller. This illustrates the origin of the name *needle variation* in a vivid manner

constraints. Therefore we first repeat the proof of the Weierstrass–Erdmann conditions (see p. 219) for the optimal control problem to the point, where it is derived that the variation have to be zero at the varied time $\delta\tilde{t}$ and the varied state $\delta\tilde{x}$ at $\tilde{t}$. Inspecting this argument carefully we shall see that this can only be done under the assumption that with admissible variations $\delta\tilde{t}$ and $\delta\tilde{x}$ also the negative variations are admissible, which is obvious if there are no further restrictions on these variations. But in our case the mixed path and pure state constraints restrict the set of admissible variations and we therefore carefully inspect the subsequent proof for mixed path and pure state constraints, separately.

Thus let us start considering the value function, defined as

$$\mathbb{L} := \int_0^T \tilde{g}(x, \dot{x}, \dot{v}, \dot{\rho}, t)\mathrm{d}t$$
$$:= \int_0^T \left(g(x(t), \dot{v}(t), t) + \dot{\rho}(t)\left(f(x(t), \dot{v}(t), t) - \dot{x}(t)\right)\right) \mathrm{d}t,$$

with

$$y := (x, v, \rho), \quad \text{and} \quad \mathbb{H}(y, \dot{y}, t) := \tilde{g}(y, \dot{y}, t) - \dot{y}\tilde{g}_{\dot{y}}(y, \dot{y}, t).$$

Then the reader may check that for the new variables we derive

$$\delta\mathbb{L}(\delta\tilde{y}, \delta\tilde{t}) = \left(\tilde{g}_{\dot{y}}(\tilde{t}^-) - \tilde{g}_{\dot{y}}(\tilde{t}^+)\right)\delta\tilde{y}$$
$$+ \left(\tilde{g}(\tilde{t}^-) - \tilde{g}_{\dot{y}}(\tilde{t}^-)\dot{y}^*(\tilde{t}^-) - g(\tilde{t}^+) + \tilde{g}_{\dot{y}}(\tilde{t}^+)\dot{y}^*(\tilde{t}^+)\right)\delta\tilde{t}.$$

This is equal to (4.47) where we only considered the terms containing variations at the time $\tilde{t}$.

Using the results of the proof of the local Maximum Principle in the previous subsection we finally find

$$\delta\mathbb{L}(\delta\tilde{x}, \delta\tilde{t}) = \left(\mathcal{H}(\tilde{t}^-) - \mathcal{H}(\tilde{t}^+)\right)\delta\tilde{t} + \left(\lambda(\tilde{t}^+) - \lambda(\tilde{t}^-)\right)\delta\tilde{x}, \tag{4.62}$$

where $\delta\tilde{x}$ and $\delta\tilde{t}$ denote the variations of the state and time at $\tilde{t}$. Then by the first part of Theorem 4.32 the necessary optimality condition becomes

$$\left(\mathcal{H}(\tilde{t}^-) - \mathcal{H}(\tilde{t}^+)\right)\delta\tilde{t} + \left(\lambda(\tilde{t}^+) - \lambda(\tilde{t}^-)\right)\delta\tilde{x} \leq 0. \tag{4.63}$$

At this point only the inequality in (4.63) can be assured since it is not guaranteed that with admissible variations $(\delta\tilde{x}, \delta\tilde{t})$ also $(-\delta\tilde{x}, -\delta\tilde{t})$ are admissible. This is caused by the fact that the constraints pose further restrictions on the variations $\delta\tilde{x}$, $\delta\tilde{u}$ and, $\delta\tilde{t}$ which we shall subsequently analyze. This analysis brings forward the principal differences between mixed path and pure state constraints and will therefore be presented separately (cf. McIntyre & Paiewonsky, 1967).

Mixed Constraint

In the case of the mixed path constraints the variations at $\tilde{t}$ have to satisfy

$$c(x^*(\tilde{t}) + \varepsilon\delta\tilde{x}, u^*(\tilde{t}) + \varepsilon\delta\tilde{u}, \tilde{t} + \varepsilon\delta\tilde{t}) \geq 0$$

for every $\varepsilon \geq 0$ small enough with $c(x^*(\tilde{t}), u^*(\tilde{t}), \tilde{t}) = 0$. Thus using the Taylor theorem, we find the inequality

$$0 \leq c(x^*(\tilde{t}) + \varepsilon\delta\tilde{x}, u^*(\tilde{t}) + \varepsilon\delta\tilde{u}, \tilde{t} + \varepsilon\delta\tilde{t})$$
$$= c_x(x^*(\tilde{t}), u^*(\tilde{t}), \tilde{t})\varepsilon\delta\tilde{x} + c_u(x^*(\tilde{t}), u^*(\tilde{t}), \tilde{t})\varepsilon\delta\tilde{u} + c_t(x^*(\tilde{t}), u^*(\tilde{t}), \tilde{t})\varepsilon\delta\tilde{t} + o(\varepsilon).$$

Dividing now by $\varepsilon > 0$ and letting ε converge to zero finally yield further restrictions on $\delta\tilde{x}$, $\delta\tilde{u}$ and $\delta\tilde{t}$ given by

$$c_x(x^*(\tilde{t}), u^*(\tilde{t}), \tilde{t})\delta\tilde{x} + c_u(x^*(\tilde{t}), u^*(\tilde{t}), \tilde{t})\delta\tilde{u} + c_t(x^*(\tilde{t}), u^*(\tilde{t}), \tilde{t})\delta\tilde{t} \geq 0. \quad (4.64)$$

Thus every admissible variation $(\delta\tilde{x}, \delta\tilde{t})$ has to satisfy (4.64), which can be rewritten as

$$c_x(x^*(\tilde{t}), u^*(\tilde{t}), \tilde{t})\delta\tilde{x} + c_t(x^*(\tilde{t}), u^*(\tilde{t}), \tilde{t})\delta\tilde{t} \geq -c_u(x^*(\tilde{t}), u^*(\tilde{t}), \tilde{t})\delta\tilde{u}. \quad (4.65)$$

Let us assume that $(\delta\tilde{x}, \delta\tilde{u}, \delta\tilde{t})$ satisfy (4.65). Since the constraint qualification $c_u(x^*(\tilde{t}), u^*(\tilde{t}), \tilde{t}) \neq 0$ holds we find $\delta\tilde{u}_2$ such that (4.65) is satisfied for $(-\delta\tilde{x}, \delta\tilde{u}_2, -\delta\tilde{t})$. This implies that the inequality of (4.63) can be replaced by the equality sign and each of the terms has to be zero, i.e.,

$$\mathcal{H}(\tilde{t}^-) - \mathcal{H}(\tilde{t}^+) = 0, \quad \lambda(\tilde{t}^+) - \lambda(\tilde{t}^-) = 0.$$

This proves that for mixed path constraints, given that the constraint qualification is satisfied, the costate λ and the Hamiltonian $\mathcal{H}$ are continuous at the junction time $\tilde{t}$ (see Seierstad and Sydsaeter 1986, p. 278 for an example, in which the constraint qualification fails).

Remark 4.39. Intuitively this proves that in the case of mixed path constraints the decision-maker has freedom enough in choosing the control to adjust the system smoothly from an unconstrained to a constrained state or vice versa.

Pure State Constraint

Next, we analyze the case of pure state constraints $h(x^*(t), t) \geq 0$. Analogously to the mixed path constraints this imposes the following restrictions on the variations $\delta\tilde{x}$ and $\delta\tilde{t}$ at $\tilde{t}$

$$h_x(x^*(\tilde{t}), \tilde{t})\delta\tilde{x} + h_t(x^*(\tilde{t}), \tilde{t})\delta\tilde{t} \geq 0. \quad (4.66)$$

Obviously with variations $(\delta\tilde{x}, \delta\tilde{t}) \neq 0$ satisfying (4.66) the negative variations $(-\delta\tilde{x}, -\delta\tilde{t})$ do not satisfy (4.66) and therefore equality in (4.63) cannot be guaranteed. Rewriting (4.66) and (4.63) in vector notation implies that

$$\text{for any} \quad \begin{pmatrix} \delta\tilde{x} \\ \delta\tilde{t} \end{pmatrix} \quad \text{satisfying} \quad (\delta\tilde{x}, \delta\tilde{t}) \begin{pmatrix} h_x(x^*(\tilde{t}), \tilde{t}) \\ h_t(x^*(\tilde{t}), \tilde{t}) \end{pmatrix} \geq 0$$

also

$$(\delta\tilde{x}, \delta\tilde{t}) \begin{pmatrix} \lambda(\tilde{t}^-) - \lambda(\tilde{t}^+) \\ \mathcal{H}(\tilde{t}^+) - \mathcal{H}(\tilde{t}^-) \end{pmatrix} \geq 0$$

has to hold. This implication is fundamentally the second statement of the Farkas lemma (Theorem A.36) and it can therefore be concluded that there exists $\eta \geq 0$ such that

$$\begin{pmatrix} h_x(x^*(\tilde{t}), \tilde{t}) \\ h_t(x^*(\tilde{t}), \tilde{t}) \end{pmatrix} \eta = \begin{pmatrix} \lambda(\tilde{t}^-) - \lambda(\tilde{t}^+) \\ \mathcal{H}(\tilde{t}^+) - \mathcal{H}(\tilde{t}^-) \end{pmatrix}.$$

But these last identities are exactly the corner conditions (4.61), concluding the proof.

Remark 4.40. Contrary to the case of mixed path constraints, in this case the decision-maker cannot influence the system directly by choosing the control to adjust the system smoothly from an unconstrained to a constrained state or vice versa.

Exercises

4.1. Solve the problem

$$\begin{aligned} &\min_{(x,y)} x^2 + y^2 + 3xy + 6x + 19y \\ \text{s.t.} \quad &3y + x = 5. \end{aligned}$$

4.2. Consider the problem

$$\begin{aligned} &\min_{(x,y)} \frac{1}{2}\alpha (x-1)^2 - x - y \\ \text{s.t.} \quad &x \geq y^2 \\ &x^2 + y^2 \leq 1. \end{aligned}$$

Find the region of α where the extremal point satisfies the Karush–Kuhn–Tucker conditions. Draw the contour lines of the objective function and the constraints to interpret the influence of the parameter α.

4.3. Consider the problem

$$\begin{aligned} &\min_{(x,y)} x^2 + y^2 \\ \text{s.t.} \quad &(x-1)^3 - y^2 \geq 0. \end{aligned}$$

Try to find the extremals of this problem. What problem arises? Draw the admissible region to clarify the problem. Does a point exist satisfying the Fritz John conditions?

4.4. Given the problem

$$\begin{aligned} &\max_{(x_1,\dots,x_n)} \sum_{i=1}^{n} \frac{c_i}{x_i} \\ \text{s.t.} \quad &\sum_{i=1}^{n} a_i x_i = b \\ &x_i \geq 0, \quad i = 1,\dots,n, \end{aligned}$$

with $a_i, c_i \geq 0$, $i = 1,\dots,n$, show that the maximum of the objective function

$$g^* = \frac{1}{b}\left(\sum_{i=1}^{n} \sqrt{c_i a_i}\right)^2.$$

Hint. Consider $\sum_{i=1}^{n} x_i \mathcal{L}_{x_i} = 0$, *where* $\mathcal{L}$ *is the Lagrangian.*

4.5. Given the problem

$$\begin{aligned} &\max_{(x,y)} 4x + 2y \\ \text{s.t.}\quad & x\log(x) - x + 1 \geq 0 \\ & x \geq 0 \\ & 3x - 2y^2 \geq 1. \end{aligned}$$

Show that there exists no point $(\tilde{x}, \tilde{y})$ satisfying the Karush–Kuhn–Tucker conditions. Why is that so? Does there exist a point satisfying the conditions of the weak Lagrange–Karush–Kuhn–Tucker theorem without rank condition?

Hint. Consider the assumption of Lagrange–Karush–Kuhn–Tucker theorem.

4.6. Prove that the constraint qualification stated in Lemma 4.9 is equivalent to the full rank of (4.11).

4.7 (Homogeneity). Prove that the first variation is homogeneous of the first degree, i.e., for $\mu \in \mathbb{R}$

$$\delta G(X^*, \mu\delta S) = \mu\delta G(X^*, \delta S).$$

Hint. Consider the definition of the first variation

$$\delta G(X^*, \mu\delta S) = \frac{\mathrm{d}}{\mathrm{d}\varepsilon} G\left(X^* + h\mu\delta S\right)\big|_{\varepsilon=0^+}.$$

4.8 (Beltrami Identity). Prove the *Beltrami identity*

$$-\dot{x}(t) + \frac{\mathrm{d}}{\mathrm{d}t}\left(g(t) - \dot{x}(t)g_{\dot{x}}(t)\right) = 0.$$

Hint. Consider the total time derivative

$$\frac{\mathrm{d}}{\mathrm{d}t} g(x, \dot{x}, t) = \dot{x}(t)g_x(t) + \ddot{x}(t)g_{\dot{x}}(t) + g_t(t),$$

together with the Euler equation.

4.9 (Brachistochrone Problem). Geometrically the brachistochrone (shortest time) problem corresponds to finding the shape of a (differentiable) curve joining two points in the plane $P_a(a, 0)$ and $P_b(b, y_b)$, with $a \neq b$ and $y_b \neq 0$, along which a mass point under the influence of gravity moves frictionlessly from P_a to P_b in the shortest possible time.

Formally this problem becomes

$$\begin{aligned} &\min_{y(\cdot)} \int_a^b \sqrt{\frac{1 + y'(x)}{2gy(x)}}\,\mathrm{d}x \\ \text{s.t.}\quad & y(a) = 0, \quad y(b) = y_b, \end{aligned}$$

where g is the gravitational constant. Find all extremals of the brachistochrone problem.

Hint. Since $f(y, y', x)$ does not explicitly depend on x, one can use the Beltrami identity in the form $f - y'f_{y'} = C$, where C is some constant, instead of the full Euler equation.

4.10 (Brachistochrone Problem with Friction). Consider the same problem formulation as in Exercise 4.9 but with kinetic friction included. Then the problem becomes

$$\min_{y(\cdot)} \int_a^b \sqrt{\frac{1+y'(x)}{2gy(x)-\mu x}}\,\mathrm{d}x$$
$$\text{s.t.}\quad y(a)=0,\quad y(b)=y_b,$$

where μ is the friction constant. Solve the problem using the Euler equation.

4.11. Formulate the following optimal control problem as a problem of the calculus of variations:

$$\max_{u(\cdot)} x_0(T)$$
$$\text{s.t.}\quad \dot{x}_0 = \left(1-u^2\right)^2$$
$$\dot{x}_1 = u,$$
$$\dot{x}_2 = 1,$$
$$x_0(0)=x_1(0)=x_2(0)=0,\quad x_1(T)=x_2(T)=1.$$

Solve the problem under the restriction $|u| \le 1/2$.

Hint. Set $x_2 = \tau$, where τ can be interpreted as a new time variable.

4.12 (Regularity Assumption). Prove that if $x^*(\cdot)$ is an optimal solution of the problem (4.36) with a kink at $0 < \tilde{t} < T$ and satisfying the regularity assumption (4.38); then $x^*(\cdot)$ is two times continuously differentiable on each of the intervals $[0,\tilde{t}]$ and $[\tilde{t},T]$.

Hint. Show that with $\delta x(\cdot) \in C^1([0,\tilde{t}])$

$$\int_0^{\tilde{t}} g\delta x - g_{\dot{x}}\dot{\delta x}\,\mathrm{d}t = 0,$$

then use the Dubois–Reymond lemma (Lemma A.140) to show that $g_{\dot{x}}$ is continuously differentiable with respect to the time. Finally consider the total time derivative

$$\frac{\mathrm{d}}{\mathrm{d}t}g_{\dot{x}} = g_{\dot{x}t} + g_{\dot{x}x}\dot{x} + g_{\dot{x}\dot{x}}\ddot{x}$$

to conclude the proof. Repeat the argumentation for the interval $[\tilde{t},T]$.

4.13 (Transversality Condition). Prove that for problem (4.37) with free terminal time the following transversality conditions have to hold

$$g_{\dot{x}}(x(T),\dot{x}(T),T) = 0$$
$$g(x(T),\dot{x}(T),T) - \dot{x}(T)g_{\dot{x}}(x(T),\dot{x}(T),T) = 0.$$

Hint. Use the time transformation

$$\tau(t,\varepsilon) := \frac{t}{T+\varepsilon\delta T}T,\quad 0 \le t \le T+\varepsilon\delta T$$

and the varied path

$$y(\tau(t,\varepsilon)) := x^*(\tau(t,\varepsilon)) + \varepsilon\delta x(\tau(t,\varepsilon)).$$

Then consider the first variation

$$\frac{\mathrm{d}}{\mathrm{d}\varepsilon}\int_0^{T+\varepsilon\delta T} g(x(\tau(t,\varepsilon)),\dot{x}(\tau(t,\varepsilon)),t)\,\mathrm{d}t\bigg|_{\varepsilon=0^+}$$

and follow the lead of the proof on p. 219.

Notes and Further Reading

In this chapter we had to handle the trade-off between presenting the theory of optimization intuitively enough to give the reader an insight into the underlying principles, but also rigorously enough to avoid making the use of mathematics a farce. What this approach lacks in "exactness" from a mathematical point of view is hopefully compensated for by the concentration on the basic concepts of the Maximum Principle and its contribution to intuitive understanding. By the way, it is not the mathematical formalism as such that complicates things, but rather the problem of investing these formal terms with meaningful content. The mathematical notation, if it is well adapted to the problem, helps to present results compactly and clearly. But to use this formal language in an efficient and helpful way it is necessary to understand the underlying concepts, and it was the aim of this chapter to provide the reader with these concepts and to enable him or her to work with and apply the derived formulas of optimal control theory.

There exists a huge range of literature on finite-dimensional optimization. Selecting three that are representative of many others for the presentation of the theory of nonlinear optimization, we relied on the presentations given in Avriel (1976); Fletcher (1987), and Léonard and Long (1992). For the original proof of the Fritz John necessary conditions under equality and inequality constraints, we refer the reader to Mangasarian and Fromovitz (1967).

The classical references for the presentation of the theory of optimization in a general setting are Ioffe and Tichomirov (1979) and Neustadt (1976), but the reader should be alerted that their approach needs a rather well-founded knowledge of mathematical concepts. The reader who is interested in general results from optimization is referred to Halkin and Neustadt (1966), which can be downloaded for free as a reprint.

For an enhanced presentation of the Fritz John conditions and a general interpretation of the Lagrange multipliers, even in the case where multiple multipliers exist or the value function is nondifferentiable see Bertsekas, Ozdaglar, and Tseng (2006) and Penot (1997).

The question of differentiability of the value function is discussed within a very general framework in Penot (2004).

Cesari (1983) bridges the gap between the calculus of variations and optimal control theory. For an excellent exposition of the connection and differences between the calculus of variations and optimal control theory from a historical point of view, see Sussmann and Willems (1997, 2002) and Dreyfus (1965). In Girsanov (1972) the classical problems of optimization, "mathematical nonlinear programming," "calculus of variations" and "optimal control theory" are studied in the framework of the general Dubovitsky–Miljutin theory (Dubovickii & Miljutin, 1965).

The techniques needed to derive the principles of the theory of the calculus of variations can be found, e.g., in the classical textbooks by Bliss (1946) and Sagan (1969). The German speaking reader we refer to the excellently written lecture note on the calculus of variations in Oberle (2006). Variational principles are also the backbone of the classical reference of the Maximum Principle by Pontryagin et al. (1962). In contrast to this original approach, we profited from the presentation in Canon, Cullum, and Polak (1970), where the theory of optimal control was presented as a mathematical programming problem. It is a mathematically rigorous exposition, and its direct comparison of the discrete- and continuous-time Maximum Principle warns one of the difficulty of trying to prove the continuous case via the discrete problem in an exact way.

5

Multiple Equilibria, Points of Indifference, and Thresholds

This chapter addresses the interesting and important topics of multiplicity and history-dependence of optimal solutions. Multiplicity means that for given initial states there exist multiple optimal solutions; thus the decision-maker is indifferent about which to chose. This explains why such initial states are called points of indifference. In contrast, history-dependence occurs when the optimal solution depends on the problem's temporal history.

The existence of multiple equilibria has been long-recognized in physics, and more recently has provided an important enrichment of economic control models. In policy-making, it may be crucial to recognize whether or not a given problem has multiple stable optimal equilibria and, if so, to locate the thresholds separating the basins of attraction surrounding these different equilibria. At such a threshold different optimal courses of actions are separated. Thus, in general, starting at a threshold, a rational economic agent is indifferent between moving toward one or the other equilibrium. Small movements away from the threshold can destroy the indifference and motivate a unique optimal course of action. Among the economic consequences of such an unstable threshold is history-dependence (also denoted as path-dependence): the optimal long-run stationary solution toward which an optimally controlled system converges can depend on the initial conditions.

In the following section we present general results on discounted, autonomous problems, which are applied to a typical problem in the subsequent section. Here multiplicity and history-dependence are explained by means of a simple one-state model that already exhibits many of the interesting features connected to indifference points. In the next section we introduce a definition of multiplicity and history-dependence for optimal control problems with an arbitrary number of states.

Therefore we are mainly concerned with discounted, autonomous models over an infinite time horizon (DAM), already introduced as:

$$\max_{u(\cdot)} \int_0^\infty e^{-rt} g(x(t), u(t))\, dt \tag{5.1a}$$

$$\text{s.t.} \quad \dot{x}(t) = f(x(t), u(t)) \tag{5.1b}$$

$$x(0) = x_0, \tag{5.1c}$$

where f and g are assumed to be continuously differentiable with respect to their arguments. Both functions do not depend on time t and for any admissible solution $(x(\cdot), u(\cdot))$ the integral (5.1a) shall converge.

5.1 Occurrence of Multiple Equilibria

Multiple equilibria and history-dependent optimal solutions are important in diverse economic models and are typically related to the presence of market imperfections, expectations, and the like. Skiba (1978) and Dechert and Nishimura (1983) explored these points of indifference for the first time when they considered a special class of economic models formulated as optimal control problems, namely the one-sector problem of optimal growth with a nonconvex production function. Singular models with multiple optimal solutions had already been analyzed by Sethi (1977, 1979a). In recognition of the studies by Sethi, Skiba, Dechert, and Nishimura, these points of indifference are denoted as *DNSS (Dechert–Nishimura–Sethi–Skiba)* or *Skiba points*.

In this book we show that DNSS points can also arise in efficient deterministic dynamic optimization models, and we explore various mechanisms that may generate multiple optimal equilibria. While most of the existing literature refers to one-dimensional state space models, we also present examples of two-dimensional optimal control problems exhibiting DNSS curves.

The following analysis covers all these cases of multiple equilibria and threshold behavior, for the special class of discounted, autonomous models over an infinite time horizon. The focus on infinite time horizon models is not a serious restriction, moreover it is the natural class of models, for which the notion of history-dependence and long-run optimal behavior only makes sense. Otherwise it is trivial, since in general the optimal transient behavior will necessarily differ for different initial states.

For these optimal control models Proposition 3.83 stated that saddle point stability[1] is the "most stable" behavior of the long-run equilibrium solutions. While stability of the equilibria of the canonical system can be excluded, with a discount rate $r > 0$, unstable equilibria may occur.[2]

Multiple long-run equilibria exist if the phase portrait of the canonical system exhibits that the isoclines have more than one intersection. According

[1] Saddle point stability concerns the canonical system in the state–costate space, which corresponds to stability in the optimized dynamical system.

[2] The possibility of instability was observed in one of the earliest economic applications of optimal control contributed by Kurz (1968).

to the continuity of the vector field, the quality of neighboring equilibria cannot be the same (see, e.g., Wagener, 2003). This implies that in such a case unstable equilibria occur.

We start with a short introduction to important aspects of the optimal vector field and multiple optimal solutions, emphasizing optimal control problems of infinite time horizon.

5.2 The Optimal Vector Field

In optimal control theory, especially as applied in the economic literature, it has become common to concentrate on the canonical system and to describe the optimal paths as solution trajectories of this $2n$-dimensional system. This approach is appealing because the costate has an immediate economic interpretation as a shadow price. Nevertheless, it causes some terminology, such as saddle point stability (see Remark 2.49), to collide with the terminology of dynamical systems, wherein a saddle point is by definition unstable. Shifting the perspective to the optimal vector field may improve understanding and avoid terminological vagueness.

In the subsequent subsections we introduce the concept of an optimal state dynamics, shedding light on the process of determining the optimal solution. As will be seen, the optimal state dynamics for a discounted, autonomous infinite time horizon problem becomes itself an autonomous vector field, making it accessible to the theory of dynamical systems. Moreover, since by Pontryagin's Maximum Principle the optimal solution corresponds to a solution of the canonical system, we shall find the rule for choosing the corresponding optimal initial costate (the *optimal costate rule*) that proves useful to describe a possible indifference point. For working out the difference between models over a finite and infinite time horizon we start with a simple example, letting us determine the important concepts analytically.

5.2.1 Finite vs. Infinite Time Horizon Models

To illustrate the difference in the description of the optimal state dynamics we start with the following model:

$$\max_{u(\cdot)} \int_0^T \mathrm{e}^{-rt}\left(-x(t)^2 - cu(t)^2\right) \mathrm{d}t \tag{5.2a}$$

$$\text{s.t.} \quad \dot{x}(t) = x(t) + u(t) \tag{5.2b}$$

$$x(t) \geq 0, \quad t \geq 0 \tag{5.2c}$$

where $r \geq 0$ is the discount rate and x is the stock of some bad such as the number of drug users, corrupt officials or terrorists, or even the level of pollution in an environmental engineering context. The control u is some activity affecting the stock. Since there is no restriction on the control values, it can in principle have either an exacerbating or an abating effect. As will be seen, applying the control only as an abatement will be optimal. The costs, interpreted as negative utility, are taken to be quadratic in the state as well as in the control.

Using Pontryagin's Maximum Principle we have to consider the Hamiltonian

$$\mathcal{H}(x, u, \lambda) = -x^2 - cu^2 + \lambda\,(x + u)\,.$$

(In Exercise 5.3.5.3 the reader may prove that the problem is also normal, i.e., $\lambda_0 = 1$, for an infinite time horizon.)

The Hamiltonian is strictly concave in u

$$\mathcal{H}_{uu}(x, u, \lambda) = -2c < 0,$$

yielding a unique optimal control value u^* with

$$u^* = \frac{\lambda}{2c}. \tag{5.3}$$

Pasting this value for u yields the corresponding canonical system

$$\dot{x} = x + \frac{1}{2c}\lambda \tag{5.4a}$$

$$\dot{\lambda} = \lambda\,(r - 1) + 2x. \tag{5.4b}$$

Lastly, the transversality condition

$$\lambda(T) = 0 \tag{5.5}$$

provides a further necessary condition. Moreover the Hamiltonian is jointly strictly concave in x and u for all λ and therefore the necessary conditions are also sufficient (see Theorem 3.29).

To work out the correspondence between the occurrence of multiple optimal solutions and the existence of multiple costate solutions $\lambda(\cdot)$ for the canonical system let us consider the dynamics (5.4a). Then the costate value $\lambda(t)$ at time t is replaced by an appropriate function $\mathcal{P}$, which, as will subsequently turn out, in general depends on time t, the initial state x_0 and the time horizon T. For an infinite time horizon this dependence of the function $\mathcal{P}$ will reduce only to a dependence on state $x(t)$ causing the optimal dynamics to be an autonomous ODE. Let us now start analyzing the canonical system (5.4).

As is illustrated in Fig. 5.1a there exists a whole range of solutions $x(\cdot), \lambda(\cdot)$ for the canonical system but only one trajectory (black curve) satisfies the transversality condition (5.5). This solution implicitly depends on the initial state x_0 as well as the time horizon T. Thus the corresponding costate value can be written as a function

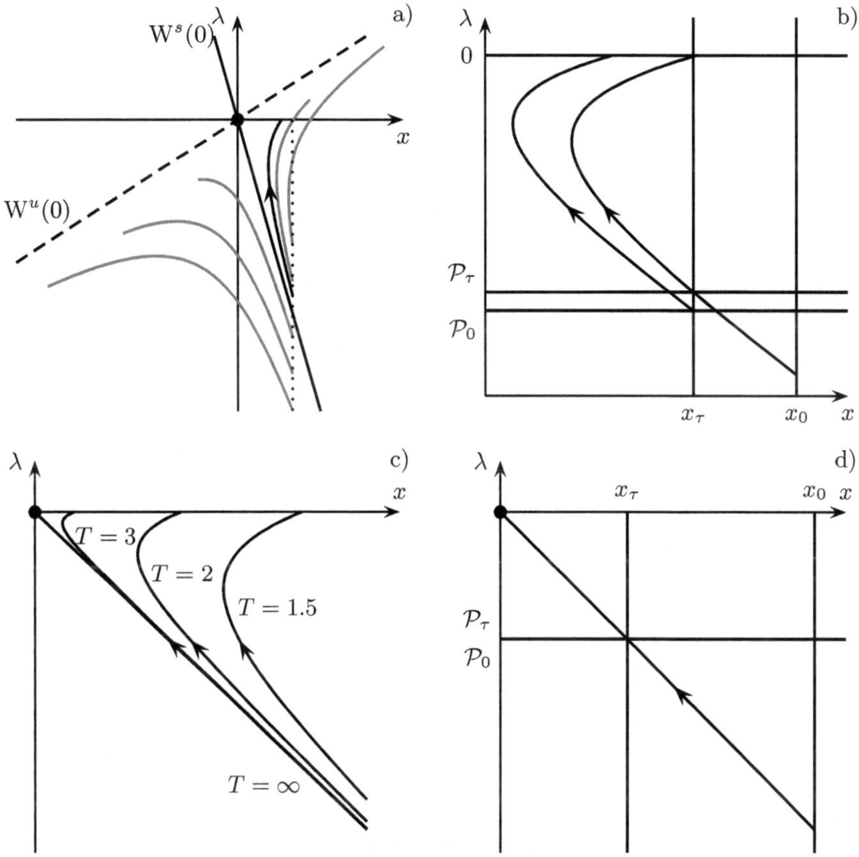

Fig. 5.1. Panel (**a**) depicts the phase portrait of the canonical system (5.4), where the *black curve* is the optimal solution for $T = 1$ starting at $x(0) = 1$. In panel (**b**) the solutions for the initial states 1 and 0.8 are displayed, revealing that $\mathcal{P}(x_0, \tau, 1) \neq \mathcal{P}(x_\tau, 0, 1)$, with $\mathcal{P}_0 = \mathcal{P}(x_\tau, 0, 1)$ and $\mathcal{P}_\tau = \mathcal{P}(x_0, \tau, 1)$. Panel (**c**) shows that for increasing T the optimal solution converges to the stable manifold. For $T = \infty$ panel (**d**) depicts that the optimal solution is time invariant exhibiting $\mathcal{P}(x_0, \tau, \infty) = \mathcal{P}(x_\tau, 0, \infty)$

$$\lambda(t) := \mathcal{P}(x_0, t, T) \tag{5.6}$$

yielding the optimal dynamics

$$\dot{x}(t) = x(t) + \frac{1}{2c}\mathcal{P}(x_0, t, T). \tag{5.7}$$

For a finite time horizon $T < \infty$ this is a nonautonomous ODE as is illustrated in Fig. 5.1b. Since for a time-shift τ the optimal solution starting at $x(0) = x^*(\tau)$ is different to the optimal trajectory $x^*(t)$, $t \in [\tau, T]$ of the primary problem. In terms of the function $\mathcal{P}$ this writes as $\mathcal{P}(x^*(\tau), 0, T) \neq \mathcal{P}(x_0, \tau, T)$.

Consider the model for an infinite time horizon $T = \infty$ the optimal solution is the unique trajectory starting at x_0 and converging to the equilibrium at the origin. This is depicted in Fig. 5.1c, where for an increasing time horizon T the optimal trajectory approaches the stable manifold $\mathrm{W}^s(0)$ and lying in the stable manifold for the infinite time horizon.

Next we derive an explicit representation of $\mathcal{P}(x_0, t, \infty)$. Therefore we note that owing to the linearity of the canonical system the stable manifold is analytically given. It is the line crossing the origin in direction of the eigenvector $\nu_s = (\nu_{1s}, \nu_{2s})'$ corresponding to the eigenvalue $\xi_s < 0$. To ease the formulas we choose the eigenvector with its first coordinate equal to one, i.e., $\nu_{1s} = 1$. Then the stable manifold is given by

$$\mathrm{W}^s(0) = \{(x, \lambda) : \lambda = x\nu_{2s},\ x \in \mathbb{R}\}.$$

Thus for $x(0) = x_0$ the state and costate trajectories exhibit the simple form

$$\begin{aligned} x^*(t) &= x_0 \mathrm{e}^{\xi_s t} \\ \lambda(t) &= \mathcal{P}(x_0, t, \infty) = \lambda(0)\mathrm{e}^{\xi_s t} \end{aligned}$$

with

$$\lambda(0) = x_0 \nu_{2s}.$$

Next we show that the explicit dependence of $\mathcal{P}(x_0, t, \infty)$ on time t can be replaced by only a dependence on the actual state $x(t)$. Therefore we consider the optimal trajectories for the problem starting at $x = x^*(\tau) = x_0 \mathrm{e}^{\xi_s \tau}$ (see Fig. 5.1d). Then we find the optimal costate as

$$\begin{aligned} \lambda(t) = \mathcal{P}(x(t), t, \infty) &= \nu_{s2} x(0)\mathrm{e}^{\xi_s t} \\ &= \nu_{s2} x_0 \mathrm{e}^{\xi_s \tau} \mathrm{e}^{\xi_s t} \\ &= \mathcal{P}(x_0, t + \tau, \infty). \end{aligned}$$

Setting $t = 0$ proves that the initial optimal costate only depends on the initial state x. Therefore we define the *optimal costate rule*

$$\mathrm{P}(x) := \mathcal{P}(x, 0, \infty).$$

Hence the optimal state dynamics for the infinite time horizon problem can be written as

$$\dot{x}(t) = x(t) + \frac{1}{2c}\mathrm{P}(x(t)), \tag{5.8}$$

which is an autonomous vector field, also called the *optimal vector field.*

This result is generally true for discounted, autonomous models over an infinite time horizon as will be proved in the next section.

5.2.2 Discounted Autonomous Models for an Infinite Time Horizon

Assume that $(x^*(\cdot), u^*(\cdot))$ is an optimal solution of *DAM* (5.1) with the initial condition $x(0) = x_0$. The following lemma shows that for these specific models the optimal costate rule is of a simpler form, since it will only depend on the actual state $x(t)$ and not on the time point t. Subsequently this property will be used to define the phenomenon of multiplicity and history-dependence:

Lemma 5.1. *The optimal solutions of* DAM *(5.1) are invariant under a positive time shift* τ.

Remark 5.2. This means that if one starts at some point of the optimal state trajectory $x^*(\cdot)$, i.e., for $\tau \geq 0$ we have $x(0) = x^*(\tau)$, the optimal solution is given by $(x^*(t), u^*(t))$ with $t \geq \tau$.

Naturally Lemma 5.1 is not satisfied for finite time problems, since in such cases $u^*(t)$ is given only on the interval $[0, T]$ and will not be defined on the interval $[\tau, T + \tau]$ for $\tau > 0$.

Proof. First, we introduce the functions

$$\begin{aligned} u_\tau(t) &:= u^*(t + \tau) \\ x_\tau(t) &:= x^*(t + \tau) \end{aligned}$$

and note that $x_\tau(\cdot)$ satisfies the state dynamics

$$\begin{aligned} \dot{x}(t) &= f\left(x(t), u_\tau^*(t)\right) \\ x_\tau(0) &= x^*(\tau). \end{aligned}$$

Next we show that the time shifted solution is optimal for the given initial state. Assume, to the contrary, that $(u^*(t+\tau), x^*(t+\tau))$ is not optimal; then there exists an admissible solution $(\tilde{u}(\cdot), \tilde{x}(\cdot))$ satisfying

$$\int_0^\infty \mathrm{e}^{-rt} g\left(\tilde{u}(t), \tilde{x}(t)\right) \mathrm{d}t > \int_0^\infty \mathrm{e}^{-rt} g\left(u^*(t+\tau), x^*(t+\tau)\right) \mathrm{d}t.$$

But this implies

$$\mathrm{e}^{-r\tau} \int_\tau^\infty \mathrm{e}^{-rt} g\left(\tilde{u}(t-\tau), \tilde{x}(t-\tau)\right) \mathrm{d}t > \mathrm{e}^{-r\tau} \int_\tau^\infty \mathrm{e}^{-rt} g\left(u^*(t), x^*(t)\right) \mathrm{d}t,$$

and therefore the solution $(u^*(\cdot), x^*(\cdot))$ could be improved on $[\tau, \infty]$, contradicting its optimality and finishing the proof. □

Denoting the set of optimal state trajectories emanating from x_0 as

$$\mathcal{S}(x_0) = \{x^*(\cdot) : \; x^*(0) = x_0\},$$

we define the *optimal costate rule*, in analogy to the previous section as

$$\mathrm{P}(x) = \{\lambda(0) : \lambda(\cdot) \text{ is a costate trajectory of } x^*(\cdot) \in \mathcal{S}(x_0)\} \subset \mathbb{R}^n.$$

Owing to the time invariance of the solution paths for problems *DAM* (5.1) the optimal state dynamics

$$\dot{x}(t) = \mathcal{H}_\lambda(x(t), \lambda(t))$$

can be written as

$$\dot{x}(t) = \mathcal{H}_\lambda(x(t), \mathrm{P}(x(t))).^3$$

Under appropriate regularity assumptions we will prove that $\mathrm{P}(x)$ is unique apart from the initial state $x(0)$, whereas $\mathrm{P}(x(0))$ may be multivalued. In that case one can choose one of these costates and consider the corresponding uniquely given autonomous ODE. The corresponding vector field is then called the *optimal vector field* and is denoted by

$$\dot{x}(t) = f^*(x(t)) \tag{5.9a}$$

$$\text{s.t.} \quad x(0) = x_0. \tag{5.9b}$$

It is now justified to use the theory of autonomous dynamical systems to analyze (5.9). For this optimal vector field, stable equilibria may exist, given by the projections of the (optimal) equilibria of the canonical system into the state space.

Moreover, we are now able to define the so-called *asymptotic solution set* by

$$\mathcal{S}^\infty(x_0) = \{x(x_0, \infty) : x(\cdot) \in \mathcal{S}(x_0)\},$$

where $x(x_0, \infty)$ is the limit set (see Definition 2.21), corresponding to the state trajectory $x(\cdot)$.

5.3 A Typical Example

To illustrate these concepts we slightly change the state dynamics (5.2a) of the model presented in Sect. 5.2.1, i.e., we assume logistic increase of the state instead of exponential increase. Thus we end up with the following model:

$$\max_{u(\cdot)} \int_0^\infty \mathrm{e}^{-rt} \left(-x(t)^2 - cu(t)^2\right) \mathrm{d}t \tag{5.10a}$$

$$\text{s.t.} \quad \dot{x}(t) = x(t)(1 - x(t)) + u(t) \tag{5.10b}$$

$$x(t) \geq 0, \quad t \geq 0 \tag{5.10c}$$

where the interpretation of the state x and the control u are analogous to the model (5.2). To simplify calculations the cost parameter is fixed at $c = 3$ and

[3] Since the set $\mathrm{P}(x)$ can contain more than one element the above expression may not be defined in the usual sense but rather denote a so-called *differential inclusion*, where $\dot{x} \in f(x, t)$ and f is a multivalued function.

$r \geq 0$ is free. In Sect. 5.5 this restriction on c will be removed and the model is analyzed in the total of its parameter space (r, c). This model is typical inasmuch as it exhibits many of the characteristics of the models presented in this book. Thus the optimal solutions are equilibria of the canonical system and the (stable) paths converging to these equilibria. Furthermore the model is simple enough to analytically compute at least the equilibria and bifurcation points (curves).

Using Pontryagin's Maximum Principle yields the canonical system

$$\dot{x} = x(1-x) + \frac{1}{6}\lambda$$
$$\dot{\lambda} = \lambda\,(r + 2x - 1) + 2x,$$

together with the transversality condition

$$\lim_{t\to\infty} \mathrm{e}^{-rt}\lambda(t) = 0.$$

The main candidates for optimal solutions are the saddles of the canonical system and their stable manifolds. For the one-dimensional case other limit sets, such as limit cycles, are excluded. The transversality condition does not rule out the existence of a diverging optimal solution, as long as $\lambda(t)$ diverges more slowly than e^{rt}. We must therefore explicitly show that diverging paths are only suboptimal.

Let us first compute the equilibria and their stability properties.

5.3.1 Existence and Stability of the Equilibria

After some basic computations we find the explicit formulas for the equilibria $(\hat{x}, \hat{\lambda})$ as

	$\hat{x}$	$\hat{\lambda}$
E_1	0	0
E_2	$\frac{1}{4}(3-r+w)$	$\frac{3}{4}(r-1)(1+r-w)-1$
E_3	$\frac{1}{4}(3-r-w)$	$\frac{3}{4}(r-1)(1+r+w)-1$

with $w = \sqrt{(r+1)^2 - 8/3}$.

Next, we have to determine the regions of existence for these three equilibria. The equilibrium at the origin $(0,0)$ exists for every r. In contrast $E_{2,3}$ only exist if w is a real number, i.e., if the radicand is positive, meaning

$$(r+1)^2 - \frac{8}{3} \geq 0 \quad \text{implying} \quad r \geq \frac{2}{3}\sqrt{6} - 1.$$

In the following we abbreviate the minimum value of r, for which the equilibria $E_{2,3}$ exist, as

$$r_0 := \frac{2}{3}\sqrt{6} - 1.$$

Since the state also has to be positive, i.e., $\hat{x} \geq 0$,

$$3 - r + w \geq 0 \quad \text{and} \quad 3 - r - w \geq 0$$

have to be satisfied too. A short calculation proves that in the first case $\hat{x} \geq 0$ holds true for all $r \geq 0$, whereas in the latter case $0 \leq r \leq 4/3$ is a necessary condition.

Finally, we determine the stability properties of the equilibria, which are characterized by the corresponding Jacobian matrix $\hat{J}$ (see Sect. 2.6.2)

$$\hat{J} = \begin{pmatrix} \frac{\partial \dot{x}}{\partial x} & \frac{\partial \dot{x}}{\partial \lambda} \\ \frac{\partial \dot{\lambda}}{\partial x} & \frac{\partial \dot{\lambda}}{\partial \lambda} \end{pmatrix} = \begin{pmatrix} 1 - 2\hat{x} & \frac{1}{6} \\ 2(\hat{\lambda} + 1) & r - 1 + 2\hat{x} \end{pmatrix}$$

the values of the trace

$$\tau = \operatorname{tr} \hat{J} = r,$$

the determinant

$$\Delta = \det \hat{J} = (1 - 2\hat{x})(r - 1 + 2\hat{x}) - \frac{1}{3}\left(\hat{\lambda} + 1\right),$$

and the discriminant

$$D = \tau^2 - 4\Delta = r^2 - 4(1 - 2\hat{x})(r - 1 + 2\hat{x}) + \frac{4}{3}\left(\hat{\lambda} + 1\right).$$

We next compute these values separately for each of the three equilibria.

The Origin E_1

Here the Jacobian matrix $\hat{J}$ reduces to

$$\hat{J} = \begin{pmatrix} 1 & \frac{1}{6} \\ 2 & r - 1 \end{pmatrix},$$

giving

$$\Delta = r - 1 - \frac{1}{3}$$

$$D = (r - 2)^2 + \frac{4}{3} > 0.$$

Hence for $r < 4/3$ the origin is a saddle, whereas for $r > 4/3$ it is an unstable node.

The Outer Equilibrium E_2

For E_2 the Jacobian matrix $\hat{J}$ becomes

$$\hat{J} = \begin{pmatrix} \frac{1}{2}(r-1-w) & \frac{1}{6} \\ \frac{3}{2}(r-1)(1+r-w) & \frac{1}{2}(r+1+w) \end{pmatrix},$$

together with

$$\Delta = \frac{1}{4}w(r-3-w).$$

Obviously $\Delta < 0$ for all $r < 3$ and hence for all r, for which the outer equilibrium exists. Therefore it is a saddle point.

The Inner Equilibrium E_3

Similarly to the last case, the Jacobian matrix $\hat{J}$ is given by

$$\hat{J} = \begin{pmatrix} \frac{1}{2}(r-1+w) & \frac{1}{6} \\ \frac{3}{2}(r-1)(1+r+w) & \frac{1}{2}(r+1-w) \end{pmatrix},$$

yielding

$$\Delta = \frac{1}{4}w(3-r-w)$$
$$D = r^2 - w(3-r-w).$$

A simple calculation shows that $\Delta \geq 0$ for all $r \leq 4/3$, and therefore on the interval, where E_3 exists. To compute the zeros of D we have to solve a quartic equation, yielding two real-valued solutions

$$\underline{r} \approx 0.6442, \quad \text{and} \quad \bar{r} \approx 0.9935$$

satisfying

$$D \begin{cases} < 0 & \text{for} \quad \underline{r} < r < \bar{r} \\ > 0 & \text{for} \quad r_0 \leq r < \underline{r}, \ \bar{r} < r \leq 4/3. \end{cases}$$

Thus the inner equilibrium is either an unstable node or an unstable focus.

5.3.2 Determining the Optimal Vector Field and the Optimal Costate Rule

Let us now illustrate, on the basis of our typical model, the terms and *optimal costate rule*. We specify two different cases, with the specific parameter values $r = 0.4$ and $r = 0.7$, giving rise to a unique optimal solution in the first case, and to an indifference point in the latter case.

A Unique Optimal Solution for $r = 0.4$

By the previous analysis for $r = 0.4$ the origin E_1 is the only equilibrium and it is a saddle with an associated stable manifold $W^s(E_1)$. Considering Fig. 5.2, which depicts the phase diagram for the canonical system, we discover that the $\dot{x}$- and $\dot{\lambda}$-isoclines divide the state–costate space into four regions (I, II, III, IV), wherein the arrows reflect the direction of the vector field.

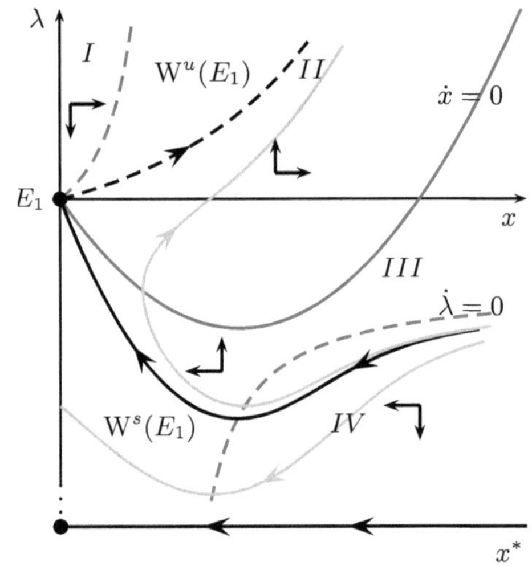

Fig. 5.2. The phase portrait is plotted together with the $\dot{x}$- and $\dot{\lambda}$-isoclines and the (un)stable manifold of the saddle E_1 for $r = 0.4$, where the stable manifold is the unique optimal solution. At the lower axis the corresponding direction of the optimal vector field $\dot{x} = f^*(x)$ is depicted

In the following we shall identify all trajectories that are ruled out as optimal solutions. Considering the quadratic costs of the control in the objective function (5.10a) and the linear occurrence of u in the state dynamics (5.10b), it becomes clear that *no* solution lying in region II and above the x-axis can be optimal. Since trajectories in this region cannot leave it (they cannot cross the $\dot{x}$-isocline), they will therefore diverge to infinity in x as well as in λ, with

$$u^*(t) = \frac{\lambda(t)}{6}.$$

Hence, if t_0 is the time point where $\lambda(\cdot)$, $(u(\cdot))$ crosses the x-axis, we have $\lambda(t) \geq 0$ for all $t \geq t_0$. Choosing $u(t) = 0$ for $t \geq t_0$ is then a better alternative, since it slows down the increase of $x(\cdot)$ and obviously has lower control costs.

Since every solution $(x(\cdot), \lambda(\cdot))$ with initial point $(x(0), \lambda(0))$ lying above the stable manifold $W^s(E_1)$ ends up in this region, we have proved that only the stable manifold and the solutions starting beneath it have to be considered.

The other trajectories can immediately be eliminated simply because those solutions cross the λ-axis for some $t_0 > 0$ and $\lambda(t_0) < 0$. And choosing $u(t) = 0$ for $t \geq t_0$ will be superior to these solutions. Thus, summing up, we have identified the stable manifold $W^s(E_1)$ as the unique optimal solution.

Regarding the stable manifold $W^s(E_1)$ as a function in x, this function is obviously the optimal costate rule $P(x)$, and thus we have

$$W^s(E_1) = \{(x, P(x)) : x \in [0, \infty)\}.$$

Moreover, the optimal vector field $f^*(x)$ is given by

$$\dot{x} = f^*(x) = x(x-1) + \frac{P(x)}{6},$$

which is depicted at the bottom of Fig. 5.2.

An Indifference Point for $r = 0.7$

For the parameter values $r = 0.7$ and $c = 5$, there exist three equilibria. The origin E_1 and outer equilibrium E_3 are saddles and the inner equilibrium E_2 is an unstable focus. Thus associated with E_1 and E_3 are the stable manifolds $W^s(E_1)$ and $W^s(E_3)$, spiraling out of the focus, as can be seen in Fig. 5.3.

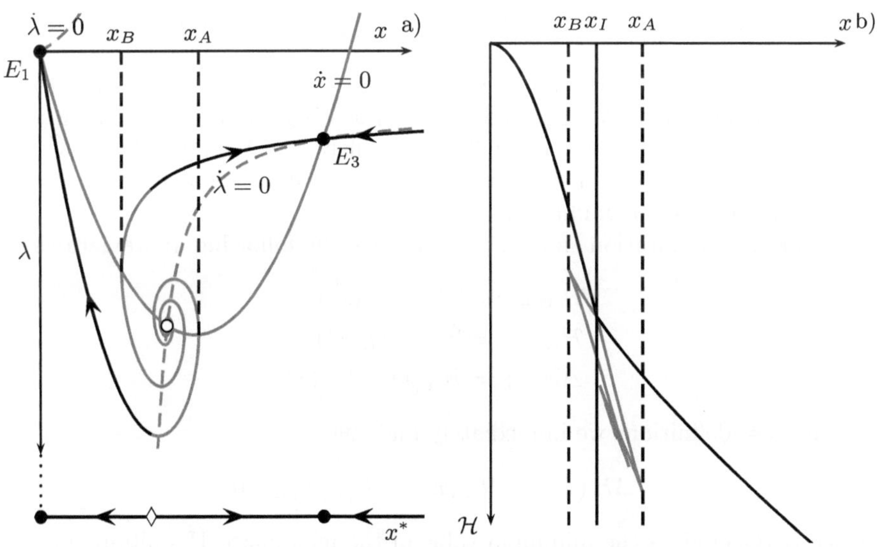

Fig. 5.3. In (**a**) the phase portraits for the canonical and the optimal system are plotted in case of an indifference point. Moreover, the direction of the optimal vector field is depicted in the *lower part of panel* (**a**). In (**b**) the intersection of the Hamiltonians for the two extremals is displayed, implying the existence of a point of indifference

By an analogous argument to that in the previous case, the two stable manifolds are identified as the only candidates for an optimal solution. Since both stable manifolds spiral out of the unstable focus, we can use a general argument to prove the existence of a unique point x_I, where both trajectories starting for $x(0) = x_I$ on the stable manifolds $\mathrm{W}^s(E_1)$ or $\mathrm{W}^s(E_3)$ are equally optimal.

In the following computations we need two general results from optimal control theory. First, Proposition 3.75 enables us to compute the objective value for an extremal solution $(\tilde{x}(\cdot), \tilde{u}(\cdot))$ starting with $x(0) = x_0$ as the value of the Hamiltonian at the initial point. Second, Proposition 3.23 reveals that the Hamiltonian achieves its minimum at the $\dot{x}$-isocline. (Note that the assumptions made in this proposition are satisfied since $\mathcal{H}_{uu} = -2c < 0$ and $f_u = 1 \neq 0$ hold.)

Result 5.3.1. *For problem (5.10) with parameter values $r = 0.7$ and $c = 3$ there exists a unique point x_I such that the problem exhibits two optimal solutions for $x(0) = x_I$.*

Proof. If we consider Fig. 5.3a, it is obvious that there exists a maximal interval $[x_A, x_B]$ where the stable manifolds have non-empty intersections in the state variables. Moreover, by the strict convexity of the Hamiltonian with respect to the costate λ (see Proposition 3.23), there exist for every $x \in [x_A, x_B]$ two costate values, $\lambda_A(x)$ and $\lambda_B(x)$, satisfying

$$(x, \lambda_A(x)) \in \mathrm{W}^s(E_3) \quad \text{and} \quad (x, \lambda_B(x)) \in \mathrm{W}^s(E_1),$$

where the maximized Hamiltonian at $(x, \lambda_A(x))$ is greater compared to all other points $(x, \lambda) \in \mathrm{W}^s(E_3)$ and at $(x, \lambda_B(x))$ is greater compared with the other points in $\mathrm{W}^s(E_1)$ (see Fig. 5.3b). Obviously $(x_A, \lambda(x_A))$ and $(x_B, \lambda(x_B))$ lie on the $\dot{x}$-isocline; if they do not, the interval could be extended, contradicting its assumed maximality.

To keep the notation simple, we introduce the following abbreviations

$$\begin{aligned}
\mathcal{H}_A(x) &:= \mathcal{H}^*\left(x, \lambda_A(x)\right) \\
\mathcal{H}_B(x) &:= \mathcal{H}^*\left(x, \lambda_B(x)\right) \\
\Delta\mathcal{H}(x) &:= \mathcal{H}_A(x) - \mathcal{H}_B(x).
\end{aligned}$$

From these definitions we immediately find that

$$\Delta\mathcal{H}\left(x_A\right) = \mathcal{H}_A\left(x_A\right) - \mathcal{H}_B\left(x_A\right) < 0,$$

since $\mathcal{H}_A(x_A)$ gives the minimum value of the maximized Hamiltonian at x_A and is therefore smaller than $\mathcal{H}_B(x_A)$. An analogous argument yields

$$\Delta\mathcal{H}\left(x_B\right) = \mathcal{H}_A\left(x_B\right) - \mathcal{H}_B\left(x_B\right) > 0.$$

But since $\Delta\mathcal{H}(x)$ is continuous on the compact interval $[x_A, x_B]$, it achieves its minimum at some point $x_I \in (x_A, x_B)$. Thus two points, $(x_I, \lambda_A(x_I))$

$\in W^s(E_3)$ and $(x_I, \lambda_B(x_I)) \in W^s(E_1)$, exist and exhibit the same objective value; the corresponding solutions are therefore equally optimal.

Lastly, we have to prove the uniqueness of x_I. Therefore we assume the existence of a further indifference point $\tilde{x}_I$, where we can assume $x_I < \tilde{x}_I$. Starting at the solution converging to E_3, we cross $\tilde{x}_I$. Since this is an indifference point, we could change the actual control to $u(\tilde{x}_I, \lambda_B(\tilde{x}_I))$, giving another optimal solution. But in the state–costate space we would jump to the stable manifold $W^s(E_1)$ exhibiting a discontinuous costate, which is excluded and therefore yields a contradiction.

Finally, we have found a unique point x_I where, if one starts at this point, two optimal solutions exist. What does this mean in terms of the optimal vector field and optimal costate rule? To answer this question we extend the definition of λ_A and λ_B to

$$\begin{aligned} \lambda_B(x) &= \lambda(x), \quad \text{satisfying } (x, \lambda(x)) \in W^s(E_1), \text{ for } 0 \le x < x_A \\ \lambda_A(x) &= \lambda(x), \quad \text{satisfying } (x, \lambda(x)) \in W^s(E_3), \text{ for } x > x_B. \end{aligned}$$

Now we can write the optimal costate rule $P(x)$ as

$$P(x) = \begin{cases} \lambda_B(x) & 0 \le x < x_I \\ \{\lambda_A(x_I), \lambda_B(x_I)\} & x = x_I \\ \lambda_A(x) & x > x_I, \end{cases}$$

with the corresponding optimal vector field

$$f^*(x) = \begin{cases} f(x, \lambda_B(x)) & 0 \le x \le x_I \\ f(x, \lambda_A(x)) & x \ge x_I. \end{cases}$$

Summing up, we have detected a point x_I, with $|P(x_I)| = 2$ and a corresponding multivalued optimal vector field $f^*(x)$ (see Fig. 5.3a). □

Remark 5.3 (Nondifferentiable Value Function). In Fig. 5.3b we see that the Hamiltonian, evaluated along an optimal solution, exhibits a kink at the DNSS point x_I. Since for the optimal solution $(x^*(\cdot), u^*(\cdot))$ with $x^*(0) = x$ the value function is given by

$$V^*(x) = \frac{1}{r}\mathcal{H}(x, u^*(0), P(x))$$

the nondifferentiability of the Hamiltonian at x_I also denotes the nondifferentiability of the value function at the DNSS point (see also Example (3.81)). The reason that the value function is nondifferentiable at a DNSS point becomes obvious, when considering that at points where $V^*(\cdot)$ is differentiable

$$\lambda(0) = P(x) = V_x^*(x)$$

holds. Thus in a neighborhood of x_I we find two sequences $(x_j^{(i)})_{i\ge 0}$, $j = 1, 2$ converging to x_I and satisfying

$$\lim_{i\to\infty} \mathrm{P}(x_1^{(i)}) \neq \lim_{i\to\infty} \mathrm{P}(x_2^{(i)})$$

by definition of a DNSS point. Therefore

$$\lim_{i\to\infty} V_x^*(x_1^{(i)}) \neq \lim_{i\to\infty} V_x^*(x_2^{(i)}),$$

proving the nondifferentiability at x_I.

Remark 5.4 (Cusp Points Along the Maximized Hamiltonian). Considering Fig. 5.3b the Hamiltonian, evaluated along an extremal solution, exhibits cusp points at turning points of the stable path. This nondifferentiability of the Hamiltonian can easily be explained. Therefore suppose $\hat{x}$ and $\hat{\lambda}$ to be a turning point of the stable path W^s. Then for a sequence $(x^{(i)})_{i\geq 0}$ with $\lim_{i\to\infty} x^{(i)} = \hat{x}$, there exist two distinct sequences $(\lambda_j^{(i)})_{i\geq 0}$ satisfying $\lim_{i\to\infty} x_j^{(i)} = \hat{\lambda}$, $j = 1, 2,$. But since

$$\hat{\lambda} = V_x^*(\hat{x}) = \mathcal{H}_x^*(\hat{x}, \hat{\lambda})$$

we find the two branches of the Hamiltonian satisfying

$$\hat{\lambda} = \lim_{i\to\infty} \mathcal{H}_x^*(\hat{x}^{(i)}, \hat{\lambda}_j^{(i)}).$$

Thus the two branches of the Hamiltonian exhibit the same tangent at the turning point $(\hat{x}, \hat{\lambda})$, and therefore being a cusp point. In the calculus of variations these points are also known as *conjugate points*.

The situation described here is the usual phenomenon of a multivalued optimal solution occurring in one-state models of the given type. Moreover this proof can be applied whenever there exists an overlap of the stable manifolds on a finite interval. In the next section we give exact definitions for the general case.

5.4 Defining Indifference and DNSS Points

We have now gathered a great deal of information concerning the multiplicity of optimal solutions. In the last section we proved in Result 5.3.1 the existence of a point where one is indifferent as to which solution is chosen. This section is devoted to the formalization of this phenomenon and to revealing some immediate consequences of the definitions used. We start by presenting a further example of multiple optimal solutions. This time it is simple enough to do all the calculations analytically; doing so shows the advantage of concentrating on the characterizing elements. Subsequently we present the definitions.

5.4.1 Multiplicity and Separability

In the last section we presented an example that, although simple enough to determine the canonical system and most of its properties analytically, required computing the optimal solution (stable manifolds) numerically. To elaborate the principles characterizing a DNSS point, we recall the Example (3.81) from Sect. 3.4.2:

$$\begin{aligned} &\max_{u(\cdot)} \int_0^\infty \mathrm{e}^{-rt} x(t)u(t)\,\mathrm{d}t \\ \text{s.t.}\quad &\dot{x}(t) = -x(t) + u(t) \\ &x(0) = x_0 \in \mathbb{R} \\ &u \in [-1, 1]. \end{aligned}$$

In Example (3.81) we have shown that the optimal state trajectories are given by

$$\mathcal{S}(x_0) = \begin{cases} -1 + \mathrm{e}^{-t}(x_0 + 1) & x_0 < 0 \\ \pm 1 \mp \mathrm{e}^{-t} & x_0 = 0 \\ 1 + \mathrm{e}^{-t}(x_0 - 1) & x_0 > 0, \end{cases}$$

and therefore

$$\mathcal{S}^\infty(x_0) = \begin{cases} -1 & x_0 < 0 \\ \pm 1 & x_0 = 0 \\ 1 & x_0 > 0 \end{cases}$$

(see Fig. 5.4a). This is one of the simplest examples exhibiting multiple optimal solutions, and it reveals the two main properties that a DNSS point has to satisfy: multiplicity and separability.

At $x = 0$ the set $\mathcal{S}(0)$ contains two elements (multiplicity), while in every neighborhood of $x = 0$ there exist solutions converging to a different limit set $\{\pm 1\}$. These observations anticipate our definition of a DNSS point and will be formalized in the following section.

From an application-oriented point of view the property of multiplicity seems not very interesting since it occurs for a negligible set compared to the entire state space (a point on an interval, a curve in a plane). But the relevance for real-world applications becomes obvious when we consider the separation property. Therefore, assume that the model (3.69) describes some real process and that some mechanism is implemented for measuring the state and consequently calculating the optimal control. Since measurements are never perfectly accurate, starting near zero can lead to a strategy that is the exact opposite of what is optimal, because if $x(0) > 0$ but small, due to some measuring error, the measured $x(0)$ could be negative; hence the corresponding control $u = -1$ is chosen instead of $u = 1$. The situation can get even worse if some feedback mechanism is implemented, whereby after some time the actual state is measured and the corresponding optimal control

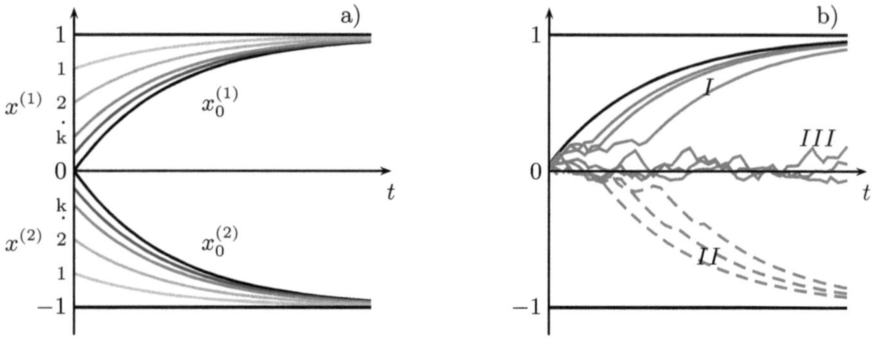

Fig. 5.4. In (**a**) the optimal trajectories of Example (3.81) are depicted for different initial points $x_k^{(1,2)}(0)$, $k = 1, 2, \dots$ converging to 0, with the corresponding optimal trajectories $x_k^{(1,2)}(\cdot)$, $k = 1, 2, \dots$ converging to $\mathcal{S}(0) = \{x_0^{(1)}(\cdot), x_0^{(2)}(\cdot)\}$.
In (**b**) different optimal (feedback) solutions with measurement errors starting at $x(0) = 0.05 > 0$ are depicted. In the extreme case chattering around the DNSS point can occur as in case III (the probability of this case persisting near 0 as t gets larger tends to zero), or the opposite strategy can be chosen as in case II. Case I exhibits the correct optimal behavior

is recalculated (see Fig. 5.4b). In the optimal control setting this feedback strategy leads to the same optimal solution (principle of optimality) if the state is measured exactly. In our real-world scenario this could result in some "chattering" behavior of the process around zero (see Fig. 5.4b)

5.4.2 Definitions

Let us now return to the question of how to define points of indifference. Reconsidering the previous example, we have to formalize the concepts of multiplicity and separability. Thus we define points of indifference as follows:

Definition 5.5 (Indifference Point). *Let $\mathcal{S}(x_0)$ be the solution set of an optimal control problem* OC *(3.3). If there exist $x_1^*(\cdot), x_2^*(\cdot) \in \mathcal{S}(x_0)$ and $t \in [0, T]$ satisfying*

$$x_1^*(t) \neq x_2^*(t),$$

then x_0 is called an indifference point. *If the solution set $\mathcal{S}(x_0)$ has cardinality $k < \infty$, then x_0 is called of* order k*; otherwise it is of* infinite order.

Remark 5.6. Note that the optimal state trajectories are continuous. Thus if they differ in a single time point t, they are already different on an open interval.

Note that Definition 5.5 is stated for a general optimal control problem, whereas for the next definition we explicitly refer to discounted, autonomous models of infinite horizon *DAM* (5.1):

Definition 5.7 (Threshold Point). *Let us consider a problem* DAM *(5.1) with* $x(0) = x_0$. *Then* x_0 *is called a* threshold point *if for every neighborhood* U *of* x_0 *there exist* $x_{10}, x_{20} \in U$, *satisfying*

$$\mathcal{S}^\infty(x_{10}) \cap \mathcal{S}^\infty(x_{20}) = \emptyset, \ \mathcal{S}^\infty(x_{i0}) \neq \emptyset, \ i = 1, 2.$$

Remark 5.8. Hence a threshold point x_0 is characterized by the property that in every neighborhood of x_0 there exist solutions converging to distinct limit sets.

The two definitions formalize the concepts of multiplicity and separability and can now be used to define the phenomenon of DNSS points often found in economic literature:

Definition 5.9 (DNSS Point). *Let us consider a problem* DAM *(5.1) with* $x(0) = x_0$. *Then* x_0 *is called a* DNSS point *if it is both an indifference point and a threshold point.*

If x_0 *is a threshold point but not an indifference point, it is called a* weak DNSS point.

Remark 5.10. Not only DNSS points separate different basins of attraction, but only at DNSS points does the decision-maker get to make a choice about how to proceed. Weak DNSS points do not create such options.

Remark 5.11. We call a weak DNSS point "weak" because as a practical matter, they are places that give the decision-maker choices about where to go in the long-run if the decision-maker is willing to pay even an infinitesimally small premium for the privilege of having that flexibility.

To further illustrate the difference between a DNSS point (multiplicity) and a weak DNSS point (history-dependence), let us analyze the following example:

$$\min_{u(\cdot)} \int_0^\infty (x(t) + u(t))^2 \, \mathrm{d}t \tag{5.11a}$$

$$\text{s.t.} \quad \dot{x}(t) = u(t)\left(u(t)^2 - 1\right) \tag{5.11b}$$

$$x(0) = x_0.$$

From the cost function (5.11a) it readily follows that $u^* = -x$. Substituting this optimal control into (5.11b) yields

$$x^*(t) = \begin{cases} \pm\left(1 - \mathrm{e}^{-2t}\left(1 - 1/x_0^2\right)\right)^{-1/2} & x_0 \gtrless 0 \\ 0 & x_0 = 0. \end{cases}$$

Thus in the long run we find

$$x^*(\infty) = \begin{cases} \pm 1 & x_0 \gtrless 0 \\ 0 & x_0 = 0. \end{cases}$$

Hence $x_0 = 0$ serves as a threshold separating the two long-run solutions ± 1, whereas at $x_0 = 0$ the unique optimal solution $u^* \equiv 0$ exists. Therefore $x_0 = 0$ satisfies the condition of separability but not that of multiplicity, and so it is a weak DNSS point.

For one-state infinite time horizon problems, Fig. 5.5 depicts the usual case for a DNSS point and a weak DNSS point, respectively. In terms of the canonical system derived from Pontryagin's Maximum Principle the characterizing element of a DNSS point is an overlap of the extremal solutions over a finite interval in the state space (see Fig. 5.5a,b). Such an overlap can occur in the case of an unstable focus or an unstable node. If no such overlap in the neighborhood of an unstable node exists we have the case of a weak DNSS point (see Fig. 5.5c). The actual characteristic (DNSS point or weak DNSS point) therefore depends on the topology of the trajectories near the unstable node (see Proposition 5.17).

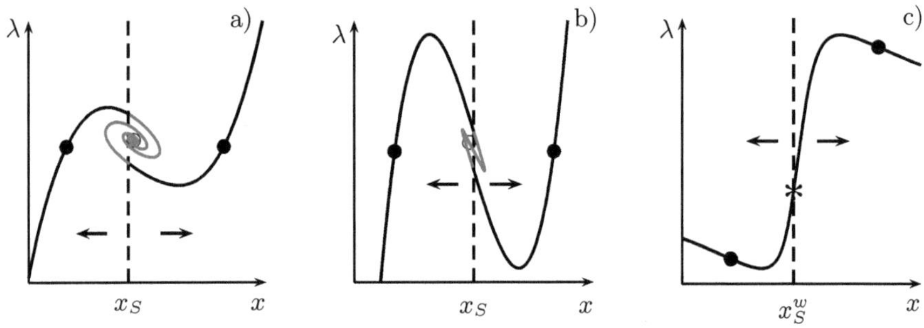

Fig. 5.5. The three cases for one-dimensional systems are depicted in the state–costate space. Case (**a**) shows a DNSS point in the neighborhood of an unstable spiral. In (**c**) the unstable node is a weak DNSS point. Owing to the overlap of the stable manifolds in state space, there exists a DNSS point near the unstable node in case (**b**)

5.4.3 Conclusions from the Definitions

Subsequently we make the following assumptions.

Assumption 5.1. For every initial state $x \in \mathbb{R}^n$ there exists at least one bounded optimal solution, with the corresponding optimal vector field

$$\dot{x}(t) = f^*(x(t)). \tag{5.12}$$

Assumption 5.2. The Hamiltonian is strictly concave in u.

Assumption 5.3. The matrix $f_u(x^*(t), u^*(t))$ has full rank along an optimal solution $(x^*(\cdot), u^*(\cdot))$.

Note that the cardinality of $\mathrm{P}(x_0)$ denotes the number of initial costates for optimal trajectories emanating from the state x_0. Under the given assumptions the following lemma holds:

Lemma 5.12. *Let* $(x^*(\cdot), u^*(\cdot))$ *be an optimal solution of* DAM *(5.1). If Assumptions 5.2 and 5.3 are satisfied; then the set* $\mathrm{P}(x^*(t))$ *with* $t > 0$ *reduces to a single point.*

Proof. The proof follows from the continuity of the costate and the uniqueness and continuity of the control and costate. Therefore the adjoint dynamics and hence the costate is uniquely determined by the initial costate at $t = 0$. □

Hence we find:

Corollary 5.13. *Under Assumptions 5.1–5.3 the number of optimal solutions is equal to the cardinality of* $\mathrm{P}(x_0)$.

Proof. From Lemma 5.12 we know that for $t > 0$ the set $\mathrm{P}(x^*(t))$ is single-valued. Thus if there exist n optimal solutions, by the uniqueness of the solution of the canonical system, n initial costates have to exist corresponding to the n optimal solutions, concluding the proof. □

Remark 5.14. In general Cor. 5.13 may not be true. Consider the following example:

$$\begin{aligned}
&\max_{u(\cdot)} \int_0^\infty -\mathrm{e}^{-rt} u(t)^2 \, \mathrm{d}t \\
\text{s.t.} \quad &\dot{x}(t) = x(t) + u(t)^3, \\
&x(0) = 0.
\end{aligned}$$

Since the integral does not depend on the state x, it is evident that the minimum is achieved for $u \equiv 0$. Thus Assumption 5.2 ($\mathcal{H}^*_{uu} = -2 < 0$) is satisfied but not Assumption 5.3 ($f^*_u = 0$). By Pontryagin's Maximum Principle we find the adjoint equation given as

$$\dot{\lambda} = (r - 1)\lambda,$$

yielding

$$\lambda(t) = \lambda(0)\mathrm{e}^{(r-1)t}.$$

Hence if $r < 1/2$, every $\lambda(0) \in \mathbb{R}$ satisfies the transversality condition, which is a necessary condition since the assumptions of Proposition 3.74 are satisfied. In that case

$$\mathrm{P}(0) = \mathbb{R},$$

which is obviously not representing the number of optimal solutions.

From the definition of a DNSS point we therefore find the following corollary:

Corollary 5.15. *Let a model* DAM *(5.1) satisfy the Assumptions 5.1–5.3 and* x_0 *be a DNSS point; then* $\mathrm{P}(x_0) \geq 2$.

We can now give a characterization of a weak DNSS point in terms of the optimal vector field:

Proposition 5.16. *Given the optimal vector field (5.12), the solution starting at a weak DNSS point* $x_0 \in \mathbb{R}^n$ *does not converge to a stable limit set of (5.12). For one-state models a weak DNSS point* x_0 *is a repelling or semistable equilibrium.*

Proof. From the definition of a weak DNSS point we know that for every neighborhood of x_0 there exist at least two solutions exhibiting different limit sets. Then Lemma A.99 assures us that for a sequence of initial points converging to x_0 the corresponding solutions converge to the solution starting at x_0, and by assumption the limit set $x(x_0, \infty) \neq \emptyset$ exists. Thus if the limit set $x(x_0, \infty) \neq \emptyset$ is stable, any solution starting in the neighborhood of x_0 converges to this limit set, contradicting the definition of a weak DNSS point and proving the first part of the proposition.

For one-state models the only limit sets are equilibria. Moreover, only three classes of equilibria are possible – namely stable, repelling, and semistable equilibria – and from the first part of the proof we can immediately exclude the stable equilibrium, since in that case x_0 is the limit set for every solution starting in a small enough neighborhood. □

For the one-state case we can provide necessary conditions for the occurrence of a weak DNSS point. This has been proved in Feichtinger and Wirl (2000) and will be restated in the following proposition:

Proposition 5.17. *Consider a one-state and one-control model* DAM *(5.1). Let the Assumptions 5.1–5.3 be satisfied and the optimized Hamiltonian* $\mathcal{H}^*$ *be strictly concave in the state* x *on an open convex set covering the equilibria of the canonical system. Then a necessary condition for the existence of an unstable equilibrium* $\hat{x}$ *of the optimal vector field is*

$$\frac{\mathrm{d}f^*(x)}{\mathrm{d}x} = f_x - f_u \left(\mathcal{H}_{ux}/\mathcal{H}_{uu}\right) > 0,$$

which can be achieved through

$$r > \mathcal{H}^*_{x\lambda} > 0.$$

If such an equilibrium $\hat{x}$ *exists, it is optimal and a weak DNSS point.*

Proof. By assumption there exists at least one equilibrium $(\hat{x}, \hat{u})$ of the canonical system, and the equilibria obviously satisfy the necessary conditions of Pontryagin's Maximum Principle. Thus by the concavity assumptions and Theorem 3.70 $(\hat{x}, \hat{u})$ is the unique optimal solution for the given problem with

$x(0) = \hat{x}$. Now assume that $(\hat{x}, \hat{u})$ is a hyperbolic equilibrium and not a saddle. In this case $\hat{x}$ is an equilibrium of the corresponding optimal vector field $f^*(\hat{x})$, satisfying

$$\frac{\mathrm{d}}{\mathrm{d}x} f^*(\hat{x}) > 0.$$

Under the given assumptions and using the implicit function theorem, we can differentiate the control $u^* = u(x, \lambda)$ in respect to x and λ, satisfying

$$\frac{\mathrm{d}u^*}{\mathrm{d}x} = -\frac{\mathcal{H}_{ux}}{\mathcal{H}_{uu}}.$$

Hence we immediately find

$$\frac{\mathrm{d}}{\mathrm{d}x} f^*(\hat{x}) = f_x + f_u \frac{\mathrm{d}u^*}{\mathrm{d}x} = f_x - f_u \frac{\mathcal{H}_{ux}}{\mathcal{H}_{uu}}.$$

This also proves that $\hat{x}$ is a weak DNSS point, since in every interval around $\hat{x}$ there exist solutions converging to (two) different limit sets (equilibria).

Next, we want to analyze the properties that an optimal unstable equilibrium of the canonical system has to satisfy. Therefore we only have to investigate the Jacobian $\hat{J}$ at $(\hat{x}, \hat{\lambda})$, satisfying

$$\begin{pmatrix} \mathcal{H}^*_{x\lambda} & \mathcal{H}^*_{\lambda\lambda} \\ -\mathcal{H}^*_{xx} & r - \mathcal{H}^*_{\lambda x} \end{pmatrix},$$

where $\mathcal{H}^*_{x\lambda} = \mathcal{H}^*_{\lambda x}$. A necessary condition for the equilibrium not to be a saddle is

$$\det \hat{J} = \mathcal{H}^*_{x\lambda}\left(r - \mathcal{H}^*_{x\lambda}\right) + \mathcal{H}^*_{\lambda\lambda}\mathcal{H}^*_{xx} > 0.$$

Due to Proposition 3.23 $\mathcal{H}^*_{\lambda\lambda} > 0$, and the assumption $\mathcal{H}^*_{xx} < 0$ we have

$$\mathcal{H}^*_{\lambda\lambda}\mathcal{H}^*_{xx} < 0.$$

Thus to assure the positivity of the $\det \hat{J}$,

$$r > \mathcal{H}^*_{x\lambda} > 0$$

has to be satisfied. To exclude unstable spirals we exhibit $r^2 - 4\det(\hat{J}) \geq 0$. This follows from the quadratic term in r

$$r^2 - 4r\mathcal{H}^*_{x\lambda} + 4\left(\mathcal{H}^*_{x\lambda}\right)^2 - 4\mathcal{H}^*_{\lambda\lambda}\mathcal{H}^*_{xx},$$

which achieves its minimum $-4\mathcal{H}^*_{\lambda\lambda}\mathcal{H}^*_{xx} > 0$ at $r = 2\mathcal{H}^*_{x\lambda}$. □

Remark 5.18. In Feichtinger and Wirl (2000) the slightly stronger assumption of concavity of the Hamiltonian $\mathcal{H}$ with respect to x and u has been made, where $\mathcal{H}_{uu} < 0$ is assumed. This yields the negative definiteness of the matrix

$$\begin{pmatrix} \mathcal{H}_{uu} & \mathcal{H}_{ux} \\ \mathcal{H}_{ux} & \mathcal{H}_{xx} \end{pmatrix}.$$

Under this assumption the necessary conditions stated in Proposition 5.17 can be refined to

$$r > f_x > 0 \quad \text{growth}$$

or

$$f_u \mathcal{H}_{ux} > 0 \quad \text{positive state–control interactions.}$$

Moreover, the concavity assumption covering *all* equilibria cannot be relaxed, as can be shown by a counter-example (see Exercise 5.2).

5.5 Revisiting the Typical Example

Having introduced exact terminology for indifference points and (weak) DNSS points, we now return to our typical example (5.10) focusing on the question of uniqueness and multiplicity of the optimal solution. Subsequently we shall consider the discount rate r as well as the cost parameter c as a variable and determine the regions with *different* dynamical behavior, i.e., doing a bifurcation analysis and calculating the corresponding bifurcation curves. Since most of the calculations are similar to those in Sect. 5.3.1, the reader is invited to complete the necessary calculations (see Exercise 5.4.5). After elementary but lengthy calculations the two fold bifurcation curves $\delta = \delta_1 \cup \delta_2$ and $\eta = \eta_1 \cup \eta_2$ can explicitly be computed and are depicted in Fig. 5.6.[4] Each of these curves is differentiated by an index one and two, referring to the fact that these parts have to be distinguished in respect to the optimal solution, which will be explained below.

The curves δ and η are given by

$$\delta := \left\{(c,r) : \ c = \frac{1}{r-1}, \ r \in (1, \infty)\right\}$$

$$\eta := \left\{(c,r) : \ c = \frac{8}{r^2+2r+1}, \ r \in [0, 3]\right\},$$

where δ characterizes a saddle-node bifurcation at the outer equilibrium and η a transcritical bifurcation at the origin.

The third curve $\beta = \beta_1 \cup \beta_2$ (see Fig. 5.6) is given by

$$\beta_1 := \left\{(c,r) : \ c = \frac{4(\Sigma_1 + \Sigma_2)}{(x+2)^2(x^2-2/3)}, \ r \in (\sqrt{2/3}, 1]\right\}$$

$$\beta_2 := \left\{(c,r) : \ c = \frac{4(\Sigma_1 - \Sigma_2)}{(x+2)^2(x^2-2/3)}, \ r \in [0, 1]\right\},$$

[4] To clarify the depiction the region between $r = 1$ and $r = 3$ is compressed.

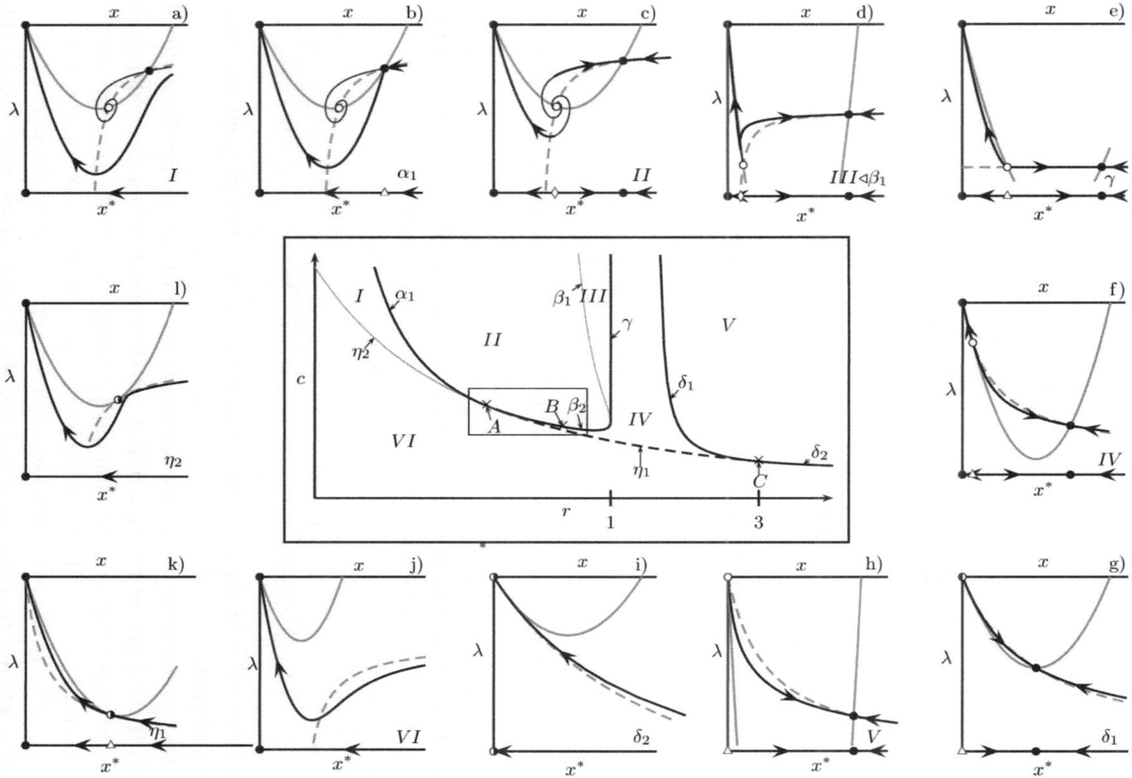

Fig. 5.6. The central figure depicts the regions for the canonical system of model (5.10) with different dynamical and optimal behavior. Around the central figure characteristic phase portraits of the canonical and optimal system are displayed, exemplifying these regions. To avoid overloading the figure the elements are explained in the text of Sect. 5.5

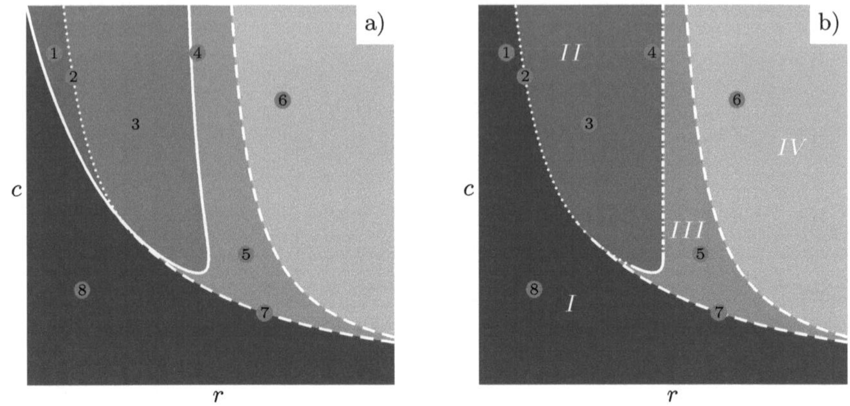

Fig. 5.7. Panel (**a**) points out the different topologically equivalent regions of the canonical system in the parameter space (r, c). In panel (**b**) the regions of different optimal behavior are depicted. The numbers are those of Fig. 5.6 and highlight the differences across the regions in the dynamical and optimal behavior

with

$$\Sigma_1 := 3r^2 + 10r - 7, \quad \text{and} \quad \Sigma_2 := (r-3)\sqrt{(r-1)(r+3)}.$$

This curve is not a bifurcation curve, but denotes the transformation of the inner equilibrium from an unstable focus to an unstable node.

The bifurcation/transformation curves δ, η and β denote local bifurcations and are analytically given. In contrast the curve α_1 (see Fig. 5.7a) depicts the case of a global bifurcation, namely a heteroclinic bifurcation, which can only be computed numerically. (Section 7.8 explains how this is done.)

Finally the curve

$$\gamma := \{(r, c) : \; r = 1, \; c \geq 2.75\}$$

denotes a bifurcation of the optimal vector field, where a DNSS point becomes a weak DNSS point.

After this preparatory work we are ready to start analyzing the optimal behavior of these different regions. In Fig. 5.6 the considered cases are depicted as well as phase portraits of the canonical systems and of the optimal vector field. The central panel of Fig. 5.6 shows the (r, c)-parameter space together with the already-mentioned bifurcation curves and transformation curves.

Arranged around this central panel are the typical phase portraits in the state–costate space together with the corresponding optimal dynamics. These phase portraits are drawn for each of the different regions and for hairline cases delimiting these regions.

In Figs. 5.6 and 5.8 the $\dot{x}$-isocline (—) and $\dot{\lambda}$-isocline (- -) together with the saddles (●), repelling equilibria (○) and non-hyperbolic equilibria

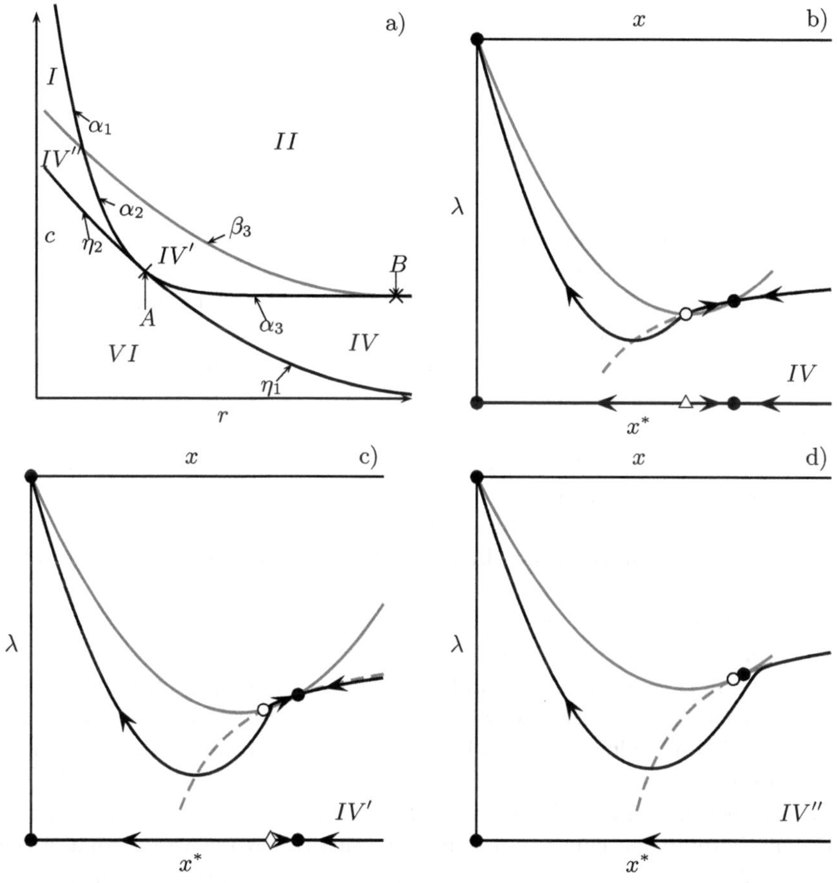

Fig. 5.8. The region denoted by the *rectangle* in Fig. 5.6 is blown up to show the details. Panel (**a**) shows (schematically) the regions in the parameter space and for regions IV, IV' and IV'' the phase portraits are depicted in the panels (**b**), (**c**) and (**d**)

(◑) are depicted. For every saddle the corresponding stable paths (—) and optimal paths (**—**) are drawn.

The phase portraits of the optimal vector field at the bottom of each of the figures denote the direction of the optimal path, together with stable equilibria (●), unstable equilibria (△), and DNSS points (◊).

Occurrence of a DNSS Point

Panels a–c of Fig. 5.6 depict the situation typical for the occurrence of a DNSS point. From a local perspective, these regions cannot be distinguished, since the occurring equilibria are all of the same type and the canonical systems are topologically equivalent at these equilibria. We can consider this sequence of panels from two points of view. The first one is the usual way of thinking about the canonical system, whereas the second tells the story from the perspective of the optimal system. Let us start with the canonical system. Here we are confronted with the problem of multiple equilibria, where a repelling equilibrium lies between two saddles. Hence, both saddles have to be considered as long-run optimal solutions. To answer the question of optimality, one has to compute the corresponding stable paths, where in region I we see that one saddle path originates from the unstable equilibrium, and the other comes from infinity. In that case the unbounded path is superior, since by Proposition 3.23 we know that the Hamiltonian is strictly convex in λ and therefore is strictly less at the outer equilibrium E_3 compared to the value at the stable path with the same x-coordinate. This implies that the saddle path of the origin is the unique optimal solution, being always superior to the saddle path of E_3.

By contrast in region II, both saddle paths spiral out of the unstable focus. Following the argumentation already given on p. 249, we find a DNSS point separating the initial values, where it is optimal to move to the origin or to the outer equilibrium, i.e., being indifferent, when starting at the DNSS point.

The intermediate situation between these two cases arises when the saddle path of the origin neither comes from infinity nor spirals out of the unstable focus, but coincides with the unstable path of the outer equilibrium, constituting a heteroclinic connection between these two saddles. Since the heteroclinic connection is unstable,[5] i.e., vanishes if one of the parameters is changed, we find a curve in the parameter space separating regions I and II. This heteroclinic connection is a global phenomenon since it depends on the saddle paths, and can therefore be calculated only numerically. Owing to our definitions, E_2 is a DNSS point since in every neighborhood two optimal solutions with different limit sets, E_1 and E_3, exist.

Changing the perspective, we now consider the optimal vector field and interpret the results in terms of this system. Thus in region I only one stable equilibrium at 0 exists. If we keep the parameter c fixed and increase r, a semistable equilibrium at the x-coordinate of E_3 arises, bifurcating into a DNSS point and a stable equilibrium at E_3. Hence in the optimal vector field the heteroclinic bifurcation of the canonical system corresponds to a bifurcation of the optimal vector field, which has no counterpart in the usual bifurcation theory of ODEs. In that sense we shall call this bifurcation an indifference bifurcation. For a more detailed description of bifurcation of the optimal vector field see Kiseleva and Wagener (2008).

[5] The heteroclinic connection is constituted by a stable and an unstable path connecting both equilibria. It is geometrically evident that a (generic C^1) perturbation will break up this connection (for a proof in the homoclinic case see Kuznetsov, 1998).

Transformation into a Weak DNSS Point

Next, we consider the panels d–f. Having the canonical system in mind, it becomes obvious that from the dynamical point of view regions III and IV are equivalent to regions I and II, since the only difference is that the unstable focus is replaced by an unstable node. But what happens to the optimal solution? Let us start with region IV, lying between $r = 1$ and the transcritical bifurcation curve δ_1. As the reader may prove, we immediately find that the assumptions of Proposition 3.23 are satisfied and thus the occurrence of DNSS points is excluded. This implies the usual case of history-dependent solutions and the existence of a weak DNSS point at the x-coordinate of the inner equilibrium E_2, where one stays put if starting exactly at E_2 or moves to the left or to the right when deviating from E_2.

Contrary to the former behavior in region III, the saddle paths have an overlap of the x-values near the unstable node; using the same argumentation as in the case of an unstable focus, we find there exists a DNSS point and the unstable node is no longer optimal. Note that since the existence of a DNSS point is a global phenomenon, this overlap can only be proved numerically. This shows that the conditions in Proposition 3.23 are sufficient but not necessary to exclude the existence of a DNSS point. This becomes obvious when we consider the region with $r < 1$ and lying between β_2 and η as is depicted in Fig. 5.8. In respect to the optimal dynamics, the curve γ separating regions III and IV denotes a demarcation curve, where the DNSS point transforms into a weak DNSS point.

From History-Dependence to Uniqueness

Finally, we consider the remaining panels g–l. Moving from region IV to region V, the transcritical bifurcation curve δ_1 is crossed and the origin becomes an unstable node, whereas the second saddle has a negative x-value and therefore does not satisfy the positivity assumption $x \geq 0$ and is dropped. In that case the origin becomes a weak DNSS point, for any other initial value of x it is optimal to converge to the outer equilibrium E_3. In Exercise 5.4 the reader is asked to compute the optimal solution at the transcritical bifurcation curve δ_1.

When crossing the saddle-node bifurcation curve η_1, the origin remains as a unique equilibrium, whereas we have already proved in Sect. 5.3.2 that its saddle path is the optimal solution.

At last the hairline case at the saddle-node bifurcation curve δ_1 has to be considered. Here it turns out that collision of the inner and outer equilibrium leaves an unstable equilibrium remain, which is a weak DNSS point.

Taking a Closer Look

In Fig. 5.8 the region including the points A and B (see Fig. 5.6) is depicted in more detail. This closer look reveals that region IV, enclosed by η and β (and δ), can be separated into IV, IV' and IV''. As we have already seen, region IV exhibits three equilibria, where an unstable node exists between two saddles. Considering the global saddle paths we see that in region IV'' (Fig. 5.8d) the saddle path exists for all $x \geq 0$ and lies beneath that of the second saddle. Following the arguments for region I we find that the origin is the unique long-run optimal solution. Contrary to this situation in region IV' (see Fig. 5.8c) both saddle paths have an overlap in their state values. Following the argumentation of region II, this gives rise to the existence of a DNSS point. Finally for region IV we already know that the state value of the unstable node is a weak DNSS point. These regions are separated by the curves α_2 and α_3 as illustrated in Fig. 5.8a.

Figure 5.7 summarizes the behavior of the system from the perspective of the canonical system panel (a) and that of the optimal dynamics panel (b).

5.6 Eradication vs. Accommodation in an Optimal Control Model of a Drug Epidemic

In this section we revisit the optimal control model of a drug epidemic which is discussed earlier and analyzed partly in Sect. 3.9. Here we focus on scenarios in which a DNSS point occurs to illustrate for the reader how the concepts introduced in this chapter can be applied.

For that purpose, let us first recall the bifurcation diagram for the social-cost parameter ρ (see Fig. 3.8). From that analysis we concluded that for low or high enough values of ρ it will always be optimal to approach the high or low equilibrium, respectively. However, for some range of intermediate levels of ρ we found two saddle points with an unstable focus in between. In these cases we may expect to find a DNSS point separating the basins of attraction of the two saddle points.

Figure 5.9 depicts such a case. In Fig. 5.9a the phase portrait is plotted in the (A, λ)-space, where we find both the $\dot{A}$- and $\dot{\lambda}$-isoclines and the stable manifolds of the saddles, which emanate from the unstable focus in between. The DNSS point is computed by comparing and intersecting the Hamiltonians along the two extremal solutions, as illustrated in Fig. 5.9b. More precisely, in Fig. 5.9b we plot the maximized Hamiltonians divided by the discount rate r to obtain the utility functional values as functions of the initial state A_0, for each of the two candidate solutions.

Finally, Fig. 5.9c depicts the optimal policy (i.e., u^* as a function of A) resulting from this analysis. The policy interpretation is as follows. The optimal control model of a drug epidemic as described above may have two optimal equilibrium solutions. One is at a low level $\hat{A}_1 = 0$, and the other is at a

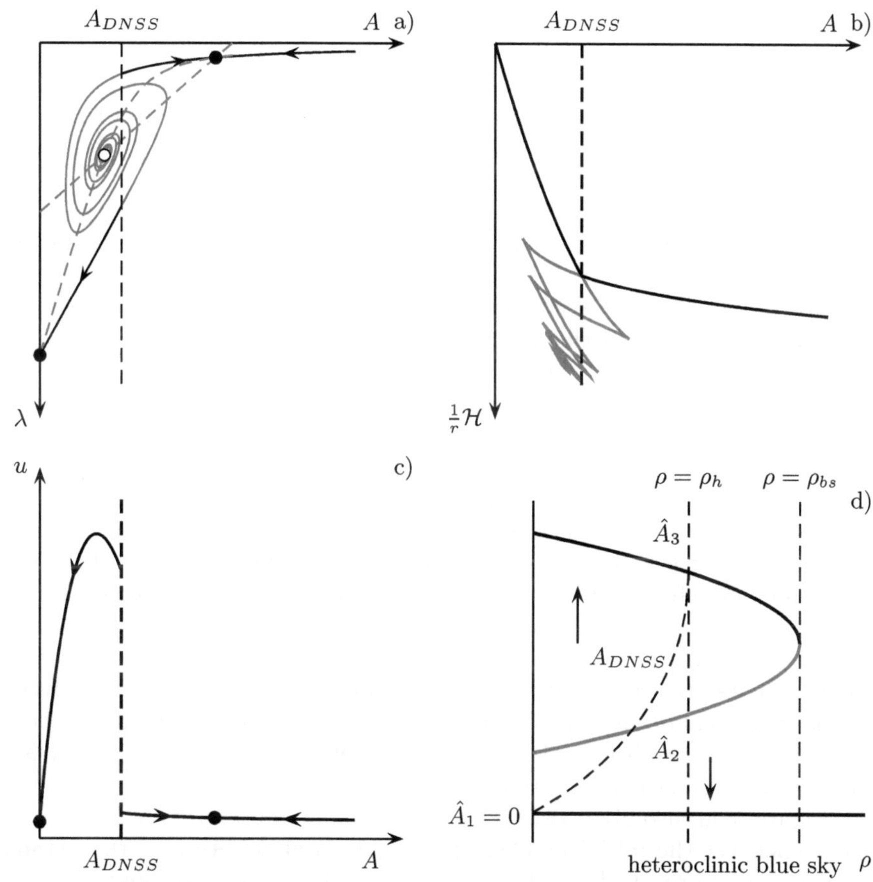

Fig. 5.9. Panel (**a**) depicts the phase diagram and the optimal paths in the (A, λ)-space. The DNSS point A_{DNSS} separates the basins of attraction of the two saddle points. In panel (**b**) the utility functional values along the saddle point paths as a function of the initial state A_0 are computed as $\frac{1}{r}H(A_0, u(0), \lambda(0))$. The point of intersection provides the DNSS point A_{DNSS}. Panel (**c**) shows the control spending u along the optimal paths ("optimal policy"). Massive treatment spending is optimal when approaching the low equilibrium ("eradication" policy), whereas only rather moderate levels of spending are used along the stable manifold of the high equilibrium ("accommodation" policy). Panel (**d**) illustrates a bifurcation diagram for ρ, keeping all other parameters constant. The DNSS point A_{DNSS} (*dashed curve*) exists iff $\rho \leq \rho_h$, where ρ_h is the location of the heteroclinic bifurcation

high level of $\hat{A}_3$ users. We showed that there exists a DNSS point, A_{DNSS} users, such that if initially there are fewer than that critical number of users it is optimal to drive use down to the low-use equilibrium (an "eradication strategy"), whereas if there are already more than that number of users, the best strategy is simply to delay but not prevent growth toward the high-level equilibrium (an "accommodation strategy").

In other words, if control begins before the problem has grown beyond the DNSS point, then it is optimal to use massive control to push it back down to a lower level of use. However, if the problem has already grown beyond that threshold, then the accommodation strategy with relatively little control spending is optimal. In the latter case, even if the eradication strategy was technically possible, it would be too expensive for it to be the optimal strategy. This is a classic DNSS point acting as a "tipping point."

The final part of the analysis of this model addresses the question for which values of the social cost parameter ρ we find a DNSS point. In Fig. 5.9d we display another bifurcation diagram for ρ, which we augment with the location of the DNSS point, A_{DNSS}, whenever it exists. We find that a DNSS point occurs for $\rho \in [0, \rho_h]$, where ρ_h is a positive value of ρ at which we find a heteroclinic bifurcation. As $\rho_h < \rho_{bs}$, we conclude that for all ρ between ρ_h and ρ_{bs} we have multiple steady states but no DNSS point, so for all initial numbers of users the optimal policy is to drive use down to the low equilibrium at $\hat{A}_1 = 0$ despite the existence of another saddle at the high level of $\hat{A}_3$ users. In mathematical terms, this rather simple example of a one-state model shows that the existence of multiple saddle points separated by an unstable steady state is not a sufficient condition for the occurrence of DNSS points.

Figure 5.9d also gives rise to a nice economic interpretation. First recall that whenever the initial number of users A_0 is above A_{DNSS}, the optimal policy is to approach the high equilibrium at $\hat{A}_3$, while below and for social costs above ρ_h it is optimal to approach the low equilibrium at $\hat{A}_1$ as indicated by the arrows in Fig. 5.9d. Starting with the lowest possible value of $\rho = 0$, the DNSS point coincides with $\hat{A}_1$, so for all positive A_0 the high equilibrium is approached. As discussed earlier, this is not at all surprising; if $\rho = 0$, no social costs occur from drug use, so the objective functional is minimized by setting the control equal to zero throughout, which results in the uncontrolled dynamics with the highest possible steady state level of users in the long run. However, A_{DNSS} is strictly positive as soon as ρ is positive, so even for very small values of the social costs, there exists some range of initial numbers of users for which it is optimal to eradicate drug use. This range is small when ρ is small, but it is increasing convexly with ρ. In other words, the larger the social costs, the larger is the basin of attraction of the low equilibrium at $\hat{A}_1$. We also observe that the high equilibrium level $\hat{A}_3$ is decreasing in ρ, which results from higher levels of control spending for increasing social costs. Finally, the DNSS point disappears at the critical level $\rho = \rho_h$, so the eradication of drug use is optimal for all values of ρ larger than ρ_h, irrespective of the initial number of users.

There is yet one more nice economic story to tell. In a remark at the end of Sect. 3.9 there was a brief discussion about the influence of the relative sizes of the discount rate r and $r_0 = k\bar{A} - \mu$ on the qualitative shape of the bifurcation diagram. A careful look at the bifurcation diagram here (Fig. 5.9d) and the one used back in Sect. 3.9 (Fig. 3.8) reveals that the location of the horizontal line representing $\hat{A}_1$ is different. The reason is that $r \in \left[\frac{r_0}{2}, 2r_0\right]$ in Fig. 3.8, while for Fig. 5.9d a value of r below $\frac{r_0}{2}$ was used. In economic terms, the decision maker is less farsighted in the old figure than in the new one presented here. That is interesting because we find that a more farsighted decision maker has a broader range of social cost values for which the saddle point at $\hat{A}_1$ exists. While only two paragraphs above we concluded that the existence of a saddle point does not imply its optimality, it can indeed be shown that the more farsighted a decision maker is, the broader is the range of parameters for which eradication is the optimal strategy as opposed to the accommodation strategy. This is probably not so much surprising, but it is definitely in line with results presented in Behrens, Caulkins, Tragler, and Feichtinger (2002).

This example ends our presentation of multiple optimal solutions and history-dependence. Even though the phenomenon of multiplicity in an economic framework has been analyzed for nearly three decades, few theoretical results are known so far. In that respect the approach taken by Wagener (2003) and Kiseleva and Wagener (2008) seems promising and opens the field for further research.

Exercises

5.1 (Gould's Second Diffusion Model). The following model is probably the first one analyzed in which a DNSS point occurs.

In Exercise 3.5 we presented a model in which advertising influences those who are "not-yet-buyers." In another scenario dealt with by Gould (1970) people learn of a product by talking with others who are knowledgeable. In particular the customers of a product inform other potential customers by word-of-mouth information diffusion. Assume that the potential market for a product is m people, of whom $x(t)$ know of the product and buy it. Consider a single firm that can influence the contact rate $a(t)$ at which people discuss the firm's product. Then the x customers inform xa people, of whom a fraction $1 - x/m$ will be newly informed. Knowledgeable people are assumed to forget at constant rate δ, e.g., by switching brands.

Assume that purchases generate concave profits $\pi(x)$. Moreover, it is reasonable to assume that the contact rate increases with advertising. Denoting the convex cost of achieving effect $a(t)$ via advertising as $c(a)$ and get

$$\max_{a(\cdot)} \int_0^\infty e^{-rt} \left(\pi(x) - c(a)\right) dt$$

$$\text{s.t.} \quad \dot{x} = ax(1 - x/m) - \delta x$$

$$x(0) = x_0 \in [0, m].$$

Show that there exist two interior long-run equilibria and one equilibrium at the boundary. Show further that the "middle" equilibrium is an unstable focus. Carry out a phase portrait analysis and interpret the optimal solutions. Discuss the role of the DNSS threshold.

5.2. To prove the necessity of the concavity assumption for Proposition 5.17, compute the optimal solution of the following model:

$$\max_{u(\cdot)} \int_0^\infty \mathrm{e}^{-rt} \left(au + bx - 1/2\left(\alpha u^2 + \beta ux - 1/2\gamma x^2\right) - \theta x^3\right) \mathrm{d}t$$

$$\text{s.t.} \quad \dot{x} = (A - \delta)\, x - 1/2x^2 - u.$$

Use the parameter values:

r	A	γ	a	α	b	β	δ	θ
2	2	1	0.01	1	0.01	0.5	0.1	1

5.3. Prove that the problem (5.2) is normal, i.e., $\lambda_0 = 1$.

5.4. For the typical example (5.10):

1. Prove that the problem is normal, i.e., $\lambda_0 = 1$.
2. Prove that the transversality condition has to hold.
3. Perform the explicit calculations to determine the stability properties of the equilibria.
4. Prove that the stable manifolds are the only candidates for an optimal solution ($r = 0.5$, $c = 5$).
5. Determine the equilibria and stability properties for the model with r *and* c variable.

Hint. Prove 1 by contradiction, and then use the linearity in u. For 2 show that the assumptions of Proposition 3.74 are satisfied.

5.5. Calculate the quadratic approximation of the center manifold for the canonical system of the typical example (5.10) at the equilibrium $(0, 0)$ and for the bifurcation parameter $c = 8/(r^2 + 2r + 1)$.

Hint. Use the procedure presented, e.g., in Kuznetsov (1998, p. 172).

5.6 (Optimal Growth with a Convex–Concave Production Function). Skiba (1978) extended Ramsey's neoclassical growth model to an S-shaped production function. This provided an early analysis of indifference or DNSS points. Consider the optimal capital-accumulation model presented in Exercise 3.11 but replace the concavity assumption of the production function by a convex–concave shape:

$$F(0) = 0, \quad F'(K) > 0, \quad F''(K) \begin{Bmatrix} > \\ = \\ < \end{Bmatrix} 0 \text{ for } K \begin{Bmatrix} < \\ = \\ > \end{Bmatrix} \bar{K}. \tag{5.13}$$

Show that if we assume the validity of the Inada-conditions (see Exercise 3.11), (5.13) implies the existence of two interior equilibria (as well as a boundary equilibrium $\hat{K} = 0$).

Prove that the "middle" equilibrium is an unstable focus, while the "upper" and the "boundary" equilibria have saddle properties. Can a node be excluded? Sketch a phase portrait and give an economic interpretation of the optimal consumption path. Use Lagrangian techniques described in Sect. 3.6.1 to cope with the mixed path constraint. Note that the left branch of the trajectory was presented incorrectly by Skiba (1978) (see Feichtinger and Hartl 1986, pp. 418–420 for a correct proof).

5.7 (Moving to Opportunity). One of the targets of US housing policy is to deconcentrate poverty. The *Moving to Opportunity for Fair Housing Program* directed by the US Department of Housing and Urban Development attempts to place poor families in middle-class neighborhoods.

Denote the proportion of middle-class families at time t by $X(t)$. The policy variable is the rate $u(t)$ at which poor families are placed in the neighborhoods.

The state dynamics of the housing mobility program,

$$\dot{X} = aX(1 - X) - \beta u + \gamma X u \tag{5.14}$$

consists of three flows

- An autonomous growth term assumed as logistic growth
- A "middle-class flight" term proportional to the inflow of poor people[6]
- An "assimilation" term,[7] $\gamma X u$

The objective is to place a compromise between placing poor families (u) and retain middle-class residents (X) as socially beneficial, and tax payers. Assuming quadratic moving costs, the target is

$$\max_{u(\cdot)\geq 0} \int_0^\infty \mathrm{e}^{-rt}(u - cu^2 + \rho X)\mathrm{d}t$$

s.t. (5.14), an initial condition $X(0) = X_0 \in (0, 1)$, and a pure state constraint $0 \leq X(t) \leq 1$.

Show the existence of a DNSS point separating initial conditions, in which the optimal policy leads to substantial middle-class flight, from those conditions in which the optimal policy leads to a stronger middle class population; see Caulkins, Feichtinger, Johnson, Tragler, and Yegorov (2005) for details of this model of controlled migration.

---

[6] That term addresses the lack of tolerance of social groups. Schelling (1971) was perhaps the first who wrote about (racial) segregation and the propensity of residents to flee neighborhoods.

[7] This term refers to the influence the existing stock of middle-class residents exerts on the incoming poor families to "assimilate."

Notes and Further Reading

The neoclassical optimal growth model of Cass (1965) and Koopmans (1965) predicts that countries will converge to a common standard of living. Empirical evidence, however, suggests diverse growth paths. The heterogeneity in growth patterns can be modeled by including the possibility of multiple equilibria, indifference points, and history-dependence.

Skiba (1978) did this by extending the Ramsey model to include a convex–concave production function, obtaining an unstable focus and a threshold separating two saddle point equilibria. Compare also Brock and Malliaris (1989, Chap. 6), in which the threshold was called a "Skiba point." (See Exercise 5.6.)

Skiba's analysis had some deficiencies. The first exact proof of the existence of a "Skiba point" was given by Dechert and Nishimura (1983); compare also Dechert (1983). Independently, Sethi (1977, 1979a) studied multiple equilibria in the context of most rapid approach paths. Other early references on multiple equilibria are Brock (1983) and Brock and Dechert (1985).

Multiple equilibria may provide an explanation for the existence of poverty traps and the development of "miracles." (See the endogenous-growth literature initiated by Lucas, 1988 and Romer, 1990.)

If there is an externality, rational agents will forecast its evolution. Depending upon the initial conditions, this can give rise to different expectations and long-run outcomes. This point was first made in Krugman (1991). A more recent application to CO_2 permits can be found in Liski (2001).

It is now recognized that multiple equilibria occur in many other contexts as will subsequently be shown. For example Brock and Starrett (1999) considered the dynamics and optimal management of a shallow lake. Internal loading of phosphorus in shallow lakes causes nonlinearities, multiple equilibria, and DNSS points. Their paper has been extended by including a number of communities that use the lake as a resource and waste sink. Mäler, Xepapadeas, and de Zeeuw (2003) showed that the initial level of accumulated phosphorus determines whether a lake will end up in a turbid state. Note that although the analysis focused on a shallow lake, the methodology applies to all models that are driven by convex–concave relations.

In the context of addiction, Becker and Murphy (1988) noted the general possibility of thresholds separating multiple equilibria. However, the linear–quadratic framework they used precluded their occurrence. That limitation was overcome by the model of Orphanides and Zervos (1998), who used a generalized nonlinear framework with convex–concave preferences. Here, three equilibria exist, the middle one being unstable. At the lower equilibrium, there is no drug consumption. At the higher one, there is addiction. In response to small shocks in drug consumption or to the impact of enforcement policies, the system can converge toward one or the other of these two equilibria. The threshold separating the optimal trajectories leading to either the lower or the higher stable equilibrium does not necessarily coincide with the middle unstable one. For a recent related contribution, see Gavrila, Feichtinger, Tragler, Hartl, and Kort (2005).

Schelling (1967, 1973) provided an interesting early analysis of multiple equilibria and history-dependence. The Nobel laureate assumed that the probability that an agent engages in an illegal transaction increases with the total number of agents that also engage in the transaction. This results in three equilibrium points, two stable boundary ones – corresponding, respectively, to a "clean" and a "dirty society"

– and an unstable interior tipping point. In this context Andvig (1991) introduced what he called a Schelling diagram to explain observed variations in corruption frequency, and gave several other examples of multiple equilibria in the context of the economics of crime.

In a certain sense Chap. 5 may be conceived of as a dynamic extension of Schelling's static considerations. The appearance of ratios of variables in a model may lead to multiple equilibria. For example, the effect of enforcement depends on the amount of law enforcement effort relative to the size of the population of offenders, i.e., on the per capita enforcement effort. This mechanism has been named *enforcement swamping* in the context of crime and illicit drug consumption; see Kleiman (1993), Caulkins (1993), Caulkins et al. (2000), Feichtinger, Grienauer, and Tragler (2002), and Tragler, Caulkins, and Feichtinger (2001). This dependency implies multiple equilibria, unstable nodes or focuses, and weak DNSS points. The result is fairly general. The use in the objective function of "per capita" quantities, generically defined as a control variable divided by a state variable, usually generates a convexity of the Hamiltonian with respect to the state and may easily lead to multiple equilibria.

Another interesting field of application of the "per capita" threshold-generating mechanism relates to adjustment costs. See the framework in Feichtinger, Hartl, Kort, and Wirl (2001) and Hartl, Kort, Feichtinger, and Wirl (2004).

Usually nonconcavity is considered to be the property that causes the long-term behavior to depend on the initial state. This history-dependence due to "increasing returns" or "positive feedbacks" plays a central role in many policy-related discussions, ranging from the choice of a technology to differences in economic development.

However, this traditional road is not the only route to multiple equilibria, since a strictly concave framework does not rule out history-dependent outcomes. This result may appear surprising, and it has been largely overlooked in the economic literature; compare, however, the early contributions of Kurz (1968) and Liviatan and Samuelson (1969), and, more recently, Feichtinger and Wirl (2000), Feichtinger et al. (2002), and Wirl and Feichtinger (2005).

A survey on multiple equilibria and history-dependence, including thresholds in concave models, is given by Deissenberg, Feichtinger, Semmler, and Wirl (2004), but let us briefly mention a few more examples.

Caulkins et al. (2006) examined optimal spending for drug-substitution programs in the context of a dynamic epidemic model of both drug use and drug use-related infections. They showed that the optimal spending for drug-substitution programs may depend on such initial conditions as the number of drug users and the number of infected users. It turned out that the optimal long-run solution may be characterized by a relatively large amount spent for drug-substitution programs and by a small number of drug users, or vice versa.

While there exist abundant applications with one-state variables, there are only a few studies using *two-state* models. Feichtinger and Steindl (2006) investigated the bifurcation behavior of an production/inventory model close to a Hamilton–Hopf bifurcation. They found different types of DNSS curves separating either the domain of attraction of the steady and oscillatory solutions or the trajectories to the same periodic solution. This discovery of *multiple DNSS curves* delivers a new family of optimal production policies. The existence of threshold indifference points, from which three different paths emanate exhibiting the same minimal value of the discounted cost stream, illustrates the complex structure of the stable manifolds and

DNSS curves. It is remarkable that such a complex behavior occurs in a "standard" model of production planning, the so-called *intensity-splitting* model, which is separable and has only a nonconcavity resulting from concave–convex production costs; see Feichtinger and Sorger (1986) and Feichtinger, Kistner, and Luhmer (1988).

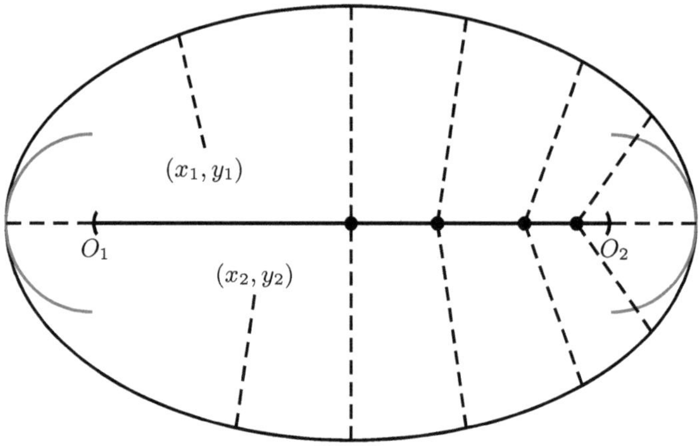

Fig. 5.10. The problem depicted is to determine the directions of minimal distance from points to an ellipse. The corresponding connections are given by the *dashed lines.* For points lying on the major axis between the center of the osculation circles $O_{1,2} = \left(\pm(a^2 - b^2)/a, 0\right)$ (shown on the *right side*) two such directions exist and therefore constitute a Maxwell set. In contrast, for every other point a unique direction exists, pointed out for the points (x_i, y_i), $i = 1, 2$. As this problem can be formulated as an optimal control problem, where the optimal trajectories are exactly the connecting lines and the optimal controls are the directions, the Maxwell set coincides with the set of DNSS points. Note that $O_{1,2}$ are not DNSS points

Hartl, Kort, and Feichtinger (2003) studied the tradeoff between the benefits and costs of preventing offenses and treating offenders. Starting with an age-structured epidemiological model (see Sect. 8.3.2), they analyzed a two-state compartment model in which multiple equilibria were identified: a "law-and-order" equilibrium (with no offenders), a "conservative" equilibrium (with few offenders), and a "liberal" equilibrium (with many offenders). Remarkably, the authors derived a kind of indifference property for this finite time horizon problem.

Asking why politics makes strange bedfellows, Caulkins, Hartl, Tragler, and Feichtinger (2001) computed DNSS curves in a more straightforward way than usual. The curves show an interesting spiral structure.

Caulkins, Hartl, Kort, and Feichtinger (2007) tried to explain why there are fashion cycles. They considered the problem of a fashion trend-setter confronting an imitator who could produce the same product at lower cost. Remarkably, the authors derived an analytic expression for a DNSS curve.

Hof and Wirl (2008) analyzed a multiple equilibria version of the Ramsey model.

For higher-dimensional problems there may exist a whole set of DNSS points. In Wagener (2006) and Pampel (2000) it was proved, at least in a special case, that under convenient assumptions these sets can (locally) be classified as DNSS curves (two-dimensional state space) or DNSS manifolds (higher-dimensional state space). Besides these numerical results, only a few theoretical propositions on the existence and appearance of DNSS points exist (see, e.g., Wagener, 2003) in the optimal control literature. Note that according to Wagener's conjecture, in the two-dimensional case there exists generically no indifference point of higher multiplicity than three.

Although there exists no comprehensive theory analyzing DNSS points in the optimal control literature, Arnold, Goryunov, Lyashko, and Vasiliev (1993) studied the problem of multiple maximum (minimum) points in detail for the theory of smooth manifolds, where, e.g., points of minimal energy (physics) or minimal distance (geometry) are considered. In this context these sets of multiple solutions are called *Maxwell sets*. For an example see Fig. 5.10. But a full mathematical comparison of the concepts of DNSS points and Maxwell points has not yet been carried out as far as we know.

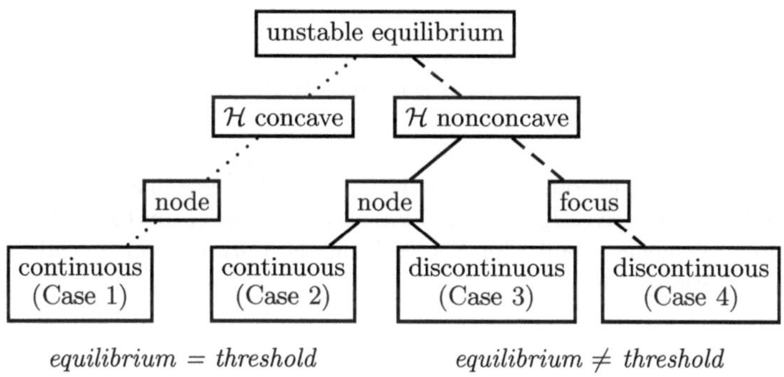

Fig. 5.11. Possible cases with respect to the unstable equilibrium; case 1 is Wirl and Feichtinger (2005), case 4 is the well-known scenario and the cases 2 and 3 are scenarios discovered by Hartl et al. (2004)

Hartl et al. (2004) derived an interesting tree diagram showing the relation between the (non)concavity of the Hamiltonian, the instability of nodes and foci, and the possibility of jumps (see Fig. 5.11)

If the Hamiltonian is concave in an unstable state, this equilibrium is a node, the function describing the initial control in respect to the initial state (*policy function*) is continuous, and the threshold coincides with the equilibria (see the dotted branch in Fig. 5.11). If the unstable equilibrium is situated in the nonconcave domain of the Hamiltonian, it can either be a node or a focus. In the literature, an unstable equilibrium is mostly assumed to be a focus, which leads to a discontinuous policy function and to a threshold different from the unstable equilibrium; see the dashed branch in Fig. 5.11. However, Hartl et al. (2004) show that the unstable equilibrium can also be a node and a further and rather subtle differentiation has to be made. In particular, a node in the nonconcave domain can sometimes exhibit characteristics similar to the node in the concave domain, i.e., continuity of the policy function and no point of indeterminancy. This contrasts with many claims found in the literature.

But such a node can also be associated also with a discontinuous policy function, while losing its equilibrium property.

To summarize, of the four possible outcomes shown at the bottom in Fig. 5.11, only one is found in the literature. Note that case 3 refers to the existence of a node with an overlapping region and a discontinuity (compare also Fig. 5.5b). Furthermore, the differentiation between concave vs. nonconcave Hamiltonians seems not to be the appropriate one and neither is the one between node and focus. The proper classification is to differentiate between continuous and discontinuous policies. Continuous policies, which require the unstable equilibrium to be optimal (an equilibrium), are ensured by concavity but are possible in nonconcave models too.

We have to admit that the definition presented here of a DNSS point may not be the end of the story. In fact, this could be seen as the initial point for further and deeper investigations, because the mathematical claim of soundness requires a definition encompassing even degenerate cases. However this multiplicity is well-known in applications where degenerate cases are of minor interest and mathematical sophistication does not necessarily lead to a better understanding for students. Hence our somewhat less formal approach suits our needs and, we believe, most of the problems appearing in the economic literature. What the present definition really lacks is verification of its mathematical significance and a connection with other analytical properties of the solution sets that would provide new insights into the phenomenon of history-dependent solutions.

We wish to thank Florian Wagener and Vladimir Veliov for providing their own results on the phenomenon of critical points. The formulations discussed here originate from their investigations and intensive discussions on this subject. We also owe Florian Wagener thanks for his work on the optimal vector field and on the DNSS bifurcation.

Part III

Advanced Topics

6

Higher-Dimensional Models

The theory of optimal control is wonderful. Now, how does one actually apply it? In particular, how does one compute the solutions numerically, including for higher-dimensional systems (since solving these systems can substantially be harder than solving one-dimensional models)? This third part of the book sheds light on the practical side of applying optimal control theory.

By "practical side" we still mean mathematical calculations, not political or organizational issues associated with persuading decision-makers to implement a solution or even statistical issues associated with data collection and model parameterization. Too often, however, texts on optimal control tell the reader *what* to do but not *how* or even *when* and *why* to do it.

The "practical side" of how to solve optimal control problems involves writing computer programs because few models have analytic solutions. The "when and why" questions concern how to organize all of the components of an overall analysis. Given a particular mathematical formulation, what does one do first? What second? What does one do when one analytic strategy hits a dead end? We illustrate how to answer such questions with three innovative examples that are worked in depth.[1] We offer one example each from the three main application areas discussed in this book: drug control, corruption, and counter-terror.

This chapter presents the model formulations and meta-analytic strategies employed to analyze them. Points in the analysis that require nontrivial computations are flagged, with a reference forward to the following chapter on numerical methods. In that subsequent Chap. 7, the discussion walks the reader step by step through the details of how to do computations of that sort, including references to the computer code available on the companion Web site for performing these numerical calculations.

[1] The example in Sect. 6.1 is also partially empirically validated.

6.1 Controlling Drug Consumption

This section illustrates the application of Pontryagin's Maximum Principle and the analytical investigation of the quality of the long-run equilibrium with a real-world policy problem pertaining to control of illicit drugs.[2]

6.1.1 Model of Controlled Drug Demand

A fundamental question of drug policy is how scarce resources should be allocated between different drug control programs, e.g., source country control, interdiction, or different forms of domestic control (such as prevention, treatment or domestic enforcement). Hence there is ongoing interest in understanding how much we can save (in terms of lives, grams of consumption, or cost to the society) per dollar invested in each of these control programs. The trouble is, however, that (illicit) drug use and associated problems change over time, so no single, *static* strategy always saves more lives, averts more grams consumed, or avoids more cost to society (or the government) than any other, and, thus, is always "best." Rather the optimal mix of interventions should *vary over time*. Behrens et al. (1999, 2000b) sought to help inform such thinking by starting with the LH-model of heterogeneous drug demand discussed in Sect. 2.7 and augmenting it to include two demand side controls representing spending on drug prevention and treatment, respectively.

1. Spending on prevention (denoted by w) such as school-based prevention programs, after school programs, Red Ribbon weeks, etc., is assumed to reduce initiation into drug use, as defined by (2.37), down to some fraction ψ of its baseline level, $I(L, H) = \tau + sL\mathrm{e}^{-q\frac{H}{L}}$. Even the very best programs only cut initiation by a modest amount (depending on the substance, reductions are typically on the order of one-sixth). Furthermore, if policy can target first the groups at highest risk of initiating drug use, one would expect the first dollars invested in prevention to produce bigger effects than later dollars. That is one would expect ψ to be a smooth convex function of prevention spending w. A simple smooth function that captures such diminishing returns to scale is an exponential decay approaching an asymptotic value h

$$\psi(w) = h + (1-h)\,\mathrm{e}^{-mw}, \tag{6.1}$$

   where
   - h is the minimum percentage to which initiation can be cut down by prevention.
   - m is a constant measuring the efficiency of prevention spending.

   Based on Caulkins et al. (1999), Behrens et al. (2000b) estimated the parameter values $h = 0.84$ and $m = 2.37 \times 10^{-9}$.

[2] The model is parametrized for cocaine use in the US for 1967–1992; 1996.

2. As in the one state drug control model discussed in Sects. 2.9 and 3.9, treatment is modeled as increasing the outflow from drug use, in this case the outflow from heavy use, H, at a per capita rate that is a concave function of treatment spending u per (heavy) user. In particular,

$$\beta(H, u) = c\left(\frac{u}{H+\varepsilon}\right)^d \tag{6.2}$$

- c is a constant measuring the efficiency of treatment.
- d is a constant measuring the extent to which expansions in treatment spending retain that efficiency as opposed to suffering from diminishing returns.

To be consistent with parallel work Tragler, Caulkins, and Feichtinger (2001) and Behrens et al. (2000b) set the diminishing returns to treatment parameter to $d = 0.6$. Based on Rydell, Caulkins, and Everingham (1996) they estimate $c = 5 \times 10^{-4}$. The constant $\varepsilon = 10^{-5}$ is a mathematical convenience that avoids the possibility of dividing by zero; its specific value has essentially no effect on the results at all. (Note: since for our parameter values the long-run equilibrium is located comfortably within the admissible range for state and control variables, one can even use $\varepsilon = 0$.)

The policy-maker or regulating authority is modeled as wanting to minimize the sum of the social costs caused by illicit drug use and the monetary costs of the control measures. Heavy users generate more social costs per capita than do light users, so social costs are assumed to be proportional to consumption measured in grams rather than to the total number of users. In particular, a constant social cost per gram consumed (estimated to be $\kappa = 113$ dollars per gram[3]) is multiplied by the total quantity consumed, denoted by Q, which is computed as the weighted sum of the number of light and heavy users,

$$Q = k_L L + k_H H, \tag{6.3}$$

with weights equal to the average annual consumption rates of light and heavy users. Rydell et al. (1996) reported those to be $k_L = 16.42$ and $k_H = 118.93$ grams per year, respectively. So the decision-maker can be modeled as seeking to minimize the entire discounted stream of costs associated with illicit drug use

$$V(u(\cdot), w(\cdot)) = \int_0^\infty \mathrm{e}^{-rt}\left(\kappa Q + u + w\right) \mathrm{d}t, \tag{6.4}$$

where $u(t)$ and $w(t)$ denote the expenditures on treatment and prevention programs at time t, respectively, $r = 0.04$ is the discount rate, and Q denotes total annual consumption in grams (6.3).

Ideally the government would be free to choose whatever controls $u(\cdot)$ and $w(\cdot)$ minimize (6.4), but public budgeting is sometimes reactive, responding to

[3] This is a political parameter ranging for different states from \$50 to \$500 per gram.

existing problems, not proactive. This tendency to respond to the problem of the day may imply that society allocates drug-control resources in proportion to the current magnitude of the drug problem. Therefore we consider the drug-control budget in (6.4) to be proportional to total current consumption, i.e.,

$$u + w = \gamma Q. \tag{6.5}$$

Behrens et al. (2000b) estimate that $\gamma = 5.31$ dollars are spent on both treatment and prevention per gram consumed. Thus the total drug-control budget is not assumed to be constant and thus frozen at a particular level, but rather is fixed in terms of being proportional to the current drug demand, γQ. The control budget's allocation between treatment and prevention can, however, be varied at each instant of time.[4]

With budget rule (6.5) we can replace prevention spending with "non-treatment spending," $w = \gamma Q - u$, and the optimization problem becomes a nonlinear control problem with a single scalar control, u, and two states, L and H, where the policy-maker is modeled as wanting to solve:

$$\max_{u(\cdot)} \left\{ -(\kappa + \gamma) \int_0^\infty \mathrm{e}^{-rt} Q \, \mathrm{d}t \right\} \tag{6.6a}$$

$$\text{s.t.} \quad \dot{L} = \psi(w)\, I(L, H) - (a + b)L, \quad L(0) = L_0, \tag{6.6b}$$

$$\dot{H} = bL - gH - \beta(H, u)H, \quad H(0) = H_0 \tag{6.6c}$$

$$u \geq 0, \tag{6.6d}$$

$$\gamma Q - u \geq 0 \tag{6.6e}$$

with initiation function

$$I(L, H) = \tau + sL\mathrm{e}^{-q\frac{H}{L}}$$

as defined in the uncontrolled case, (2.37) and Q defined by (6.3).

Remark 6.1. From a numerical point of view it is advisable to replace the constraint (6.6d) with

$$u \geq k_0 > 0,$$

where k_0 is some positive constant, since at $u = 0$ the dynamics of the control (6.11b) exhibits a singularity and will therefore entail numerical difficulties. Decreasing k_0 to zero approximates the solution for $k_0 = 0$.

[4] The original analysis reported in Behrens (1998) and Behrens et al. (2000b) also analyzed two other budget rules, including unconstrained control spending. This represented a sort of structural sensitivity analysis with respect to the consequences of different budgeting strategies. While the results are quite interesting for substantive purposes, those extra analyzes are not needed here to illustrate how to solve optimal control problems of this sort, and so we confine ourselves to this one budget allocation model.

6.1.2 Deriving the Canonical System

Since we have to consider mixed path constraints as defined by (6.6d) and (6.6e), we analyze the form of the canonical system for control values lying in the interior and at the boundary of the control set separately.

Control Values in the Interior

The analysis proceeds as described in Chap. 3, where $\mathcal{H}$ denotes the Hamiltonian and λ_1 and λ_2 denote the costate variables with respect to L and H, respectively, all in current-values

$$\mathcal{H} = \lambda_0(\kappa + \gamma)\left(-k_L L - k_H H\right) + \lambda_1 \dot{L} + \lambda_2 \dot{H}.$$

Remark 6.2. We restrict our analysis to the normal case, i.e., $\lambda_0 = 1$, even though we have to admit the $\lambda_0 = 0$ cannot principally excluded (see Exercise 6.1).

Remark 6.3. Since the derivatives of the (negative) cost function in (6.6a) with respect to the states are both negative along the optimal path, i.e.,

$$-\frac{\partial(\kappa+\gamma)\left(k_L L + k_H H\right)}{\partial L} < 0, \quad \text{and} \quad -\frac{\partial(\kappa+\gamma)\left(k_L L + k_H H\right)}{\partial H} < 0,$$

the economic interpretation of the costates as imputed values or shadow prices of an additional light and heavy user, respectively, and (3.11) tell us that λ_1 and λ_2 are negative (see Theorem 3.54 on the signs of the costate variables). This means that even though the optimal values for L and H, and thus optimally controlled prevalence, may increase over time, an additional user is always "bad" in terms of the objective because its "value" is negative.

The Hamiltonian maximizing condition for optimal interior control values, $u^* = u^*(L, H, \lambda_1, \lambda_2)$, is given by

$$\mathcal{H}_u = \lambda_1 I \psi_u - \lambda_2 H \beta_u = 0, \tag{6.7}$$

together with the Legendre–Clebsch condition

$$\mathcal{H}_{uu} = \lambda_1 I \psi_{uu} - \lambda_2 H \beta_{uu} \le 0. \tag{6.8}$$

An immediate calculation proves that for $h, d < 1$, $\lambda_1, \lambda_2 < 0$, and $L, H > 0$ (6.8) satisfies the strict inequality for all u, and thus a unique interior optimal control value for (6.7) exists.

Remark 6.4. Equation (6.7) reveals that the intertemporal optimal drug control requires that at any instant of time the value that the decision-maker assigns to the change in incidence (due to prevention) just balances the value that the decision-maker assigns to the change in the number of heavy users (due to treatment).

The following two differential equations determine the evolution of the costates λ_1 and λ_2 (which can be interpreted as the changes in the values of an additional light and heavy user, respectively), where the notation is simplified by

$$\begin{aligned}
&\Xi(L,H,u^*) := I_L\psi + I\psi_L - (a+b)\\
&\Sigma(H,u^*) := g + (1+d)\beta > 0\\
&\Pi(L,H,u^*) := I_H\psi + I\psi_H < 0, \text{ yielding}
\end{aligned}$$

$$\dot{\lambda}_1 = r\lambda_1 - \mathcal{H}_L = k_L(\kappa+\gamma) + (r - \Xi(L,H,u^*))\lambda_1 - b\lambda_2 \tag{6.9a}$$

$$\dot{\lambda}_2 = r\lambda_2 - \mathcal{H}_H = k_H(\kappa+\gamma) - \Pi(L,H,u^*)\lambda_1 + (r + \Sigma(H,u^*))\lambda_2. \tag{6.9b}$$

The optimal control value u^* is only implicitly determined by (6.7) and cannot be replaced by a closed-form representation. This implies that the canonical system (6.6b), (6.6c), (6.9a) and (6.9b) is also only implicitly given. A way to avoid this inconvenience is to transfer the canonical system from the state–costate space into the state-(costate-)control space, or in our case from the $(L, H, \lambda_1, \lambda_2)$-space, into the (L, H, λ_1, u)-space using the following procedure (see also Sect. 7.3). We start by determining the total time derivative of the Hamiltonian maximizing condition (6.7) and replacing λ_2 by $\lambda_1\zeta$, where

$$\zeta := \frac{I\psi_u}{H\beta_u}. \tag{6.10}$$

Solving the resulting equation for $\dot{u}$ yields a differential equation for the control variable, which allows us, together with $\lambda_2 = \zeta\lambda_1$ to replace (6.9a) and (6.9b) by

$$\dot{\lambda}_1 = k_L(\kappa+\gamma) + (r - \Xi - b\zeta)\lambda_1 \tag{6.11a}$$

$$\dot{u} = \frac{1}{\zeta_u}\left(\frac{k_H - k_L\zeta}{\lambda_1}(\kappa+\gamma) - \Pi + (b\zeta + \Sigma + \Xi)\zeta - \zeta_L\dot{L} - \zeta_H\dot{H}\right). \tag{6.11b}$$

Remark 6.5. The continuous differentiability of $u(\cdot)$ is assured as long as the strict Legendre–Clebsch condition is satisfied. Since in that case the formula for implicit differentiation provides the continuous derivative for $u(\cdot)$ (see also the regularity assumption in Theorem 4.33 of the calculus of variations).

Remark 6.6. We cannot prove that the necessary conditions are sufficient. Therefore, when proceeding with the analysis, we keep in mind this limitation when it comes to interpretation.

Control Values at the Boundary

To determine the form of the canonical system for solutions exhibiting a boundary arc (see Sect. 3.6.1), we have to consider the Lagrangian

$$\mathcal{L} = \mathcal{H} + \mu_1 u + \mu_2 \left(\gamma \left(k_L L + k_H H\right) - u\right).$$

The constraint qualification (3.48) is satisfied, since the corresponding matrix,

$$\begin{pmatrix} 1 & u & 0 \\ -1 & 0 & \gamma \left(k_L L + k_H H\right) - u \end{pmatrix},$$

has full rank. Thus we can use Pontryagin's Maximum Principle Theorem 3.60 to derive the necessary conditions.

Obviously the control constraints cannot be simultaneously active as long as $L,\ H > 0$. We can therefore consider both cases separately. From

$$\mathcal{L}_u = 0$$

we find explicit representations of the Lagrange multipliers as follows

$$\begin{aligned} \mu_1 &= -\mathcal{H}_u \\ \mu_2 &= \mathcal{H}_u. \end{aligned}$$

Hence for $u^* = 0$ the canonical systems in the state–costate space reads as

$$\dot{L} = \psi\left(\gamma\left(k_L L + k_H H\right)\right) I(L,H) - (a+b)L \tag{6.12a}$$

$$\dot{H} = bL - gH \tag{6.12b}$$

$$\dot{\lambda}_1 = k_L\left(\kappa+\gamma\right) + \left(r - \varXi\left(L,H,0\right)\right)\lambda_1 - b\lambda_2 \tag{6.12c}$$

$$\dot{\lambda}_2 = k_H\left(\kappa+\gamma\right) - \varPi\left(L,H,0\right)\lambda_1 + \left(r + \varSigma\left(H,0\right)\right)\lambda_2, \tag{6.12d}$$

and for $u^* = \gamma\left(k_L L + k_H H\right)$ as

$$\begin{aligned} \dot{L} &= I(L,H) - (a+b)L \\ \dot{H} &= bL - gH - \beta(H,u^*) \\ \dot{\lambda}_1 &= k_L\left(\kappa+\gamma\right) + \left(r - \varXi\left(L,H,u^*\right)\right)\lambda_1 - b\lambda_2 \\ \dot{\lambda}_2 &= k_H\left(\kappa+\gamma\right) - \varPi\left(L,H,u^*\right)\lambda_1 + \left(r + \varSigma\left(H,u^*\right)\right)\lambda_2. \end{aligned}$$

Remark 6.7. Note that a transition into the (L,H,λ_1,u^*)-space is not necessary here, because at the boundary arc u^* is explicitly be given (either $u^* = 0$ or $u^* = \gamma\left(k_L L + k_H H\right)$).

Additionally, the slackness conditions

$$\mu_1 u^* \geq 0, \quad \text{and} \quad \mu_2\left(\gamma\left(k_L L + k_H H\right) - u^*\right) \geq 0,$$

and nonnegativity conditions

$$\mu_1 \geq 0, \quad \text{and} \quad \mu_2 \geq 0,$$

have to be satisfied.

Table 6.1. Set of base-case parameter values chosen by Behrens et al. (1999, 2000b) in consideration of Caulkins (1996); Office of National Drug Control Policy (1996); Rydell et al. (1996) and Rydell and Everingham (1994) to model the US cocaine epidemic

a	b	g	s	q	τ	c	d	h	m	r	γ	κ
0.163	0.024	0.062	0.61	7.00	5×10^4	5×10^{-4}	0.60	0.84	2.37×10^{-9}	0.04	5.31	1.13×10^2

6.1.3 The Endemic Level of Drug Demand

As is commonly the case, it is useful to start investigating the dynamics of a system by looking for equilibria of the canonical system. One can determine these equilibrium values by solving the nonlinear algebraic equations obtained by setting the differential equations of the canonical system to zero. In doing this one should try to proceed with the analysis as far as possible without specifying the parameter values. The next section on corruption gives a good example of when this is fruitful. However, the complex functional forms needed to adequately represent real world problems often make it impossible to follow this analytical track very far. Here that is the case. Therefore, we proceed with the numerical problem for parameter values given by Table 6.1.

Determining the Equilibrium

Finding roots numerically can be tricky (see Sect. 7.4.1). In this case the system (6.6b), (6.6c), (6.11a) and (6.11b) yields the following equilibrium in the positive section of the state–control-space:

$$\hat{E} = \begin{pmatrix} \hat{L} \\ \hat{H} \\ \hat{\lambda}_1 \\ \hat{u}^* \end{pmatrix} = \begin{pmatrix} 347,474 \\ 124,354 \\ -36,863 \\ 5,890,747 \end{pmatrix}.$$

The eigenvalues ξ_i, $i = 1, 2, 3, 4$, of the linearized system around this equilibrium are found to be conjugate complex, one pair having positive, one having negative real parts. The reader is invited to check this result numerically in Exercise 6.1. Hence $\hat{E}$ is hyperbolic and of saddle-type, exhibiting transient oscillations. Since the values of parameters are never known with certainty, hyperbolicity is of importance. This assures that modest changes in parameter values do not alter the stability properties of the equilibrium (see Sect. 2.6.2). Note that the equilibrium shadow price of an additional heavy user,λ_2, and equilibrium treatment spending, $\hat{w}^*$, can be computed using (6.10) and (6.5), respectively

$$\hat{\lambda}_2 = \frac{I(\hat{L},\hat{H})\psi_u\left(\gamma\left(k_L\hat{L}+k_H\hat{H}\right)\right)}{\hat{H}\beta_u(\hat{w}^*,\hat{H})}\hat{\lambda}_1 = -11,499$$

$$\hat{w}^* = \gamma\left(k_L\hat{L}+k_H\hat{H}\right) - \hat{u}^* = 102,937,557.$$

Comparing the Result with the "Real World" Problem

Having calculated the equilibrium values, it is natural to compare those values with current values observed from the system in the real world. In this case the levels of equilibrium drug use are far less than contemporary levels in the US. Likewise, equilibrium prevention spending $\hat{w}^*$ is quite small relative to current prevention, and treatment spending per capita $\hat{u}^*$ is also slightly below current rates. Hence, in the model's long-run equilibrium, it is optimal to spend less per user on demand-side control than is being spent now. Thus the first conclusion is that in this model it is never optimal to use prevention and treatment to push the final state of the epidemic (i.e., its endemic level) to a place very different from where it would go "naturally."

If control is not what pushes drug use below current levels, what does? Recall that in this model initiation can be tempered by a bad reputation for a drug if most current users are heavy or dependent users (cf. Sect. 2.7). Once this feedback effect of heavy use on initiation is included, the system gravitates toward a relatively low level of equilibrium drug use on its own. That equilibrium is fairly "stubborn" (in part because of the constant inflow τ of initiation by "innovators"), and so it is not worth trying to use treatment or prevention to suppress it much further; at least not if the social cost per gram consumed is equal to $\kappa = 113$. We can examine how characteristics of the equilibrium depend on the other model parameter values; but because little control is used in an equilibrium, the results are not so different from those reported in Sect. 2.7.

The values ($\hat{u}^*$, $\hat{w}^*$) are assumed as the optimal controls for the initial states (L_0, H_0) = ($\hat{L}$, $\hat{H}$). Strictly speaking its optimality has to be proved, since the equilibrium only satisfies the necessary conditions (see Remark 6.6). In what follows we assume its optimality and determine paths converging to this long-run optimal solution starting at different initial positions.

6.1.4 Optimal Dynamic Policy away from the Endemic State

That a control plays a minor role in an equilibrium does not imply that it is generally unimportant. On the contrary – control could still play a crucial role in determining the transient path leading toward the equilibrium. One way to test this proposition is to assess the effect on the objective function of beginning optimal control at different points in the drug epidemic.

Therefore, we calculate the total discounted cost caused by the drug epidemic as a function of T_0, where T_0 denotes the time when prevention and treatment interventions begin. To compute this graph, we run the *uncontrolled model* for T_0 years, leading to a particular and uniquely defined state $(L(T_0), H(T_0))$ at time T_0, keeping track of the discounted amount of drug use and, hence, social cost along the (uncontrolled) way. Next, starting with that state, $(L(T_0), H(T_0))$, as the initial condition, we run the optimally controlled allocation problem with the standard infinite planning-horizon assumption, also keeping track of discounted social cost plus cost of control.

Computing the Path Leading to the Endemic State

The specific question to answer is, how to solve the optimal control problem (6.6) for the initial states $(L_0, H_0) = (L(T_0), H(T_0))$, because "running the optimal control model" differs from "running the uncontrolled model." Whereas in the uncontrolled case we have two differential equations and two initial conditions, in the optimally controlled model we have four differential equations plus information on the two initial states and also the terminal conditions, that the solution converges to the equilibrium. Thus we solve a BVP, where the infinite time horizon is replaced by some finite horizon t_e and the terminal conditions are replaced by asymptotic boundary conditions, which assure that the solution lies time t_e at the local stable manifold of the equilibrium, as explained in Sect. 7.4.1. Therefore the following steps have to be accomplished.

Determining the Asymptotic Boundary Condition

First we have to find a condition guaranteeing that we reach the stable eigenspace $\mathrm{E}^s(\hat{E})$ of the equilibrium $\hat{E}$. Owing to Proposition 7.20 we therefore have to determine the eigenvectors of the transposed matrix $\hat{J}'$ for the eigenvalues with positive real part, where $\hat{J}$ is the Jacobian evaluated at the equilibrium $\hat{E}$. In our case there exist two conjugate complex eigenvectors ν and $\bar{\nu}$. Therefore we only have to consider the real and imaginary part of one of these eigenvectors, yielding

$$\nu = \begin{pmatrix} -0.0108 - 0.0846\mathrm{i} \\ 0.1399 + 0.3950\mathrm{i} \\ 0.9039 \\ -0.0002 - 0.0002\mathrm{i} \end{pmatrix}.$$

Then the matrix

$$F = \begin{pmatrix} \operatorname{Re}\nu' \\ \operatorname{Im}\nu' \end{pmatrix} = \begin{pmatrix} -0.0108 & 0.1399 & 0.9039 & -0.0002 \\ -0.0846 & 0.3950 & 0 & -0.0002 \end{pmatrix},$$

determines the stable eigenspace $\mathrm{E}^s(\hat{E})$ by

$$\mathrm{E}^s(\hat{E}) = \{X \in \mathbb{R}^4 : F(X - \hat{E}) = 0\},$$

with $X = (L, H, \lambda_1, u^*)$. The condition at infinity, that the trajectory converges to the equilibrium $\hat{E}$, is replaced by the condition $X(t_e) \in \mathrm{E}^s(\hat{E})$ for the finite time t_e, which can always be normalized to 1 (see Sect. 7.1.4)

$$F(X(1) - \hat{E}) = 0.$$

Denoting the dynamics of the canonical system for interior control values by $f^I(X)$ the BVP becomes

$$\begin{aligned} \dot{X} &= t_e f^I(X),\ t \in [0,\, 1] \\ X_1(0) &= L_0,\ X_2(0) = H_0 \\ F(X(1) &- \hat{E}) = 0. \end{aligned}$$

Carrying out the Continuation of the Optimal Solution

Next we want to answer, how to proceed, if we want to find the optimal path starting, e.g., at

$$A_1 = \begin{pmatrix} L_0 \\ H_0 \end{pmatrix} = \begin{pmatrix} 2 \times 10^6 \\ 1 \times 10^5 \end{pmatrix}.$$

The only solution for the BVP, that we already established, is the "trivial" equilibrium solution. Therefore we numerically solve the BVP, starting at the equilibrium $\hat{E}$ and continuing the solution, by means of one of the continuation algorithms presented in Sect. 7.2, along the line $l(\gamma)$, connecting the state values of the equilibrium $\hat{E}$ and A_1 (see Fig. 6.1a), i.e.,

$$A_\gamma = l(\gamma) = (1-\gamma)\begin{pmatrix} L_0 \\ H_0 \end{pmatrix} + \gamma \begin{pmatrix} \hat{L} \\ \hat{H} \end{pmatrix}, \quad \text{with} \quad \gamma \in [0,\, 1].$$

During these continuation steps we always check the admissibility of the solution. For $\gamma_0 \approx 0.3579$ the state trajectory starts at A_{γ_0} (see Fig. 6.1a). For this initial state the corresponding control is zero (see Fig. 6.1b) and continuing the solution for $\gamma > \gamma_0$ the control would become negative. At this point the algorithm stops since it has detected an exit point of a boundary arc with $u = 0$. If we continue the solution along the line l for $\gamma > \gamma_0$ we have to take into account, that we start at the boundary arc ($u = 0$) and that at some time $\bar{t}$ an exit point exists, where we switch to the interior arc (see Fig. 6.1c).

Carrying out the Continuation of an Optimal Solution Exhibiting an Exit Point

To continue the solution for $\gamma > \gamma_0$ we use the algorithm described in Sect. 7.6.3. We therefore have to consider the canonical systems for the boundary and the interior arc. Furthermore we know that there exists an exit time $\bar{t}$. At the time $\bar{t}$ the solution path is connected continuously in the states and

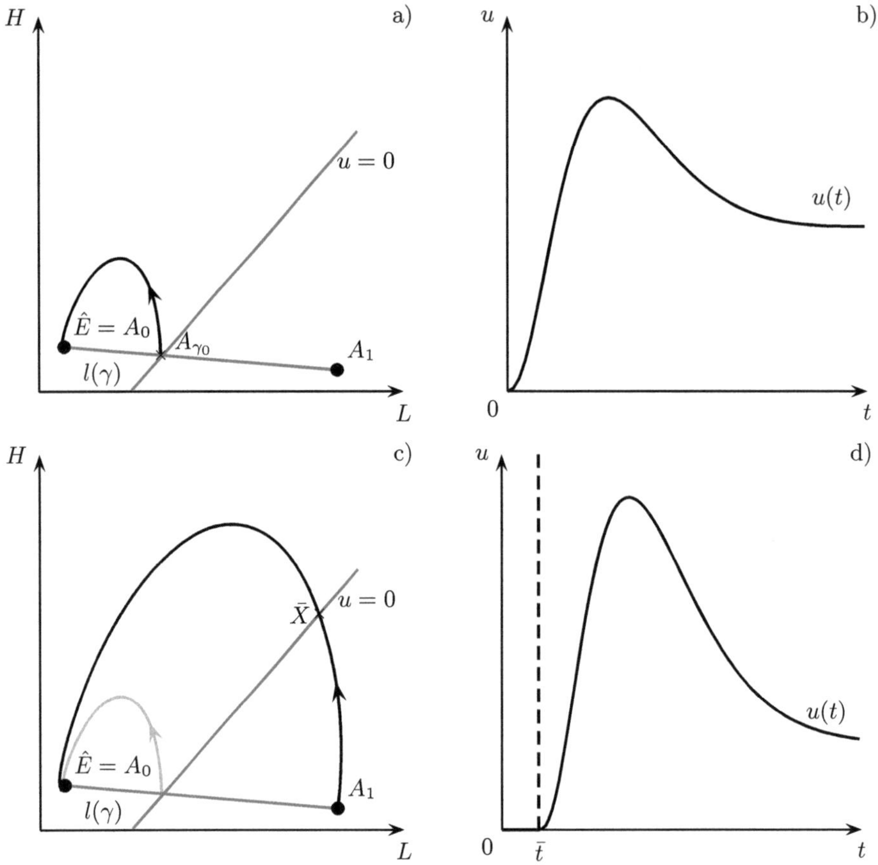

Fig. 6.1. The continuation process of the solution from $\hat{E}$ to A_1 along the connecting line l is depicted. In panel (**a**) the state trajectory $X(\cdot)$ is depicted starting at $X(0) = A_{\gamma_0}$. For this initial state the corresponding control value is zero at time $t = 0$ and greater than zero later on, as illustrated in (**b**). In panel (**c**) the state trajectory starting at $X(0) = A_1$ is depicted with an exit point $\bar{X}$ at $\bar{t}$. The corresponding control $u^*(\cdot)$ is shown in panel (**d**). In that case $u^*(\cdot)$ is zero until time $\bar{t}$ and greater than zero for $t \geq \bar{t}$

the costates and the control is zero. These conditions suffice to state a well-defined BVP. The dynamical systems for the interior and the boundary arc are normalized with respect to time and considered on the time interval $[0, 1]$ (see Sect. 7.6.3).

Denoting the interior arc by $X^I(\cdot)$, the boundary arc by $X^B(\cdot)$, and the corresponding dynamics by f^I and f^B, respectively, the BVP becomes:

$$\dot{X}^I = t_e f^I(X^I), \quad t \in [0, 1] \tag{6.14a}$$

$$\dot{X}^B = \bar{t} f^B(X^B), \quad t \in [0, 1] \tag{6.14b}$$

$$\begin{pmatrix} X_1^B(0) \\ X_2^B(0) \end{pmatrix} = A_\gamma \tag{6.14c}$$

$$X^I(0) = X^B(1) \tag{6.14d}$$

$$X_4^I(1) = 0 \tag{6.14e}$$

$$F\left(X^I(1) - \hat{E}\right) = 0, \tag{6.14f}$$

where t_e is the previously fixed terminal time and $\bar{t}$ the unknown exit time.

Thus we solve an optimal control problem of terminal time $t_e + \bar{t}$, satisfying the initial condition (6.14c), the terminal condition (6.14f) and the corner conditions (6.14d) and (6.14e). The BVP (6.14) is well-posed since the number of unknowns equals the number of equations to be satisfied.

Remark 6.8. Note that $X^I = (L, H, \lambda_1, u)'$, whereas $X^B = (L, H, \lambda_1, \lambda_2)'$.

Remark 6.9. This solution finding strategy can in principle be extended for an arbitrary number of junction points. At each time, when a junction point is reached the BVP is augmented by the corresponding dynamics and corner conditions. Then the continuation process is started with the last detected solution as described before.

To start the continuation process for the BVP (6.14) at $\gamma = \gamma_0$ we initialize a BV-Solver with the "trivial" solution $\bar{t} = 0$

$$X^I(t) = X(t), \quad t \in [0, 1]$$
$$X^B(t) = X(0), \quad t \in [0, 1],$$

where $X(t)$ is the last detected solution starting at $(X_1(0), X_2(0))' = A_{\gamma_0}$. Continuing this solution we finally find the solution for the initial state A_1 (see Fig. 6.1c,d).

Processing the Effect of Delaying Control by T_0 Years

Having now derived the controlled trajectory "connecting" the initial point $(L(T_0), H(T_0), \lambda_1(T_0), u^*(T_0))$ with the equilibrium $\hat{E} = (\hat{L}, \hat{H}, \hat{\lambda}_1, \hat{u}^*)$, we multiply the absolute value of the resulting optimal objective functional by e^{-rT} to discount those costs back to the original starting time and add them to the social costs resulting from the uncontrolled trajectory over period $[0, T_0]$. The such computed total costs $C(T_0)$ are given by

$$C(T_0) = \int_0^{T_0} e^{-rt}\kappa\,(k_L L + k_H H)\,dt + \int_{T_0}^{\infty} e^{-rt}(\kappa+\gamma)\,(k_L L^* + k_H H^*)\,dt$$

$$\text{s.t.}\quad \dot{L} = \begin{cases} I(L,H) - (a+b)L & t \in [0,\,T_0] \\ \psi(w^*)I(L^*,H^*) - (a+b)L^* & t > T_0 \end{cases}$$

$$\dot{H} = \begin{cases} bL - gH & t \in [0,\,T_0] \\ bL^* - gH^* - \beta(H^*,u^*)H^* & t > T_0, \end{cases}$$

where $(u^*(\cdot), w^*(\cdot))$ is the optimal control for the time shifted problem (6.6) starting at $(L(T_0),\, H(T_0))$. The uncontrolled dynamics on the interval $[0,\, T_0]$ is that of Sect. 2.7.

As Fig. 6.2 illustrates, one could avert as much as half of the total costs associated with the drug problem by starting control early. Note that total discounted cost $C(T_0)$ of delaying control reaches a maximum at the same time that light use peaks. Starting control later than that causes lower values of $C(T_0)$ because heavy use is already giving the drug a bad reputation, and one merely needs to optimally support the decline of the epidemic, instead of proactively driving the levels of use toward the equilibrium state.

For the actual computations, depicted in Fig. 6.2, we solved the uncontrolled model starting at $L_0 = 1,010,000$ and $H_0 = 70,000$ (these are the estimated numbers of light and heavy users by Everingham and Rydell, 1994) yielding an uncontrolled trajectory $(L(t),\, H(t))$ with $t \in [0,\, 24]$, where $t = 0$ corresponds to 1967. Then we solved the optimal control problem taking each of the points $(L(t),\, H(t))$ as an initial point and added the total costs as described above.

6.1.5 Optimal Policies for Different Phases of a Drug Epidemic

Having established that control during the transient phase of a drug epidemic can be important, it is next natural to ask what the control spending should look like. To investigate how spending patterns respond to the time (or phase) of the drug epidemic, we calculate trajectories "connecting" the equilibrium value, $\hat{E}$, with data on drug prevalence observed for US cocaine in a particular year, $(L(year),\, H(year))$ (for the actual calculation technique see Sect. 7.5.1 and Remark 6.9). Four such examples are shown by Fig. 6.3.

For illustrative purposes we focus on further investigating and discussing the "1967-trajectory," which should help us to develop a better understanding of drug control over the entire course of a drug epidemic (see Fig. 6.4). Analyzing the other trajectories completes the picture, but for this particular model the qualitative results do not dramatically differ from the ones described below for the "1967-time-path." Note that throughout the discussion in the remainder of this chapter the years will appear in quotation marks, because they

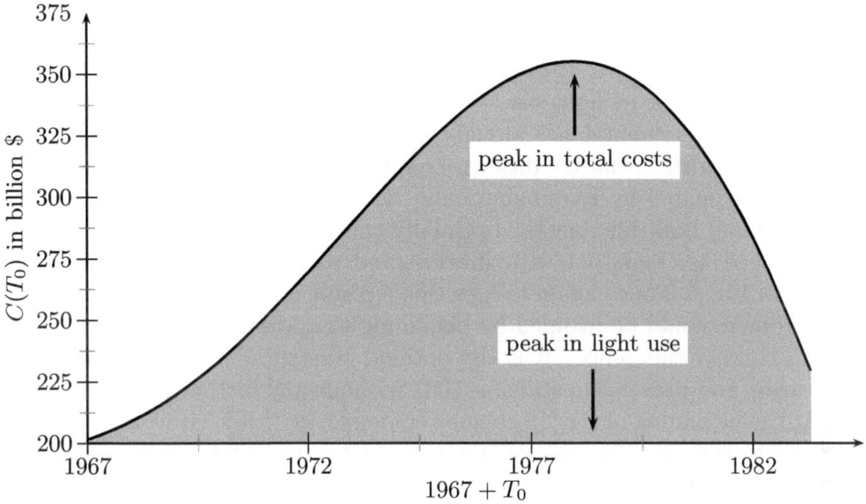

Fig. 6.2. Totals costs, $C(T_O)$, of delaying control as a function of T_O, where T_O denotes the time when government starts control. Calculation initiated with data observed in 1967 (corresponding to $t = 0$)

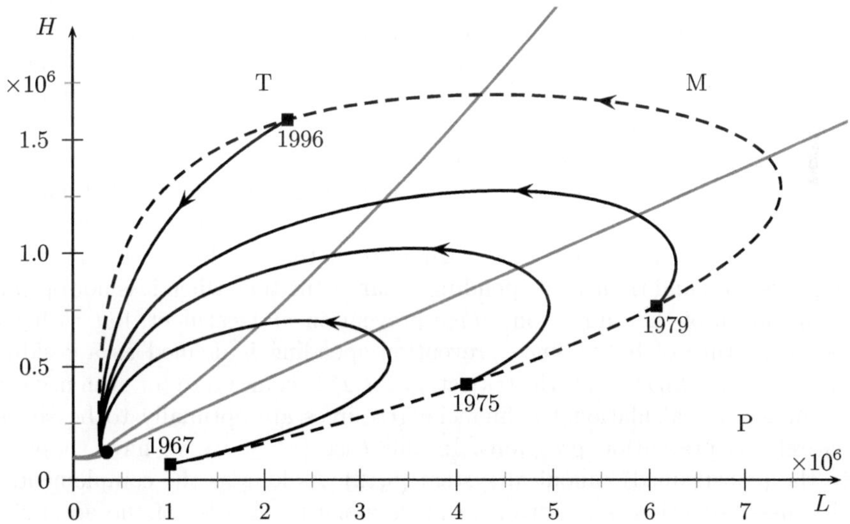

Fig. 6.3. Projections of the controlled trajectories into the (L, H)-plane for initial data from various years of the uncontrolled modeled epidemic (where the uncontrolled epidemic follows approximately the *dashed line*). The *gray lines* separate the regions P of (L, H) values for which treatment is optimally zero, M where a mixture of treatment and prevention spending is optimal and T where treatment is set to maximum absorbing the entire drug control budget

refer not only to particular years but also, more importantly, to particular "phases of the (US cocaine) epidemic." "1967," for instance, means "at the onset of an epidemic." "1975" and "1979" correspond to phases "before" or "close to the peak in light use," whereas "1996" refers to a later phase, in which the drug epidemic has already stared to ebb on its own accord.

Starting with initial conditions, (L_0, H_0), that reflect US cocaine use in 1967 (as estimated by Everingham and Rydell, 1994), Fig. 6.3 shows (in the (L, H)-plane) how different the optimally controlled *cocaine epidemics* would have looked as compared with its observed path (indicated by the dashed line).[5] In Fig. 6.3 once again last section's result is emphasized on how much of a problem could be avoided by beginning to address it early. What causes such a massive difference? It is the optimal allocation of the budget to drug treatment and prevention starting 1967 without any further delay.

At the beginning of the US cocaine epidemic, in "1967," it would have been optimal to put all drug-control resources (determined by γ dollars times the quantity currently consumed $(k_L L + k_H H)$) into prevention (see Fig. 6.4b). No money should have been spent on treatment until shortly after the peak in optimally controlled light use was observed at a level of 3.1 million (only 9 years after starting control). At this point there would have been a very rapid changeover from all prevention to all treatment (see Fig. 6.4). This transition would have been completed in just 6 years. Treatment spending would then have quickly risen to a peak and decayed slowly as the amount of use fell (due to a decline in heavy use). Then in "2020" prevention would begin to kick in again, taking over nearly the entire (much smaller) drug-control budget approaching the equilibrium state replacing some of the drug's bad reputation (which is not bad enough anymore to have $w^* = 0$).

The basic recommendation is prevention first, then treatment, then back to mostly prevention as an epidemic approaches its equilibrium, with very abrupt changes from one control regime to another (cf. Fig. 6.4b). The kinks in prevention and treatment spending occur at the time when it is not optimal to spend all of the budget on *either* prevention *or* treatment, but rather to use a mixture of both. Since prevention spending is defined as a residual, $w^* = \gamma(k_L L + k_H H) - u^*$, the trajectory for u^* becomes zero (or even negative in numerical calculations) if financial resources are optimally to be shifted entirely to prevention programs. In this case ($u^* \leq 0$) we have to switch to the (constrained) canonical system (6.12). As long as the complementary slackness condition is positive, we move along the border of the admissible control space ($u^* = 0$, $w^* = \gamma(k_L L + k_H H)$). If the complementary slackness condition again becomes zero, the control variable u^* becomes positive and optimal prevention spending is again defined by $w^* = \gamma(k_L L + k_H H) - u^*$.

With optimal control, the proportion of all users who are heavy users, an indicator of the severity of the drug problem, would peak in terms of

[5] The corresponding evolution of controlled and uncontrolled light and heavy users over time is depicted by Fig. 6.4a.

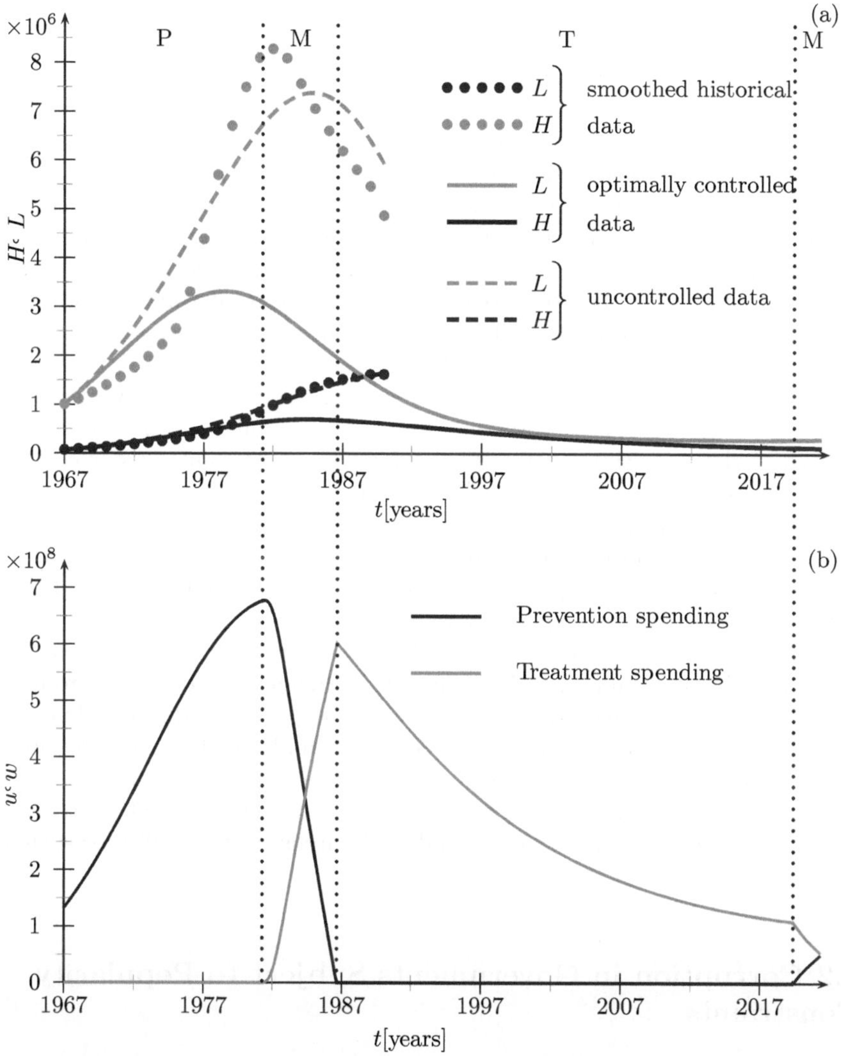

Fig. 6.4. In panel (**a**) time paths of controlled and uncontrolled cocaine use and smoothed historical data (Everingham and Rydell, 1994) are depicted; start of optimal budget allocation in 1967. Panel (**b**) shows the optimal allocation of the drug control budget in million dollars. The dotted lines correspond to the lines in Fig. 6.3 separating the all Prevention region (P) from the all Treatment region (T), and the region where the Mix is optimal (M).

Fig. 6.4a in "1998" at roughly 40%, then decrease to its equilibrium value of 26%. This low proportion of heavy users in equilibrium partially explains why treatment's share of all control spending is so small at the equilibrium. The other factor is that since heavy users help to suppress initiation by serving as a negative example, it may be optimal to have at least some of them around to prevent a recurrence of the epidemic cycle.

A logical next step in the analysis would be to solve the optimal control model starting with initial conditions reflecting other levels of use. Technically this is done in exactly the same way done so far, except for starting with a different initial state. For this particular model the results are not dramatically different. We therefore omit them here and refer the interested reader to Behrens (1998) and for Behrens et al. (2000b).

We have learned a lot about dynamic drug policy. Both prevention and treatment are helpful in suppressing drug consumption – but not necessarily applied at the same time. In fact the period when both demand side controls should be implemented is strikingly brief. This is an important insight, but a thorough OR-study would not stop here. A next step is to ask whether the optimal drug control policy and its timing would look very different and whether the equilibrium approached would be very different from $\hat{E}$, if total prevention and treatment spending were *not limited* to being proportional to the "size of the current drug problem." This could answer questions about how much valuable it would be to be able to shift financial resource to problems before they are perceived to be problems by the public, and how valuable it would be to be flexible with respect to recruiting additional financial resources at all. This would yield a control model with two states L and H and two controls u and w, but no budget rule apart from $u, w \geq 0$. The interested reader may consult Behrens (1998) and for Behrens et al. (2000b) for such an analysis.

6.2 Corruption in Governments Subject to Popularity Constraints

To combat corruption and improve the well-being of a society, we need to understand politicians' motivation for being honest or dishonest. Drawing heavily on the work of Feichtinger and Wirl (1994) the normative model presented here seeks to find conditions under which self-interested (rational) officials do or do not want to abuse their power. By analyzing the behavior of a rational politician who derives benefits from both being popular and corrupt, we aim to identify situations or scenarios in which either being honest or being crooked would be in the politician's self-interest. Knowing this could help with the design of appropriate counter-measures, such as passing sunshine laws that make information available to the public.

6.2.1 The Modeled Incentive for Being Corrupt

As public opinion poll numbers show, a politician's popularity evolves according to a dynamic process. For present purposes we assume that a central dynamic is that an official's popularity suffers when evidence of corruption piles up and gradually recovers over periods when there are no new reports of corruption or scandal. Thus the public responds to a cumulative level of awareness of current and past corruption, not just to isolated observations of corruption today. It seems reasonable that these features should be incorporated into a model that aims at explaining the incentives for being a corrupt official.

We suppose that the public's memory (or level of awareness) of recent and past corruption (represented by the state variable C) increases if politicians are acting in corrupt ways. The decision to be corrupt is not a one-time, binary choice. Rather, it is modeled as an ongoing level of participation in shady activities. So at each instant of time t the politician's decision variable (or control variable) u represents this level of current engagement in corrupt activities. This control variable is positive when the politician is engaging in corrupt practices (taking bribes), but it can also become negative if the politician – in order to promote his or her popularity to stay in office – engages in a crusade against corruption, since that requires scarce human resources and may alienate the bureaucracy, which retaliates with red tape.

The accumulated level of awareness, C, does not, however, remain at one fixed level forever. The public's memory fades. We assume that the public forgets past knowledge at a rate $\delta \geq 0$, which corresponds to an exponentially declining memory. Thus the evolution of the public's memory of recent and past corruption C can be modeled as

$$\dot{C} = u - \delta C, \qquad C(0) = C_0, \tag{6.15}$$

where

C ... accumulated awareness (knowledge) of past corruption

u ... extent of corruption (politician's control variable)

δ ... rate of forgetting past corruption

The accumulated knowledge of corruption is just one influence on a politician's popularity. If word of mouth is crucial to maintaining the public's goodwill, then aside from the effects of corruption, the politician's popularity (represented by the second state variable P) may grow according to a diffusion process. This suggests using a logistic law or some other concave function $g(P)$ where $g'' < 0$.

The effect of awareness or memory of current or past corruption, C, on the politician's popularity P is clearly negative. It is not uncommon when modeling corruption to assume that cumulative reports of corruption (or the public's memory of current and past corruption) are necessary to trigger opposition and resistance. One explanation seems to be that people are quite aware that corruption is to some degree unavoidable or at least irrationally expensive to uproot. Put another way, in at least some jurisdictions, a modest level of shady dealing is not out of the ordinary. Hence, a low-level reputation for corruption might have quite modest effects on popularity, since throwing the current politician out of office might lead to a replacement who is every bit as bad. However, as the perception of the extent of corruption grows, there might be less and less tolerance for such behavior. These considerations suggest that if the function $f(C)$ measures the loss of popularity caused by the awareness of current and past corruption C, then $f' > 0$ and quite plausibly that $f'' \geq 0$ as well. Given these considerations, the evolution of a politician's popularity P can be modeled by the following differential equation

$$\dot{P} = g(P) - f(C), \qquad P(0) = P_0, \tag{6.16}$$

where

P	...	politician's popularity
C	...	accumulated awareness (knowledge) of past corruption
g	...	growth function of popularity
f	...	function measuring the loss of popularity caused by C

Note that u influences C directly, and has an indirect negative impact on P via $f(C)$ as indicated by Fig. 6.5. Formally, the politicians face an intertemporal trade-off between the benefits associated with being popular (for example, being confirmed in office), $U_1(P)$, and the benefits resulting from bribery and fraud, $U_2(u)$. Even if the politicians do not personally accept any bribes, they benefit from the support of the bureaucrats and the public. While tolerance of corruption may secure support among the bureaucracy, it hurts public support. Therefore, we assume that the two types of benefits are to be modeled as being separable, $U_1(P)+U_2(u)$, and that both utility functions are increasing and concave

$$U_1' > 0, \quad U_1'' \leq 0, \quad U_2' > 0, \quad U_2'' < 0.$$

We proceed by analyzing a continuous-time optimization problem in which a politician seeks to maximize the discounted stream of benefits coming from being honest and from being dishonest. So the intertemporal utility functional, V, is given by the following expression

$$V(u(\cdot)) = \int_0^\infty \mathrm{e}^{-rt} \left(U_1(P) + U_2(u)\right) \mathrm{d}t. \tag{6.17}$$

The politician seeks to maximize benefits (6.17), subject to the two dynamic constraints (6.15) and (6.16).

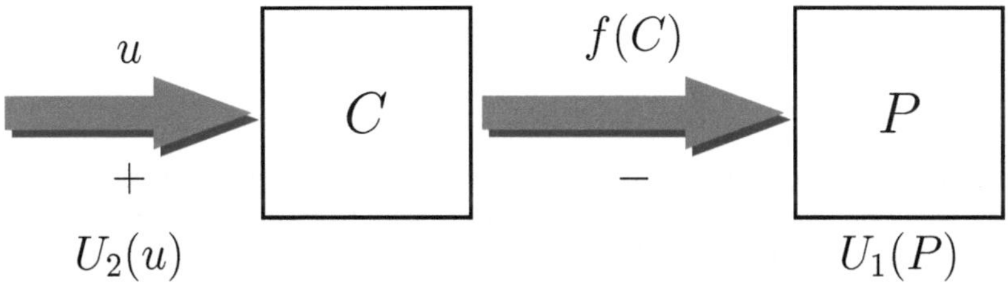

Fig. 6.5. Effect of corruption on the two state variables in the corruption model

6.2.2 Optimality Conditions

Following Pontryagin's Maximum Principle we state the current-value Hamiltonian function

$$\mathcal{H} = \lambda_0 \left(U_1\left(P\right) + U_2\left(u\right)\right) + \lambda_1 \dot{P} + \lambda_2 \dot{C},$$

where λ_1 and λ_2 denote the costates of the states C and P, respectively.

Remark 6.10. An immediate argument proves that the problem is normal and therefore $\lambda_0 = 1$. Suppose to the contrary that $\lambda_0 = 0$, then the Hamiltonian maximizing condition yields $\lambda_2(t) = 0$ for all t. Since otherwise the maximum of $\mathcal{H}$ is achieved for $u = \infty$ or $u = -\infty$ depending on the sign of λ_2. This implies that $\dot{\lambda}_2(t) = -\mathcal{H}_C = \lambda_1(t) f'(C(t)) = 0$ yielding $\lambda_1(t) = 0$ due to $f' > 0$. But this contradicts the condition that the vector$(\lambda_0, \lambda_1(t), \lambda_2(t))$ is nonzero for all t.

This Hamiltonian is concave in both states and control because the objective function, $U_1(P) + U_2(u)$, and the state transition equations, $\dot{P}$ and $\dot{C}$, are concave. The adjoint variable λ_1 must be positive because the derivative of the objective function, $U_1(P) + U_2(u)$, with respect to P is larger than zero. The concavity implies that the sufficient optimality conditions (see Sect. 3.3.5) are satisfied if additionally the limiting transversality conditions are satisfied

$$\lim_{t\to\infty} \mathrm{e}^{-rt}\lambda_1 P = 0$$
$$\lim_{t\to\infty} \mathrm{e}^{-rt}\lambda_2 C = 0.$$

The Hamiltonian maximizing condition for control values lying in the interior is given by

$$\mathcal{H}_u = U_2'\left(u^*\right) + \lambda_2 = 0, \tag{6.18}$$

which is already the general case owing to the strict concavity of the Hamiltonian with respect to u

$$\mathcal{H}_{uu} = U_2''(u) < 0.$$

Using the inverse function theorem we see that the inverse function

$$h(\lambda_2) := \left(U_2'\right)^{-1}(\lambda_2)$$

exists, satisfying

$$\mathcal{H}_u(C, P, h(\lambda_2), \lambda_1, \lambda_2) = 0.$$

Intertemporal optimality requires that the marginal utility of being corrupt, $U_2'(u)$, just balances the negative shadow price, λ_2, of the stock of corruption. The following two differential equations determine the evolution of the costates λ_1 and λ_2

$$\dot{\lambda}_1 = (r - g'(P))\,\lambda_1 - U_1'(P) \tag{6.19a}$$

$$\dot{\lambda}_2 = (r + \delta)\,\lambda_2 + \lambda_1 f'(C). \tag{6.19b}$$

6.2.3 Insights About the Incentive to Be Corrupt

To produce results that are as general as possible, in this subsection we do not yet specify the precise form of the functions. The necessary conditions (6.18)–(6.19b) deliver the following canonical system

$$\dot{P} = g(P) - f(C) \tag{6.20a}$$

$$\dot{C} = h(\lambda_2) - \delta C \tag{6.20b}$$

$$\dot{\lambda}_1 = (r - g'(P))\,\lambda_1 - U_1'(P) \tag{6.20c}$$

$$\dot{\lambda}_2 = (r + \delta)\,\lambda_2 + \lambda_1 f'(C). \tag{6.20d}$$

First we consider the properties of an equilibrium $(\hat{P}, \hat{C}, \hat{\lambda}_1, \hat{\lambda}_2)$ of the canonical system, which are described by the corresponding Jacobian matrix:

$$\hat{J} = \begin{pmatrix} g'(\hat{P}) & -f'(\hat{C}) & 0 & 0 \\ 0 & -\delta & 0 & -\dfrac{1}{U_2''(\hat{u}^*)} \\ -\dfrac{g''(\hat{P})U_1'(\hat{P})}{r - g'(\hat{P})} - U_1''(\hat{P}) & 0 & r - g'(\hat{P}) & 0 \\ 0 & \dfrac{f''(\hat{C})U_1'(\hat{P})}{r - g'(\hat{P})} & f'(\hat{C}) & r + \delta \end{pmatrix}.$$

The eigenvalues of this matrix are crucial for characterizing the local dynamics of the linear ODE that approximates the canonical equations (6.20) at the equilibrium point. Using the formula (7.28a) on p. 345 the eigenvalues become

$$\xi_{3,4}^{1,2} = \frac{r}{2} \pm \sqrt{\frac{r^2}{4} - \frac{K}{2} \pm \frac{1}{2}\sqrt{K^2 - 4\det \hat{J}}}, \tag{6.21}$$

where the coefficient K for our "corrupt politician problem" yields

$$K = g'(\hat{P})\left(r - g'(\hat{P})\right) - \delta\,(r + \delta) + \frac{f''(\hat{P})U_1'(\hat{P})}{U_2''(\hat{u}^*)(r - g'(\hat{P}))}. \tag{6.22}$$

The determinant of the Jacobian evaluated at the equilibrium is given by

$$\det \hat{J} = -g'\delta\,(r-g')\,(r+\delta) + \frac{g''U_1'f'^2}{U_2''(r-g')} + \frac{f'^2U_1''}{U_2''} + \frac{g'f''U_1'}{U_2''}. \qquad (6.23)$$

Using the indicator K and $\det \hat{J}$ above, we can use Table 7.1 as a kind of menu to look up the long-run system behavior once the parameters are specified. That includes understanding how the long-run system behavior would change if those parameters are altered by counter corruption measures:

- If $g'(\hat{P}) \leq 0$, then the long-run equilibrium is a saddle point. This result follows directly from (6.23), since $g' \leq 0$ implies that $\det \hat{J} > 0$ and $K < 0$. Therefore, exactly two eigenvalues must have negative real parts. This local property does not, however, exclude transient and damped oscillations. In fact, damped oscillations are optimal in many cases.

More complex types of behavior are possible for $g'(\hat{P}) > 0$, as the second main result states:

- If $0 < g'(\hat{P}) < r$, then all the different possible cases of long-run system behavior can occur: saddle point stability (including local monotonicity and damped oscillations), locally unstable spirals, and instability such that convergence to the equilibrium is restricted to a one-dimensional set of initial conditions. In particular, the transition from a domain of stable to locally unstable spirals may give birth to limit cycles according to the Poincaré–Andronov–Hopf theorem.

The existence part of the Poincaré–Andronov–Hopf theorem (see Sect. 2.10) is proved below after the functional forms for the objective and the constraints are specified.

Obviously, $g' = 0$, or equivalently $\tilde{P}$, separates the domain of stable policies from the domain where complexities may (but need not) arise. What is the reason for this result? Arithmetically, the supposition of growth, $g' > 0$ for $P < \tilde{P}$, is crucial here. An economic and intuitive explanation follows. A diffusion process g with one, and only one, point $\tilde{P}$ such that $g'(\tilde{P}) = 0$ implies that the time path of popularity (i.e., integrating g) consists of a convex segment (if $P < \tilde{P}$) and a concave segment (if $P > \tilde{P}$) with respect to time. In other words, the domain of low popularity ($P < \tilde{P}$) exhibits increasing returns and the domain of high popularity ($P > \tilde{P}$) is characterized by diminishing returns. It is plausible that diminishing returns lead to stable equilibria, whereas increasing returns to popularity favor complexities (in particular cycles). The reason is that a low popularity level may increase to a certain threshold so that it may be rational for the politician to sacrifice his/her good reputation because it is "easy" to replenish the public's goodwill.

Figure 6.6 highlights that a large weight on popularity – such that stationary popularity exceeds $\tilde{P} := \operatorname{argmax} g(P)$ – is sufficient (but not necessary) to stabilize corruption. However, this stable level of corruption may be quite high.

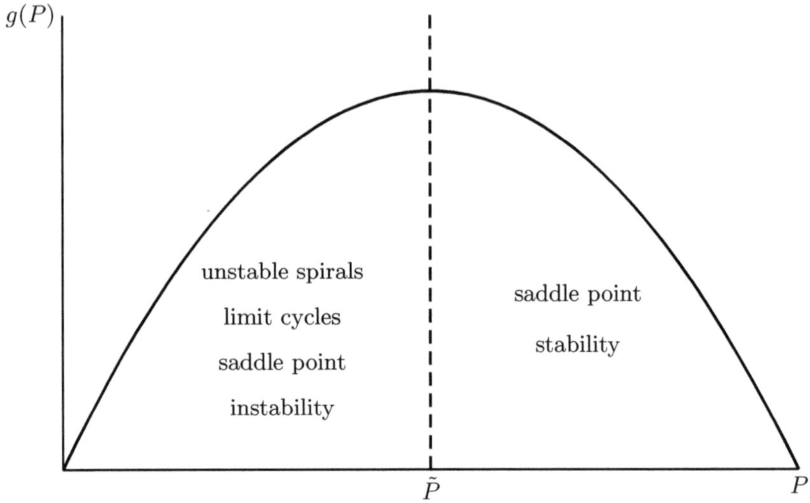

Fig. 6.6. Properties of equilibria depending on popularity

6.2.4 Is Periodic Behavior Caused by Rational Optimization?

Model Specifications

Assuming that the benefits of popularity are proportional to its current level yields the benefit function (6.24a). The growth of the benefits associated with the current accumulated level of corruption is, however, not unrestricted but rather reaches a maximum level. Thus we specify the functional forms occurring in (6.15)–(6.17) as follows

$$U_1(P) = \beta_1 P, \quad \beta_1 > 0 \tag{6.24a}$$

$$U_2(u) = \alpha_1 u - \frac{1}{2}\alpha_2 u^2, \quad \alpha_i > 0,\ i = 1,2 \tag{6.24b}$$

$$g(P) = P(1-P) \tag{6.24c}$$

$$f(C) = \gamma C, \quad \gamma > 0. \tag{6.24d}$$

Equations (6.24c) and (6.24d) represent the fact that a maximum level of popularity exists toward which P grows in the absence of corruption, while the decline in popularity is proportional to the accumulated level of awareness of corruption C.

Assuming that the forgetting rate of the accumulated level of awareness with respect to corruption is equal to zero, i.e., $\delta = 0$, yields $\hat{u}^* = 0$. That is, in the long-run, current corruption will be wiped out if the public never forget past wrong-doing. Then (6.23), i.e., the determinant of the Jacobian of the associated linearized system and K, see (6.22), can be simplified to

$$\det \hat{J} = \frac{f'^2(\hat{P})}{U_2''(\hat{u}^*)}\left(\frac{g''(\hat{P})U_1'(\hat{P})}{r - g'(\hat{P})}\right) = \frac{2r\alpha_1\gamma}{\alpha_2} \tag{6.25}$$

and

$$K = g'(\hat{P})\left(r - g'(\hat{P})\right) = \frac{\beta_1\gamma(r^2\alpha_1 - \beta_1\gamma)}{\alpha_1^2 r^2}. \tag{6.26}$$

Poincaré–Andronov–Hopf Bifurcation

The Poincaré–Andronov–Hopf theorem gives sufficient conditions for the existence of limit cycles of nonlinear ODEs. Informally, we can think of this theorem as requiring that the equilibrium must suddenly change from a sink to a source with variation of a parameter. Arithmetically this requires that a pair of purely imaginary eigenvalues exists for a particular value of the bifurcation parameter and that the real part of this pair of eigenvalues smoothly changes its sign as the parameter is altered from below its actual value to above (see Sect. 2.10). These two arithmetic conditions guarantee the existence of limit cycles for a one-sided neighborhood of the critical value of the bifurcation parameter.

Thus we have to analyze the eigenvalues given by (6.21) and specified for (6.25) and (6.26) in more detail. For any equilibrium satisfying $0 < g'(\hat{P}) < r$, (6.25) as well as (6.26) is positive. By the classification scheme in Sect. 7.4.1 we see that the existence of purely imaginary roots requires the following relation

$$\det \hat{J} - \left(\frac{K}{2}\right)^2 - r^2\frac{K}{2} = 0. \tag{6.27}$$

(The reader may verify this condition for herself/himself by substituting (6.27) into (6.21).)

For our computation we specify the parameter values as given in Table 6.2.

Table 6.2. Parameter values

α_1	α_2	γ	r	δ
1	1	0.071	1	0

Now we investigate the system's structure with respect to variations of the parameter β_1. For the given parameter values we find a unique equilibrium at

$$\hat{E}(\beta_1) = \left(\hat{P}, \hat{C}, \hat{\lambda_1}, \hat{\lambda_2}\right) = \left(\frac{7}{200}\beta_1,\ \frac{1}{2}\beta_1 - \frac{7}{400}\beta_1^2,\ \frac{100}{7},\ -1\right).$$

After some tedious but straightforward calculations, (6.27) becomes a quartic equation in β_1

$$\frac{7}{50} - \frac{7}{200}\beta_1 + \frac{49}{40000}\beta_1^2 + \frac{343}{2000000}\beta_1^3 - \frac{2401}{400000000}\beta_1^4 = 0,$$

which can explicitly be solved yielding

$$\left(\beta_1^{PAH}\right)_{1,2}^{3,4} = 6.6910;\ 7.5947;\ -15.4403;\ 29.7260.$$

Since β_1 is assumed as positive and $\hat{P} \in (0,\, 1)$ only the first two values of β_1 have to be considered. At these critical parameter values both K and $\det \hat{J}$ are positive, so that one pair of purely imaginary roots exists. Therefore, both small and large values of β_1 imply a saddle point, while intermediate values, $\beta_1 \in (6.6910,\, 7.5947)$, induce complex eigenvalues, all with positive real parts.

We will now numerically calculate a limit cycle at the PAH-bifurcation for β_1 and continue the limit cycles up to the upper bound for β_1.

Finding and Continuing a Limit Cycle

First we set β_1 equal to $\beta_1^{PAH} = 6.6910$ yielding for the eigenvalue $\xi = 0.3528\mathrm{i}$ the eigenvector

$$\tilde{\nu} = \begin{pmatrix} -0.0161 + 0.0121\mathrm{i} \\ -0.0610 + 0.1730\mathrm{i} \\ 0.9807 + 0\mathrm{i} \\ -0.0610 - 0.0215\mathrm{i} \end{pmatrix}.$$

Next we use the procedure presented on p. 347 approximating the limit cycle by

$$\Gamma_\varepsilon(t) = 2\varepsilon\left(\nu_R \cos\omega_0 t - \nu_I \sin\omega_0 t\right), \tag{6.28}$$

where $\varepsilon > 0$ is some arbitrarily chosen parameter, the angular velocity ω_0 is given by the imaginary part of the eigenvalue ξ, and $\nu = \nu_R + \mathrm{i}\nu_I$ additionally satisfying

$$\langle \nu_R, \nu_R \rangle + \langle \nu_I, \nu_I \rangle = 1,\ \langle \nu_R, \nu_I \rangle = 0. \tag{6.29}$$

By Remark 7.15 on p. 348 we have to find some $c \in \mathbb{C}$ such that $\nu = c\tilde{\nu}$ satisfies the normalization conditions (6.29). Using the abbreviations $\tilde{\nu}_R = \operatorname{Re}\tilde{\nu}$ and $\tilde{\nu}_I = \operatorname{Im}\tilde{\nu}$ and setting $c = c_1 + \mathrm{i}c_2$ the conditions read as

$$\begin{aligned} (c_1^2 + c_2^2)(A + B) &= 1 \\ (c_1^2 - c_2^2)C + c_1 c_2 (A - B) &= 0, \end{aligned}$$

with

$$A = \langle \tilde{\nu}_R, \tilde{\nu}_R \rangle,\ B = \langle \tilde{\nu}_I, \tilde{\nu}_I \rangle,\ C = \langle \tilde{\nu}_R, \tilde{\nu}_I \rangle.$$

Solving these equations in c_1 and c_2 yields four symmetric solutions, where we choose $c = -0.0101 + \mathrm{i}0.9999$. For this choice the associated eigenvector becomes

$$\nu = \begin{pmatrix} -0.0162 + 0.0119\mathrm{i} \\ -0.0628 + 0.1724\mathrm{i} \\ 0.9806 + 0.0099\mathrm{i} \\ -0.0608 - 0.0222\mathrm{i} \end{pmatrix}.$$

To locate the limit cycle we consider the BVP (see Sect. 7.4.2)

$$\dot{X} = \Theta f(X)$$
$$X(0) = X(1)$$
$$\psi(X) = 0,$$

where $X = (P, C, \lambda_1, \lambda_2)'$ and f is the dynamics of the canonical system.

Using the cycle defined by (6.28), where we choose[6] $\varepsilon = 7.5^{-3}$ we can initialize the BVP (6.30) (see Fig. 6.7a). Now we can continue this initial limit cycle for increasing β_1, which is illustrated in Fig. 6.7b.

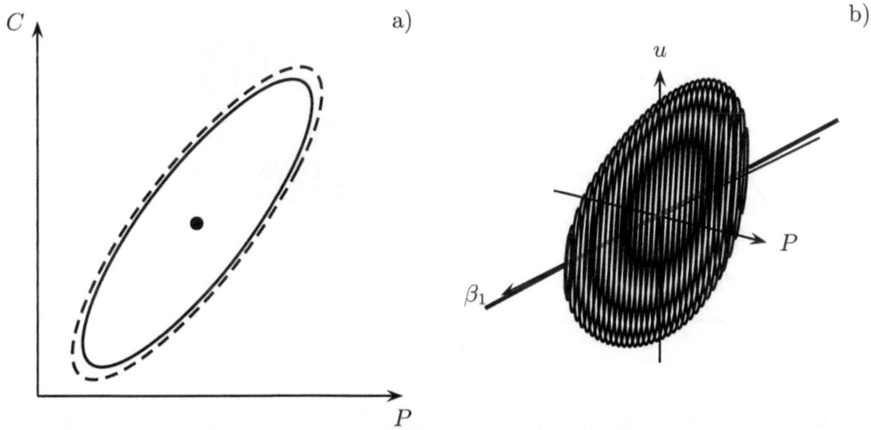

Fig. 6.7. Panel (**a**) depicts the approximated (*dashed line*) and the actual limit cycle (*solid line*) for $\beta_1 = 6.6910$. In panel (**b**) the continuation of the limit cycles in the (P, u)-plane are shown for varying parameter β_1

Determining the Stability of a Limit Cycle

As an example we consider the limit cycle Γ with period $\Theta = 17.8201$ for the parameter value $\beta_1 = 7.2$ and use the approach presented on p. 348 to determine its stability.

Therefore we compute the monodromy matrix M (see p. 81) at some point $x_0 \in \Gamma$. The monodromy matrix is the solution of the variational equation

[6] To find a limit cycle crucially depends on the choice of ε. Thus, one often has to try a wide range of different values for ε.

$$\dot{Y}(t) = \begin{pmatrix} \mathcal{H}^*_{\lambda_1 x}(\Gamma(t)) & \mathcal{H}^*_{\lambda_1\lambda_1}(\Gamma(t)) \\ -\mathcal{H}^*_{xx}(\Gamma(t)) & r\mathbb{I}^{(n)} - \mathcal{H}^*_{x\lambda_1}(\Gamma(t)) \end{pmatrix} Y(t),$$

along the periodic solution $\Gamma(\cdot)$, solved for the initial condition $Y(0) = \mathbb{I}^{(n)}$ on the interval $[0, \Theta]$, where $\Theta = 17.8201$.

Since we already calculated the limit cycle and we can take any point $x_0 \in \Gamma$. Thus we can numerically solve the extended system containing the canonical system as well as the variational equation. But due to the numerical errors integrating this system on $[0, \Theta]$ only provides an inaccurate solution (see Fig. 6.8a). But using this result as an initial solution, we can solve the corresponding BVP yielding an accurate solution of M exhibiting the eigenvalues

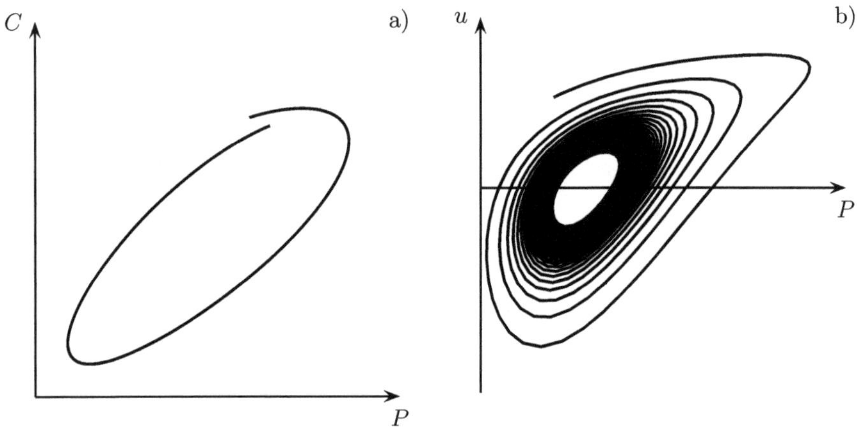

Fig. 6.8. Panel (**a**) shows the error when integrating the canonical system for one period of the limit cycle, starting at x_0 a point lying numerically on the limit cycle. Panel (**b**) depicts an optimal trajectory in the state–control space converging to the limit cycle

$$\xi^{3,4}_{1,2} = 1;\ 0.9863;\ 5.5612 \times 10^7;\ 5.4850 \times 10^7.$$

This numerically proves the existence of a two-dimensional stable manifold of the limit cycle and a "strong" unstable manifold, explaining the inaccurate results of the IVP approach.

Interpretation of the Results

Using the parameter values as specified in Table 6.2 Fig. 6.9a shows the phase portrait of a politician's cyclical strategy in the (P, u)-plane. We observe for the model specified according to (6.24) and parameter values given by Table 6.2 that optimal corruption u^* and the optimal popularity level P^* move clockwise around a popularity level of approximately 23.5% (see Fig. 6.9a). The amplitude is small because β_1 is close to its critical value, $\beta_1^{PAH} = 6.6910$, but the amplitude would increase for parameter values further away from the critical value (see Fig. 6.7b). Four regimes, labeled I–IV, characterize this cycle:

$$\begin{aligned} \text{I: } \dot{P} > 0, &\quad \text{and} \quad \dot{C} > 0, \\ \text{II: } \dot{P} > 0, &\quad \text{and} \quad \dot{C} < 0, \\ \text{III: } \dot{P} < 0, &\quad \text{and} \quad \dot{C} < 0, \\ \text{IV: } \dot{P} < 0, &\quad \text{and} \quad \dot{C} > 0. \end{aligned}$$

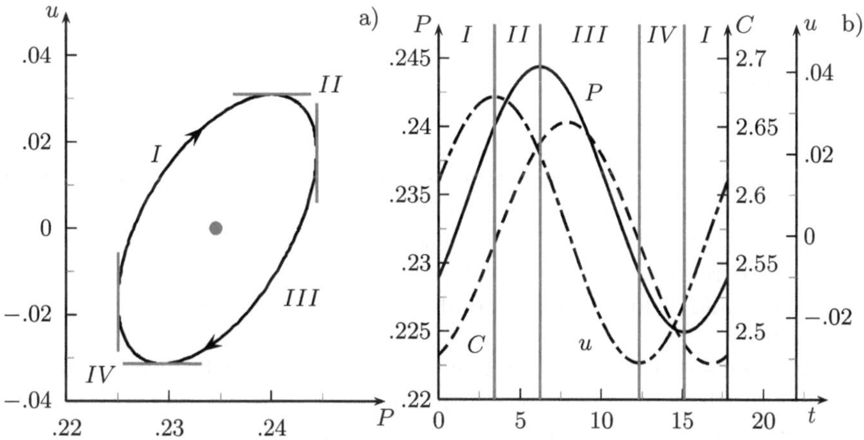

Fig. 6.9. The cyclical strategy of the corrupt politician for the base parameter values is depicted in (**a**) in the (P, u)-plane and in (**b**) in the time domain

Another way to characterize the regimes is to differentiate between "give" (first half of Phase I, second half of Phase III, Phase IV) and "take" (second half of Phase I, Phase II, first half of Phase III). The following paragraphs explain the behavior embodied in Fig. 6.9a and describe the associated optimal behavior of the politician. General conclusions should not be drawn from this particular illustration, with the parameter values taken from Table 6.2 and $\beta_1 = 6.691$.

Suppose that we start with the minimum level of public approval. Phase I begins with a fight against corruption ($u^* < 0$), but at a diminishing rate ($\dot{u} > 0$). This crusade purges the memory of past corruption, thereby replenishing goodwill, and once there is sufficient popularity corruption returns and continues to rise. Corruption declines while popularity is still rising to its peak (Phase II). This entire Phase II, plus the end of Phase I and the beginning of Phase III, may be labeled the "skimming period," where the politician exploits the previously acquired public goodwill. The resulting accumulated history of corruption now begins to adversely affect popularity; hence, corruption must be lowered and eventually a crusade against corruption is launched to halt this decline of popularity (Phase III). Finally, the fight against corruption is slightly relaxed while popularity completes its downward trend (Phase IV). This phase plus neighboring segments from III and I paint the politician as "Saint George fighting a dragon called corruption."

On the one hand, Fig. 6.9b highlights how corruption and later the crusade against corruption run ahead of popularity while public awareness C lags behind. The reason is that public perception of contained corruption increases the politician's popularity, and he/she can skim off the benefits acquired through active corruption, given the inherent dynamics and inertia of diffusion. On the other hand, it takes quite some time to purge the public's memory of historic mismanagement, so the public remains quite skeptical, even if the current level of corruption is low or even if corruption is actively being fought.

Two of these four phases dominate the picture both in the phase portrait and in the time domain. More precisely, positive correlations (Phases I and III) dominate the other two segments where corruption and popularity are negatively correlated. This is the expected pattern as higher corruption should lower popularity. One important consequence of this analysis is that cross-sectional regressions drawing on data generated from such complex underlying processes could yield misleading results if the data come from certain parts of this cycle.

Politicians or other officials may consider bribes to be like a consumption good, which is disliked by the public. Thus, any government is subject to popularity constraints (at least if reelection is desired). If popularity (in absence of corruption) grows too quickly toward its carrying capacity, a rational decision-maker may become a corrupt (at least periodically) to exploit this popularity for personal gain. That is, if the drop in popularity which is associated with corruption is easily counter-acted, it is optimal for the politician to accepts bribes. A public that forgives and forgets too readily is likely repeatedly victimized.

6.3 Is It Important to Manage Public Opinion While Fighting Terrorism?

There is a growing literature on counter-terror policy that uses a state variable to model the size or strength of a terrorist organization. The model here, described by Caulkins, Feichtinger, Grass, and Tragler (2007b), supplements that approach with a second state variable R, for reputation, representing the level of public sympathy for the counter-terror forces (because force strength is not all that matters in unconventional or asymmetric warfare). The battles are fought as much in the court of world opinion as they are in conventional firefights, a concept reflected in Arquilla and Ronfeldt (1999) about *noopolitik.*[7]

6.3.1 What One Should Know when Fighting Terrorism

The state variable S denoting the size of the terrorist organization has inflows for recruitment of new terrorists and outflows due to both counter-terror operations and also "natural outflow" at a constant per capita rate, μ. As in the *fire-and-water model* introduced in Sect. 2.5 we include both a constant recruitment term, τ, and an inflow term that is a power function in S.

Outflow due to controlled counter-terror operations (denoted by u) is proportional to the level of those operations. It is concave in S, because the more terrorists there are, the more targets there are for counter-terror operations (but the relationship is concave, not linear, because counter-terror operations are often driven by intelligence leads, not just by random search).

The distinctive feature of this model is that this outflow also increases (and is concave) with the positive reputation of, or sympathy for, the counter-terror forces (denoted by R). The dependence on both S and R is modeled by a power function. Power functions are convenient, increasing concave functions. Indeed modeling a production level (in this case the number of terrorists eliminated) as the product of power functions of the input factors (R, S, and u in this case) is common enough to have a special name (the so-called Cobb–Douglas production function). With this approach, the first-state dynamic equation can be written as

$$\dot{S} = \tau + kS^{\alpha} - \mu S - \eta u S^{\beta} R^{\gamma}. \tag{6.31}$$

On the one hand, public sympathy R is presumed to tend toward a baseline b, but when terrorists are strong (large S), that raises support for the decision-maker (like a regulating authority or state). Here that rate of increase is assumed to be proportional to S.

On the other hand, counter-terror operations sometimes create collateral damage to innocent parties that erodes respect for the authorities. Caulkins et al. (2007b) modeled that erosion as being convex in the intensity of counter-terror operations, the reasoning being that overzealous measures can erode public sympathy more than proportionally. For convenience, here the outflow is taken to be proportional to the square of the intensity of counter-terror operations.

Hence the state equation for the world's regard for the counter-terror authority's legitimacy, R, can be written

$$\dot{R} = \delta S - \rho u^2 + \kappa \left(b - R \right).$$

The objective is simply to minimize a discounted (at rate r) sum of the terrorists' strength and the control costs. Control costs are modeled as being

[7] Noopolitik is stated in contrast to realpolitik and is based on ethics and ideas instead.

proportional to the square of the control intensity, for the usual diminishing-returns arguments. Hence the model becomes:

$$\begin{aligned}
&\min_{u(\cdot)} \int_0^\infty \mathrm{e}^{-rt}\left(cS + \frac{u^2}{2}\right) \mathrm{d}t \\
\text{s.t.}\quad & \dot{S} = \tau + kS^\alpha - \mu S - \eta u S^\beta R^\gamma \\
& \dot{R} = \delta S - \rho u^2 + \kappa\,(b - R) \\
& S(0) = S_0 \geq 0, R(0) = R_0 \geq 0 \\
& u \geq 0.
\end{aligned}$$

Note that we keep the original notation as a minimization problem.

6.3.2 Derivation of the Canonical System

Applying Pontryagin's Minimum Principle gives the Hamiltonian

$$\begin{aligned}
\mathcal{H} = \lambda_0 &\left(cS + \frac{u^2}{2}\right) + \lambda_1\left(\tau + kS^\alpha - \mu S - \eta u S^\beta R^\gamma\right) \\
&+ \lambda_2\left(\delta S - \rho u^2 + \kappa\,(b - R)\right).
\end{aligned}$$

Even though the abnormal case ($\lambda_0 = 0$) cannot be excluded for this model from the outset, we restrict our considerations to the normal case ($\lambda_0 = 1$).

From the Hamiltonian minimizing condition we find

$$\mathcal{H}_u = u - \lambda_1 \eta S^\beta R^\gamma - 2\rho\lambda_2 u = 0 \tag{6.32a}$$

$$\mathcal{H}_{uu} = 1 - 2\lambda_2\rho. \tag{6.32b}$$

Provided that (6.32b) satisfies the strict Legendre–Clebsch condition (see the next remark and note that for a minimization problem $\mathcal{H}_{uu} \geq 0$ has to be satisfied) (6.32a) yields the (interior) optimal control value

$$u^* = \frac{\lambda_1 \eta S^\beta R^\gamma}{1 - 2\rho\lambda_2}. \tag{6.32c}$$

Remark 6.11. A heuristic argument establishes that for the economically meaningful cases the first costate λ_1 will be positive, whereas the second costate λ_2 will be negative. Therefore we consider the economic interpretation of the costate as shadow price. On the one hand, obviously a small increase in the terrorist strength S implies an increase of the objective function and thus $\lambda_1 \geq 0$. On the other hand, increasing the public sympathy R results, due to (6.31), in a decrease of the terrorist strength and hence of the objective function, yielding $\lambda_2 \leq 0$.

Thus for the economically relevant cases, the Legendre–Clebsch condition (6.32b) will be satisfied and since $\lambda_1 \geq 0$ the nonnegativity of the control is guaranteed. This is only heuristic reasoning, showing what can be expected, and has to be verified for the concrete calculation.

Next, we have to establish the adjoint equations, yielding

$$\dot{\lambda}_1 = \lambda_1(-k\alpha S^{\alpha-1} + \mu + \eta u^* \beta S^{\beta-1} R^{\gamma} + r) - c - \lambda_2 \delta$$
$$\dot{\lambda}_2 = \lambda_1 \eta u^* S^{\beta} \gamma R^{\gamma-1} + \lambda_2(\kappa + r),$$

where u^* has to be replaced by (6.32c). Obviously it is not possible to find equilibria of the state–costate equations analytically. Hence we resort to numerical methods.

Remark 6.12. Note that if the constant inflow of terrorist strength, τ, is zero, we immediately find the equilibrium $\hat{S} = 0$, $\hat{R} = b$ and $\hat{\lambda}_2 = 0$. Unfortunately the first costate $\hat{\lambda}_1$ can become infinite if $\alpha < 1$ (which is inconvenient for numerical purposes). To circumvent this problem we therefore consider a small τ keeping that equilibrium $\hat{S}$ near zero but away from the possible singularity. Letting τ converge to zero can then help to determine what the optimal solution would be for τ equal to zero.

Thus for the base-case we apply the parameter values taken from Table 6.3.

Table 6.3. The specified parameter values for the base-case

r	γ	α	b	β	c	δ	η	k	κ	μ	ρ	τ
0.01	1	0.8	1	0.5	1	0.25	0.085	0.05	0.05	0.05	1	10^{-5}

6.3.3 Numerical Calculations

For these base-case parameter values the following three equilibria exist:

$$\hat{E}_l = \begin{pmatrix} 0.0001 \\ 0.9613 \\ 74.7315 \\ -0.0363 \end{pmatrix}, \quad \hat{E}_m = \begin{pmatrix} 0.0155 \\ 0.7061 \\ 147.2660 \\ -3.5342 \end{pmatrix}, \quad \hat{E}_h = \begin{pmatrix} 0.0226 \\ 0.7379 \\ 95.1430 \\ -2.7760 \end{pmatrix},$$

where the computation of the eigenvalues for the corresponding Jacobian matrices reveals that $\hat{E}_l$ (low) and $\hat{E}_h$ (high) exhibit a two-dimensional and $\hat{E}_m$ (medium) exhibits a one-dimensional stable manifold.

To analyze the model's behavior we start calculating the one-dimensional stable manifold of $\hat{E}_m$ using the IVP approach presented on p. 350 in Sect. 7.5.1, which is depicted in Figs. 6.10a and 6.11a as the gray line. Given the existence of multiple equilibria, we have to determine whether one of the equilibria is the unique optimal solution in the long run, or whether there exists a DNSS curve separating regions, where in the long run for initial points lying on the DNSS curve either the low or high equilibrium is optimal. Therefore we continue the optimal solutions, using a BVP approach (see on p. 352 in Sect. 7.5.1) along the connecting line from $\hat{E}_l$ to $\hat{E}_h$ and vice versa. In both cases this continuation process ends at the one-dimensional stable manifold. This result, as projected into the (R, λ_2)-plane, is shown in Fig. 6.10b. It suggest the existence of a weak DNSS point. This weak DNSS point lies on the one-dimensional stable manifold and starting exactly at this point the optimal solution is to move to the medium equilibrium $\hat{E}_m$.

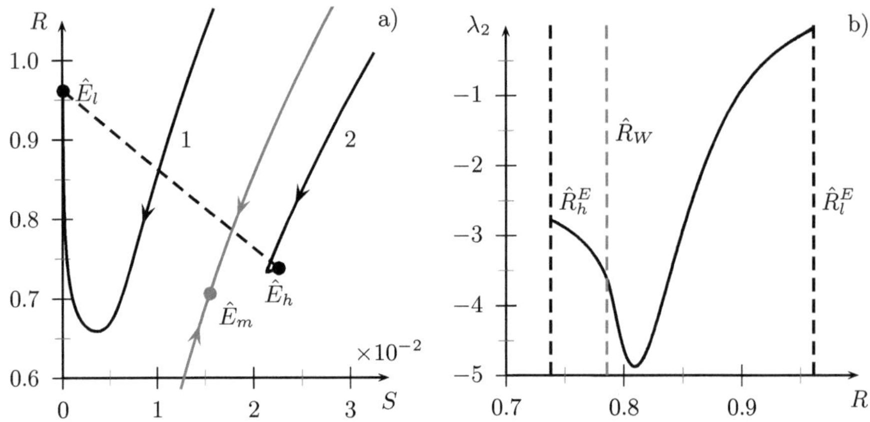

Fig. 6.10. Panel (**a**) depicts the neighborhood of the equilibria, with the one-dimensional stable manifold of $\hat{E}_m$ (*gray line*) and two solution paths (*dark line*). The *dashed line* shows the line along which the solution is continued from $\hat{E}_h$ to $\hat{E}_l$ and vice versa. The result, projected into the (R, λ_2)-plane, is displayed in panel (**b**), where the numerical results suggest the existence of a weak DNSS point (S_W, R_W), lying on the one-dimensional stable manifold

Next we try to find out if the one-dimensional stable manifold serves as a DNSS curve in the state space, separating the regions where it is optimal to move to the high equilibrium inside, move to the low equilibrium outside, or move to the medium equilibrium when starting exactly at the one-dimensional stable manifold. Therefore the two solutions starting at the initial states A and B (see Fig. 6.11a) are continued to the opposite point. I.e., the solution starting at A is continued to B and vice versa. The numerical result reveals that the continuation can be processed further the one-dimensional stable manifold from both sides. Therefore an overlap along the connecting line exists (see Fig. 6.11b). Considering the corresponding Hamiltonian we find a DNSS point for which two optimal solutions exist.

For the numerical computation of the DNSS point and subsequently the DNSS curv the following BVP is stated:

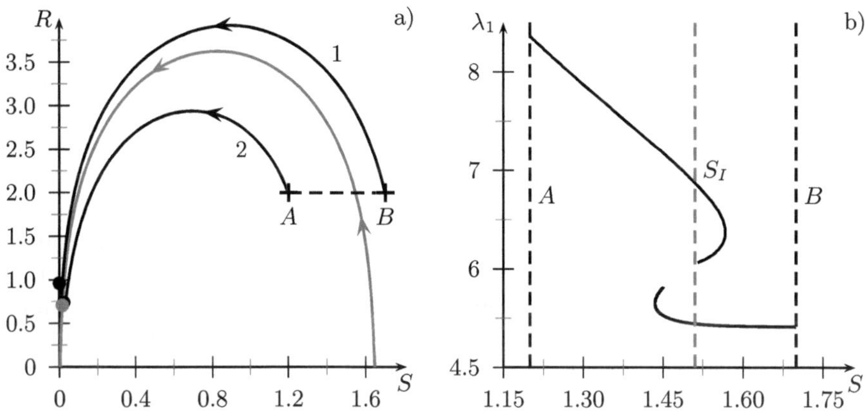

Fig. 6.11. Panel (**a**) depicts the global behavior of the one-dimensional stable manifold of $\hat{E}_m$ (*gray line*), together with two optimal solutions (*dark line*). Along the *dashed line* the solutions starting at the initial points A and B are continued. In panel (**b**) the slice manifolds (see Definition 7.25), i.e., the state–costate values at time zero for the stable paths starting with initial states on the connecting line, are depicted, revealing an overlap, which numerically proves the existence of a DNSS point

$$\dot{X}_l = Tf(X_l), \quad t \in [0, 1] \tag{6.33a}$$

$$\dot{X}_h = Tf(X_h), \quad t \in [0, 1] \tag{6.33b}$$

$$X_l^1(0) = X_h^1(0) = S_0 \tag{6.33c}$$

$$X_l^2(0) = X_h^2(0) \tag{6.33d}$$

$$F_l(X_l(1) - \hat{E}_l) = 0 \tag{6.33e}$$

$$F_h(X_h(1) - \hat{E}_h) = 0 \tag{6.33f}$$

$$\mathcal{H}(X_l(0)) - \mathcal{H}(X_h(0)) = 0, \tag{6.33g}$$

where $X_l = X_h = (S, R, \lambda_1, \lambda_2)'$ and T is some fixed finite time. The first two equations (6.33a) and (6.33b) denote the dynamics of the two different paths, converging to the low and high equilibrium, respectively. The next two equations (6.33c) and (6.33d) cause the first coordinate at time $t = 0$ to be fixed at some value S_0, whereas along the second coordinate the DNSS point is searched for. Equation (6.33e) and (6.33f) are the usual asymptotic boundary conditions (see, e.g., p. 288) assuring that the solutions end up at the stable manifold of the equilibria $\hat{E}_l$ and $\hat{E}_h$, respectively. The last equation (6.33g) finally states the usual DNSS point condition, that the objective value (determined by the Hamiltonian) of both solutions are the same.

Thus we finally find the situation shown in Fig. 6.12b, where part of the one-dimensional stable manifold is a weak DNSS curve, and at some connecting point (a weak DNSS point) this weak part passes over to a DNSS curve.

6.3.4 Optimal Strategy for a Small Terror Organization

The terrorist organization is much stronger in one of the optimal equilibria than in the other ($\hat{S}_h = 0.023$ vs. $\hat{S}_l = 0.0001$). Since the focus is on terror, we refer to these states as the high and low equilibria, respectively, even though the second state variable, the reputation, is lower ($\hat{R}_h = 0.73$ vs. $\hat{S}_l = 0.961$) in the high equilibrium. That is, there is less respect for the counter-terror authorities when the terrorists are stronger because larger terror organizations require a more aggressive control program, and those efforts undermine public support for the authorities. At the low equilibrium, terrorism has been all but eradicated, so only very modest efforts ($u = 0.044$) are needed to hold it in check. This lets the authorities' reputation return nearly to the constant level (of unity) that would pertain in the absence of terror-related influences.

In between the two optimal equilibria there is also an unstable equilibrium $(\hat{S}_m, \hat{R}_m) = (0.016, 0.706)$ with a one-dimensional stable manifold m_s. This situation is reminiscent of the one-dimensional counter-drug model explored in Sect. 2.9. When two stable equilibria are separated by an unstable equilibrium, one should be on the lookout for separating thresholds such that on one "side" of the threshold one should go toward one stable equilibrium, while on the other "side" one should approach the other equilibrium, and on the threshold one is indifferent as to which direction one moves.

Here, however, we have a two-dimensional state space, so that there are no "sides" and the threshold is in general mot a point but a curve. In some two-dimensional models the threshold curve will be more or less a vertical line. One can then still speak of choosing to move to the left or right from the threshold. However, this example shows that the separating thresholds can have complicated shape and hence lead to complicated policy prescriptions.

A numerically computed curve Φ divides the state space into two regions. The curve Φ is composed of parts of the one-dimensional stable path of $\hat{E}_m$ and the set of DNSS points (see Fig. 6.12a). Both parts are connected by a point P_W (denoted by $\otimes$ in Fig. 6.12a). This point is part of the weak DNSS curve, and not a DNSS point itself (see, e.g., the geometric example of a DNSS set Fig. 5.10, where the points $O_{1,2}$ correspond to the point P_W). Starting exactly on the curve Φ left of P_W, one is on the "weak" part of the DNSS curve and hence remain on that curve and move toward the node $\hat{E}_m$. In contrast, starting to the right of P_W, the decision-maker has two optimal strategies, one leading to the lower equilibrium and the other leading to the higher equilibrium. Subsequently we refer to the curve Φ as weak DNSS curve, even though it consists of a "strong" part of DNSS points.

For any initial state outside the region limited by the weak DNSS curve in Fig. 6.12a, the optimal trajectory approaches the higher equilibrium $\hat{E}_h$, whereas for any initial state in the interior of this region, the optimal trajectory approaches the lower equilibrium $\hat{E}_l$.

The shape and direction of the weak DNSS curve makes intuitive sense. The greater the initial level of sympathy, the more likely it is to be optimal to

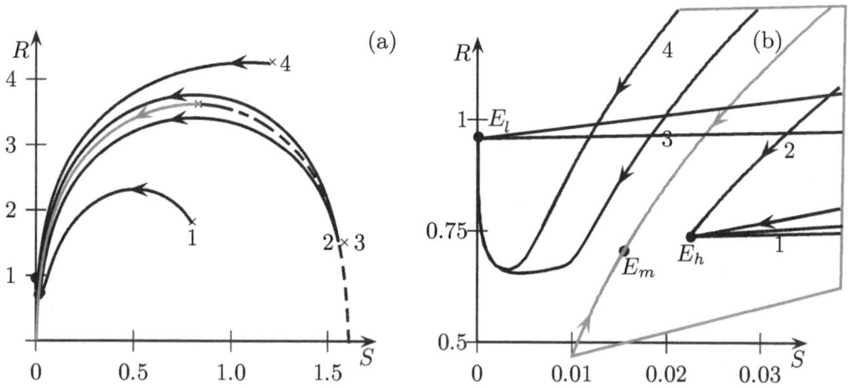

Fig. 6.12. In panel (**a**) four optimal paths (*black solid curves*), denoted by 1, 2, 3, 4, are depicted. Path 1 and 2 converge to the high equilibrium E_h and the paths 3 and 4 move to the low equilibrium E_l. The *gray solid line* is a weak DNSS curve approaching the medium equilibrium E_m. The *dashed black curve* is a DNSS curve and the paths 2 and 3 are two equally optimal solutions starting at one of DNSS points. The weak DNSS curve and DNSS curve meet at point ⊗, which is the last weak DNSS point. In panel (**b**) the trajectories 1–4 and weak DNSS curve are depicted in the neighborhood of the equilibria

drive the number of terrorists down to the low equilibrium. It would appear that sympathy acts like a capital stock that is drawn down in order to drive the number of terrorists close to "extinction." Once the number of terrorists has been reduced, the intensity of control is low, and sympathy rebounds as the lower equilibrium is approached.

Likewise, for any given initial level of sympathy, $R(0)$, if the initial number of terrorists is smaller than (to the left of) the weak DNSS curve (see Fig. 6.12a,b) then it is optimal to drive the number of terrorists down to the lower equilibrium. But if the initial number of terrorists is "too large," then the best one can do is to moderate growth in the number of terrorists toward the larger equilibrium. Such "eradicate or accommodate" choices have appeared before in optimal dynamic control models of "bad stocks" whose inflow is increasing in the level of the stock (see, e.g., Sect. 3.9).

That tidy interpretation does not, however, hold up if one moves away from the origin. Figure 6.12b parallels Fig. 6.12a, but for S-values up to almost two, it shows that the weak DNSS curve that was upward sloping reaches a maximum, then bends back down all the way to the horizontal axis. That the weak DNSS curve Φ may reach a maximum is not so surprising. It says that if sympathy is large enough, it is not only possible but also optimal to use counter-terror operations to drive the number of terrorists down to the low equilibrium, no matter how many terrorists there are initially.

That the weak DNSS curve bends back down to the axis is more surprising. This says that for initial numbers of terrorists $S(0)$ around 1.5 and initial sympathy levels that are not high (e.g., $R < 3$), the policy prescription is reversed. If the initial number of terrorists is very large (to the right of the weak DNSS curve), it is optimal to scale the number of terrorists back to very low levels. But if there are not so many terrorists initially, then the optimal strategy is to let them persist in the long run in greater numbers; because neither the intensity of the terror problem nor the public sympathy is high enough admitting the usage of large control to reduce the number of terrorists near to "extinction."

Clearly, if one could instantly move to either equilibrium at no cost, one would prefer the lower equilibrium. Therefore if it is optimal to approach the higher equilibrium, the trajectory to that equilibrium must be better in the short run. That is the case here. When $S(0)$ is to the left of the right-hand side of the weak DNSS curve, the best way to reach the higher equilibrium is to quickly drive down the number of terrorists. When the initial number of terrorists is larger, specifically to the right of the weak DNSS curve, the number of terrorists will fall relatively quickly of its own accord because it greatly exceeds the uncontrolled equilibrium number of $\hat{S} = 1$. The optimal policy in that case is not to deploy counter-terror operations too aggressively at first, but instead to build up the stock of public sympathy. Once that stock has grown, then it becomes optimal to deploy counter-terror operations aggressively. Furthermore, given the accumulation of public sympathy, those counter-terror operations can and should be used to drive the number of terrorists down to the lower equilibrium.

With the base-case parameters, larger initial levels of public sympathy $R(0)$ always increase the range of initial numbers of terrorists for which it is optimal to essentially eradicate terrorism. That is, the weak DNSS curve bends back down, but it does not turn back on itself. Is that result robust?

It turns out that the answer is no. Modest changes in parameter values can lead to a backward bending right-hand side of the weak DNSS curve. For example, this occurs if κ is reduced from 0.05 to 0.02.

Following the examples in this chapter step-by-step the reader should have gotten a deeper understanding of how optimal control problems can be applied to real world problems (and how to *apply* the theory). Of course the precise description of the numerical steps are brief, keeping in mind that the next chapter is devoted to this topic only.

Exercises

6.1 (Endemic Level of US Cocaine Epidemic). Determine the equilibrium and the stability properties for the canonical system for the abnormal case of problem (6.6). Determine the equilibrium and the stability properties for the canonical system (normal case) of problem (6.6) for the parameter values given in Table 6.1.

6.2 (Rational Addiction and Bingeing). Becker and Murphy (1988) and Dockner and Feichtinger (1993) considered the following rational addiction model:

$$\begin{aligned} \max_{c(\cdot)} & \int_0^\infty \mathrm{e}^{-rt} U(c, S, W)\, dt \\ \text{s.t.} \quad & \dot{S} = c - \delta S, \quad S(0) = S_0 \geq 0 \\ & \dot{W} = c - \alpha W, \quad W(0) = W_0 \geq 0, \end{aligned}$$

where $c(t)$ denotes the consumption rate at time t, S the accumulated consumption, W the weight or, more generally, the health status of a person, and δ, $\alpha > 0$ constant depreciation rates. The utility function $U(c, S, W)$ is assumed to be strictly concave in c, S, and W. While $U_{SW} = 0$, it is assumed that the marginal consumption utility increases with past consumption

$$U_{cS} = \frac{\partial}{\partial S} \frac{\partial U}{\partial c} > 0.$$

There are at least two interpretations of the model, namely dieting–overweighting and binge drinking. Show that stable limit cycles may occur as stable solutions for sufficiently positive values of U_{cS} and high discount rates r. Becker (1992) has characterized *addiction* by these properties. Discuss and interpret *bingeing*, i.e., alternate periods of high and low consumption.

6.3 (Harm Reduction). A heated debate in drug policy concerns the relative merits of "harm reduction" (e.g., reducing drug-related HIV/AIDS transmission) vs. "use reduction" (controlling drug use per se). The following two-state model investigates whether shifting emphasis between these goals over the course of a drug epidemic might reduce social costs (compare Caulkins, Feichtinger, Tragler, & Wallner, 2007).

Denote by $A(t)$ the number of drug users at time t, and by $S(t)$ the number of nonusers (susceptibles). The control variable $v(t)$ is the percentage reduction in harmfulness of drug use at time t. Social costs are the product of A and a baseline social cost per user per unit of time when there is no harm reduction. The harmfulness without harm reduction is, without loss of generality, normalized to 1. Then $1 - v$ is the proportion of harm that is not averted via harm reduction policies.

This leads to the following problem

$$\begin{aligned} \min_{v(\cdot)} & \int_0^\infty \mathrm{e}^{-rt} \left(A(1-v) + c(v)\right) dt \\ \text{s.t.} \quad & \dot{S} = k - \delta S - f(A) S h(v) \\ & \dot{A} = f(A) S h(v) - \mu A \\ & 0 \leq v \leq 1, \end{aligned}$$

where k denotes the inflow rate, δ the outflow rate, and μ a death or ceasing rate, all three of which are assumed to be constant. Moreover, $f(A)$ is assumed a convex function measuring the dependence of drug initiation on the number of users, whereas $h(v)$, which is assumed to be a convex increasing function with $h(0) = 1$, and measures the impact of harm reduction on initiation.

Determine the long-run equilibria in the (A, S)-plane and carry out a stability analysis. Use the functions $c(v) = cv^2$, as well as $f(A) = c_1 A^\alpha$ and $h(v) = 1 + \beta v$, where the parameter c denotes the costs of the percentage decrease in harm, c_1 and α determine the strength of the influence of the users, and β describes how much any reduction of harm influences the flow from susceptibles to users (compare Seidl,

2008). Show that for the parameter constellation $c = 8$, $r = 0.04$, $k = 1$, $\delta = 0.05$, $c_1 = 0.01$, $\alpha = 1.75$, $\beta = 0.17$, and $\mu = 0.1$ there exist three long-run equilibria and try to calculate a (weak) DNSS curve. Try to interpret the results for an evaluation of drug policy.

6.4 (Multiple Drug Use). Reconsider the drug model from Sect. 3.9 with the single state A representing the number of users of some given drug. Assume now that we have two different drugs denoted simply by 1 and 2, and let A_1 and A_2 represent the numbers of users consuming drug 1 and 2, respectively. Assume further that, at any given time, a user may consume only drug 1 or drug 2, but allow for the users to change their drug of choice. Then, we may formulate the following two-state model:

$$\min_{u_1(\cdot),u_2(\cdot)} \int_0^\infty \mathrm{e}^{-rt}\left(\rho_1 A_1 + \rho_2 A_2 + u_1 + u_2\right) \mathrm{d}t$$

$$\text{s.t.}\quad \dot{A}_1 = k_1 A_1\left(\bar{A}_1 - A_1\right) - c_1 u_1^{z_1} A_1^{1-z_1} - \mu_1 A_1 - \gamma_1 A_1 + \gamma_2 A_2$$

$$\dot{A}_2 = k_2 A_2\left(\bar{A}_2 - A_2\right) - c_2 u_2^{z_2} A_2^{1-z_2} - \mu_2 A_2 + \gamma_1 A_1 - \gamma_2 A_2,$$

where the control variables u_1 and u_2 represent treatment spending for drugs 1 and 2, respectively, γ_1 and γ_2 are the rates at which users switch from one drug to the other, and the other parameters are to be interpreted as in the original model formulation.

It is obvious that for the special case $\gamma_1 = \gamma_2 = 0$, this model decomposes into two fully uncoupled problems as given by the original model. In that case, one may draw a phase diagram in the (A_1, A_2)-plane with a fourfold indifference point, from which one may approach four different equilibria (cf. Brock and Dechert, 1983). First, analyze this model in a fully symmetric scenario, where all parameters are the same for the two populations, and take values as provided in Sect. 3.9, but allow $\gamma_1 = \gamma_2$ to be not only zero but also positive. Once you gain sufficient insight into the behavior of the model, consider also a heterogeneous setting, where parameters are different for the two populations. For instance, drug 1 may be less costly than drug 2 (i.e., $\rho_1 < \rho_2$), drug 2 may be more attractive and more readily available than drug 1 (i.e., $k_2 > k_1$ and $\bar{A}_2 > \bar{A}_1$), drug 2 is more costly and harder to treat than drug 1 (i.e., $\rho_1 < \rho_2$ and $c_1 > c_2$).

Other examples of the A_1A_2-paradigm are optimal growth of disparate regions, pollution, economic growth, and lobbying.

6.5 (An Extended Heterogeneous Drug Model). In the Sects. 3.9 and 6.1 we analyzed a model of drug demand that embodied two different levels of consumption, light and heavy use. "Light" users were envisioned as suffering few adverse consequences and hence helping to spread drug use, while "heavy" users were envisioned as suffering substantially more harm and thus, when there are relatively many heavy users, dampening the rate of initiation into drug use.

This example introduces an autonomous three-state, single-control model to explore how best to control epidemics of drug use when initiation is both contagious (transmitted from existing users) and moderated by the *memory of past experiences* of drug use, as suggested by Musto (1987). This extension has obvious appeal. All knowledge of the negative experiences of a heavy user is unlikely to disappear the very moment the individual leaves the population, particularly if his/her exit is due to physical death from drug use (as opposed to ceasing use or moving out of the area). Thus we assume that the drug's reputation is governed by the relative number of light users (denoted by the state variable L) and a decaying memory of people who have ever been heavy users (denoted by the state variable E). The flow into this state is the same as the flow into the number of current heavy users (denoted by the state variable H). The outflow is a simple exponential decay governed by a memory parameter δ. When this parameter is small, memories of heavy users are long-lived; when δ is large, the dampening effect of heavy users' problems on initiation dissipates rapidly. Hence, we model initiation as

$$I(L,\, E) = \tau + sL\mathrm{e}^{-q\frac{E}{L}},$$

where

- τ = rate of "spontaneous initiation"
- s = annual rate at which light users attract nonusers when a drug's reputation is benign
- q = constant which measures the deterrent effect of heavy use

Drug treatment (denoted by the control variable $u(t)$) is the only drug control intervention concerned and is modeled according to (6.2). The objective is assumed to minimize the total drug related cost. Thus we seek values of u that maximize the integral

$$\max_{u(\cdot)} \int_0^\infty \mathrm{e}^{-rt} \left(-\kappa \left(\mu_L L - \mu_H H\right) - u\right) \mathrm{d}t$$

$$\text{s.t.} \quad \dot{L} = I\left(L, E\right) - (a+b)L, \quad L(0) = L_0$$

$$\dot{H} = bL - \left(g + \beta\left(H, u\right) H, \quad H(0) = H_0\right.$$

$$\dot{E} = bL - \delta E, \quad E(0) = E_0 = H_0.$$

Determine the necessary conditions for the problem sketched above. Determine the equilibrium point and the Jacobian evaluated at the equilibrium. Draw a bifurcation diagram for δ for the following set of parameter values: $r = 0.04$, $\kappa = 113$, $\mu_L = 16.42$, $\mu_H = 118.93$, $a = 0.163$, $b = 0.024$, $s = 0.61$, $q = 7.25$, $d = 0.6$, $c = 5 \times 10^{-4}$, $\tau = 50,000$. Is recurrent behavior likely to occur if δ varies? What about the discount rate? Is the parameter value r capable of producing periodic solutions (i.e., is it optimal to repeat the past (epidemics) if the future is not highly valued (r large))?

6.6 (Methadone Maintenance Treatment). In order to determine how much should be spent methadone maintenance treatment (MMT), consider the following optimal control model (compare Caulkins et al., 2006; Pollack, 2001). The state variables N and I define the total number of illicit drug users (IDU) and the number of them who are HCV infected, respectively. Authorities try to control the illicit drug use and the spreading of HCV infection (caused by needle sharing) by installing MMT programs. In the model, M defines the number of IDUs undergoing methadone treatment.

The parameter r denotes the discount rate and the other exogenous parameters of the model are:

- θ exogenous increase of IDUs due to initiation or immigration

- δ per capita outflow of IDUs in the absence of treatment
- μ exit rate of IDUs due to treatment
- γ proportion of those exiting due to treatment who do not relapse
- κ risk of infection in case of sharing a needle with an infected IDU
- ψ frequency of needle sharing
- Ω fraction of those IDUs who share needles

C^M, C^N, and C^I model the costs caused by methadone treatment, illicit drugs use, and HCV infection. (Note that the rate of new HCV infections is $\kappa\psi\,(\Omega N - I)\,\frac{I}{\Omega N}$ in the absence of an MMT program. Methadone treatment reduces this rate by the proportionality factor $(1 - \frac{M}{N})$.)

Hence, consider the following optimal control model, where the aggregated overall costs are minimized:

$$\begin{aligned}
&\min_{M(\cdot)} \int_0^\infty \mathrm{e}^{-rt}\left(C^M(M) + C^N(N) + C^I\left(\kappa\psi(1-\frac{M}{N})(\Omega N - I)\frac{I}{\Omega N}\right)\right)\mathrm{d}t \\
&\text{s.t. } \dot{N} = \theta - \delta\,(N - M) - \mu\gamma M, \\
&\quad \dot{I} = \kappa\psi\left(1 - \frac{M}{N}\right)(\Omega N - I)\,\frac{I}{\Omega N} - \delta I\left(1 - \frac{M}{N}\right) - \mu\gamma I\frac{M}{N}, \\
&\quad N(0) = N_0 \ge 0, \quad I(0) = I_0 \in [0,\,\Omega N_0] \\
&\quad 0 \le M \le N.
\end{aligned}$$

The model can be simplified by replacing the state variable I by $P = I/N$ and the control variable M by $U = M/N$, and grouping parameters $a = \mu\gamma - \delta$, $\beta_1 = \kappa\psi$, $\beta_2 = \frac{\kappa\psi}{\Omega}$. Verify the adapted model has the following form:

$$\begin{aligned}
&\min_{U(\cdot)\in[0,1]} \int_0^\infty \mathrm{e}^{-rt}\left(C^M(UN) + C^N(N) + C^I\left((\beta_1 - \beta_2 P)(1-U)NP\right)\right)\mathrm{d}t \\
&\text{s.t.} \quad \dot{N} = \theta - \delta N - aUN, \\
&\quad \dot{P} = P\left((1-U)\,(\beta_1 - \beta_2\,P) - \frac{\theta}{N}\right), \\
&\quad N(0) = N_0, \quad P(0) = P_0 = \frac{I_0}{N_0} \in [0,\,\Omega].
\end{aligned}$$

Assume now that the treatment intensity U constant. Compute the equilibrium of the system dynamics in case of absence of HCV infections ($P = 0$). Analyze the local stability of this equilibrium.

Hint. Distinguish between the cases $\delta < \beta_1$ and $\delta > \beta_1$.

Prove that there are equilibria with positive P only if $U < (\beta_1 - \delta)/(\beta_1 + a)$. As a result, there exists no equilibrium in case of $\delta > \beta_1$ regardless of what policy is implemented.

Define $C^M(M) = \alpha_1 M + \alpha_2 M^2$ quadratically, and $C^N(N) = \rho N$ and $C^I(x) = \nu x$ linearly. Determine and maximize the Hamiltonian (take care that $u \in [0,1]$). Derive the dynamics of the costate variables λ_1 and λ_2. Compute equilibria of this state costate dynamics in the absence of any infection. ($P = 0$). To investigate further the equilibria, reduce the system of four nonlinear equations $\dot{N} = \dot{P} = \dot{\lambda}_1 = \dot{\lambda}_2 = 0$ to a single equation $g(N) = 0$ in the single variable N.

The equation $g(N) = 0$ is too tricky to investigate it analytically. To do this job numerically parameter specifications are needed. Start your investigations with the following parameter specification: $r = 3/100$, $\theta = 183$, $\delta = 183/2,000$, $\mu = 0.9125, \gamma = 2/10$, $\kappa = 4/100$, $\psi = 52$, $\Omega = 3/10$; moreover $\rho = 6,000$, $\alpha_1 = 4,014$, $\alpha_2 = 1$. The specification of ν is a more complicated; estimates of the costs of an HCV infected person vary between some thousands of USD up to more than 100K USD (depending especially on whether indirect costs, like reduction of economic productivity, are included or not).

Vary ν in the interval $[2000, 11000]$ and produce a two-dimensional plot containing the U values of the equilibria. (Remark: U and ν are the axes.) Investigate the local stability of these equilibria. Fix ν at 70K. Now vary $\sigma := \mu\gamma$ within the values $\sigma \in [11/10\,\delta, 23/10\,\delta]$ and produce a two-dimensional plot containing the U values of the equilibria. (Remark: U and σ are the axes.) Investigate the local stability of these equilibria.

6.7 (A Two-State Capital Accumulation Model). Consider the following capital accumulation model with the capital stock K and the investment rate I as state variables, and the change of investment rate v as control (compare Haunschmied, Kort, Hartl, & Feichtinger, 2003):

$$\max_{v(\cdot)} \int_0^\infty \mathrm{e}^{-\rho t} \left(R(K) - c(I) - \frac{\alpha}{2} v^2 \right) \mathrm{d}t,$$

$$\text{s.t.} \quad \dot{K} = I - \delta K,$$

$$\dot{I} = v.$$

The revenue function $R(K)$ is monotonously increasing and features a convex segment, i.e., it has a concave–convex–concave shape. Moreover $R(0) = 0$ and the limits satisfy $\lim_{K\to 0} R'(K) = \infty$, $\lim_{K\to\infty} R(K) = 0$, and $\lim_{K\to\infty} R'(K) = 0$. (Note: R' decreases from infinity to a positive minimum, increases to a maximum and finally decreases to zero.[8])

The function

$$c(I) = c_1 I + \frac{c_2}{2} I^2$$

denotes the investment costs.

Derive the necessary optimality conditions. Prove that there are at least one and at most three equilibria fulfilling the necessary optimality conditions. Show that in case of three equilibria the local stability analysis results in one equilibrium with a one-dimensional stable invariant manifold, and two equilibria with a two-dimensional stable invariant manifold. The latter two equilibria are saddle points with transient oscillations if

$$(\alpha\delta(\rho + \delta) - c_2)^2 + 4R''(K_i)\alpha < 0;$$

otherwise they are saddle points with real eigenvalues. (Note: K_i are the equilibrium values of K.)

Specify the revenue function by

$$R(K) = k_1 \sqrt{K} - k_3 \frac{K}{1 + k_2 K^4}.$$

[8] For an economic explanation see Haunschmied et al. (2003).

Use a new time scaling $\tau = \delta t$ and the parameter grouping

$$\tilde{k}_2 = \sqrt[4]{k_2},\ \bar{\rho} = \frac{\rho}{\delta},\ a_1 = \frac{k_3}{k_1\sqrt{\tilde{k}_2}},\ a_2 = \frac{c_1\delta}{k_1\sqrt{\tilde{k}_2}},\ a_3 = \frac{c_2\delta^2}{k_1\tilde{k}_2\sqrt{\tilde{k}_2}},\ a_4 = \frac{\alpha\delta^4}{k_1\tilde{k}_2\sqrt{\tilde{k}_2}}.$$

Transform the model variables as follows

$$x(\tau) = k_2' K\left(\frac{\tau}{\delta}\right),\quad y(\tau) = \frac{\tilde{k}_2}{\delta} I\left(\frac{\tau}{\delta}\right),\quad u(\tau) = \frac{\tilde{k}_2}{\delta^2} v\left(\frac{\tau}{\delta}\right).$$

Show that the optimal control problem can be written in a more simplified shape:

$$\max_{u(\cdot)} \int_0^\infty \mathrm{e}^{-\bar{\rho}\tau}\left(\sqrt{x} - a_1\frac{x}{1+x^4} - a_2 y - \frac{a_3}{2}y^2 - \frac{a_4}{2}u^2\right)\mathrm{d}\tau,$$
$$\text{s.t.}\quad \dot{x} = y - x, \qquad \dot{y} = u.$$

Use the simplified version of the optimal control model to analyze the model numerically. For this purpose specify

$$\tilde{k}_2 = 0.329,\quad \bar{\rho} = 0.160,\quad a_1 = 0.872,\quad a_2 = 0.163,\quad a_3 = 0.414,\quad a_4 = 0.124.$$

Derive the adapted necessary optimality conditions. Derive the two equilibria with a two-dimensional stable invariant manifold. Try to compute numerically at least one point in the state space, where one is indifferent to control the system optimally to one or the other of these two equilibria. Finally verify numerically that it is not possible to control the system by fulfilling the necessary optimality conditions in a way starting at the state values of one equilibrium and finally converging to the state values of the other equilibrium.

6.8 (A Technology Investment Decision Problem). Consider a single product firm that optimizes discounted and aggregated profits (sale revenues minus investment costs). The state variables are sales volume C and the technology content T of the product (relative to a baseline). The firm controls the investment in improving the technology content of the product (compare Haunschmied, Feichtinger, Kort, & Hartl, 2005).

$$\max_{I(\cdot)\geq 0} \int_0^\infty \mathrm{e}^{-rt}(\alpha C - a(I))\,\mathrm{d}t$$

$$\begin{aligned}\text{s.t.}\quad & \dot{C} = \gamma\left(f(T) - C\right) - k\,C\,I,\\ & \dot{T} = h(T)I - \delta T,\\ & C(0) = C_0 > 0,\quad T(0) = T_0 > 0.\end{aligned}$$

The parameters r, α, γ, k, δ are positive, $a(\cdot)$ is monotonously increasing and convex, whereas $f(\cdot)$ is monotonously increasing and concave; $a(0) = f(0) = 0$. Moreover, postulate various assumptions on the effectiveness $h(T)$ of technology investments:

A_1: The effectiveness of technology investments increases from 0 at $T = 0$ and decreases to 0 at infinity and it is unimodal with a maximum at T_{max}; additionally $\lim_{T\to 0^+} h(T)/T = 0$.

$\widetilde{A_1}$: The marginal effectiveness of technology investments ($h'(T)$) monotonously increases in the interval $[0, T_1)$, decreases until T_2 (of course $T_1 < T_{max} < T_2$) and finally increases to zero at infinity.

A_2: The "technology investment effectiveness elasticity" $\frac{h'(T)}{h(T)} T$ decreases monotonically from a positive value for $T = 0$ to a negative value for $T \to \infty$.

Determine and maximize the current-value Hamiltonian (take care that $I \geq 0$). Derive the dynamics of the costate variables λ_1 and λ_2. The system dynamics has a trivial equilibrium at $C = T = I = 0$. Compute the relevant costate values. To investigate further equilibria reduce the system of four nonlinear equations $\dot{C} = \dot{T} = \dot{\lambda}_1 = \dot{\lambda}_2 = 0$ to a single equation $G(T) = 0$ in the single variable T. Prove that there are at most three equilibria.

Specify

$$a(I) = a_1 I + a_2 I^2, \quad f(T) = f_1 T, \quad h(T) = \frac{h_1 T^2}{1 + \left(\frac{T}{h_2}\right)^3}.$$

Start your investigations with the following parameter specification

$$r = 0.05,\ \delta = \frac{1}{24},\ \alpha = 2,\ \gamma = 0.0625,\ f_1 = 1,\ a_1 = 1,\ a_2 = \frac{1}{3},\ h_1 = \frac{1}{2700},\ h_2 = 75.$$

Vary parameter k in the interval $[0.002, 0.014]$ and investigate the local stability of the computed equilibria. You should find a special equilibrium, where the eigenvalues of the local linearization of the state costate dynamics are purely imaginary (PAH-bifurcation point.)

Employ a bifurcation analysis program to compute limit cycles emanating from this bifurcation point by decreasing k. Verify (with the aid of the bifurcation analysis program) that these limit cycles are unstable.

Decrease k further to the point where the stable limit cycle merges with another limit cycle and then for even smaller k the limit cycles disappear (limit point bifurcation).

Now start from the limit point bifurcation, where you face a semistable limit cycle and increase k, but now concentrate on the development of the stable limit cycle.

Note that in the four-dimensional state costate space these cycles are not fully stable but feature a two-dimensional stable invariant manifold. Fix $k = 0.00852$ and compute some trajectory on this manifold.

Hint. Use the monodromy matrix to compute points on this manifold next to the limit cycle.

Try to find a set of initial values C_0 and T_0, where one is indifferent between controlling the system in a way that the solution path converges to the origin or to the limit cycle.

Notes and Further Reading

Corruption is a perennial phenomenon. The political scientist Friedrich wrote that "politics needs all these dubious practices, it cannot be managed without corruption"

(Friedrich, 1972). The evolution of corruption within a society – its emergence and expansion but also its uncovering, prosecution, and deterrence – is often complex and apparently spontaneous.

Economic analysis of the supply and demand of bribes was pioneered by Rose-Ackerman (1978) (for recent applications see Chander & Wilde, 1992 on illegal tax evasion, Hillman & Katz, 1987 on the distribution of bribes within hierarchical bureaucracies, and Shleifer & Vishny, 1993 for a survey).

The model of corruption in governments subject to popularity constraints analyzed in Sect. 6.2 traces back to Feichtinger and Wirl (1991, 1994) and is remarkable for at least two reasons. First, it admits various interesting interpretations ("the two sides of a medal"). One of them is optimal consumption or production under environmental constraints, see Wirl (1999). Second, the model provides probably the simplest optimal control framework in which *optimal stable limit cycles* occur. Note that the model, also called *Wirl's paradigm*, is not only separable (i.e., no interaction occurs), but also is strictly concave; compare also Wirl (1992).

Just as economics is divided into micro- and macro-level analysis, so too are there multiple levels of mathematical modeling of substance abuse issues. At the lowest unit of analysis there is a medical/scientific literature addressing the pharmacokinetics of drug molecules binding with receptors, being broken down into metabolites, and possibly being detected via assays. This level of analysis is omitted in this text because it requires a substantial time investment to understand the underlying biochemistry and biophysics. However, advances in brain science and investments in treatment research, including innovations such as vaccines that can interdict drug molecules after ingestion but before they cross the blood-brain barrier (Harwood & Myers, 2003) make this an exciting domain of mathematical modeling.

The next level of analysis focuses on explaining individual behavior. The bulk of work at this unit of analysis is empirical and statistical, but Becker and Murphy (1988) introduced the notion of explaining certain stylized facts concerning addictive behavior via rational actor (economic) models that included a state variable representing an individual's accumulated past history of consumption, the so-called *consumption stock*. As perhaps was Becker and Murphy's intent, this "rational addiction theory" (RAT) was controversial and stimulated considerable follow-on research. For example, Dockner and Feichtinger (1993) demonstrated that consumption behavior may end up in persistent oscillations (stable limit cycles). This may explain binges that continue to cycle often throughout an agent's lifetime.

Becker (1992) stressed that a key idea, underpinning these models of *habit formation* and *addiction*, is that past consumption influences current behavior. In this literature, addiction means that greater past consumption raises the marginal utility of present consumption, although other parameters are also important for modeling the development of strong habits, including, for instance, the rate of discount on future utilities. To the extent that this tradition regards addiction as just a strong habit, the fact that drugs bind directly with neuroreceptors rather than operating through the five senses is irrelevant. RAT thus creates a bridge between drug use modeling and an older economic literature on habit formation, including, e.g., the important contribution made by Ryder and Heal (1973) who anticipated persistent oscillatory consumption behavior as a result of the degree of complementarity between past and current consumption.

Most of the drug control examples discussed in this text come from a third and higher level of aggregation, namely studying change over time in the population-level prevalence of drug use and drug-related problems. This level of analysis draws on two distinct traditions: the literatures in epidemiology and mathematical biosciences modeling the spread of contagious diseases and the literatures in marketing and management modeling "viral" or "word of mouth" diffusion of innovation and new product adoption.

Earlier modeling was primarily descriptive or confined to static optimization (e.g., Baveja, Batta, Caulkins, & Karwan, 1993; Behrens et al., 1999; Caulkins, 1993; Gardiner & Schreckengost, 1987; Homer, 1993a; Levin et al., 1975; Rossi, 1999; Rydell et al., 1996; Rydell & Everingham, 1994). Behrens et al. (2000b) and Tragler et al. (2001) were the first to apply optimal dynamic control theory to these epidemic models. The former is the basis for the LH-drug control model discussed in this chapter, and the latter being the basis for the A-model discussed earlier.

So-called SIR-models of contagious diseases often model explicitly not only people who currently have the condition/use drugs (I for "infected" individuals), but also to track the number who are susceptible (S for "susceptible") to initiation. Recent work has been extending the drug epidemic models to also consider explicitly individuals who are not currently using but who are susceptible to initiation. In particular, Caulkins et al. (2007) use such a model to explore implications of varying a country's drug control objectives between reducing drug use and reducing drug-related harm even if use *per se* is not released. Use reduction is the dominant policy in the US, but Australia and a few European countries (including the UK and the Netherlands) make an explicit objective of reducing the harmfulness of drug use. Both sides seem to have convincing arguments. Many harm reduction advocates focus on harm suffered by users, notably the risk of overdose and HIV/AIDS. Many advocates of use reduction focus on harm to nonusers such as drug-related crime. Caulkins et al. (2007) discussed the trade-off that efforts to reduce harmfulness will spur greater use; compare also MacCoun (1998) and MacCoun, Reuter, and Schelling (1996).

Many dependent users have used more than one substance and are willing to alter their drug of choice in response to price and availability. Likewise, it is common for careers of drug use to begin with certain substances (e.g., cannabis), with some progressing on to use other substances (e.g., heroin or cocaine). So it is natural to want to extend these drug control models to address explicitly interactions between users of different drugs, e.g., to create an A_1A_2-model with one state variable for the number of current users of each of two different drugs. An early analysis of a model with this sort of structure was given by Brock and Dechert (1983). The multiple drug use model of Exercise 6.4 is part of a PhD thesis by Zeiler (2008) that substantially extends this line of analysis. There seem to be many applications of the A_1A_2-model paradigm in various other fields, including optimal economic growth of different regimes and the interaction between pollution and economic growth.

Likewise, there are any number of two-state models relevant to crime and delinquency. For example, Caulkins, Feichtinger, Tragler, and Veliov (2007) analyzed a two-state model of cycles of violence in which oscillations are generated when surges in lethal violence shrink the pool of active violent offenders. The analysis includes finding the optimal dynamic trajectory of incarceration and violence prevention interventions.

In some countries, terrorists try to hurt the country income from the tourism industry by violent actions against tourists. Feichtinger, Hartl, Kort, and Novak (2001) attempted to model the interaction of tourists and terrorists as predator-prey relation. They analyze a two-state optimal control model, the controls being the investment in the touristic infrastructure as well as in counter-terroristic measures. For reasonable parameter values, the optimal trajectory exhibits a cyclical strategy. The interpretation is that, after starting out with a low number of tourists and terrorists, tourism investments are undertaken to increase tourism. This attracts terrorists reducing the effect of tourism investments. Therefore, investment declines and so does the number of tourists. This makes it less attractive for terrorists to act, so we are back in the original situation, where the whole thing starts again.

Illegal drug use is a relatively recent concern, dating primarily to the late nineteenth century, but terrorism has been around for centuries. Still, terrorism has particular potency in the modern era of electronic media and global interdependence. Whereas in the past terror tactics might have been employed to instill fear in the populace in a particular region, now terrorists can strive for global visibility and impact.

The September 11th attacks in the US ushered in a period of greater attention to terrorism and a willingness, even a determination, to take a multi-disciplinary approach (see, e.g., Kaplan, Mintz, Mishal, & Samban, 2005; Keohane & Zeckhauser, 2003) to thinking about terror control. Before September 11th, analyzing terror issues was primarily the province of political scientists, regional studies experts, and military analysts. Now a much broader range of disciplines is involved, including Operations Research, as evidenced by the recent issue of the journal *Interfaces* that was devoted to homeland security (vol. 36(6), 2006). Likewise annual conferences that have been launched to present and promote mathematical analysis of counter-terror, including the MAPUSE series, which will continue under the new name of INESS, and the series of conferences held on Mathematical Methods in Counterterrorism, held most recently at the Rochester Institute of Technology in the US.

The importance of the contribution of mathematical modeling applied to the field of terrorism is not without controversy. It is therefore appropriate to close by noting some would disagree with the familiar perception of mathematics as a neutral tool – a view summarized by statistician Jerzy Neyman's statement (see Høyrup, 1994): "*I prove theorems, they are published, and after that I don't know what happens to them.*" In particular, we refer the reader to Booß-Bavnbek and Høyrup (2003); Forman and Sánchez-Rón (1996); Høyrup (1994) for discussion of mathematical methods applied to warfare from different and often controversial perspectives.

Brito (1999) characterized the local dynamics of a three-state control model.

7

Numerical Methods for Discounted Systems of Infinite Horizon

In the previous chapters we presented both the theoretical background of optimal control theory and some interesting examples from the application fields of drugs, corruption, and terror. What remains is the question of how to actually compute the optimal solutions. How should we apply the theoretical results to retrieve algorithms for numerical calculations? A broad range of numerical algorithms can be used to solve optimal control problems, and presenting the underlying theory is far beyond the scope of this book. We therefore restrict our considerations to the special class of autonomous, discounted infinite time horizon problems. We concentrate on this restricted class of optimal control models because they are the most commonly investigated problems in an economic context. Furthermore, we provide a collection of MATLAB files (`OCMat` toolbox)[1] enabling the numerical calculations of such optimal control problems.

Several approaches can be chosen to solve optimal control problems. The method presented here uses Pontryagin's Maximum Principle to establish the corresponding canonical system. In its essence, solving an optimal control problem is translated to the problem of analyzing the canonical system (see Definition 3.6). Before we go into further detail we have to introduce some notational specifics and general techniques that are used throughout this chapter.

7.1 General Remarks

This section addresses the problem formulation under consideration in this book and the notational conventions used specifically for this chapter. In particular we present a general multi-point boundary value problem (BVP) in the framework of optimal control theory and its transformation to a two-point BVP as well as the important technique of continuing an already established

[1] `OCMat` is available via `http://www.eos.tuwien.ac.at/OR/OCMat`.

solution. The section helps us to avoid having to explain the same procedures in several places.

7.1.1 Problem Formulation and Assumptions

For this section on numerical methods we establish that the problems of concern are of the following type (OCN):

$$V^*(x_0) := \max_{u(\cdot)} \int_0^\infty \mathrm{e}^{-rt} g(x(t), u(t), \mu)\, \mathrm{d}t \tag{7.1a}$$

$$\text{s.t.} \quad \dot{x}(t) = f(x(t), u(t), \mu), \quad t \in [0, \infty) \tag{7.1b}$$

$$x(0) = x_0 \tag{7.1c}$$

$$c(x(t), u(t), \mu) \geq 0, \quad \text{for all} \quad t \in [0, \infty) \tag{7.1d}$$

$$h(x(t), \mu) \geq 0, \quad \text{for all} \quad t \in [0, \infty), \tag{7.1e}$$

where $\mu \in \mathbb{R}^p$ and the discount rate $r \geq 0$ are exogenous parameters of the model, and the functions g, f, c, and h are two times continuously differentiable with respect to their arguments. The integral (7.1a) is finite for any admissible pair $(x(\cdot), u(\cdot))$.

To simplify notation we omit μ wherever we do not explicitly refer to this dependence. If we are analyzing the change in only one parameter, we also use the variable μ, tacitly assuming that the other variables are kept fixed. For the necessary optimality conditions for infinite time horizon problems of type (7.1) we refer the reader to Sect. 3.8.

In addition, the following assumptions hold for all parameter values μ:[2]

Assumption 7.1. The problem OCN (7.1) is normal, i.e., $\lambda_0 = 1$.

Assumption 7.2. For any $x \in \mathbb{R}^n$ and $\lambda \in \mathbb{R}^n$ there exists a unique $\hat{u}$ satisfying

$$\mathcal{H}_u(x, \hat{u}, \lambda, \mu) = 0, \quad \text{and} \quad \mathcal{H}_{uu}(x, \hat{u}, \lambda, \mu) \quad \text{negative definite.}$$

Assumption 7.3. For any x satisfying (7.1e) and $\lambda \in \mathbb{R}^n$

$$\operatorname*{argmax}_{u \in \Omega(x)} \mathcal{H}(x, u, \lambda, \mu) \neq \emptyset$$

with $\Omega(x) = \{u : c(x, u, \mu) \geq 0\}$.

Assumption 7.4. The pure state constraint (7.1e) is of order one in each of its coordinate functions, and not more than one constraint is active at any time t (see Definition 3.56).

---

[2] Most of the assumptions are stated to simplify the presentation, and are no principle restrictions for the application of the here presented methods.

Assumption 7.5. For the mixed path constraints (7.1d) and the pure state constraints (7.1e) the constraint qualifications (3.48) and (3.57) are satisfied for all t (see Sect. 3.6).

Assumption 7.6. For any $x_0 \in \mathbb{R}^n$ satisfying (7.1e) there exists an optimal solution of *OCN* (7.1).

Assumption 7.7. If not otherwise stated, the equilibria and limit cycles we consider are hyperbolic (see Sect. 2.6.2). For notational reasons, we assume that the eigenvectors are ordered so that the first n_- eigenvectors correspond to the stable directions.

We do not tackle the questions of existence and asymptotic behavior of the optimal solution but instead refer the reader to Carlson et al. (1991), where those topics are considered. We also have to admit that for many problems we only identify an extremal and owe the exact proof for its optimality.

7.1.2 Notation

In this chapter we use superscripts for the coordinates. This allows us to refer to specific coordinates of a point already characterized by a subscript, e.g., x_0^I or x_s^j. It is often necessary to denote specific coordinates $I = \{i_1, \ldots, i_k\} \subset \{1, \ldots, n\}$ of a variable $x = (x^1, \ldots, x^n)$. Thus throughout this chapter we shall write in shorthand

$$x^I := (x^{i_1}, \ldots, x^{i_k}),$$

with the specific definition

$$x^{\emptyset} := \emptyset.$$

Another notational problem arises when we have to consider BVPs for different systems of ODEs, e.g., when we have to distinguish between interior and boundary arcs. In that case we denote the corresponding states and functions by left-side superscripts, e.g.,

$$\begin{aligned} {}^1\dot{x} &= {}^1f({}^1x), \quad {}^1x^I(0) = {}^1x_0^I \\ {}^2\dot{x} &= {}^2f({}^2x), \quad {}^2x^J(0) = {}^2x_0^J. \end{aligned}$$

This notation may seem disconcerting at first, but it will allow us to keep the formulation compact. So as not to overload this compact notation, we restrict the presentation to the case in which at most two different dynamics are considered.

In most of the cases we do not refer to the following specific form of the canonical system

$$\begin{aligned} \dot{x}(t) &= \mathcal{H}_\lambda(x(t), u^*(t), \lambda(t)) \\ \dot{\lambda}(t) &= r\lambda(t) - \mathcal{H}_x(x(t), u^*(t), \lambda(t)). \end{aligned}$$

Therefore we often summarize the state and costate vector as one vector of dimension $2n$, denoted, if there is no ambiguity, by the variable x. For the corresponding dynamics we mostly use the letter f. In any case, the reader should not be confused since the meaning becomes clear from the context.

7.1.3 Numerical Methods for Solving Optimal Control Problems

There exists a huge literature on and various approaches to the topic of numerical methods for solving optimal control problems. For a short survey see, e.g., the Notes p. 382. In this classification schema the method presented here is referred to as an *indirect* method, in which the necessary conditions are derived from Pontryagin's Maximum Principle. In contrast to the indirect approach the *direct* methods transform, by time discretization, the optimal control problem into a finite-dimensional nonlinear program, which can then be solved by standard SQP methods. These methods are highly efficient and can be used for real-time implementations (see, e.g., Büskens & Maurer, 2000) and for large-scale systems such as those used in engineering and aeronautics.

Compared with applications originating from engineering models, economic problems are characterized by only a small number of states and controls and the consideration of an infinite time horizon. Thus we are mostly interested in the long-run optimal behavior of the given systems. Moreover, the autonomous structure of the models *OCN* (7.1) under consideration already suggests the application of the theory of dynamical systems to optimal control problems not least because the costate exhibits a special economic interpretation as shadow price. This gives strong evidence for analyzing the canonical system derived from Pontryagin's Maximum Principle and yielding a two-point BVP.

But the most convincing argument supporting our approach is the occurrence of limit sets (equilibria, limit cycles) of the canonical system as long-run optimal solutions. These limit sets serve as first "trivial" solutions of the optimal control problem, which can then be *continued* in order to derive the optimal solutions for arbitrary initial states. A further advantage of this approach is the application of bifurcation theory to explain changes in the optimal strategy, when one is varying the parameter values of the model. This approach becomes especially important in the case of multiple optimal solutions (see Chap. 5). Thus the models presented here suggest in a "natural way" the formulation as a BVP problem, which can then be analyzed by continuation methods, which we introduce in the subsequent Sect. 7.2.

7.1.4 Boundary Value Problems from Optimal Control

At this point we remind the reader that Pontryagin's Maximum Principle defines a BVP given by the canonical system (see Definition 3.6), together with the condition for the initial state and some transversality condition. For the infinite time horizon problems and under the assumption that the optimal solution converges to a limit set (equilibrium or limit cycle) the transversality condition can be replaced by a so-called asymptotic boundary condition. In what follows we refer to these asymptotic boundary conditions at the terminal point T by

$$\Sigma\left(x(T), \omega, \mu\right) = 0,$$

where ω is the limit set of the canonical system. For examples see the previous Chap. 6.

So in general we are confronted with a BVP of the following form, where some of the conditions can be empty:

$$
\begin{aligned}
{}^1\dot{x} &= {}^1\!f\left({}^1x, \mu\right), \quad t \in [0, T_1],\ {}^1x \in \mathbb{R}^{n_1} && \text{(7.2a)}\\
{}^2\dot{x} &= {}^2\!f\left({}^2x, \mu\right), \quad t \in [T_2, T_3],\ {}^2x \in \mathbb{R}^{n_2} && \text{(7.2b)}\\
{}^1x^{I_1}(0) &= {}^1x_0 \in \mathbb{R}^{q_1} && \text{(7.2c)}\\
{}^2x^{I_2}(T_2) &= {}^2x_0 \in \mathbb{R}^{q_2} && \text{(7.2d)}\\
\Psi\left({}^1x(T_1), {}^2x(T_2), \mu\right) &= 0 && \text{(7.2e)}\\
{}^1\Sigma\left({}^1x(T_1), {}^1\omega, \mu\right) &= 0 && \text{(7.2f)}\\
{}^2\Sigma\left({}^2x(T_3), {}^2\omega, \mu\right) &= 0. && \text{(7.2g)}
\end{aligned}
$$

Here (7.2a–7.2b) denote the underlying dynamics given by maybe different representations of the canonical system (see Sect. 7.6). In addition (7.2c–7.2d) provide the initial conditions and (7.2e) summarizes all the conditions the system has to satisfy connecting both dynamics (corner conditions). Finally, (7.2f–7.2g) denote the asymptotic boundary conditions for infinite time horizon problems, specified for an equilibrium in Proposition 7.20 and for a limit cycle in Proposition 7.27. All these equations may depend on some exogenously given parameter values summarized in μ.

As an example consider, e.g., the problem of p. 290, where $n_1 = n_2 = 4$, $T_1 = T_3 = 1$, $T_2 = 0$, $q_1 = 2$, (7.2e) is given by $X_4^I(1) = 0$, the asymptotic boundary condition (7.2f) is given by $F(X^I(1) - \hat{E}) = 0$, and (7.2d) and (7.2g) are empty.

The reader should be aware that this is a multi-point BVP. Using the procedure presented in Sect. 2.12.2, we can rewrite this problem as a standard-type two-point BVP. This is precisely what we aim at doing (and describing) now with problem (7.2). We therefore normalize the time intervals to $[0, 1]$, yielding the dynamics in the form

$$
\begin{aligned}
{}^1\dot{x} &= T_1\ {}^1\!f\left({}^1x, \mu\right), \quad t \in [0, 1]\\
{}^2\dot{x} &= (T_3 - T_2)\ {}^2\!f\left({}^2x, \mu\right), \quad t \in [0, 1].
\end{aligned}
$$

Setting

$$x := \begin{pmatrix} {}^1x \\ {}^2x \end{pmatrix}, \quad f := \begin{pmatrix} T_1\ {}^1\!f \\ (T_3 - T_2)\ {}^2\!f \end{pmatrix}, \quad x_0 := \begin{pmatrix} {}^1x_0 \\ {}^2x_0 \end{pmatrix}, \quad \text{and} \quad \omega := \begin{pmatrix} {}^1\omega \\ {}^2\omega \end{pmatrix}$$

with

$$\tilde{\Psi}\left(x(0), x(1), \mu\right) := \Psi\left({}^1x(T_1), {}^2x(T_2), \mu\right)$$
$$\tilde{\Sigma}\left(x(1), \omega, \mu\right) := \begin{pmatrix} {}^1\Sigma\left({}^1x(T_1), {}^1\omega, \mu\right) \\ {}^2\Sigma\left({}^2x(T_3), {}^2\omega, \mu\right) \end{pmatrix},$$

we have reduced the problem (7.2) to the form:

$$\dot{x} = f(x, \mu), \quad t \in [0, 1], \ x \in \mathbb{R}^n, \ n = n_1 + n_2 \tag{7.3a}$$
$$x^I(0) = x_0 \in \mathbb{R}^q, \quad I = I_1 \cup I_2, \quad q = q_1 + q_2 \tag{7.3b}$$
$$\tilde{\Psi}\left(x(0), x(1), \mu\right) = 0 \tag{7.3c}$$
$$\tilde{\Sigma}\left(x(1), \omega, \mu\right) = 0, \tag{7.3d}$$

where we subsequently omit the tilde-sign. The practical use of these transformations will become clear in the following sections.

Next, we introduce continuation as a strong numerical tool for finding solutions to a problem with varying parameter values.

7.2 Numerical Continuation

For the numerical analysis of dynamical systems, especially when one is studying the behavioral changes for varying parameters, *continuation* methods are the tool of choice (see, e.g., Krauskopf, Osinga, & Galán-Vioque, 2007; Kuznetsov, 1998). Continuation means continuing an already detected solution while varying a model-specific parameter value. In the context of BVPs this method has applications in many fields, not least in optimal control theory. To introduce the reader to this topic we present a simple example, that already exhibits the main ideas.

Let us consider the problem:

$$F(x, \mu) = 0$$

with the $x \in \mathbb{R}^n$ and $\mu \in \mathbb{R}$ and a specific solution x_s for μ_s being known; then the problem of *continuation* is to find a continuous solution curve $x(\gamma)$ satisfying

$$F(x(\mu), \mu) = 0$$

for $\mu \in [\mu_s, \mu_e]$.

The numerical task of a *continuation process* is to provide an algorithm allowing the successive computation of points $x(\mu_i)$, $i = 1, \ldots, N$, approximating the solution curve $x(\mu)$ with $\mu_N = \mu_e$.

Remark 7.1. The continuation problem can be stated not only for the finite-dimensional case $\mathbb{R}^n$ but also more generally for the infinite-dimensional case of normed vector spaces (see, e.g., Krauskopf et al., 2007, Chap. 1).

We introduce a simple continuation algorithm, actually used for the `OCMat` toolbox, illustrated by a simple example.

7.2.1 Continuation Algorithms

Let us consider the problem

$$F(x, \mu) = 0 \tag{7.4}$$

with the state variable $x \in \mathbb{R}^n$ and the parameter variable $\mu \in \mathbb{R}^p$. The function $F : \mathbb{R}^n \times \mathbb{R}^p \to \mathbb{R}^n$ is continuously differentiable. Suppose a solution x_s is established for the specific parameter values μ_s, satisfying

$$\operatorname{rk} F_x(x_s, \mu_s) = n.$$

Then the problem is to find a solution to (7.4) for arbitrarily given parameter values $\mu_e \neq \mu_s$.

A possible solution procedure is as follows:

Reparameterization : We reparameterize the problem by introducing a scalar continuation variable $\gamma \in [0, 1]$ setting

$$\begin{aligned}\mu(\gamma) &:= \mu_s + \gamma(\mu_e - \mu_s)\\ &= \mu_s(1-\gamma) + \gamma\mu_e, \quad \gamma \in [0, 1],\end{aligned} \tag{7.5}$$

with $\mu(0) = \mu_s$ and $\mu(1) = \mu_e$.
Substituting (7.5) into (7.4) yields the reparameterized problem:

$$\tilde{F}(x, \gamma) = 0 \tag{7.6}$$

with

$$\tilde{F}(x, \gamma) := F\left(x, \mu(\gamma)\right)$$

satisfying the rank condition

$$\operatorname{rk} \tilde{F}_x(x_s, 0) = \operatorname{rk} F_x(x_s, \mu_s) = n, \tag{7.7}$$

at the specific solution $F(x_s, 0) = 0$.

Initialization $0 \le i \le j$: We define some $j \in \mathbb{N}$ and positive constant $0 < \sigma_0 \le \frac{1}{j+1}$, to repeat the following steps j times. Thus we determine at step $i + 1 \le j$ the solution of (7.4) for

$$\gamma_{i+1} = \gamma_i + \sigma_0, \tag{7.8}$$

with $x_0 = x_s$ and $\gamma_0 = 0$. Since the rank condition (7.7) is satisfied, there exist j solutions $(x_0, \ldots, x_j)$ at the distinct parameter values $0 \le \gamma_1, \ldots, \gamma_j \le 1$ for σ_0 small enough.

Continuation Step $i > j$: The existence of a solution relies on the assumption that the rank condition is satisfied. But even in simple cases (see, e.g., the example (7.13), in which the solution curve exhibits turning points) this condition is violated. To tackle this kind of problem we augment problem (7.6) by adding

$$\Phi(x, \gamma, x_i, \dots, x_{i-j+1}, \gamma_i, \dots, \gamma_{i-j+1}, \sigma) = 0, \quad j \geq 0, \ i \geq j, \tag{7.9}$$

where Φ is a scalar function relying on the solutions $(x_k, \gamma_k)_{k=i-j+1}^{i}$ detected at the previous steps $i-j+1, \dots, i$ and σ is some positive constant, satisfying the following conditions:

$$\Phi(x_i, \gamma, x_i, \dots, x_{i-j+1}, \gamma_i, \dots, \gamma_{i-j+1}, 0) = 0$$

$$\operatorname{rk} \Phi_{(x,\gamma)}(x_i, \gamma_i, x_i, \dots, x_{i-j+1}, \gamma_i, \dots, \gamma_{i-j+1}, 0) = \begin{cases} n+1 & j > 0 \\ 1 & j = 0. \end{cases}$$

Then the implicit function theorem assures the existence of a solution $(x_{i+1}(\sigma), \gamma_{i+1}(\sigma))$ for σ small enough, independently of the rank of $\tilde{F}_x(x, \gamma)$. Subsequently we present different functional forms of (7.9).
This step can be repeated until $\gamma \geq 1$ or some stopping condition is reached. To find the actual solution x_{i+1}, a prediction step can be applied, which we present next.

Prediction Step : In general the numerical detection of a solution requires that an approximation $(\tilde{x}_{i+1}, \tilde{\gamma}_{i+1})$ for the correct (unknown) solution (x_{i+1}, γ_{i+1}) be provided. Therefore the approximated solution is linearly extrapolated from the two previous solutions, (x_{i-1}, γ_{i-1}) and (x_i, γ_i), yielding

$$\tilde{x}_{i+1} = x_i + \alpha\,(x_i - x_{i-1}) = x_i(\alpha + 1) - \alpha x_{i-1} \tag{7.10a}$$
$$\tilde{\gamma}_{i+1} = \gamma_i + \alpha\,(\gamma_i - \gamma_{i-1}) = \gamma_i(\alpha + 1) - \alpha \gamma_{i-1}. \tag{7.10b}$$

The constant α is determined, depending on the current and previous step size given by the ratio

$$\alpha = \frac{\sigma_{i+1}}{\sigma_i}.$$

Remark 7.2. The actual zero-finding process of the initialization and continuation step is either done by an algorithm solving nonlinear equations in the finite-dimensional case or used to continue the solution of a BVP by a BV-Solver. There exist numerous algorithms and software packages on this topic; for an overview the reader is referred to Kuznetsov (1998, App. 3) and Krauskopf et al. (2007). For our calculations we used the MATLAB implementations `fsolve` (Optimization Toolbox) to solve nonlinear equations and the BV-Solver `bvp4c` for solving BVPs, (see Kierzenka & Shampine, 2001).

Remark 7.3. In an actual application it may be convenient to consider the continuation not only along [0, 1] but also for an arbitrary interval [a, b], with $a, b \in \mathbb{R}$.

Remark 7.4. The constant σ of the continuation step can be made dependent on information about the numerical quality of the solution process and can therefore be considered as a sequence $(\sigma_i)_{i\geq j}$.

Remark 7.5. The properties of the added function (7.9) assures the existence of a solution $(x_{i+1}(\sigma), \gamma_{i+1}(\sigma))$ for σ small enough. Denoting the corresponding value of the variable σ at step i by σ_i, we can distinguish different scenarios for the sequence of corresponding continuation parameter values $(\gamma_i)_{i\geq j}$. Here we present three important cases from an applied point of view:

1. There exists some $N \in \mathbb{N}$ with $\gamma(\sigma_N) \geq 1$.
2. $\lim_{i\to\infty} \gamma(\sigma_i) = \gamma_{crit} < 1$.
3. There exists some $\gamma_{crit} < 1$ and $N \in \mathbb{N}$ such that $\gamma(\sigma_i) \leq \gamma_{crit}$ for all i and $\gamma(\sigma_i) > \gamma(\sigma_{i+1})$ for $i \geq N$.

In the first case we can solve the problem (see, e.g., Fig. 7.1a,b or the example of p. 337). In the second case the solution curve has a limit point at $\gamma = \gamma_{crit} < 1$ (see, e.g., Fig. 7.1c). And in the last case the solution curve exhibits a turning point (see, e.g., Fig. 7.1d).

Exogenous Continuation $j = 0$

In the case of exogenous continuation $j = 0$, the solution at step $i + 1$ does not depend on the previous state(s) and the simplest functional form of (7.9) is given by

$$\Phi(\gamma, \gamma_i, \sigma) = \gamma - \gamma_i - \sigma. \tag{7.11}$$

This simply represents (7.8) of the initialization step, which is well adapted as long as the rank condition is satisfied.

For this specification of Φ the continuation variable γ is exogenously given at each step i by (7.11). Therefore this continuation algorithm is also called the *exogenous continuation.*

Another algorithm, which does not exhibit the drawback of an exogenously given step width, is presented next.

Endogenous Continuation

For the endogenous approach the function Φ explicitly depends on the unknown variable x. Therefore (7.6) denotes a coupled system of equations, in which the continuation variable is not exogenously given. Hence this algorithm is called the *endogenous continuation.*

We use the following two specifications for the function Φ with $j = 1$ and $j = 2$, respectively,

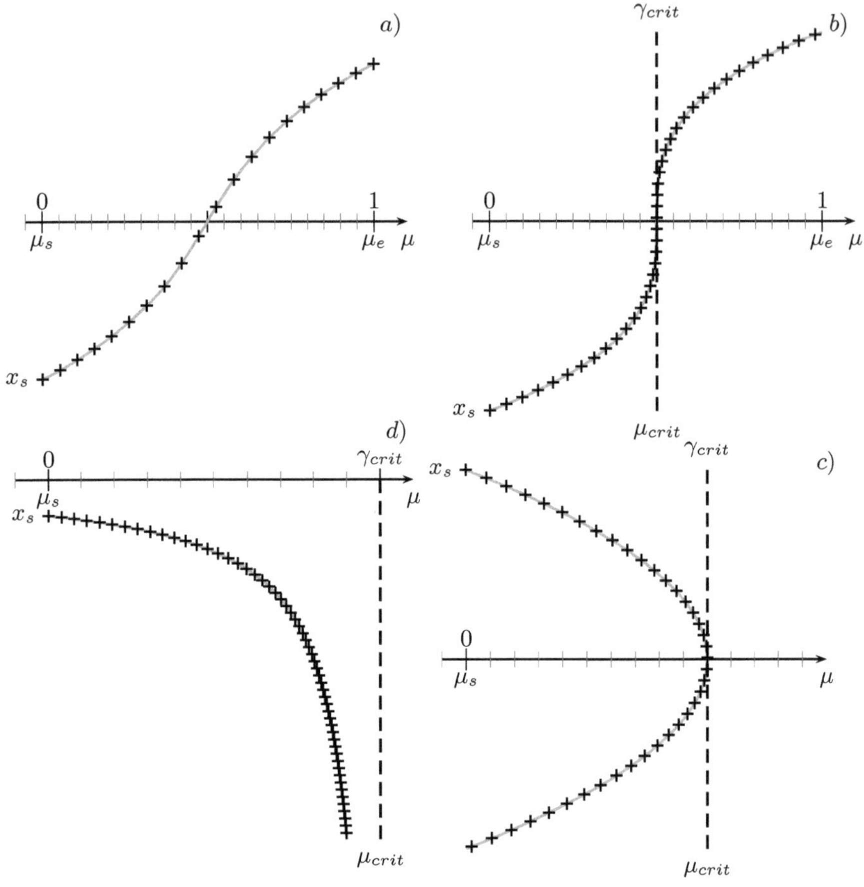

Fig. 7.1. In panel (**a**) the continuation process is depicted for $x(x^2+1)-\mu=0$, starting at the solution for $\mu_s=-1$. In (**b**) the solution curve of $x^3-\mu=0$ is shown, for which the rank condition is violated at $\mu_s=0$. Contrary to the previous case the critical parameter value $\mu_{crit}=0$ for the problem $x^2-\mu=0$ in (**c**) denotes a turning point. And in (**d**) the continuation process converges to $\mu_{crit}=0$ for the equation $x^{-1}-\mu=0$

$$\Phi(x,\gamma,x_i,\gamma_i,\sigma) := \|x-x_i\|^2+(\gamma-\gamma_i)^2-\sigma^2, \tag{7.12a}$$

$$\Phi(x,\gamma,x_i,x_{i-1},\gamma_i,\gamma_{i-1},\sigma) := \begin{pmatrix}\Delta x_i\\ \Delta\gamma_i\end{pmatrix}' \begin{pmatrix}x-x_i\\ \gamma-\gamma_i\end{pmatrix} - \sigma\left\|\begin{pmatrix}\Delta x_i\\ \Delta\gamma_i\end{pmatrix}\right\|^2, \tag{7.12b}$$

$$\Delta x_i = x_i - x_{i-1},\ \Delta\gamma_i = \gamma_i-\gamma_{i-1},$$

where $x_k = x(\gamma_k)$, $k=i-1,i$ are previously detected solutions and $\sigma>0$ is a given constant, assuring that the new solution differs from the previous solution. Geometrically (7.12a) describes a circle of radius σ around the solution at step i (see Fig. 7.2a), whereas (7.12b) ascribes a line perpendicular to the direction of the linear extrapolation of the last two detected solutions (see Fig. 7.2b).

Remark 7.6. For both cases the new solution is given by the intersection of the circle or line, respectively, with the (searched for) solution curve. Therefore it is evident that in the first case there exist two intersection points, which can yield numerical inconveniences and therefore the second approach is preferred.

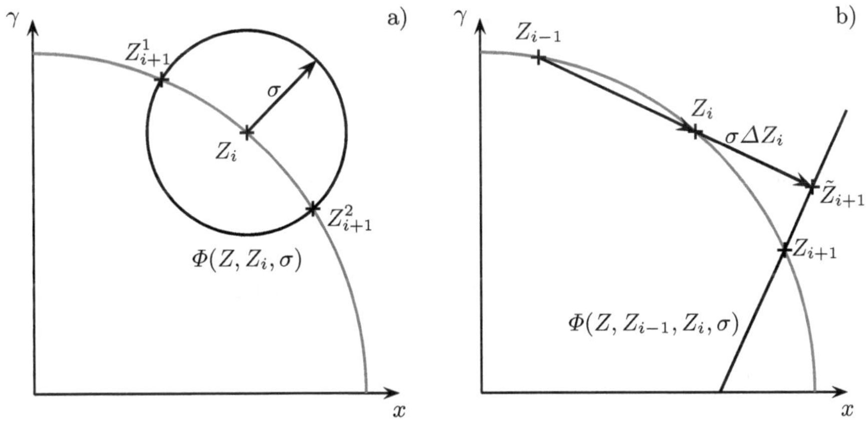

Fig. 7.2. Panel (**a**) depicts the geometric representation of (7.12a), and panel (**b**) that of (7.12b), where $Z = (x, \gamma)$

A Simple Example

As a simple example of (7.4) we consider the cubic function

$$F(x, \mu) := x(x^2 - 1) + \mu. \tag{7.13}$$

Then we want to find a continuous curve $x(\mu)$ with $\mu \in [\mu_s, \mu_e]$ satisfying

$$F(x(\mu), \mu) = 0,$$

with a specific solution $x(\mu_s) = x_s$ given for $\mu_s = -1$ and $x_s = 1.3247$. The problem (7.13) satisfies the rank condition

$$F_x(x_s, \mu) = 3x_s^2 - 1 \neq 0. \tag{7.14}$$

Thus for the given x_s the implicit function theorem assures the existence of a unique solution curve $x(\mu)$ of (7.13), with $0 < |\mu + 1| < \varepsilon$. Note that for $x_s \pm \frac{\sqrt{3}}{3}$ the rank condition of (7.14) is violated. These points correspond to the turning points of the solution curve (see Fig. 7.3).

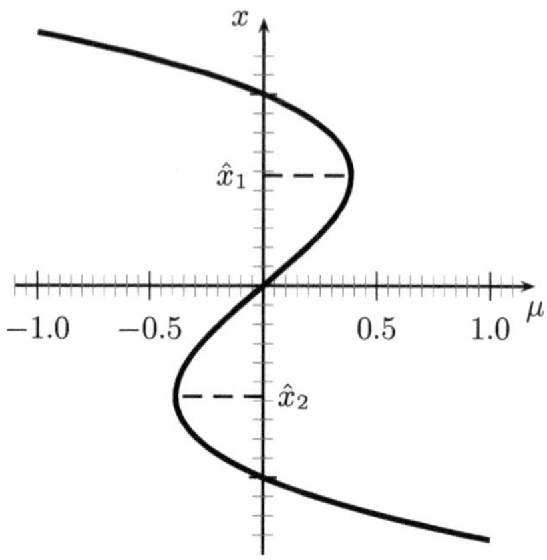

Fig. 7.3. The solution curve of (7.13) is depicted for $\mu \in [-1, 1]$. At the critical points $\hat{x}_{1,2} = \pm\frac{\sqrt{3}}{3}$ the rank condition (7.14) is not satisfied

Next we normalize the interval $[-1, 1]$ to $[0, 1]$ which yields

$$\tilde{F}(x, \gamma) = x(x^2 - 1) + \mu_s + \gamma(\mu_e - \mu_s) = 0,$$

where for

$$\mu = \mu(\gamma) := \mu_s + \gamma(\mu_e - \mu_s)$$

we find $x(\mu(0)) = x(\mu_s) = x_s$.

Next, we apply the exogenous and endogenous approaches for the numerical computation of the solution curve $x(\mu(\gamma))$, $\gamma \in [0, 1]$.

Applying the exogenous continuation to our problem (7.13), we find that the continuation process will fail if μ exceeds $2\sqrt{3}/9$ (see Fig. 7.4a), since for this parameter value the solution curve exhibits a turning point and cannot be continuously extended by increasing the parameter value.

In Fig. 7.4b the result of the endogenous continuation process for the example (7.13) is depicted, showing that the solution curve was followed beyond its turning points.

7.2.2 Continuing the Solution of a BVP

In this subsection we apply the continuation technique to the problem of continuing solutions of BVPs. In the context of a BVP we are interested not only in continuing a solution for varying model parameters but also in continuing a solution along varying initial conditions $x(0) = x_0$. From a theoretical point of view this does not make any difference. To verify that, we add the following artificial dynamics and initial conditions to the system (7.3)

$$\dot{\mu} = 0, \quad t \in [0, 1]$$
$$\mu(0) = \mu_0 \in \mathbb{R}^p.$$

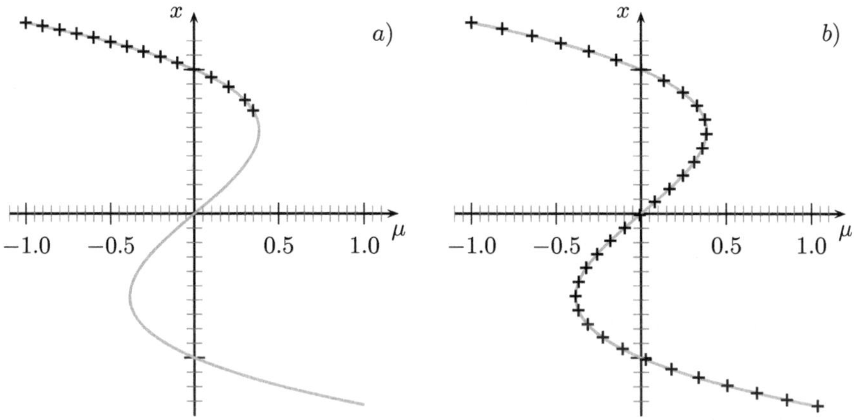

Fig. 7.4. Panel (**a**) depicts the continuation process (+) for an exogenously given step width σ aborting at a turning point of the (*gray*) solution curve $x(\mu)$. In panel (**b**) the continuation problem is augmented by the continuation variable γ allowing one to follow the solution curve beyond its turning points

Introducing the extended state variable $\tilde{x}$ and dynamics $\tilde{f}$

$$\tilde{x} := \begin{pmatrix} x \\ \mu \end{pmatrix}, \quad \tilde{f} := \begin{pmatrix} f \\ 0 \end{pmatrix}, \quad \tilde{x}_0 := \begin{pmatrix} x_0 \\ \mu_0 \end{pmatrix},$$

together with

$$\begin{aligned} \tilde{\Psi}\left(\tilde{x}(0), \tilde{x}(1)\right) &:= \Psi\left(x(0), x(1), \mu\right) \\ \tilde{\Sigma}\left(\tilde{x}(1), \omega\right) &:= \Sigma\left(x(1), \omega, \mu\right) \\ \tilde{I} &:= I \cup \{q+1, \ldots, q+p\}, \end{aligned}$$

we find that the augmented problem is a usual BVP without exogenous parameter values, i.e.,

$$\dot{\tilde{x}} = \tilde{f}(\tilde{x}), \quad t \in [0,\, 1],\ \tilde{x} \in \mathbb{R}^{\tilde{n}},\ \tilde{n} = n + p \tag{7.15a}$$

$$\tilde{x}^{\tilde{I}}(0) = \tilde{x}_0 \in \mathbb{R}^{\tilde{q}}, \quad \tilde{q} = q + p \tag{7.15b}$$

$$\tilde{\Psi}\left(\tilde{x}(0), \tilde{x}(1)\right) = 0 \tag{7.15c}$$

$$\tilde{\Sigma}\left(\tilde{x}(1), \omega\right) = 0, \tag{7.15d}$$

where we subsequently omit the tilde-sign to simplify the notation. Thus the new problem (7.15) does not exhibit explicit parameter values.

In this context we are often confronted with the question of how to find a solution satisfying

$$x^I(0) = x_e \neq x_s$$

if we already established a solution of (7.15) that meets the initial condition

$$x^I(0) = x_s.$$

This question can be seen as a continuation problem, wherein we have to continue a solution from x_s to x_e.

Using the method of the previous subsection, we can try to find the solution along the line connecting x_s and x_e, i.e., the solution trajectory $x(\cdot)$ satisfying

$$x^I(0) = x_s(1-\gamma) + \gamma x_e, \quad 0 \le \gamma \le 1,$$

where γ is the continuation parameter.

Repeating the arguments above, we see that γ can be considered as an additional state variable with the dynamics

$$\dot{\gamma} = 0$$

added to system (7.15a).

Since this increases the number of states by one, we also need an additional boundary condition to get a well-defined BVP. The results of the previous section suggest a (scalar) boundary condition of the form

$$\Phi\left(x(0), \gamma, x_i(0), \dots, x_{i-j+1}(0), \gamma_i, \dots, \gamma_{i-j+1}, \sigma_{i+1}\right) = 0, \quad j \ge 0,\ i \ge j,$$

where $x_k(\cdot)$ and γ_k, $k = i-j+1, \dots, i$, are solutions of j previous steps. Thus several functional forms for Φ can be specified:

$$\Phi\left(x(0), \gamma, \gamma_i, \sigma\right) := \gamma - \gamma_i - \sigma \tag{7.16a}$$

$$\Phi\left(x(0), \gamma, x_i(0), \gamma_i, \sigma\right) := \|x(0) - x_i(0)\|^2 + (\gamma - \gamma_i)^2 + \sigma^2, \tag{7.16b}$$

or

$$\Phi\left(x(0), \gamma, x_i(0), x_{i-1}(0), \gamma_i, \gamma_{i-1}, \sigma\right) :=$$
$$\begin{pmatrix} \Delta x_i(0) \\ \Delta\gamma_i \end{pmatrix}' \begin{pmatrix} x(0) - x_i(0) \\ \gamma - \gamma_i \end{pmatrix} - \sigma \left\| \begin{pmatrix} \Delta x_i(0) \\ \Delta\gamma_i \end{pmatrix} \right\|^2, \tag{7.16c}$$
$$\text{with} \quad \Delta x_i(0) = x_i(0) - x_{i-1}(0),\ \Delta\gamma_i = \gamma_i - \gamma_{i-1},$$

where $\sigma > 0$ denotes some step width. For notational simplicity we omit most of the arguments of Φ and simply write

$$\Phi(x(0), \gamma).$$

The BVP for the continuation process can therefore be written as

$$\begin{aligned}
&\dot{x} = f(x), \quad t \in [0,\, 1],\ \tilde{x} \in \mathbb{R}^n \\
&\dot{\gamma} = 0 \\
&x^I(0) = \gamma x_e + (1-\gamma)x_s \in \mathbb{R}^q \\
&\Phi(x(0), \gamma) = 0 && (7.17a) \\
&\Psi\left(x(0), x(1)\right) = 0 \\
&\Sigma\left(x(1), \omega\right) = 0, && (7.17b)
\end{aligned}$$

where (7.17a) exhibits one of the functional forms ascribed in (7.16).

Continuing the Solution of a Simple BVP

In this section we illustrate the usage of the continuation method for BVPs by means of the following simple example. Given the linear ODE

$$\dot{x} = \begin{pmatrix} \cos\frac{\pi}{4} & 0 & -\sin\frac{\pi}{4} \\ 0 & 1 & 0 \\ \sin\frac{\pi}{4} & 0 & \cos\frac{\pi}{4} \end{pmatrix} \begin{pmatrix} -1 & -1 & 0 \\ 1 & -1 & 0 \\ 0 & 0 & 1 \end{pmatrix} x =: Jx \tag{7.18a}$$

we want to find the solution $x(\cdot)$ lying on the stable manifold of the origin for (7.18a) and satisfying

$$x^{\{1,2\}}(0) = x_0 \in \mathbb{R}^2, \tag{7.18b}$$

where $x_0 \neq 0$ is some fixed point.

Since J exhibits two eigenvalues with negative real parts and one positive eigenvalue, the stable manifold $\mathrm{W}^s(0)$ of the origin is a plane spanned by the corresponding "stable" eigenvectors. Using Proposition A.51, we find that this plane is given by

$$\mathrm{W}^s(0) = \{x \in \mathbb{R}^3 : \langle b_u, x\rangle = 0\},$$

where b_u is the unstable eigenvector of the transposed matrix J'.

Considering the ODE (7.18a) on a finite time interval $[0, T]$, we add the boundary condition

$$\langle b_u, x(T)\rangle = 0 \tag{7.18c}$$

to the system (7.18), which assures that the solution lies on the stable manifold of the equilibrium at the origin.

Thus the equations (7.18) determine a BVP to find a solution converging to the origin and withe initial condition (7.18b).

Owing to the linearity of the ODE (7.18a), the stable manifold is analytically given and the application of a continuation algorithm is superfluous. But its illustration for this simple case may help the reader to adapt it to more involved cases. Thus in Fig. 7.5 the problem is depicted for the case in which the first two coordinates of a point A are given and the third coordinate has to be computed, so that the corresponding solution converges to the origin. Since the equilibrium solution $x(\cdot) \equiv 0$, trivially satisfies the BVP (7.18), we start a continuation process in which the solution is continued for initial points lying on the (gray) line connecting the origin and $A^{\{1,2\}}$ (see Fig. 7.5a). At each step the trajectory satisfying the BVP (7.18) for the initial state $x_0 = \gamma A^{\{1,2\}}$ is detected (see Fig. 7.5b) until $A^{\{1,2\}}$ is reached for $\gamma = 1$.

Remark 7.7. Although this example may be considered trivial, it presents the main ideas used throughout this chapter, namely to truncate the integration interval to $[0, T]$, to formulate a so-called asymptotic boundary condition (7.18c), and to start the continuation of the BVP at a trivial solution, as it is given by an equilibrium or limit cycle.

This ends our general introduction. We shall now address the specific problems and questions that occur when we solve optimal control problems.

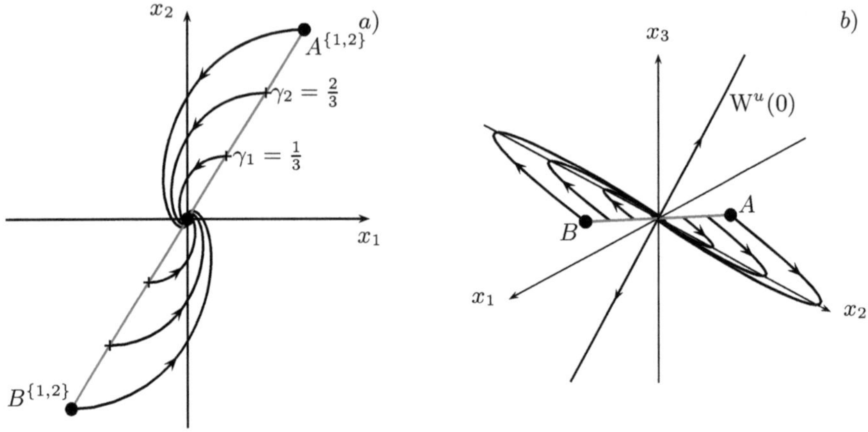

Fig. 7.5. To find the solution of (7.18a) lying in the stable manifold of the origin, where the first two initial states are given by $A^{\{1,2\}}$ or $B^{\{1,2\}}$, a continuation process is used. The intermediate results of the continuation process for the steps γ_i, $i = 1, 2$ are depicted, projected into the (x_1, x_2)-space in (**a**), whereas in (**b**) the orbits are shown in $\mathbb{R}^3$

7.3 The Canonical System Without Active Constraints

We start by considering the canonical system for solutions, where no constraint becomes active. Then Assumptions 7.2 and 7.3 implies that the uniquely given optimal control value u^* satisfies

$$\mathcal{H}_u(x, u^*, \lambda) = 0, \quad \text{and} \quad \mathcal{H}_{uu}(x, u^*, \lambda) \quad \text{negative definite.} \tag{7.19}$$

Thus by the implicit function theorem we find that the optimal control variable can be considered as a function of x and λ with $u^*(x, \lambda)$, which is continuously differentiable with respect to x and λ. Then the canonical system is given by

$$\dot{x} = f(x, u^*(x, \lambda)) = \mathcal{H}_\lambda(x, u^*(x, \lambda), \lambda) \tag{7.20a}$$

$$\dot{\lambda} = r\lambda - \mathcal{H}_x(x, u^*(x, \lambda), \lambda). \tag{7.20b}$$

Using the implicit differentiability of $u^*(x, \lambda)$, we may consider the total time derivative

$$\dot{u}^*(t) = u^*_x\left(x(t), \lambda(t)\right) \dot{x}(t) + u^*_\lambda\left(x(t), \lambda(t)\right) \dot{\lambda}'(t). \tag{7.21}$$

In our applications it is often possible to find an analytic expression for $u^*(x, \lambda)$. But what can be done if no such analytic expression exists, as, e.g., in the drug model of Sect. 6.1? Assume that there exist $l \leq n$ control coordinates[3] $u_i^*(x, \lambda)$, $i = 1, \dots, l$, for which no closed-form representation exists. If $(f_{u_i})_{i=1}^l$ has full rank[4] l, then

[3] For simplicity these are assumed to be the first l coordinates.

[4] For notational clarity we assume the first l row vectors of $(f_{u_i})_{i=1}^l$ to be linearly independent.

$$\mathcal{H}_{u_i}(x,u,\lambda) = g_{u_i}(x,u) + \lambda f_{u_i}(x,u) = 0, \quad i = 1,\dots,l$$

can be solved explicitly for the first l costates λ_i, $i = 1,\dots,l$. Thus the first l costate variables can be expressed as functions

$$\lambda_i\left(x, u_1,\dots,u_l,\lambda_{l+1},\dots,\lambda_n\right), \quad i = 1,\dots,l\,. \tag{7.22}$$

(The reader should write these equations down for the special cases of $n = 3$ and $l = 2$.)

Setting $v = (u_1,\dots,u_l)'$ and using (7.21), we find

$$\begin{aligned} 0 = \frac{\mathrm{d}}{\mathrm{d}t}\mathcal{H}_v(x,u,\lambda) &= \dot{v}'\mathcal{H}_{vv} + \dot{x}'\mathcal{H}_{vx} + \dot{\lambda}\mathcal{H}_{v\lambda} \\ &= \dot{v}'\mathcal{H}_{vv} + f'\mathcal{H}_{vx} + (r\lambda - H_x)\, f_v. \end{aligned}$$

Since $\mathcal{H}_{vv}$ is a negative definite matrix and therefore invertible, the last equation yields

$$\dot{v} = -\left(\mathcal{H}_{xv} f + f_v'\left(r\lambda' - H_x'\right)\right)\mathcal{H}_{vv}^{-1}. \tag{7.23}$$

Replacing the first l costate variables by (7.22) and the $n-l$ control variables by their analytic expressions, we can finally replace the first l adjoint equations with (7.23), yielding together with the state equations a system of $2n$ differential equations in the variables $(x, u_1,\dots,u_l,\lambda_{l+1},\dots,\lambda_n)$.

Remark 7.8. This transformation is also of general interest, since from an applied point of view the representation in the state–control space has an immediate economic interpretation. Attention has also to be drawn to the derivative f_v, which has to be invertible; otherwise singularities in the transformed dynamics may occur, which are only a spurious result of an improper transformation.

Remark 7.9. In the case that Assumption 7.2 is not satisfied, there may exist multiple control values $u^1,\dots,u^k$ satisfying (7.19), where in general the number k depends on the actual state x and costate λ. Then we have to consider each of the corresponding functions $u^1(x,\lambda),\dots,u^k(x,\lambda)$ separately, and the actual control value has to be determined by the Hamiltonian maximizing condition.

Next, we analyze the canonical system with respect to long-run optimal solutions.

7.4 Calculating Long-Run Optimal Solutions

Since we are considering problems with infinite time horizons, we are interested in the long-run behavior of the canonical system, where the most common phenomena characterizing the (long-run) behavior are equilibria and limit cycles of the canonical system (see Chap. 2). In the following subsections we therefore analyze equilibria and limit cycles in more detail.

7.4.1 Equilibria

The most straightforward elements characterizing the behavior of a dynamical system are equilibria $(\hat{x}, \hat{\lambda})$ of the canonical system where (7.20) becomes zero, i.e.,

$$\mathcal{H}_\lambda(\hat{x}, u^*(\hat{x}, \hat{\lambda}), \hat{\lambda}, \mu) = 0 \tag{7.24a}$$

$$r\lambda - \mathcal{H}_x(\hat{x}, u^*(\hat{x}, \hat{\lambda}), \hat{\lambda}, \mu) = 0. \tag{7.24b}$$

Locating Equilibria

In general the algebraic equations (7.24) are nonlinear and cannot be solved analytically. Thus one often has to resort to numerical calculations to find roots of (7.24). There exist powerful algorithms, implemented in mathematical software packages such as MATLAB, for finding the roots of nonlinear functions. So it is not the place here to go into details about these algorithms; and the reader is referred to Kuznetsov (1998, Sect. 10.8) for a more thorough discussion of this topic.

Given that an equilibrium has been located for a specific set of parameter values, μ, continuation (see Sect. 7.2) can be used to find an equilibrium for a different set of parameter values.

In Sect. 2.6.2 we have seen that the local stability properties of an equilibrium are given by the properties of the corresponding Jacobian $\hat{J}$ evaluated at the equilibrium. Owing to the specific structure of the dynamics (7.20), a general result can be derived for the number of stable eigenvectors. This is subsequently shown.

Stability of Equilibria

Let $(\hat{x}, \hat{\lambda})$ be an equilibrium of (7.20); then the corresponding Jacobian becomes

$$\hat{J}(\hat{x}, \hat{\lambda}) = \begin{pmatrix} \mathcal{H}^*_{\lambda x} & \mathcal{H}^*_{\lambda\lambda} \\ -\mathcal{H}^*_{xx} & r\mathbb{I}^{(n)} - \mathcal{H}^*_{x\lambda} \end{pmatrix}, \tag{7.25}$$

where $\mathcal{H}^* := \mathcal{H}(\hat{x}, u^*(\hat{x}, \hat{\lambda}), \hat{\lambda})$ is the maximized Hamiltonian.

To figure out the stability of the equilibrium we have to compute the eigenvalues of (7.25), which is done by finding the roots ξ_i, $i = 1, \ldots, 2n$ of the characteristic polynomial, given by

$$\det \begin{pmatrix} \xi\mathbb{I}^{(n)} - \mathcal{H}^*_{\lambda x} & -\mathcal{H}^*_{\lambda\lambda} \\ \mathcal{H}^*_{xx} & (\xi - r)\mathbb{I}^{(n)} + \mathcal{H}^*_{x\lambda} \end{pmatrix} = 0. \tag{7.26}$$

Note that the determinant (7.26) can be written in symmetrical form as

$$\det \begin{pmatrix} \left(\xi - \frac{r}{2}\right)\mathbb{I}^{(n)} - \mathcal{H}^*_{\lambda x} + \frac{r}{2}\mathbb{I}^{(n)} & -\mathcal{H}^*_{\lambda\lambda} \\ \mathcal{H}^*_{xx} & \left(\xi - \frac{r}{2}\right)\mathbb{I}^{(n)} + \mathcal{H}^*_{x\lambda} - \frac{r}{2}\mathbb{I}^{(n)} \end{pmatrix} = 0. \tag{7.27}$$

Using the symmetries of (7.27) yields the following theorem (a proof can be found in Appendix B.8):

Theorem 7.10. *Let $\hat{J}$ be the Jacobian evaluated at an equilibrium $(\hat{x}, \hat{\lambda})$ of the canonical system (7.20). Then the corresponding eigenvalues $\xi_i, i = 1, \dots, 2n$, are symmetric around $r/2$ and the dimension of the (local) stable manifold is at most n.*

Remark 7.11. Theorem 7.10 implies that for one- and two-state models, the generic asymptotically stable optimal solutions converging toward an equilibrium are a one-dimensional curve or lie in a two-dimensional surface, respectively. The numerical computation of the paths lying in the stable manifold is the subject of Sect. 7.5.

Remark 7.12. As a consequence from Theorem 7.10 it follows that for $r > 0$ no stable equilibria exist. This can also be seen by considering that $\operatorname{tr} \hat{J} = nr > 0$, which proves that the occurring equilibria cannot be stable, since for a stable equilibrium $\operatorname{tr} \hat{J} < 0$ has to hold.

Equilibrium Properties of Two-State Control Models

For the special case of two-state optimal control models the long-run (equilibrium) behavior has been fully characterized by Dockner (1985) and Dockner and Feichtinger (1991). Solving (7.27), we can explicitly calculate the eigenvalues of the Jacobian matrix J as

$$\xi_{3,4}^{1,2} = \frac{r}{2} \pm \sqrt{\frac{r^2}{4} - \frac{K}{2} \pm \frac{1}{2}\sqrt{K^2 - 4 \det J}}, \tag{7.28a}$$

where the coefficient K can be expressed as the sum of determinants of the following submatrices of the Jacobian J

$$K = \begin{vmatrix} \frac{\partial \dot{x}_1}{\partial x_1} & \frac{\partial \dot{x}_1}{\partial \lambda_1} \\ \frac{\partial \dot{\lambda}_1}{\partial x_1} & \frac{\partial \dot{\lambda}_1}{\partial \lambda_1} \end{vmatrix} + \begin{vmatrix} \frac{\partial \dot{x}_2}{\partial x_2} & \frac{\partial \dot{x}_2}{\partial \lambda_2} \\ \frac{\partial \dot{\lambda}_2}{\partial x_2} & \frac{\partial \dot{\lambda}_2}{\partial \lambda_2} \end{vmatrix} + 2 \begin{vmatrix} \frac{\partial \dot{x}_1}{\partial x_2} & \frac{\partial \dot{x}_1}{\partial \lambda_2} \\ \frac{\partial \dot{\lambda}_1}{\partial x_2} & \frac{\partial \dot{\lambda}_1}{\partial \lambda_2} \end{vmatrix}. \tag{7.28b}$$

Remark 7.13. Equations (7.28) are sometimes referred to as *Dockner's formula.*

Note that the term K is composed of the determinants of the hypothetical one-state models (x_1, λ_1), and (x_2, λ_2), as well as some mixed interaction term. Using the results of Sect. 2.6.2, we are able to characterize the local stability properties of the equilibrium in terms of K and $\det \hat{J}$, depicted in Fig. 7.6 and presented in Table 7.1.

Table 7.1. Classification of the equilibria according to K and $\det J$, where the regions are depicted in Fig. 7.6

Region/curve	Type	$\dim W^s(\hat{x}, \hat{\lambda})$	Local behavior
I	Saddle-node	2	Monotonic
II	Saddle-focus	2	Transient oscillation
III	Focus	0	Unstable
IV	Focus/node	0	Unstable
V	Saddle	1	Diverging except stable path
α	PAH-bifurcation	?	?

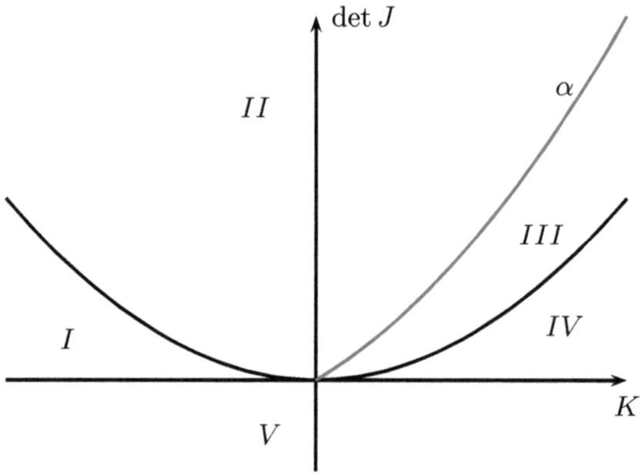

Fig. 7.6. The different regions characterizing the stability properties at an equilibrium for a two-state model are depicted in terms of $\det J$ and K. The *black curve* is given by $\left(\frac{K}{2}\right)^2$ and the *gray curve* α by $\left(\frac{K}{2}\right)^2 + r^2 \frac{K}{2}$ for $r = 1$

7.4.2 Limit Cycles

In Proposition 3.83 it has been stated that, for discounted autonomous models with $r > 0$, cyclic behavior can be excluded. Hence limit cycles may occur only for models with at least two states; for an example see Sect. 6.2. In general the numerical effort to find limit cycles is much greater than that of calculating equilibria, especially if they are neither attracting nor repelling.

Locating a Limit Cycle

Let us consider the following autonomous system:

$$\dot{x} = f(x, \mu), \quad x \in \mathbb{R}^n, \; n \geq 2.$$

From the Definition 2.20 of a limit cycle Γ with period Θ we find the characterizing property

$$x(t+\Theta) = x(t), \quad \text{for all} \quad t.$$

By a time scaling $t \to t/\Theta$ the problem becomes a BVP:

$$\dot{x} = \Theta f(x, \mu) \tag{7.29a}$$

$$\text{s.t.} \quad x(0) = x(1), \tag{7.29b}$$

where the trajectory $x(\cdot)$ and the period Θ have to be determined. Since (7.29b) only provides n boundary conditions, we have to specify an additional condition for identifying Θ.

This can also be seen as a problem of identifying a specific trajectory among all *phase-shifted* periodic solutions, representing the limit cycle Γ, since every solution with $x(0) = x_\Gamma \in \Gamma$ satisfies the BVP (7.29). Therefore a scalar functional $\psi(x(\cdot)) = 0$ is introduced, which fixes the phase-shift, and is therefore called a *phase condition*. Different functional forms for ψ are conceivable and may be more or less well adapted to the specific situation. A simple and easy-to-implement condition is presented here.

To find a limit cycle we assume that we already know the approximate position of the limit cycle. Then we fix some point $p \notin \Gamma$ and have to find $x_\Gamma \in \Gamma$ satisfying

$$f(p)(x_\Gamma - p) = 0.$$

Thus we fix the solution crossing the hyperplane lying orthogonally to the direction $f(p)$. If p is near enough to the limit cycle, such a solution exists.

Therefore the phase condition becomes

$$\psi(x(\cdot)) := f(p)\,(x(0) - p)\,, \tag{7.29c}$$

delivering together with (7.29a) and (7.29b) a well-defined BVP.

Remark 7.14. Having located a limit cycle, a continuation process can be used to follow the limit cycle for varying parameters. A natural choice for the point p in the phase condition (7.29c) is a point $x_i \in \Gamma_i$ from the previous limit cycle calculation, and $f(p)$ can be replaced by $\dot{x}_i$, the velocity at x_i from the previous step. We refer the reader to `MatCont`, which provides an efficient algorithm for the continuation and detection of limit cycles (see also Kuznetsov, 1998, p. 472).

Initializing a Limit Cycle

The simplest and also often the only way to locate a periodic solution is via the PAH-bifurcation, where the Poincaré–Andronov–Hopf theorem allows computing an approximation of the cycle at the bifurcation value μ_0. For this parameter value the Jacobian $\hat{J}$ evaluated at the associated equilibrium exhibits two purely imaginary eigenvalues $\pm i\omega_0$ with $\omega_0 > 0$ and two corresponding eigenvectors, ν and its complex conjugate $\bar{\nu}$. Then the limit cycle can be approximated by (see Kuznetsov, 1998, p. 489)

$$\Gamma_\varepsilon(t) = 2\varepsilon\left(\nu_R \cos\omega_0 t - \nu_I \sin\omega_0 t\right),$$

where $\varepsilon > 0$ is some arbitrary constant, $\nu_R = \operatorname{Re}\nu$, and $\nu_I = \operatorname{Im}\nu$, where ν has to satisfy

$$\langle \nu, \nu\rangle = 1,\ \langle \nu_R, \nu_I\rangle = 0$$

or, separated into the real and imaginary parts, these conditions become:

$$\langle \nu_R, \nu_R\rangle + \langle \nu_I, \nu_I\rangle = 1,\ \langle \nu_R, \nu_I\rangle = 0. \tag{7.30}$$

Remark 7.15. The conditions (7.30) are necessary to determine the eigenvector ν uniquely. Since for any complex number $c = c_1 + ic_2 \in \mathbb{C}$, $c\nu$ is also an eigenvector of $\hat{J}$ for $i\omega_0$. Thus for an arbitrary eigenvector $\tilde{\nu}$ we have to specify two conditions for c_1 and c_2, such that $\nu = c\tilde{\nu}$ satisfies (7.30).

Stability of Limit Cycles

In Sect. 2.12.1 we have shown that the stability of a limit cycle Γ is determined by the monodromy matrix $\mathrm{M} = Y(\Theta)$, where Y is the solution of the corresponding variational equation

$$\dot{Y}(t) = f_x(\Gamma(t))Y(t),$$

with $Y(0) = \mathbb{I}^{(n)}$ and $\Gamma(\cdot)$ is a periodic solution representing the limit cycle. Note that this is a non-autonomous ODE.

For the calculation of the monodromy matrix M of a limit cycle Γ at a point $x_\Gamma \in \Gamma$, the following BVP has to be solved:

$$\dot{x} = \Theta f(x) \tag{7.31a}$$
$$\dot{Y} = \Theta f_x(x)Y \tag{7.31b}$$
$$\text{s.t.}\quad x(0) = x(1) \tag{7.31c}$$
$$\psi\left(x(\cdot)\right) = 0 \tag{7.31d}$$
$$Y(0) = \mathbb{I}^{(n)}, \tag{7.31e}$$

where $\mathrm{M} = Y(1)$ is the sought solution and $\psi(x)$ is the phase condition.

Remark 7.16. Alternatively, if a limit cycle has already been detected, the monodromy matrix M at a point $x_\Gamma \in \Gamma$ can be computed by an IVP approach. Therefore, we have to solve the ODE (7.31a) and (7.31b) for the initial conditions $x(0) = x_\Gamma$ and (7.31e). The quality of this IVP approach relies heavily on the approximation of the limit cycle by the trajectory when starting at x_Γ. In the case of a saddle-type limit cycle one often has to do the calculations with a high degree of accuracy.

for a numerical example see Sect. 6.2.

Limit Cycles of the Canonical System

To determine the stability of a limit cycle occurring as an optimal solution of the problem *OCN* (7.1) we use (7.20), for which the corresponding variational equation becomes

$$\dot{Y}(t) = \begin{pmatrix} \mathcal{H}^*_{\lambda x}(\Gamma(t)) & \mathcal{H}^*_{\lambda\lambda}(\Gamma(t)) \\ -\mathcal{H}^*_{xx}(\Gamma(t)) & r\mathbb{I}^{(n)} - \mathcal{H}^*_{x\lambda}(\Gamma(t)) \end{pmatrix} Y(t), \tag{7.32}$$

with $Y(0) = \mathbb{I}^{(n)}$ and $\Gamma(\cdot)$ is a periodic solution representing the limit cycle. Now Liouville's formula (see Proposition 2.76)

$$W(t) = W(0)\mathrm{e}^{\int_0^t \operatorname{tr} \hat{J}(s)\,\mathrm{d}s},$$

where $W(t) = \det Y(t)$ and

$$\hat{J}(\cdot) = \begin{pmatrix} \mathcal{H}^*_{\lambda x}(\Gamma(\cdot)) & \mathcal{H}^*_{\lambda\lambda}(\Gamma(\cdot)) \\ -\mathcal{H}^*_{xx}(\Gamma(\cdot)) & r\mathbb{I}^{(n)} - \mathcal{H}^*_{x\lambda}(\Gamma(\cdot)) \end{pmatrix}$$

is the Jacobian evaluated along the trajectory $\Gamma(\cdot)$, allows one to exclude the existence of stable limit cycles:

Theorem 7.17. *Let Γ be a limit cycle of (7.20) with $r > 0$; then Γ is unstable.*

Proof. From (7.32) we find $\operatorname{tr} \hat{J}(t) = nr > 0$ for all t. Applying the formula of Liouville, together with $\det W(0) = 1$, yields

$$W(\Theta) = \det \mathrm{M} = \mathrm{e}^{nr\Theta} > 1.$$

By Cor. 2.87 this proves the instability of the limit cycle and concludes the proof. □

Thus the occurring limit cycles are repelling or of saddle-type; in the latter case the trajectories lying in the stable manifold are candidates for optimal solutions.

7.5 Continuing the Optimal Solution: Calculating the Stable Manifold

In the last section we identified equilibria and limit cycles as important candidates for the long-run optimal solutions of optimal control problems. In Sect. 2.6.2 we have seen that in the case of equilibria/limit cycles of saddle-type a stable manifold exists, which consists of the points from which the solution converges to these limit sets. For infinite horizon problems stable paths are candidates for optimal solutions.

In general it is not possible to calculate the stable manifolds explicitly; therefore efficient algorithms have to be provided to do the computations numerically. The following subsections address this topic.

7.5.1 Stable Manifold of an Equilibrium

Given a hyperbolic equilibrium $\hat{x}$ of saddle-type, the Hartman–Grobman theorem assures that the system is equivalent to its linear approximation in a (small) neighborhood of $\hat{x}$. We know from the manifold theorem for flows that the local stable manifold is tangential to the eigenspace $\mathrm{E}^s(\hat{x})$ and exhibits the same dimension n_-, which is the number of eigenvalues ξ satisfying $\operatorname{Re}\xi < 0$. In other words the linear space $\mathrm{E}^s(\hat{x})$ approximates the stable manifold in a neighborhood of $\hat{x}$.

From these considerations two numerical approaches can be derived. Both make use of the property that every trajectory starting at the stable manifold finally ends up at the local stable manifold, which is approximately given by the stable eigenspace; i.e., there exists a local representation of the stable manifold of the form

$$\mathrm{W}^s_{loc}(\hat{x}) = \{x : x = \hat{x} + \sum_{i=1}^{n_-} c_i \nu_i + o(\nu_i),\ \operatorname{Re}\xi_i < 0,\ c_i \in \mathbb{R}\}. \tag{7.33}$$

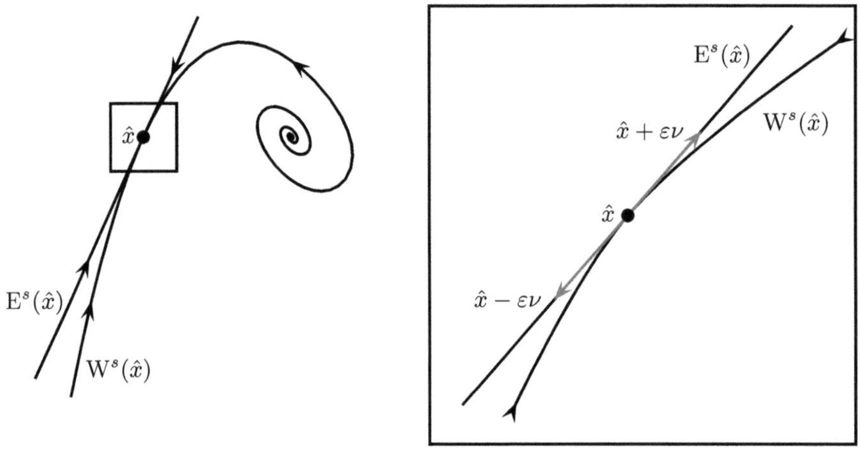

Fig. 7.7. In panel (**a**) the stable eigenspace $\mathrm{E}^s(\hat{x})$ and the global stable manifold $\mathrm{W}^s(\hat{x})$ are depicted, where the IVP approach for the calculation of the stable manifold has been used. Panel (**b**) shows the initial points for the calculation of the global stable manifold, approximated by $\hat{x} \pm \varepsilon\nu$

IVP Approach

In the IVP approach (see Fig. 7.7b) the linear approximation of (7.33) is used to calculate points x_s lying on the linearized stable manifold near the equilibrium $\hat{x}$ given by

$$x_s = \hat{x} + \sum_{i=1}^{n_-} c_i \nu_i, \tag{7.34}$$

with $\|\sum_{i=1}^{n_-} c_i \nu_i\| \leq \varepsilon$ and ε is "small." If we assume that ε is small enough that the quadratic terms of the approximation can be omitted, the trajectory

$$x(t) = \varphi^{-t} x_s, \quad 0 \leq t \leq T < \infty,$$

with $T > 0$, lies in the neighborhood of the stable manifold. Thus, to calculate points of the (approximated) stable manifold, one has to specify some initial point x_s satisfying (7.34) and solve the IVP in reversed time, i.e., for $[0, -T]$.

Remark 7.18. Note that the actual values of ε for the neighborhood of $\hat{x}$ and T for the integration time depend on the problem.

For the case of a one-dimensional stable manifold, i.e., $n_- = 1$, this simply reduces to the problem of solving the IVP for

$$x_s^{(1,2)} = \hat{x} \pm \varepsilon \nu,$$

where ν is the eigenvector corresponding to the eigenvalue ξ satisfying $\operatorname{Re} \xi < 0$. If ε is small enough, the orbit of the solution gives a good approximation of the stable manifold.

Remark 7.19. The IVP approach is easy to implement and well adapted for the computation of one-dimensional manifolds. For higher-dimensional manifolds the numerical effort increases considerably if, e.g., one of the eigenvalues dominates the others significantly in size. In that case one has to calculate with high accuracy to attain qualitatively good results. In principle it would also be possible to reduce the initial approximation error by using a quadratic or higher local approximation of the stable manifold (see, e.g., Ushiki, 1980; Xue, Teo, Lu, & Mei, 2006), which is not followed here.

However, the IVP approach exhibits another drawback for higher-dimensional problems. From the setup of an optimal control problem we are interested in the optimal solution, starting at some initial state x_0. (Note that here x_0 denotes an initial value for the state in the state–costate space of the optimal control problem.) Thus the problem becomes finding a point $(x_s, \lambda_s) \in \mathrm{E}^s(\hat{x}, \hat{\lambda})$ such that

$$x_0 = \mathrm{P}\, \varphi^{-T}(x_s, \lambda_s),$$

where P denotes the projection into the state space; i.e.,

$$\mathrm{P}(x, \lambda) = x,$$

which describes a BVP. Therefore the IVP approach can be seen as part of some *shooting method* for solving the corresponding BVP.

Summing up, it can be said that the IVP algorithm is well-suited to the case of finding a one-dimensional stable manifold. But for the higher-dimensional case a BVP approach is often better adapted to the problem described above.

BVP Approach

To introduce the BVP approach, let us start with the reformulation of an optimal control problem, where it is assumed that the stable manifold of the equilibrium $(\hat{x}, \hat{\lambda})$ is of dimension n and is the long-run optimal solution. Then, given an initial state $x(0) = x_0 \in \mathbb{R}^n$, we have to find a trajectory $(x(\cdot), \lambda(\cdot))$ that satisfies the ODEs of the canonical system and converges to the equilibrium $(\hat{x}, \hat{\lambda})$. Using the definition of the local stable manifold the last statement can be reformulated so that for some T

$$(x(T), \lambda(T)) \in \mathrm{W}^s_{loc}(\hat{x}, \hat{\lambda}),$$

or approximating $\mathrm{W}^s_{loc}(\hat{x}, \hat{\lambda})$ by its linearization $\mathrm{E}^s(\hat{x}, \hat{\lambda})$,

$$(x(T), \lambda(T)) \in \mathrm{E}^s(\hat{x}, \hat{\lambda}). \tag{7.35}$$

Thus the problem is reduced to a BVP, where initial condition $x(0) = x_0$ and terminal condition (7.35) are given.

General Problem

We now return to the general problem of solving a BVP of the form:

$$\dot{x} = f(x, \mu) \tag{7.36a}$$

$$\text{s.t.} \quad x^{N_-}(0) = x_0 \in \mathbb{R}^{n_-} \tag{7.36b}$$

$$x(T) \in \mathrm{E}^s\, \hat{x}(\mu), \tag{7.36c}$$

where $N_- = \{1, \ldots, n_-\}$ and $T > 0$ is some fixed (problem-specific) number and $\hat{x}(\mu)$ is the equilibrium in dependence of the parameter value μ. To solve this problem we have to find an equation describing (7.36c), which is given by the following proposition (where for notational simplicity we omit the dependence on the parameter values μ):

Proposition 7.20 (Asymptotic Boundary Condition at an Equilibrium). *Let $\hat{x}$ be a hyperbolic equilibrium of (7.36a), with an n_--dimensional stable manifold ($n_- > 0$). Then $(x - \hat{x}) \in \mathrm{E}^s(\hat{x})$ iff $x - \hat{x}$ is orthogonal to every eigenvector b of the adjoint problem*

$$\dot{x} = -f_x(\hat{x})' x,$$

where b corresponds to an eigenvalue ξ of the Jacobian at $\hat{x}$ with $\mathrm{Re}\,\xi > 0$. *Then*

$$\mathrm{E}^s(\hat{x}) = \{x : F'(x - \hat{x}) = 0\}, \tag{7.36d}$$

with F an $n_+ \times n$ matrix constituted of all eigenvectors b_j corresponding to $\mathrm{Re}\,\xi_j > 0$, *and normalized such that $b_j' \nu_j = 1$, $j = n_- + 1, \ldots, n$. The condition (7.36d) is called an* asymptotic boundary condition.

Remark 7.21. Note that F has full-rank n_+; therefore the number of independent boundary conditions from (7.36b) and (7.36d) sum to n.

Remark 7.22. In a more general setting it is proved in Pampel (2000) that for $T \to \infty$ the solution of (7.36) converges to the corresponding stable path.

Remark 7.23. To calculate paths of the unstable manifold the reversed dynamics

$$\dot{x} = -f(x, \mu)$$

has to be considered.

If we replace the condition (7.36c) with (7.36d), we have to solve the following BVP:

$$\dot{x} = f(x, \mu) \tag{7.37a}$$

$$\text{s.t.} \quad x^{N_-}(0) = x_0 \in \mathbb{R}^{n_-} \tag{7.37b}$$

$$\Sigma(x(T), \hat{x}(\mu), \mu) = 0, \tag{7.37c}$$

with $\Sigma(x(T), \hat{x}(\mu), \mu) = F(\mu)' (x - \hat{x}(\mu))$.

Remark 7.24. If a continuation process, as described in Sect. 7.2, is used to calculate the solution for a varying parameter μ, the equilibrium $\hat{x}(\mu)$ and the matrix $F(\mu)$ have to be recalculated during the continuation process. This may increase the numerical effort considerably (for details the reader is referred to Beyn, Pampel, and Semmler 2001).

When analyzing an optimal control problem one often has to solve a BVP of the form (7.37) for different initial states x_0. Given that we already established a solution $x_1(\cdot)$ of (7.37) with initial value $x_1^{N_-}(0) = x_s$ and that we want to find the solution $x_2(\cdot)$ with $x_2^{N_-}(0) = x_e$, we can use one of the continuation algorithms presented in Sect. 7.2.2. Therefore we continue the solution along a line connecting x_s and x_e by varying the continuation parameter γ. During this process we find trajectories $x(\cdot, \gamma)$:

Definition 7.25 (Slice Manifold). *Let $x(\cdot, \gamma)$ be a solution of the BVP (7.37) satisfying*

$$x^{N_-}(0, \gamma) = (1 - \gamma)x_s + \gamma x_e, \quad L_1 \le \gamma \le L_2;$$

then the function

$$\eta(\gamma) := (x(0, \gamma))$$

is called the slice manifold.

In the one-dimensional case the slice manifold coincides with the stable manifold, whereas in the higher-dimensional case it yields the cut through the stable manifold along the line from the starting point $x(0, L_1)$ to the endpoint $x(0, L_2)$.

Remark 7.26. The slice manifold plays an important role for optimal control problems. For these problems the state variable x contains the state as well as the costate variable of the optimal control problem. Then Proposition 3.75 states that the objective value $V^*(x_0)$ of an extremal solution with initial condition $x(0) = x_0$ only depends on the initial state and costate by

$$V^*(x_0) = \frac{1}{r}\mathcal{H}^*\left(x^*(0), \lambda(0)\right).$$

Thus

$$\frac{1}{r}\mathcal{H}^*\left(\eta(\gamma)\right), \quad L_1 \leq \gamma \leq L_2,$$

is the value function for an optimal control problem with initial state $x_0(\gamma) = (1-\gamma)x_s + \gamma x_e$.

How, then, to start the numerical computation of the BVP (7.37)?

Initialization

To initialize a BV-Solver we have to provide an initial solution for the BVP. A trivial solution for (7.37) with $x^{N_-}(0) = \hat{x}^{N_-}$ is the equilibrium $\hat{x}$ itself. Thus a continuation algorithm of Sect. 7.2 can be used to continue this trivial solution to an arbitrarily given point x_e.

Another possibility is to use the IVP approach p. 350 for calculating a first solution and starting the continuation process for this initial solution.

In the next subsection we consider the computation of the stable manifold of a limit cycle.

7.5.2 Stable Manifold of Limit Cycles

In Sect. 2.12.1 we have seen that the stable manifold at a point x_Γ of the limit cycle Γ is tangential to the stable eigenspace of the associated monodromy matrix at x_Γ. Thus an analogous approach to the case of an equilibrium can be used for calculating the stable manifold of a limit cycle. Again an IVP approach or a BVP procedure can be used for the numerical calculations. But the BVP approach is more tricky in the case of a limit cycle, as the sought solution converges to a set (the orbit of the limit cycle) and not just to a single point.

In the hyperbolic case in which the number n_- of eigenvalues ξ corresponds to stable directions, these are the eigenvalues satisfying $|\mathrm{Re}\,\xi| < 1$, and the number n_+ of unstable directions satisfying $|\mathrm{Re}\,\xi| > 1$ sum to $n = n_- + n_+ + 1$ (see Sect. 2.12.1). Thus the dimension of the stable manifold is given by $n_- + 1$.

IVP Approach

To start the IVP approach we have to choose a point $x_\Gamma \in \Gamma$ of the limit cycle and calculate the corresponding monodromy matrix M by solving problem

(7.31). Then the n_- eigenvectors ν_i corresponding to eigenvalues with $|\mathrm{Re}\,\xi_i| < 1$ have to be determined.

Specifying some arbitrary time T and $\varepsilon > 0$, c_i, $i = 1,\dots,n_-$ with $\|\sum_{i=1}^{n_-} c_i\nu_i\| < \varepsilon$, one can determine a point x_s lying on the linear approximation of the stable manifold by

$$x_s = x_\Gamma + \sum_{i=1}^{n_-} c_i\nu_i. \tag{7.38}$$

Solving the ODE (7.31a) with $x(0) = x_s$ backward in time $[0, -T]$ yields a solution, approximating a path lying on the stable manifold.

This approach suffers from the same deficiency as its equilibrium counterpart, which is mainly the problem of calculating a solution starting from a specific initial point. This becomes more striking in the case of constraints, as we shall see in Sect. 7.6, since the IVP approach does not make use of the intrinsically underlying BVP. Nonetheless, it is an easy-to-implement algorithm, and the solution of the IVP problem can, e.g., be used as an initial solution for the BVP approach.

BVP Approach

Let us now state the underlying problem in full detail. We consider the ODE

$$\dot{x}(t) = f(x(t),\mu),$$

exhibiting a limit cycle $\Gamma(\mu)$ (depending on μ) of period Θ. Recall that the limit cycle $\Gamma(\mu)$ can be represented by any phase-shifted periodic solution $\Gamma(\cdot,\varphi,\mu)$ (see p. 346).

Hence the problem to find a path converging to the limit cycle becomes:

$$\dot{\Gamma}(t,\varphi,\mu) = \Theta(\mu) f\left(\Gamma(t,\varphi,\mu),\mu\right) \tag{7.39a}$$
$$\Gamma(0,\varphi,\mu) = \Gamma(1,\varphi,\mu)$$
$$\dot{x} = \Theta(\mu) f(x,\mu)$$
$$x(T) \in \mathrm{W}^s_{loc}\left(\Gamma(\mu),\mu\right). \tag{7.39b}$$

Next we state an asymptotic boundary condition replacing (7.39b). In the following proposition we omit the dependence on the parameter μ:

Proposition 7.27 (Asymptotic Boundary Condition at a Limit Cycle). *Let $\Gamma(\cdot,\varphi_0)$ be a periodic solution of (7.39a) for a fixed phase-shift φ_0 and $x_\Gamma = \Gamma(0,\varphi)$. The corresponding limit cycle Γ is hyperbolic with $n_- > 0$ stable eigenvectors. Then $(x - x_\Gamma) \in \mathrm{E}^s(\Gamma)$ at x_Γ iff*

$$X(0)\,(x - x_\Gamma) = 0, \tag{7.40}$$

where $X(0) \in \mathbb{R}^{(n_+ +1)\times n}$ is a solution of the adjoint variational matrix equation

$$\begin{aligned} &\dot{X}(t) = -X(t)\Theta f_x\left(\Gamma(t,\varphi)\right)', \\ \text{s.t.}\quad &X(1) = \Lambda X(0), \end{aligned} \tag{7.41}$$

where Λ is a matrix with eigenvalues ξ satisfying $|\mathrm{Re}\,\xi| > 1$.

For the proof see Appendix B.9.2.

Remark 7.28. Specifically the matrix $X(0)$ can be chosen as the adjoint eigenvectors of the monodromy matrix M at x_Γ corresponding to eigenvalues ξ with $|\mathrm{Re}\,\xi| > 1$ (see Appendix B.9.2).

Remark 7.29. Note that

$$F = X(0)',$$

the matrix describing the asymptotic boundary condition, explicitly depends on the phase shift φ. Hence, in the following we indicate this by writing $F(\varphi)$.

Since we have now solved the problem of describing the asymptotic boundary condition (7.40), we can replace the condition (7.39b) with

$$F(\varphi,\mu)\left(\Gamma(T,\varphi,\mu) - x(T)\right),$$

where for reasons of simplicity we assume $T \in \mathbb{N}$ yielding

$$F(\varphi,\mu)\left(\Gamma(0,\varphi,\mu) - x(T)\right),$$

since by the time-scaling the limit cycle is of period one.

Summing up, we have to consider the following BVP for $T \in \mathbb{N}$:

$$\dot{\Gamma}(t,\varphi,\mu) = \Theta(\mu) f\left(\Gamma(t,\varphi,\mu),\mu\right) \tag{7.42a}$$
$$\dot{x} = \Theta(\mu) f(x,\mu) \tag{7.42b}$$
$$\text{s.t.}\quad x^{N_-}(0) = x_s \in \mathbb{R}^{n_-} \tag{7.42c}$$
$$\Gamma(0,\varphi,\mu) = \Gamma(1,\varphi,\mu) \tag{7.42d}$$
$$\psi\left(\Gamma(\cdot,\varphi,\mu),\varphi\right) = 0 \tag{7.42e}$$
$$\Sigma\left(x(T),\Gamma(\mu),\mu\right) = 0, \tag{7.42f}$$

where

$$\Sigma\left(x(T),\Gamma(\mu),\mu\right) = F(\varphi,\mu)\left(\Gamma(0,\varphi,\mu) - x(T)\right)$$

and $F(\varphi)$ is derived from (7.41).

Examples for the phase-fixing functional $\psi\left(\Gamma(\cdot,\varphi,\mu)\right)$ are given below.

Remark 7.30. To admit a general $T \geq 0$ we have to change the dynamics of (7.41) to

$$\dot{X}(t) = -X(t)\Theta(\mu) f_x(\varphi, t + T \bmod 1)'$$

(which coincides with (7.41) if $T \in \mathbb{N}$).

Assuming that we have already established a solution that satisfies the BVP (7.42), we can use one of the continuation algorithms to continue the solution along a line analogous to the equilibrium case. But solving the BVP (7.42) for a new initial value x_s or changed parameter value μ is numerically expensive, since the phase-shift may change and therefore needs a recalculation of $F(\varphi)$. Thus to reduce the computational costs the so-called *boundary corrector method* can be used; Pampel (2000) proved that this method provides the same numerical results as the original problem. The boundary corrector method includes the following steps:

1. The matrix $F(\varphi_i)$ is known from a preceding solution step.
2. The BVP (7.42) is solved for the fixed $F(\varphi_i)$.
3. $F(\varphi_{i+1})$ is recalculated from (7.41) using the solution $z(t)$ from the preceding BVP.
4. Return to point 1.

In the case that the parameter values μ are fixed and only the initial condition x_s changes, the problem can be further simplified, as we subsequently show. But first we consider the problem of a specific phase-fixing functional.

Phase-Fixing Functional ψ

Note that (7.42f) explicitly refers to a free phase-shift. This is necessary because the reference point x_Γ on the limit cycle for the stable manifold may vary during the solution process. We therefore have to specify a phase-fixing functional $\psi(z,\varphi)$. As presented in Beyn et al. (2001), different functional forms are possible, such as

$$\psi(z,\varphi) := \dot{\Gamma}_0(0,0)' \left(z(0) - \Gamma_0(0,\varphi)\right)$$

or

$$\psi(z,\varphi) := f\left(\Gamma_0(0,0)\right)' \left(z(0) - \varphi f(\Gamma_0(0,0))\right),$$

where $\Gamma_0(\cdot,\varphi)$ is an already known periodic solution of the limit cycle. But these specifically chosen functions are only applicable for the case of varying model-specific parameters. In the case that the stable manifold is continued for fixed model parameters, Beyn et al. (2001) propose another functional $\psi(z,\varphi)$. It is assumed that a two-dimensional stable manifold in a four-dimensional space is analyzed. Then an arbitrary point $\bar{x} = (\bar{x}_1, \bar{x}_2)$ is chosen lying in the interior of the projected limit cycle. Now we can define

$$\psi(z,\varphi) := \sin\left(2\pi(\varphi+\varphi_0)\right)\left(\bar{x}_1 - z_1(0)\right) - \cos\left(2\pi(\varphi+\varphi_0)\right)\left(\bar{x}_2 - z_2(0)\right), \tag{7.43}$$

where $\psi(z,\varphi)$ denotes the angular change (see Fig. 7.8) relative to some initially given point x_Γ, satisfying

$$\psi(x_\Gamma, 0) = 0.$$

Next, we present a method that allows avoiding the problem of a changing phase-shift.

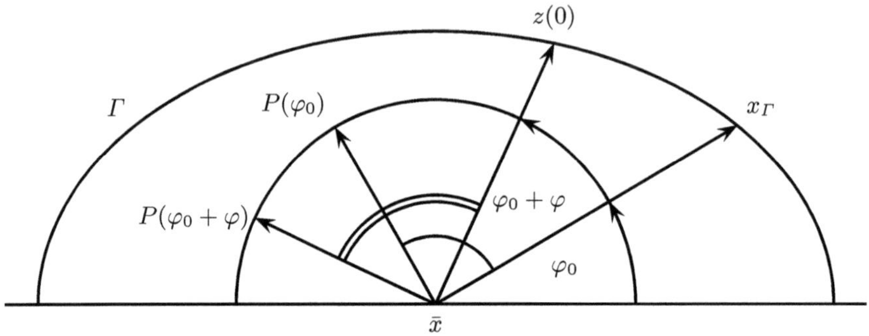

Fig. 7.8. The phase-fixing function $\psi(z, \varphi)$ defined in (7.43) is an orthogonality relation, between the vector $\bar{x} - z(0)$ and $P(\varphi_0 + \varphi) = (\sin(\varphi_0 + \varphi), -\cos(\varphi_0 + \varphi))$

Simplification for Fixed Parameter Values μ

Let us consider the problem of solving the BVP (7.42) for different initial states $x^{N_-}(0)$. In that case we can reduce the computational costs considerably if we can assure that we always end up near the same reference point x_Γ. Therefore we free the integration time T and add the new constraint

$$f(x_\Gamma)(x_\Gamma - x(T)) = 0.$$

Then the general problem (7.42) can be specified as a BVP on the time interval [0, 1]

$$\dot{x} = Tf(x) \tag{7.44a}$$
$$\text{s.t.} \quad x^{N_-}(0) = x_s \in \mathbb{R}^{n_-} \tag{7.44b}$$
$$f(x_\Gamma)(x(T) - x_\Gamma) = 0 \tag{7.44c}$$
$$\Sigma\left(x(1), \Gamma\right) = 0, \tag{7.44d}$$

with

$$\Sigma\left(x(1), \Gamma\right) = F\left(x_\Gamma - x(1)\right),$$

where F is derived from the monodromy matrix at x_Γ (see Remark 7.28).

This approach has the advantage that the matrix F has to be calculated only once and does not change during a continuation process. Moreover, the problem of recalculating the limit cycle is avoided. Thus, instead of solving the general problem (7.42), it is easier to solve (7.44) as long as the parameter values do not change.

Initialization

The question to be resolved is how to find an initial solution. We therefore compute a trajectory of the limit cycle on the time interval $[0, T]$ with $T = n\Theta$, $n \in \mathbb{N}$. Thus we solve the BVP (7.29) with the boundary condition

$$\Gamma(0) = \Gamma(T),$$

and use this trajectory as a first trivial solution.

Remark 7.31. In the case of a general time $T \geq 0$ we use the boundary condition

$$\Gamma(T \bmod 1) = \Gamma(T).$$

As a further possibility we can solve the IVP for a point given by (7.38) and use the corresponding trajectory as an initial solution for the BVP.

7.6 Optimal Control Problems with Active Constraints

In Sect. 7.3 we considered solutions of *OCN* (7.1), where no constraint becomes active. Here we analyze the case in which constraints in the form of mixed path constraints (7.1d) or pure state constraints (7.1e) become active. Therefore we restate the necessary conditions for a maximizer provided by Pontryagin's Maximum Principle Theorem 3.60:

$$\mathcal{H}(x^*, u^*, \lambda) = \max_u \mathcal{H}(x^*, u, \lambda) \tag{7.45a}$$

$$\mathcal{L}_u(x^*, u^*, \lambda) = 0 \tag{7.45b}$$

$$\dot{\lambda} = -\mathcal{L}_x(x^*, u^*, \lambda) \tag{7.45c}$$

together with the complementary slackness conditions

$$\mu(t) \geq 0, \quad \mu c(x^*, u^*) = 0 \tag{7.45d}$$

$$\nu(t) \geq 0, \quad \nu h(x^*) = 0. \tag{7.45e}$$

Furthermore, at a junction time $\tilde{t}$ the following corner conditions have to hold:

$$\lambda(\tilde{t}^+) = \lambda(\tilde{t}^-) + \eta(\tilde{t}) h_x(\tilde{t}), \tag{7.45f}$$

$$\mathcal{H}(\tilde{t}^+) = \mathcal{H}(\tilde{t}^-) - \eta(\tilde{t}) h_t(\tilde{t}),$$

with $\eta(t) \geq 0$ and $\eta(t)h(t) = 0$. The Lagrangian $\mathcal{L}$ is given by

$$\mathcal{L}(x, u, \lambda, \mu, \nu) = \mathcal{H}(x, u, \lambda) + \mu(t)c(x, u) + \nu(t)h(x).$$

By Assumption 7.5, the constraint qualification is satisfied (see Sect. 3.6).

To completely analyze a system that includes constraints, one has to consider the possible combinations of constraints and the corresponding forms of the representations of the canonical system. Then each of these systems has to be analyzed separately by locating the equilibria and limit cycles, respectively, and computing the corresponding stable paths. During these calculations the continued solutions might reach points, for which some necessary condition is violated. These points are so-called *junction points* (see Sect. 3.6). At these junction points the system has to be switched. From an applied point of view this leads to a multi-point BVP. The implementation of these steps in the concrete case is the subject of the following subsections. To simplify the presentation we consider mixed path and pure state constraints separately.

7.6.1 The Form of the Canonical System for Mixed Path Constraints

In the case that mixed path constraints are given, only (7.45a)–(7.45d) have to be considered. We assume that the constraint $c(x,u)=0$ holds,[5] then the following conditions have to be satisfied:

$$\begin{aligned} &c(x,u)=0 \\ &\mathcal{L}_u(x,u,\lambda,\mu)=0 \qquad (7.46a) \\ &\mu(\cdot)\geq 0, \quad \mu c(x,u)=0 \\ &c_u(x,u) \quad \text{is invertible.} \qquad (7.46b) \end{aligned}$$

For a boundary arc the control value is given by a continuously differentiable function $u^*(x)$. This follows from the constraint qualification (7.46b) together with the implicit function theorem. Equations (7.46a) and (7.46b) yield for the Lagrange multiplier $\mu(t)$

$$\mathcal{L}_u=0 \quad \text{iff} \quad \mu=-\mathcal{H}_u^* c_u^{-1}.$$

Thus the corresponding canonical system is given by

$$\dot{x}=f\left(x,u^*(x,\lambda)\right) \qquad (7.47a)$$

$$\dot{\lambda}=r\lambda-\mathcal{H}_x^*+\mathcal{H}_u^* c_u^{-1} c_x. \qquad (7.47b)$$

Remark 7.32. The Jacobian of (7.47),

$$\hat{J}(\hat{x},\hat{\lambda})=\begin{pmatrix} \mathcal{L}_{\lambda x}^* & \mathcal{L}_{\lambda\lambda}^* \\ -\mathcal{L}_{xx}^* & r\mathbb{I}^{(n)}-\mathcal{L}_{x\lambda}^* \end{pmatrix},$$

exhibits the same structure as in the unconstrained case. Thus the restriction for the dimension of the stable manifold, Theorem 7.10, and the instability of limit cycles, Theorem 7.17, also holds true for the system (7.47).

7.6.2 The Form of the Canonical System for Pure State Constraints

In the case that only the pure state constraint $h(x)=0$ is active,[6] the following conditions are satisfied:

$$\begin{aligned} &h(x)=0 \qquad (7.48) \\ &\mathcal{L}_u(x,u,\lambda,\nu)=0 \\ &\nu(\cdot)\geq 0, \quad \nu h(x)=0 \\ &d_u(x,u)\neq 0 \end{aligned}$$

---

[5] If only some of the mixed path constraints are active, we agree in denoting these active constraints by the same variable c.

[6] If only some of the pure state constraints are active, we agree in denoting those active constraints by the same variable h.

where $d_u(x,u)$ is the total time derivative of $h(x)$ (see Definition 3.56).

Since the pure state constraint (7.1e) do not explicitly depend on the control variable u, the equation

$$0 = \mathcal{L}_u = \mathcal{H}_u$$

does not contain the Lagrange multiplier ν. Thus, to derive an explicit expression for the multiplier $\nu(\cdot)$, we consider the total time derivative of $\mathcal{L}_u$, yielding

$$\frac{\mathrm{d}}{\mathrm{d}t}\mathcal{L}_u(x,u,\lambda) = \frac{\mathrm{d}}{\mathrm{d}t}\mathcal{H}_u(x,u,\lambda) = 0.$$

This can explicitly be written as

$$\begin{aligned} 0 = \frac{\mathrm{d}}{\mathrm{d}t}\mathcal{H}_u &= \frac{\mathrm{d}}{\mathrm{d}t}g_u + \lambda\frac{\mathrm{d}}{\mathrm{d}t}f_u + \dot{\lambda}f_u \\ &= \frac{\mathrm{d}}{\mathrm{d}t}g_u + \lambda\frac{\mathrm{d}}{\mathrm{d}t}f_u + \left(r\lambda - \mathcal{H}_x - \nu h_x\right)f_u \\ &= \frac{\mathrm{d}}{\mathrm{d}t}g_u + \lambda\frac{\mathrm{d}}{\mathrm{d}t}f_u + \left(r\lambda - \mathcal{H}_x\right)f_u - \nu h_x f_u \\ &= \frac{\mathrm{d}}{\mathrm{d}t}g_u + \lambda\frac{\mathrm{d}}{\mathrm{d}t}f_u + \left(r\lambda - \mathcal{H}_x\right)f_u - \nu d_u. \end{aligned} \tag{7.49}$$

By Assumption 7.4 the state constraint is of order one and satisfies the constraint qualification

$$d_u(x,u) \neq 0, \quad \text{for all} \quad t \in [\underline{t},\ \bar{t}].$$

Using (7.49), we can therefore express the Lagrange multiplier by

$$\nu = \left(\frac{\mathrm{d}}{\mathrm{d}t}g_u + \lambda\frac{\mathrm{d}}{\mathrm{d}t}f_u + f_u\left(r\lambda - \mathcal{H}_x\right)\right)d_u^{-1}.$$

By the implicit function theorem, and Assumptions 7.4 and 7.5, it is assured that at the time interval $(\underline{t},\ \bar{t})$ the kth coordinate of the optimal control value u^* can be written as a function of x and is differentiable with respect to x. Using the chain rule, this proves that $\dot{u}$ exists on the interval $(\underline{t},\ \bar{t})$, yielding

$$\begin{aligned} \frac{\mathrm{d}}{\mathrm{d}t}g_u &= g_{uu}\dot{u} + g_{ux}\dot{x} \\ \frac{\mathrm{d}}{\mathrm{d}t}f_u &= f_{uu}\dot{u} + f_{ux}\dot{x}. \end{aligned}$$

Hence we have finally found an explicit representation of the canonical system

$$\begin{aligned} \dot{x} &= f\left(x, u^*(x,\lambda)\right) \\ \dot{\lambda} &= r\lambda - \mathcal{H}_x^* - \nu h_x. \end{aligned}$$

Now we turn to the important question of joining interior and boundary arcs at junction points.

7.6.3 Solutions Exhibiting Junction Points

In the numerical analysis of a system exhibiting an interior as well as a boundary arc, the focus lies on the junction point, where the switching between the boundary and the interior arc takes place or vice versa. Pontryagin's Maximum Principle Theorem 3.60 for problems with constraints provides further conditions, which have to be satisfied at these points, resulting in a multi-point BVP. Thus we have to analyze a system of the following structure, where we assume an entry point $\underline{x}$ for reasons of notational simplicity. The following arguments also hold true for an exit point; only the order of interior and boundary arc changes. Let $0 < \underline{t} < \infty$ be the entry time; then the following system has to be considered (note that the first n coordinates of ${}^{i}x$, $i = 1, 2$ denote the states and the last n coordinates the costates of the optimal control problem):

$$
\begin{aligned}
{}^{1}\dot{x} &= {}^{1}f\left({}^{1}x\right), \quad t \in [0, \underline{t}], \ {}^{1}x \in \mathbb{R}^{2n} && (7.50a)\\
{}^{2}\dot{x} &= {}^{2}f\left({}^{2}x\right), \quad t \in (\underline{t}, \infty), \ {}^{2}x \in \mathbb{R}^{2n} && (7.50b)\\
{}^{1}x^{N}(0) &= x_0 \in \mathbb{R}^{n}, \quad N = \{1, \dots, n\} && (7.50c)\\
\Psi &\left({}^{1}x(\underline{t}), {}^{2}x(\underline{t})\right) = 0 && (7.50d)\\
\Sigma &\left({}^{2}x(T), \omega\right) = 0, && (7.50e)
\end{aligned}
$$

where (7.50a) is the canonical system for the interior arc, (7.50b) is the dynamics at the boundary arc, (7.50c) denotes the initial condition, (7.50d) characterizes the corner conditions (see Sect. 3.6.2) at the entry point, which are subsequently specified in more detail, and finally (7.50e) is the usual asymptotic boundary condition.

Corner Conditions and the Two-Point BVP

Under the Assumptions 7.1–7.6, system (7.50) yields the following multi-point BVP:

$$
\begin{aligned}
&{}^{1}\dot{x} = {}^{1}f\left({}^{1}x\right), \quad t \in [0, \underline{t}]\\
&{}^{2}\dot{x} = {}^{2}f\left({}^{2}x\right), \quad t \in [\underline{t}, T]\\
\text{s.t.}\quad &{}^{1}x^{N}(0) = x_0 \in \mathbb{R}^{n}\\
&\Psi\left({}^{1}x(\underline{t}), {}^{2}x(\underline{t})\right) = 0\\
&\Sigma\left({}^{2}x(T), \omega\right) = 0,
\end{aligned}
$$

where T is the truncation time and Σ the usual asymptotic boundary condition. For specifying the corner conditions Ψ at an entry (junction) point we distinguish between the mixed path and pure state constraints.

Corner Conditions for Mixed Path Constraints

In the case of mixed path constraints the corner conditions simply reduce to the postulation of continuity for both the state and the costate at the entry time $\underline{t}$ as well as the continuity of the Hamiltonian (see Sect. 4.4), yielding

$$\begin{aligned} &{}^1x^N(\underline{t}) = {}^2x^N(\underline{t}) \\ &{}^1x^{N^c}(\underline{t}) = {}^2x^{N^c}(\underline{t}), \quad N^c = \{n+1,\dots,2n\} \\ &\mathcal{H}^*\left({}^1x(\underline{t})\right) = \mathcal{H}^*\left({}^2x(\underline{t})\right). \end{aligned} \tag{7.51}$$

Thus the corner condition Ψ becomes

$$\Psi\left({}^1x(\underline{t}), {}^2x(\underline{t})\right) := \begin{pmatrix} {}^2x^N(\underline{t}) - {}^1x^N(\underline{t}) \\ {}^2x^{N^c}(\underline{t}) - {}^1x^{N^c}(\underline{t}) \\ \mathcal{H}^*\left({}^1x(\underline{t})\right) - \mathcal{H}^*\left({}^2x(\underline{t})\right) \end{pmatrix}. \tag{7.52}$$

The equation for the continuity of the Hamiltonian at an entry (junction) point allows us to determine the entry time $\underline{t}$, which is a free variable of the corresponding BVP.

Corner Conditions for Pure State Constraints

In the case of pure state constraints the costates as well as the Hamiltonian may exhibit a discontinuity at the entry time $\underline{t}$ of the form (7.45f) (see Sect. 4.4), yielding

$$\begin{aligned} &{}^1x^{N^c}(\underline{t}) = {}^2x^{N^c}(\underline{t}) + \eta h_x(\underline{t}), \quad N^c = \{n+1,\dots,2n\} \\ &\mathcal{H}^*\left({}^1x(\underline{t})\right) = \mathcal{H}^*\left({}^2x(\underline{t})\right) - \eta h_t(\underline{t}), \end{aligned}$$

with $\eta \geq 0$. But in our case the possible discontinuity of the Hamiltonian reduces to continuity since, by assumption, the state constraint does not explicitly depend on time (see (7.48)).

Contrary to the problem with mixed path constraints, we have to consider an additional variable η. Thus to state a well-defined BVP, an additional condition has to be provided. Therefore we recall that the states have to be continuous, i.e.,

$${}^1x^N(\underline{t}) = {}^2x^N(\underline{t})$$

yielding

$$h\left({}^1x^N(\underline{t})\right) = 0. \tag{7.53}$$

This last condition states that at the entry time $\underline{t}$ the state constraint has to hold also for the interior arc.

Summarizing these equations, we find the following corner conditions

$$\Psi\left({}^1x(\underline{t}), {}^2x(\underline{t})\right) := \begin{pmatrix} {}^2x^N(\underline{t}) - {}^1x^N(\underline{t}) \\ {}^2x^{N^c}(\underline{t}) - {}^1x^{N^c}(\underline{t}) + \eta h_x(\underline{t}) \\ \mathcal{H}^*\left({}^1x(\underline{t})\right) - \mathcal{H}^*\left({}^2x(\underline{t})\right) \\ h\left({}^1x^N(\underline{t})\right). \end{pmatrix}. \tag{7.54}$$

Stating the Two-Point BVP of (7.50)

For the specified corner conditions in the form (7.52) or (7.54) the BVP (7.50) becomes a well-defined multi-point BVP. This can be transformed into a two-point BVP as shown in Sect. 7.1.4, finally yielding:

$$\begin{aligned} & {}^1\dot{x} = \bar{t}\, {}^1\!f\left({}^1x\right), \quad t \in [0,1] \\ & {}^2\dot{x} = (T - \bar{t})\, {}^2\!f\left({}^2x\right), \quad t \in [0,1] \\ \text{s.t.}\quad & {}^1x^N(0) = x_0 \in \mathbb{R}^n \\ & \Psi\left({}^1x(1), {}^2x(0)\right) = 0 \\ & \Sigma\left({}^2x(1), \omega\right) = 0 \end{aligned}$$

where Ψ denotes the corner conditions and Σ denotes the asymptotic conditions for converging to the limit set ω.

Remark 7.33. In our presentation of the corner conditions we considered the special case of an entry point. But the results also hold true for an exit point, where only the succession of interior and boundary arcs interchange. Thus the condition (7.53) has to be replaced by

$$h\left({}^2x^N(\bar{t})\right) = 0.$$

Remark 7.34. The case of only one junction point, presented here, can immediately be generalized to the case of $i \in \mathbb{N}$ junction points. Therefore only the additional dynamics

$${}^j\dot{x} = {}^j\!f\left({}^jx\right), \quad j = 1, \dots, i+1$$

with the corresponding corner conditions have to be considered.

Remark 7.35. If Assumption 7.2 is strengthened so that the Hamiltonian satisfies $\mathcal{H}_{uu} < 0$ for all u, and the constraint qualification Assumption 7.5 is satisfied, then the corner condition (7.51) for mixed path constraints reduces to

$$c\left({}^1x^N(\underline{t})\right) = 0, \quad \text{entry time } \underline{t}$$

or

$$\mu\left({}^1x^N(\bar{t})\right) = 0, \quad \text{exit time } \bar{t}.$$

In the case of pure state constraints the costates are continuous, yielding $\eta = 0$ and therefore the continuity condition of the Hamiltonian is superfluous and the conditions on the costates can be replaced by

$${}^2x^{N^c}(\underline{t}) = {}^1x^{N^c}(\underline{t}), \quad \text{entry time } \underline{t}$$

or

$$\nu\left({}^1x^N(\bar{t})\right) = 0, \quad \text{exit time } \bar{t}.$$

Locating a Junction Point

For reasons of simplicity we now consider the case of an exit point and assume that the Hamiltonian is negative definite for all u. Then the corner conditions can be replaced by those stated in Remark 7.35.

The usual way of encountering an exit point is during a continuation process, in which we continue a solution until a constraint is violated.

Let us therefore suppose that at step $i > 1$ of a continuation process we have found the solution $x_i(\cdot)$, with $x_i(0) = x_{i,0} \in \mathbb{R}^n$, satisfying the constraints $\Upsilon(x_{i+1}(0)) \geq 0$. But at the next step one of these conditions is violated, i.e., $\Upsilon(x_{i+1}(0)) < 0$, where Υ is a mixed path or pure state constraint. By a continuity argument we can assume that in the neighborhood of $x_{i+1}(0)$ there exists a solution $x(\cdot)$ satisfying

$$\Upsilon(x(0)) = 0. \tag{7.55}$$

Therefore a straightforward way to find this solution is to free one of the variables of x^N, say x^j, and search along the jth coordinate for a solution satisfying (7.55) and $x^{N_{\{j\}}}(0) = x_0^{(j)}$, where $N_{\{j\}} = N \setminus \{j\}$.

Remark 7.36. For the more general case Assumption 7.2 it may occur that the maximum of the Hamiltonian is achieved for an interior control value u^*_{int} as well as for a boundary value u^*_{bound}, satisfying $c(u^*_{bound}, x) = 0$. Thus also the maximum condition on the Hamiltonian has to be verified at each continuation step.

Finding a Curve of Junction Points

The previous method for locating a junction point can easily be adapted to find a curve of junction points, i.e., to calculate an entire curve $l(\gamma) \in \mathbb{R}^n$ and $\gamma \in [L_1, L_2]$ satisfying $\Upsilon(l(\gamma)) = 0$ for all γ. Therefore one only has to use one of the continuation algorithms in which, e.g., one coordinate serves as the continuation parameter.

Continuing a Solution from a Junction Point

Let us assume that during a continuation process we have computed a solution $x(\cdot)$ satisfying the (interior) dynamics

$$\dot{x} = f_{inter}(x, u^*(x)), \ [0, \infty)$$

at time zero exhibiting a point, where a constraint becomes active. The canonical system representing the system for this active constraint is denoted as f_{bound}. Defining ${}^2x(\bar{t} + \cdot) = x(\cdot)$ then ${}^2x(\bar{t}) = x(0)$ denotes the values of the interior arc at exit time $\bar{t}$. Setting ${}^1x \equiv \bar{x}$, we have constructed a solution for the BVP (7.50) with $\bar{t} = 0$. This solution can then be continued by one of the continuation processes described in Sect. 7.2.

7.7 Retrieving DNSS Sets

In Chap. 5 we scrutinized the phenomenon of multiple or history-dependent solutions. In general a point exhibiting multiple optimal solutions points exhibiting multiple optimal solutions can only be computed numerically. The underlying algorithms are presented in the following sections.

7.7.1 Locating a DNSS Point

A DNSS point x_I was characterized (see Definition 5.9) by the property that there exist two different trajectories $(x_i(\cdot), \lambda_i(\cdot))$, $i = 1, 2$, with $x_{1,2}(0) = x_I$ converging to different limit sets $\omega_1 \neq \omega_2$ and satisfying

$$V^*\left(x_1(0)\right) = V^*\left(x_2(0)\right).$$

Using Proposition 3.75, we can rewrite the last condition as

$$\mathcal{H}\left(x_1(0), \lambda_1(0)\right) = \mathcal{H}\left(x_2(0), \lambda_2(0)\right). \tag{7.56}$$

Remark 7.37. Note that if $\omega_1 = \omega_2$ the corresponding point x_I is an indifference but not a DNSS point. Anyhow, the following argumentation also holds true, and from a computational point of view we shall not distinguish between these cases.

Formulating the BVP

Setting

$$\begin{aligned}
&{}^i x(\cdot) := (x_i(\cdot), \lambda_i(\cdot)) \\
&{}^i \omega := \omega_i, \ i = 1, 2 \\
&\Psi\left({}^1x(0), {}^2x(0)\right) := \mathcal{H}\left(x_1(0), \lambda_1(0)\right) - \mathcal{H}\left(x_2(0), \lambda_2(0)\right) \\
&N := \{1, \dots, n\}, \ \ N_{\{i\}} := N \setminus \{i\}, \ \ 1 \le i \le n
\end{aligned}$$

and denoting the corresponding canonical system as f, we can formulate the problem as a BVP of the following form:

$$\begin{aligned}
{}^1\dot{x} &= f\left({}^1x\right), \quad t \in [0, T_1] && (7.57a)\\
{}^2\dot{x} &= f\left({}^2x\right), \quad t \in [0, T_2] && (7.57b)\\
\text{s.t.} \quad {}^1x^{N_{\{i\}}}(0) &= {}^2x^{N_{\{i\}}}(0) = x_0^{N_{\{i\}}} \in \mathbb{R}^{n-1} && (7.57c)\\
{}^1x^i(0) - {}^2x^i(0) &= 0 && (7.57d)\\
\Psi\left({}^1x(0), {}^2x(0)\right) &= 0 && (7.57e)\\
\Sigma_1\left({}^1x(T_1), {}^1\omega\right) &= 0 && (7.57f)\\
\Sigma_2\left({}^2x(T_2), {}^2\omega\right) &= 0. && (7.57g)
\end{aligned}$$

The first two equations (7.57a–7.57b) define the dynamics of the corresponding paths where T_1 and T_2, respectively, are the truncated time intervals. The third equation (7.57c) fixes $n-1$ of the initial state variables for both ${}^1x^i(0)$ and ${}^2x^i(0)$ at $x_0^{N\{i\}}$, whereas (7.57d) frees the ith coordinate of the initial state variables but assures that both paths start from the same initial state. The next equation (7.57e) provides the usual DNSS point condition, i.e., that both solutions exhibit the same objective value. The last equations (7.57f) and (7.57g) denote the asymptotic boundary conditions.

In the vein of Sect. 7.1.4 the multi-point BVP (7.57) can be transformed into a two-point BVP:

$$
\begin{aligned}
& {}^1\dot{x} = T_1 f\left({}^1x\right), \quad t \in [0,1] && (7.58a)\\
& {}^2\dot{x} = T_2 f\left({}^2x\right), \quad t \in [0,1] && (7.58b)\\
\text{s.t.}\quad & {}^1x^{N\{i\}}(0) = {}^2x^{N\{i\}}(0) = x_0^{N\{i\}} \in \mathbb{R}^{n-1} && (7.58c)\\
& {}^1x^i(0) - {}^2x^i(0) = 0 && (7.58d)\\
& \Psi\left({}^1x(0), {}^2x(0)\right) = 0 && (7.58e)\\
& \Sigma_1\left({}^1x(1), {}^1\omega\right) = 0 && (7.58f)\\
& \Sigma_2\left({}^2x(1), {}^2\omega\right) = 0. && (7.58g)
\end{aligned}
$$

Remark 7.38. The BVP (7.58) can easily be adapted to problems in which constraints have to be considered. Therefore only the corresponding system dynamics and corner conditions have to be added.

Initializing the BVP

After the problem formulation an important step is to provide an initial solution for the BV-Solver. We present the case of a one- and higher-dimensional model separately, although we do this only for the sake of convenience and not because of theoretical need.

One-Dimensional Models

For one-state models the existence of at least two saddles is a necessary condition for the existence of a DNSS point. For simplicity we assume two saddles. Thus to locate a DNSS point we first have to compute the stable manifolds for these saddles using the IVP or BVP approach. If there exists a region in the state space where the stable manifolds of both equilibria exist, we have to compare the corresponding Hamiltonians evaluated along the stable manifolds. If these curves intersect, the intersection point satisfies (7.56) and (if we assume there is no other superior solution) is therefore a DNSS point. The intersection of the Hamiltonian of the stable manifolds can be realized by some interpolation algorithm, or the solutions near such an intersection point can be used as an initial solution for the BVP (7.58), which is then solved.

Two-Dimensional Models

For two-dimensional models the optimal solution may not only converge to an equilibrium but also to a limit cycle. Assuming that there exist two limit sets ω_i, $i = 1, 2$, of saddle-type with a two-dimensional stable manifold, we can use a similar strategy as for the one-dimensional case.

Therefore we consider two states $\hat{x}_i \in \omega_i$ from each of the limit sets and continue the stable manifold of ω_1 with reference point $\hat{x}_1$ to the point $\hat{x}_2$ and vice versa. If there exists a region at the connecting line from $\hat{x}_1$ to $\hat{x}_2$ where the stable manifold exists for both limit sets, we can compare the Hamiltonians evaluated along the corresponding slice manifolds (see Definition 7.25). If the corresponding curves intersect, the intersection point x_I satisfying (7.56) yields a DNSS point (assuming there is no other superior solution). The solutions starting at the intersection point x_I provide an initial solution for a continuation problem considered in the next subsection.

Remark 7.39. Assuming that for a model of dimension $n > 2$ only equilibria and limit cycles appear as long-run optimal solutions, the method presented here can also be applied to this higher-dimensional case.

7.7.2 Continuing a DNSS Point

If there exists a DNSS point x_I in a two-dimensional model, generically there exists a DNSS curve in some neighborhood of x_I (see, e.g., Beyn et al., 2001). Using the solutions starting at x_I, which are calculated during the DNSS point search, one can use a continuation algorithm to calculate a DNSS curve from BVP (7.58). For higher-dimensional models ($n > 2$) this algorithm can be used to compute curves lying in the DNSS hyper-surface.

7.8 Retrieving Heteroclinic Connections

Let us consider the system

$$\dot{x}(t) = f(x(t), \mu_0), \quad x \in \mathbb{R}^{2n}, \ \mu \in \mathbb{R}, \tag{7.59}$$

where it is assumed that (7.59) exhibits two equilibria $\hat{x}_1$ and $\hat{x}_2$, that both are saddles having n-dimensional stable and unstable manifolds, respectively, and that both exhibit a heteroclinic connection of the equilibria. Subsequently we shall formulate the corresponding BVP, which will allow us to compute the heteroclinic connection and continue it in the parameter space.

7.8.1 Locating a Heteroclinic Connection

Let us assume that we do not know the exact parameter value μ_0, for which the heteroclinic connection exists. Then we have to find μ_0 such that there exists some $x_0 \in \mathbb{R}^{2n}$ satisfying

$$\lim_{t\to\infty} \varphi^t x_0 = \hat{x}_1 \tag{7.60a}$$

$$\lim_{t\to-\infty} \varphi^t x_0 = \hat{x}_2 \tag{7.60b}$$

(see Definition 2.53).

To solve this problem we augment to the ODE (7.59) the μ as a new variable with the dynamics

$$\dot{\mu} = 0.$$

Then we consider the following BVP:

$$\begin{aligned} & {}^1\dot{x} = f\left({}^1x\right) && (7.61a)\\ & {}^2\dot{x} = -f\left({}^2x\right) && (7.61b)\\ & \dot{\mu} = 0 && (7.61c)\\ \text{s.t.}\quad & {}^1x^{N_{\{i\}}}(0) = {}^2x^{N_{\{i\}}}(0) && (7.61d)\\ & {}^1x^i(0) = {}^2x^i(0) = x_0^i \in \mathbb{R}, && (7.61e) \end{aligned}$$

where the solutions ${}^1x(\cdot)$ and ${}^2x(\cdot)$ satisfy the conditions (7.60) and x_0^i is some fixed value.

Applying the usual truncation method, we can transform the problem (7.61) into a multi-point BVP, which can finally be restated as the following two-point BVP:

$$\begin{aligned} & {}^1\dot{x} = T_1 f\left({}^1x\right), \quad t \in [0,\, 1]\\ & {}^2\dot{x} = -T_2 f\left({}^2x\right), \quad t \in [0,\, 1]\\ & \dot{\mu} = 0\\ \text{s.t.}\quad & {}^1x^{N_{\{i\}}}(0) = {}^2x^{N_{\{i\}}}(0)\\ & {}^1x^i(0) = {}^2x^i(0) = x_0^i \in \mathbb{R}\\ & \Sigma_1({}^1x(1),\, {}^1\omega, \mu)\\ & \Sigma_2({}^2x(1),\, {}^2\omega, \mu) \end{aligned}$$

where Σ_i, $i = 1, 2$ are the asymptotic boundary conditions for (7.60).

7.8.2 Continuing a Heteroclinic Connection in Parameter Space

To continue an already detected heteroclinic connection, it is necessary that the number of parameters p be greater than one. In that case we can fix $p-2$ parameter values and keep the two others μ^{i_1} and μ^{i_2} free. Then we can apply one of the continuation algorithms described in Sect. 7.2 to find the curve in the $(\mu^{i_1},\, \mu^{i_2})$-plane where a heteroclinic connection exists.

7.9 Numerical Example from Drug Control

The following model has already been introduced as an exercise in Chap. 6. For an interpretation of this model we therefore refer the reader to Exercise 6.6 or Caulkins et al. (2006). In this section we use the model as an example of some of the algorithms presented in this chapter. The model is given by:

$$\max_{U(\cdot)} \int_0^\infty \mathrm{e}^{-rt} \left(-\alpha NU - \beta(NU)^2 - \rho N - \nu PN \left(b - fP\right)\left(1 - U\right)\right) \mathrm{d}t$$

$$\text{s.t.} \quad \dot{N} = \theta - \delta N - aUN \qquad (7.62a)$$

$$\dot{P} = P\left(\left(1 - U\right)\left(b - fP\right) - \theta/N\right) \qquad (7.62b)$$

$$0 \le U \le 1 \qquad (7.62c)$$

$$P(0) = P_0 > 0, \quad N(0) = N_0 > 0, \qquad (7.62d)$$

and the base-case parameters are summarized in Table 7.2.

Table 7.2. Set of base-case parameters for model (7.62)

r	a	α	b	β	δ	f	ν	ρ	θ
0.03	0.09125	4014	2.08	1	0.09125	6.93	2000	6000	183

7.9.1 Stating the Necessary Conditions

We only consider the normal case, $\lambda_0 = 1$, as is done in Caulkins et al. (2006), and therefore derive the Hamiltonian

$$\begin{aligned}\mathcal{H}\left(N, P, U, \lambda_1, \lambda_2\right) = &-\alpha NU - \beta(NU)^2 - \rho N - \nu PN\left(b - fP\right)\left(1 - U\right) \\ &+\lambda_1\left(\theta - \delta N - aUN\right) \\ &+\lambda_2\left(P\left(\left(1 - U\right)\left(b - fP\right) - \theta/N\right)\right),\end{aligned} \qquad (7.63)$$

and the Lagrangian

$$\mathcal{L}\left(N, P, U, \lambda_1, \lambda_2, \mu_1, \mu_2\right) = \mathcal{H}\left(N, P, U, \lambda_1, \lambda_2\right) + \mu_1 U + \mu_2\left(1 - U\right).$$

From (7.63) we find

$$\mathcal{H}_{UU} = -2\beta N > 0,$$

as long as $N > 0$, which is guaranteed by the state dynamics (7.62a) and the initial condition (7.62d). Thus the optimal control value in the interior of the control region [0, 1] is uniquely given by $\mathcal{H}_U = 0$, yielding

$$U^*(N, P, \lambda_1, \lambda_2) = -\frac{\alpha N + a\lambda_1 N + b\lambda_2 P - bN\nu P - f\lambda_2 P^2 + fN\nu P^2}{2\beta N^2}. \qquad (7.64)$$

From the derivative of the control constraints with respect to the control U we see that the matrix

$$\begin{pmatrix} 1 & u & 0 \\ -1 & 0 & 1-u \end{pmatrix}$$

has full rank, validating the constraint qualification. Thus the Lagrange multipliers μ_1 and μ_2 can be derived from $\mathcal{L}_U = 0$, yielding

$$\mu_1 = \alpha N - \nu PN\left(b - fP\right) + \lambda_1 aN - \lambda_2 P\left(-b + fP\right)$$
$$\mu_2 = -\alpha N - 2\beta N^2 + \nu PN\left(b - fP\right) - \lambda_1 aN + \lambda_2 P\left(-b + fP\right).$$

Next, we consider the representations of the canonical system for every possible combination of active constraints. Since both control constraints cannot become active at the same time, we find the three cases $U = 0$, $U \in (0, 1)$, and $U = 1$, which are analyzed subsequently.

For an interior arc the canonical system is written as

$$\dot{N} = \theta - \delta N - aU^* N \tag{7.65a}$$

$$\dot{P} = P\left(\left(1 - U^*\right)\left(b - fP\right) - \frac{\theta}{N}\right) \tag{7.65b}$$

$$\dot{\lambda}_1 = r\lambda_1 + \rho - \lambda_2 P\frac{\theta}{N^2} + \nu\left(bP - fP^2\right)\left(1 - U^*\right) + \alpha U^* + 2\beta N\left(U^*\right)^2 - \lambda_1\left(-\delta - aU^*\right) \tag{7.65c}$$

$$\dot{\lambda}_2 = r\lambda_2 - \lambda_2\left(-\frac{\theta}{N} - fP\left(1 - U^*\right) + \left(b - fP\right)\left(1 - U^*\right)\right) + \nu\left(bN - 2fNP\right)\left(1 - U^*\right), \tag{7.65d}$$

with U^* given by (7.64).

For the boundary arc with $U = 0$ the canonical system becomes

$$\dot{N} = \theta - \delta N \tag{7.66a}$$

$$\dot{P} = P\left(b - fP - \frac{\theta}{N}\right) \tag{7.66b}$$

$$\dot{\lambda}_1 = r\lambda_1 + \rho - \lambda_2 P\frac{\theta}{N^2} + \nu\left(bP - fP^2\right) + \delta\lambda_1 \tag{7.66c}$$

$$\dot{\lambda}_2 = r\lambda_2 - \lambda_2\left(-\frac{\theta}{N} - fP + \left(b - fP\right)\right) + \nu\left(bN - 2fNP\right), \tag{7.66d}$$

and for the canonical system for $U = 1$ we find

$$\dot{N} = \theta - \delta N - aN \tag{7.67a}$$

$$\dot{P} = P\left(-\frac{\theta}{N}\right) \tag{7.67b}$$

$$\dot{\lambda}_1 = r\lambda_1 + \rho - \lambda_2 P\frac{\theta}{N^2} + \alpha + 2\beta N - \lambda_1\left(-\delta - a\right) \tag{7.67c}$$

$$\dot{\lambda}_2 = r\lambda_2 + \lambda_2\frac{\theta}{N}. \tag{7.67d}$$

Remark 7.40. From a theoretical point of view writing (7.66) and (7.67) seems to duplicate work, since these equations are already contained within (7.65). But this notation helps one to keep track when one is stating the BVP moreover, this schema is better adapted to the situation when the Hamiltonian is not strictly concave with respect to U.

7.9.2 Equilibria of the Canonical System

Next, we calculate the equilibria for the three representations of the canonical system.

Setting the dynamics (7.65) to zero, we get from (7.65c) and (7.65a) explicit formulas for the variables λ_1 and λ_2 with respect to the states N and P; i.e.,

$$\hat{\lambda}_1 = \lambda_1(N,P), \quad \text{and} \quad \hat{\lambda}_2 = \lambda_2(N,P).$$

Substituting these expressions into (7.65b), we can find the following values for $\hat{P}$

$$\begin{aligned} \hat{P}^1 &= 0 \\ \hat{P}(N) &= \frac{abN + b\delta N - a\theta - b\theta}{f\,(aN + \delta N - \theta)}. \end{aligned} \tag{7.68}$$

For $\hat{P}^1$ the corresponding stationary state $\hat{N}^1$ and costates $\hat{\lambda}^1_{1,2}$ can explicitly be calculated, a task that is left as an exercise for the reader (see Exercise 7.7).

Substituting P for (7.68) in the functional forms of $\lambda_{1,2}(N,P)$ and inserting these expressions into (7.65d) yields an equation for the state N, (in Exercise 7.7 this equation is denoted as $\Omega(N)$). This equation cannot be solved analytically; therefore the corresponding roots have to be calculated numerically.

For the equilibria at the boundary of the control region the reader is invited to find their explicit expressions (see Exercise 7.7).

After this preparatory work we can start analyzing the model numerically. But first we refer the reader to our implicit assumption, which is, in accordance with Caulkins et al. (2006), that an optimal solution of the model converges to an equilibrium, which will not be proved here. Thus strictly speaking, any conclusion about the models optimal solution is stated under the premise that the assumption is valid.

7.9.3 Numerical Analysis

We consider two different cases by changing the parameter value ν. Thus we start with the base-case ($\nu = 2,000$) and compare it with $\nu = 12,000$. The canonical systems for both of these two parameters are locally topological orbital equivalent (see Sect. 2.4.3), i.e., they exhibit the same number and type of equilibria for each representation. From Tables 7.3 and 7.4 we infer that the equilibria at the boundary of the control region drop can be excluded since the corresponding Lagrange multipliers are negative. The equilibrium at the interior region $\hat{E}_I^1$ also drops out, since the corresponding optimal control is larger than one. Thus only $\hat{E}_I^i$, $i = 2, \ldots, 5$, remain as possible candidates.

From these remaining four equilibria $\hat{E}_I^3$ exhibits only a one-dimensional stable manifold whereas the others exhibit a two-dimensional stable manifold. $\hat{E}_I^5$ can only be reached if we already start at some $P(0) = 0$ (see Exercise 7.7). Thus the main candidates for long-run optimal solutions are $\hat{E}_I^2$ and $\hat{E}_I^4$.

Table 7.3. Equilibria and their properties for $\nu = 2,000$. The values, which are crossed out, denote the violation of either the nonnegativity condition of the Lagrange multipliers or the control constraint

Descr.	$\hat{E}_I^1$	$\hat{E}_I^2$	$\hat{E}_I^3$	$\hat{E}_I^4$	$\hat{E}_I^5$	$\hat{E}_0^1$	$\hat{E}_0^1$	$\hat{E}_1^1$
$\hat{N} \times 10^3$	0.9240	1.0503	1.0801	1.7450	1.7547	2.0055	2.0055	1.0027
$\hat{P}$	0.4677	0.0226	0.1296	0.2824	0.0000	0.0000	0.2870	0.0000
$\hat{\lambda}_1 \times 10^4$	−5.7304	−5.6114	−5.5834	−4.9576	−4.9485	−4.9485	−4.9536	−5.6562
$\hat{\lambda}_2 \times 10^7$	0.5308	−1.5213	−0.1108	0.6425	0.7591	0.8519	0.7540	0
$\hat{U}$	~~1.1705~~	0.9094	0.8567	0.1492	0.1429	0.0000	0.0000	1.0000
$\mathrm{Re}\,\hat{\xi}_1$	−1.3264	−0.1217	−0.1710	1.6856	−1.6485	−1.9588	0.1213	0.2125
$\mathrm{Re}\,\hat{\xi}_2$	1.3564	−0.1217	0.0150	−1.6556	−0.0912	−0.0912	2.0187	−0.1825
$\mathrm{Re}\,\hat{\xi}_3$	−0.1862	0.1517	0.0150	−0.0905	0.1212	0.1213	−1.9888	−0.1825
$\mathrm{Re}\,\hat{\xi}_4$	0.2162	0.1517	0.2010	0.1205	1.6785	1.9888	−0.0912	0.2125
$\hat{\mu}_1 \times 10^6$	0.0000	0.0000	0.0010	0.0000	0.0000	~~−1.0057~~	~~−1.0278~~	0.0000
$\hat{\mu}_2 \times 10^5$	0.0000	0.0000	0.0000	0.0000	0.0000	0.0000	0.0000	~~−0.8605~~

In the following subsections we analyze the optimal vector field for the two cases. Every step in the solution process accomplished for the first time will be written down in full detail with reference to the corresponding sections, where the reader can find the theoretical background.

7.9.4 Optimal Vector Field for ν = 4,000

First, we try to continue the stable paths converging to $\hat{E}_I^2$ along the line connecting $\hat{E}_I^2$ and $\hat{E}_I^4$, and vice versa, using the BVP approach presented in Sect. 7.5.1. Thus we fix the truncation time, $T = 1,000$, and finally we want to solve the BVP with interior dynamics:

$$\dot{x} = 1,000 f(x), \quad x = (N, P, \lambda_1, \lambda_2)' \tag{7.69a}$$

Table 7.4. Equilibria and their properties for $\nu = 12,000$. The values, which are crossed out, denote the violation of either the nonnegativity condition of the Lagrange multipliers or the control constraint

Descr.	$\hat{E}_I^1$	$\hat{E}_I^2$	$\hat{E}_I^3$	$\hat{E}_I^4$	$\hat{E}_I^5$	$\hat{E}_0^1$	$\hat{E}_0^1$	$\hat{E}_1^1$
$\hat{N} \times 10^3$	0.8721	1.0475	1.1558	1.7240	1.7547	2.0055	2.0055	1.0027
$\hat{P}$	0.4012	0.0053	0.2139	0.2818	0.0000	0.0000	0.2870	0.0000
$\hat{\lambda}_1 \times 10^4$	−5.7792	−5.6141	−5.5121	−4.9774	−4.9485	−4.9485	−4.9640	−5.6562
$\hat{\lambda}_2 \times 10^7$	1.3591	−6.5026	0.7691	1.8995	2.2772	2.5555	2.2620	0.0000
$\hat{U}$	~~1.2996~~	0.9145	0.7351	0.1633	0.1429	0.0000	0.0000	1.0000
$\mathrm{Re}\,\hat{\xi}_1$	−1.6532	−0.1293	0.0150	1.6352	−1.6485	−1.9588	0.1213	0.2125
$\mathrm{Re}\,\hat{\xi}_2$	1.6832	−0.1293	0.0150	−1.6052	−0.0912	−0.0912	2.0187	−0.1825
$\mathrm{Re}\,\hat{\xi}_3$	−0.1844	0.1593	−0.2078	−0.0887	0.1212	0.1213	−1.9888	−0.1825
$\mathrm{Re}\,\hat{\xi}_4$	0.2144	0.1593	0.2378	0.1187	1.6785	1.9888	−0.0912	0.2125
$\hat{\mu}_1 \times 10^6$	0.0000	0.0000	0.00100	0.0000	0.0000	~~−1.0057~~	~~−1.0720~~	0.0000
$\hat{\mu}_2 \times 10^5$	0.0000	0.0000	0.0000	0.0000	0.0000	0.0000	0.0000	~~−0.8605~~

given by (7.65) satisfying the initial condition

$$x_1(0) = \hat{N}_I^4, \quad x_2(0) = \hat{P}_I^4 \tag{7.69b}$$

and the asymptotic boundary condition

$$F' \left(\begin{pmatrix} x_1(1) \\ x_2(1) \\ x_3(1) \\ x_4(1) \end{pmatrix} - \begin{pmatrix} \hat{N}_I^2 \\ \hat{P}_I^2 \\ \hat{\lambda}_{1I}^2 \\ \hat{\lambda}_{2I}^2 \end{pmatrix} \right). \tag{7.69c}$$

To find the matrix F we take the eigenvectors of the transposed Jacobian matrix at $\hat{E}_I^2$ corresponding to the positive eigenvalues (see Sect. 7.5.1) yielding

$$F' = \begin{pmatrix} -0.0000176788 & -0.9999999654 & 0.0002624966 & 0.0000000034 \\ 0.0019074544 & 0.9999981807 & 0.0000142733 & -0.0000005043 \end{pmatrix}.$$

Even though this matrix lacks mathematical beauty, it does the job. Next, the BVP (7.69) has to be solved. But until now we only have information about the equilibria. Thus we set

$$x_0(\gamma) = (1-\gamma) \begin{pmatrix} \hat{N}_I^2 \\ \hat{P}_I^2 \end{pmatrix} + \gamma \begin{pmatrix} \hat{N}_I^4 \\ \hat{P}_I^4 \end{pmatrix}$$

and add

$$\dot{\gamma} = 0 \tag{7.70}$$

to the dynamics (7.69a) and solve the augmented system for the initial conditions

$$\gamma(0) = \gamma_i, \quad i \geq 0$$
$$x^{1,2}(0) = x_0(\gamma),$$

where $\gamma_i = \gamma_{i-1} + \sigma$, $i > 0$, with a fixed σ and the initial value $\gamma_0 = 0$ (see the exogenous continuation algorithm Sect. 7.2). But for this new BVP $x \equiv \hat{E}_I^2$ is a trivial solution and a BV-Solver can start the continuation process. The result of this computation is depicted in Fig. 7.9a, where the solid line $x^{1,2}(\cdot, 1)$ is the state path converging to $\hat{E}_I^2$. We have therefore numerically proved that there exists an extremal state trajectory $x(\cdot)$ converging to $\hat{E}_I^2$ when starting at a point, which coincides with the state values of $\hat{E}_I^4$. Comparing the Hamiltonians of the equilibrium $\hat{E}_I^4$ and $x(0)$, we find the latter to be larger. Thus we have numerically proved that the trajectory converging to $\hat{E}_I^2$ is superior to the equilibrium solution $\hat{E}_I^4$. Therefore $\hat{E}_I^4$ can be excluded as a long-run optimal solution.

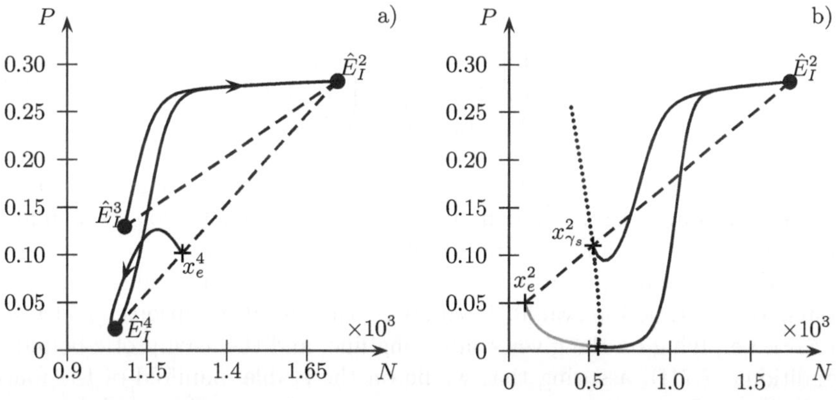

Fig. 7.9. In panel (**a**) the paths (*solid curves*) projected into the state space and lying in the stable manifold of the corresponding equilibria are depicted. These paths are solutions of a continuation process along the *dashed lines*. Panel (**b**) shows the solution trajectory starting at $x_{\gamma_s}^2$, where the *gray curve* denotes the boundary arc and the *black curve* the interior arc of the solution. This curve is the result of a continuation process along the *dashed line*, where at $x_{\gamma_s}^2$ the BVP for the continuation has to be augmented for including an exit point

The same procedure depicted in Fig. 7.9a for the connecting line from $\hat{E}_I^2$ to $\hat{E}_I^3$ excludes the third equilibrium as an optimal solution. This shows that the second equilibrium is the only long-run optimal solution, provided that every optimal solution converges to an equilibrium.

Next, we analyze the optimal solution for some other initial point. For this we choose the arbitrary point of the state space $N_e = 100$ and $P_e = 0.05$ and continue the solution along the connecting line by the same approach as before (see Fig. 7.9b). The algorithm yields admissible results until the continuation parameter $\gamma_s = 0.74273$ is reached. At this step control of the corresponding solutions trajectory $x(\cdot, \gamma_s)$ becomes $U = 1.00001$, violating the control constraint. Thus we expect that the solution for $\gamma > \gamma_s$ starts with maximum control until an exit point is reached, where the optimal control switches to the interior control region. Using the approach presented in Sect. 7.6.3, we formulate a new BVP by doubling the number of variables. In this BVP the first four variables stand for the boundary arc and the other four variables for the interior arc. This can explicitly be written as

$$
\begin{aligned}
&{}^1\dot{x} = \bar{t}\ {}^1f\left({}^1x\right), \quad t \in [0,\ 1] && (7.71a)\\
&{}^2\dot{x} = \left(T - \bar{t}\right)\ {}^2f\left({}^2x\right), \quad t \in [0,\ 1] && (7.71b)\\
&\dot{\gamma} = 0 && (7.71c)\\
\text{s.t.}\quad &{}^1x^{1,2}(0) = x_0^{1,2}(\gamma) && (7.71d)\\
&\gamma(0) = \gamma_i,\ i > 0 && (7.71e)\\
&F'\left(\begin{pmatrix} {}^2x_1(1)\\ {}^2x_2(1)\\ {}^2x_3(1)\\ {}^2x_4(1)\end{pmatrix} - \begin{pmatrix} \hat{N}_I^2\\ \hat{P}_I^2\\ \hat{\lambda}_{1I}^2\\ \hat{\lambda}_{2I}^2\end{pmatrix}\right), && (7.71f)
\end{aligned}
$$

where ${}^1f$ is given by (7.65) and ${}^2f$ is given by (7.67), T is fixed at 1,000, F is the matrix from before, ${}^{1,2}x$ denote the states and costates for the boundary and interior system, and γ is the continuation parameter.

In this formulation we have to find a solution of an eight-dimensional system on the time interval $[0,\ 1]$ satisfying the initial conditions, (7.71d) and (7.71e), i.e., lying on the given connecting line, and the asymptotic boundary conditions (7.71f), assuring that we lie on the stable manifold of the fourth equilibrium. So far these two state–costate vectors are disjointed from each other. But from theory (see Sect. 7.6.3) we know that the two arcs have to satisfy corner conditions at the exit points ${}^1x(1)$ and ${}^2x(0)$.

For our model these corner conditions read as continuity of the states and costates at the exit time, i.e.,

$$ {}^1x(1) = {}^2x(0), \qquad (7.71g) $$

and continuity of the control, yielding

$$ \alpha N + a\lambda_1 N + b\lambda_2 P - bN\nu P - f\lambda_2 P^2 + fN\nu P^2 + 1 = 0 \qquad (7.71h) $$

by using the equation for the optimal control value (7.64), where

$$ (N,\ P,\ \lambda_1,\ \lambda_2) = \left({}^2x_1(0),\ {}^2x_2(0),\ {}^2x_3(0),\ {}^2x_4(0)\right). $$

For $\gamma = \gamma_s$ and $\bar{t} = 0$ the trajectory

$$^1x(\cdot) = x(1, \gamma_s)$$
$$^2x(\cdot) = x(\cdot, \gamma_s)$$

from the last continuation step is trivially a solution of the BVP (7.71). Thus for this augmented system the continuation process can be continued, finally reaching $N_e = 100$ and $P_e = 0.05$, as is depicted in Fig. 7.9b.

7.9.5 Optimal Vector Field for $\nu = 12{,}000$

From Table 7.4 we see that the initial situation, as compared to the previous case with $\nu = 4,000$, is the same. Again the equilibria $\hat{E}_I^2$ and $\hat{E}_I^4$ are the main candidates for the long-run optimal solutions. Therefore we continue the stable paths from the second to the fourth equilibrium and vice versa along the connecting line. In Fig. 7.10a the result of this continuation is depicted, and reveals that we have to consider an exit point for the path converging to $\hat{E}_I^4$.

All the necessary computational steps have already been described in the previous section. But, unlike before, the paths cannot be continued to the opposite equilibrium and thus none of the long-run solutions is always superior to the other. Therefore we can expect a DNSS point to exist on the connecting line. To prove that, we evaluate the Hamiltonians along the slice manifolds (see Definition 7.25) for both continuation processes, where the result is shown in Fig. 7.10b. This reveals the existence of a DNSS point (N_I, P_I) at the crossing of the Hamiltonians. Next, the solutions for both equilibria are continued to this DNSS point, shown in Fig. 7.10c. From the existence of the DNSS point we can expect a DNSS curve at least in a neighborhood of (N_I, P_I).

To compute this DNSS curve we use the approach of Sect. 7.7. Therefore we set the truncation times $T = T_1 = T_2 = 1000$ and have to compute the matrices $F_{1,2}$ for the asymptotic boundary conditions at the corresponding equilibria, yielding

$$F_1' = \begin{pmatrix} -0.0000075574 & 1.0000000000 & -0.0000000508 & -0.0000000001 \\ 0.0000030801 & 0.0000000000 & 0.0000010213 & 0.0000000000 \end{pmatrix}$$
$$F_2' = \begin{pmatrix} 0.0000197999 & 0.9999999960 & -0.0000871293 & -0.0000000012 \\ 0.0018115151 & 0.9999983591 & 0.0000143135 & -0.0000001593 \end{pmatrix}.$$

For the dynamics we have to consider that one solution trajectory exhibits an exit point. Thus the boundary conditions for the solution converging to $\hat{E}_I^4$ become

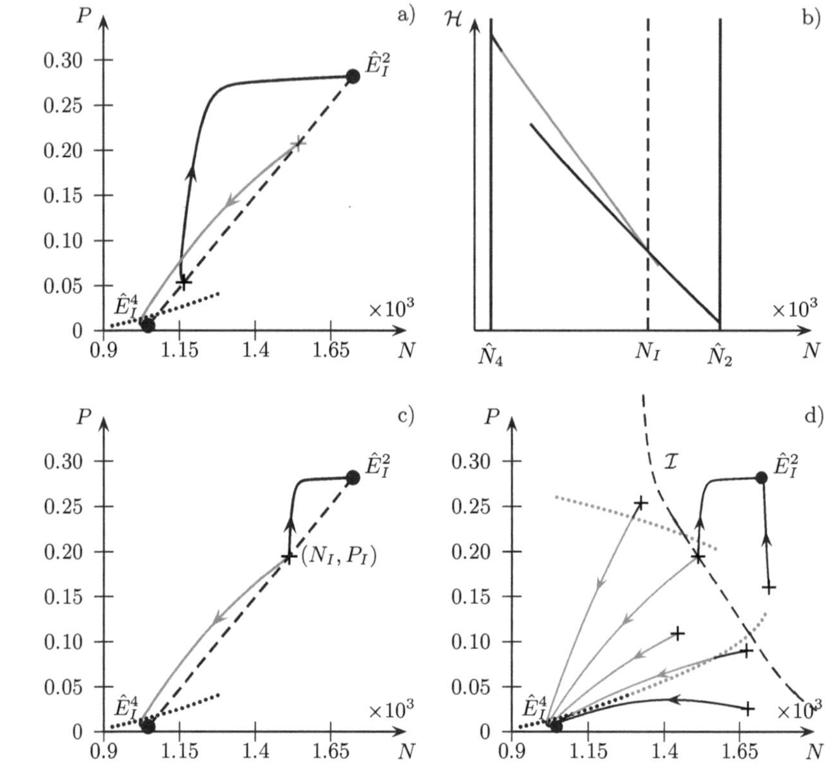

Fig. 7.10. Panel (**a**) depicts the solutions of two continuation processes resulting in the solution curves converging to $\hat{E}_I^2$ and $\hat{E}_I^4$. The *dotted line* shows the curve of exit points for solutions converging to the fourth equilibrium. Panel (**b**) reveals that there exists a DNSS point on the connecting line for the two equilibria and in panel (**c**) the corresponding solutions are drawn. In panel (**d**) regions of different optimal behaviors are depicted. The curve $\mathcal{I}$ is a DNSS curve and the *gray dotted lines* denote entry points for solutions moving to $\hat{E}_I^4$. For each region a characteristic solution path is shown

$$
\begin{aligned}
&{}^1\dot{x} = \bar{t}\ {}^1\!f\left({}^1x\right), \quad t \in [0, 1] && \text{(7.72a)}\\
&{}^2\dot{x} = (T - \bar{t})\ {}^2\!f\left({}^2x\right), \quad t \in [0, 1] && \text{(7.72b)}\\
\text{s.t.}\quad &{}^1x(1) = {}^2x(0) && \text{(7.72c)}\\
&\alpha N + a\lambda_1 N + b\lambda_2 P - bN\nu P - f\lambda_2 P^2 + fN\nu P^2 + 1 = 0 && \text{(7.72d)}\\
&F_1'\left(\begin{pmatrix} {}^2x_1(1)\\ {}^2x_2(1)\\ {}^2x_3(1)\\ {}^2x_4(1)\end{pmatrix} - \begin{pmatrix}\hat{N}_I^4\\ \hat{P}_I^4\\ \hat{\lambda}_{1I}^4\\ \hat{\lambda}_{2I}^4\end{pmatrix}\right), && \text{(7.72e)}
\end{aligned}
$$

with

$$(N,\,P,\,\lambda_1,\,\lambda_2) = \left({}^2x_1(0),\,{}^2x_2(0),\,{}^2x_3(0),\,{}^2x_4(0)\right),$$

${}^1f$ the boundary dynamics (7.67) and ${}^2f$ the interior dynamics (7.65).

The BVP for the solution converging to $\hat{E}_I^2$ is of the simpler form:

$$ {}^3\dot{x} = T\ {}^3f\left({}^3x\right), \quad t \in [0,\,1] \tag{7.72f}$$

$$\text{s.t.}\quad F_2'\left(\begin{pmatrix} {}^3x_1(1) \\ {}^3x_2(1) \\ {}^3x_3(1) \\ {}^3x_4(1) \end{pmatrix} - \begin{pmatrix} \hat{N}_I^2 \\ \hat{P}_I^2 \\ \hat{\lambda}_{1I}^2 \\ \hat{\lambda}_{2I}^2 \end{pmatrix}\right), \tag{7.72g}$$

where ${}^3f$ denotes the interior dynamics (7.65). Next, we have to provide the conditions assuring that both trajectories start at a DNSS point. Therefore the states have to be equal; i.e.,

$$\begin{pmatrix} {}^1x_1(0) \\ {}^1x_2(0) \end{pmatrix} = \begin{pmatrix} {}^3x_1(0) \\ {}^3x_2(0) \end{pmatrix},$$

and the Hamiltonians for both initial points have to be equal, yielding

$$\mathcal{H}\left({}^1x(0), U^*\left({}^1x(0)\right)\right) - \mathcal{H}\left({}^3x(0), 1\right) = 0. \tag{7.72h}$$

To continue the already detected DNSS point we introduce some continuation parameter γ to keep the first state coordinate fixed for a value specified by γ and search for the DNSS point along the second state coordinate. Thus we finally find the conditions

$$ {}^1x_1(0) = N_I + \gamma_i, \quad i \geq 0 \tag{7.72i}$$

$$ {}^3x_1(0) = N_I + \gamma_i, \quad i \geq 0 \tag{7.72j}$$

$$ {}^1x_2(0) = {}^3x_2(0), \tag{7.72k}$$

where $\gamma_i = \gamma_{i-1} + \sigma$, $i > 0$ for some fixed σ and $\gamma_0 = 0$. Since we have already computed the solutions starting at $(N_I,\,P_I)$, this can be taken as an initial solution for the BVP (7.72) and $\gamma_0 = 0$, which can then be continued for positive and negative σ. The result of this process is depicted in Fig. 7.10d.

In fact the here described continuation process only returns the DNSS curve $\mathcal{I}$ to between the gray dotted curves. These dotted lines denote entry points, where control constraints become active. Therefore the BVP has to be adapted to this situation. This does not add any new strategy to the solution process. One only has to consider a fourth dynamics for (7.72) and the corresponding corner conditions for an entry point. The explicit calculations are therefore left as an exercise for the interested reader. With this last example we conclude the chapter and encourage the reader to use the here presented methods for many different models, thereby becoming acquainted with the strengths and weaknesses of this method.

Exercises

7.1 (Model of Bridge Building). Consider the following model developed by Caulkins, Feichtinger, Grass, and Tragler (2007a):

$$\min_{u(\cdot)} \int_0^\infty \mathrm{e}^{-rt} \left(\left(x^2 - 1\right)^2 + cu^2 \right) \mathrm{d}t$$
$$\text{s.t.} \quad \dot{x} = x^3 - x + u,$$

with $r,\, c \geq 0$.

This very simple model reflects the challenges and benefits of building bridges by standing at the edge of one's home organization and reaching out to the external world. It describes how various strategies are preferred as a function of one's level of patience (discount rate) and the cost of adjusting one's social position:

1. Establish the canonical system
2. Determine the equilibria and their stability properties
3. Find the bifurcation curves
4. Choose parameters for every region with different stability properties of the equilibria and:
   a) Calculate the stable and unstable manifolds, using the IVP and BVP approach
   b) In case of multiple saddles determine whether a DNSS point exists
   c) Find the heteroclinic bifurcation curve

7.2 (Fire-and-Water). Consider the one-dimensional terror model with constant controls u, v of Sect. 2.5 as a dynamic optimization problem, where the total costs caused by a terror organization as well as the counter-terror operations have to be minimized; i.e.,

$$\min_{u(\cdot),v(\cdot)} \int_0^\infty \mathrm{e}^{-rt} \left(S + u^2 + v^2\right) \mathrm{d}t$$

given the state dynamics

$$\dot{S} = \tau + (1 + \rho v)kS^\alpha - \mu S - \beta \ln(1 + u)\, S^\theta - \gamma \ln(1 + v)\, S,$$

and the control constraints

$$u(t) \geq 0, \quad v(t) \geq 0.$$

Then:

1. Establish the canonical system and the functional forms of the Lagrange multipliers
2. Using the parameter values given in Table 7.5:
   a) Find the equilibrium/equilibria of the canonical system
   b) Compute the stable manifolds
   c) Find the entry and exit points and compute the corresponding extremal solutions
   d) If multiple saddles exist, prove or refute the existence of a DNSS point
3. Analyze the system when the parameter values change

Table 7.5. The specified parameter values for the base case

r	α	β	c	k	μ	γ	ρ	θ	τ
0.05	0.75	0.01	1	0.05	0.05	0.1	1	0.1	10^{-5}

7.3 (One-Dimensional Corruption). Consider the corruption-model of Sect. 2.3 with constant control u as a dynamic optimization model with the objective function to be minimized, i.e.,

$$\min_{u(\cdot)} \int_0^\infty \mathrm{e}^{-rt} \left(x + \frac{1}{2} u^2 \right) \mathrm{d}t,$$

and the state dynamics

$$\dot{x} = k \left(wx - u \right), \quad k,\, w \geq 0,$$

together with the state constraints

$$0 \leq x \leq 1.$$

Then:

1. Establish the canonical system together with the functional form of the Lagrange multiplier for the state constraints
2. Choose different parameter values for r, w, and k and compute the optimal solution

7.4 (*LH*-model). Consider the drug model (6.6) of Sect. 6.1. Reproduce the canonical system for the interior and boundary control regions; then:

- Find the corresponding equilibria
- Find the curves of entry and exit points in the state space for the optimal solutions
- Increase and decrease the discount parameter r and compare the results. How do the boundary curves change? Interpret the result

7.5 (Corrupt Government and Popularity). Reproduce the results for the corruption model of Sect. 6.2.

7.6. Calculate the DNSS curve for the terror model of Sect. 6.3.

7.7 (Drug Substitution Program). Consider the model (7.62); then:

1. Find the expression for $\Omega(N)$
2. Find the equilibrium at $\hat{P}^1 = 0$
3. Find the equilibria at the boundaries of the control region
4. Prove that an equilibrium exhibiting $\hat{P} = 0$ can only be reached from an initial state $P(0) = 0$

Notes and Further Reading

Roughly speaking, one can distinguish between three different approaches to the computational methods for solving optimal control problems. The first method relies on the principle of dynamic programming (Bellman, 1957, 1961) and uses the HJB equation. A recent presentation of this approach can be found in Bertsekas (2005) or, specifically for economic applications, in Luenberger (1997). For the special case of infinite time horizon problems we refer the reader to Dolcetta (1983); Falcone (1987), and Grüne (1997). The two other approaches are referred to as the *direct* and *indirect methods* (see, e.g., Kraft, 1994; Pytlak, 1999; von Stryk & Bulirsch, 1992). For the direct method the objective function, state dynamics, and given constraints are first discretized in time and then solved as a nonlinear programming problem. This method is especially useful when one is considering large-scale problems, i.e., problems with a huge number of states, which often appear in the field of engineering (see, e.g., Barclay, Gill, & Rosen, 1997), or when considering second-order conditions (Maurer, Büskens, Kim, & Kaya, 2005; Maurer & Oberle, 2002). For infinite time horizon problems, direct methods are provided by Alemdar, Sirakaya, and Hüsseinov (2006); Mercenier and Philippe (2001).

These direct methods have the advantage that one does not have to provide an approximation of the adjoint equation, which is in general hard to provide.

The indirect approach uses Pontryagin's Maximum Principle and the canonical system thereby derived to formulate a BVP, as has been presented in this chapter. Depending on the underlying algorithm, one distinguishes between shooting methods (Fraser-Andrews, 1999; Oberle, 1986) and collocation methods (Goffe, 1993), with the special application of infinite time horizon problems discussed in Beyn et al. (2001) and Kunkel and von dem Hagen (2000).

As we have already stated, one of the most critical points concerning the indirect approach is the provision of some initial solution. But for infinite time horizon problems and under the assumption that the optimal solution converges to some limit set, this limitation is of only minor importance, since the long-run optimal solution already determines a solution, which can be continued by some continuation process (see, e.g., Kuznetsov, 1998). To circumvent the problem of solving a BVP for an infinite time interval, one can choose either two distinct strategies. Most of the existing algorithms approximate the solution by truncating the problem to a finite time interval (de Hoog & Weiss, 1980). Another strategy is to transform the infinite time interval into the unit interval.

An important disadvantage of this continuation technique is that the number of ODEs in the optimality system is increased by $2n$ with each entry or exit point. For the case when optimal control is bang-bang, Kaya and Noakes (1996, 2003), and Kaya, Lucas, and Simakov (2004) propose computational techniques that do not augment the optimality system.These techniques are used by Kaya et al. (2004) for finding optimal bang-bang constrained controls for the LH-model. One of these techniques was implemented by Maurer et al. (2005) in the verification of second-order sufficient conditions for bang-bang controls.

In any direct method for optimal control problems, it is essential to know at least roughly the structure of the switching and the places of the entry and exit points. It is therefore often useful to solve a less accurate discretized version of the problem by employing some finite-dimensional optimization technique, to get an idea about the structure of the optimal trajectories and control. Doing so provides no guarantee that the structure will be a correct one, but can it be mentioned as a possible starting point before one applies an indirect method (see, e.g., Maurer et al., 2005; Weiser & Deuflhard, 2007).

The method presented here relies on methods presented in Beyn et al. (2001). In Pampel (2000) the convergence of the solution for the truncated problem to the solution of the infinite time problem has been proved. We have, moreover, extended the formulation of the corresponding BVP to include path constraints. For these constrained problems it is not necessary to know a priori the structure of the interior and boundary arcs. This structure becomes apparent along the continuation process. Within the same framework it is also possible to consider multi-stage optimal control problems as described in Chap. 8.

Furthermore, we provide a collection of MATLAB files (`OCMat`), which allows the numerical analysis of discounted infinite time horizon problems. This `OCMat` is an implementation of the indirect method and takes advantage of the inherently given BVP structure of the problem. Using this toolbox, it is possible to compute the optimal solutions compounded of interior and boundary arcs for mixed- or pure-path constraints exhibiting an arbitrary number of exit (entry) points. It is also possible to calculate the boundaries of the regions separating interior and boundary regions. Moreover, this toolbox allows the detection of DNSS points and computation of DNSS curves, and, in the parameter space, heteroclinic bifurcation lines can be computed.

8

Extensions of the Maximum Principle

In the preceding seven chapters we explored the basic principles of optimal control theory applied to problems typically arising in economics and management science. In particular we illustrated how the interplay of analytical and numerical methods can be used to obtain insight when fighting drugs, corruption, and terror. Before concluding our tour we should briefly sketch several important extensions of "standard-type" optimal control theory.

Usually, in optimal control theory, systems evolve continuously in time, but in reality sudden discontinuous changes may happen at certain time points. Those changes may pertain not only to the model's parameter values but also to sudden modifications of the model's functional forms. In Sect. 8.1 we give a short introduction into the important and growing field of *multi-stage models.*

Section 8.2 provides a brief introduction to the fundamentals of *differential games.* The Nash and the Stackelberg concepts are introduced. Examples from the fields of corruption and terrorism are provided to illustrate the flavor of differential games.

The homogeneity of economic agents is admittedly a fiction. There are several avenues to introduce heterogeneity. One of them has been discussed in Chap. 6, namely multi-compartment models. Partial differential equations (PDEs) are another powerful tool for distinguishing individuals according to various characteristics evolving over time.[1] In Sect. 8.3 we present some basic facts about *distributed parameter control.*

Finally, in Sect. 8.4 we mention a number of other important topics in optimal control modeling, including stochastic models, impulse control, delayed systems, and nonsmooth systems.

[1] Overlapping generations models can be seen as a connecting link between compartment models and PDE models.

8.1 Multi-Stage Optimal Control Problems

The previous chapters illustrated that optimal control methods have been successfully applied to systems that evolve continuously over time. In many decision situations arising in economics and Operations Research, however, abrupt changes occur. For example, all of a sudden new drugs emerge on the market (or disappear from it), or terror organizations may conduct a massive attack that triggers a qualitatively different phase of counter-terror operations. The discontinuity is modeled as a switch between alternative and consecutive regimes, where in this context we understand a *regime* as the specification of a system dynamics and an objective functional prevailing during a certain time interval. The timing of such a switch may either be determined exogenously or depend on how the process develops (over time). In what follows we consider multi-stage optimal control problems, in which the moment of switching between the regimes is optimally determined.

In Sect. 8.1.1 we present conditions to manage n-stage optimal control processes with $n = 2$. To cope with the switching instants between two consecutive regimes, particular "matching" conditions both of the adjoint variable(s) and the Hamiltonian have to be included in the analysis. In the following two subsections we present two simple examples of two-stage processes. Whereas the first one deals with an illicit drug market disruption generated by an exogenous shock and the optimal switching from use reduction to harm reduction goals, respectively, the second one refers to two consecutive phases of counter-terror interventions, where the switching time is after an event like September 11th, 2001 (compare Exercise 8.6).

8.1.1 Necessary Optimality Conditions for Two-Stage Control Problems

We present a set of necessary optimality conditions for a specific family of two-stage models, in which we can switch at time t_s between two different regimes. The switching time t_s is either given exogenously or can be determined to maximize the objective function value. Then, the objective function may be written as

$$\max_{u(\cdot)} \left\{ \int_0^{t_s} \mathrm{e}^{-rt} g_1(x,u,t)\,\mathrm{d}t + \mathrm{e}^{-rt_s} S\left(x(t_s)\right) + \int_{t_s}^{\infty} \mathrm{e}^{-rt} g_2(x,u,t_s,t)\,\mathrm{d}t \right\},$$

where $S(x(t_s))$ denotes the switching costs

The system state equation is given by

$$\dot{x} = \begin{cases} f_1(x,u,t) & \text{for } 0 \le t < t_s \\ f_2(x,u,t_s,t) & \text{for } t_s < t \end{cases}$$

with $x(0) = x_0$.

Using the current-value Hamiltonians

$$\mathcal{H}_1 = g_1(x,u,t) + \lambda_1 f_1(x,u,t)$$
$$\mathcal{H}_2 = g_2(x,u,t_s,t) + \lambda_2 f_2(x,u,t_s,t),$$

we find that the necessary optimality conditions are the usual conditions

$$\mathcal{H}_i(x^*,u^*,\lambda_i,t) = \max_u \mathcal{H}_i(x^*,u,\lambda_i,t), \quad i=1,2$$
$$\dot{\lambda}_i = r\lambda_i - \mathcal{H}_{ix}, \quad i=1,2,$$

and the matching conditions are read as

$$\lambda_1(t_s) + S_x(x(t_s)) = \lambda_2(t_s), \tag{8.1}$$
$$\mathcal{H}_1(t_s) + \int_{t_s}^{\infty} \mathrm{e}^{-r(t-t_s)} \frac{\partial \mathcal{H}_2}{\partial t_s}\,\mathrm{d}t - rS(x(t_s)) = \mathcal{H}_2(t_s). \tag{8.2}$$

The matching condition (8.2) is an extension of the result of Tomiyama and Rossana (1989) to the infinite time horizon problems, which can be proved by variational principles analogously to Makris (2001) (see also Sect. 4.4.1). The above optimality conditions have nice economic interpretations; they apply to $0 < t_s < \infty$ (compare Tomiyama & Rossana, 1989).

Note that corner solutions may occur, e.g., immediate switching, $t_s = 0$, or sclerosis, $t_s = \infty$ (see, e.g., Boucekkine, Saglam, & Vallée, 2004).

Remark 8.1. Numerically multi-stage problems can be considered analogous to the switching between interior and boundary arcs as described in Sect. 7.6. Where the corner conditions (7.45d) and (7.45e), have to be replaced by the switching conditions (8.1) and (8.2). Note that the latter condition can be formulated as a corresponding differential equation.

8.1.2 Two-Stage Models of Drug Control

In earlier sections of the book we studied the question of how efficient drug policies should evolve over the course of a drug epidemic (see, e.g., Sect. 6.1). Now we ask questions like the following:

1. Given that a certain program is cost-effective during "normal" times, what should be done if a drug is temporarily in short supply?
2. At what time over the course of a drug epidemic should the policy objective switch from use reduction to harm reduction?

Both situations are characterized by continuous changes *and* abrupt discontinuities. Whereas in case (1) the market disruption is exogenously given, in case (2) the decision-maker has to choose the switching time in an optimal manner. Nonetheless, both problems fit into the framework of two-stage (or multi-stage) processes. Let us briefly describe these situations.

ad(i) Markets for illicit drugs are frustratingly resilient, but over the last three decades every important illicit drug has experienced at least one significant supply shock, such as recently observed during the Australian "heroin drought." It seems plausible that there will be more such disruptions in the future, and therefore it is worth asking how, if at all, policy should adapt to take advantage of a forthcoming market disruption. For instance, we have to answer the question whether a market disruption, as discussed above, is a good time to expand treatment programs, because the disruption produces an extra incentive to quit drug use. In other words, does the moment of market weakness create opportunities for controlling supply to affect changes that it cannot affect when the market is more robust?
For market disruptions, long-run equilibrium models are not appropriate, but multi-stage optimal control models provide a powerful tool for analyzing such *disequilibrium cases*. For instance, there are some promising first results from a two-stage optimal control problem in which drug prices are abnormally high in the first stage and the policy planner is allowed to adjust the level of drug control funding over time (see Bultmann et al., 2007, and Bultmann, Caulkins, Feichtinger, & Tragler, 2008).

ad(ii) There is a heated debate in drug policy over the relative merits of "harm reduction" (reducing, e.g., drug-related disease transmission) vs. "use reduction" (controlling drug use per se). In the past, harm reduction has been embraced by some countries (e.g., Australia) and shunned by others (e.g., the US). Reducing harmfulness of drug use may have an ambiguous impact on total harm, since making an activity safer may encourage greater use (compare Caulkins, Feichtinger, Tragler, & Wallner, 2007). To build a two-stage model, we consider use reduction in stage 1 with conventional controls such as prevention, demand-side enforcement, etc.; stage 2 would be a harm reduction regime with special forms of treatment. Note that the number of users has a higher penalty in stage 1 but a lower rate of initiation, whereas after the switch the situation is just the opposite. In contrast with case (i), the transition time, in which one switches from use reduction to harm reduction, is now a choice variable. The situation is described in more detail in Exercise 8.3; compare also Exercise 6.3.

8.1.3 Counter-Terror Measures in a Multi-Stage Scenario

Another two-stage system that may be of interest is the planning of counter-terror measures. September 11th changed the conflict between international terrorism and possible target countries from a low-intensity "police investigation" to essentially a war. There are two phases of that conflict. From the perspective of an international terror organization the timing of the phase change was a decision variable. The terrorists chose to launch the attacks that elicited a response that turned the conflict into open warfare. From the likely target country's perspective, the timing of the change was a random variable. In the second (current) phase, the likely target countries drastically changed the set of instruments employed, and the terrorists' visibility greatly increased, as did their ability to inspire recruits. The Israeli–Palestinian conflicts, for instance, also exhibit phase changes between active phases (Intifada in Palestine) and less violent phases. Even the active phase can be divided into constituent phases.

To be precise, consider the following extension of our Fire-and-Water model (see Sect. 2.5). Assume that at time $t = 0$ a terror attack takes place that initiates active hostilities (e.g., September 11th). Then the government can choose an optimal time $t = t_s$ after which it implements aggressive, anti-terror measures ("fire tactics"), which have the side effect of increasing the inflow of recruits to the terrorists while combating terrorism more efficiently. In the phase before the switching time t_s the government reacts to terror with only targeted anti-terror measures ("water tactics"). One interesting question this model can address is under what circumstances (if any) it is optimal to respond to a terrorist attack very aggressively from the outset ($t_s = 0$) and when it is advantageous to pursue some preparatory phase in which such aggressive tactics are disavowed. Thus, we consider a *two-stage* process, in which the transition between these two stages can be optimally determined by the government.

Let us denote by $x(t)$ the number of terrorists at time t, $u(t)$ the "water strategy," and $v(t)$ the "fire strategy" at time t. The model reads as follows:

Stage 1: After a terrorist attack, counter measures are modest. Only water operations u are applied, but information for more efficient use of fire strategies is gathered.

$$\int_0^{t_s} \mathrm{e}^{-rt}(cx + u^2)\,\mathrm{d}t$$

$$\text{s.t.} \quad \dot{x} = \tau + kx^{\alpha} - \mu x - \beta u x^{\theta}, \quad x(0) = x_0.$$

Stage 2: At time t_s an additional counter-terror measure v (fire strategy) is used. The efficiency of the fire strategy depends on the switching time t_s: the later v is applied, the more efficient it is.

$$\int_{t_s}^{\infty} \mathrm{e}^{-rt}(cx + u^2 + v^2)\,\mathrm{d}t$$

$$\text{s.t.} \quad \dot{x} = \tau + k(1 + \rho v)x^{\alpha} - \mu x - \beta u x^{\theta} - \left(\gamma_0 - \frac{\gamma_0 - \varepsilon}{1 + t_s}\right) v x,$$

where $\gamma_0 > \varepsilon$.

Parameter values are given in Table 8.1. For brevity we omit here the analysis of the model.

The optimal path in the state–costate space and the optimal controls for $x_0 = 0.2$ are shown in Fig. 8.1a,b, respectively. The optimal switching time is $t_s = 8.3135$.

Table 8.1. Parameters for the two-stage fire-and-water model

Variables	Description	Value
r	Discount rate	0.05
c	Costs per unit of terrorists	10
τ	Constant inflow	0
ρ	Contribution of fire control to recruitment	0.2
k	Normalization factor	0.05
α	Influence of actual state on recruitment	0.5
μ	"Natural" per capita outflow	0.05
β	Efficiency of water operations	0.01
θ	Diminishing returns from water operations	0.5
γ_0	Maximum efficiency of fire operations	0.1
ε	Minimal efficiency	0

During the first stage the terrorist organization is allowed to grow, but water operations are used to slow its growth. From time $t = t_s$ onward fire strategies are applied aggressively and the number of terrorists is driven down toward its equilibrium value $\hat{x}$. However, a moderate level of water strategies is still used (see Fig. 8.1a, b).

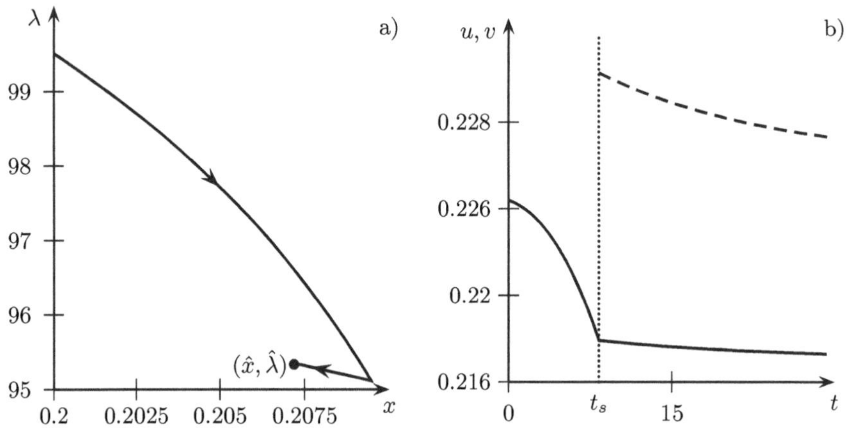

Fig. 8.1. Panel (**a**) depicts the optimal path in the state–costate space for $x_0 = 0.2$. The number of terrorists grows during the first stage peaks at the switching time $t_s = 8.3135$ and converges to $(\hat{x}, \hat{\lambda})$. In panel (**b**) the corresponding optimal controls $u(\cdot)$ (*solid curve*) and $v(\cdot)$ (*dashed curve*) are shown

A so-called *anticipation effect*, known from capital accumulation models, may be relevant; in this case one expects the investment in the control to be reduced before the optimal time for switching. This would mean that the special tactics are reduced before the government begins fighting back with aggressive measures.

In a nutshell, in Sect. 8.1 we expanded the range of formulations that could be addressed to deal with changes at abrupt point in time in the "environment" in which the drug users, corrupt politicians, terrorists, etc., live. The next section expands the range of formulations further by adding another important ingredient of the decision-making processes that are focus of this book.

8.2 Differential Games

So far we have presented intertemporal optimization models dealing with illicit drug problems, corruption, and terrorism in which a decision-making authority is confronted with the behavior of offenders. Yet, real-world processes usually involve more than one decision-maker. Therefore, sometimes accurately modeling processes that aim to control deviant behavior requires including *strategic* considerations and interactions among the decision-makers involved. This can be the case when drug users and drug dealers, bribers and those taking bribes, terrorists and non-terrorists not only react to (the optimally designed) control measures of an authority, but also actively decide how to act. Game theory has proved to be a useful tool for conceptualizing situations in which there are many (rational) decision-makers and for predicting the outcome of their competition or cooperation. Our discussion focuses, however, on a particular type of game.

We consider here differential games. So what is a differential game? Imagine that a conflict situation is such that an arbitrary number of decision-makers (e.g., the government, police authorities, drug dealers, drug users) interact in an environment (such as a drug market, a particular country, or a society) that evolves over time in a way that is affected by the decision-makers' choices. If this environment is then modeled as a continuous-time dynamical system, we speak of a *differential game.*[2] Therefore, one could envisage a differential game formulation of a problem to be something like an optimal control formulation with additional decision-makers – keeping in mind that the theory of differential games is not just a further development of control theory, but rather comes from a different field of research.

Therefore it should not be such a surprise that differential game solution techniques are not as nicely or as comprehensively developed as optimal control techniques (given the richness of possible types of interaction and information available). They provide solutions for only specific classes of differential games. In other words, while we "*are exploring an ocean of possible applications for optimal control theory in economics and management science,*

[2] If time is discrete, we speak of a *difference game.*

with differential games we are still sailing along its shores."[3] What has been established so far is, however, very useful (see, e.g., Fudenberg & Tirole, 1991). Drawing on the work of, e.g., Başar and Olsder (1999), Dockner, Jørgensen, Long, and Sorger (2000), Engwerda (2005), and Jørgensen and Zaccour (2004), in what follows we give a very brief introduction to the fundamentals of differential games, complementing the theory with two examples from the control of deviant behavior.

8.2.1 Terminology

Depending on how decision-makers (from now on called *players*) interact (whether they collaborate or compete, whether they behave rationally or boundedly rational, etc.), different types of (differential) games are appropriate for modeling the resulting situation. Note that it is the richness of possible types of interaction and information available to the players at the moment of choice that accounts for the fact that differential games are harder to solve than optimal control problems. Therefore, we focus discussion on behavior that is most likely to occur in explaining and controlling deviant behavior.

Since players in the fields of illicit drug use, corruption, and terrorism do not have recourse to civil courts to enforce contracts or resolve disputes they may most accurately be modeled as so-called noncooperative (differential) games. As the name indicates, in this type of game the players are unable or unwilling to cooperate, i.e., to make binding agreements among each other, but aim at independently optimizing their own performance indices. Thus if we have N decision-makers, we also have N different objectives. A classical example is the model of a military conflict. An entire class of game theoretic models assumes that, for $N = 2$, the gain of one player exactly equals the loss of the other player. This assumption may be appropriate for a model of war (even though students often remark that war can be negative sum in the sense that no one wins), but this assumption does not apply to models of deviant behavior, since the sum of objective function values is not (necessarily) equal to zero. Society, for instance, does not win exactly what a drug dealer loses when picked up by the police. In this case society may profit much more from getting rid of all the adverse consequences of persistent drug-trafficking. Therefore, in what follows we focus on noncooperative, non-zero-sum differential games, starting with their formal definition.

Let N players interact in a way that can be modeled by a *finite-time noncooperative (non-zero-sum) differential game*. In such a game all N players seek to maximize their individual objective functions over a finite planning horizon $[0, T]$, where the time variable is denoted by t. Let player i then decide about his/her action at time t, represented by the *control variable* $u^i(t) \in \Omega^i \subset \mathbb{R}^{m^i}$, where $i = 1, \dots, N$, Ω^i represents the set of player i's

[3] Such a statement was made by the French Operations Researcher Jacques Lesourne.

admissible control variables,[4] and $m^i \geq 1$ is the dimension of the column vector $u^i(t)$.

As in optimal control models, it is assumed that all relevant influences of past decisions are adequately summarized in a state variable $x(t) \in X \subset \mathbb{R}^n$. Over time this state variable evolves according to the differential equation

$$\dot{x} = f(x, u^1, \ldots, u^N, t), \quad x(0) = x_0,$$

where the initial state, x_0, is known by all players.

When at time t each player i chooses his/her control variable, u^i, he/she receives a *payoff rate* $g^i(x, u^1, \ldots, u^N, t)$, where $i = 1, \ldots, N$. This yields a total discounted payoff (i.e., a total objective function value) given by

$$V^i(u^1, \ldots, u^N) = \int_0^T \mathrm{e}^{-r^i t} g^i(x, u^1, \ldots, u^N, t)\,\mathrm{d}t + \mathrm{e}^{-r^i T} S^i(x(T)), \qquad (8.3)$$

where r^i is the ith player's rate of time preference and $S^i(x(T))$ is his/her salvage value.[5] By choosing an optimal control path for $t \in [0, T]$, every player i seeks to maximize his/her individual payoff functional (8.3). Note that the strategic interdependence among all players' choices is indicated by the dependence of the ith player's payoff on the control variables (=choices) of the $N-1$ opponents.

Remark 8.2. The number of players, their payoffs, and the sets of strategies available to them are called the *rules of the game.* An essential assumption of game theory is that all players know the rules of the game and each player knows that his/her opponents know the rules as well. Moreover each player knows that each player knows that the opponents knows ....

When solving a differential game, it is essential to specify what kind of information is available to the players when at time t their decisions have to be made. Suppose each player chooses his/her control variable according to a *strategy,* φ^i, that is a decision rule determining an action as a function of some set of available information. The choice of the decision rule is made at time $t = 0$ and the player commits to follow the strategy for the entire duration of the game. This sounds like a very limiting concept, but whether it is or not depends on the *information structure* underlying the design of the decision rule. Here we present the two most common types of information pattern. Other concepts can be found in, e.g., Başar and Olsder (1999, p. 221).

---

[4] More generally, the set of admissible control values Ω^i may depend on time t, the state variable $x(t)$, and the other players' control variables $u^j(t)$ for $j \neq i$.

[5] Note that player i's ($i = 1, \ldots, N$) present-value payoff for an infinite horizon problem is given by

$$V^i(u^1, \ldots, u^N) = \int_0^\infty \mathrm{e}^{-r^i t} g^i(x, u^1, \ldots, u^N, t)\,\mathrm{d}t. \qquad (8.4)$$

Markovian or Feedback Information Pattern

Using a *Markovian strategy,* (also known as a feedback or *closed-loop strategy*) each player i, $i = 1, \dots, N$, observes the system's position as embodied in (x, t), and chooses his/her action according to

$$u^i(t) = \varphi^i(x(t), t).$$

The players then behave in a way that the current state (but no memory of past states) serves as the informational basis of their decisions. However, when the rate of change in the state of the environment, f, and the payoff rates, g^i, do not explicitly depend on time, and the game is played over an infinite time horizon, it is usual to confine the interest to stationary Markovian strategies, $u^i(t) = \varphi^i(x(t))$.

Open-Loop Information Pattern

An *open-loop strategy* is a decision rule in which the controls depend only on time:[6]

$$u^i(t) = \varphi^i(t).$$

An open-loop strategy is most appropriately applied if the players disregard the information embodied in the state variable when taking their actions, perhaps because they cannot observe the state vector. Using an open-loop strategy means that at time $t = 0$ a player commits to a fixed time path for his/her actions for the entire duration of the game. Engwerda (2005), for instance, related the open-loop pattern to a situation in which at time $t = 0$ all players submit their strategies to some authority that is then obliged to carry them out (until $t = T$).

Remark 8.3. For $T = \infty$, one has to be precise when using the term "optimality" (see Sect. 3.7.1).

8.2.2 Nash Equilibria

A fundamental game theoretic solution concept is the *Nash equilibrium.* Here none of the simultaneously acting players has an incentive to deviate from his/her own Nash equilibrium strategy as long as no other players does. This leads to the following definition:

Definition 8.4 (Nash Equilibrium). *Any N-tuple $(\varphi^1, \dots, \varphi^N)$ of strategies constitutes a Nash equilibrium if*

$$V^i(\varphi^1, \dots, \varphi^N) \geq V^i(\varphi^1, \dots, \varphi^{i-1}, u^i, \varphi^{i+1}, \dots, \varphi^N)$$

for all $u^i \in \Omega^i$, $i = 1, \dots, N$.

[6] Since open-loop strategies depend also on the initial state x_0, sometimes they are written as $u^i(t) = \varphi^i(t, x_0)$. Note that in the open-loop case there is no need to distinguish between u^i and φ^i.

This is a very general equilibrium concept; only in exceptional cases does a game exhibit a unique Nash equilibrium.

How can one compute such a Nash equilibrium? If all $N-1$ opponents of player i use Markovian strategies, $u^j(t) = \varphi^j(x,t)$, $j \neq i$, then player i faces an optimal control problem of the form discussed in Chap. 3. In this case player i's decision problem can be rewritten as

$$\max_{u^i(\cdot)\in\Omega^i} \int_0^T \mathrm{e}^{-r^i t} g^i(x, u^i, \varphi^{-i}(x,t), t)\,\mathrm{d}t + \mathrm{e}^{-r^i T} S^i(x(T)) \tag{8.5a}$$

$$\text{s.t.}\quad \dot{x} = f(x, u^i, \varphi^{-i}(x,t), t), \quad x(0) = x_0, \tag{8.5b}$$

where

$$\varphi^{-i}(x,t) = (\varphi^1(x,t), \dots, \varphi^{i-1}(x,t), \varphi^{i+1}(x,t), \dots, \varphi^N(x,t)).$$

So far Definition 8.4 embodies information only about the timing of the players' choices. Nothing is said about the information that is available for the players when making their decision. Let us assume that only the current state is available as the informational basis for the players' choices. This leads us to the definition of a Markovian Nash equilibrium:

Definition 8.5 (Markovian Nash Equilibria (MNE)). *Any N-tuple $(\varphi^1, \dots, \varphi^N)$ of functions*

$$\varphi^i : X \times [0,T) \to \mathbb{R}^{m^i}, \quad i = 1, \dots, N$$

is a Markovian Nash equilibrium (MNE) if for every player i there exists an optimal control path of the problem (8.5) that is generated by the Markovian strategy $u^i(t) = \varphi^i(x,t)$.

Finding an MNE amounts to solving N optimal control problems. If we replace $\varphi^i(x,t)$ by $\varphi^i(t) = u^i(t)$, Definition 8.5 becomes the characterization of an *open-loop Nash equilibrium solution (OLNE)* because an OLNE is a degenerate MNE, but clearly not vice versa.

The following result solves the optimal control problem (8.5) by using Pontryagin's Maximum Principle:[7]

Theorem 8.6. *Let $(\varphi^1, \dots, \varphi^N)$ be a given N-tuple of functions*

$$\varphi^i : X \times [0,T] \to \mathbb{R}^{m^i}, \quad i = 1, \dots, N, \quad T < \infty,$$

and assume that there is a unique, continuous solution $x(\cdot) \in X$ of the initial value problem

$$\dot{x} = f(x, \varphi^1(x,t), \dots, \varphi^N(x,t), t), \quad x(0) = x_0.$$

[7] The theorem specifies sufficient conditions for an MNE. Omitting the concavity assumptions made, provides necessary optimality conditions.

Moreover, assume that the state space, X, is convex and the functions representing the salvage values S^i, $i = 1, \dots, N$, are concave. Let the Hamiltonians be then defined by

$$\mathcal{H}^i(x, u^i, \lambda^i, t) = g^i(x, u^i, \varphi^{-i}(x,t), t) + \lambda^i f(x, u^i, \varphi^{-i}(x,t), t)$$

and the maximized Hamiltonian by

$$\mathcal{H}^{i^*}(x, \lambda^i, t) = \max_{u^i(\cdot)\in\Omega^i} \mathcal{H}^i(x, u^i, \lambda^i, t).$$

Suppose that for $i = 1, \dots, N$ there exist N continuous functions $\lambda^i(\cdot)$: $[0, T] \to \mathbb{R}^n$ such that

1. *The Hamiltonian maximizing condition,*
$$\mathcal{H}^i(x, \varphi^i(x,t), \lambda^i, t) = \mathcal{H}^{i^*}(x, \lambda^i, t)$$
holds,
2. *The n adjoint equations*
$$\dot{\lambda}^i = r^i \lambda^i - \mathcal{H}^{i^*}_x(x, \lambda^i, t) \tag{8.6}$$
are satisfied for almost all $t \in [0, T]$, and
3. *The N transversality conditions for $T < \infty$,*
$$\lambda^i(T) = S^i_x(x(T))$$
hold for all $i = 1, \dots, N$,

3′. *Or the limiting transversality conditions for $T = \infty$*
$$\lim_{t\to\infty} \mathrm{e}^{-r^i t}\lambda^i(t)\tilde{x}(t) = 0 \tag{8.7}$$
hold for all admissible (i.e., for all admissible but not necessarily optimal) state trajectories $\tilde{x}(t)$ and $i = 1, \dots, N$.

Moreover, the functions $\mathcal{H}^{i^*}$, $i = 1, \dots, N$, are continuously differentiable in x and concave in x for all $t \in [0, T]$.

Then $(\varphi^1, \dots, \varphi^N)$ is an MNE.

Remark 8.7. The adjoint equation (8.6) reveals that generally it is much more difficult to determine an MNE than an OLNE. (One exception is for state-separable games.) Since each nondegenerate Markovian strategy φ^j, $j = 1, \dots, i-1, i+1, \dots, N$ depends on x, the maximized Hamiltonian $\mathcal{H}^{i^*}$, $i \neq j$ depends – via any φ^j, $i \neq j$ – also on x. An infinitesimal change of x causes the opponents to change their strategies φ^j, $j = 1, \dots, i-1, i+1, \dots, N$ by $\partial\varphi^j/\partial x$, $j \neq i$. Since $\partial\mathcal{H}^{i^*}/\partial\varphi^j \neq 0$ for $j \neq i$, those opponents' reactions influence player i's payoff, and hence also his/her shadow price, λ^i. The terms $\partial\mathcal{H}^{i^*}/\partial\varphi^j$ and $\partial\varphi^j/\partial x$ show player i how the competitors react to a change of the state variable. Note that for open-loop strategies the derivatives $\partial\varphi^j/\partial x$, vanish making the solution of the adjoint equation much simpler.

8.2.3 Tractable Game Structures

Analytical solutions of differential games are scarce (numerical solutions being the rule), but they allow an understanding of the true "nature" of the players' optimal strategies. Therefore, before we discuss another fundamental game theoretic (equilibrium) solution concept useful for modeling conflicts involving deviant behavior, we shall summarize important facts about two classes of differential games for which we are able to derive analytical characterizations of open-loop Markovian Nash equilibria.

The first class of tractable differential games consists of *linear–quadratic games*. They are characterized by the property that the state dynamics is a first-order polynomial and the objective functions are second-order polynomial functions with respect to the state and the control variables. If the state dynamics includes an additional constant, the game is called *affine quadratic.* The corresponding solutions are given by, e.g., Başar and Olsder (1999), Dockner et al. (2000), Engwerda (2005), and Jørgensen and Zaccour (2004).

The second class of tractable differential games is the class of *state-separable games*. They were introduced by Dockner, Feichtinger, and Jørgensen (1985), and Dockner et al. (2000, Sect. 7.2) also denote them as *linear state games.* This class consists of games for which the state equation and the objective function are linear in the state variables and which have no (multiplicative) interaction between control variables and state variables, i.e.,

$$\mathcal{H}^i_{xx} = 0, \qquad \text{and} \quad \mathcal{H}^i_{u^i x} = 0 \quad \text{for} \quad \mathcal{H}^i_{u^i} = 0.$$

State-separability is important for at least two reasons. First, these games have the property that their open-loop Nash equilibria qualify as a Markovian solution.[8] Second, state-separable games are "tractable" also in the case of hierarchical moves.[9] (One such differential game in the context of international terrorism is presented in Sect. 8.2.6.)

The following section aims at improving understanding of Nash equilibria by presenting the analysis of a differential game on corruption. Drawing heavily on Wirl, Novak, Feichtinger, and Dawid (1997), the game describes the strategic interactions between a corrupt politician, his/her hidden corruption, and the revealing efforts of investigative journalism.

8.2.4 A Corrupt Politician vs. the Tabloid Press

Whereas in Sect. 6.2 we examined a politician's decision whether or not to engage in corrupt behavior (yielding an optimal control model), the model presented here focuses on the strategic interaction between the corrupt official

[8] Note that this property is stated for Nash games. The coincidence of open-loop and Markovian strategies for any other solution concept may or may not occur.

[9] Note that, in the case of optimal control models, state-separability implies that the saddle point paths are horizontal in the phase portraits.

(player 1) and the press (player 2).[10] A magazine with market power attracts customers and thus increases its profit by uncovering the corrupt practices of the "filthy" politician. The more popular the politician is, the more readers an expose of his/her corruption is likely to attract. Revealing corruption lowers the politician's popularity. Uncovering a less popular official attracts fewer additional readers than revealing the hidden corruption of a more popular person.

The Model

To keep the analysis as simple as possible, we restrict ourselves to a one-state differential game, with the politician's level of popularity being the state variable, denoted by x. Popularity, which is continuously assessed by public polls, increases, but at a decreasing rate. This is embodied in a concave (popularity) growth function $g(x)$. The impact of disclosed corruption depends on both the politician's intensity of corruption, v, and the newspaper editor's intensity of pursuing investigative journalism, u. Thus the dynamics of popularity growth can be written as

$$\dot{x} = g(x) - \delta(u, v)x, \tag{8.8}$$

with $x(0) = x_0$ as the initial popularity level (which is known by both players). On the politician's side, increased corruption, u, harms popularity: a greater corruption increases the likelihood of exposure by the journalists, and it also implies a disproportionally greater loss of popularity. Thus, $\delta_u > 0$ and $\delta_{uu} > 0$. If the newspaper increases its expenses for investigative efforts, v, the discovery rate of the corrupt practices tends to increase, everything else being equal, and this harms the politician's public support, $\delta_v > 0$. By assumption, these expenses satisfy the law of diminishing returns, $\delta_{vv} < 0$. Finally, the loss of (or gain in) popularity itself depends on the politicians current level of popularity, x, because exposing evidence of corruption is much more harmful to popular politicians (who are perceived to be honest) than to non-popular politicians (who are suspected of engaging in various nefarious activities). This dependence of the change in the politicians popularity on x yields a strategic

[10] Note that analyzing the corrupt politician's optimal control problem presented in Sect. 2.3 helps us to understand an offender's motivation for misconduct and, consequently, helps authorities to remove incentives for acting so. Analyzing a differential game between a politician and a superior authority would go beyond this analysis and explicitly ask for the appropriate counter-corruption measures at a time t to remove these incentives. Thus the control problem itself can shed valuable insight into an offender's motivation for a particular kind of behavior, while the corresponding game is capable of delivering an intertemporal strategy for eliminating the incentives for a rational offender to act in a corrupt manner. Note, however, that the game presented here describes a rather different situation. The press does not really aim to wipe out corruption, but rather to expose it. Therefore, this game is more similar to a "farmer–cow relationship" than to an "exterminator–vermin relationship."

element for the press, which may feel tempted to selfishly exploit this dynamic dependence. That is because the newspaper's gain from demolishing popular public figures is greater than from exposing already unpopular politicians.

The politician's benefit from being popular is assumed to be proportional to his/her current level of popularity, σx. But, the politician also derives a benefit from engaging in corrupt activities. This type of benefit is embodied in the concave utility function $U(u)$. Taking the present value, using the discount rate r^1, leads to player 1's objective,

$$V^1(u,v) = \int_0^\infty \mathrm{e}^{-r^1 t} \left(\sigma x + U(u)\right) \mathrm{d}t. \tag{8.9}$$

The newspaper editor's benefit is assumed to be proportional to the loss of the politicians popularity, which translates into readers and profits, $\delta(u,v)x$. The cost of the investigation is assumed to increase linearly in the investigative effort. This leads to player 2's objective,

$$V^2(u,v) = \int_0^\infty \mathrm{e}^{-r^2 t} \left(\delta(u,v)x - av\right) \mathrm{d}t. \tag{8.10}$$

For simplicity and since it would not be easy to specify salvage values for both players we consider a game of infinite duration.

The reader may enjoy thinking about how the formulation could be modified to capture the dynamics at play when the tabloids expose embarrassing personal information about movie stars and other celebrities.

Stability Analysis

Our analysis focuses on the OLNE of the game because the politician's degree of popularity cannot be sufficiently known at any time t to admit a Markovian solution. To facilitate the analytical calculations and to simplify the numerical computations, we specify the forms of the functions g, δ, and U in (8.8), (8.9), and (8.10) as follows

$$g(x) = \rho x, \quad U(u) = C - \frac{b\eta}{1-\eta} u^{\eta-1},$$
$$\delta(u,v) = u^{\varepsilon} v^{\pi}, \quad \rho,\, b,\, C > 0, \quad \eta,\, \pi \in (0,1), \quad \varepsilon > 1.$$

For simplicity we assume that the politicians degree of popularity grows exponentially. The revelation rate δ is specified as a power function, where the parameters ε and π are chosen in a way that all assumptions stated above are satisfied. This yields the following differential game:

$$\max_{u(\cdot)} \int_0^\infty \mathrm{e}^{-r^1 t} \left(\sigma x + C - \frac{b\eta}{1-\eta} u^{\eta-1}\right) \mathrm{d}t$$
$$\max_{v(\cdot)} \int_0^\infty \mathrm{e}^{-r^2 t} \left(u^{\varepsilon} v^{\pi} x - av\right) \mathrm{d}t$$
$$\text{s.t.} \quad \dot{x} = (\rho - u^{\varepsilon} v^{\pi})x, \quad x(0) = x_0.$$

The OLNE is then characterized by the property that each player's strategy, as a function of time (u, v, $t \geq 0$), is a best response to the opponent's exogenously given strategy, and in an equilibrium both strategies are simultaneously best-response strategies. This means that we are solving two optimal control problems, in which the respective control variable of the opponent $j \neq i$ is arbitrary but fixed. Then, the current-value Hamiltonians of the players, $i = 1, 2$, are defined as

$$\begin{aligned}\mathcal{H}^1 &= \sigma x + C - \frac{b\eta}{1-\eta}u^{\eta-1} + \lambda\left(\rho - u^{\varepsilon}v^{\pi}\right)x \\ \mathcal{H}^2 &= u^{\varepsilon}v^{\pi}x - av + \mu\left(\rho - u^{\varepsilon}v^{\pi}\right)x,\end{aligned}$$

where λ and μ denote the current values of the adjoint variables (or shadow prices) of x for player 1 and player 2, respectively.[11] Since popularity is an asset for the politician, clearly $\lambda > 0$. The sign of μ, however, is ambiguous.

$\mathcal{H}^1$ is concave in u since $\lambda > 0$, and $\mathcal{H}^2$ is concave in v whenever $\mu < 1$. Under these conditions the optimal strategies can be calculated in explicit form

$$u^* = \left(\frac{b\eta}{x\lambda\varepsilon v^{\pi}}\right)^{\frac{1}{\varepsilon-\eta+1}} \tag{8.11a}$$

$$v^* = \left(\frac{a}{\pi u^{\varepsilon}x(1-\mu)}\right)^{\frac{1}{\pi-1}}. \tag{8.11b}$$

The adjoint variables must satisfy the following differential equations

$$\dot{\lambda} = \lambda r^1 - \mathcal{H}^1_x, \qquad \dot{\mu} = \mu r^2 - \mathcal{H}^2_x.$$

After substitution of the optimal controls, given by (8.11), into the equations for the adjoint variables, the following canonical system (a three-dimensional system of first-order differential equations) in the variables (x, λ, μ) results

$$\begin{aligned}\dot{x} &= \left(\rho - u^{\varepsilon}v^{\pi}\right)x \\ \dot{\lambda} &= \lambda(r^1 - \rho + u^{\varepsilon}v^{\pi}) - \sigma \\ \dot{\mu} &= \mu\left(r^2 - \rho + u^{\varepsilon}v^{\pi}\right) - u^{\varepsilon}v^{\pi}.\end{aligned} \tag{8.12}$$

The equilibrium of the dynamical system, (8.12), is unique and can be explicitly computed as

$$\begin{aligned}\hat{x} &= \left(\rho^{(1-\eta)(1-\pi)+\varepsilon}\left(\frac{a}{\pi(1-\frac{\rho}{r^2})}\right)^{\pi(1-\eta)}\left(\frac{b\eta r^1}{\varepsilon\sigma}\right)^{-\varepsilon}\right)^{\frac{1}{\pi(1-\eta)-\varepsilon}} \\ \hat{\lambda} &= \frac{\sigma}{r^1}, \qquad \hat{\mu} = \frac{\rho}{r^2}, \qquad \hat{u}^{\varepsilon}\hat{v}^{\pi} = \rho.\end{aligned}$$

---

11 Note that both players act simultaneously. Thus the numbering of the players does not indicate any hierarchy in decision-making.

For a comprehensive stability analysis of the canonical equations (8.12) we refer to Wirl et al. (1997). There we find that calculating the Jacobian evaluated at the equilibrium, together with applying the Poincaré–Bendixson theorem with ρ as the bifurcation parameter, yields the model's main result:[12]

There exists a positive value ρ_{crit} such that either for all ρ near ρ_{crit} with $\rho < \rho_{crit}$ or for all ρ near ρ_{crit} with $\rho > \rho_{crit}$ there exists a pair of periodic functions, $u \geq 0$ and $v \geq 0$, that satisfy the necessary conditions of an OLNE. If the cycle appears for $\rho < \rho_{crit}$, it is stable and the long-run behavior of any Nash equilibrium solution starting in the neighborhood of the (limit) cycle exhibits recurrent behavior.

Denoting the pair of complex eigenvalues of the Jacobian by $\xi_{2,3}(\rho) = \alpha(\rho) \pm \mathrm{i}\beta(\rho)$, we can easily see that $\xi_{2,3}(\rho_{crit}) = \pm\mathrm{i}\beta(\rho_{crit})$, and that $\partial\alpha(\rho)/\partial\rho < 0$ holds. By Theorem 2.71 this implies that cycles will appear either for $\rho < \rho_{crit}$ or for $\rho > \rho_{crit}$ and that a cyclical solution of the canonical equations (8.12) appearing for $\rho < \rho_{crit}$ will be stable (corresponding to a supercritical PAH-bifurcation, see Sect. 2.10).

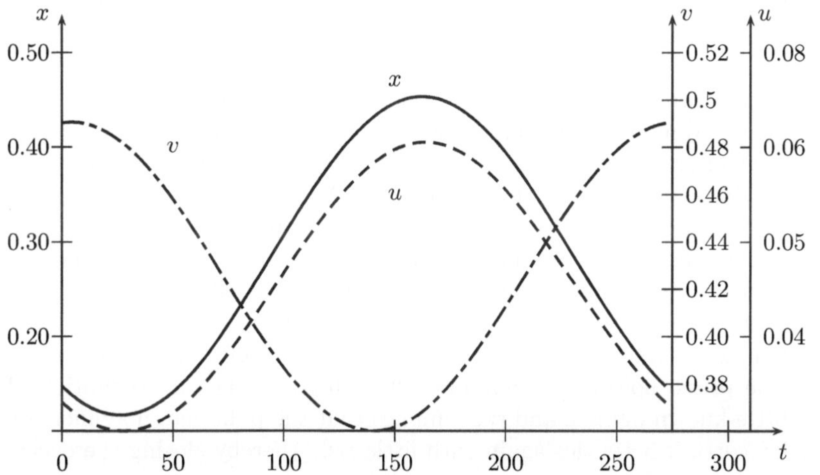

Fig. 8.2. Time paths of state and control variables along one period of the periodic solution. Note that the journalists' efforts "follow" essentially the politician's degree of popularity, whereas the politician behaves "anti-cyclically"

Using a numerical simulation, one can illustrate that the emerging cycle may truly be attracting for the set of parameter values collected in Table 8.2.

[12] The real parts of the roots of the characteristic polynomial, which is cubic, determine the stability properties of the canonical system (8.12).

Table 8.2. Set of base-case parameter values for the corruption game

r_1	r_2	a	b	C	σ	π	ε	η	ρ
0.008	0.100	0.018	0.700	5.000	0.150	0.450	1.200	0.700	0.09263

A detailed analysis shows that for the occurrence of stable limit cycles, the discount rate of the press, r^2, has to be larger than that of the politicians, r^1. Thus the politicians would have to be more farsighted than the press to generate persistent oscillations. The (corresponding) periodic time paths of the state and the control variable are depicted in Fig. 8.2. Why such a situation may lead to the occurrence of a limit cycle has been explained by Wirl et al. (1997, p. 131), who describes the following pattern:

> In a situation where the corruption rate of the politicians is high but their popularity is very low, a farsighted politician knows that he has to build up a stock of popularity to gain a secure income. He will therefore give up some of his income from corruption until he has attained some popularity. The press gains only little income from its effort in such a situation and will therefore curb its efforts at exposure. As the politician becomes more popular, he will become more and more interesting to the press and the journalists will increase their efforts to expose him. After some time the press discovers the continuing corruption of the politician. A farsighted way for the press to react would be to reveal some of the corruption, but not too much, so that the politician remains popular. We assume, however, that the press reacts myopically and immediately reveals all of the politician's corruption – which yields a high instant income for the newspaper but lowers its future income, as the politician loses all his popularity. The press, however, is not interested in revealing the corruption of little-known figures, and that implies that the politician may increase his corrupt activities again with little risk, thereby closing the cycle.

Multiple Open-Loop Nash Equilibria

In addition to the occurrence of recurrent optimal strategies, the corruption game has another remarkable property: there exists a pair of eigenvalues with negative real parts implying multiple OLNE. If two eigenvalues of the Jacobian have negative real parts, then the corresponding two-dimensional manifold Φ in the $\mathbb{R}^3$ allows convergence toward the equilibrium (see Fig. 8.3). Now, intersecting this manifold Φ with the plane Π corresponding to the initial condition $x = x_0$ results in a one-dimensional manifold of initial conditions (λ_0, μ_0) in this plane, i.e., it results in a curve in the three-dimensional space such that all paths starting at this curve, denoted as Γ, reach the equilibrium.

Since all these solutions satisfy the canonical equations (8.12) and obviously a transversality condition, these curves constitute a Nash equilibrium, at least, if the sufficient optimality conditions are met.

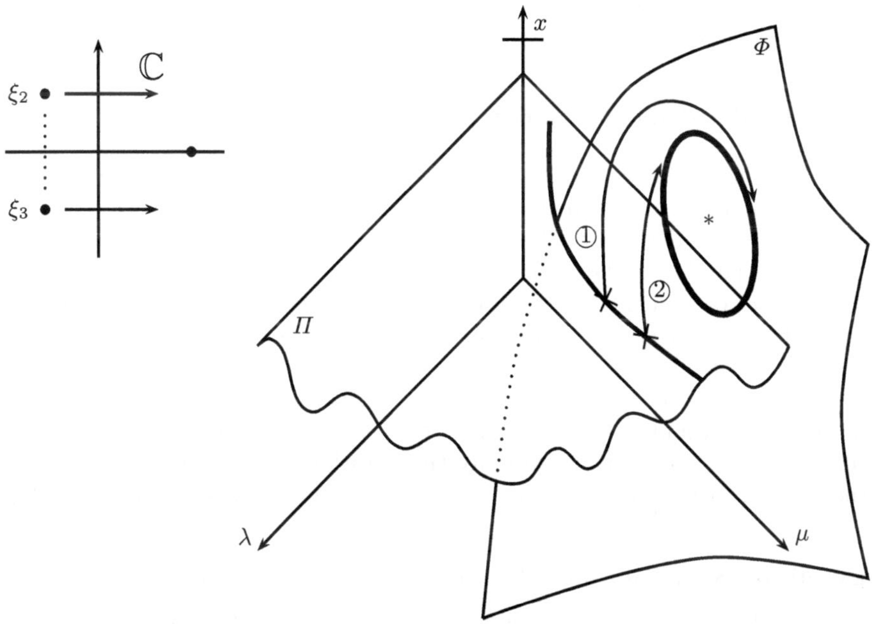

Fig. 8.3. Limit cycle in the politician–press game; indeterminacy of open-loop equilibrium. Two OLNE are shown as ① and ②; Π denotes the plane corresponding to the initial condition $x(0) = x_0$, while Φ is the two-dimensional manifold for the stationary point $(\hat{x}, \hat{\lambda}, \hat{\mu})$

The intersection of Φ and Π defines generally a curve Γ of infinitely many initial conditions $(x_0,\ \lambda_0,\ \mu_0)$ that allow for convergence toward a Nash equilibrium solution. The PAH-bifurcation, i.e., the crossing of the pair of complex conjugate eigenvalues ξ_2 and ξ_3 of the imaginary axis in the complex plane $\mathbb{C}$, is also depicted in the upper-left corner of Fig. 8.3.

Let us summarize the main results of this game. First, an OLNE may exist. An entire one-dimensional manifold (in the three-dimensional space of state and costates) describes the initial conditions allowing for convergence. Second, within this domain of multiple equilibria, a stable limit cycle may describe the long-run behavior. The existence of (stable) limit cycles means that the (corrupt) politician has to be significantly more farsighted in his/her decision planning than the newspaper editor has to be.

Remark 8.8. A variant of the corrupt politician vs. tabloid press model in which the stock of popularity grows exponentially, and the term $\delta(u, v)x$ occurring in (8.8) and (8.10) is replaced by $\delta(u, v)$ alone, i.e., without the factor x, serves as a nice example of a state-separable game; see also Exercise 8.10 and Feichtinger and Novak (2008).

The following section deals with differential games with hierarchical play.

8.2.5 Leader–Follower Games

The Nash solution concept, as illustrated in the last section, assumes that all players decide about their actions *simultaneously*. We now turn to a class of two-player games in which one player, the *leader*, has the opportunity to move first, i.e., *before* the opponent, the *follower*, makes his/her decision. This hierarchical or sequential situation is called a *leader–follower* or *Stackelberg* game. For simplicity we restrict our analysis to open-loop Stackelberg equilibria (OLSE).

To describe the stepwise procedure to derive such an equilibrium solution we assume without loss of generality that the first player is the leader and the second the follower. To simplify the notation we denote the control and the adjoint variable of player 1 by u and λ, respectively, and for player 2 by v and μ:

Definition 8.9 (Open-loop Stackelberg Equilibrium).

Step 1: *The leader, i.e., player 1, announces his/her strategy $u(\cdot)$.*

Step 2: *Taking this path as given, the follower selects $v(\cdot)$ so as to maximize his/her objective function V^2 (compare (8.3) or (8.4)). Thus the follower solves a standard-type optimal control problem. The resulting strategy $v(\cdot)$ is denoted as his/her* reaction function

$$v = R^2(x, u, \mu, t), \tag{8.13}$$

where $\mu(\cdot)$ denotes the adjoint variable of the follower's optimal control problem, i.e., his/her shadow price of an infinitesimal change in the state variable x.

Step 3: *The leader uses the follower's reaction function (8.13) to maximize his/her own objective function V^1. It is important to note that in the leader's optimization problem not only x appears as a state variable, but also μ resulting from the follower's optimization problem.*

The control paths of the leader and the follower in open-loop form are

$$\varphi^1 = u, \quad \text{and} \quad \varphi^2 = v,$$

respectively. Next, we describe the formal derivation of an open-loop Stackelberg equilibrium.

Assume $x \in \mathbb{R}^n$, $u \in \mathbb{R}^{m^1}$, $v \in \mathbb{R}^{m^2}$ and the state dynamics

$$\dot{x} = f(x, u, v, t), \quad x(0) = x_0. \tag{8.14}$$

At time $t = 0$ the leader (player 1) announces his/her control path $u(\cdot)$ for the entire duration of the game, i.e., for the finite planning horizon $[0, T]$.[13] Taking this path as given, the follower (player 2) selects his/her control trajectory $v(\cdot)$ so as to maximize the stream of discounted profits,

$$V^2 = \int_0^T \mathrm{e}^{-r^2 t} g^2(x, u, v, t)\,\mathrm{d}t + \mathrm{e}^{-r^2 T} S^2(x(T)),$$

where $r^2 > 0$ is the follower's discount rate, g^2 denotes his/her instantaneous profit function, and S^2 the salvage value function. Given the trajectory $u(\cdot)$, the follower faces a standard-type optimal control problem. To solve this, denote by $\mu(\cdot)$ the vector of adjoint variables. Then the follower's current-value Hamiltonian is given by

$$\mathcal{H}^2(x, u, v, \mu, t) = g^2(x, u, v, t) + \mu f(x, u, v, t).$$

Given the time path $u(\cdot)$, the optimality conditions of the follower's problem may be written in well-known form

$$\mathcal{H}^2_v(x, u, v, \mu, t) = g^2_v(x, u, v, t) + \mu f_v(x, u, v, t) = 0, \tag{8.15a}$$

$$\dot{\mu} = r^2 \mu - \mathcal{H}^2_x(x, u, v, \mu, t), \tag{8.15b}$$

$$\mu(T) = S^2_x(x(T)). \tag{8.15c}$$

If the Hamiltonian of the follower is jointly concave in x and v, the conditions (8.14), (8.15a)–(8.15c) are sufficient for the optimality of $v(\cdot)$. If $\mathcal{H}^2$ is strictly concave in $v(\cdot)$, then (8.15a) determines v as a function of x, u, μ, and t,

$$v = R^2(x, u, \mu, t). \tag{8.16}$$

The function R^2 is the follower's best response to the announced time path $u(\cdot)$ of the leader. Substituting (8.16) for (8.14) and (8.15b), the follower has to solve a two-point boundary value problem to get $v^*(\cdot)$ as his/her best reply to $u(\cdot)$.

Let us turn now to the leader's optimization problem. Player 1 knows the follower's best response R^2, determined by (8.16), to each control trajectory

[13] Note that the open-loop Stackelberg equilibrium solution may be imagined to be valid if the leader makes binding commitments about future policy actions where the opponents rational reactions are anticipated. This implies that both players base their actions only on the initial state, x_0. Hence, the open-loop Stackelberg equilibrium solution is derived in analogy to open-loop Nash – with the additional assumption of an asymmetric information structure.

$u(\cdot)$ that the leader may announce. Thus the leader chooses $u(\cdot)$, maximizing his/her discounted profit stream

$$V^1 = \int_0^T \mathrm{e}^{-r^1 t} g^1(x, u, R^2(x, u, \mu, t), t)\,\mathrm{d}t + \mathrm{e}^{-r^1 T} S^1(x(T))$$

subject to

$$\dot{x} = f(x, u, R^2(x, u, \mu, t), t), \quad x(0) = x_0,$$

as well as (8.15b) and (8.15c). Note that in the leader's optimization problem, not only x appears as a state variable but also the adjoint variable μ from the follower's optimization problem.[14] The current-value Hamiltonian of the leader is given by

$$\mathcal{H}^1(x, u, \mu, \lambda, \psi, t) = g^1(x, u, R^2, t) + \lambda f(x, u, R^2, t) + \psi k^2(x, u, \mu, t),$$

where λ and ψ denote the adjoint variables of x and μ, respectively, and k^2 denotes the right-hand side of (8.15b). Then, the Maximum Principle delivers

$$\mathcal{H}^1_u(x, u, \mu, \lambda, \psi, t) = 0, \tag{8.17a}$$
$$\dot{\lambda} = r^1\lambda - \mathcal{H}^1_x(x, u, \mu, \lambda, \psi, t), \tag{8.17b}$$
$$\dot{\psi} = r^1\psi - \mathcal{H}^1_\mu(x, u, \mu, \lambda, \psi, t), \tag{8.17c}$$
$$\lambda(T) = S^2_x(x(T)), \tag{8.17d}$$
$$\psi(0) = 0. \tag{8.17e}$$

Note that to simplify the derivation of the transversality condition (8.17d), we have assumed a zero salvage value for the follower; i.e., $S^2 = 0$. Note also that (8.17e) refers to a free initial state $\mu(0)$ of F (see also Chap. 5.2 in Dockner et al., 2000 about time inconsistency).

If $\mathcal{H}^1$ is jointly concave in the states x, μ, and the control u, then the conditions (8.14), (8.15b), and (8.17a)–(8.17e) are sufficient for the optimality of u.

Remark 8.10. Note that in state-separable games the costate of the follower has no influence on the optimization problem of the leader. The corresponding second costate of the leader neither appears in the dynamics of the other costates and state variables nor in the optimal control variables. Under the assumption of no control–state interaction in the state dynamics and in the objective functional of the follower, the leader's control does not depend on his/her second costate variable ψ. If additionally the Hamiltonian of the follower is linear in the state, then the second costate variable ψ also does not enter the dynamics of the first costate λ.

[14] Note that the leader faces a nonclassical optimal control problem taking into account the dynamics of the optimal decisions of the followers which are expressed by an additional costate equation.

Remark 8.11. An important feature in noncooperative game theory is *time consistency*. Omitting details (see, e.g., Dockner et al., 2000), a *subgame* of a differential game played in $[0, T]$ is its restriction to a time interval $[t, T]$ having the initial condition $x(t) = x$, where x is fixed, but arbitrary in X. An equilibrium solution of a differential game is time consistent if it is an equilibrium solution of any subgame that starts out of the equilibrium trajectory. It is well known that every Markovian Nash equilibrium is time consistent (for a proof see, e.g., Dockner et al., 2000, Sect. 4.3). A stronger property than time consistency is *subgame perfectness* meaning that the strategy φ^i represents optimal behavior not only along the equilibrium state trajectory but also *off* this path (see, e.g., Dockner et al., 2000, Sect. 4.4, for details). A Markovian Nash equilibrium that is subgame perfect is called a *Markov perfect equilibrium*. An important fact is that OLSE are in general *time inconsistent* (compare, e.g., Dockner et al., 2000, Example 5.1, for an illustrative justification).

Nondegenerate Markovian Stackelberg equilibria can be defined, but their analysis may lead to considerable technical difficulties (see Dockner et al., 2000, Sect. 5.3).

Our example from the field of international terrorism will show that, in terms of payoff, the player who makes the first move in a leader–follower game is better off when playing a Stackelberg game. Thus both players prefer to play a Stackelberg rather than Nash game, a property that is denoted as *Stackelberg dominance*.

8.2.6 A Post September 11th Game on Terrorism

The model presented here is based upon the description of the evolution of a stock of terrorists over time discussed in Sect. 2.5. Thus all arguments given there carry over to the model presented here. There is, however, one significant difference. Whereas the *terrorism model* in Sect. 2.5 has only one decision-maker, here we consider the strategic interaction of two decision-makers with opposing objectives.

We shall refer to the decision-maker on the terrorist side as *ITO*, an abbreviation for some *I*nternational *T*error *O*rganization. The ITO's opponent is assumed to be the government of a country that is at high risk of being a target of a future terror attack; for ease of exposition referred to as "the target country." Both the ITO and the target country have access to (at least) one instrument for altering the status quo. The ITO can choose the rate at which it commits terror attacks; the target country can choose the rate at which it counterattacks. In times of "war," attacks by both sides reduce the stock of terrorists in contrast to "peacetime," when neither side is making attacks.

The Model

In a post September 11th scenario, it seems plausible that the mere existence of terrorists is perceived as being a perpetual threat to any likely target country. Thus, at any instant of time, both the ITO and the target country have to decide whether or not to launch an attack in the "terror war." The state variable of the resulting (modeled) conflict corresponds to the number of terrorists (denoted by x).

We suppose that new terrorists are recruited by existing terrorists, and that the ITO grows exponentially in the absence of controls. Translating this into an equation, we suppose that the number of terrorists at time t, $x(t)$, evolves according to

$$\dot{x} = \rho x, \quad x(0) > 0, \tag{8.18}$$

where ρ denotes the endogenous growth rate of the ITO.

The ITO's attacks (denoted by v) reduce the number of ITO members. It is obvious that suicide attacks reduce the stock but even non-suicide attacks will tend to reduce the size of the ITO because every attack exposes the organization to law enforcement risks and its operatives to an increased likelihood of imprisonment or death. We recognize this fact by adding an outflow term to (8.18) that is proportional to the number of attacks, i.e., νv.

Terror-control activities pursued with intensity u (=control variable of the target country) kill, capture, or incapacitate terrorists; that is their purpose. The greater the intensity of terror-control interventions, the more resources there are that can be devoted to investigating the aftermath of an attack. These interventions may in turn provide information about other ITO operatives, so that subsequent attackers can be effectively stopped. Therefore, the greater the target country's intensity of terror-control measures, the higher is the probability of finding and arresting ITO operatives. This is approximated by $f(u) = \beta u$, where the parameter β denotes the ratio of ITO operatives lost per successful attack when the target country is on full counter-offensive, ($u = 1$) vs. none at all.[15] As the number of ITO attacks declines with an increasing probability of arresting ITO operatives who knew somebody involved in an attack, we add a second outflow term to (8.18) that weighs the number of attacks v with βu.

The target country is not limited to counterattacking when the terrorists strike. The ITO's opponent is also capable of attacking terrorists at its own initiative, a condition modeled by adding an outflow term to (8.18) that is proportional to the intensity of terror-control attacks (φu). Such "direct" terror control, however, may be seen as "disproportionate," especially if persons and property not belonging to the ITO are killed or destroyed during the target country's attacks, and may generate resentment among the populations

[15] Note that even though we normalize $u = 1$ to stand for the *maximum long-run sustainable intensity* of terror-control activities, *brief* periods of "extra intensity" ($u > 1$) are possible owing to the nature and speed of modern armed conflict.

from which the ITO seeks recruits. This resentment in turn may increase the number of new terrorists, modeled by adding an inflow term that is more than proportional in u. For convenience, we designate the inflow to the ITO caused by such collateral damage as being proportional to the square of the intensity of terror-control measures.[16]

These considerations yield the following equation describing the evolution of the number of terrorists over time:

$$\dot{x} = \rho x - \varphi u + \frac{\alpha}{2}u^2 - \nu v - \beta uv, \quad x(0) > 0, \tag{8.19}$$

with

- $x \geq 0$ number of terrorists (state variable)
- $u \geq 0$ intensity of the target country's terror-control activities, relative to its maximum sustainable level (control variable of the "target country")
- $v \geq 0$ number of ITO attacks (control variable of ITO)
- $\rho \geq 0$ endogenous growth rate of the ITO
- $\varphi \geq 0$ rate at which terror-control operations would deplete the ITO if the target country were on a full counter-offensive
- $\frac{\alpha}{2} \geq 0$ growth rate of the ITO due to collateral damage induced by the target country's terror-control attacks u
- $\beta \geq 0$ ratio of ITO operatives lost per successful attack when the target country is on full counter-offensive, $(u = 1)$ vs. none at all
- $\nu \geq 0$ average number of terrorists killed or captured per attack

We assume that the target country may have up to three policy goals and thus up to three components of its objective function. The target country certainly wants to minimize the number of terrorist attacks, v, but it may also independently seek to minimize the number of terrorists (by minimizing x). The principal reason the target country may wish to minimize the number of terrorists is their potential to commit attacks in the future, which would be captured in a v-term in the objective. However, merely living under the threat of attack can be costly even if there are no attacks, because of costs

[16] It is important to realize that (in contrast to the terror model in Sect. 2.5) here we do not distinguish between fire-type interventions and water-type interventions. That is, the target country's control variable u consists of both types of interventions. Thus the terror-control attacks by the target country may have the direct benefit of eliminating current terrorists, but also the undesirable indirect effect of increasing the ITO's recruitment rate (cf. Keohane & Zeckhauser, 2003). We imagine here that the undesirable indirect effects of what is perceived as excessive and inappropriate terror-control attacks increase more than proportionally with the intensity of those attacks. That is, we imagine that in the eyes of a potential terrorist recruit, some degree of counterattacking is to be expected, but excessive levels warrant sympathy for the ITO. The terms $-(\varphi u + \beta uv)$ and $+(\alpha/2)u^2$ account for the two-edged effect of terror-control activities induced by combining water- and fire-type strategies in a single control.

associated with psychological stress, maintaining homeland security capacity, and activities (e.g., business investments) avoided because of the uncertainty created by an imminent threat.

The target country also has an interest in minimizing the number of terror-control strikes (by minimizing u). One obvious reason is that terror-control efforts cost money, just like the exercise of almost any control policy. Decision-makers in optimal control formulations (with or without a game theoretic component) are routinely described as trying to minimize a weighted sum of various quantitative objectives (x and v in our case) and the costs of efforts intended to reduce that problem (u in our case). Hence, for an infinite time horizon and a positive discount rate r^1, the target country's objective can be written as

$$\min_{u(\cdot)} \int_0^\infty \mathrm{e}^{-r^1 t} \left(c_1 x + c_2 v + c_3 u \right) \, dt. \tag{8.20}$$

The ITO, on the other side, is interested in becoming powerful (by increasing x). It may value deaths of the target country's citizens that are a consequence of its own successful attacks (by increasing v). But carrying out terror attacks is expensive. This fact is modeled by including a quadratic cost function, $(c_4/2)v^2$, in the ITO's objective function. Additionally (or alternatively), the ITO may have political objectives aimed at inducing "excessive" counterattacks by the target country (eliciting high values of u) as an indirect way of stirring up sentiments against the target country. This could, for instance, smooth the way for changes in local regimes. These considerations lead to the following objective function of ITO for an infinite time horizon and a positive discount rate r^2:

$$\max_{v(\cdot)} \int_0^\infty \mathrm{e}^{-r^2 t} \left(b_1 x + b_2 v + b_3 u - \frac{c_4}{2} v^2 \right) \, dt. \tag{8.21}$$

For

$$r^i > \rho, \qquad i = 1, 2, \tag{8.22}$$

the target country and the ITO aim at optimizing (8.20) and (8.21), respectively, subject to (8.19) and the path constraints

$$x, \; u, \; v \geq 0.$$

The final component of the model specification is the choice of the solution concept, which governs how the "game" will be played. But before we discuss the implications of this choice we describe the calculation of both the Nash and the Stackelberg equilibrium solutions.

Nash Equilibrium

In what follows we compute the stationary Nash solution. Remarkably, since the game is state-separable (see Sect. 8.2.3), any open-loop Nash solution qualifies as a Markov perfect equilibrium.

In computing the Nash equilibria we have to assume that both players act simultaneously. Both the target country and the ITO then determine the optimal controls u^* and v^*, respectively, by solving an optimal control problem with the opponent's activity as given. Denoting by λ and μ the shadow prices of x for the target country and the ITO, respectively, the mathematical analysis of the war on terror starts with the formulation of both current-value Hamiltonians,

$$\mathcal{H}^1 = -c_1 x - c_2 v - c_3 u + \lambda \left(\rho x - \left(\varphi - \frac{\alpha}{2} u \right) u - \nu v - \beta u v \right) \tag{8.23}$$

$$\mathcal{H}^2 = b_1 x + \left(b_2 - \frac{c_4}{2} v \right) v + b_3 u + \mu \left(\rho x - \left(\varphi - \frac{\alpha}{2} u \right) u - \nu v - \beta u v \right). \tag{8.24}$$

The target country's shadow price λ in (8.23) is always negative along the optimal path since adding one more terrorist is harmful to the target country. The ITO's shadow price μ in (8.24) is always positive along the optimal path since one more ITO operative is beneficial to the terrorists. Pontryagin's Maximum Principle determines the evolution of the target country's shadow price of an additional terrorist by

$$\dot{\lambda} = (r^1 - \rho)\lambda + c_1 \tag{8.25}$$

with the equilibrium

$$\hat{\lambda} = -\frac{c_1}{r^1 - \rho} < 0. \tag{8.26}$$

Analogously, we find that the ITO's shadow price μ evolves according to

$$\dot{\mu} = (r^2 - \rho)\mu - b_1$$

with the equilibrium

$$\hat{\mu} = \frac{b_1}{r^2 - \rho} > 0. \tag{8.27}$$

According to (8.26) the long-run damage to the target country implied by having one more terrorist ($\hat{\lambda}$) increases as a result of an increasing per capita cost associated with the mere existence of an ITO operative (c_1).

Note that according to Theorem 8.6 the transversality conditions (8.7) hold for all admissible state trajectories.

The analysis presented here is confined to interior solutions, $u, v > 0$. Then, the Hamiltonian maximizing condition for the intensity of the target country's terror-control interventions is given by

$$\mathcal{H}^1_u = 0 \quad \text{implies} \quad u^* = \frac{1}{\alpha} \left(\frac{c_3}{\lambda} + \varphi + \beta v \right). \tag{8.28}$$

Thus the optimal intensity of counter-terror attacks u^* increases with a rising number of ITO attacks, an increasing ratio of ITO operatives lost per successful attack if the target country is on a full counter-offensive (β), and a growing rate at which terror-control operations deplete the ITO (φ). The growth rate of the ITO induced by the target country's "low-specificity" terror-control attacks ($\alpha/2$) has a diminishing impact on the target country's intensity of conducting counter-terror measures. Note that if the cost of control is large (c_3) relative to the target country's perception of damage caused by an additional ITO operative ($\lambda < 0$), the optimal intensity u^* is low and may hit the boundary of the set of admissible controls at $u^* = 0$. In that case it is optimal for the target country to abstain from counter-terror measures. If, on the other hand, the cost of control does not matter (because its fight against terrorism has an unlimited budget), the target country's shadow price disappears from (8.28) and u^* is determined by a (strictly positive) affine response function in the number of terror attacks v.

The maximizing condition for the number of ITO attacks is determined by

$$\mathcal{H}_v^2 = 0 \qquad \text{implies} \qquad v^* = \frac{b_2}{c_4} - \frac{\mu}{c_4}(\nu + \beta u). \tag{8.29}$$

The optimal number of ITO attacks v^* decreases with an increasing average number of terrorists killed or captured per attack (ν), an increasing probability of finding and arresting ITO operatives who knew somebody involved in an attack (βu), and with an increasing shadow price μ of the ITO. Thus, if the value of an additional ITO operative increases, the number of attacks declines. On the other hand, if the benefit of an attack (b_2) increases relative to its cost (c_4), it is optimal for the ITO to increase the number of its terror attacks.

Equations (8.28) and (8.29) may be interpreted as follows: The optimally chosen intensity of terror-control measures increases with an increasing number of terror attacks, while the optimal number of attacks decreases with an increasing intensity of counterattacks.

The stationary Nash equilibrium is given by

$$\begin{aligned}\hat{u}_N &= \frac{\beta(b_2 - \hat{\mu}\nu) + c_4(\varphi + c_3/\hat{\lambda})}{c_4\alpha + \hat{\mu}\beta^2} \\ \hat{v}_N &= \frac{\alpha(b_2 - \hat{\mu}\nu) - \hat{\mu}\beta(\varphi + c_3/\hat{\lambda})}{c_4\alpha + \hat{\mu}\beta^2},\end{aligned} \tag{8.30}$$

with $\hat{\lambda}$ given in (8.26), $\hat{\mu}$ given in (8.27), and where the subscript N denotes the Nash solution. Thus the equilibrium value of the stock of terrorists is given by

$$\hat{x}_N = \frac{1}{\rho}\left(\left(\varphi - \frac{\alpha}{2}\hat{u}_N\right)\hat{u}_N + (\nu + \beta\hat{u}_N)\,\hat{v}_N\right), \tag{8.31}$$

where the optimal controls are given by (8.30).[17]

[17] Note that $\hat{x}_N$ is an unstable equilibrium, i.e., for $x_0 \neq \hat{x}_N$ the state trajectory diverges.

Note that (8.30) is a *unique* Markovian Nash equilibrium, which is quite unusual (as multiple Nash equilibria are the rule in differential games).

The explicit representation (8.30) of the stationary Nash equilibrium opens the possibility for a sensitivity analysis with respect to the model parameters. Table 8.3 summarizes the results of such a comparative static analysis for (8.22) and $c_3 = 0$. This can be argued since relative to the costs imposed by terror attacks, direct budgetary outlays on terror-control attacks (as distinct from homeland security and the invasion of a country, such as Iraq) are fairly modest. If the target country thought the only cost of employing u was budgetary, or the cost of intervention "did not matter" because the war on terror had to be fought regardless of the efforts it took, u would be a negligible part of the target country's objective (i.e., the third unit cost would be equal to zero, i.e., $c_3 = 0$). Moreover, we assume that the stationary equilibria $(\hat{u}, \hat{v})$ are interior solutions.

Table 8.3. Comparative static analysis of the interior stationary Nash equilibrium $(\hat{u}_N, \hat{v}_N)$ of the terror game (8.19)–(8.21) with respect to the model parameters for $c_3 = 0$. + means that $\partial(\cdot)/\partial\text{parameter} > 0$, − the opposite case, 0 means that the parameter has no influence on the control, and ? denotes ambiguity

Parameter/ Nash equilibrium	ρ	φ	α	β	ν	c_1	c_2	b_1	b_2	b_3	c_4	r^1	r^2
$\hat{u}_N$	−	+	−	?	−	0	0	−	+	0	?	0	+
$\hat{v}_N$	−	−	+	?	−	0	0	−	+	0	?	0	+
$\hat{x}_N$	?	?	?	?	?	0	0	−	+	0	?	0	+

The results of Table 8.3 make economic sense. Note, e.g., that according to (8.27) the stationary shadow price $\hat{\mu}$ decreases with r^2, but increases with b_1 and ρ. Thus, according to (8.30), the stationary Nash control of the terrorists decreases with increasing ρ (provided that $c_3 = 0$). In addition, in that case $\hat{u}_N$ decreases too.

The Nash equilibrium computed above reflects a scenario in which the target country and the ITO make their decisions at the same time. If, however, the ITO announced further terror attacks via the Internet or other media, a Stackelberg game with the ITO as leader would be an appropriate model of the corresponding scenario.[18] Clearly, altering the solution concept changes the results. But what in particular is the difference between the outcomes of a Nash game and a Stackelberg game? What changes if the opponent makes the first move?

[18] For the Stackelberg game with the target country as the game's leader we refer to Exercise 8.9.

The Stackelberg Equilibrium with the ITO as Leader

Let us now consider the open-loop Stackelberg game with the ITO (player 2) as leader and the target country (player 1) as follower. We assume furthermore that the cost of terror control is perceived to be negligible, i.e., $c_3 = 0$. The Stackelberg solution of the game requires the following three steps:

Step 1: The ITO announces its strategy v.

Step 2: The target country solves, for this given v, the same control problem as in the Nash case. Thus, analogously to (8.25), the target country's optimal response to v (for $c_3 = 0$) is given by

$$u^* = u^*(v) = \frac{1}{\alpha}(\varphi + \beta v). \tag{8.32}$$

As before, the adjoint variable has to follow the linear differential equation (8.25).

Step 3: Using the follower's reaction function (8.32), the leader solves the following optimal control problem:

$$\max_{v(\cdot)} \int_0^\infty \mathrm{e}^{-r^2 t}\left(b_1 x + \left(b_2 - \frac{c_4}{2}v\right)v + b_3 u^*(v)\right)\,\mathrm{d}t$$

s.t. the following two-state equations

$$\dot{x} = \rho x - \left(\varphi - \frac{\alpha}{2}u^*(v)\right)u^*(v) - \nu v - \beta u^*(v)v \tag{8.33}$$

$$\dot{\lambda} = (r^1 - \rho)\lambda + c_1 \tag{8.34}$$

with $u^*(v)$ given by (8.32). Then the Hamiltonian of player 2 in this Stackelberg case becomes equal to

$$\mathcal{H}^2 = b_1 x + \left(b_2 - \frac{c_4}{2}v\right)v + b_3 u^*(v) + \mu\dot{x} + \psi\dot{\lambda},$$

with the adjoint variables μ and ψ belonging to (8.33) and (8.34), respectively, and u^* given by (8.32).[19] Solving the first-order condition, $\mathcal{H}^2_v = 0$, with respect to v yields v^*.

Substituting player 2's optimal control in (8.32) allows for calculating the stationary Stackelberg equilibrium (with the ITO as the leader) determined by

$$\begin{aligned}\hat{u}_S &= \frac{\beta(b_2 - \hat{\mu}\nu) + c_4\varphi + b_3(\beta^2/\alpha)}{c_4\alpha + \hat{\mu}\beta^2}\\ \hat{v}_S &= \frac{\alpha(b_2 - \hat{\mu}\nu) - \beta(\hat{\mu}\varphi - b_3)}{c_4\alpha + \hat{\mu}\beta^2}\end{aligned} \tag{8.35}$$

[19] Note that ψ plays no role in the optimization procedure. This is due to the state-separability of the model (see Remark 8.10).

with $\hat{\lambda}$ given in (8.26), and where the subscript S refers to the Stackelberg solution. Thus the equilibrium value of the stock of terrorists is

$$\hat{x}_S = \frac{1}{\rho}\left(\left(\varphi - \frac{\alpha}{2}\hat{u}_S\right)\hat{u}_S + (\nu + \beta\hat{u}_S)\,\hat{v}_S\right), \tag{8.36}$$

where the optimal controls are given by (8.35). The qualitative properties of the stationary Stackelberg solution are essentially the same as the ones of the stationary Nash solutions. But not entirely. The next section summarizes the two solutions' similarities and differences.

Comparison of the Nash and Stackelberg Equilibrium Solutions

The stationary Stackelberg solution (given by (8.35)) can be expressed in terms of the stationary Nash solution (see (8.30)):

$$\hat{u}_S = \hat{u}_N + \frac{\beta}{\alpha}\varDelta, \quad \hat{v}_S = \hat{v}_N + \varDelta$$

with

$$\varDelta := \frac{b_3\beta}{c_4\alpha + \beta^2\hat{\mu}} > 0. \tag{8.37}$$

The difference between the optimal stationary Nash and Stackelberg equilibrium is driven by the term $\varDelta$ given by (8.37). The fewer ITO operatives lost per successful attack (β), the smaller is $\varDelta$. If $\beta = 0$ the Nash and Stackelberg equilibrium solutions coincide. Note that this is also the case, if we investigate a Stackelberg game in which the target country is the leader that announces its terror-control policy to the ITO(see Exercise 8.9). Moreover, if the ITO has no political objective at all ($b_3 = 0$), then the Nash and Stackelberg equilibrium solutions also coincide. If b_3 is positive, however, the ITO announces a number of attacks, v_S, such that the target country responds with a high intensity of control, u_S. This in turn fuels recruitment and increases x, which allows the ITO to carry out more terror attacks.

Since it follows from a comparison of (8.35) and (8.30) that

$$\hat{u}_S > \hat{u}_N, \qquad \text{and} \qquad \hat{v}_S > \hat{v}_N$$

the war on terror will be more intense if the ITO has a first mover advantage (*and* a political objective) and announces the number of terror attacks to be carried out to the target country (compared to the case where both players act at the same time). Thus the ITO being the Stackelberg-leader, leads to a higher number of terror attacks and more intensive counter-terror interventions, and, thus, a more intensive conflict.

Since both the Stackelberg leader and follower increase their efforts in contrast with the players in the Nash equilibrium, it is interesting to analyze the effect of $\hat{u}_S > \hat{u}_N$ and $\hat{v}_S > \hat{v}_N$ on the equilibrium.The difference between the equilibrium values (8.31) and (8.36),

$$\hat{x}_S - \hat{x}_N > 0,$$

is positive, and therefore we can conclude that the ITO being the leader yields an increase in the size of the ITO, $\hat{x}_S > \hat{x}_N$.

We conclude the comparison of the results of the two solution concepts with a comparison of their objective function values. Since the state equation is linear, $x(t)$ can explicitly be solved, yielding

$$x_N(t) = x_{N0}e^{\rho t} + \hat{x}_N(1 - e^{\rho t})$$
$$x_S(t) = x_{S0}e^{\rho t} + \hat{x}_S(1 - e^{\rho t}).$$

Then the objective function values of the leader (ITO) for both solution concepts (using stationary controls) can be calculated as

$$V_N^2 = \int_0^\infty e^{-r^2 t}\left(b_1 x + (b_2 - \frac{c_4}{2}\hat{v}_N)\hat{v}_N + b_3\hat{u}_N\right) dt$$
$$= b_1 \frac{r^2 x_{N0} - \rho \hat{x}_N}{r^2\,(r^2 - \rho)} + \frac{2b_2\hat{v}_N - c_4\hat{v}_N^2 + 2b_3\hat{u}_N}{2r^2},$$

and

$$V_S^2 = \int_0^\infty e^{-r^2 t}\left(b_1 x + (b_2 - \frac{c_4}{2}\hat{v}_S)\hat{v}_S + b_3\hat{u}_S\right) dt$$
$$= b_1 \frac{r^2 x_{S0} - \rho \hat{x}_S}{r^2\,(r^2 - \rho)} + \frac{2b_2\hat{v}_S - c_4\hat{v}_S^2 + 2b_3\hat{u}_S}{2r^2}.$$

Since the difference between the objective function values,

$$V_S^2 - V_N^2 = \frac{b_3\beta\Delta}{2r^2\alpha} > 0,$$

is positive, the ITO is better off leading when playing the Stackelberg strategy than when playing the Nash strategy.

Inasmuch as being a Stackelberg leader involves committing up front to a course of action, whereas the Nash concept involves simultaneous and hence more interactive decision-making, we have uncovered a logical reason why an ITO might want to cultivate a reputation for being fanatically devoted to a course of action. Simply put, the ITO achieves a better outcome (objective function value) if it can convince the target country to play a Stackelberg game in which the ITO's fanatical (superficially "irrational") favor gives it the first-mover advantage.

Together with Exercise 8.9, the above results provide an informative picture of three possible "war on terror" scenarios and the impact of the many possible types of interaction on the results. This is remarkable because the model is stunningly simple (while allowing for analytical calculations). With these pieces of information decision-makers can gain an understanding of the interaction between terrorists and likely target countries (both striking back and attacking) and insight into the consequences of policy-making. Better-informed policy-makers can then make better policy.

Differential games "extend" standard-type optimal control problems with respect to the number of decision-makers. The next subsection returns to the one-decision-maker assumption, but allows for an explicit dependence of the fundamentals on age.

8.3 Age-Structured Models

A drawback of the models presented so far is the assumption of homogeneous agents. In Chap. 6 we considered multi-compartment models, e.g., the LH-model in Sect. 6.1, to cope with heterogeneities. The present section considers age and duration as a source of heterogeneous behavior.

A usual framework for including those variables in economic problems is provided by overlapping generations models. In the present context, however, partial differential equations (PDEs) are introduced to deal with age-specific processes.

According to (Keyfitz, 1977, Sect. 5.7), there are *four* ways of modeling the evolution in time of an age-structured population: the classical Lotka integral equation, the Leslie matrix, the renewal difference equation approach, and the McKendrick PDE. More than eighty years ago, McKendrick (1926) used the latter for his studies on mathematical epidemiology (compare also Hadeler, 1984, Dietz, 1997). Mathematicians working on nonlinear population models have rediscovered McKendrick's formulation and used it to cope with time-dependent and interacting populations (compare, e.g., Webb, 1985). In the simplest case the PDE reduces to a well-known renewal integral equation.

Denoting by $x = x(t, a)$ the density of a population of age a at time t, McKendrick's PDE may be written as

$$\frac{\partial x}{\partial t} + \frac{\partial x}{\partial a} = -\mu(t, a)x(t, a), \tag{8.38}$$

where $\mu(t, a)$ is the force of mortality or instantaneous death rate of an individual of age a at t. Equation (8.38) represents the dynamics in the interior of the so-called *Lexis diagram* (see Fig. 8.4), named after W. Lexis (1837–1914). This diagram summarizes the basic logic of population dynamics:[20] from any age an individual can go to the next age or die, and at certain ages $a \in (\alpha, \beta)$ a woman can give birth to a child aged zero. For a more detailed description, compare Keyfitz and Keyfitz (1997), and Keyfitz (1977, pp. 139–140).

The behavior along the coordinate axes is described by the initial and boundary conditions

[20] We restrict our analysis to closed one-sex populations.

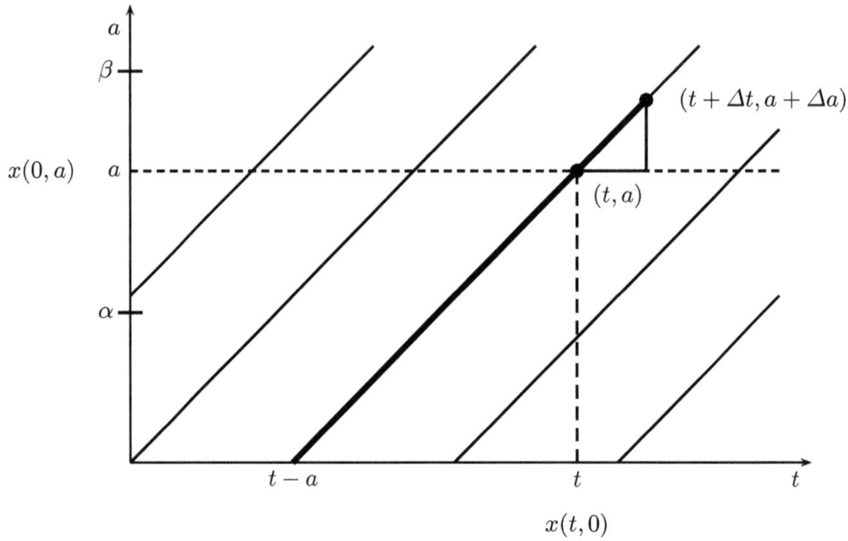

Fig. 8.4. Lexis diagram

$$x(0, a) = x_0(a), \quad \text{at } t = 0,\ a \geq 0 \tag{8.39}$$

$$x(t, 0) = \int_{\alpha}^{\beta} m(t, a)x(t, a)\, \mathrm{d}a, \tag{8.40}$$

where $m(t, a)$ denotes the age-specific fertility rate at time t, and $[\alpha, \beta]$ the reproductive interval, $[\alpha,\ \beta] \subset [0,\ \omega]$, ω representing the maximal possible age (possibly infinite).

A substantial difference between the boundary condition (8.40) and the boundary conditions usually arising in mathematical physics (e.g., for the classical transport equation, which has the same form as (8.38)) is that the right-hand side of (8.40) depends on the density $x(t, \cdot)$. In epidemiological models similar *non-local* terms as in (8.40) also appear in the right-hand side of (8.38).

Recently optimal control problems for age-structured systems have generated increasing interest. There are many applications in various fields of population dynamics, including birth control, harvesting, and epidemiology. For a non-exhaustive list see Feichtinger, Tragler, and Veliov (2003). Many of those studies present optimality conditions for particular models, usually in the form of Pontryagin's Maximum Principle. A Maximum Principle for McKendrick's systems has been derived by Brokate (1985). In what follows we sketch a Maximum Principle derived in Feichtinger et al. (2003) for a fairly general model of an age-structured control system with nonlocal dynamics and nonlocal boundary conditions.

8.3.1 A Maximum Principle for Distributed Parameter Systems

Let us consider the following optimal control problem:

$$\max_{u(t,a)\in\Omega} \int_0^T \int_0^\omega g(x(t,a), q(t), u(t,a))\,\mathrm{d}a\,\mathrm{d}t \tag{8.41a}$$

$$\text{s.t.} \quad \left(\frac{\partial}{\partial t} + \frac{\partial}{\partial a}\right) x(t,a) = f(x(t,a), u(t,a)) \tag{8.41b}$$

$$q(t) = \int_0^\omega h(x(t,a), u(t,a))\,\mathrm{d}a, \tag{8.41c}$$

the initial condition (8.39) and the boundary condition

$$x(t,0) = \varphi(t, q(t)). \tag{8.42}$$

Here t is the time, running in a given interval $[0,\ T]$, where T can also be infinite, $a \in [0,\ \omega]$ denotes age, $x(t,a) \in \mathbb{R}^n$, and $q(t) \in \mathbb{R}^r$ are the states of the system, $u(t,a) \in \Omega \subset \mathbb{R}^m$ are distributed controls.

Remark 8.12. To simplify our considerations, we omit the possibility of initial and boundary controls. Moreover, we assume the existence of optimal solutions and omit the technical properties of the model functions.

The following theorem refers to necessary optimality. By using the classical Weierstrass method in the calculus of variations, Feichtinger et al. (2003) derive a *global* Maximum Principle.

For the solution of the optimal control with distributed parameter a we define the (distributed) Hamiltonian

$$\mathcal{H}(x, u, \lambda, \eta) = g(x,u) + \lambda f(x,u) + \eta h(x,u).$$

The adjoint system for the adjoint variables (λ, η) is given by

$$\left(\frac{\partial}{\partial t} + \frac{\partial}{\partial a}\right) \lambda(t,a) = -H_x(x, u, \lambda, \eta) \tag{8.43a}$$

$$\lambda(T,a) = 0, \quad a \in [0,\ \omega] \tag{8.43b}$$

$$\lambda(t,\omega) = 0 \tag{8.43c}$$

$$\eta(t) = \lambda(t,0)\nabla_q \varphi + \int_0^\omega \lambda(t,a)\nabla_q f\,\mathrm{d}a. \tag{8.43d}$$

Provided with these definitions, we can formulate the following necessary optimality conditions for distributed parameter control models of the type (8.39), (8.41a)–(8.42):

Theorem 8.13 (Maximum Principle for Distributed Parameter Models). *Assume that there exists an optimal solution and that certain regularity conditions are satisfied. Then the adjoint system (8.43) has unique solutions* (λ, η), *and for almost every* $t \in [0,\ T]$, $a \in [0, \omega]$ *it holds that*

$$\mathcal{H}_u(x, u, \lambda, \eta) = 0.$$

8.3.2 Age-Structured Drug Initiation

The following model for drug initiation extends the traditional models, see, e.g., Sects. 2.9 and 3.9, by considering explicitly the age distribution of the users. Drug use is contagious, i.e., most users are introduced by members of a reference group. The experience of others can be instrumental in shaping perceptions of the risk of using drugs, and those perceptions influence initiation.

Let us assume the existence of only two types of individuals, nonusers and users. To simplify, mortality and migration are neglected, and a constant birth rate and an upper age limit are assumed. The user population consists of current users and individuals who have ever used drugs (former users). Here, we consider the nonuser population, focusing on the transition of nonusers denoted as $x(t, a)$ to ever users (current or former users). Denoting by $\mu(t, a)$ the initiation rate, the McKendrick dynamics

$$\left(\frac{\partial}{\partial t} + \frac{\partial}{\partial a}\right) x(t, a) = -\mu(t, a)x(t, a) \tag{8.44}$$

states that the rate of change of nonusers of any age a at time t equals the negative per capita initiation rate times $x(t, a)$. The initial population of nonusers is given by (8.39), while the boundary condition at age $a = 0$ is assumed to be constant. By choosing this constant k, we can interpret $x(t, a)$ as the proportion of nonusers:

$$x(t, 0) = k. \tag{8.45}$$

The initiation rate incorporates three factors:

$$\mu(t, a) = \bar{\mu}(t, a)\Theta(x(t, a))\Psi(w(t, a)), \tag{8.46}$$

where $\bar{\mu}(t, a)$ denotes the basic age-specific initiation intensity of a nonuser who starts consuming drugs. The term $\Theta(x(t, a))$ represents the influence of the reputation of the drug on the initiation of nonusers of age a.[21] Finally, the prevention factor $\Psi(w(t, a))$ refers to the effect of age-specific prevention programs $w(t, a)$, especially school-based programs that are targeted at certain age groups. For a prevention efficiency function, recall the function introduced in (6.1) for the LH-model given by

$$\Psi(w) = (1 - c)\mathrm{e}^{-\varepsilon w} + c, \tag{8.47}$$

where $(1 - c) \in (0, 1)$ measures the maximal proportional reduction in initiation and ε reflects the efficiency of prevention spending. (8.47) states that initiation decreases with increasing prevention expenditures w, but with diminishing efficiency and up to a maximal amount of less than 100%.

[21] Here, for simplicity, it is assumed that nonusers are influenced only by users of the *same* age group. In reality, the interaction of individuals is distributed among the ages. This effect is discussed in detail in Almeder, Caulkins, Feichtinger, and Tragler (2004).

The objective is to minimize the stream of discounted social costs of drug consumption and also to minimize the expenditures on prevention

$$V = \int_0^T \mathrm{e}^{-rt} \int_0^\omega (\rho(a)(k - x(t,a)) + w(t,a)) \, \mathrm{d}a \, \mathrm{d}t, \tag{8.48}$$

where $\rho(a)$ denotes the age-specific social costs of a person who has ever consumed drugs.[22] For a specification of the model functions and parameters, see Almeder et al. (2004).

The following result follows from Theorem 8.13 and states the necessary optimality conditions. To simplify notation, we mostly omit the arguments:

Theorem 8.14. *Assume that $w(t,a)$ is the optimal control for the model (8.39), (8.44)–(8.48). Then there exists an adjoint variable $\lambda(t,a)$ and a state trajectory $x(t,0)$ such that*

$$\left(\frac{\partial}{\partial t} + \frac{\partial}{\partial a}\right) \lambda = -\rho + r\lambda + \bar{\mu}\Psi(w) \left(x\Theta'(x) + \Theta(x)\right) \lambda \tag{8.49}$$

together with

$$\lambda(t,\omega) = 0 \quad \text{for} \quad 0 \le t \le T$$
$$\lambda(T,a) = 0 \quad \text{for} \quad 0 \le a \le \omega.$$

For the optimal control $w(t,a), (t,a) \in [0,\, T] \times [0,\, \omega]$ we have

$$w = \begin{cases} 0 & \text{for } (1-c)\varepsilon\bar{\mu}\lambda x\Theta(x) \le 1 \\ \frac{1}{\varepsilon} \ln\left((1-c)\varepsilon\bar{\mu}\lambda x\Theta(x)\right) & \text{otherwise.} \end{cases} \tag{8.50}$$

Proof. The proof uses a Maximum Principle that is simpler than the one stated in Theorem 8.13, which can be found in Derzko, Sethi, and Thompson (1980) or Muzicant (1980).

The present-value Hamiltonian function is given by

$$\tilde{\mathcal{H}} = -\mathrm{e}^{-rt}\rho(k - x) - \mathrm{e}^{-rt}w + \tilde{\lambda}\left(-x_a - \bar{\mu}\Theta(x)\Psi(w)x\right).$$

The adjoint equation obeys

$$\left(\frac{\partial}{\partial t} + \frac{\partial}{\partial a}\right) \tilde{\lambda} = -\mathrm{e}^{-rt}\rho + \tilde{\lambda}\bar{\mu}\Psi(w) \left(x\Theta'(x) + \Theta(x)\right).$$

For the current-value adjoint variable $\lambda = \mathrm{e}^{rt}\tilde{\lambda}$, this yields (8.49).

To maximize the Hamiltonian, we consider only those terms that depend on w, i.e.,

$$F(w) := -w - \bar{\mu}\lambda x\Theta(x)\Psi(w).$$

[22] Another performance measure might include costs of initiation.

According to (8.47) we have

$$F'(w) = -1 + (1-c)\varepsilon\bar{\mu}\lambda x\Theta(x)\mathrm{e}^{-\varepsilon w}$$
$$F''(w) = -(1-c)\varepsilon^2\bar{\mu}\lambda x\Theta(x)\mathrm{e}^{-\varepsilon w}.$$

Solving $F'(w) = 0$ gives the optimal control (8.50). To verify that it is indeed a maximum, we have to determine the sign of λ and distinguish between the cases $\lambda > 0$ and $\lambda \leq 0$ as follows:

$\lambda > 0 : F'' < 0$, w is an interior maximum
$\lambda \leq 0 : F' < 0$, $w = 0$.

□

Finally, note that the change of the marginal value of a nonuser given by, $\lambda_t + \lambda_a$ in (8.49), equals the sum of the following three terms, which makes economic sense:

- $-\rho + r\lambda$, i.e., the effects of social costs and the discount rate
- $\bar{\mu}\Psi(w)\Theta(x)\lambda$, i.e., the effect of the additional initiation $\bar{\mu}\Psi(w)\Theta(x)$ valued with λ, because an additional nonuser is also a potential new user
- $\bar{\mu}\Psi(w)\Theta'(x)x\lambda$, i.e., the effect of the change of the initiation rate due to the additional nonuser weighted with λ

8.4 Further Optimal Control Issues

The purpose of this brief concluding section is to mention a few additional methodological avenues of optimal control theory. Although they play an increasing role in economics and management science, they have not been presented and applied in this book mainly owing to the lack of space. Nevertheless, we do not want to finish without at least referring to them and to where they can be studied further.

8.4.1 Delayed Systems

In all models dealt with in this book it is assumed that the system's reaction to a control is immediate. In many systems, however, there is a *delay* with respect to the impact of the control; i.e., the present state of the system changes at time t in a manner affected by the value of some variable at a time $t - \tau$. In many biological, engineering, and economic examples, besides such *discrete* delays with a fixed τ, so-called *distributed delays* occur. This means that the present state of the system changes at time t in a manner affected by an integral over all the past values of some variable. MacDonald (1989) and Kolmanovskii and Shaikhet (1996) give a readable introduction to such delay systems.

Consider, e.g., the Nerlove–Arrow model sketched in Exercise 3.4. A basic assumption of this marketing model is that any advertising message *immediately* has an impact on the goodwill stock. However, advertising a product at time s may instead cause an increase in sales in period $t = s + \tau$, for some $\tau > 0$. Even more realistically, advertising a product may affect sales at a continuum of future times, not just at a specific instant. If we assume that the *lags* are *distributed* over an interval, we get the following (distributed lag) control model:

$$\max_{u(\cdot)} \int_0^T g(x,u,t)\,\mathrm{d}t + S(x(T),T)$$

$$\text{s.t.} \quad \dot{x} = f(x,u,t) + \int_{-\infty}^{t} h(x(\tau),u(\tau),\tau,t)\,\mathrm{d}t \tag{8.51}$$

$$x(t) = \tilde{x}(t), \quad u(t) = \tilde{u}(t), \quad t \in (-\infty, 0]. \tag{8.52}$$

The state dynamics (8.51) is now a so-called *integro-differential equation*. It states that the rate of change at time t depends not only on the state and control at that time but also on the past control path and state trajectory. According to (8.52) both the state and the control path have to be known in the interval $(-\infty, 0]$, not just for a single initial condition at time zero.

It makes sense to define the Hamiltonian as follows

$$\mathcal{H}(x,u,\lambda(\cdot),t) = g(x,u,t) + \lambda(t)f(x,u,t) + \int_t^T \lambda(\tau)h(x,u,t,\tau)\,\mathrm{d}\tau, \tag{8.53}$$

where $\lambda(\cdot)$ denotes the adjoint variable and $\mathcal{H}$ depends not only on x, u, and t, but also on the function $\lambda(\tau)$, $\tau \in [t,T]$. Note that via the integral term in (8.53) future considerations influence the present. It measures the value of all future marginal change densities h in $x(\tau)$, i.e., for $\tau \geq t$. Thus the Hamiltonian represents the total profit rate.

By using (8.53), it is possible to write necessary optimality conditions similar to those in the Maximum Principle. Sethi (1974) showed that sufficiency holds if the maximized Hamiltonian is concave in x. Hartl and Sethi (1984) provided a nice interpretation of the adjoint variable of the Hamiltonian in the style of Sect. 3.3.4. For an illustrative analysis of an *advertising capital model* see Hartl (1984) and also Feichtinger and Hartl (1986, Example A.4.1). There, one can find further references.

An example from the field of illicit drugs is the delayed impact of drug prevention on initiation. Although initiation of marijuana consumption in the US peaks sharply around age 16 or 17, and the average age of cocaine initiation is about 21 years, school-based prevention programs are typically run in the 7th and 8th grades (for children of ages 12 and 13) and sometimes even as early as elementary school. Thus, whether a prevention effort pays or not in the sense of being cost effective is not observed until an average of three to eight years after the financial resources are invested in the program.

Recall that in Sect. 6.1 we addressed the question of how and when a public policy-maker should, over the course of a cocaine epidemic, devote financial resources to demand-side drug interventions. In the optimal control model (6.6) spending money on either treatment or prevention affects drug use immediately; but, at least for cocaine, there is about an eight year lag between when prevention funds are spent and when they affect cocaine initiation. That delay is not a problem if there is no constraint on the drug control budget; in that case if the model suggests spending a given amount on prevention in year t, that should be construed as implying that the amount should actually be spent on prevention programs in year $t - \tau$, for $\tau \approx 8$. However, when the control budget is assumed to be proportional to the size of the problem, denoted as $Q(t)$ and reflecting a weighted average of light and heavy users, then the control is related both to the current state (via the budget constraint) and the future state (via prevention's lagged effect). In that case we confront a true delayed system with a budget constraint written as follows, where $w(t+\tau)$ reflects the effect of prevention at shifted time $t+\tau$ that stems from spending at time t

$$u(t) + w(t + \tau) = \gamma Q(t).$$

The corresponding lagged differential optimal control problem is more challenging to solve. Contrasting this formulation with that in Sect. 6.1 offers an interesting case study in modeling. Budgets are almost always constrained to at least some extent, so that, all other things being equal, the budget-constrained formulation is more appealing. All other things are not equal, however. When there was no budget constraint we could solve a standard optimal control problem without lags, just by remembering that the optimal $w(t)$ should be interpreted as indicating how much should have been spent on prevention that had an effect at time t, which means how much should have been spent on prevention eight years before time t. Adding the budget constraint makes that approach invalid and forces one to grapple with a problem that is considerably harder to solve. The art of modeling involves developing good skill judgment as to when the benefits of a more realistic model (e.g., one with a budget constraint) justify its greater complexity, which makes the more realistic problem harder to solve.

8.4.2 Stochastic Optimal Control

In the previous chapters it was assumed that the state variables of the system were known with certainty. In many applications, however, the development of the system is represented by a controlled stochastic process rather than by deterministic modeling. Uncertainties may arise for various reasons, e.g., by exogenous random influences as in the demand or price development of drugs or other commodities, notably including stock prices in finance problems. Moreover, measurements are usually noisy in physical, medical, or engineering systems. Quite often the interaction of the model variables is only partially known or observable.

To take into consideration these stochastic influences, the system dynamics may be described by a stochastic differential equation of a type known as the *Itô equation*,[23]

$$\mathrm{d}x = f(x,u,t) + \sigma(x,u,t)\,\mathrm{d}z, \qquad x(0) = x_0, \tag{8.54}$$

where x denotes the state u the control, and f denotes the expected change of the state x. The term $\sigma \mathrm{d}z$ includes the "stochastic perturbation," whereas $\mathrm{d}z$ denotes "white noise" which formally is the derivative of a Wiener process (Brownian motion). Note that the stochastic differential equation (8.54) is a short notation of *Itô's integral equation*,

$$x(t) = \int_0^t f(x(s),u(s),s)\,\mathrm{d}s + \int_0^t \sigma(x(s),u(s)\mathrm{d}s)\,\mathrm{d}z(s) + x_0.$$

For the mathematical calculus see, e.g., Fleming and Rishel (1975).

The decision-maker's problem is to maximize the expected utility stream

$$\max_{u(\cdot)} \mathbb{E}\left\{\int_0^T g(x,u,t)\,\mathrm{d}t + S(x(T),T)\right\}, \tag{8.55}$$

subject to (8.54). The appropriate solution procedure uses the stochastic version of the Hamilton–Jacobi–Bellman equation.

Defining the value function $V(x,T)$ as in (8.55), one obtains, after some manipulations (see, e.g., Arnold, 1974 or Karatzas & Shreve, 1998):

$$-V_t(x,t) = \max_{u\in\Omega}\{g(x,u,t) + V_x(x,t)f(x,u,t) + \frac{1}{2}V_{xx}(x,t)\sigma^2(x,u,t)\}, \tag{8.56}$$

and $\quad V(x,T) = S(x,T).$

Note that the distinctive term between the stochastic HJB equation (8.56) and the deterministic version given as (3.29a) is the addition of $\frac{1}{2}V_{xx}\sigma^2$.

8.4.3 Impulse Control and Jumps in the State Variables

In the systems analyzed until now the control affects only the time derivatives of the state variable. Thus the state variable can only change continuously.

However, in many situations in management science and economics it makes sense to allow for finite jumps in the state variables at some instants of time. Examples are orders or deliveries at discrete time points, maintenance of machinery or investments (buying a machine) at certain times, or vaccinations

[23] For more, see one of the good introductions such as Dixit and Pindyck (1994) or Huisman (2001); see also Sethi and Thompson (2000, Chap. 13), Sethi and Zhang (1994) and Sethi (1983, 1997).

in epidemiological models. In all these cases finite changes in the value of a state variable occur. To be more concrete, we consider the following extension of the standard optimal control problem (3.3):

$$\max_{u(\cdot)} \left\{ \int_0^T g(x,u,t)\,\mathrm{d}t + \sum_{i=1}^{N(T)} h(x(\tau_i^-), v(\tau_i), \tau_i) + S(x(T)) \right\} \tag{8.57a}$$

$$\text{s.t.} \quad \dot{x} = f(x(t), u(t), t) + \sum_{i=1}^{N(T)} k(x(\tau_i), v(\tau_i), \tau_i)\delta(\tau_i), \qquad x(0) = x_0. \tag{8.57b}$$

Here u denotes the ordinary control, v is an impulse control variable, which is applied at time points τ_i, and $\delta(\tau_i)$ Dirac's delta function. The solution of the problem involves the determination of the jumping times τ_i, the magnitudes of the pulses $v(\tau_i)$, as well as the number $N(T)$ of impulse points. At the times τ_i when impulse control is applied, we have

$$x(\tau_i^+) = x(\tau_i^-) + k(x(\tau_i^-), v(\tau_i), \tau_i).$$

Blaquière (1985) has derived a Maximum Principle to solve problem (8.57). Sethi and Thompson (2000, Chap. 12) and Miller and Rubinovich (2003) present some nice applications of impulse control. Bensoussan and Lions (1984) wrote an interesting book on impulse control and quasi-variational inequalities.

8.4.4 Nonsmooth Systems

In many economic problems there occur functions that are non-differentiable or even discontinuous. Well-known examples are kinks in the cost functions in production/inventory problems such as those coming from unit cost reductions when volume reaches some quantity discount thresholds. A typical example from the economics of crime (and thus relevant to drugs, corruption, and terror) is sentencing guidelines that are well modeled by a piece-wise linear function of some measure of criminal involvement, such as the quantity of drugs possessed at the time of arrest.

There is a huge literature on optimal control of nonsmooth systems. For an introduction see Clarke (1983), Clarke et al. (1998) and Loewen (1993).

Exercises

8.1 (Optimal Timing of "Cold Turkey").
In the economic modeling of addiction "cold turkey" means an immediate and total abstinence from consumption of a drug. (The symptoms have been portrayed strikingly in Otto Preminger's movie "The Man with the Golden Arm," in which

Frank Sinatra shows stereotypical cold turkey symptoms of a person dependent on heroin.)

Consider a simplified variant of the Becker–Murphy addiction model described in Exercise 6.2. Denoting by u the consumption rate of a drug, and by x the accumulated consumption (habit), the state dynamics is

$$\dot{x} = u - \delta x, \quad x(0) = x_0, \tag{8.58}$$

with $\delta > 0$ being the constant depreciation rate. Typically, the consumption utility also depends on the state. While the positive interaction of u and x (in Exercise 6.2) characterizes addiction, we simplify this to

$$\max_{u(\cdot)} \int_0^T \mathrm{e}^{-rt} \left(U(u) - cu - D(x)\right) \mathrm{d}t - \mathrm{e}^{-rT} S(x(T)), \tag{8.59}$$

$$\text{s.t.} \quad u(t) \geq 0, \quad \text{for all} \quad t \in [0, T], \tag{8.60}$$

where $U(u)$ is a concave utility function, c represents the cost of the drug, and $D(x)$ measures the disutility of accumulated consumption, assumed to be convex.

For simplicity we assume

$$U(u) = au - \frac{b}{2}u^2, \; D(x) = 0, \; S(x(T)) = Sx(T),$$

where a, b, $S > 0$. Now let us assume that cold turkey takes place at time $t_s \in [0, T]$. This means that after t_s nothing is consumed.

Formulate this as a two-stage optimal control problem where the switching time t_s has to be determined optimally.

Find an explicit formula for the optimal timing of cold turkey, t_s^*, by using the matching conditions (8.1) and (8.2) (continuity and optimality). Show that t_s^* decreases both with the salvage value S, as well as with costs c, but increases with r, δ, and the marginal utility $U'(0) = a$. Discuss the possibility of corner solutions, i.e., immediate switching and permanent consumption.

Prove that for a square-root consumption utility function $U(u) = \sqrt{u}$ it holds that $t_s^* = T$.

Remark 8.15. Note that this model may also be solved as a one-stage standard optimal control problem.

There are at least three other interpretations of the sketched scenario:

Optimal drinking behavior at a party: Gustav and Peter both attend a party to consume beer. G's drinking program is modeled by a standard one-stage control problem (8.58)–(8.59), while P intends to stop optimally at time t_s to avoid a hangover, measured by the salvage value $S(x(T))$ (as well as by the current disutility $D(x(\cdot))$. Show that both men follow the same optimal behavior. Why is it always optimal in that case to "drink until the end of the party?" (Compare also Exercise 3.16.)

Environmental pollution: If we interpret x as a stock of pollution generated by consumption u, we get a simple environmental model (in which c may be interpreted as production costs).

"De Statu Corruptionis" (Lehner, Meran, & Möller, 1980): Optimal switch from a "Saulinic" phase in which the decision-maker sins to a "Paulinic" stage, in which the person regrets sinning (or at least does not sin). The salvage value refers to the last judgment (compare also Feichtinger & Mehlmann, 1986).

8.2 (Escalation of Terror). Consider the following extension of the fire-and-water model analyzed in Sect. 2.5 dealing with the reactions of a government faced with a dramatic terrorist attack (such as that on September 11th). The situation described in Sect. 8.1.3 may be captured by the following two-stage model:

$$\min_{u(\cdot),v(\cdot),t_s} \int_0^\infty \mathrm{e}^{-rt}(x^2+u+v)\,\mathrm{d}t$$

$$\text{s.t.} \quad \dot{x} = \begin{cases} \tau + kx^\alpha - \mu x - \beta\ln(1+u)x^\theta & t \le t_s \\ \tau + (k+\rho v)x^\alpha - \mu x - \beta\ln(1+u)x^\theta - \gamma\ln(1+v)x & t > t_s \end{cases}$$

$$u(t) \ge 0, \quad v(t) \ge 0, \quad \text{for all} \quad t.$$

The parameter γ measures the efficiency of fire measures. It would make sense to assume that $\gamma = \gamma(t_s)$ depends on the switching time t_s.

8.3 (Switching to Harm Reduction). Denote by A the number of current users, and by u the treatment rate. While in the first stage of this two-stage problem treatment is the only control instrument, in the second stage another control variable, v, is introduced. It measures the percentage reduction in the harmfulness of drug use (compare Exercise 6.3). At any given time, social costs are the product of A and $(1-v)$, with the social cost per user per unit of time, when there is no harm reduction, normalized to 1. Drug use spreads via social interaction. The probability of initiation per interaction depends on the prevalence of the epidemic. The hallmark of the epidemiological approach to drug use is a concave function, $f(A)$, governing the initiation rate. While the benefit of control reduces the instantaneous social cost, it is plausible that it may increase initiation. Although there exist no empirical data on the extent of this effect, Caulkins et al. (2007) assumed a convex increasing function $h(v)$ with $h(0)=1$ and $h'(v)>0$ that multiplies the initiation term. Denoting by r the discount rate and by t_s the switching time, we consider the following two-stage optimal control model:

$$\min_{u(\cdot),v(\cdot),t_s} \left\{ \int_0^{t_s} \mathrm{e}^{-rt}(A+u)\,\mathrm{d}t + \int_{t_s}^\infty \mathrm{e}^{-rt}\left(A(1-v)+u\right)\,\mathrm{d}t \right\} \tag{8.61}$$

$$\text{s.t.} \quad \dot{A} = \begin{cases} f(A) - g(u,A) & t \le t_s \\ f(A)\left\{1 + (h(v)-1)\left(1-\mathrm{e}^{-\gamma(t-t_s)}\right)\right\} - g(u,A) & t > t_s \end{cases} \tag{8.62}$$

$$u(t) \ge 0, \quad 0 \le v(t) \le \bar{v}, \quad \text{for all} \quad t. \tag{8.63}$$

As in Sect. 3.9 the function $g(u,A)$ models how treatment u reduces drug use. The objective value (8.61) measures the discounted social and instrumental costs, while the system dynamics describes the change of the state variable A depending at stage 1 only on u, but at stage 2 also on the newly introduced harm reduction control v. Usually, $\bar{v} < 1$; i.e., full harm reduction is not possible. The exponential term in (8.62) refers to a learning effect, γ being the learning rate. Learning effects provide an example in which t_s occurs explicitly in the system dynamics or in the utility function. Formally, it is taken into consideration in the matching condition (8.2). An example in which it makes economic sense is given by Boucekkine et al. (2004). It means that harm reduction does not have an immediate impact on initiation. The objective of drug policy-making is to choose the time paths u^* and v^* so that the cost functional in (8.61) is minimized. In addition to that, the switching time, t_s^*, between the two regimes has to be determined in an optimal way.

8.4. Solve the two-stage counter-terror model presented in Sect. 8.1.3.

8.5 (Capital Accumulation and Embodied Technological Progress). Grass, Hartl, and Kort (2007) considered the following two-stage optimal control problem:

$$\max_{I(\cdot),t_s} \left\{ \int_0^{t_s} \mathrm{e}^{-rt} \left(R(K) - C(I)\right) \mathrm{d}t - \mathrm{e}^{-rt_s} S(t_s) + \int_{t_s}^{\infty} \mathrm{e}^{-rt} \left(R(K) - C(I)\right) \mathrm{d}t \right\}$$

$$\text{s.t. } \dot{K} = \begin{cases} I - \delta K & t \leq t_s \\ q(t_s)I - \delta K & t > t_s, \end{cases}$$

where t_s denotes the switching time, $K(t)$ the capital stock at time t, $I(t)$ the investment rate, $R(K)$ the return, and $C(I)$ the investment cost. The coefficient $q(\cdot)$ measures the productivity, where $q(0) = 1$, $q'(\cdot) > 0$.

Solve the problem for $R(K) = p_0 K - \frac{m}{2} K^2$, $q(t) = 1 + bt$, $b > 0$, $C(I) = I + \frac{c}{2} I^2$. $S(t_s)$ are switching costs ($S(0) = 0$, $S' > 0$).

Three cases are possible in this scenario, a given switching time t_s, stochastic t_s (use the Kamien Schwartz "trick"; compare Sect. 8.4), and t_s as determined optimally. Here we consider the third case.

Try to characterize the optimal switching time t_s^*. Check whether boundary solutions $t_s = 0$, $t_s \to \infty$ can occur or not. Apply the optimality conditions stated in Sect. 8.1 to calculate the optimal investment program. Show that there is a jump in the investment rate at t_s. Carry out a phase portrait analysis and discuss the negative anticipation effect implied by the technological progress. This means that investment drops before the switching time. Show that the steady-state capital stocks in stage 1 are always below the equilibrium in the second stage.

8.6. Carry out the stability analysis of the three-dimensional canonical system (8.12) of the differential game presented in Sect. 8.2.4.

8.7. Solve the terror game analyzed in Sect. 8.2.6 by using the HJB equation.

Hint. Apply the technique presented in Sect. 3.4.1 to differential games; see, e.g., Dockner et al. (2000).

8.8. Carry out the calculations leading to the comparative static analysis collected in Table 8.3. Then, discuss the plausibility of the various signs.

8.9 (ITO as Follower). Consider the terror game presented in Sect. 8.2.6 in a Stackelberg framework *reversed* to the one analyzed there, i.e., with the target country as leader and the ITO as follower. Carry out an analysis and show that for the stationary Stackelberg equilibrium (with $c_3 = 0$) the following controls are optimal

$$\hat{u}_S = \frac{\beta(b_2 - \hat{\mu}\nu) + c_4\varphi - \beta\hat{\mu}(\frac{c_2}{\lambda} + \nu)}{c_4\alpha + 2\beta^2\hat{\mu}}, \quad \hat{v}_S = \frac{b_2\alpha - \hat{\mu}(\alpha\nu + \beta\varphi) + b_3\beta + \frac{\beta^2\hat{\mu}^2}{c_4}(\frac{b_2}{\hat{\mu}} + \frac{c_2}{\lambda})}{c_4\alpha + 2\beta^2\mu}.$$

Try to compare this Stackelberg solution with the stationary Nash equilibrium. Carry out a comparative static analysis for the reverse Stackelberg solution. Do the results make economic sense?

Discuss parameter constellations in which the stationary Stackelberg controls are "less aggressive" than the corresponding Nash equilibria. Show that the Stackelberg leader is always better off than as a Nash player. Is the follower better or worse off than the corresponding Nash player?

8.10 (Government vs. Terrorists). The following differential game between a government and a terroristic organization is simple enough that both its Nash and its Stackelberg equilibria can be analytically determined and compared. Since the game is *state-separable*, any *open-loop* Nash solution is a *Markovian open* (*closed-loop*) Nash solution.

The first player, i.e., the government, chooses the intensity of its counter-terroristic measures, u, while the second player, i.e., the terroristic organization, controls (the number of) its attacks, v.

The stock of terrorists, x is exploited by a "harvest" function $h(u,v)$ with

$$h_u > 0, \quad h_{uu} \leq 0; \quad h_v > 0, \quad h_{vv} \geq 0; \quad h_{uv} \geq 0.$$

Hence, simply assuming exponential growth, the system dynamics is given as

$$\dot{x} = \rho x - h(u,v), \qquad x(0) = x_0 > 0.$$

The first player draws utility from the terrorists being arrested or killed, but incurs disutility both from the stock of terrorists as well as from their attacks, and bears costs related to its counter-terror measures.

The second player seeks to maximize its terrorist attacks, v, and its power, x. Thus we have

$$V^1 = \int_0^\infty e^{-r^1 t} \left(\omega h(u,v) - c_1 x - c_2 v - c_3 u\right) dt$$

$$V^2 = \int_0^\infty e^{-r^2 t} \left(b_1 x + b_2 v\right) dt,$$

where for simplicity we assume linear utilities and cost functions.

Remark 8.16. Note that the present game also admits an interpretation as a corruption game. In such a scenario player 1 is a revealing authority or the public media, while player 2 is a corrupt agent, x being his/her reputation (see Sect. 8.2.4 for a similar game).

To calculate the Nash equilibrium, first solve the adjoint equations. Note that the assumption

$$r^i > \rho, \qquad i = 1, 2$$

makes sense to assure for the steady costates $\hat{\lambda} < 0$, and $\hat{\mu} > 0$. Check whether the limiting transversality conditions stated in Theorem 8.6 are satisfied.

To proceed we specify the functions as follows

$$h(u,v) = u^\pi v^\varepsilon, \quad \text{with} \quad \pi \in (0,1), \quad \varepsilon > 1.$$

Determine the Nash equilibrium $\hat{u}$, $\hat{v}$ and $\hat{x}$, and carry out a comparative static analysis.

Calculate Stackelberg equilibria, first by considering the government as leader and the terrorist as follower, and second for the opposite case, i.e., with the terrorist organization as leader.

Restricting the analysis to the equilibrium, both Stackelberg solutions can be ascertained explicitly and compared with the Nash solution. Show that in the case in which the terrorists are acting as Stackelberg leader, both the leader and the follower reduce their effort as compared with the Nash equilibrium. Does this result change when the government is the leader?

Note that the adjoint equation of the follower plays no role as second state variable in the leader's optimization procedure. Why is this the case?

Finally, is the open-loop Stackelberg also closed-loop?

8.11 (Optimal Pilfering by a Thief). Sethi (1979b) considered a thief who chooses a continuous pilfering rate to maximize the present value of total expected gain. For this, denote by $F(\cdot)$ the probability of getting caught by time t. The hazard rate $h(u,t)$, i.e., the conditional probability of getting caught at time t provided that the thief has not yet been caught, is given by

$$h(u,t) = \dot{F}(t)/(1 - F(t)).$$

The hazard rate is not only a measure of the law enforcement activity, but also depends on the thief's pilfering activities u. Let us assume for simplicity that $h(u,t) = hu(t)$, where $h > 0$ is a constant.

Thus we get the state equation

$$\dot{F} = hu(1 - F), \quad F(0) = 0, \tag{8.64}$$

where the pilfering rate u acts as the thief's control variable.

The gain function incorporates the amount of pilfering, the one-shot penalty at the time of arrest, and the continuous punishment subsequent to arrest. Denoting by $R(u)$ the instantaneous return on pilfering, by K the penalty at the time of arrest, and by p the rate of punishment of an arrested thief, we find that the thief maximizes expected gain as follows:

$$\max_{u(\cdot)} \int_0^\infty \mathrm{e}^{-rt} \left(R(u)(1 - F) - K\dot{F} - pF \right) \mathrm{d}t$$
$$\text{s.t.} \quad 0 \le u(t) \le \bar{u}, \quad \text{and (8.64)}.$$

Solve the thief's optimal control problem for a profit-maximizer ($R'' = 0$), a risk-averter ($R'' < 0$), and a kleptomaniac ($R'' > 0$).

Feichtinger (1983) supplemented Sethi's model by including a law enforcement agency as a second player. The objective function of the police incorporates convex costs of law enforcement, a one-shot utility at the time of an offender's arrest, and a cost or utility rate per time unit after the offender is arrested. The probability that the thief is caught by time t is influenced not only by the pilfering rate but also, and now explicitly, by the law enforcement rate.

Formulate a non-zero-sum differential game focusing on a noncooperative Nash solution. Show that given the special structure of the Hamiltonians, a system of two nonlinear differential equations for the control variables of both players can be derived. The reason for that simplification is the so-called *state-separability* of the model; see Sect. 8.2.2.

Try to solve this system, assuming power functions both for the utility of pilfering and for the law enforcement costs. What kind of qualitative insights for the Nash-optimal pilfering rate and law enforcement intensity can be derived?

8.12 (Corrupt Politician vs. Newspaper Editor). Look at the game presented in Sect. 8.2.4, where a corrupt politician and the editor of a major newspaper "play" against each other:

(1) Calculate the open-loop Stackelberg solution of the game with the newspaper's editor as the leader
(2) Calculate the OLNE

Now assume that several (competitive) newspapers exist. The function

$$\delta(u, v_1, \ldots, v_l)$$

measuring the impact of disclosed corruption on the level of the politician's popularity depends on all players' efforts then. To keep things "simple," restrict the analysis to three players.

8.13 (Transboundary Pollution). Dockner et al. (2000, Examples 5.1 and 5.2) analyzed the following environmental pollution game. Let x denote the stock of pollution affecting the welfare of two countries. The control variables u and v are the countries' consumption rates, which are assumed to be proportional to their emission rates.

The state equation is

$$\dot{x} = u + v - \alpha x,$$

where α is the natural cleaning rate. Assuming zero discounting on a fixed given planning horizon T, the first player's objective functional is

$$\max_{u(\cdot)} \int_0^T (u - u^2/2 - x^2/2)\, \mathrm{d}t,$$

while the second country intends to maximize its intertemporal welfare, i.e.,

$$\max_{u(\cdot)} \int_0^T (v - v^2/2 - x^2/2)\, \mathrm{d}t.$$

The model is simple enough to enable you to calculate explicitly both the Nash and the Stackelberg equilibria. Consider also the state-separable case by replacing the quadratic disutility of the pollution by a linear function.

Hint. Use the Maximum Principle as well as the HJB equation.

8.14 (Intertemporal Sharecropping: A Principal–Agent Problem). A landlord/landlady owns land that is divided into a cultivated area and wilderness. The landlord/landlady offers a farmer a portion of the agricultural acreage for tillage and uses the rest. In return for the rights of usufruct the farmer cultivates new acreage. The landlord/landlady may also make the soil arable. Cultivated land degrades to desert at a constant rate.

Denote by $A(t)$ the agricultural acreage at time t and by δ the natural decay rate of the land. Let $u_1(t)$ be the rate of cultivation of the farmer (player 1) and $u_2(t)$ be the cultivation rate of the landlord/landlady (player 2) at time t.

Then the system dynamics is given by

$$\dot{A} = u_1 + u_2 - \delta A. \tag{8.65}$$

Player 2 allocates at each time the cultivated area. The corresponding portions are denoted by $1 - v_2$ and v_2, respectively. It is reasonable to assume that the yield is proportional to the acreage. The cultivation incurs costs that, for simplicity, are assumed to be quadratic. Moreover, a constant duration of the game, T, is assumed. With r being a nonnegative discount rate, the objective functionals for the two players can be written as:

$$V_1 = \int_0^T \mathrm{e}^{-rt}\left((1-v_2)A - \frac{c_1}{2}u_1^2\right) \mathrm{d}t$$

$$V_2 = \int_0^T \mathrm{e}^{-rt}\left(v_2 A - \frac{c_2}{2}u_2^2\right) \mathrm{d}t.$$

Although nonnegative salvage values would make sense, for simplicity we set them equal to zero.

The problem is summarized as follows:

$$\begin{aligned} &\max_{u_1(\cdot)} V_1, \qquad \max_{u_2(\cdot), v_2(\cdot)} V_2 \\ \text{s.t.} \quad &(8.65) \\ &u_1(t) \geq 0, \quad u_2(t) \geq 0; \qquad 0 \leq v_2(t) \leq 1, \quad t \in [0, T]. \end{aligned}$$

Calculate the open-loop Nash equilibrium solution. Show that the farmer's Nash profit is zero, whereas the landlord/landlady always earns a positive amount.

Calculate the open-loop Stackelberg with the landlord/landlady as leader and the farmer as follower. Show that for $c_1 < c_2$ the farmer cultivates land in an initial interval at an increasing rate u_1. Moreover, the activity u_2 of the landlord/landlady decreases monotonically. After an egoistic period in which $v_2 = 1$, the landlord/landlady switches to a singular solution $\hat{v} < 1$. Since the farmer knows that his share $1 - v_2$ will not increase after the switching point, the farmer's activity u_1 decreases thereafter.

Show that the following relation between Nash and Stackelberg cultivation rates holds:

$$\begin{aligned} 0 < u_1^N(t) < u_1^S(t) \qquad &\text{for} \quad t \in [0, T) \\ u_2^N(t) > u_2^S(t) \qquad &\text{for} \quad t \in [0, T). \end{aligned}$$

Prove that both players prefer to play Stackelberg rather than Nash. Show further that in a Stackelberg game with the farmer as leader and the landlord/landlady as follower the solution coincides with the Nash equilibrium.

Remark 8.17. The sharecropping game admits another, more academic interpretation concerning the well-known relationship between a professor and graduate assistant. The variable A may denote the value of a research project. The professor has the power to transfer a portion of the remuneration obtained for the project to the assistant. How should the principal act and the agent react?

8.15 (Cattle-Ranching Problem). Derzko et al. (1980) considered a model for the optimal management of an age-structured renewable resource, i.e., a cattle herd (see also Sethi & Thompson, 2000). Let $x(t,a)$ denote the number of cattle of age a at time t. Let $u(t,a)$ be the rate at which a-aged cattle are bought at time t, where a negative value of u denotes a sale.

The system dynamics is

$$\frac{\partial x}{\partial t} + \frac{\partial x}{\partial a} = u(t,a).$$

The boundary conditions are (8.39) and

$$x(t,0) = v(t), \quad x(0,0) = x_0(0) = v(0),$$

where $v(t)$ is a given inflow rate. Note that here $v(t)$ is exogenously specified. It could, however, be endogenously modeled as in (8.40) by allowing the breeding rate $v(t)$ to be a control variable; see also Feichtinger and Hartl (1986, pp. 524–526).

The objective functional is given as

$$\int_0^T \int_0^\omega -\left\{c(a)x(t,a) + p(t,a)u(t,a) + q\left(u(t,a) - \tilde{u}(t,a)\right)^2\right\} \mathrm{d}a\,\mathrm{d}t$$
$$+ \int_0^T R(t)x(t,\omega) + \int_0^\omega S(a)x(T,a)\,\mathrm{d}a,$$

where ω is the age at maturity at which the cattle are slaughtered, $c(a)$ denotes the age-dependent feeding costs, $p(t,a)$ denotes the purchase or selling price of an a-aged animal at time t, for $u > 0$ or $u < 0$, respectively, and $\tilde{u}(t,a)$ is a goal-level purchase/selling rate, whereby any deviation from this goal is quadratically penalized (q being a positive constant). Finally, R and S represent the returns of the cattle-ranching business.

Solve the problem by using the Maximum Principle for distributed control problems. Show that the adjoint equations can be solved explicitly. Find an expression for the optimal state trajectory and give economic interpretations for both the state and the costate paths.

Hint. Use an appropriate partition of the admissible domain $[0,T] \times [0,\omega]$.

8.16 (Health, Survival, and Consumption). In recent years most industrialized countries have allocated increasing shares of their GDP to health care. At the same time life expectancy has continued to increase. The following model investigates the socially optimal problem of consumption and health investments. The dynamics of the population is described by the McKendrick equation (see Keyfitz & Keyfitz, 1997):

$$x_t + x_a = -\mu(a, h(t,a))x(t,a) \qquad x(t,0) = B(t), \;\; x(0,a) = x_0(a), \tag{8.66}$$

where $x_0(a)$ describes the initial age distribution of the population and $B(t)$ equals the number of newborns assumed, for simplicity, to be exogenously given.

The state variable $x(t,a)$ represents the number of a-year-old individuals at time t. The age-specific mortality rate $\mu(a, h(t,a))$ depends on age a and can be reduced instantaneously by providing to the individual an age-specific amount $h(t,a)$ of health care (or other health-enhancing goods and services). For details see Kuhn, Prskawetz, Wrzaczek, and Feichtinger (2007).

The second control variable is consumption $c(t,a)$. The objective of the social planner is to maximize the social welfare, which is defined as the sum of the instantaneous utilities of all individuals (total utilitarianism).

$$\int_0^T \int_0^\omega \mathrm{e}^{-rt} u(c(t,a))x(t,a)\,\mathrm{d}a\,\mathrm{d}t, \tag{8.67}$$

where ω is the maximal age that an individual can reach and r denotes the discount rate.

We also assume that the budget constraint is balanced for each birth cohort. This is expressed by the introduction of total wealth $A(t,a)$ held by age group a at time t and the following dynamics

$$\begin{aligned}
&A_t + A_a = \rho A(t,a) + (p(a) - c(t,a) - h(t,a))x(t,a)\\
&A(t,0) = A(t,\omega) = 0, \qquad \text{for all} \quad t\\
&A(0,a) = A_0(a), A(a,T) = A_T(a), \quad \text{for all} \quad a,
\end{aligned} \tag{8.68}$$

where ρ denotes the interest rate, assumed to be exogenous to the economy and $p(a)$ denotes the income/output accruing to an a-year-old individual.

The formal problem of the social planner is to choose the age-specific schedule of consumption and health expenditure (health care) to maximize the sum of instantaneous utility of all individuals; i.e., (8.67), subject to (8.66) and (8.68).

Formulate the necessary optimality conditions by applying the maximum principle stated in Theorem 8.13.

The following adjoint variables play a role in the analysis:

$$\begin{aligned}
&\lambda^x(t,a) \quad \text{of the population stock} \quad x(t,a),\\
&\lambda^A(t,a) \quad \text{of the cohort assets} \quad A(t,a).
\end{aligned}$$

Show that the following relations hold true and try to give economic interpretations:

$$u_c(c)x = -\lambda^x \mu_h(a,h)x$$

$$c_t + c_a = \frac{u_c(c)}{u_{cc}(c)}(r-\rho).$$

According to Rosen (1988) the *social value of life* can be defined as

$$\Psi^A(t,a) = -\frac{\partial V/\partial\mu}{\partial V/\partial A},$$

where V denotes the value function, i.e., optimal social value. This formula expresses the marginal rate of substitution (MRS) between mortality and social wealth, which describes the slope of the indifference curve including all combinations of $\mu(a,h(t,a))$ and $A(t,a)$ with the same social welfare. The denominator equals the shadow price of cohort assets λ^A. For the numerator one obtains

$$\frac{\partial V}{\partial\mu} = \frac{\partial V}{\partial x}\frac{\partial x}{\partial\mu} = -\lambda^x(a)x(a).$$

Putting these two expressions together, we obtain

$$\Psi^A(t,a) = \frac{\lambda^x(t,a)x(t,a)}{\lambda^A(t,a)} = \frac{\lambda^x(t,a)x(t,a)}{u_c(c)}.$$

The value λ^x of one more a-year-old individual at time t is multiplied by the number of such individuals N, as only such individuals will benefit from a reduction of the mortality rate in this specific age group at that time. This value is divided by the marginal utility, so that the SVOL is expressed in monetary values.

In this model an exogenous number of births $B(t)$ has been assumed. If the number of newborns is considered endogenous, then the SVOL and the shadow price for population can be decomposed into two effects, where one effect is analogous to the *reproductive value* introduced by Fisher (1930) and well-known in demography (see, e.g., Keyfitz, 1977). For details see Wrzaczek, Kuhn, and Oeppen (2007).

Hint. The Maximum Principle does not allow for initial and end conditions for the states. Thus the terminal constraints have to be included by a penalty function.

Notes and Further Reading

Multi-stage processes were considered in the 1980s (Tomiyama, 1985; Tomiyama & Rossana, 1989). Astonishingly, there have been few applications of the multi-stage paradigm, although sudden changes in model assumptions seem to be ubiquitous. Recently there has been a revived interest in multi-stage modeling, (see Makris, 2001; Saglam, 2002).

Boucekkine et al. (2004) analyzed a two-stage optimal control problem to solve a technology adoption problem under conditions of technological progress. Grass et al. (2007) study a similar problem, but then within the framework of a capital accumulation problem of a firm (see Exercise 8.5).

Whereas Exercise 8.3 provides an example of a two-stage harm reduction model with one state, Caulkins et al. (2007) analyzed a two-state model in which v acts in a continual way over the whole planning horizon.

Differential games are a creation of Isaacs in the early fifties (see Breitner, 2005, for a historical development). In those days the interest focused on zero-sum games with military applications (pursuer–evader games). The monograph of Isaacs (1965) showed the relation of differential games and optimal control (see also Ho, 1970).

By far the best book on differential games is Dockner et al. (2000). Note that Chap. 3 of their monograph contains a very useful, short introduction to optimal control of economic processes. Other valuable references are Başar and Olsder (1999), Mehlmann (1988), and Jørgensen and Zaccour (2004, 2007).

Games can be divided into cooperative and noncooperative games. In the latter case all players act in their own best interest, paying no attention to their rivals. In a cooperative game the players can coordinate their actions for their mutual gains. Dockner et al. (2000) is restricted to noncooperative games; references for cooperative games are El Ouardighi (2002); Yeung and Petrosyan (2006) and Haurie (2001).

An early reference on differential games is Leitmann (1974). The problem studied there is how to find a Pareto optimal solution. The approach is the standard one, to consider an optimal control problem with an objective being a weighted sum of the individual player's objectives. This has been used in, e.g., natural resources (see Dockner et al., 2000) and marketing (see Jørgensen & Zaccour, 2004). The idea explored in this literature is how the players can design an intertemporal allocation of the total, cooperative payoff such that individual rationality is satisfied for any player at any instant of time.

Although the dynamic game sketched in Exercise 8.11 is rather simple, it provides a crude picture of the competitive situation between offenders and a law enforcement authority in an intertemporal setting. Feichtinger (1983) showed that the optimal enforcement rate increases monotonically, whereas the thief's Nash-optimal behavior depends on the parameter constellation. The thief–police game provides an example of a so-called state-separable differential game (compare also Dockner et al., 1985). In such a game, the candidates for open-loop Nash optimality qualify also as closed-loop Nash solutions. Furthermore, the ansatz (8.64) has been used in several other situations such as maintenance/replacement, market-entrance games, and R&D competition; compare Feichtinger (1982a,b); Kamien and Schwartz (1971).

An important family of differential games focuses on capital accumulation (see Dockner et al., 2000, Chap. 9). In them, a firm invests in a private physical or financial capital stock. Thus each firm has its own capital accumulation equation. However, if we consider knowledge accumulation, where knowledge is modeled as a pure public good, every player has access to all knowledge in the economy. This implies that there is only a single stock of capital, in which two or more players invest. Assuming convex (quadratic) costs of investment and concave (negative quadratic) benefits from the capital stock, one gets a model formally equivalent to those dealt with in Exercise 8.13.

Dawid, Feichtinger, and Novak (2002) studied the dynamic strategic interaction between a criminal gang extorting money from shop owners and the police force. A gang asks a shopkeeper for an amount of money and threatens to destroy the shop if the sum is not paid. The decision variables of such an extortion game are the effort of the gang to keep up the threat and the effort of the police to protect the shopkeeper. One purpose is to characterize the factors that are important in determining whether the capital stock of local shop owners continues to grow in spite of extortion or whether criminal activity leads to economic stagnation.

Dawid and Feichtinger (1996) analyzed a differential game between a drug dealer and an authority. Although the game has no special form such as linear–quadratic, stationary feedback Nash equilibria can be calculated. The obtained solution admits nice economic interpretations.

Fent, Feichtinger, and Zalesak (1999) studied the impact of an offender's prior criminal record on the punishment of a given crime. Fent, Feichtinger, and Tragler (2002) analyzed a dynamic game that models the interactions between an offender and a law enforcement authority.

In differential games, multiple-feedback Nash equilibrium equilibria can arise even in the case of a linear-quadratic game with one state variable. This results from the fact that the differential equation implied by the HJB equation lacks a boundary condition. The multiplicity of equilibria was first noted in Tsutsui and Mino (1990). In an early application, Dockner and Long (1993) argued that a proper choice of nonlinear strategies could resolve in a noncooperative way the tragedy of the commons.

The terror game studied in Sect. 8.2.6 traces back to Behrens, Caulkins, Feichtinger, and Tragler (2007). The authors tried to solve it by using a sort of incentive Stackelberg solution concept. Incentive equilibrium solutions have been considered by Ehtamo for cooperative games; compare Ehtamo and Hämäläinen (1986, 1993).

By assuming a state-separable structure of the terror game, we are able to find analytical expressions of the stationary Nash equilibrium. Our understanding of these issues has benefited from discussions with Engelbert Dockner, Andreas Novak, and Gerhard Sorger.

For another differential game on terrorism see Feichtinger and Novak (2008); compare Exercise 8.10.

Hager, Neck, and Behrens (2001) presented an algorithm for solving dynamic games; see also Behrens and Neck (2007).

Optimal control problems for age-structured systems play an increasing role in many areas of application, including harvesting, epidemiology, population economics, and vintage capital models; see, e.g., Feichtinger et al. (2003). A Maximum Principle for linear McKendrick-type PDEs has been derived by Brokate (1985); Feichtinger et al. (2003) has delivered a fairly general extension that includes nonlocal dynamics and boundary conditions. Among the various applications are vintage capital models Feichtinger, Hartl, Kort, and Veliov (2006a,b), environmental planning (Feichtinger, Hartl, Kort, & Veliov, 2005), and demographic dynamics. Vintage models have played an important role since the work of Solow (1956); compare Barucci and Gozzi (1998, 2001). To study the effects of technological progress, it is natural to distinguish between different generations of capital goods ("vintages"). An important question in that context is how decisions to adopt new technologies are affected by the prospect that superior technologies will arrive in the future (or are already available).

Early applications of distributed optimal control are in inventory control of perishable goods, such as wine or blood; see Bensoussan, Nissen, and Tapiero (1975) and Haurie, Sethi, and Hartl (1984), who provided applications in social service systems and gave nice economic interpretations of the optimality conditions. Personnel planning is another important field of application. Gaimon and Thompson (1984) analyzed a duration-dependent organization structure.

Feichtinger, Prskawetz, and Veliov (2004) considered a social planner maximizing an aggregate intertemporal utility function that depended on per capita consumption. They included age-dependent features of both the population and the capital stock. In using the Maximum Principle (8.43a)–(8.43d), one can derive interesting results for optimal migration and saving rates (both age-dependent) in an aging population.

A more recent application is the optimal recruitment and promotion policy in university systems or learned societies. Feichtinger and Veliov (2007) considered a constant-sized organization in which the intake was determined by the number of deaths and a statutory retirement age. It turns out that two conflicting goals, to keep the age structure young and guaranteeing a higher recruitment, are reached by means of a bipolar recruitment distribution.

Age and duration also plays an important role in epidemic disease control and optimal vaccination; see Müller (1999). Almeder, Feichtinger, Sanderson, and Veliov (2007) compare to prevention medication as approaches to fighting the HIV/AIDS epidemic; see also Feichtinger, Tsachev, and Veliov (2004).

While duration-specific models use the same formalism as age-structured models, the cross-classification age *and* duration is more difficult to handle.

Yaari (1965) was the first to consider life insurance in a theoretical framework. Optimal health investment was first dealt with in Grossman's seminal paper 1972. This idea was developed further in the macro model of Hall and Jones (2007) and in the life-cycle model of Ehrlich (2000).

A model similar to the ones described in Exercise 8.16 can be formulated for one individual over the life cycle. The objective function is the sum over the utility from consumption over the entire (possible) lifespan ω weighted by the survival probability. The corresponding dynamics is similar to the McKendrick equation with initial condition (8.66). The crucial difference from the social welfare model is due to the formulation of the savings (assets) dynamics, in which three cases can be distinguished. First a dynamics equal to the social welfare model with an additional nonnegativity restriction (savings must not be negative); second, an insurance that pays additional interest with a rate equal to the average mortality rate (after optimization it is equal to that of the individual), which cannot be influenced by the individual; and, third, a "perfect" insurance that is able to observe the real mortality risk of each individual, implying that the individual can influence this part of the interest rate. One might show that only the first two cases lead to differences in the social welfare model and then interpret the result. However, a difference between the social and individual models can always be obtained by including external effects (see Kuhn et al., 2007).

An interesting future-oriented research issue would be the combination of distributed parameter control with the multi-stage framework. The natural distributed parameter setup would be an age-specific feedback on drug initiation (as in Almeder et al., 2004), coupled with temporary disruptions to the market (as in Bultmann et al., 2007). Thus, for example, one could be stuck at a high-use equilibrium, but if there were then a market disruption that reduced initiation overall, perhaps one could jump on that to depress initiation long enough to create a "hole" in the age-distribution of users. If that absence of young users undercut future initiation (because older users are not relevant role models), then the use could extinguish itself over time, even if the proximate reduction in use following the market disruption were rather modest. Distributed parameter control has been applied in spatial optimal control modeling, see, e.g., Goetz and Zilberman (2000, 2007).

Yong and Zhou (1999) provided interesting remarks on the history of stochastic (as well as deterministic) optimal control theory. Bensoussan and Lions (1982) applied variational inequalities to stochastic control.

Filar and Vrieze (1997) provided a readable introduction to stochastic games.

Essential for the nonsmooth optimization are the concepts of generalized gradients, supergradients, and differential inclusions (see, e.g., Aubin and Frankowska, 1990). Optimality conditions have been derived using the above concepts (e.g., Clarke, 1976; Kaskosz & Lojasiewicz, 1985). For the numerical aspects see, e.g., Lempio and Veliov (1998).

Part IV

Appendices

A

Mathematical Background

We aim at keeping the theory presented in this textbook strictly target-oriented and therefore confine ourselves to spaces, terms, and concepts necessary to understand *nonlinear dynamics* and *optimal control theory.* For the reader searching for more information about the mathematics behind our straightforward approach we refer to additional literature on areas of expertise that go beyond the scope of this textbook. Thus this section is a concise survey of the basics, serving as a minimum standard.

A.1 General Notation and Functions

Here we review some basic material and notation used throughout the book. The notions of sets and functions are fundamental, as sets allow us to collect elements exhibiting some joint property, and functions describe relations between different sets.

We largely avoid the use of abbreviations and write logical operators in full length. The only logical abbreviation we use throughout the book is that of the term "if and only if" denoted as *iff*.

Sets and functions are used in a naive sense, where sets are denoted by capital letters A, $B, \dots$ and are formed by means of braces $\{\}$, so that

$$\{x : \text{proposition about } x\}$$

is the set of all elements x such that the properties about x are satisfied. A set $\{x\}$ containing exactly one element x is called a *singleton*. A singleton is often identified with the element itself.

If B is a *subset of* A we write $B \subset A$. To indicate that B is a *proper subset of* A, i.e., $B \subset A$ and $B \neq A$, we write $B \subsetneq A$. If B is *not a subset of* A we write $B \not\subset A$. The set

$$A \setminus B := \{x : x \in A, \quad \text{and} \quad x \notin B\}$$

denotes the *relative complement of* B *in* A.

Definition A.1. *The set*

$$\emptyset := \{x : x \neq x\}$$

is called the empty set *and is denoted by* $\emptyset$. *If* $A \neq \emptyset$, *then* A *is called a* non-empty set.

For two sets A, B *the set*

$$A \times B := \{(a, b) : \; a \in A, \quad \textit{and} \quad b \in B\}$$

is called the Cartesian product of A, B. *For* $A = B$ *the Cartesian product* $A \times A$ *is shortly written as* A^2 *or inductively defined for* $n \in \mathbb{N}$

$$A^n = \underbrace{A \times \cdots \times A}_{n-times}.$$

The usual sets we consider are those of the *natural numbers* $\mathbb{N}$, *integers* $\mathbb{Z}$, *real numbers* $\mathbb{R}$, *nonnegative real numbers* $\mathbb{R}_+$, *extended real numbers* $\bar{\mathbb{R}} = \mathbb{R} \cup \{\pm\infty\}$ and *complex numbers* $\mathbb{C}$.

Definition A.2 (Maximum, Upper Bound and Supremum). *Let* $A \subset \mathbb{R}$; *an element* $m \in A$ *is called a* maximal element *of* A *or shortly* maximum *of* A, *denoted as* $m = \max A$ *if* $x \in A$ *and* $x \geq m$ *implies* $x = m$.

An element $b \in \mathbb{R}$ *is called an* upper bound for A *if* $x \leq b$ *for all* $x \in A$.

An upper bound b *for* A *is called a* supremum of A, *denoted as* $b = \sup A$ *if* b *is the least upper bound for* A. *If no upper bound for* A *exists* $\sup A := \infty$.

If the inequalities are reversed the corresponding terms are minimum, lower bound *and* infimum.

A *function (mapping, transformation)* f describing a relation between the sets X and Y is denoted as

$$f : X \to Y,$$

and is specified by an explicit assignment

$$y = f(x), \quad \text{or} \quad x \mapsto f(x),$$

where x is called the *argument* of the function f. If there is no ambiguity, the argument of f is often omitted or the function is written as $f(\cdot)$. If $f(x)$ exhibits more than one element f is called a *multivalued* function. A "usual" function f is sometimes also referred to as a *single-valued* function.

Definition A.3. *Let* f *be a function from* X *into* Y; *then the set* X *is called the* domain *of* f *and the set* Y *is called the* codomain *of* f. *The* range of f *is defined as*

$$\operatorname{range} f = f(X) := \{f(x) : \; x \in X\}.$$

For $B \subset Y$ *the set*

$$f^{-1}(B) = \{x \in X : \; f(x) \in B\}$$

is called the preimage *of* B.

If $A \subset X$, then the function

$$f|_A : A \to Y, \quad \textit{with} \quad f|_A(x) = f(x), \textit{ for all } x \in A$$

is called the restriction *of f to A.*

The function $f(x) = x$ for $x \in X$ is called the identity function *and is denoted as* Id_X.

If the domain X of f is itself a set of functions then f is called a functional.

The function f is called injective *if for any $x_1, x_2 \in X$*

$$x_1 \neq x_2 \quad \textit{implies} \quad f(x_1) \neq f(x_2).$$

The function f is called surjective *if for any $y \in Y$ there exists an $x \in X$ satisfying $y = f(x)$. If the function f is injective and surjective, it is called* bijective.

If $f : X \to Y$ and $g : V \to W$ are two functions, satisfying $f(X) \subset V$, then the function $h : X \to W$ defined by

$$h(x) := g(f(x))$$

is called the composition function *of f and g, and is denoted as*

$$g \circ f.$$

The constant function *$f : X \to Y$ with*

$$f(x) = y_0, \quad y_0 \in Y,$$

for all $x \in X$ is denoted as $f \equiv y_0$.

From the definition of a bijective function we find the following proposition:

Proposition A.4. *Let $f : X \to Y$ be a bijective function; then there exists a unique bijective function $g : Y \to X$ satisfying*

$$f \circ g = g \circ f = \mathrm{Id}_X .$$

This unique function g is called the inverse function *of f and is denoted as f^{-1}.*

We are mostly concerned with functions $f : \mathbb{R}^n \to \mathbb{R}^m$, $n, m \in \mathbb{N}$. For $m = 1$, the function f is also called a *scalar* or *real-valued function*, as opposed to a *vector-valued* function if $m > 1$. In the latter case f will also be written as the m-tuple

$$f = \begin{pmatrix} f_1 \\ \vdots \\ f_m \end{pmatrix} \quad \text{with} \quad f(x) = \begin{pmatrix} f_1(x) \\ \vdots \\ f_m(x) \end{pmatrix}.$$

For $\mathbb{R}^n$ equipped with the usual norm (see Appendix A.2.7),

$$\|x\| = \sqrt{x_1^2 + \cdots x_n^2}, \quad x \in \mathbb{R}^n,$$

we can give the following definition:

Definition A.5 (Boundedness). *A function $f : \mathbb{R}^n \to \mathbb{R}^m$ is* bounded *if there exists $M > 0$ such that*

$$\|f(x)\| < M, \quad \textit{for all} \quad x \in \mathbb{R}^n.$$

Definition A.6 (Monotone Function). *Let $f : \mathbb{R} \to \mathbb{R}$, then f is called* increasing *or* non-decreasing *if for all $x \leq y$ one has $f(x) \leq f(y)$. If for all $x \leq y$ one has $f(x) \geq f(y)$ the function f is called* decreasing *or* non-increasing. *If the strict inequality holds f is called* strictly increasing *or* strictly decreasing, *respectively.*

A function, which is either increasing or decreasing is called a monotone *function.*

Definition A.7 (Level Set, Contour Line). *Let $f : \mathbb{R}^n \to \mathbb{R}$ and $c \in \mathbb{R}$; then the set*

$$N_f(c) := \{x : f(x) = c\}$$

is called the level set *of f for value c. For $n = 2$ a level set is also called a* contour line.

Definition A.8 (Epigraph). *Let $f : D \subset \mathbb{R}^n \to \mathbb{R}$; then the set*

$$\operatorname{epi}(f) := \{(x, r) \in \mathbb{R}^{n+1} : x \in D, \ \textit{and}\, r \geq f(x)\}$$

is called epigraph *of f.*

We often make use of the following function:

Definition A.9 (Absolute Value Function). *The function $f : \mathbb{R} \to \mathbb{R}$ defined by*

$$f(x) = \begin{cases} x & x \geq 0 \\ -x & x < 0, \end{cases}$$

is called the absolute value function *and is denoted by $|\cdot|$.*

A helpful notation for specifying the degree of approximation or convergence is the big-O and little-o notation, also known as the *Landau symbols*:

Definition A.10 (Landau Symbols). *Let $f : \mathbb{R}^n \to \mathbb{R}^m$ and $\alpha \in \mathbb{R}$; then f is called a* big-O *of $\|x\|^\alpha$, denoted as $f = O(\|x\|^\alpha)$ if there exists some $M > 0$ such that*

$$\lim_{\|x\| \to 0} \|f(x)\| / \|x\|^\alpha \leq M,$$

and f is called a little-o *of $\|x\|^\alpha$, denoted as $f = o(\|x\|^\alpha)$ if*

$$\lim_{\|x\| \to 0} \|f(x)\| / \|x\|^\alpha = 0.$$

Definition A.11 (Commutative Group). *Let G be a non-empty set and a function $+ : G \times G \to G$ defined on G satisfying:*

Associative Law: $(x + y) + z = x + (y + z)$ *for all* $x, y, z \in G$.
Neutral Element: there exists an element $e \in G$ *such that* $e + x = x + e = x$ *for all* $x \in G$.
Inverse Element: for every $x \in G$, *there exists an element* $-x \in G$ *such that* $x + (-x) = (-x) + x = e$.
Commutative Law: $x + y = y + x$ *for all* $x, y \in G$.

Then the pair $(G, +)$ *is called a* commutative group.

A.2 Finite-Dimensional Vector Spaces

In our discussion of vector space theory we focus on the real finite-dimensional case.

A.2.1 Vector Spaces, Linear Dependence, and Basis

We start by introducing the concept of a *real vector space* V:

Definition A.12 (Real Vector Space). *Let* $\mathbb{V}$ *be a set on which two operations are defined:*

Vector addition: $+ : \mathbb{V} \times \mathbb{V} \to \mathbb{V}$ *defined by*

$$x + y \in \mathbb{V}, \quad \textit{for all} \quad x, y \in \mathbb{V}. \tag{A.1a}$$

Scalar multiplication: $\cdot : \mathbb{R} \times \mathbb{V} \to \mathbb{V}$ *(the symbol* $\cdot$ *is mostly omitted)*

$$\alpha \cdot x \; (= \alpha x) \in V, \quad \textit{for all} \quad \alpha \in \mathbb{R}, x \in \mathbb{V}. \tag{A.1b}$$

Then the set $\mathbb{V}$, *together with the operations A.1a and A.1b, is called a* real vector space *if:*

1. $\mathbb{V}$ *is a commutative group with respect to vector addition.*
2. *For all* $\alpha, \beta \in \mathbb{R}$ *and* $x, y \in \mathbb{V}$ *we have*
   a) $(\alpha + \beta)x = \alpha x + \beta x$,
   b) $\alpha(x + y) = \alpha x + \beta y$,
   c) $(\alpha\beta)x = \alpha(\beta x)$,
   d) $1x = x$.

The elements of $\mathbb{V}$ *are called* vectors. *The neutral element of vector addition is called the* zero *or* null vector *and is denoted as* 0.
Let $x_i \in \mathbb{V}$, $i = 1, \ldots, m$; *then*

$$x = \sum_{i=1}^{m} \alpha_i x_i, \; \alpha_i \in \mathbb{R}$$

is called a linear combination *of the vectors* x_i.

Remark A.13. The adjective *real* refers to the fact that we consider only real numbers, α, as scalars. In a more general definition the scalars in Definition A.1b can be taken from the field of complex numbers or even any other field. Since we restrict our considerations to the real case, we omit the denotation real and simply speak about a vector space, instead of a real vector space.

Examples of vector spaces are:

Standard Space $\mathbb{R}^n$: The set $\mathbb{R}^n$ equipped with the following operations:
Vector addition: $+ : \mathbb{R}^n \times \mathbb{R}^n \to \mathbb{R}^n$ defined by

$$x + y := \begin{pmatrix} x_1 + y_1 \\ \vdots \\ x_n + y_n \end{pmatrix}, \quad \text{for all} \quad x, y \in \mathbb{R}^n. \tag{A.2a}$$

Scalar Multiplication: $\mathbb{R} \times \mathbb{R}^n \to \mathbb{R}^n$ defined by

$$\alpha x := \begin{pmatrix} \alpha x_1 \\ \vdots \\ \alpha x_n \end{pmatrix}, \quad \text{for all} \quad \alpha \in \mathbb{R}, \ x \in \mathbb{R}^n. \tag{A.2b}$$

Continuous functions: The set of real-valued continuous functions on $[0, T]$

$$C^0([0, T]) := \{f : f : [0, T] \to \mathbb{R} \quad \text{continuous}\},$$

together with the pointwise operations

$$\begin{aligned} (f + g)(x) &:= f(x) + g(x), \quad f, g \in C^0([0, T]), \\ (\alpha f)(x) &:= \alpha f(x), \quad f \in C^0([0, T]), \ \alpha \in \mathbb{R}. \end{aligned}$$

Definition A.14 (Subspace and Span). *Let $\mathbb{V}$ be a vector space. A non-empty subset $S \subset \mathbb{V}$ is called a* subspace of $\mathbb{V}$ *if the following properties hold:*

$$\begin{aligned} &x_1 + x_2 \in S, \quad \textit{for all} \quad x_1, x_2 \in S \\ &\alpha x \in S, \quad \textit{for all} \quad x \in S, \ \alpha \in \mathbb{R}. \end{aligned}$$

Let $A \subset \mathbb{V}$ then

$$\operatorname{span} A := \{x : x = \sum_{i=1}^{m} \alpha_i x_i, \ \alpha_i \in \mathbb{R}, \ x_i \in A, \ m \in \mathbb{N}\}$$

is a subspace of $\mathbb{V}$ and is called the span of A.

Given some subspace $S \subset \mathbb{V}$, one can ask: what is the minimum number of elements $x_i \in S$, $i \in I$ such that $S = \operatorname{span}\{x_i, i \in I\}$? This question gives rise to the central concept of linear dependence and independence in vector space theory:

Definition A.15. *A finite number of vectors $x_i, i = 1, \dots, m$ are called* linearly independent *if*

$$\sum_{i=1}^{m} \alpha_i x_i = 0$$

implies $\alpha_1 = \cdots = \alpha_m = 0$. Otherwise the vectors are called linearly dependent.

A subset $A \subset \mathbb{V}$ of $\mathbb{V}$ is called linear independent *if any finite collection of vectors of A is linearly independent.*

We can now introduce the important concept of a basis for a vector space $\mathbb{V}$:

Definition A.16 (Basis of a Vector Space). *Let B be a subset of the vector space $\mathbb{V}$; then B is called a* basis of the vector space $\mathbb{V}$ *if the following properties are satisfied:*

$$\mathbb{V} = \operatorname{span} B$$
$$B \quad \textit{is a linearly independent set.}$$

If the set B consists of a finite number n of elements, then the vector space $\mathbb{V}$ is called a finite *vector space of* dimension n, *written in shorthand as*

$$\dim \mathbb{V} = n.$$

Definition A.17 (Hyperplane). *Let $\mathbb{V}$ be an n-dimensional vector space; then an $n-1$-dimensional subspace is called a* (linear) hyperplane *in $\mathbb{V}$.*

Remark A.18. For two basis B and B' of a vector space $\mathbb{V}$ there exists a bijective transformation between B and B'. Thus in the finite-dimensional case the number of elements of B and B', respectively is unique.

Remark A.19. This definition justifies considering $\mathbb{R}^n$ together with vector addition (A.2a) and scalar multiplication (A.2b) as an n-dimensional vector space, since the n vectors

$$e_i = (e_i^j)_{j=1}^n = \begin{cases} 1 & j = i \\ 0 & j \neq i \end{cases},$$

$i = 1, \dots, n$, build a basis for $\mathbb{R}^n$. Indeed they form a particularly simple basis which is called the *canonical basis* of $\mathbb{R}^n$.

The importance of Definition A.16 stems from the property that any element $x \in \mathbb{V}$ can uniquely be written as a finite linear combination of elements of B.

Remark A.20. Whereas the number of vectors building a basis of a vector space is unique, the set of vectors is not. In fact, any linearly independent set of n vectors of $\mathbb{V}$ with $\dim \mathbb{V} = n$ can span the vector space.

Next, we consider the class of linear transformations $L : \mathbb{V} \to \mathbb{W}$.

A.2.2 Linear Transformations and Matrices

A linear transformation $L : \mathbb{V} \to \mathbb{W}$ is characterized by the following properties:

Definition A.21. *Let* $\mathbb{V}$ *and* $\mathbb{W}$ *be two vector spaces and* $L : \mathbb{V} \to \mathbb{W}$ *be a mapping; then* L *is called a* linear transformation *if the following properties are satisfied:*

$$L(x_1 + x_2) = L(x_1) + L(x_2), \quad \textit{for all} \quad x_1, x_2 \in \mathbb{V} \tag{A.3a}$$
$$L(\alpha x) = \alpha L(x), \quad \textit{for all} \quad x \in \mathbb{V}, \ \alpha \in \mathbb{R}. \tag{A.3b}$$

Remark A.22. The properties (A.3a) and (A.3b) assure that linear combinations in the vector space $\mathbb{V}$ are transformed by L into linear combinations in $\mathbb{W}$. Thus linear transformations preserve the vector-space structure of the sets $\mathbb{V}$ and $\mathbb{W}$ and are therefore the "natural" mappings to be considered in vector space theory.

For a linear transformation L one can show:

1. $L(\sum_{i=1}^{m} \alpha_i x_i) = \sum_{i=1}^{m} \alpha_i L(x_i)$ for all $\alpha_i \in \mathbb{R}$, $x_i \in \mathbb{R}^n$, $i = 1, \ldots, m$.
2. $L(0) = 0$ where 0 is the zero vector of the corresponding vector spaces.
3. If the transformation L is bijective, its inverse $L^{-1} : \mathbb{W} \to \mathbb{V}$ is also a linear transformation.
4. If $\mathbb{V}$ is finite-dimensional, then two linear transformations $L_1, L_2 : \mathbb{V} \to \mathbb{W}$ coinciding on a basis of $\mathbb{V}$ are identical.

Two important characteristics of a linear transformation $L : \mathbb{V} \to \mathbb{W}$ are its *kernel* and its *rank*, defined as

$$\begin{aligned} \operatorname{kern} L &:= \{x \in \mathbb{V} : \ L(x) = 0\} \\ \operatorname{rk} L &:= \dim \operatorname{range} L. \end{aligned}$$

The kernel is the set of all vectors mapped into the zero vector. The rank is the dimension of the range of L.

Definition A.23. *Let* $L : \mathbb{V} \to \mathbb{W}$ *be a bijective linear transformation; then* L *is called an* isomorphism *and* $\mathbb{V}$ *and* $\mathbb{W}$ *are called* isomorphic, *which can be written in shorthand as*

$$\mathbb{V} \cong \mathbb{W}.$$

Remark A.24. Isomorphic vector spaces are indistinguishable from the viewpoint of vector space theory.

Remark A.25. Every finite-dimensional vector space $\mathbb{V}$ with $\dim \mathbb{V} = n$ is isomorphic to the vector space $\mathbb{R}^n$, which justifies calling $\mathbb{R}^n$ the *standard space.*

Next we introduce matrices, which denote a "rectangular schema" of the form

$$A = (a_{ij}) = \begin{pmatrix} a_{11} & a_{12} & \cdots & a_{1n} \\ a_{21} & a_{22} & \cdots & a_{2n} \\ \vdots & \vdots & \ddots & \vdots \\ a_{m1} & a_{m2} & \cdots & a_{mn} \end{pmatrix}.$$

This is called an $m \times n$ *matrix*, with $m, n \in \mathbb{N}$, or a *matrix of* m *rows and* n *columns*. The set of all $m \times n$ matrices is denoted as $\mathbb{R}^{m\times n}$. The elements

$$a_j = \begin{pmatrix} a_{1j} \\ a_{2j} \\ \vdots \\ a_{mj} \end{pmatrix}, \quad j = 1, \dots, n$$

and

$$b_i = (a_{i1}, a_{i2}, \cdots, a_{in}), \quad i = 1, \dots, m$$

are called the *column vectors* and *row vectors* respectively. They are elements of $\mathbb{R}^{m\times 1}$ and $\mathbb{R}^{1\times n}$. The $m \times n$ matrix exhibiting only zeros is called the *null matrix* and denoted by 0. If $m = n$, then A is called a *square matrix of size* n; a_{ii}, $i = 1, \dots, n$ are called its *diagonal elements*, and

$$\operatorname{tr} A = \sum_{i=1}^{n} a_{ii},$$

is called the *trace of* A.

A square matrix A of the form

$$A = \begin{pmatrix} d_1 & 0 & \cdots & 0 \\ 0 & d_2 & \cdots & 0 \\ \vdots & \vdots & \ddots & \vdots \\ 0 & 0 & \cdots & d_n \end{pmatrix}, \quad d_i \in \mathbb{R}, \quad i = 1, \dots, n$$

is called a *diagonal matrix*.

The set $\mathbb{R}^{m\times n}$ together with the operations

$$\begin{aligned} A + B = (a_{ij}) + (b_{ij}) &:= (a_{ij} + b_{ij}), \quad \text{for all} \quad A, B \in \mathbb{R}^{m\times n} \\ \alpha A = \alpha(a_{ij}) &:= (\alpha a_{ij}), \quad \text{for all} \quad A \in \mathbb{R}^{m\times n}, \ \alpha \in \mathbb{R} \end{aligned}$$

is a real vector space of dimension mn.

Remark A.26. Note that we identify vector space $\mathbb{R}^n$ with $\mathbb{R}^{n\times 1}$ and a vector $x \in \mathbb{R}^n$ is therefore a column vector.

Additionally to the additive structure of matrices we can define a *matrix product* $\cdot : \mathbb{R}^{m\times n} \times \mathbb{R}^{n\times p} \to \mathbb{R}^{m\times p}$, where for matrices $A \in \mathbb{R}^{m\times n}$ and $B \in \mathbb{R}^{n\times p}$ the matrix product $A \cdot B$, which can be written more compactly as AB, is defined by the matrix C with the components

$$(c_{ij}) := \left(\sum_{k=1}^{n} a_{ik} b_{kj} \right).$$

For square matrices of size n the matrix product exhibits further properties. There exists an *identity* or *unit matrix*

$$\mathbb{I}^{(n)} := \begin{pmatrix} 1 & 0 & \cdots & 0 \\ 0 & 1 & \cdots & 0 \\ \vdots & \vdots & \ddots & \vdots \\ 0 & 0 & \cdots & 1 \end{pmatrix},$$

satisfying $A\mathbb{I}^{(n)} = \mathbb{I}^{(n)}A = A$ for all $A \in \mathbb{R}^{n\times n}$. If for a matrix $A \in \mathbb{R}^{n\times n}$ there exists a matrix $B \in \mathbb{R}^{n\times n}$ satisfying $AB = BA = \mathbb{I}^{(n)}$, then A is called *invertible* or *nonsingular* and B its *inverse matrix*. If A is not invertible it is called a *singular* matrix.

The following proposition states the important correspondence between matrices and linear transformations:

Proposition A.27. *Let $L : \mathbb{R}^n \to \mathbb{R}^m$ be a linear transformation; then there exists an $m \times n$ matrix A satisfying $L = L_A$, with*

$$L_A(x) = Ax, \quad \textit{for all} \quad x \in \mathbb{R}^n.$$

If B is an $n \times p$ matrix then

$$L_A \circ L_B = L_{AB}.$$

Given this unique correspondence between linear transformations and matrices, we can define the *kernel* and *rank* of a matrix $A : \mathbb{R}^n \to \mathbb{R}^m$ as

$$\begin{aligned} \operatorname{kern} A &= \{x \in \mathbb{R}^n : \; Ax = 0\} \\ \operatorname{rk} A &= \dim \operatorname{range} L_A. \end{aligned}$$

Moreover, it can be proved that:

$$\operatorname{rk} A = \dim \operatorname{span}\{a_j, \; j = 1, \ldots, n\} = \dim \operatorname{span}\{b_i, \; i = 1, \ldots, m\},$$

where a_j are the column vectors and b_i are the row vectors of A. Then we define:

Definition A.28 (Full Rank). *A matrix $A \in \mathbb{R}^{m\times n}$ is said to have* full rank *if*

$$\operatorname{rk} A = \min\{m, n\}.$$

Remark A.29. For an invertible matrix A with inverse B the corresponding linear transformations L_A and L_B satisfy $L_A \circ L_B = \mathrm{Id}$.

An important operation on $\mathbb{R}^{m\times n}$ is *transposition* along the main diagonal of A, which is defined as follows:

Definition A.30 (Transposition). *Let $A = (a_{ij})$ be an $m \times n$ matrix. Then the mapping $(\cdot)' : \mathbb{R}^{m\times n} \to \mathbb{R}^{n\times m}$ defined by*

$$A' := (a_{ji}) = \begin{pmatrix} a_{11} & a_{21} & \cdots & a_{m1} \\ a_{12} & a_{22} & \cdots & a_{m2} \\ \vdots & \vdots & \ddots & \vdots \\ a_{1n} & a_{2n} & \cdots & a_{mn} \end{pmatrix},$$

is called transposition *and A' is called the* transposed matrix of A.

The transposition satisfies the following properties:

1. $(\alpha A + \beta B)' = \alpha A' + \beta B'$ for all $A, B \in \mathbb{R}^{m\times n}$, $\alpha, \beta \in \mathbb{R}$.
2. $(A')' = A$ for all $A \in \mathbb{R}^{m\times n}$.
3. $(\cdot)' : \mathbb{R}^{m\times n} \to \mathbb{R}^{n\times m}$ is an isomorphism.

Definition A.31 (Definiteness, Symmetric and Skew-Symmetric). *Let A be an $n \times n$ matrix satisfying*

$$x'Ax \leq 0, \quad \textit{for all} \quad x \in \mathbb{R}^n,$$

then A is called negative semidefinite. *If strict inequality holds, it is called* negative definite. *For the opposite inequality $>$ $(\geq)$ the matrix is called* positive (semi)definite.

If A satisfies $A = A'$; then A is called a symmetric *matrix. If A satisfies $A = -A'$; then A is called a* skew-symmetric *matrix.*

A.2.3 Inverse Matrices and Linear Equations

We have seen that invertible matrices can be defined for $n \times n$-matrices. We denote the set of invertible matrices as the *general linear group*

$$\mathrm{GL}_n := \{A \in \mathbb{R}^{n\times n} : A \text{ invertible}\}.$$

The set GL_n exhibits the following properties:

1. For $A \in \mathrm{GL}_n$ there exists a *unique* inverse matrix V, denoted as $A^{-1} := V$.
2. If $A, B \in \mathrm{GL}_n$, then also $AB \in \mathrm{GL}_n$ with $(AB)^{-1} = B^{-1}A^{-1}$.
3. If $A \in \mathrm{GL}_n$, then also $A^{-1} \in \mathrm{GL}_n$ with $(A^{-1})^{-1} = A$.
4. If $A \in \mathrm{GL}_n$, then also $A' \in \mathrm{GL}_n$ with $(A')^{-1} = (A^{-1})'$.

To decide whether a square matrix A is invertible, the following criteria can be applied:

Theorem A.32 (Equivalence Theorem for Inverse Matrices). *For a matrix $A \in \mathbb{R}^{n \times n}$ the following properties are equivalent:*

1. $A \in \mathrm{GL}_n$.
2. *The mapping* $x \mapsto Ax$ *is bijective.*
3. *The mapping* $x \mapsto Ax$ *is injective.*
4. *The rows of* A *form a basis of* $\mathbb{R}^n$.
5. *The columns of* A *form a basis of* $\mathbb{R}^n$.
6. A *has full rank, i.e.,* $\operatorname{rk} A = n$.

Matrices were first introduced as a short notation for linear equations, i.e.,

$$\begin{cases} a_{11}x_1 + a_{12}x_2 + \cdots + a_{1n}x_n = b_1 \\ a_{21}x_1 + a_{22}x_2 + \cdots + a_{2n}x_n = b_2 \\ \cdots\cdots\cdots\cdots\cdots\cdots\cdots\cdots\cdots \\ a_{m1}x_1 + a_{m2}x_2 + \cdots + a_{mn}x_n = b_m \end{cases}$$

which in matrix notation can be written very concisely as

$$Ax = b, \quad \text{with} \quad A = \begin{pmatrix} a_{11} & \cdots & a_{1n} \\ \vdots & \ddots & \vdots \\ a_{m1} & \cdots & a_{mn} \end{pmatrix}, \; x = \begin{pmatrix} x_1 \\ \vdots \\ x_n \end{pmatrix}, \; b = \begin{pmatrix} b_1 \\ \vdots \\ b_m \end{pmatrix}, \tag{A.4}$$

where A and b are given and x is unknown:

Definition A.33 (Solvability). *Let* $A \in \mathbb{R}^{m \times n}$ *and* $b \in \mathbb{R}^m$. *If there exists a vector* $y \in \mathbb{R}^n$ *satisfying*

$$Ay = b;$$

then (A.4) is called solvable *and* y *is called a* solution *of (A.4).*

An important question when solving linear equations is whether there is a unique solution. The answer depends on the properties of matrix A:

Theorem A.34. *Let* $A \in \mathbb{R}^{n \times n}$*; then the following propositions are equivalent:*

1. *For every* $b \in \mathbb{R}^n$ *there exists an* $x \in \mathbb{R}^n$ *satisfying* $Ax = b$.
2. $Ax = 0$ *has the unique solution* $x = 0$.
3. $A \in \mathrm{GL}_n$.

For $A \in \mathrm{GL}_n$ *the solution of* $Ax = b$ *is uniquely given by* $x = A^{-1}b$.

An important theorem that has many extensions to more general cases, known as the *Fredholm Alternative*, can be stated as:

Theorem A.35 (Finite-Dimensional Fredholm Alternative). *Let* $A \in \mathbb{R}^{m \times n}$ *and* $b \in \mathbb{R}^m$. *Then the equation* $Ax = b$ *has a solution iff* $y'b = 0$ *for every* $y \in \mathbb{R}^m$ *satisfying* $y'A = 0$.

Here we also state the Farkas lemma (Farkas, 1902), which is an extension of the previous theorem to the case in which inequalities have to be considered.

First we introduce the notational convention that for an $m \times n$ matrix $A = (a_{ij})$

$$A \geq 0 \quad \text{iff} \quad a_{ij} \geq 0, \quad \text{for all} \quad i = 1, \dots, m, \; j = 1, \dots, n.$$

Theorem A.36 (Farkas Lemma). *Let $A \in \mathbb{R}^{m\times n}$ and $b \in \mathbb{R}^m$. Then the following propositions are equivalent:*

1. *The system of linear equations $Ax = b$ has a solution $x \in \mathbb{R}^n$ with $x \geq 0$.*
2. *If $y \in \mathbb{R}^m$ satisfies $y'A \geq 0$, then $y'b \geq 0$.*

For a proof see Appendix B.1 and for a geometric interpretation see Fig. A.1.

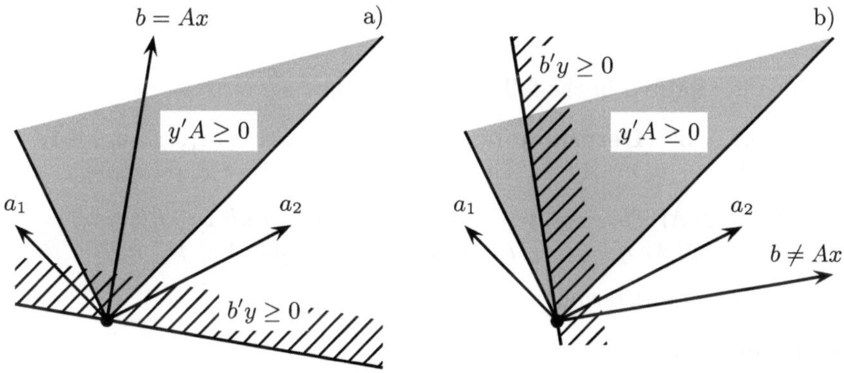

Fig. A.1. This figure depicts the geometric argument for the Farkas lemma for $n = m = 2$. Let C (*gray area*) be the positive cone $\{y : y'A \geq 0\}$, with $A = (a_1, a_2)$. In case (**a**) it is shown that if the vector b lies in the positive cone spanned by a_1 and a_2 then C is contained in the positive half-plane given by $b'z \geq 0$. In case (**b**) there exist directions y with $y'A \geq 0$ which do not satisfy $b'y \geq 0$

A.2.4 Determinants

To motivate the introduction of the important concept of a determinant, let us consider a parallelogram in $\mathbb{R}^2$ given by the vectors a, b (Fig. A.2). If we let $\mathcal{A}(a, b)$ be the area of the parallelogram a little thought shows that the function $\mathcal{A}(a, b)$ satisfied the following properties:

1. $\mathcal{A}(a + b, b) = \mathcal{A}(a, b)$ and $\mathcal{A}(a, b + a) = \mathcal{A}(a, b)$.
2. $\mathcal{A}(\lambda a, b) = \lambda\mathcal{A}(a, b)$ and $\mathcal{A}(a, \lambda b) = \lambda\mathcal{A}(a, b)$ for $\lambda \geq 0$.
3. $\mathcal{A}(a, b) = 0$ if a, b are linearly dependent.

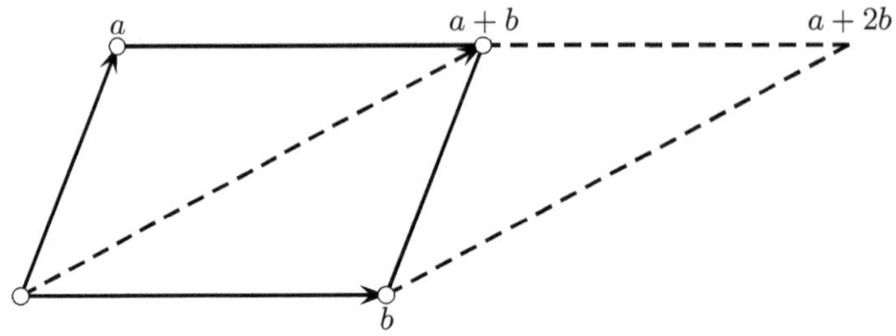

Fig. A.2. Using the geometric properties of a parallelogram we see that the areas of both parallelograms spanned by a, b and by $a+b$, b are equal. Denoting the areas as $\mathcal{A}(a,b)$ and $\mathcal{A}(a+b,b)$ this yields the identity $\mathcal{A}(a,b) = \mathcal{A}(a+b,b)$, which can be used as a defining property for the determinant. It reveals that the determinant can be interpreted as a "signed" area

4. $\mathcal{A}(e_1, e_2) = 1$.

This idea is captured in the following definition:

Definition A.37 (Determinant Function). *Let $A = (a_1, \ldots, a_n) \in \mathbb{R}^{n\times n}$, and $B = (b_1, \ldots, b_n) \in \mathbb{R}^{n\times n}$. The function $\Delta : \mathbb{R}^{n\times n} \to \mathbb{R}$ satisfying:*

1. *$\Delta(B) = \Delta(A)$ if $b_i = a_i$, $i \neq j$ and $b_j = a_j + \alpha a_k$ with $1 \le j, k \le n$, $\alpha \in \mathbb{R}$.*
2. *$\Delta(B) = \beta\Delta(A)$ if $b_i = a_i$, $i \neq j$ and $b_j = \beta a_j$ with $1 \le j \le n$, $\beta \in \mathbb{R}$.*

then Δ is called a determinant function.

Now it can be proved:

Proposition A.38. *For all $n \in \mathbb{N}$ there exists a unique determinant function*

$$\det : \mathbb{R}^{n\times n} \to \mathbb{R}$$

satisfying

$$\det \mathbb{I}^{(n)} = 1.$$

Then $\det(A)$ *also written as* $\det A$ *is called the* determinant *of matrix A.*

For all $A, B, C, D \in \mathbb{R}^{n\times n}$, α, $\beta \in \mathbb{R}$ and $x, y \in \mathbb{R}^n$ the following properties hold:

1. $\det : \mathbb{R}^{n\times n} \to \mathbb{R}$ is multilinear, i.e.,

$$\det((\ldots, \alpha x + \beta y, \ldots)) = \alpha \det((\ldots, x, \ldots)) + \beta \det((\ldots, y, \ldots)).$$

2. $\det AB = \det A \det B$.
3. $\det \alpha A = \alpha^n \det A$.
4. $\det A' = \det A$.

5.
$$\det \begin{pmatrix} A & B \\ 0 & D \end{pmatrix} = \det A \det D = \det \begin{pmatrix} A & 0 \\ C & D \end{pmatrix} \quad \text{(block structure)}.$$

6. Setting
$$e^A := \sum_{i=0}^{\infty} \frac{A^i}{i!}$$
we find
$$\det e^A = e^{\operatorname{tr} A}. \tag{A.5}$$

7. If A is invertible the identity
$$e^{A^{-1}BA} = A^{-1} e^B A$$
holds.

We can now provide a further criterion characterizing invertible matrices A:

Theorem A.39. *Let $A \in \mathbb{R}^{n \times n}$; then the following properties are equivalent:*

1. $A \in \mathrm{GL}_n$.
2. $\det A \neq 0$.

In this case we also find that
$$\det\left(A^{-1}\right) = (\det A)^{-1}.$$

A.2.5 Linear Form and Dual Space

Next we consider linear mappings from a vector space into the set, considered as the vector space, of real numbers $\mathbb{R}$:

Definition A.40. *Let $\mathbb{V}$ be a vector space and $L : \mathbb{V} \to \mathbb{R}$ be a linear transformation; then L is called a* linear form *of $\mathbb{V}$. The vector space of the linear forms of $\mathbb{V}$ is called the* dual space *of $\mathbb{V}$, denoted by $\mathbb{V}^*$.*

For the vector space $\mathbb{R}^n$ the following proposition can be proved:

Proposition A.41 (Basis of Linear Forms). *Let $a_1, \ldots, a_n$ be a basis of $\mathbb{R}^n$; then there exist linear forms $\lambda_1, \ldots, \lambda_n$ of $\mathbb{R}^n$ satisfying*
$$\lambda_i(a_j) = \begin{cases} 1 & i = j \\ 0 & i \neq j, \end{cases} \tag{A.6}$$
that build a basis of $(\mathbb{R}^n)^*$.

Definition A.42 (Dual Basis of $\mathbb{R}^n$). *The basis defined by (A.6) is called the* dual basis of $(\mathbb{R}^n)^*$ associated with $a_1, \ldots, a_n$.

From the foregoing identification of matrices and linear transformations we know that a linear form λ of $\mathbb{R}^n$ can be identified as an element of $\mathbb{R}^{1\times n}$, i.e., a row vector. Thus a corollary of Proposition A.41 is:

Corollary A.43. *Let λ be a linear form of $\mathbb{R}^n$, i.e., $\lambda \in (\mathbb{R}^n)^*$, then there exists a unique row vector $a \in \mathbb{R}^{1\times n}$ satisfying*

$$\lambda(x) = ax = \sum_{i=1}^{n} a_i x_i. \tag{A.7}$$

Identifying the linear form with its vector representation we find:

Corollary A.44. *The vector space $\mathbb{R}^n$ is isomorphic to its dual space $(\mathbb{R}^n)^*$, i.e.,*

$$\mathbb{R}^n \cong (\mathbb{R}^n)^*.$$

Since the expression (A.7) proves important, we give it the following definition:

Definition A.45 (Scalar Product). *Let x, $y \in \mathbb{R}^n$. Then the expression*

$$\langle x, y\rangle := x'y = \sum_{i=1}^{n} x_i y_i = x_1y_1 + x_2y_2 + \ldots + x_ny_n,$$

is called the scalar product *of x and y.*

The scalar product satisfies the following properties:

Bilinearity: $\langle x, y\rangle$ is linear in both x and y.
Symmetry: $\langle x, y\rangle = \langle y, x\rangle$ for all $x, y \in \mathbb{R}^n$.
Nondegeneracy: $\langle x, y\rangle = 0$ for all $y \in \mathbb{R}^n$ implies that $x = 0$.
Positivity: $\langle x, x\rangle > 0$ for all $x \in \mathbb{R}^n$ and $x \neq 0$.
Cauchy-Schwarz inequality: $\langle x, y\rangle^2 \leq \langle x, x\rangle \langle y, y\rangle$ for all x, $y \in \mathbb{R}^n$, where the equality holds iff x and y are linearly dependent.
For $A \in \mathbb{R}^{m\times n}$ and $x \in \mathbb{R}^n$, $y \in \mathbb{R}^m$ we have

$$\langle Ax, y\rangle = \langle x, A'y\rangle.$$

Definition A.46 (Half-Space). *Let $a \in \mathbb{R}^n$ with $a \neq 0$ and $\alpha \in \mathbb{R}$, then the set*

$$\{x : \langle a, x\rangle \geq \alpha\}$$

is called a half-space. *If $n = 2$ the set is called a* half-plane *and for $n = 1$ it is called a* half-line.

A.2.6 Eigenvalues and Eigenvectors

A central concept for the application of vector space theory is that of an eigenvalue and eigenvector, defined by:

Definition A.47 (Eigenvalue and Eigenvector). *Let A be an $n \times n$ matrix and $\nu \in \mathbb{R}^n$ with $\nu \neq 0$. If there exists an $\xi \in \mathbb{R}$ such that*

$$A\nu = \xi\nu, \tag{A.8}$$

then ξ is called an eigenvalue *of A, and every vector ν satisfying (A.8) is called an* eigenvector *of ξ.*
The vector space

$$\mathrm{E}^{\xi} = \mathrm{span}\{\nu : A\nu = \xi\nu\}$$

is called the eigenspace *of the eigenvalue ξ.*

From (A.8) the following characterization of an eigenvalue and eigenvector immediately follows:

Lemma A.48. *Let $A \in \mathbb{R}^{n \times n}$ and $\xi \in \mathbb{R}$, then the following propositions are equivalent:*

1. *ξ is an eigenvalue of A.*
2. $\det\left(\xi\mathbb{I}^{(n)} - A\right) = 0$.

Definition A.49. *The polynomial*

$$\chi_A(x) := \det\left(x\mathbb{I}^{(n)} - A\right)$$

is called the characteristic polynomial *of A.*

Remark A.50. In general the characteristic polynomial of $A \in \mathbb{R}^{n \times n}$ exhibits also complex roots. Thus eigenvalues with $\xi = \xi_R + \mathrm{i}\xi_I \in \mathbb{C}$ have to be considered. In that case its complex conjugate $\bar{\xi} = \xi_R - \mathrm{i}\xi_I$ is an eigenvalue and $\mathrm{E}^{\bar{\nu}} \subset \mathbb{C}^n$.

Proposition A.51. *Let A be a real $n \times n$ matrix; then A' has the same eigenvalues as A.*

It is often important to find for a given matrix A another matrix B whose representation is as simple as possible while still exhibiting the same characteristic properties. We therefore define:

Definition A.52 (Similar and Diagonalizable Matrices). *Two matrices $A, B \in \mathbb{R}^{n \times n}$ are called* similar *if there exists a matrix $W \in \mathrm{GL}_n$ such that*

$$W^{-1}AW = B.$$

If B is a diagonal matrix then A is called diagonalizable.

The following proposition shows that if the eigenvectors of a matrix form a basis for $\mathbb{R}^n$ then that matrix can be transformed into a simple form:

Proposition A.53. *Let A be an $n \times n$ matrix exhibiting n distinct real eigenvalues $\xi_1, \ldots, \xi_n$; then A is diagonalizable, satisfying*

$$UAU^{-1} = \begin{pmatrix} \xi_1 & 0 & \cdots & 0 \\ 0 & \xi_2 & \cdots & 0 \\ \vdots & \vdots & \ddots & \vdots \\ 0 & 0 & \cdots & \xi_n \end{pmatrix},$$

where the rows of the matrix U are given by the transposed eigenvectors ν_i'.

Definition A.54 (Upper Triangular Matrix). *A matrix $A \in \mathbb{R}^{n\times n}$ of the form*

$$A = \begin{pmatrix} a_{11} & a_{12} & \cdots & a_{1n} \\ 0 & a_{22} & \cdots & a_{2n} \\ \vdots & \vdots & \ddots & \vdots \\ 0 & 0 & \cdots & a_{nn} \end{pmatrix}$$

is called an upper triangular matrix. *If the diagonal elements are also zero then A is called a* strictly upper triangular matrix.

Proposition A.53 assumes that the zeros of the characteristic polynomial are distinct and real. In general this does not hold, therefore we define:

Definition A.55 (Reducible Matrix). *A matrix $A \in \mathbb{R}^{n\times n}$ is called* reducible *if its characteristic polynomial is of the form*

$$\chi_A(x) = (x - \xi_1)^{n_1} \cdot \ldots \cdot (x - \xi_m)^{n_m}, \quad m \le n, \;\; n_1 + \cdots n_m = n, \tag{A.9}$$

with distinct $\xi_i \in \mathbb{R}$, $i = 1, \ldots, m$.

The so-called *Jordan normal form* exploits this fact to generalize Proposition A.53:

Theorem A.56 (Jordan Normal Form). *Let $A \in \mathbb{R}^{n\times n}$ be a reducible matrix with a characteristic polynomial of the form (A.9). Then A is similar to a matrix J of the following type:*

$$J = \begin{pmatrix} B_1 & 0 & \cdots & 0 \\ 0 & B_2 & \cdots & 0 \\ \vdots & \vdots & \ddots & \vdots \\ 0 & 0 & \cdots & B_m \end{pmatrix},$$

where B_j is a quadratic $n_j \times n_j$ matrix for $j = 1, \ldots, m$ exhibiting the following form:

$$B_j = \xi_j \mathbb{I}^{(n_j)} + N$$

and N is a strictly upper triangular matrix.

Remark A.57. Note that if we consider the vector space $\mathbb{R}^n$ over the field of complex numbers then the characteristic polynomial is always reducible to linear factors. For this vector space the Jordan normal form exists for every matrix $A \in \mathbb{R}^{n \times n}$.

There exist powerful numerical algorithms to compute the eigenvalues and corresponding eigenvectors (see, e.g., Golub & van Loan, 1996), whereas the following recursive formula proves sometimes useful for deriving theoretical results (see Appendix B.8):

Theorem A.58 (Characteristic Polynomial). *Let A be an $n \times n$ matrix and $\sigma_k = \operatorname{tr}(A^k)$ denote the trace of A^k. Then the characteristic polynomial $\chi_A(x)$ can be written as*

$$\chi_A(x) = \sum_{j=0}^{n} (-1)^j \omega_j(A) x^{n-j}, \tag{A.10}$$

where $\omega_0(A) = 1$ and for any $1 \le j \le n$, $\omega_j(A)$ can iteratively be calculated by

$$j\omega_j(A) = \sum_{k=1}^{j} (-1)^{k+1} \sigma_k \omega_{j-k}(A).$$

The following proposition allows a simple characterization of a subspace spanned by eigenvectors:

Proposition A.59. *Let ξ_i, $i = 1, \ldots, m \le n$ be the eigenvalues of the matrix $A \in \mathbb{R}^{n \times n}$. Assume that $\xi_1 \in \mathbb{R}$ has a one-dimensional eigenspace. Then*

$$y \in \operatorname{span}\{\mathrm{E}^{\xi_i} : i \ge 2\} \quad \textit{iff} \quad b_1' y = 0,$$

where b_1 is the eigenvector of the transposed matrix A' corresponding to the eigenvalue ξ_1.

A.2.7 Euclidean Vector Space $\mathbb{R}^n$

If we want to "measure" distances between vectors, we need a well-defined concept of "length." We start developing such a "device to measure length" by introducing the concept of a norm:

Definition A.60. *Let $\|\cdot\| : \mathbb{V} \to \mathbb{R}$ be a function satisfying the following conditions:*

$$\begin{aligned} &\|x\| = 0 \quad \textit{iff} \quad x = 0 \\ &\|\alpha x\| = |\alpha| \|x\|, \quad \textit{for all} \quad \alpha \in \mathbb{R},\ x \in \mathbb{V} \\ &\|x + y\| \le \|x\| + \|y\|, \quad \textit{for all} \quad x, y \in \mathbb{V}. \end{aligned}$$

Then $\|\cdot\|$ is called a norm *of the vector space $\mathbb{V}$ and the pair $(\mathbb{V}, \|\cdot\|)$ is called a* normed vector space.

Reconsidering the properties of the scalar product for $\mathbb{V} = \mathbb{R}^n$, one can prove that the function,

$$\|x\|_s := \sqrt{\langle x, x \rangle}, \tag{A.11}$$

satisfies the axioms of a norm. Therefore we can define:

Definition A.61. *Let* $\|\cdot\|_s$ *be given by (A.11); then* $(\mathbb{R}^n, \|\cdot\|_s)$ *is called the* Euclidean vector space. *Moreover,* $\|x\|_s$ *is called the* length *of* x *and*

$$\mathrm{d}(x, y) := \|x - y\|_s$$

is called the distance *between* x *and* y. *If*

$$\langle x, y \rangle = 0,$$

then x *and* y *are called* orthogonal (normal, perpendicular), *also denoted by* $x \perp y$.
For $S \subset \mathbb{R}^n$ *the set*

$$S^{\perp} := \{x : \ x \perp s, \quad \textit{for all } s \in S\}$$

is called the orthogonal complement *of* S.

In Euclidean spaces it is possible to construct a basis exhibiting the specific property of orthonormality. We therefore define as follows:

Definition A.62. *Let* $(\mathbb{R}^n, \|\cdot\|_s)$ *be the Euclidean vector space; then the vectors* $b_1, \ldots, b_n$, *satisfying property*

$$\langle b_i, b_j \rangle = \begin{cases} 1 & i = j \\ 0 & i \neq j \end{cases}$$

are called an orthonormal basis *of* $(\mathbb{R}^n, \|\cdot\|_s)$.

Using this definition the following classical result can be proved:

Theorem A.63 (Gram-Schmidt Process). *For the Euclidean vector space* $(\mathbb{R}^n, \|\cdot\|_s)$ *there exists an orthonormal basis. For a given basis* $b_1, \ldots, b_n$ *an orthonormal basis* $\tilde{b}_1, \ldots, \tilde{b}_n$ *can be constructed as follows:*

$$d_1 = b_1, \quad \tilde{b}_1 = \frac{b_1}{\|b_1\|}$$

$$d_{j+1} = b_{j+1} - \sum_{i=1}^{j} \frac{\langle d_i, b_{j+1} \rangle}{\langle d_i, d_i \rangle} d_i, \quad \tilde{b}_{j+1} = \frac{d_{j+1}}{\|d_{j+1}\|}, \quad j = 1, \ldots, n-1.$$

Remark A.64. For an orthonormal basis $b_1, \ldots, b_n$, an arbitrary vector $x \in \mathbb{R}^n$ is represented by

$$x = \sum_{i=1}^{n} \langle b_i, x \rangle \, b_i.$$

A.3 Topology and Calculus

A.3.1 Open Set, Neighborhood, and Convergence

Next we introduce the concept of an open set for the specific case of the Euclidean vector space $(\mathbb{R}^n, \|\cdot\|_s)$. Subsequently we use $\|\cdot\|$ instead of $\|\cdot\|_s$:

Definition A.65 (Open Set and Neighborhood). *Let* $(\mathbb{R}^n, \|\cdot\|)$ *be the Euclidean vector space and* O *be a subset of* $\mathbb{R}^n$. *If for any* $x \in O$ *there exists an* $\varepsilon > 0$ *with*

$$N(x, \varepsilon) = N_\varepsilon(x) := \{y : \|y - x\| < \varepsilon\}$$

satisfying

$$N(x, \varepsilon) \subset O;$$

then U *is called an* open set *of* $\mathbb{R}^n$ *and* $N(x, \varepsilon)$ *is called an* open ball *or* ε-neighborhood. *The set*

$$\tau = \{O : O \text{ open}\}$$

is called the norm topology *of* $\mathbb{R}^n$ *and the pair* $(\mathbb{R}^n, \tau)$ *is called the corresponding* topological space.

A set U *with* $x \in U \subset \mathbb{R}^n$ *for which there exists an open set* O *with* $x \in O$ *and* $O \subset U$ *is called a* neighborhood *of* x.

From the definition of an open set the following properties of the topology τ can be derived:

Finite Intersection: If O_1, $O_2 \in \tau$ then also $O_1 \cap O_2 \in \tau$.
Arbitrary Union: If for all $i \in I$, $O_i \in \tau$, then $\bigcup_{i \in I} O_i \in \tau$.

In a general approach these properties are used to define a topology τ. It is possible to use a complementary approach:

Definition A.66 (Closed Set). *Let* O *be an open set; then the set* $C = \mathbb{R}^n \setminus O$ *is called a* closed set.
The set

$$\overline{N}(x, \varepsilon) := \{y : \|y - x\| \leq \varepsilon\}$$

is called the closed ball *of* x.

One can immediately prove the following properties:

1. If C_1, C_2 are closed, then $C_1 \cup C_2$ is also closed.
2. If for all $i \in I$, C_i is closed, then $\bigcap_{i \in I} C_i$ is closed.
3. The set

   $$\overline{N}(x, \varepsilon) := \{y : \|y - x\| \leq \varepsilon\}$$

   is closed for the norm topology.

We now define the terms interior, closure, and boundary for an arbitrary set S:

Definition A.67. *Let S be a subset of the topological space $(\mathbb{R}^n, \tau)$; then the set*

$$S^\circ := \bigcup_{O \subset S} O, \quad O \text{ open}$$

is called the interior *of S, the set*

$$\overline{S} := \bigcap_{S \subset C} C, \quad C \text{ closed}$$

is called the closure *of S, and the set*

$$\partial S = \overline{S} \setminus S^\circ$$

is called the boundary *of S.*

Another important concept is that of compactness:

Definition A.68 (Compactness). *Let $K \subset \mathbb{R}^n$; then K is called* compact *if for any open cover $(O_i)_{i \in I}$ of K, i.e., $K \subset \bigcup_{i \in I} O_i$, there exists a finite subset $F \subset I$ such that $K \subset \bigcup_{i \in F} O_i$ is satisfied.*

Theorem A.69 (Heine–Borel). *The set $K \subset \mathbb{R}^n$ is compact iff K is closed and bounded, i.e., $K = \overline{K}$ and there exists $x \in K$ and $r > 0$ with $K \subset N(x, r)$.*

We can now provide a precise definition of *convergence* in $\mathbb{R}^n$:

Definition A.70 (Convergence in $\mathbb{R}^n$). *A sequence $(x_i)_{i \in \mathbb{N}}$ with $x_i \in \mathbb{R}^n$ is said to* converge *to $\hat{x} \in \mathbb{R}^n$ (abbreviated by $\lim_{i \to \infty} x_i = \hat{x}$) if for every $\varepsilon > 0$ there exists an $M \in \mathbb{N}$, in general depending on ε, such that for all $i \geq M$*

$$x_i \in N(\hat{x}, \varepsilon).$$

Then $\hat{x}$ is called the limit *of the sequence $(x_i)_{i \in \mathbb{N}}$.*

Theorem A.71 (Bolzano–Weierstrass Theorem). *Let $(x_i)_{i \in \mathbb{N}} \subset \mathbb{R}^n$ be a bounded sequence; then there exists a convergent subsequence, i.e., $\hat{x} \in \mathbb{R}^n$ and $i_j \in \mathbb{N}$ with $i_{j+1} > i_j$ for $j \in \mathbb{N}$ such that*

$$\lim_{j \to \infty} x_{i_j} = \hat{x}.$$

Given this introduction to some topological concepts, we now introduce the basic concepts of calculus.

A.3.2 Continuity and Differentiability

The topological structure of $\mathbb{R}^n$ allows one to tackle the important questions of continuity and differentiability:

Definition A.72 (Continuity). *A function $f : D \subset \mathbb{R}^n \to \mathbb{R}^m$, with D open, is* continuous *at $\hat{x} \in D$ if for every $\varepsilon > 0$ there exists a $\delta > 0$ such that*

$$\|x - \hat{x}\| < \delta$$

implies

$$\|f(x) - f(\hat{x})\| < \varepsilon.$$

The function f is called continuous *in $D \subset \mathbb{R}^n$ if it is continuous for all $x \in D \subset \mathbb{R}^n$.*
The set of all continuous functions of $f : D \subset \mathbb{R}^n \to \mathbb{R}^m$ is denoted as

$$C^0(D, \mathbb{R}^m) \quad or \quad C^0(D), \quad or\ even \quad C^0,$$

if there is no ambiguity concerning the codomain $\mathbb{R}^m$ or the domain D.

In terms of limits it can easily be proved that this definition is equivalent to a formulation with sequences:

Proposition A.73. *Let $f : D \subset \mathbb{R}^n \to \mathbb{R}^m$, with D open; then f is continuous at $\hat{x}$ iff for every sequence $(x_i)_{i\in\mathbb{N}}$ satisfying*

$$\lim_{i\to\infty} x_i = 0$$

such that $\hat{x} + x_i \in D$

$$\lim_{i\to\infty} f(\hat{x} + x_i) = f(\hat{x})$$

holds.

Remark A.74. The reader may also verify that Definition A.72 is equivalent to the requirement that

$$N(\hat{x}, \delta) \subset f^{-1}\left(N\left(f(\hat{x}), \varepsilon\right)\right).$$

Since only the concept of neighborhood is used, continuity can be defined for arbitrary topological spaces and not only for normed spaces.

Proposition A.75 ($C^0(\mathbb{R}, \mathbb{R}^n)$ as a Normed Vector Space). *The following pair $(C^0(\mathbb{R}, \mathbb{R}^n), \|\cdot\|_\infty)$ with*

$$\|f\|_\infty := \sup_{x\in\mathbb{R}} \|f(x)\|, \quad for \quad f \in C^0(\mathbb{R}, \mathbb{R}^n)$$

is a normed vector space and $\|f\|_\infty$ is called the supremum norm *of f.*

The following type of continuity proves important for existence and uniqueness results for ODEs:

Definition A.76 (Lipschitz Continuity). *A function $f : D \subset \mathbb{R}^n \to \mathbb{R}^m$, with D open, is* Lipschitz continuous *if there exists a constant $K \geq 0$ such all $x, y \in D$ satisfy*

$$\|f(x) - f(y)\| \leq K\|x - y\|.$$

Definition A.77 (Uniform Continuity). *A function $f : D \subset \mathbb{R}^n \to \mathbb{R}^m$, with D open, is* uniformly continuous *in D if for every $\varepsilon > 0$ there exists a $\delta > 0$ such that for all $x, y \in D$ with*

$$\|x - y\| < \delta$$

also

$$\|f(x) - f(y)\| < \varepsilon$$

holds.

Remark A.78. In the definition of continuity δ may depend on ε as well as on $\hat{x}$. In the case of uniform continuity δ only depends on ε.

For functions with a scalar argument we introduce the concept of right- and left-hand continuity:

Definition A.79 (Right- and Left-Hand Continuity). *Let $f : (a, b) \subset \mathbb{R} \to \mathbb{R}^m$; we say that the* right-hand limit *of f at a is $f(a^+)$ (or* left-hand limit *of f at b is $f(b^-)$), and we write,*

$$\lim_{x \to a^+} f(x) = f(a^+) \quad \left(or \quad \lim_{x \to b^-} f(x) = f(b^-) \right),$$

if there exists $y \in \mathbb{R}$ such that for every $\varepsilon > 0$ there exists a $\delta > 0$ such that

$$\|f(x) - y\| < \varepsilon$$

whenever $x \in (a, b)$ and $x - a < \delta$ (or $b - x < \delta$). We then set $f(a^+) := y$ (or $f(b^-) := y$).

Suppose that f is defined on $[a, b]$. Then f is called right continuous *at a (or* left continuous *at b) if*

$$\lim_{x \to a^+} f(x) = f(a) \quad \left(or \quad \lim_{x \to b^-} f(x) = f(b) \right).$$

An immediate consequence of this definition is the following corollary:

Corollary A.80. *Let $f : (a, b) \subset \mathbb{R} \to \mathbb{R}^m$, $\hat{x} \in (a, b)$; then f is continuous at $\hat{x}$ iff it is left and right continuous at $\hat{x}$.*

Definition A.81 (Piecewise Continuity). *Let $f : D \to \mathbb{R}^m$ with $D = [a, b] \subset \mathbb{R}$. Then f is called* piecewise continuous *on D if there exist a finite number of points $x_0 = a < x_1 < \cdots < x_n = b$, where f is continuous on every interval (x_{i-1}, x_i), $i = 1, \ldots, n$. At a point of discontinuity the right- and left-hand side limits exist and the function exhibits a so-called* jump discontinuity.

The set of piecewise continuous functions on D is denoted as $C_p^0(D, \mathbb{R}^m)$.

A stronger property is that of absolute continuity:

Definition A.82 (Absolute Continuity). *Let $f : D \subset \mathbb{R} \to \mathbb{R}^m$; then f is called* absolutely continuous *if for every $\varepsilon > 0$ there exists a $\delta > 0$ such that if for every finite sequence of points $(x_i)_{i=1}^{2k} \subset D$, $k \geq 1$ satisfying*

$$\sum_{j=1}^{k} |x_{2j} - x_{2j-1}| < \delta$$

then

$$\sum_{j=1}^{k} \|f(x_{2j}) - f(x_{2j-1})\| < \varepsilon$$

holds.

Differentiability is another important property of a function $f : \mathbb{R}^n \to \mathbb{R}^m$:

Definition A.83 (Differentiability). *Let $f : D \subset \mathbb{R}^n \to \mathbb{R}^m$, with D open and $\hat{x} \in D$; then f is called* differentiable *at $\hat{x}$ if there exists a matrix $L : \mathbb{R}^n \to \mathbb{R}^m$ such that*

$$\lim_{\substack{x \to \hat{x} \\ x \neq \hat{x}}} \frac{\|f(x) - f(\hat{x}) - L(x - \hat{x})\|}{\|x - \hat{x}\|} = 0.$$

The matrix L is then called the derivative *of f at $\hat{x}$ and is denoted as*

$$\frac{\mathrm{d}f(\hat{x})}{\mathrm{d}x} = f_x(\hat{x}) = f'(\hat{x}) := L.$$

Otherwise f is called nondifferentiable *at $\hat{x}$.*

If the derivative exists for every $\hat{x} \in D$, then f is said to be differentiable *in D with* derivative

$$\frac{\mathrm{d}f}{\mathrm{d}x}, \quad f_x, \quad or \quad f'.$$

If the derivative

$$\frac{\mathrm{d}f}{\mathrm{d}x} : D \to \mathbb{R}^{n \times m}$$

is continuous in D, then f is called continuously differentiable *in D and the set of continuously differentiable functions in D is denoted as $C^1(D, \mathbb{R}^m)$.*

The following properties are satisfied:

1. The derivative $f'(\hat{x})$ is uniquely determined.
2. If the function f is differentiable at $\hat{x}$, it is continuous at $\hat{x}$.
3. If f and g are differentiable at $\hat{x}$, then $f + g$ and αf with $\alpha \in \mathbb{R}$ are also differentiable at $\hat{x}$.

Proposition A.84 ($C^1(\mathbb{R}, \mathbb{R}^n)$ as a Normed Vector Space). *The following pair $(C^1(\mathbb{R}, \mathbb{R}^n), \|\cdot\|_{C^1}$ with*

$$\|f\|_{C^1} := \sup_{x \in \mathbb{R}} \|f(x)\| + \sup_{x \in \mathbb{R}} \|f'(x)\|, \quad for \quad f \in C^1(\mathbb{R}, \mathbb{R}^n)$$

is a normed vector space and $\|f\|_{C^1}$ is called the C^1 norm *of f.*

Proposition A.85 (De L'Hospital's Rule). *Let $f : \mathbb{R} \to \mathbb{R}$ and $g \mathbb{R} \to \mathbb{R}$ be continuously differentiable at $\hat{x}$. If $\lim_{x\to\hat{x}} f(x) = \lim_{x\to\hat{x}} g(x) = 0$ and*

$$\lim_{x\to\hat{x}} \frac{f(x)}{g(x)}, \quad g(x) \neq 0, \;\; x \neq \hat{x}$$

exists; then

$$\lim_{x\to\hat{x}} \frac{f(x)}{g(x)} = \lim_{x\to\hat{x}} \frac{f'(x)}{g'(x)}.$$

Definition A.86 (Right and Left Side Derivative). *Let $f : [a, b] \subset \mathbb{R} \to \mathbb{R}^m$; then f is called* differentiable from the right *at a (or* differentiable from the left *at b) if there exists a matrix $L : \mathbb{R} \to \mathbb{R}^m$ such that*

$$\lim_{\substack{x\to a^+ \\ x\neq a}} \frac{\|f(x) - f(a) - L(x-a)\|}{x-a} = 0 \left(\text{or} \lim_{\substack{x\to b^- \\ x\neq b}} \frac{\|f(x) - f(b) - L(x-b)\|}{x-b} = 0 \right).$$

The matrix L is then called the right-hand side derivative *of f at a (or* left-hand side derivative *of f at b) and is denoted as*

$$\frac{\mathrm{d}f(\hat{x}^{\pm})}{\mathrm{d}x} = f_x(\hat{x}^{\pm}) = f'(\hat{x}^{\pm}) := L.$$

Definition A.87 (Piecewise Continuous Derivative). *Let $f : D \subset \mathbb{R} \to \mathbb{R}^k$ with $D = [a, b] \subset \mathbb{R}$. Then f is called* piecewise continuously differentiable *on F if f is continuous on D and there exist points $x_0 = a < x_1 < \cdots < x_n = b$, where f is continuously differentiable on every interval (x_{i-1}, x_i), $i = 1, \dots, n$. At a point where the derivative is not continuous but the left and right-hand side derivatives exist, the function f exhibits a so-called* kink.

The set of piecewise continuously differentiable functions on D is denoted as $C_p^1(D, \mathbb{R}^k)$.

Functions which are continuous and piecewise continuously differentiable are denoted as $C_p^{0,1}(D, \mathbb{R}^k)$.

For the composition of two differentiable functions we find:

Theorem A.88 (Chain Rule). *Let $f : D \subset \mathbb{R}^n \to \mathbb{R}^m$ be differentiable at $\hat{x}$ and $g : V \subset \mathbb{R}^m \to \mathbb{R}^k$ be differentiable at $\hat{y} = f(\hat{x})$ with D, V open, $\hat{x} \in D$ and $f(\hat{x}) \in V$. Then $g \circ f$ is defined in an open neighborhood of $\hat{x}$ and is differentiable at $\hat{x}$, satisfying*

$$\frac{\mathrm{d}\,(g \circ f)\,(\hat{x})}{\mathrm{d}x} = \frac{\mathrm{d}g(\hat{y})}{\mathrm{d}y} \frac{\mathrm{d}f(\hat{x})}{\mathrm{d}x}.$$

A further concept is that of partial derivatives:

Definition A.89 (Partial Derivative). *Let $f : D \subset \mathbb{R}^n \to \mathbb{R}^m$, with D open, and $\hat{x} = (\hat{x}_1, \dots, \hat{x}_n)' \in D$. Let $j = 1, \dots, n$ then f is said to be* partially differentiable *at the jth coordinate if the function*

$$g_j(h) := f(\hat{x}_1, \dots, \hat{x}_{j-1}, \hat{x}_j + h, \hat{x}_{j+1}, \dots, \hat{x}_n)$$

is differentiable at $h = 0$. The corresponding derivative is then called the jth partial derivative *of f at $\hat{x}$ and is denoted as*

$$\frac{\partial f(\hat{x})}{\partial x_j}, \quad or \quad f_{x_j}(\hat{x}).$$

Using partial derivatives we find:

Proposition A.90 (Jacobian). *Let the function $f : D \subset \mathbb{R}^n \to \mathbb{R}^m$, with D open, be differentiable at $\hat{x} \in D$. Then the matrix $f_x(\hat{x})$ is given by*

$$J(\hat{x}) = \begin{pmatrix} \frac{\partial f_1}{\partial x_1}(\hat{x}) & \cdots & \frac{\partial f_1}{\partial x_n}(\hat{x}) \\ \vdots & \ddots & \vdots \\ \frac{\partial f_m}{\partial x_1}(\hat{x}) & \cdots & \frac{\partial f_m}{\partial x_n}(\hat{x}) \end{pmatrix},$$

where $J(\hat{x})$ is called the Jacobian matrix *of f at $\hat{x}$.*

For scalar-valued functions the partial derivative can be generalized to:

Definition A.91 (Directional Derivative). *Let $f : D \subset \mathbb{R}^n \to \mathbb{R}$, with D open, and $\hat{x} \in D$, $v \in \mathbb{R}^n$, $\|v\| = 1$. If the limit*

$$\frac{\partial f(\hat{x})}{\partial v} := \lim_{\substack{h \to 0 \\ h \neq 0}} \frac{f(\hat{x} + hv) - f(\hat{x})}{h}$$

exists, then it is called the directional derivative *of f in direction v at $\hat{x}$.*

Definition A.92 (Gradient). *Let $f : D \subset \mathbb{R}^n \to \mathbb{R}$, with D open, be partially differentiable at $\hat{x} \in \mathbb{R}^n$. Then the vector*

$$\nabla f(\hat{x}) := f_x(\hat{x}) = (f_{x_1}(\hat{x}), \dots, f_{x_n}(\hat{x}))$$

is called the gradient *of f at $\hat{x}$, and ∇ is called the* Nabla operator.

As a row vector the gradient of f can be interpreted as an element of the dual space of $\mathbb{R}^n$ and is therefore a linear form (Fig. A.3). This interpretation is stressed by the following theorem:

Proposition A.93. *Let $f : D \subset \mathbb{R}^n \to \mathbb{R}$, with D open, be differentiable at $\hat{x}$ and $v \in \mathbb{R}^n$, $\|v\| = 1$; then*

$$\frac{\partial f(\hat{x})}{\partial v} = (\nabla f(\hat{x}))v.$$

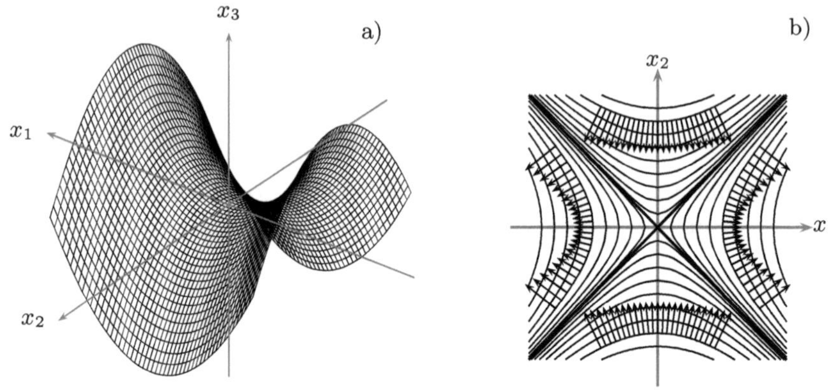

Fig. A.3. Panel (**a**) shows a plot of the hyperbolic function $x_3 = f(x_1, x_2) = x_1^2 - x_2^2$. And in the *right panel* (**b**) some of the gradients $\nabla f(x_1, x_2) = (2x_1, -2x_2)$ are depicted in a contour plot

Proposition A.94. *Let $f : D \subset \mathbb{R}^n \to \mathbb{R}$, with D open, be differentiable at $\hat{x}$ with $f_x(\hat{x}) \neq 0$. Then the gradient $\nabla f(\hat{x})$ denotes the direction with the largest directional derivative of f in norm with corresponding value $\|\nabla f(\hat{x})\|$.*

We now extend the definition of differentiability to higher orders:

Definition A.95. *Let $f : D \subset \mathbb{R}^n \to \mathbb{R}^m$, with D open, be differentiable on D. If the derivative $f_x(\cdot)$ is differentiable at $\hat{x}$, then f is said to be* twice *(or* two times*)* differentiable *at $\hat{x}$ and the derivative of $f_x(\cdot)$ at $\hat{x}$ is called the* second derivative *and is denoted as*

$$\frac{\mathrm{d}^2 f(\hat{x})}{\mathrm{d}x^2} = f_{xx}(\hat{x}) = f''(\hat{x}) := \frac{\mathrm{d}f_x(\hat{x})}{\mathrm{d}x}.$$

If $f_x(\cdot)$ is differentiable in D, then f is called twice (two times) differentiable *in D.*

Remark A.96. Higher-order derivatives can inductively be defined, where the ith derivative at $\hat{x}$ is denoted as

$$\frac{\mathrm{d}^i f(\hat{x})}{\mathrm{d}x^i}.$$

Remark A.97. For functions $f : \mathbb{R} \to \mathbb{R}^n$, where the argument can be interpreted as time, the *derivative* is often abbreviated by $\dot{f}$ and $\ddot{f}$, $\dddot{f}, \dots$ for higher order derivatives.

Analogously to the set of all continuous functions, we denote the set of i-times continuously differentiable functions $f : D \subset \mathbb{R}^n \to \mathbb{R}^m$ as

$$C^i(D, \mathbb{R}^m) \quad \text{or} \quad C^i(D), \quad \text{or even} \quad C^i$$

and the set of functions, which are arbitrarily often differentiable are denoted as

$$C^\infty(D,\mathbb{R}^m) := \bigcap_{i=0}^{\infty} C^i(D,\mathbb{R}^m).$$

Proposition A.98 (Hessian). *Let $f : D \subset \mathbb{R}^n \to \mathbb{R}$, with D open, be twice continuously differentiable at $\hat{x}$. Then the second-order derivative at $\hat{x}$ is given by the matrix*

$$f_{xx}(\hat{x}) = \begin{pmatrix} \frac{\partial^2 f(\hat{x})}{\partial x_1^2} & \cdots & \frac{\partial^2 f(\hat{x})}{\partial x_1 \partial x_n} \\ \vdots & \ddots & \vdots \\ \frac{\partial^2 f(\hat{x})}{\partial x_n \partial x_1} & \cdots & \frac{\partial^2 f(\hat{x})}{\partial x_n^2} \end{pmatrix},$$

which is called the Hessian matrix *of f at $\hat{x}$, denoted by $H(\hat{x})$. Moreover, $H(\hat{x})$ is symmetric.*

Next we state a lemma considering the continuous dependence of the solutions of an ODE with respect to its initial conditions

Lemma A.99. *Let $(x^{(i)}(\cdot))$, $i \in \mathbb{N}$ be a sequence of solutions of the ODE*

$$\dot{x}(t) = f(x(t)), \tag{A.12}$$

with $x^{(i)}(0) = x_0^{(i)} \in \mathbb{R}^n$ and f continuously differentiable in x. If

$$\lim_{i\to\infty} x_0^i = x_0,$$

then the corresponding flows of (A.12) satisfy

$$\lim_{i\to\infty} \varphi^t x^i = \varphi^t x_0, \quad \textit{for all}\, t \geq 0.$$

For a proof see, e.g., Jost (2005, Theorem 5.11).

A.3.3 Maximization of Real-Valued Functions in $\mathbb{R}^n$

Definition A.100 (Global and Local Maximum). *Let $f : X \subset \mathbb{R}^n \to \mathbb{R}$, and $f(X)$ has a maximal element; then $\hat{x}$ is called a* (global) maximizer *of f if $f(\hat{x}) = \max f(X)$. The maximal element of $f(X)$ is called the* (global) maximum *of f and the set of maximizers of f is denoted by*

$$\operatorname*{argmax}_{x\in X} f(x).$$

In case that no maximizer exists $\operatorname{argmax}_{x\in X} f(x) := \emptyset$. If $\operatorname{argmax}_{x\in X} f(x)$ is a singleton then $\hat{x}$ is called a strict (global) maximizer *of f and $f(\hat{x})$ the* strict (global) maximum *of f.*

If there exists an open neighborhood $D \subset \mathbb{R}^n$ of $\hat{x}$ such that

$$\hat{x} \in \underset{x \in D \cap X}{\operatorname{argmax}} f(x),$$

then $\hat{x}$ *is called a* local maximizer *of* f *in* D *and* $f(\hat{x})$ *is called a* local maximum *of* f. *If* $\operatorname{argmax}_{x \in D} f(x)$ *is a singleton then* $\hat{x}$ *is called a* strict local maximizer *of* f *and* $f(\hat{x})$ *the* strict local maximum *of* f *at* D. *These definitions can be formulated in a straight forward way for a* (local) minimum *and a* (local) minimizer. *An element* $\hat{x}$ *being a (local) maximizer or minimizer is called a* (local) optimizer *and the corresponding (local) maximum or minimum is called the* (local) optimum.

Remark A.101. The maximum (minimum) of a function f may not exist, whereas the supremum (infimum) of $f(X)$ always exists in $\bar{\mathbb{R}}$. Thus in optimization theory it is crucial to guarantee the existence of a maximizer (minimizer):

Theorem A.102 (Existence of an Optimizer). *Let* $f : K \subset \mathbb{R}^n \to \mathbb{R}$, *with* K *be compact and* f *be continuous; then*

$$\underset{x \in K}{\operatorname{argmax}} f(x) \neq \emptyset, \quad \textit{and} \quad \underset{x \in K}{\operatorname{argmin}} f(x) \neq \emptyset.$$

Theorem A.103 (Necessary Conditions for an Optimizer). *Let* $\hat{x} \in D$, *with* D *open, be a local maximizer (or minimizer) of* $f : D \subset \mathbb{R}^n \to \mathbb{R}$, *and let* f *be partially differentiable at* $\hat{x}$. *Then* $f_x(\hat{x}) = 0$.

Theorem A.104 (Second Order Necessary Conditions). *Let* $\hat{x} \in D$, *with* D *open, be a local maximizer of* $f : D \subset \mathbb{R}^n \to \mathbb{R}$, *and let* f *be twice continuously differentiable at* $\hat{x}$. *Then* $f_{xx}(\hat{x})$ *is negative semidefinite.*

Theorem A.105 (Sufficient Conditions). *Let* $f : D \subset \mathbb{R}^n \to \mathbb{R}$, *with* D *open, be twice continuously differentiable. Assume that for* $\hat{x} \in D$

$$f_x(\hat{x}) = 0.$$

If the Hessian matrix $f_{xx}(\hat{x})$ *is negative definite then* f *has a strict local maximum at* $\hat{x}$.

In many applications the function f also depends on exogenously given parameter values $\mu \in \Gamma \subset \mathbb{R}^p$, then we define:

Definition A.106 (Value Function). *Let* $f : X \times \mathbb{R}^p \to \mathbb{R}$, *with* $X \subset \mathbb{R}^n$; *then the function* $f^* : \Gamma \subset \mathbb{R}^p \to \bar{\mathbb{R}}$ *given by*

$$f^*(\mu) := \begin{cases} f(x^*(\mu), \mu) & x^*(\mu) \in \operatorname{argmax}_{x \in X} f(x, \mu) \\ \infty & \operatorname{argmax}_{x \in X} f(x, \mu) = \emptyset \end{cases}$$

is called the value function *of the parameterized maximization problem*

$$\max_{x \in X} f(x, \mu), \quad \mu \in \Gamma.$$

A.3.4 Convex Analysis

Sets in $\mathbb{R}^n$ can exhibit a special structure that is especially important for optimization theory:

Definition A.107 (Convex Set). *$C \subset \mathbb{R}^n$ is called a* convex set, *if for all $\theta \in [0, 1]$ and for all $x, y \in C$*

$$\theta x + (1 - \theta)y \in C.$$

Remark A.108. Convexity is an important property assuring that whenever x and y are contained in a set C, the line segment connecting these two points is contained in C. In other words, convexity excludes holes and indentations of a set.

For a convex set the following properties hold:

Lemma A.109. *Let $C \subset \mathbb{R}^n$ be a convex set; then the sets C° and $\overline{C}$ are convex.*

We can now define concave functions f given on a convex set C:

Definition A.110 (Concave Function). *Let $C \subset \mathbb{R}^n$ be a convex set; then the function $f : \mathbb{R}^n \to \mathbb{R}$ is called* concave *in C if for all $\theta \in [0, 1]$ it holds that*

$$\theta f(x) + (1 - \theta)f(y) \leq f(\theta x + (1 - \theta)y), \quad \textit{for all} \quad x, y \in C.$$

If strict inequality holds for all $\theta \in (0, 1)$, then the function f is called strictly concave. *If the opposite inequality holds, the function f is called a* (strictly) convex *function.*

An equivalent characterization can be given in terms of the epigraph:

Proposition A.111. *A function $f : C \subset \mathbb{R}^n \to \mathbb{R}$ is concave iff the epigraph* $\mathrm{epi}(-f) \in \mathbb{R}^{n+1}$ *is a nonempty convex set.*

The following proposition is an immediate result of Definition A.110:

Proposition A.112. *Let $f : C \subset \mathbb{R}^n \to \mathbb{R}$, with C a convex set, be continuously differentiable and concave; then for $x_1, x_2 \in C$ the following inequality holds*

$$f(x_1) - f(x_2) \leq f_x(x_2)(x_1 - x_2).$$

Maximizers of a concave function are characterized by:

Theorem A.113 (Sufficient and Necessary Maximum Condition). *Let $f : C \subset \mathbb{R}^n \to \mathbb{R}$, with C a convex set, be continuously differentiable and concave; then x^* is maximizer of f on C iff*

$$f_x(x^*)(x^* - x) \geq 0, \quad \textit{for all} \quad x \in C.$$

Definition A.114 (Supergradient). *Let $f : C \subset \mathbb{R}^n \to \mathbb{R}$, with C a convex set and $\hat{x} \in C$; then a vector $a \in \mathbb{R}^n$ is called a* supergradient *of f at $\hat{x}$ if*

$$f(x) - f(\hat{x}) \leq \langle a, x - \hat{x} \rangle, \quad \textit{for all} \quad x \in C.$$

Definition A.115 (Quasiconcave Function). *Let $C \subset \mathbb{R}^n$ be a convex set; then the function $f : \mathbb{R}^n \to \mathbb{R}$ is called* quasiconcave *in C if for all $\theta \in [0, 1]$ it holds that*

$$\min\{f(x),\, f(y)\} \leq f(\theta x + (1 - \theta) y), \quad \textit{for all} \quad x, y \in C.$$

Definition A.116 (Convex and Positive Cone). *A set $C \subset \mathbb{R}^n$ is called a* convex cone *if $\alpha x + \beta y \in C$ for every $\alpha \geq 0$, $\beta \geq 0$ and x, $y \in C$. A set $C \subset \mathbb{R}^n$ is called a* positive cone *if $x \in C$ implies $\alpha x \in C$ for all $\alpha \geq 0$.*

Definition A.117 (Convex Hull). *Let $C \subset \mathbb{R}^n$ then the set*

$$\text{con}\, C := \{x : x = \sum_{i=1}^{k} \alpha_i x_i,\; x_i \in C,\; \alpha_i \geq 0,\; i = 1, \ldots, n,\; k \in \mathbb{N}\}$$

is a convex cone called the convex hull *of C.*

Next we formulate different separation theorems:

Theorem A.118 (Separation of a Point and Closed Convex Set). *Let $C \subset \mathbb{R}^n$ be a closed convex set, with $0 \notin C$; then there exists a vector $a \in \mathbb{R}^n$ with $a \neq 0$ such $\langle a, x \rangle > 0$ for all $x \in C$.*

Theorem A.119 (Separation of a Point and Convex Set). *Let $C \subset \mathbb{R}^n$ be a convex set with $C^\circ \neq \emptyset$ and $v \notin C^\circ$; then there exists a vector $a \in \mathbb{R}^n$ with $a \neq 0$ satisfying $\langle a, x \rangle > \langle a, v \rangle$ for all $x \in C$.*

Theorem A.120 (Separation of a Point and Closed Convex Cone). *Let $C \subset \mathbb{R}^n$ be a closed convex cone and $v \in \mathbb{R}^n$ with $v \notin C$; then there exists a vector $a \in \mathbb{R}^n$ satisfying $\langle a, x \rangle \geq 0 > \langle a, v \rangle$ for all $x \in C$.*

A consequence of Theorem A.119 is:

Proposition A.121 (Existence of a Supergradient). *Let $f : C \subset \mathbb{R}^n \to \mathbb{R}$, with C convex, be a concave function and $\hat{x} \in C^\circ$; then there exists a supergradient a of f at $\hat{x}$.*

A classical reference to convex analysis is Rockafellar (1970), for a more recent presentation the reader is referred to Bertsekas, Nedic, and Ozdaglar (2003).

A.3.5 Taylor Theorem and Implicit Function Theorem

Since we are now familiar with the basic definitions of *continuity* and *differentiability*, we recapitulate some well-known and important results from calculus:

Theorem A.122 (Mean Value Theorem). *Let $f : D \subset \mathbb{R}^n \to \mathbb{R}$ be differentiable on D, where D is an open and convex set, and let the points $\hat{x}$ and $\hat{x} + h$ be elements of D. Then there exists a real-value θ, with $0 \leq \theta \leq 1$, such that*

$$f(\hat{x} + h) - f(\hat{x}) = f_x(\hat{x} + \theta h)h$$

holds.

The so-called *Taylor theorem*, generalizes this to $\mathbb{R}^m$. It allows the approximation of a differentiable function f by a polynomial whose coefficients are given by the derivatives of f. This theorem is frequently used (at least implicitly) and is presented here for the common case of an at least twice continuously differentiable vector-valued function f:

Theorem A.123 (Taylor Theorem). *Let $f \in C^2(D, \mathbb{R}^m)$ with $D \subset \mathbb{R}^n$ open and $\delta > 0$ with $N(\hat{x}, \delta) \subset D$. Then for $\|z\| < \delta$ we have*

$$f(\hat{x} + z) = f(\hat{x}) + f_x(\hat{x})z + o(\|z\|). \tag{A.13}$$

Remark A.124. Omitting the $o(\|z\|)$ term from the Taylor theorem allows one to approximate a differentiable function by a polynomial (A.13), the so-called *(truncated) Taylor polynomial.* An example of this is depicted in Fig. A.4a, where at the origin $x = 0$, the function $f(x) = \cos x$ is approximated by Taylor polynomials of orders one and two, where the fit improves with the order of the polynomial. But as is shown in Fig. A.4b for the function $f(0) = 1$ and $f(x) = 1 + \mathrm{e}^{-1/x^2}$ for $x \neq 0$ the Taylor polynomials do not approximate the function in a neighborhood of zero. In other words, the $o(|x|^k)$-term cannot be omitted for any order $k \in \mathbb{N}$ because at the origin the function e^{-1/x^2} is as flat as the constant function $y \equiv 0$.

Another important tool from calculus is the so-called implicit function theorem, which assures an explicit representation of an implicitly given function near a point $\hat{x}$:

Theorem A.125 (Implicit Function Theorem). *Let $f : D \subset \mathbb{R}^n \to \mathbb{R}^m$, with D open, with $m < n \in \mathbb{N}$ be a continuously differentiable function on D and $\hat{z} = (\hat{x}, \hat{y})$ with $\hat{x} \in \mathbb{R}^{n-m}$ and $\hat{y} \in \mathbb{R}^m$ be a point with $f(\hat{z}) = 0$. It is assumed that the derivative of f at $\hat{z}$ exists and that $f_y(\hat{z})$ has rank m. Then there exist open neighborhoods $N(\hat{x}, \varepsilon) \subset \mathbb{R}^{n-m}$ of $\hat{x}$ and $N(\hat{y}, \delta) \subset \mathbb{R}^m$ of $\hat{y}$, and a continuously differentiable function $g : N(\hat{x}, \varepsilon) \to N(\hat{y}, \delta)$, with $\hat{y} = g(\hat{x})$ and*

$$f(x, g(x)) = 0 \tag{A.14}$$

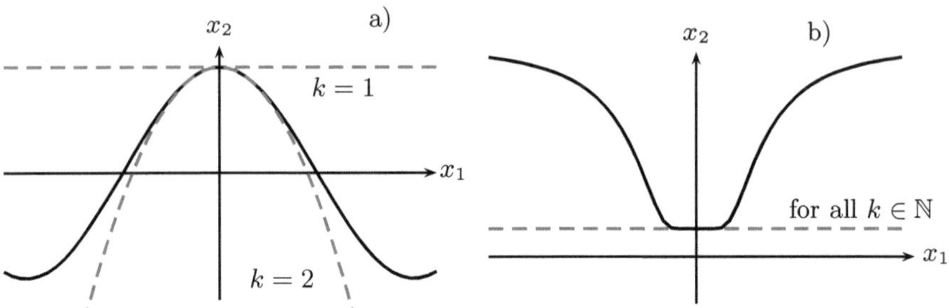

Fig. A.4. Panel (**a**) shows the function $f(x) = \cos(x)$ together with the Taylor polynomials up to second order at point $x = 0$. In panel (**b**) the case of the function $f(x) = 1 + e^{-1/x^2}$ for $x \neq 0$ and $f(0) = 1$ is depicted, which, although infinitely often differentiable, cannot be approximated by Taylor polynomials around $x = 0$ as $d^k f/dx^k(0) = 0$ for all $k \in \mathbb{N}$

for all $x \in N(\hat{x}, \varepsilon)$. The derivative of g evaluated at $\hat{x}$ is given by

$$g_x(\hat{x}) = -f_y^{-1}(\hat{z}) f_x(\hat{z}).$$

Furthermore, for every $x \in N(\hat{x}, \varepsilon)$, $g(x)$ is the only solution of (A.14) in $N(\hat{y}, \delta)$.

A direct consequence of the implicit function theorem is the following:

Theorem A.126 (Inverse Function Theorem). *Let $f : D \subset \mathbb{R}^n \to \mathbb{R}^n$, with D open, be a continuously differentiable function on D and $\hat{x} \in D$. Let the derivative of f at $\hat{x}$ be invertible. Then there exists an open neighborhood $U \subset D$ of $\hat{x}$ and an open neighborhood $V \subset \mathbb{R}^n$ of $\hat{y} = f(\hat{x})$, such that f maps U bijectively onto V and the inverse function $g = f^{-1} : V \to U$ is continuously differentiable, where its derivative at $\hat{y}$ is given by*

$$g_y(\hat{y}) = (f_x(g(\hat{y})))^{-1} = (f_x(\hat{x}))^{-1}.$$

In connection with invertible functions the following definitions are useful:

Definition A.127 (Homeo- and Diffeomorphism). *Let $f : \mathbb{R}^n \to \mathbb{R}^n$ be invertible (bijective) on an open set $U \subset \mathbb{R}^n$. Then f is called a* homeomorphism *if f as well as f^{-1} are continuous on U and $f(U)$, respectively; in that case U and $f(U)$ are called* homeomorph. *Likewise f is called a* diffeomorphism *if f as well as f^{-1} are continuously differentiable on U and $f(U)$, respectively; in that case U and $f(U)$ are called* diffeomorphic.

The implicit function theorem gives rise to the notion of a differentiable manifold (see, e.g., Chillingworth, 1976). The here presented definition is only a special case of a more general definition for differentiable manifolds. Anyhow, it satisfies our needs and we define:

Definition A.128 (Differentiable Manifold). *Let $f : \mathbb{R}^{n+k} \to \mathbb{R}^n$, $k \geq 0$ be continuously differentiable, and put $M = f^{-1}(0)$. If $\operatorname{rk} f_z(z) = k$ for all $z \in M$; then M is called an n-*dimensional differentiable manifold *and*

$$T_z M := \operatorname{span}\{\operatorname{grad} f(z)\}^{\perp}$$

is called the tangent space *of M at z.*

Remark A.129. For every $z = (x, y) \in M$ the implicit function theorem assures the existence of a continuously differentiable function $g : U \subset \mathbb{R}^n \to V \subset \mathbb{R}^k$, such that $y = g(x)$ iff $f(x, y) = 0$. Thus the function $\varphi : (U \times V \cap M \to U$ given by

$$\varphi(x, g(x)) := x$$

is bijective, justifying the denotation of $x \in U$ as the coordinates of the n-dimensional manifold M.

A.3.6 Integration Theory

Besides the operation of differentiation, integration is a further fundamental operation. At this place we only introduce the Riemann–Stieltjes integral and its properties instead of the more general Lebesgue integral:

Definition A.130 (Subdivision and Refinement). *Let $[a, b]$ be a closed interval in $\mathbb{R}$. Then any finite set*

$$\Delta = \{a = x_0 < x_1 < \cdots < x_N = b\}$$

is called a finite partition *of $[a, b]$, denoted by $\Delta = (x_i)_{i=0}^{N}$, and*

$$|\Delta| := \max_i \{|x_{i+1} - x_i| : i = 0, \ldots, N-1\}$$

is called the norm *of Δ.*

A finite partition Δ' with $\Delta \subsetneq \Delta'$ is called a refinement *of Δ.*

Let f and g be real-valued functions on $[a, b]$ and $\Delta = (x_i)_{i=0}^{N}$ be a finite partition. Then for an arbitrary sequence y_i, $i = 0, \ldots, N-1$ with $y_i \in (x_i, x_{i+1})$ the sum

$$\sum_{i=0}^{N-1} f(y_i)\,(g(x_{i+1}) - g(x_i))$$

is called a Riemann–Stieltjes sum *for the partition Δ.*

Definition A.131 (Riemann–Stieltjes Integral). *Let f and g be real-valued functions on $[a, b]$ and $\Delta = (x_i)_{i=1}^{N}$ be a finite partition of $[a, b]$. If for any sequence of $\Delta^{(j)} = (x_i^{(j)})_{i=0}^{N(j)}$, $j \in \mathbb{N}$ of refinements of Δ with $\lim_{j\to\infty} |\Delta^{(j)}| = 0$ the sequence of corresponding Riemann–Stieltjes sums*

$$\sum_{i=0}^{N(j)-1} f(y_i^{(j)}) \left(g\left(x_{i+1}^{(j)}\right) - g\left(x_i^{(j)}\right)\right), \quad y_i^{(j)} \in \left(x_i^{(j)}, x_{i+1}^{(j)}\right)$$

converges to some $I \in \mathbb{R}$, *then* f *is called* Riemann–Stieltjes integrable (RS-integrable) *with respect to* g *over* $[a, b]$, *with* integral I *denoted as*

$$I = \int_a^b f(x)\,\mathrm{d}g(x).$$

If $g = \mathrm{Id}_{\mathbb{R}}$ *then* f *is called* Riemann integrable (R-integrabel) over $[a, b]$ *with* integral I *denoted as*

$$I = \int_a^b f(x)\,\mathrm{d}x.$$

Remark A.132. It can be shown that the definition of integral I does not depend on the initially chosen partition $\Delta = (x_i)_{i=1}^N$.

Remark A.133. If for a vector-valued function $f = (f_1, \ldots, f_n)' : [a, b] \to \mathbb{R}^n$ each function f_i, $i = 1, \ldots, n$ is RS-integrable with respect to some function g, then

$$\int_a^b f(x)\,\mathrm{d}g(x) := \begin{pmatrix} \int_a^b f_1(x)\,\mathrm{d}g(x) \\ \vdots \\ \int_a^b f_n(x)\,\mathrm{d}g(x) \end{pmatrix}$$

is the RS-integral of f with respect to g over $[a, b]$.

For Riemann integrals we can formulate:

Theorem A.134 (Fundamental Theorem of Calculus). *Let* $f : [a, b] \to \mathbb{R}$ *be a continuous function and let*

$$F(x) := \int_a^x f(y)\,\mathrm{d}y,$$

then F *is differentiable on* (a, b) *and the left and right side derivative exist at* a *and* b *satisfying*

$$F'(x) = f(x),\ x \in [a, b].$$

Theorem A.135. *Let the function* $f : [a, b] \to \mathbb{R}$ *have a continuous or R-integrable derivative* $f' : [a, b] \to \mathbb{R}$ *then*

$$f(b) = f(a) + \int_a^b f'(x)\,\mathrm{d}x.$$

Remark A.136. These theorem tells us that for a special class of functions, differentiation and integration are inverse operations and allows therefore the computation of the integral without considering limits of the Riemann sums.

For the Riemann integral the following rules hold:

Proposition A.137 (Integration by Substitution). *Let $[a, b] \subset \mathbb{R}$ and $[c, d] \subset \mathbb{R}$ be closed intervals, $h : [a, b] \to [c, d]$ be a continuously differentiable function, and $f : [c, d] \to \mathbb{R}$ be continuous; then*

$$\int_a^b f(h(x))\, h'(x)\, \mathrm{d}x = \int_{h(a)}^{h(b)} f(y)\, \mathrm{d}y.$$

Proposition A.138 (Integration by Parts). *Let f and g be continuously differentiable functions on $[a, b]$; then*

$$\int_a^b f(x) g'(x)\, \mathrm{d}x = f(b)g(b) - f(a)g(a) - \int_a^b f'(x) g(x)\, \mathrm{d}x.$$

Proposition A.139 (Leibniz Integral Rule). *Let $F(x,t)$ and $F_x(x,t)$ be continuous in both x and t. If $f(x)$ and $g(x)$ are continuously differentiable on (a, b); then*

$$\frac{\mathrm{d}}{\mathrm{d}x} \int_{f(x)}^{g(x)} F(x,t)\, \mathrm{d}t = F(x, g(x)) \frac{\mathrm{d}g(x)}{\mathrm{d}x} - F(x, f(x)) \frac{\mathrm{d}f(x)}{\mathrm{d}x} + \int_{f(x)}^{g(x)} \frac{\mathrm{d}}{\mathrm{d}x} F(x,t)\, \mathrm{d}t. \tag{A.15}$$

for $x \in (a, b)$.

The following results prove important for the calculus of variations:

Lemma A.140 (Dubois–Reymond Lemma). *If $f \in C^0([a, b])$ and*

$$\int_a^b f(x) h'(x)\, \mathrm{d}x = 0$$

for all $h \in C^1([a, b])$ with $h(a) = h(b) = 0$, then it is necessary that for some constant c,

$$f(x) = c,$$

for all $x \in [a, b]$.

As a corollary we find:

Corollary A.141. *If $f, g \in C^0([a, b])$ and*

$$\int_a^b \left(f(x)h(x) + g(x)h'(x)\right) \mathrm{d}x = 0$$

for all $h \in C^1([a, b])$ with $h(a) = h(b) = 0$; then g is differentiable with

$$g'(x) = f(x), \quad x \in [a, b].$$

Another important consequence of Dubois–Reymond lemma is the so-called:

Theorem A.142 (Fundamental Theorem of the Calculus of Variations). *If* $f \in C^0([a,\, b])$ *and*

$$\int_a^b f(x)h(x)\,\mathrm{d}x = 0$$

for all $h \in C^1([a,\, b])$ *with* $h(a) = h(b) = 0$*; then*

$$f(x) = 0$$

for all $x \in [a,\, b]$.

To consider the question of whether a Riemann–Stieltjes integral exists we define functions of bounded variation:

Definition A.143 (Functions of Bounded Variation). *Let* $f : [a,\, b] \to \mathbb{R}$*; then the function* f *is said to be of* bounded variation *if it satisfies the following condition: there exists a real number* $M \geq 0$ *such that for every finite partition* $(x_i)_{i=0}^N$ *of* $[a,\, b]$

$$\sum_{i=0}^{N-1} |f(x_{i+1}) - f(x_i)| < M.$$

A vector-valued function $f : [a,\, b] \to \mathbb{R}^n$ *is said to be of* bounded variation *if this property holds for every each* f_i, $i = 1, \ldots, n$. *The set of functions of bounded variations is denoted as* $BV([a,\, b])$.

functions of bounded variation exhibit the following property:

Theorem A.144. *Let* $f \in BV([a,\, b])$, *then* f *has finite right- and left-hand limits at all points of* $[a,\, b]$, *and* f *is continuous except at a countable set of points in* $[a,\, b]$.

Now the following theorem can be proved:

Theorem A.145 (Existence of Riemann–Stieltjes Integral). *Let* f *be a continuous function and* g *a function of bounded variation on* $[a,\, b]$*; then* f *is RS-integrable with respect to* g *over* $[a,\, b]$.

If f *is R-integrable over* $[a,\, b]$ *and* g *is differentiable on* $(a,\, b)$, *where the derivative* g' *is R-integrable over* $[a,\, b]$*; then the RS-integral becomes*

$$\int_a^b f(x)\,\mathrm{d}g(x) = \int_a^b f(x)g'(x)\,\mathrm{d}x.$$

Theorem A.146 (Integration by Parts). *Let* $f \in C^0([a,\, b])$ *and* $g \in BV([a,\, b])$*; then the following formula holds:*

$$\int_a^b f(x)\,\mathrm{d}g(x) = f(b)g(b) - f(a)g(a) - \int_a^b g(x)\,\mathrm{d}f(x).$$

A.3.7 Distributions

An important concept for the theory of partial differential equations is that of distributions introduced by Schwartz (1950). Therefore we define:

Definition A.147 (Functions with Compact Support). *Let* $\varphi : \mathbb{R}^n \to \mathbb{R}$*; then the set*

$$\operatorname{supp}\varphi := \overline{\{x : \varphi(x) \neq 0\}}$$

is called the support of φ. *And the elements of the set*

$$\mathcal{D}(\mathbb{R}^n) := \{\varphi \in C^\infty : \operatorname{supp}\varphi \text{ is compact}\}$$

are called C^∞ functions with compact support *or* test functions.

Without going into any details and referring the reader instead to Friedlander and Joshi (1998) we note that $\mathcal{D}(\mathbb{R}^n)$ can be equipped with a topology τ making the pair $(\mathcal{D}(\mathbb{R}^n), \tau)$ to a topological space and therefore the following definition can be given:

Definition A.148 (Distributions). *The elements of the dual space* $\mathcal{D}^*(\mathbb{R}^n)$ *of* $(\mathcal{D}(\mathbb{R}^n), \tau)$ *are called* distributions of $\mathbb{R}^n$.

Remark A.149. For a topological vector space, like $\mathcal{D}(\mathbb{R}^n)$, it is also claimed that the linear forms of the corresponding dual space are continuous, which extends Definition A.40.

As a specific example we consider the case $n = 1$ and define the derivative of a distribution of $\mathbb{R}$ as:

Definition A.150 (Derivative of a Distribution). *Let* $F \in \mathcal{D}^*(\mathbb{R})$*; then* F' *given by*

$$F'(\varphi) := -F(\varphi'), \quad \textit{for all} \quad \varphi \in \mathcal{D}(\mathbb{R})$$

is called the derivative of the distribution F.

Remark A.151. Note that $\varphi \in \mathcal{D}(\mathbb{R})$ iff $\varphi' \in \mathcal{D}(\mathbb{R})$.

Remark A.152. Definition A.150 is motivated by the consideration that for a function $f \in C^1(\mathbb{R})$ the products $f\varphi$ and $f'\varphi$ with $\varphi \in \mathcal{D}(\mathbb{R})$ are R-integrable on $(-\infty, \infty)$. Moreover f gives rise to elements $T_f \in \mathcal{D}^*(\mathbb{R})$ and $T_{f'} \in \mathcal{D}^*(\mathbb{R})$ by

$$T_f(\varphi) := \int_{-\infty}^{\infty} f(x)\varphi(x)\,\mathrm{d}x$$

$$T_{f'}(\varphi) := \int_{-\infty}^{\infty} f'(x)\varphi(x)\,\mathrm{d}x.$$

Then by partial integration the latter integral can be written as

$$T_{f'}(\varphi) = \lim_{x\to\infty} f(x)\varphi(x) - \lim_{x\to-\infty} f(x)\varphi(x) - \int_{-\infty}^{\infty} f(x)\varphi'(x)\,\mathrm{d}x$$
$$= -\int_{-\infty}^{\infty} f(x)\varphi'(x)\,\mathrm{d}x = -T_f(\varphi').$$

Identifying $T_{f'}$ with the derivative T_f' this relation finally motivates Definition A.150.

Definition A.153 (Heaviside Function). *The function* $H : \mathbb{R} \to \mathbb{R}$ *given by*

$$H(x) := \begin{cases} 0 & x < 0 \\ 1 & x \geq 0 \end{cases}$$

is called Heaviside function.

Then

$$F_H(\varphi) := \int_{-\infty}^{\infty} H(x)\varphi(x)\,\mathrm{d}x, \quad \text{for all} \quad \varphi \in \mathcal{D}(\mathbb{R}) \tag{A.16}$$

is a distribution of $\mathbb{R}$. We now define:

Definition A.154 (Dirac Delta Function). *Let* $H : \mathbb{R} \to \mathbb{R}$ *be the Heaviside function and* F_H *the corresponding distribution defined by (A.16); then the derivative* F_H' *is called the* Dirac delta function *and is denoted as* δ.

The Dirac delta function δ satisfies:

$$\begin{aligned}\delta(\varphi) &= F_H'(\varphi) = -F_H(\varphi') \\ &= -\int_{-\infty}^{\infty} H(x)\varphi'(x)\,\mathrm{d}x \\ &= -\int_{0}^{\infty} \varphi'(x)\,\mathrm{d}x = -\lim_{x\to\infty} \varphi(x) + \varphi(0) \\ &= \varphi(0).\end{aligned}$$

Remark A.155. The last identity is the property which is often used in a loosely introduction of the Dirac Delta Function by

$$\delta(x) := \begin{cases} \infty & x = 0 \\ 0 & x \neq 0, \end{cases}$$

satisfying the identity

$$\int_{-\infty}^{\infty} \delta(x)\,\mathrm{d}x = 1.$$

Such a function does not exist in the usual sense but should satisfy the characteristic equation

$$\int_{-\infty}^{\infty} \delta(x)\varphi(x)\,\mathrm{d}x = \varphi(0),$$

in a formal sense, which has rigorously been shown by the concept of distributions.

B

Derivations and Proofs of Technical Results

This appendix summarizes technicalities and proofs which may be of interest to the reader but would have interrupted the flow of exposition in the main text.

B.1 Separation Theorems, Farkas Lemma and Supergradient

First we proof the separation theorem A.118:

Proof. Since C is not empty and closed, there exists an $r > 0$ such that $K = N_r(0) \cap C \neq \emptyset$ is a compact set. Considering the problem of minimizing the distance between the origin and the convex set C is therefore equivalent to

$$\min_{x \in C} \|x\|^2 = \min_{x \in K} \|x\|^2 > 0.$$

This minimizing problem exhibits a minimizer $x^* \neq 0$, since the norm $\|\cdot\|$ is continuous and K is compact (see Theorem A.102).

Let $x \in C$ then $\theta x + (1-\theta)x^* \in C$ for $0 < \theta \leq 1$ satisfies

$$\begin{aligned}
&\|\theta x + (1-\theta)x^*\|^2 \geq \|x^*\|^2 \\
&\theta^2 \langle x - x^*, x - x^* \rangle + 2\theta \langle x - x^*, x^* \rangle + \langle x^*, x^* \rangle \geq \langle x^*, x^* \rangle \\
&\theta^2 \langle x - x^*, x - x^* \rangle + 2\theta \langle x - x^*, x^* \rangle \geq 0 \\
&\lim_{\theta \to 0^+} \theta \langle x - x^*, x - x^* \rangle + 2 \langle x - x^*, x^* \rangle = 2 \langle x - x^*, x^* \rangle \geq 0
\end{aligned}$$

yielding

$$\langle x, x^* \rangle \geq \langle x^*, x^* \rangle > 0.$$

Setting $a := x^*$ therefore finishes the proof. □

The separation theorem A.119 follows immediately from separation theorem A.118:

Proof. First the vector v is shifted to the origin and we note that the shifted set

$$C' := \{x' : x' = x - v,\ x \in C\}$$

is convex and $C \subset \overline{C}$. Since $v \notin C$ we find $0 \notin C'$. Thus either $0 \in \partial C'$ or $0 \notin \overline{C'}$. In the latter case applying separation theorem A.118 yields a vector $a \neq 0$ satisfying for all $x' \in C'$, $\langle a, x' \rangle > 0$. Using the definition of C' yields

$$\langle a, x' \rangle = \langle a, x - v \rangle > 0 \quad \text{iff} \quad \langle a, x \rangle > \langle a, v \rangle$$

for all $x \in C$.

In case of $0 \in \partial C'$ we have $v \in \partial C$ and using the properties of a boundary we find a sequence $(v_i)_{i \in \mathbb{N}}$ satisfying

$$\lim_{i \to \infty} v_i = v, \quad \text{and} \quad v_i \notin \overline{C}.$$

Then by the previous consideration there exists a sequence $(a_i)_{i \in \mathbb{N}}$ with

$$\langle a_i, x \rangle > \langle a_i, v_i \rangle, \quad i \in \mathbb{N},\ x \in C.$$

Since $a_i \neq 0$ we can, without loss of generality, assume $\|a_i\| = 1$, $i \in \mathbb{N}$. Then by the Bolzano–Weierstrass theorem (Theorem A.71) we find a subsequence of $(a_i)_{i \in \mathbb{N}}$ converging to some vector $a \in \mathbb{R}^n$ with $\|a\| = 1$ satisfying, by the continuity of the scalar product,

$$\langle a, x \rangle \geq \langle a, v \rangle$$

for all $x \in C$, which concludes the proof. □

Next we prove separation theorem A.120:

Proof. Analogous to the proof of separation theorem A.118 we consider the problem of minimizing the distance between the vector v and the cone C, i.e.,

$$\min_{x \in C} \|x - v\|^2.$$

By the same arguments this minimizing problem exhibits a solution x^*.

Since C is a cone $\alpha x^* \in C$ for all $\alpha \geq 0$. Thus the function

$$g(\alpha) := \|\alpha x^* - v\|^2 = \langle \alpha x^* - v, \alpha x^* - v \rangle,$$

achieves its minimum at $\alpha = 1$. Since g is continuously differentiable and $\alpha = 1$ is in the interior of $[0, \infty)$ it has to satisfy the necessary condition

$$\frac{dg(1)}{d\alpha} = 0.$$

yielding

$$\langle x^*, x^* - v \rangle = 0. \tag{B.1}$$

Repeating the arguments of the proof of separation theorem A.118 we find for $\theta \in (0,\, 1)$ and $x \in C$

$$\begin{aligned}
&\|\theta(x - x^*) + x^* - v\|^2 \geq \|x^* - v\|^2 \\
&\theta^2 \|x - x^*\|^2 + 2\theta \langle x - x^*, x^* - v \rangle \geq 0 \\
&\lim_{\theta \to 0^+} \theta \|x - x^*\|^2 + 2 \langle x - x^*, x^* - v \rangle \geq 0 \\
&\langle x - x^*, x^* - v \rangle = \langle x, x^* - v \rangle \geq 0,
\end{aligned} \tag{B.2}$$

where for the last equality we used (B.1).

Setting $a := x^* - v$ and using (B.1), we find

$$\langle v, a \rangle = \langle v - x^*, a \rangle = - \langle a, a \rangle < 0. \tag{B.3}$$

Since $v \notin C$ and thus $a \neq 0$ the inequalities (B.2) and (B.3) conclude the proof. □

We can now prove the Farkas lemma (Theorem A.36):

Proof. Suppose that the first assertion of the Farkas lemma holds and the second assertion is violated. Then there exists a y satisfying

$$y'A \geq 0 \tag{B.4}$$

and $y'b < 0$. But if (B.4) holds we find $x \geq 0$ satisfying $Ax = b$; but then

$$\begin{aligned}
&y'Ax \geq 0 \\
&y'b \geq 0
\end{aligned}$$

contradicts $y'b < 0$. Therefore the second assertion has to hold.

To prove the other implication we consider the set

$$C := \{c : \ c = Ax,\, x \geq 0\}\,, \quad \text{with} \quad A = (a_1, \ldots, a_n),$$

which is a closed convex cone. Assume that the second assertion of the Farkas lemma (Theorem A.36) holds but the first assertion is not satisfied, implying that $b \notin C$. Then by the separation theorem A.119 there exists a vector y separating C and b, i.e., $y'c \geq 0$ for all $c \in C$ and $y'b < 0$. Since $a_i \in C$, $i = 1, \ldots, n$, there is a vector $y \in \mathbb{R}^m$, satisfying $y'A \geq 0$ and $y'b < 0$ contradicting the second assertion and finishing the proof. □

Finally we prove the existence of a supergradient for a concave function Proposition A.121

Proof. By Proposition A.111 the concavity of f is equivalent to the convexity of the epigraph of $-f$

$$C' := \operatorname{epi}(-f) = \{(x,r) \in \mathbb{R}^{n+1} : x \in C, \text{ and } r \leq f(x)\}.$$

Then for $\hat{x} \in C^\circ$, $(\hat{x}, f(\hat{x})) \notin C'^\circ$, where $C'^\circ \subset \mathbb{R}^{n+1}$ is convex. Applying separation theorem A.119 we therefore find $b = (b_1, \ldots, b_n, b_{n+1}) \in \mathbb{R}^{n+1}$ and $b \neq 0$, such that for all $x \in C$ and $r \geq f(x)$

$$\langle b, (x,r)\rangle \geq \langle b, (\hat{x}, f(\hat{x}))\rangle$$
$$\left\langle \bar{b}, x\right\rangle + b_{n+1} r \geq \langle b, \hat{x}\rangle + b_{n+1} f(\hat{x}) \tag{B.5}$$

with $\bar{b} = (b_1, \ldots, b_n) \in \mathbb{R}^n$. Next we show that $b_{n+1} < 0$. First assume that $b_{n+1} = 0$, then (B.5) yields for every $x \in C$

$$\langle b, x - \hat{x}\rangle \geq 0. \tag{B.6}$$

Since $\hat{x} \in C^\circ$ we find $y \in \mathbb{R}^n$ with $y \neq 0$ such that $\hat{x} + y \in C$ and $\hat{x} - y \in C$. But then (B.6) yields

$$\langle b, y\rangle = 0,$$

and therefore also $\bar{b} = 0$ contradicting that $b \neq 0$.

Next we assume that $b_{n+1} > 0$. Thus for $r < f(\hat{x})$ we find

$$b_{n+1}(r - f(\hat{x})) < 0.$$

But this contradicts (B.5) which especially holds for $(\hat{x}, r)$ and therefore yielding

$$b_{n+1}(r - f(\hat{x})) \geq 0.$$

Thus we finally showed that

$$a := -\frac{\bar{b}}{b_{n+1}}$$

is a supergradient since from (B.5)

$$f(x) - f(\hat{x}) \leq \langle a, x - \hat{x}\rangle$$

follows, which concludes the proof. □

B.2 Proof of the Michel Theorem

For the proof of Theorem 3.71 presented in Michel (1982) the existence of the indefinite integral (3.64a) and the independence of the functions g and f from the time variable are of crucial importance. This allows a twofold extension of the usual proof for the infinite time horizon problem in Halkin (1974). First of all the finite objective value allows the introduction of a salvage value for a truncated problem. Whereas secondly a new state z and linear control v, denoting a strictly increasing time transformation, allow the derivation of a transversality condition. Since Theorem 3.71 is of great importance for the models presented in this book we present the proof in full detail.

B.2.1 Augmented and Truncated Problem

Let us consider some fixed and finite time T. Then we formulate the augmented problem:

$$\begin{aligned}
\max_{u(\cdot),v(\cdot)} & \int_0^{z(T)} \mathrm{e}^{-r\tau} g\left(x(\tau), u(\tau)\right) \mathrm{d}\tau + S\left(z(T) - T\right) \qquad \text{(B.7)}\\
\text{s.t.} \quad & \dot{x}(\tau) = f\left(x(\tau), u(\tau)\right)\\
& \dot{z}(\tau) = v(\tau)\\
& x(0) = x_0, \quad x(z(T)) = x^*(T), \quad z(0) = 0\\
& v(\tau) \geq \frac{1}{2}, \quad \text{for all} \quad \tau \in [0,\, z(T)],
\end{aligned}$$

where $S(y) = \int_{T+y}^{\infty} \mathrm{e}^{-rs} g\left(x^*(s-y), u^*(s-y)\right) \mathrm{d}s$. Note that $v \equiv 1$ yields $z(t) = t$ and therefore the objective value of (B.7) equals that of the original problem at the optimal solution.

Due to the function $z(T)$ occurring in (B.7) this problem is not of standard type, but using integration by substitution we find:

$$\max_{\tilde{u}(\cdot),v(\cdot)} \int_0^T v(t) \mathrm{e}^{-rz(t)} g(\tilde{x}(t), \tilde{u}(t))\, \mathrm{d}t + S\left(z(T) - T\right) \qquad \text{(B.8a)}$$

$$\text{s.t.} \quad \dot{\tilde{x}}(t) = v(t) f\left(\tilde{x}(t), \tilde{u}(t)\right) \qquad \text{(B.8b)}$$

$$\dot{z}(t) = v(t) \qquad \text{(B.8c)}$$

$$\tilde{x}(0) = x_0, \quad \tilde{x}(T) = x^*(T), \quad z(0) = 0 \qquad \text{(B.8d)}$$

$$v(t) \geq \frac{1}{2}, \quad \text{for all} \quad t \in [0,\, T], \qquad \text{(B.8e)}$$

with $\tilde{x}(t) = x\left(z(t)\right)$ and $\tilde{u}(t) = u\left(z(t)\right)$.

B.2.2 Optimal Solution of Problem (B.8)

First we show that

$$(\tilde{x}^*(t), z^*(t), \tilde{u}^*(t), v^*(t)) = (x^*(t), t, u^*(t), 1), \quad t \in [0,\, T] \qquad \text{(B.9)}$$

is an optimal solution of (B.8).

Obviously this solution is admissible, then suppose on the contrary that it is not optimal. Hence a solution $(\hat{x}(\cdot), \hat{z}(\cdot), \hat{u}(\cdot), \hat{v}(\cdot))$ exists satisfying

$$\int_0^T \hat{v}(t) \mathrm{e}^{-r\hat{z}(t)} g(\hat{x}(t), \hat{u}(t))\, \mathrm{d}t + S\left(\hat{z}(T) - T\right) > \int_0^\infty \mathrm{e}^{-rt} g(x^*(t), u^*(t))\, \mathrm{d}t.$$

Using the definition of the salvage value therefore yields

$$\int_0^T \hat{v}(t) \mathrm{e}^{-r\hat{z}(t)} g(\hat{x}(t), \hat{u}(t))\, \mathrm{d}t > \int_0^{z(T)} \mathrm{e}^{-rt} g(x^*(t), u^*(t))\, \mathrm{d}t. \qquad \text{(B.10)}$$

Next we note that due to (B.8c) the function $z: [0, T] \to [0, \tilde{T}]$ is strictly increasing and thus invertible. Moreover its inverse function is differentiable with

$$\frac{\mathrm{d}z^{-1}(\tau)}{\mathrm{d}\tau} = \frac{1}{v(z^{-1}(\tau))}.$$

Applying the substitution rule to the left side of (B.10) for $t = z^{-1}(s)$ we find

$$\int_0^{z(T)} \mathrm{e}^{-rs} g(\hat{x}(z^{-1}(s)), \hat{u}(z^{-1}(s)))\,\mathrm{d}s > \int_0^{z(T)} \mathrm{e}^{-rt} g(x^*(t), u^*(t))\,\mathrm{d}t.$$

But then

$$x^{**}(t) := \begin{cases} \hat{x}(z^{-1}(t)) & t \in [0,\, z(T)] \\ x^*(t) & t > z(T) \end{cases}, \quad u^{**}(t) := \begin{cases} \hat{u}(z^{-1}(t)) & t \in [0,\, z(T)] \\ u^*(t) & t > z(T) \end{cases}$$

is an admissible solution of the infinite time horizon problem yielding

$$\begin{aligned}\int_0^\infty \mathrm{e}^{-rt} g(x^{**}(t), u^{**}(t))\,\mathrm{d}t &= \int_0^{z(T)} \mathrm{e}^{-rt} g(\hat{x}(z^{-1}(t)), \hat{u}(z^{-1}(t)))\,\mathrm{d}t \\ &\quad + \int_{z(T)}^\infty \mathrm{e}^{-rt} g(x^*(t), u^*(t))\,\mathrm{d}t \\ &> \int_0^\infty \mathrm{e}^{-rt} g(x^*(t), u^*(t))\,\mathrm{d}t.\end{aligned}$$

Thus we found a solution of the original infinite time problem contradicting the optimality of $(x^*(\cdot), u^*(\cdot))$. Therefore we proved that (B.9) constitutes an optimal solution of the finite time problem.

B.2.3 Necessary Conditions for Problem (B.8)

From Pontryagin's Maximum Principle we find the following necessary conditions for problem (B.8). There exist λ_0^T and piecewise continuously differentiable functions $\lambda^T(t), \mu^T(t)$, with

$$\left(\lambda_0^T, \lambda^T(t), \mu^T(t)\right) \neq 0 \quad \text{for all} \quad 0 \le t \le T \tag{B.11a}$$

$$\tilde{\mathcal{H}}(x^*, t, u^*, 1, \lambda^T, \mu^T, \lambda_0^T) = \max_{(\tilde{u}, v)} \tilde{\mathcal{H}}(\tilde{x}^*, z^*, \tilde{u}, v, \lambda^T, \mu^T, \lambda_0^T) \tag{B.11b}$$

$$\dot{\lambda}^T = -\lambda_0^T \mathrm{e}^{-rt} g_x(x^*, u^*) - \lambda^T f_x(x^*, u^*) \tag{B.11c}$$

$$\dot{\mu}^T = \lambda_0^T r \mathrm{e}^{-rt} g(x^*, u^*) \tag{B.11d}$$

$$\lambda^T(T) \quad \text{free} \tag{B.11e}$$

$$\mu^T(T) = \lambda_0^T S_y(0) = -r\lambda_0^T \int_T^\infty \mathrm{e}^{-rt} g(x^*, u^*)\,\mathrm{d}t, \tag{B.11f}$$

with the Hamiltonian

$$\tilde{\mathcal{H}}(\tilde{x}, z, \tilde{u}, v, \lambda^T, \mu^T) = \lambda_0^T v \mathrm{e}^{-rz} g(\tilde{x}, \tilde{u}) + \lambda^T v f(\tilde{x}, \tilde{u}) + \mu^T v. \tag{B.12}$$

Exploiting the fact that we already know the optimal solution $(x^*(t), t)$ and $(u^*(t), 1)$, we can state the necessary conditions (B.11) more precisely.

Since the control v appears linearly in $\tilde{\mathcal{H}}$ the maximum of the Hamiltonian (B.12) with respect to v is achieved at one of the endpoints of the interval $[1/2, \infty)$, whenever $\tilde{\mathcal{H}}_v \neq 0$. But $v^* \equiv 1$, therefore $\tilde{\mathcal{H}}_v(t) = 0$ has to hold, yielding

$$\lambda_0^T \mathrm{e}^{-rt} g\left(x^*(t), u^*(t)\right) + \lambda(t)^T f\left(x^*(t), u^*(t)\right) + \mu(t)^T = 0. \tag{B.13}$$

Since $v > 0$ we see that the maximum of the Hamiltonian (B.12) with respect to u is independent of v and also does not depend on the term $\mu^T v$. Thus

$$\underset{\tilde{u}}{\operatorname{argmax}}\, \tilde{\mathcal{H}}\left(x^*(t), z(t), \tilde{u}, v(t), \lambda^T(t), \mu^T(t)\right) = \underset{u}{\operatorname{argmax}}\, \mathcal{H}\left(x^*(t), u, \lambda^T(t), \lambda_0^T\right)$$

with

$$\mathcal{H}\left(x, u, \lambda^T, \lambda_0^T\right) = \lambda_0^T \mathrm{e}^{-rz} g\left(x, u\right) + \lambda^T f\left(x^*, u\right)$$

yields

$$u^*(t) \in \underset{u}{\operatorname{argmax}}\, \mathcal{H}\left(x^*(t), u, \lambda^T(t), \lambda_0^T\right). \tag{B.14}$$

Finally we show that (B.11a) can be strengthened to $(\lambda_0^T, \lambda^T(t)) \neq 0$ for all $t \in [0, T]$. Otherwise a $t_0 \in [0, T]$ exists with $\left(\lambda_0^T, \lambda^T(t_0)\right) = 0$. But owing to (B.11f) and (B.11d) this also implies $\mu^T(t_0) = 0$, and hence contradicts (B.11a). Note that especially $(\lambda_0^T, \lambda^T(0)) \neq 0$ has to hold, which can be reformulated, without loss of generality, as

$$\|(\lambda_0^T, \lambda^T(0))\| = 1. \tag{B.15}$$

B.2.4 Limit of Solutions for Increasing Time Sequence

In a final step we consider an increasing time sequence $(T_i)_{i \in \mathbb{N}}$ satisfying that $\lim_{i \to \infty} T_i = \infty$. For each of these times T_k we can apply the results of the previous subsection. Thus, using (B.15), for every T_i there exists a vector $(\lambda_0^{(i)}, \lambda^{(i)}(t))$ satisfying

$$\left\|\left(\lambda_0^{(i)}, \lambda^{(i)}(0)\right)\right\| = 1.$$

Then from the Bolzano–Weierstrass theorem (Theorem A.71) we know that every bounded sequence has a convergent subsequence. For notational simplicity we denote this convergent subsequence by the same indices yielding the existence of $(\lambda_0, \lambda(0))$ with

$$\lim_{i\to\infty} \lambda_0^{(i)} = \lambda_0, \quad \lim_{i\to\infty} \lambda^{(i)}(0) = \lambda(0), \quad \|(\lambda_0, \lambda(0))\| = 1.$$

Then a general result of linear ODEs, see, e.g., Hartman (1982), assures the existence of a unique solution $\lambda(\cdot)$ of (B.11c) where $\lambda(0)$ is given by the limit of $\lambda^{(i)}(0)$. Since this solution continuously depends on the initial value we also find

$$\lim_{i\to\infty} \lambda^{(i)}(t) = \lambda(t), \quad \text{for all} \quad t \geq 0.$$

Similar arguments prove the existence of a function $\mu(\cdot)$ satisfying

$$\lim_{i\to\infty} \mu^{(i)}(t) = \mu(t), \quad \text{for all} \quad t \geq 0.$$

For these functions the necessary conditions become

$$\lambda_0 \geq 0, \quad (\lambda_0, \lambda(t)) \neq 0, \quad \text{for all } t$$

$$\dot{\lambda} = -\tilde{\mathcal{H}}_x(x^*, z^*, u^*, v^*, \lambda, \mu, \lambda_0) \tag{B.16a}$$

$$\dot{\mu} = \lambda_0 r \mathrm{e}^{-rt} g(x^*, u^*) \tag{B.16b}$$

$$\lim_{i\to\infty} \mu(T_i) = 0 \tag{B.16c}$$

$$-\mu(t) = \lambda_0 \mathrm{e}^{-rt} g(x^*, u^*) + \lambda f(x^*, u^*), \tag{B.16d}$$

where the last identity follows from (B.13) and the others are a direct result of the necessary conditions (B.11).

Using the definition of the Hamiltonian of the original problem *DAM* (3.64)

$$\mathcal{H}(x, u, \lambda, \lambda_0) = \lambda_0 \mathrm{e}^{-rt} g(x, u) + \lambda f(x, u),$$

together with (B.14) yields the Hamiltonian maximizing condition for the original problem

$$\mathcal{H}(x^*(t), u^*(t)\lambda(t), \lambda_0) = \max_u \mathcal{H}(x^*(t), u, \lambda(t), \lambda_0), \quad \text{for all} \quad t \geq 0.$$

The identity

$$\tilde{\mathcal{H}}_x(x^*, z^*, u^*, v^*, \lambda, \mu, \lambda_0) = \mathcal{H}_x(x^*, u^*, \lambda, \lambda_0)$$

together with (B.16a) yields the usual adjoint equation

$$\dot{\lambda} = -\mathcal{H}_x(x^*, u^*, \lambda, \lambda_0).$$

Furthermore (B.16d) and (B.16c) yield

$$-\mu(t) = \mathcal{H}(x^*, u^*, \lambda, \lambda_0)$$

and

$$\lim_{t\to\infty} \mathcal{H}(x^*(t), u^*(t), \lambda(t), \lambda_0) = 0.$$

Finally (B.16b) verifies

$$\mu(t_1) - \mu(t_0) = \lambda_0 r \int_{t_0}^{t_1} \mathrm{e}^{-rt} g(x^*, u^*)\,\mathrm{d}t,$$

yielding

$$\mathcal{H}(x^*(t_0), u^*(t_0), \lambda(t_0), \lambda_0) = \lambda_0 r \int_{t_0}^{\infty} \mathrm{e}^{-rt} g(x^*, u^*)\,\mathrm{d}t,$$

which concludes the proof. □

B.3 Proof of the Transversality Condition in Proposition 3.74

We next follow up with the proof of the necessity of the transversality condition stated in Proposition 3.74.

Proof. The proof uses the following inequality

$$\begin{aligned}
-\mu(t) &= r\lambda_0 \int_t^{\infty} \mathrm{e}^{-rs} g(x^*, u^*)\,\mathrm{d}s \\
&= \lambda_0 \mathrm{e}^{-rt} g(x^*(t), u^*(t)) + \lambda(t) f(x^*(t), u^*(t)) \\
&\geq \lambda_0 \mathrm{e}^{-rt} g(x^*(t), u) + \lambda(t) f(x^*(t), u) \\
&\geq \lambda(t) f(x^*(t), u),
\end{aligned} \tag{B.17}$$

where for the first inequality we use the Hamiltonian maximizing condition and for the last inequality we use the nonnegativity of the function g.

Equation (B.16c) says that $\lim_{t\to\infty} \mu(t) = 0$, implying by (B.17) that the product $\lambda(t) f(x^*(t), u) \leq 0$ for t large enough. Since this inequality holds for arbitrary $u \in \mathbb{R}^m$ the somewhat opaque assumption

$$\{f(x^*, u) : u \in \mathbb{R}^m\} \supset (-\kappa, \kappa),\ \kappa > 0,\ \text{for all } t \geq T_0 \geq 0$$

guarantees that the product and moreover the factor $\lambda(t)$ converges to zero.

The exact proof is done by contradiction. Therefore the bounded variable $\hat{\lambda}$ is defined by

$$\hat{\lambda}(t) = \frac{\lambda(t)}{\max\{1, \|\lambda(t)\|\}}.$$

Thus $\|\hat{\lambda}\| \leq 1$ and hence the following limit exists

$$l = \lim_{t\to\infty} \sup\{\|\hat{\lambda}(s)\| : s \geq t\}.$$

If $l = 0$, we are finished; otherwise we can assume $l > 0$ and a sequence $(t_i)_{i=0}^{\infty}$ converging to infinity and $\|\hat{\lambda}(t_i)\| > l/2$. Since $\kappa > 0$, an ε can be chosen that satisfies $\varepsilon 4/l^2 < \kappa$. Using (B.16c) we especially find an $N \in \mathbb{N}$ such that for all $j \geq N$, $-\varepsilon < -\mu(t_j) < \varepsilon$. Moreover for every t_j a $u_j \in \mathbb{R}^m$ exists with

$$f(x^*(t_j), u_j) = \frac{\varepsilon 4}{l^2 \hat{\lambda}(t_j)},$$

yielding

$$\begin{aligned} -\mu(t_j) &\geq \lambda(t_j) f(x^*(t_j), u_j) = \max\{1, \|\lambda(t)\|\} \frac{\varepsilon 4/l^2}{\|\hat{\lambda}(t_j)\|^2} \\ &\geq \frac{\varepsilon 4}{l^2 \|\hat{\lambda}(t_j)\|^2} > \varepsilon, \end{aligned}$$

which contradicts $-\mu(t_j) < \varepsilon$ and proves the proposition. □

B.4 The Infinite Horizon Transversality Condition Revisited

Let us therefore restate the transversality condition for a problem formulated as a problem of the calculus of variations. Thus we consider

$$\max_{x(\cdot)} \int_0^T g(t, x(t), \dot{x}(t))\, \mathrm{d}t.$$

Using the results of Pontryagin's Maximum Principle we find the corresponding transversality condition

$$g_u\left(t, x(t), u(t)\right)\big|_{t=T} = g_{\dot{x}}\left(t, x(t), \dot{x}(t)\right)\big|_{t=T} = 0$$

and hence for the infinite horizon case

$$\lim_{t \to \infty} g_u\left(t, x(t), u(t)\right) = 0. \tag{B.18}$$

We now restate the example from Halkin (1974) presented in Sect. 3.8.1 under this aspect and note that the problem

$$\begin{aligned} &\max_{u(\cdot)} \int_0^\infty (1 - x)\, u\, \mathrm{d}t \\ \text{s.t.} \quad &\dot{x} = (1 - x)\, u, \\ &x(0) = 0, \quad u \in [0,\ 1], \end{aligned}$$

can easily be transformed in a problem of the calculus of variations by setting

$$\begin{aligned} &\max_{x(\cdot)} \int_0^\infty \dot{x}(t)\, \mathrm{d}t \\ \text{s.t.} \quad &0 \leq \dot{x} \leq (1 - x), \\ &x(0) = 0. \end{aligned}$$

With $g(t, x, \dot{x}) = \dot{x}$ we immediately see (what we already know) that the transversality condition (B.18) is violated since $g_u = 1$. But why does this condition fail in that case? Therefore we directly apply the variational technique and consider a slightly disturbed solution

$$x_\varepsilon(t) := x^*(t) + \varepsilon \delta x(t),$$

where x^* is the optimal solution together with

$$\delta I(\varepsilon) = \lim_{t \to \infty} \left(\int_0^t g(t, x^*, \dot{x}^*) \, \mathrm{d}s - \int_0^t g(t, x_\varepsilon, \dot{x}_\varepsilon) \, \mathrm{d}s \right).$$

Assumed that $\delta I(\varepsilon)$ is differentiable and differentiation and integration can be interchanged we find by the general necessary conditions of a maximizer (see Theorem 4.32):

$$\frac{\mathrm{d}}{\mathrm{d}\varepsilon} \delta I(0) = \lim_{t \to \infty} \left(\int_0^t g_x^* \delta x + g_u^* \dot{\delta x} \, \mathrm{d}s \right) \geq 0.$$

In our case this simply reduces to

$$\lim_{t \to \infty} g_u^* \delta x(t) = \lim_{t \to \infty} \delta x(t) \geq 0. \tag{B.19}$$

But in this form we immediately see, that to be allowed to deduce the transversality condition (B.18) from (B.19) the set of admissible variations $\delta x(\cdot)$ has to be rich enough. One of these conditions is that with $\delta x(\cdot)$ also $-\delta x(\cdot)$ is admissible, allowing to replace the inequality by an equality condition. The other condition has to assure that variations exist satisfying $\lim_{t \to \infty} |\delta x(t)| \geq c > 0$ to be able to deduce

$$\lim_{t \to \infty} g_u^* = 0.$$

But these conditions are easily identified as the property in Proposition 3.74 requiring that the set of admissible velocities contains a neighborhood of zero.

For our example already the first condition fails. To see that we only have to remind that the optimal solution is given for $u \equiv 1$ yielding

$$\dot{x} = 1 - x.$$

Since the varied solutions $x_\varepsilon(\cdot)$ have to satisfy

$$\dot{x}_\varepsilon \leq 1 - x_\varepsilon,$$

we find

$$\begin{aligned} \dot{x} + \varepsilon \dot{\delta x} &\leq 1 - \delta x \\ \varepsilon \dot{\delta x} &\leq -\delta x. \end{aligned} \tag{B.20}$$

Thus if we consider some variation $\delta x(\cdot)$ satisfying (B.20), which is not the zero variation, i.e., $\delta x \not\equiv 0$, its negative counterpart $-\delta x(\cdot)$ cannot satisfy (B.20). But therefore only the condition in the form (B.19) can be deduced and not the stronger transversality condition (B.18).

These considerations can be accomplished in a more general setting and show once more the importance of the set of admissible variations for the derivation of necessary conditions.

Remark B.1. This part on the transversality condition for infinite time horizon problems dates back to the ideas of Florian Wagener, to whom we are grateful for this insight.

B.5 Monotonicity of the Solution Path

The Proposition 3.85 is an immediate consequence of the fact that for an autonomous model of infinite horizon, the optimal solution does not depend on the initial time, but only on the initial state x_0, i.e., the optimal dynamics is an autonomous system. This fact will be proved later in Lemma 5.1 and is depicted in Fig. B.1. Here, we present a proof by constructing a further optimal solution contradicting the assumption of uniqueness. Therefore let us assume that the optimal state trajectory is not monotone and then there exists a $t_0 \geq 0$ and $\tau > 0$, such that $x(t_0) = x(t_0 + \tau)$.

Thus we can define other admissible solutions as

$$(\tilde{u}(t), \tilde{x}(t)) := \begin{cases} (u(t), x(t)) & \text{for} \quad 0 \leq t \leq t_0 \\ (u(t+\tau), x(t+\tau)) & \text{for} \quad t > t_0 \end{cases}$$

$$(\hat{u}(t), \hat{x}(t)) := \begin{cases} (u(t), x(t)) & \text{for} \quad 0 \leq t \leq t_0 + \tau \\ (u(t-\tau), x(t-\tau)) & \text{for} \quad t > t_0 + \tau \end{cases} .$$

To keep the notation simple we use the abbreviations

$$\begin{aligned} g(t) &:= g\left(x(t), u(t)\right) \\ \tilde{g}(t) &:= g\left(\tilde{x}(t), \tilde{u}(t)\right) \\ \hat{g}(t) &:= g\left(\hat{x}(t), \hat{u}(t)\right). \end{aligned}$$

By the optimality of $(x(\cdot), u(\cdot))$ we have

$$V(u^*(\cdot)) = \int_0^\infty \mathrm{e}^{-rt} g(t)\, \mathrm{d}t > \int_0^\infty \mathrm{e}^{-rt} \tilde{g}(t)\, \mathrm{d}t,$$

yielding

$$\begin{aligned} \int_{t_0}^\infty \mathrm{e}^{-rt} g(t)\, \mathrm{d}t &> \int_{t_0}^\infty \mathrm{e}^{-rt} g(t+\tau)\, \mathrm{d}t \\ &= \mathrm{e}^{r\tau} \int_{t_0+\tau}^\infty \mathrm{e}^{-rt} g(t)\, \mathrm{d}t, \end{aligned}$$

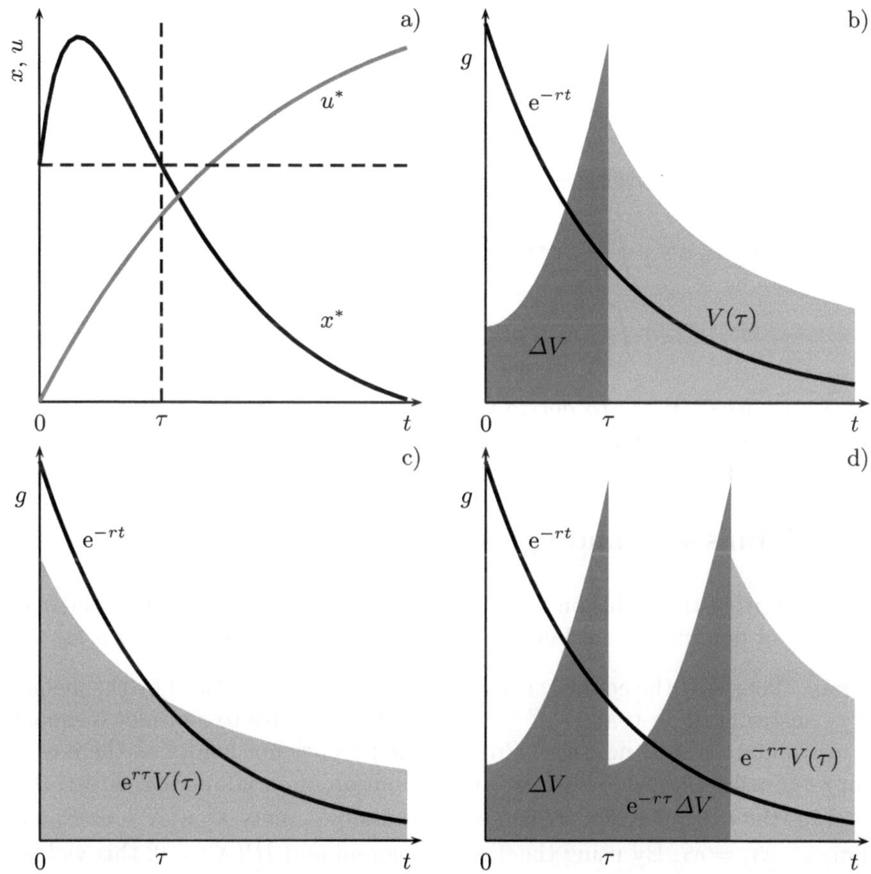

Fig. B.1. The main idea for the proof of Proposition 3.85 is graphically depicted with $t_0 = 0$. Panel (**a**) shows optimal trajectories $x^*(\cdot)$ and $u^*(\cdot)$, with $x^*(0) = x^*(\tau)$. In panel (**b**) the cost function along the optimal path together with the depreciation function is illustrated, where ΔV denotes the total costs for the time interval $[0, \tau]$ and $V(\tau)$ gives the costs for $t \geq \tau$. Then the composition of the costs are depicted in panel (**c**) for the admissible path $(\tilde{u}(\cdot), \tilde{x}(\cdot))$ and in (**d**) for $(\hat{u}(\cdot), \hat{x}(\cdot))$

and

$$\int_{t_0}^{t_0+\tau} \mathrm{e}^{-rt} g(t)\,\mathrm{d}t > (\mathrm{e}^{r\tau} - 1) \int_{t_0+\tau}^{\infty} \mathrm{e}^{-rt} g(t)\,\mathrm{d}t. \tag{B.21}$$

Comparing now the objectives corresponding to $(x(\cdot), u(\cdot))$ and $(\hat{x}(\cdot), \hat{u}(\cdot))$ we find

$$
\begin{aligned}
\Delta V &= \int_0^\infty \mathrm{e}^{-rt} g(t)\,\mathrm{d}t - \int_0^\infty \mathrm{e}^{-rt} \hat{g}(t)\,\mathrm{d}t \\
&= \int_{t_0+\tau}^\infty \mathrm{e}^{-rt} g(t)\,\mathrm{d}t - \int_{t_0+\tau}^\infty \mathrm{e}^{-rt} g(t-\tau)\,\mathrm{d}t \\
&= \int_{t_0+\tau}^\infty \mathrm{e}^{-rt} g(t)\,\mathrm{d}t - \mathrm{e}^{-r\tau} \int_{t_0}^\infty \mathrm{e}^{-rt} g(t)\,\mathrm{d}t \\
&= \left(1 - \mathrm{e}^{-r\tau}\right) \int_{t_0+\tau}^\infty \mathrm{e}^{-rt} g(t)\,\mathrm{d}t - \mathrm{e}^{-r\tau} \int_{t_0}^{t_0+\tau} \mathrm{e}^{-rt} g(t)\,\mathrm{d}t \\
&< \left(1 - \mathrm{e}^{-r\tau}\right) \int_{t_0+\tau}^\infty \mathrm{e}^{-rt} g(t)\,\mathrm{d}t - \mathrm{e}^{-r\tau}\left(\mathrm{e}^{r\tau} - 1\right) \int_{t_0+\tau}^\infty \mathrm{e}^{-rt} g(t)\,\mathrm{d}t = 0,
\end{aligned}
$$

where we used (B.21) to derive the inequality. Hence the contradiction and the proof is completed.

B.6 Admissible and Quasi-Admissible Directions

First we proof the inclusion $\mathbb{A} \subset \mathbb{A}_q$ stated in Proposition 4.8, then under the constraint qualification of Lemma 4.9 we show the converse inclusion $\mathbb{A}_q \subset \mathbb{A}$.

Proof. Note that the equality constraint $F = 0$ can be replaced by the inequality constraints $F \geq 0$ and $-F \geq 0$. Thus we only have to consider inequality constraints. Assume now that Proposition 4.8 does not hold, i.e., there exists an $i \in \mathcal{I}$ with $H^i_X(\hat{X})\delta S < 0$. But the definition of an admissible direction δS assures the existence of a sequence of admissible points $X_j = \hat{X} + \theta_j \delta S_j$ with $\lim_{j\to\infty} \delta S_j = \delta S$. By using the Taylor theorem and $H^i(\hat{X}) = 0$, this yields

$$0 \leq H^i(X_j) = \theta_j H^i_X(\hat{X})\delta S_j + o(\theta_j).$$

Dividing this equation by $\theta_j > 0$ and considering the limit, we get the contradiction

$$0 \leq \lim_{j\to\infty} H^i_X(\hat{X})\delta S_j + o(\theta_j)/\theta_j = H^i_X(\hat{X})\delta S < 0,$$

finishing the proof. □

Proof. First we consider the case of pure equality constraints, and then we consider the general case with inequality constraints.

Case 1 ($H \equiv 0$): To keep the notation as simple as possible, let us introduce the following conventions. Assume that the coordinates are ordered in such a way that the derivative of F for the last k coordinates has full rank, and therefore denote $X = (X^1, X^2)$, with $X^1 \in \mathbb{R}^{n-k}$ and $X^2 \in \mathbb{R}^k$ and any admissible direction δS is written as $\delta S = (\delta S^1, \delta S^2)$. Furthermore, we omit the arguments of functional terms whenever there is no ambiguity and denote the evaluation of function F at $\hat{X}$ by $\hat{F}$. Note furthermore that due to the full rank of $F_X(\hat{X})$ the inequality $k \le n$ has to hold.

We now prove that for $\delta S \in \mathbb{A}_q$ also $\delta S \in \mathbb{A}$ follows. Therefore we take some arbitrary $\delta S \in \mathbb{A}_q$. From the definition of a quasi-admissible direction we find $\hat{F}_X \delta S = 0$, which can be rewritten as $\hat{F}_{X^1}\delta S^1 + \hat{F}_{X^2}\delta S^2 = 0$, and from the assumed ordering of the coordinates, together with the full-rank condition of $\hat{F}_{X^2}$, we find

$$\delta S^2 = -(\hat{F}_{X^2})^{-1}\hat{F}_{X^1}\delta S^1. \tag{B.22}$$

Furthermore, we know from the implicit function theorem that a continuously differentiable function $P : N(X^1, \varepsilon) \to \mathbb{R}^k$ exists with

$$F(X^1, P(X^1)) = 0, \quad \text{and} \quad \hat{X}^2 = P(\hat{X}^1).$$

I.e., for every $X^1 \in N$ the point $(X^1, P(X^1))$ is admissible. Furthermore, the formula of the implicit derivative yields

$$\hat{P}_{X^1} = -(\hat{F}_{X^2})^{-1}\hat{F}_{X^1},$$

and together with (B.22) the identity

$$\delta S^2 = \hat{P}_{X^1}\delta S^1$$

is proved.

Now we have to define a sequence $\theta_i > 0$ and δS_i with $i \in \mathbb{N}$, such that $\lim_{i\to\infty} \delta S_i = \delta S$ (definition of admissible sets). Therefore we use the continuous differentiability of P at X^1 and the property that a κ small enough exists with $X^1 + \theta\delta S^1 \in N$ for all $\theta \le \kappa$. Using the Taylor theorem, we find

$$X_i^2 = P(X^1 + \theta\delta S^1) = \hat{P} + \theta\hat{P}_{X^1}\delta S^1 + o(\theta).$$

We now define a sequence $\theta_i < \kappa$, $i \in \mathbb{N}$ with $\lim_{i\to\infty}\theta_i = 0$ and $\delta S_i = (\delta S^1, \delta S_i^2)$ where

$$\delta S_i^2 := (X_i^2 - \hat{X}^2)/\theta_i.$$

From this construction it is evident that $\hat{X} + \theta_i\delta S_i$ is admissible. Finally, we have to prove that $\lim_{i\to\infty}\delta S_i = \delta S$ holds, by:

$$\begin{aligned}\lim_{i\to\infty}\delta S_i &= (\lim_{i\to\infty}\delta S^1, \lim_{i\to\infty}\delta S_i^2)\\ &= (\delta S^1, \hat{P}_{X^1}\delta S^1)\\ &= (\delta S^1, \delta S^2) = \delta S,\end{aligned}$$

which concludes the proof for $H \equiv 0$.

Case 2 ($H \geq 0$): For $\delta S \in \mathbb{A}_q$ we find $F_X^{j_1}\delta S = 0$ for all $j_1 = 1, \dots, m$, $H_X^{j_2}\delta S = 0$ for $j_2 \in \mathcal{I}_1 \subseteq \mathcal{I}$ and $H_X^{j_3}\delta S > 0$ for $j_3 \in \mathcal{I}_2 \subseteq \mathcal{I}$, where $\mathcal{I}_1 \cap \mathcal{I}_2 = \emptyset$. Applying the construction algorithm of Case 1, we can find a sequence $\theta_i > 0$ and δS_i and corresponding points $X_i = \hat{X} + \theta_i \delta S_i$ satisfying $F^{j_1}(X_i) = 0$ for $j_1 = 1, \dots, m$ and $H^{j_2}(X_i) = 0$ for $j_2 \in \mathcal{I}_1$. Since $\lim_{i\to\infty} \delta S_i = \delta S$ there exists an $N \in \mathbb{N}$ such that for all $i \geq N$ the inequality $H_X^{j_3}\delta S_i > 0$ for all $j_3 \in \mathcal{I}_2$ holds. But then a possibly larger index $M \geq N$ exists with

$$H^{j_3}(X_i) = H^{j_3}(\hat{X}) + \theta_i H_X^{j_3}\delta S_i + o(\theta_i^2) > 0$$

for all $i \geq M$ and $j_3 \in \mathcal{I}_2$. Therefore the subsequence θ_i and δS_i with $i \geq M$ satisfies the conditions of the approximating sequence for δS, the definition of an admissible direction, which finishes the proof. □

B.7 Proof of the Envelope Theorem

Next we prove the envelope theorem for constrained maxima.

Proof. To keep notation simple we assume $\mu \in \mathbb{R}$ and $H \equiv 0$, i.e., only one external parameter and no inequality constraints.

From the first-order necessary condition and the equality constraints we derive

$$G_X(X^*(\mu), \mu) + \Lambda F_X(X^*(\mu), \mu) = 0 \tag{B.23}$$
$$F(X^*(\mu), \mu) = 0, \tag{B.24}$$

where $X^*(\mu)$ denotes the maximizer depending on the parameter μ.

For notational clearness we omit the arguments in the following. If we now consider the total change in the constraints F this yields

$$\frac{\mathrm{d}F}{\mathrm{d}\mu} = \frac{\partial F}{\partial \mu} + F_X \frac{\partial X^*}{\partial \mu}.$$

But as the changed solution $X^*(\mu + \mathrm{d}\mu)$ also has to satisfy (B.24), the total change $\mathrm{d}F/\mathrm{d}\mu = 0$. Hence we get the equivalence relation at $X^*(\mu)$

$$\frac{\partial F}{\partial \mu} = -F_X \frac{\partial X^*}{\partial \mu}. \tag{B.25}$$

From the first-order necessary condition (B.23) we derive at $X^*(\mu)$

$$G_X = -\Lambda F_X. \tag{B.26}$$

Finally, the total change in the objective function G is given by

$$\frac{\mathrm{d}G^*}{\mathrm{d}\mu} = \frac{\partial G}{\partial \mu} + G_X \frac{\partial X^*}{\partial \mu}. \tag{B.27}$$

This reflects the fact that the maximized objective function G^* also depends on μ in its argument X.

Substituting now (B.25) and (B.26) in (B.27)

$$\begin{aligned}\frac{\mathrm{d}G^*}{\mathrm{d}\mu} &= \frac{\partial G}{\partial \mu} - \Lambda F_X \frac{\partial X^*}{\partial \mu} \\ &= \frac{\partial G}{\partial \mu} + \Lambda \frac{\partial F}{\partial \mu} \\ &= \frac{\partial \mathcal{L}}{\partial \mu},\end{aligned}$$

proves the theorem. □

B.8 The Dimension of the Stable Manifold

In this section we prove Theorem 7.10, where it is stated that the dimension of the stable manifold of an equilibrium of the canonical system is at most n. Therefore we consider the corresponding eigenvalue problem which can be stated in the symmetric form

$$\det \begin{pmatrix} \left(\xi - \frac{r}{2}\right)\mathbb{I}^{(n)} - \mathcal{H}^*_{\lambda x} + \frac{r}{2}\mathbb{I}^{(n)} & -\mathcal{H}^*_{\lambda\lambda} \\ \mathcal{H}^*_{xx} & \left(\xi - \frac{r}{2}\right)\mathbb{I}^{(n)} + \mathcal{H}^*_{x\lambda} - \frac{r}{2}\mathbb{I}^{(n)} \end{pmatrix} = 0. \qquad \text{(B.28)}$$

Thus the matrix

$$\begin{pmatrix} -\mathcal{H}^*_{\lambda x} + \frac{r}{2}\mathbb{I}^{(n)} & -\mathcal{H}^*_{\lambda\lambda} \\ \mathcal{H}^*_{xx} & \mathcal{H}^*_{x\lambda} - \frac{r}{2}\mathbb{I}^{(n)} \end{pmatrix}$$

exhibits the following structure

$$\begin{pmatrix} A & B \\ C & -A' \end{pmatrix}, \qquad \text{(B.29)}$$

where B and C are symmetric. To analyze the characteristic polynomial of a matrix of this form, we prove the following lemmas:

Lemma B.2. *Let M be a matrix of the form (B.29); then for $n \in \mathbb{N}$ the matrix*

$$M^{2n} = \begin{pmatrix} \bar{A}_n & \bar{B}_n \\ \bar{C}_n & \bar{A}'_n \end{pmatrix}, \qquad \text{(B.30)}$$

with $\bar{B}_n$ and $\bar{C}_n$ being skew-symmetric.

Proof. First, we prove the conclusion for $n = 1$, i.e., M^2, yielding

$$\begin{pmatrix} A & B \\ C & -A' \end{pmatrix}^2 = \begin{pmatrix} AA + BC & AB - BA' \\ CA - A'C & A'A' + CB \end{pmatrix}.$$

Direct inspection verifies

$$
\begin{aligned}
(A'A' + CB)' &= AA + B'C' = AA + BC \\
(AB - BA')' &= -AB' + B'A' = -(AB - BA') \\
(CA - A'C)' &= -C'A + A'C' = -(CA - A'C)\,.
\end{aligned}
$$

In a further step we show that the product of two matrices M_1 and M_2, where both are of the form (B.30), and which are commutative with respect to the matrix product, exhibit the same structure (B.30). Therefore consider

$$
\begin{pmatrix} A_1 & B_1 \\ C_1 & A_1' \end{pmatrix} \begin{pmatrix} A_2 & B_2 \\ C_2 & A_2' \end{pmatrix} = \begin{pmatrix} A_2 & B_2 \\ C_2 & A_2' \end{pmatrix} \begin{pmatrix} A_1 & B_1 \\ C_1 & A_1' \end{pmatrix}
$$

$$
\begin{pmatrix} A_1A_2 + B_1C_2 & A_1B_2 + B_1A_2' \\ C_1A_2 + A_1'C_2 & C_1B_2 + A_1'A_2' \end{pmatrix} = \begin{pmatrix} A_2A_1 + B_2C_1 & A_2B_1 + B_2A_1' \\ C_2A_1 + A_2'C_1 & C_2B_1 + A_2'A_1' \end{pmatrix}.
$$

Using these identities, we show

$$
\begin{aligned}
(C_2B_1 + A_2'A_1')' &= (B_1'C_2' + A_1''A_2'')' \\
&= B_1'C_2' + A_1A_2 \\
&= A_1A_2 + B_1C_2.
\end{aligned}
$$

The other properties are verified analogously.

Finally, Lemma B.2 is proved by induction. The case $n = 1$ has explicitly been shown. And the identity $M^{2(1+n)} = M^{2(n+1)} = M^{2n}M^2 = M^2M^{2n}$ finishes the proof. □

Lemma B.3. *Let M_1 be a matrix of the form (B.29) and M_2 of the form (B.30); then* $\operatorname{tr}(M_1M_2) = 0$.

Proof. First consider a symmetric matrix $S = S'$ and a skew symmetric matrix $F = -F'$. In that case $\operatorname{tr}(SF) = 0$ holds. This follows from

$$
\begin{aligned}
\operatorname{tr}(FS) &= \sum_{k=1}^{n}\sum_{j=1}^{n} f_{kj}s_{jk} = \sum_{k=2}^{n}\sum_{j=1}^{k-1}(f_{kj}s_{jk} + f_{jk}s_{kj}) + \sum_{k=1}^{n} f_{kk}s_{kk} \\
&= \sum_{k=2}^{n}\sum_{j=1}^{k-1}(f_{kj}s_{jk} - f_{kj}s_{jk}) = 0,
\end{aligned}
$$

where we used the fact, that the diagonal elements of a skew symmetric matrix are zero.

Using the identities $\operatorname{tr}(AB) = \operatorname{tr}(BA)$ and $\operatorname{tr}(A') = \operatorname{tr}(A)$ for all square matrices A and B we are almost finished. The block structure of M_1 and M_2 yields

$$
\begin{aligned}
\operatorname{tr}(M_1M_2) &= \operatorname{tr}\begin{pmatrix} A_1A_2 + B_1C_2 & * \\ * & C_1B_2 - A_1'A_2' \end{pmatrix} \\
&= \operatorname{tr}(A_1A_2) + \operatorname{tr}(B_1C_2) + \operatorname{tr}(C_1B_2) + \operatorname{tr}(-A_1'A_2'),
\end{aligned}
$$

with $B_1 = B_1'$, $C_1 = C_1'$ and $B_2 = -B_2'$, $C_2 = -C_2'$. Therefore

$$\operatorname{tr}(B_1C_2) = \operatorname{tr}(C_1B_2) = 0$$

and

$$\operatorname{tr}(A_1A_2) + \operatorname{tr}(-A_1'A_2') = \operatorname{tr}(A_1A_2) - \operatorname{tr}(A_2A_1) = 0,$$

concludes the proof. □

Thus we can prove Theorem 7.10:

Proof. We mainly refer to the recursive structure of the characteristic polynomial presented in Theorem A.10

$$\chi_J(x) = \sum_{j=0}^{n}(-1)^j\omega_j(J)x^{n-j},$$

where $\omega_0(A) = 1$ and for any $1 \leq j \leq n$

$$j\omega_j(J) = \sum_{k=1}^{j}(-1)^{k+1}\sigma_k\omega_{j-k}(J), \quad \sigma_k = \operatorname{tr}(J^k).$$

From Lemmas B.2 and B.3

$$\sigma_{2i+1} = \operatorname{tr}(J^{2i+1}) = 0 \quad \text{for} \quad i \geq 0$$

immediately follows. Next we prove by induction that

$$\omega_{2i+1}(J) = 0.$$

For $i = 0$ this is evident using $\omega_1(J) = \sigma_1\omega_0(J) = 0$ since $\sigma_1 = 0$. Assuming that $\omega_{2i+1}(J) = 0$ for $i \leq m$, we use the recursive definition of $\omega_i(J)$ to verify the conclusion for $i = m + 1$. In that case we find

$$\begin{aligned}
(2m+3)\omega_{2m+3}(J) &= \sum_{k=1}^{2m+3}(-1)^{k+1}\sigma_k\omega_{2m+3-k}(J) \\
&= \sum_{k=1}^{2m+1}(-1)^{k+1}\sigma_k\omega_{2m+1-k}(J) \\
&\qquad + \sigma_{2m+2}\omega_1(J) + \sigma_{2m+3}\omega_0(J) \\
&= (2m+1)\omega_{2m+1}(J) + 0 + 0 = 0.
\end{aligned}$$

Thus we proved that the characteristic polynomial for (B.28) is given by

$$\chi_J(x) = \sum_{j=0}^{n}(-1)^{2j}\omega_{2j}(J)\tilde{x}^{2(n-j)}$$

or setting $y = x^2$ and using $(-1)^{2j} = 1$ this identity simplifies to

$$\chi_J(y) = \sum_{j=0}^{n} \omega_{2j}(J)\tilde{y}^{n-j}.$$

The last polynomial exhibits n roots $\tilde{\xi}_i,\ i = 1, \dots, n$. Thus the eigenvalues $\xi_k, k = 1, \dots, 2n$ are given by

$$\xi_{2i-1} = \frac{r}{2} + \sqrt{\tilde{\xi}_i},\ \xi_{2i} = \frac{r}{2} - \sqrt{\tilde{\xi}_i}, \quad i = 1, \dots, n.$$

These eigenvalues are symmetric around $\frac{r}{2}$, verifying that at least n eigenvalues have nonnegative real part, which proves that at most n eigenvalues have negative real part, which finishes the proof. □

B.9 Asymptotic Boundary Condition

In this section we proof the propositions about the asymptotic boundary conditions for the case of an equilibrium Proposition 7.20 and limit cycle Proposition 7.27.

B.9.1 Equilibrium

The proof for Proposition 7.20:

Proof. Assume that the first n_- eigenvectors correspond to the stable eigenvalues. Then a point x lying in the linear variety given by the stable eigenspace at $\hat{x}$ satisfies

$$x = \hat{x} + \sum_{i=1}^{n_-} c_i \nu_i \quad \text{iff} \quad x - \hat{x} = \sum_{i=1}^{n_-} c_i \nu_i.$$

From Proposition A.51 we know that $n_+ = n - n_-$ adjoint eigenvectors b_j corresponding to the eigenvalues $\{\xi_j : j = n_- + 1, \dots, n\}$ exist. And in Proposition A.59 it has been proved that b_j is an adjoint eigenvector iff it is orthogonal to the subspace given by $\operatorname{span}\{\nu_i : i \neq j\}$ or equivalently written as

$$b_j' \sum_{i \neq j} c_i \nu_i = 0.$$

Since

$$\mathrm{E}^s\, \hat{x} = \bigcap_{j=n_-+1}^{n} \operatorname{span}\{\nu_i : i \neq j\},$$

this is identical with

$$b_j' \sum_{i \neq j} c_i \nu_i = 0$$

for all $j = n_- + 1, \ldots, n$. Setting

$$\tilde{b}_j = b_j/(b_j'\nu_j)$$

proves the lemma with

$$F = \left(\tilde{b}_{n_-+1}, \ldots, \tilde{b}_n\right).$$

□

B.9.2 Limit Cycle

The proof for Proposition 7.27

Proof. From Theorem 2.78 we know that any fundamental solution $Y(\cdot)$ of (7.39) can be represented by

$$Y(t) = C(t)\mathrm{e}^{Rt},$$

where $C(\cdot)$ is periodic with period 1 and $R \in \mathbb{R}^{n\times n}$ is a constant matrix. Thus the monodromy matrix M is given by

$$\mathrm{M} = Y(1) = \mathrm{e}^{R},$$

since $Y(0) = C(0) = C(1) = \mathbb{I}^{(n)}$. The matrix Q built from a basis of (generalized) eigenvectors of R (and therefore also of M) satisfies

$$Q^{-1}\mathrm{M}\,Q = \mathrm{e}^{D} \quad \text{iff} \quad \mathrm{M}\,Q = Q\mathrm{e}^{D}, \tag{B.31}$$

where D is of block form satisfying

$$D = \begin{pmatrix} D_+ & 0 \\ 0 & D_- \end{pmatrix},$$

with $D_+ \in \mathbb{R}^{(n_++1)\times(n_++1)}$ and $D_- \in \mathbb{R}^{n_-\times n_-}$, denoting the matrices corresponding to the nonnegative and negative eigenvalues of R.

Since the adjoint variational equation

$$\begin{aligned} \dot{Z} &= -Z\Theta f_x\left(\Gamma(t,\varphi)\right)' \\ \text{s.t.} \quad Z(0) &= \mathbb{I}^{(n)} \end{aligned}$$

satisfies $Z(1) = Y^{-1}(1) = \mathrm{M}^{-1}$, we derive from (B.31)

$$Q^{-1}Z(1) = \mathrm{e}^{-D}Q^{-1}.$$

Partitioning the matrices Q^{-1} into the matrices $Q_+^{-1} \in \mathbb{R}^{(n_++1)\times n}$ and $Q_-^{-1} \in \mathbb{R}^{n_-\times n}$, we define $X(t) = Q_+^{-1}Z(t)$. Now owing to the block form of e^{-D} we find

$$\dot{X} = -X\Theta f_x\left(\Gamma(t,\varphi)\right)',$$

with $X(1) = \mathrm{e}^{-D_+} X(0)$ and

$$X(0)Q_- = 0.$$

The latter identity follows from

$$X(0)Q_- = Q_+^{-1} Z(0) Q_- = Q_+^{-1} Q_-,$$

using $Z(0) = \mathbb{I}^{(n)}$ and the block matrix identity

$$\begin{pmatrix} Q_-^{-1} \\ Q_+^{-1} \end{pmatrix} (Q_- \; Q_+) = \begin{pmatrix} Q_-^{-1}Q_- & Q_-^{-1}Q_+ \\ Q_+^{-1}Q_- & Q_+^{-1}Q_+ \end{pmatrix} = \mathbb{I}^{(n)}.$$

In a last step we prove that instead of the specific matrix e^{-D_+} any matrix Λ can be chosen if only it satisfies $|\mathrm{Re}\,\xi| > 1$ for all eigenvalues ξ of Λ. Since in that case an invertible matrix $\tilde{Q}$ exists with

$$\Lambda = \tilde{Q}\mathrm{e}^{-D_+},$$

and therefore

$$\tilde{X} = \tilde{Q}X$$

suffices (7.41) and finishes the proof. □

References

Abraham, R. H. & Shaw, C. D. (1982). *Dynamics – The geometry of behavior*. The Visual Mathematics Library. Santa Cruz, CA: Aerial.

Alemdar, N. M., Sirakaya, S., & Hüsseinov, F. (2006). Optimal time aggregation of infinite horizon control problems. *Journal of Economic Dynamics and Control*, *30*(4), 569–593.

Almeder, C., Caulkins, J. P., Feichtinger, G., & Tragler, G. (2004). An age-structured single-state drug initiation model – cycles of drug epidemics and optimal prevention programs. *Socio-Economic Planning Science*, *38*(1), 91–109.

Almeder, C., Feichtinger, G., Sanderson, W. C., & Veliov, V. M. (2007). Prevention and medication of HIV/AIDS: The case of Botswana. *Central European Journal of Operations Research*, *15*(1), 47–62.

Andronov, A. A. (1929). Les cycles limites de Poincaré et la théorie des oscillations autoentretenues. *Comptes Rendus de l'Académie des Sciences de Paris*, *189*, 559–561.

Andvig, J. C. (1991). The economics of corruption: A survey. *Studi economici*, *43*(1), 57–94.

Annemans, L., Vanoverbeke, N., Tecco, J., Hariga, F., Carpentier, C., & Hartnoll, R. (2000). Macro-economic analysis of heroin markets in the EU and the impact of substitution treatment. EMCDDA Scientific Report EMCDDA/EPI/CT.99.EP.05B/2000, EMCDDA.

Apostol, T. M. (1977). *Mathematical analysis* (2nd ed.). Reading, MA: Addison-Wesley.

Arnold, L. (1974). *Stochastic differential equations: Theory and applications*. New York: Wiley.

Arnold, V. I. (1983). *Geometrical methods in the theory of ordinary differential equations*, volume 250 of *Grundlehren der mathematischen Wissenschaften*. New York: Springer.

Arnold, V. I., Goryunov, V. V., Lyashko, O. V., & Vasiliev, V. A. (1993). *Dynamical system VIII: Singularity theory II – Applications*, volume 39 of *Encyclopaedia of Mathematical Sciences*. Berlin: Springer.

Arquilla, J. & Ronfeldt, D. (1999). *The emergence of noopolitik: Toward an American information strategy.* Santa Monica, CA: RAND.

Arrow, K. J., Karlin, S., & Scarf, H. E. (1958). *Studies in the mathematical theory of inventory and production.* Stanford, CA: Stanford University Press.

Arrow, K. J. & Kurz, M. (1970). *Public investment, the rate of return, and optimal fiscal policy.* Baltimore: The Johns Hopkins University Press.

Arrowsmith, D. K. & Place, C. M. (1990). *An introduction to dynamical systems.* New York: Cambridge University Press.

Arutyunov, A. V. & Vinter, R. B. (2004). A simple "finite approximations" proof of the Pontryagin maximum principle under reduced differentiability hypotheses. *Journal of Set Valued Analysis, 12*(1–2), 5–24.

Ascher, U. M., Mattheij, R. M. M., & Russell, R. D. (1995). *Numerical solution of boundary value problems for ordinary differential equations.* Philadelphia, PA: Society for Industrial and Applied Mathematics.

Aubin, J. P. & Cellina, A. (1984). *Differential inclusions: Set-valued maps and viability theory.* New York: Springer.

Aubin, J. P. & Frankowska, H. (1990). *Set valued analysis.* Boston: Birkhäuser.

Avriel, M. (1976). *Nonlinear programming: analysis and methods.* Automatic computations. Englewood Cliffs, NJ: Prentice-Hall.

Başar, T. & Olsder, G. J. (1999). *Dynamic noncooperative game theory* (2nd ed.). Philadelphia: Society for Industrial and Applied Mathematics.

Barclay, A., Gill, P., & Rosen, J. (1997). SQP methods and their application to numerical optimal control. Numerical Analysis Report 97–3, Department of Mathematics, University of California, San Diego, La Jolla, CA.

Barron, E. N. & Jensen, R. (1986). The Pontryagin maximum principle from dynamic programming and viscosity solutions to first-order partial differential equations. *Transactions of the American Mathematical Society, 298*(2), 635–641.

Barucci, E. & Gozzi, F. (1998). Investment in a vintage capital model. *Research in Economics, 52*(2), 159–188.

Barucci, E. & Gozzi, F. (2001). Technology adoption and accumulation in a vintage capital model. *Journal of Economics, 74*(1), 1–38.

Baveja, A., Batta, R., Caulkins, J. P., & Karwan, M. H. (1993). Modeling the response of illicit drug markets to local enforcement. *Socio-Economic Planning Sciences, 27*(2), 73–89.

Baveja, A., Feichtinger, G., Hartl, R. F., Haunschmied, J. L., & Kort, P. M. (2000). A resource-constrained optimal control model for crackdown on illicit drug markets. *Journal of Mathematical Analysis and Applications, 249*(1), 53–79.

Becker, G. S. (1992). Habits, addictions, and traditions. *Kyklos, 45*(3), 327–346.

Becker, G. S. & Murphy, K. M. (1988). A theory of rational addiction. *Journal of Political Economy, 96*(4), 675–700.

Behrens, D. A. (1998). *The US cocaine epidemic: An optimal control approach to heterogeneous consumption behavior.* PhD thesis, Vienna University of Technology.

Behrens, D. A., Caulkins, J. P., Feichtinger, G., & Tragler, G. (2007). Incentive Stackelberg strategies for a dynamic game on terrorism. In Jørgensen, S., Quincampoix, M., & Thomas, V. L. (Eds.), *Advances in dynamic game theory,* volume 9 of *Annals of the International Society of Dynamic Games* (pp. 459–486). Boston: Birkhäuser.

Behrens, D. A., Caulkins, J. P., Tragler, G., & Feichtinger, G. (2000a). Memory, contagion, and capture rates: Characterizing the types of addictive behavior that are prone to repeated epidemics. Research Report 251, Institute for Mathematical Methods in Economics.

Behrens, D. A., Caulkins, J. P., Tragler, G., & Feichtinger, G. (2000b). Optimal control of drug epidemics: Prevent and treat – but not at the same time? *Management Science, 46*(3), 333–347.

Behrens, D. A., Caulkins, J. P., Tragler, G., & Feichtinger, G. (2002). Why present-oriented societies undergo cycles of drug epidemics. *Journal of Economic Dynamics and Control, 26*(6), 919–936.

Behrens, D. A., Caulkins, J. P., Tragler, G., Haunschmied, J. L., & Feichtinger, G. (1999). A dynamic model of drug initiation: Implications for treatment and drug control. *Mathematical Biosciences, 159*(1), 1–20.

Behrens, D. A. & Neck, R. (2007). OPTGAME: An algorithm approximating solutions for multi-player difference games. In Elleithy, K. (Ed.), *Advances and innovations in systems, computing sciences and software engineering* (pp. 93–98). Dodrecht: Springer.

Bell, D. J. & Jacobson, D. H. (1975). *Singular optimal control problems,* volume 117 of *Mathematics in Science and Engineering.* London: Academic.

Bellman, R. (1957). *Dynamic programming.* Princeton, NJ: Princeton University Press.

Bellman, R. (1961). *Adaptive control processes: A guided tour.* Princeton, NJ: Princeton University Press.

Bensoussan, A., Hurst Jr., E. G., & Näslund, B. (1974). *Management applications of modern control theory.* Amsterdam: North-Holland.

Bensoussan, A. & Lions, J. L. (1982). *Application of variational inequalities in stochastic control.* Amsterdam: North-Holland.

Bensoussan, A. & Lions, J. L. (1984). *Impulse control and quasi-variational inequalities.* Paris: Bordas.

Bensoussan, A., Nissen, G., & Tapiero, C. S. (1975). Optimum inventory and product quality control with deterministic and stochastic deterioration – An application of distributed parameter control. *IEEE Transactions on Automatic Control, 20*(3), 407–412.

Bertsekas, D. P. (2005). *Dynamic programming and optimal control* (3rd ed.). Belmont, MA: Athena Scientific.

Bertsekas, D. P., Nedic, A., & Ozdaglar, A. E. (2003). *Convex analysis and optimization.* Belmont, MA: Athena Scientific.

Bertsekas, D. P., Ozdaglar, A. E., & Tseng, P. (2006). Enhanced Fritz John conditions for convex programming. *SIAM Journal on Optimization, 16*(3), 766–797.

Beyn, W. J., Pampel, T., & Semmler, W. (2001). Dynamic optimization and Skiba sets in economic examples. *Optimal Control Applications and Methods, 22*(5–6), 251–280.

Blaquière, A. (1985). Impulsive optimal control with finite or infinite time horizon. *Journal of Optimization Theory and Applications, 46*(4), 431–439.

Bliss, G. A. (1925). *Calculus of variations.* Number 1 in Carus Mathematical Monograph. Chicago: Open Court.

Bliss, G. A. (1946). *Lectures on the calculus of variations.* Chicago: University of Chicago Press.

Boltyanski, V. G. (1994). The maximum principle: How it came to be. Report 526, Mathematisches Institut, Technische Universität, München.

Boltyanski, V. G., Gamkrelidze, R. V., & Pontryagin, L. S. (1956). On the theory of optimal processes. *Doklady Akademii Nauk SSSR, 110*(1), 7–10.

Booß-Bavnbek, B. & Høyrup, J. (Eds.). (2003). *Mathematics and war.* Basel: Birkhäuser.

Boucekkine, R., Saglam, H. C., & Vallée, T. (2004). Technology adoption under embodiment: A two-stage optimal control approach. *Macroeconomic dynamics, 8*(2), 250–271.

Breakwell, J. V. (1964). Minimum impulse transfer. In Szebehely, V. G. (Ed.), *Celestial mechanics and astrodynamics. Progress in astronautics and aeronautics,* volume 14 (pp. 583–589). New York: Academic.

Breitner, M. (2005). The genesis of differential games in light of Isaacs' contributions. *Journal of Optimization Theory and Applications, 124*(3), 523–559.

Brito, P. M. B. (1999). Local dynamics for optimal control problems of three-dimensional ODE systems. *Annals of Operations Research, 89*(0), 195–214.

Brock, W. A. (1983). Pricing, predation and entry barriers in regulated industries. In D. S. Evans (Ed.), *Breaking Up Bell* (pp. 191–229). New York: North-Holland.

Brock, W. A. & Dechert, W. D. (1983). The generalized maximum principle. Working Paper 8316, Social Science Research Institute, University of Wisconsin.

Brock, W. A. & Dechert, W. D. (1985). Dynamic Ramsey pricing. *International Economic Review, 26*(3), 569–591.

Brock, W. A. & Malliaris, A. G. (1989). *Differential equations, stability and chaos in dynamic economics.* Amsterdam: North-Holland.

Brock, W. A. & Starrett, D. (1999). Nonconvexities in ecological management problems. Working Paper, University of Wisconsin.

Brokate, M. (1985). Pontryagin's principle for control problems in age-dependent population dynamics. *Journal of Mathematical Biology, 23*(1), 75–101.

Bryson, A. E. & Ho, Y. C. (1975). *Applied optimal control: Optimization, estimation, and control.* New York: Hemisphere Publishing.

Bultmann, R. (2007). The impact of supply shocks on optimal dynamic drug policies. Master's thesis, Vienna University of Technology.

Bultmann, R., Caulkins, J. P., Feichtinger, G., & Tragler, G. (2007). How should drug policy respond to market disruptions? forthcoming in *Contemporary Drug Problems.*

Bultmann, R., Caulkins, J. P., Feichtinger, G., & Tragler, G. (2008). Modeling supply shocks in optimal control models of illicit drug consumption. forthcoming in *Lecture Notes in Computer Science, 4818*, 275–282.

Bushaw, D. W. (1952). *Differential equations with a discontinuous forcing term.* PhD thesis, Princeton University, Department of Mathematics.

Büskens, C. & Maurer, H. (2000). SQP-methods for solving optimal control problems with control and state constraints: adjoint variables, sensitivity analysis and real-time control. *Journal of Computational and Applied Mathematics, 120*(1), 85–108.

Byrd, W. & Ward, C. (2004). Drugs and development in Afghanistan. Social Development Papers – Conflict Prevention & Reconstruction 18, The World Bank.

Canon, M. D., Cullum, C. D., & Polak, E. (1970). *Theory of optimal control and mathematical programming.* New York: McGraw-Hill Book Company.

Caputo, M. R. (2005). *Foundations of dynamic economic analysis.* Cambridge, UK: Cambridge University Press.

Carathéodory, C. (1926). Über das Schwarzsche Lemma bei analytischen Funktionen von zwei komplexen Veränderlichen. *Mathematische annalen, 97*(1), 76–98.

Carathéodory, C. (1935). Exemples particuliers et théorie générale dans le calcul des variations. *L'Enseigement Mathématique, 34*, 255–261.

Carlson, D. A., Haurie, A., & Leizarowitz, A. (1991). *Infinite horizon optimal control: deterministic and stochastic systems* (2nd ed.). New York: Springer.

Caroff, N. & Frankowska, H. (1996). Conjugate points and shocks in nonlinear optimal control. *Transactions of the American Mathematical Society, 348*(8), 3133–3153.

Carr, J. (1981). *Applications of center manifold theory.* New York: Springer.

Cass, D. (1965). Optimum growth in an aggregative model of capital accumulation. *Review of Economic Studies, 32*(3), 233–240.

Cass, D. (1966). Optimum growth in an aggregative model of capital accumulation: A turnpike theorem. *Econometrica, 34*(4), 833–850.

Castillo-Chavez, C. & Song, B. (2003). Models of the transmission dynamics of fanatic behaviors. In Banks, H. T. & Castillo-Chavez, C. (Eds.), *Bioterrorism: Mathematical modeling applications in Homeland Security*, volume 28 of *Frontiers in applied mathematics* (pp. 155–172). Philadelphia: Society for Industrial and Applied Mathematics.

Caulkins, J. P. (1993). Local drug markets' response to focused police enforcement. *Operations Research, 41*(5), 848–863.

Caulkins, J. P. (1996). What does mathematical modeling tell us about harm reduction? *Drug and Alcohol Review, 15*(3), 231–235.

Caulkins, J. P. (2005). Models pertaining to how drug policy should vary over the course of a drug epidemic. In Lingren, B. & Grossman, M. (Eds.), *Substance use: Individual behavior, social interactions, markets, and politics*, volume 16 of *Advances in Health Economics and Health Services Research* (pp. 407–439). Amsterdam: Elsevier.

Caulkins, J. P., Behrens, D. A., Knoll, C., Tragler, G., & Zuba, D. (2004). Markov chain modeling of initiation and demand: The case of the US cocaine epidemic. *Health Care Management Science, 7*(4), 319–329.

Caulkins, J. P., Dietze, P., & Ritter, A. (2007). Dynamic compartmental model of trends in Australian drug use. *Health Care Management Science, 10*(2), 151–162.

Caulkins, J. P., Dworak, M., Feichtinger, G., & Tragler, G. (2000). Price-raising drug enforcement and property crime: A dynamic model. *Journal of Economics, 71*(3), 227–253.

Caulkins, J. P., Feichtinger, G., Gavrila, C., Greiner, A., Haunschmied, J. L., Kort, P. M., & Tragler, G. (2006). Dynamic cost-benefit analysis of drug substitution programs. *Journal of Optimization Theory and Applications, 128*(2), 279–294.

Caulkins, J. P., Feichtinger, G., Grass, D., & Tragler, G. (2007a). Bifurcating DNS thresholds in a model of organizational bridge building. *Journal of Optimization Theory and Applications, 133*(1), 19–35.

Caulkins, J. P., Feichtinger, G., Grass, D., & Tragler, G. (2007b). Optimal control of terrorism and global reputation. In submission.

Caulkins, J. P., Feichtinger, G., Johnson, M., Tragler, G., & Yegorov, Y. (2005). Skiba thresholds in a model of controlled migration. *Journal of Economic Behavior & Organization, 57*(4), 490–508.

Caulkins, J. P., Feichtinger, G., Tragler, G., & Veliov, V. M. (2007). Cycles of violence: A dynamic control analysis. *European Journal of Operational Research, 181*(1), 350–361.

Caulkins, J. P., Feichtinger, G., Tragler, G., & Wallner, D. (2007). When in a drug epidemic should the policy objective switch from use reduction to harm reduction? In submission.

Caulkins, J. P., Gragnani, A., Feichtinger, G., & Tragler, G. (2006). High and low frequency oscillations in drug epidemics. *International Journal of Bifurcation and Chaos, 16*(11), 3275–3289.

Caulkins, J. P., Hartl, R. F., Kort, P. M., & Feichtinger, G. (2007). Explaining fashion cycles: Imitators chasing innovators in product space. *Journal of Economic Dynamics and Control, 31*(5), 1535–1556.

Caulkins, J. P., Hartl, R. F., Tragler, G., & Feichtinger, G. (2001). Why politics makes strange bedfellows: Dynamic model with DNS curves. *Journal of Optimization Theory and Applications, 111*(2), 1573–2878.

Caulkins, J. P., Rydell, C. P., Peter, C., Everingham, S. S., James, C., & Shawn, B. (1999). *An ounce of prevention, a pound of uncertainty: The cost-effectiveness of school-based drug prevention programs.* Santa Monica, CA: RAND.

Cesari, L. (1983). *Optimization – Theory and applications, problems with ordinary differential equations.* New York: Springer.

Chander, P. & Wilde, L. (1992). Corruption in tax administration. *Journal of Public Economics, 49*(3), 333–349.

Chiang, A. C. (1992). *Elements of dynamic optimization.* New York: McGraw-Hill.

Chiarella, C. (1988). The cobweb model: Instability and the onset of chaos. *Economic modelling, 5*(4), 377–384.

Chillingworth, D. R. J. (1976). *Differential topology with a view to applications.* London: Pitman.

Clarke, F. H. (1976). The maximum principle under minimal hypotheses. *SIAM Journal on Control and Optimization, 14*(6), 1078–1091.

Clarke, F. H. (1983). *Optimization and nonsmooth analysis.* New York: Wiley.

Clarke, F. H., Ledyaev, Y., Stern, R. J., & Wolenski, P. R. (1998). *Nonsmooth analysis and control theory.* New York: Springer.

Crandall, M. G. & Lions, P. L. (1983). Viscosity solutions of Hamilton-Jacobi equations. *Transactions of the American Mathematical Society, 277*(1), 1–42.

Cullum, J. (1969). Discrete approximations to continuous optimal control problems. *SIAM Journal on Control and Optimization, 7*(1), 32–49.

Dawid, H. & Feichtinger, G. (1996). Optimal allocation of drug control efforts: A differential game analysis. *Journal of Optimization Theory and Applications, 91*(2), 279–297.

Dawid, H., Feichtinger, G., & Novak, A. J. (2002). Extortion as an obstacle to economic growth: A dynamic game analysis. *European Journal of Political Economy, 18*(3), 499–516.

de Hoog, F. R. & Weiss, R. (1980). An approximation theory for boundary value problems on infinite intervals. *Computing, 24*(2-3), 227–239.

Dechert, W. D. (1983). Increasing returns to scale and the reverse flexible accelerator. *Economics Letters, 13*(1), 69–75.

Dechert, W. D. & Nishimura, K. (1983). A complete characterization of optimal growth paths in an aggregated model with a non-concave production function. *Journal of Economic Theory, 31*(2), 332–354.

Deissenberg, C., Feichtinger, G., Semmler, W., & Wirl, F. (2004). Multiple equilibria, history dependence, and global dynamics in intertemporal optimization models. In W. A. Barnett, C. Deissenberg, & G. Feichtinger (Eds.), *Economic Complexity: Non-linear Dynamics, Multi-agents Economies and Learning* (pp. 91–122). Amsterdam: Elsevier Science.

Derzko, N. A., Sethi, S. P., & Thompson, G. L. (1980). Distributed parameter systems approach to the optimal cattle ranching problem. *Optimal Control Applications and Methods, 1*(1), 3–10.

Dietz, K. (1997). Introduction to McKendrick (1926), Applications of mathematics to medical problems. In S. Kotz & N. L. Johnson (Eds.), *Breakthroughs in Statistics* (pp. 17–26). Berlin: Springer.

Dixit, A. K. & Pindyck, R. S. (1994). *Investment under uncertainty.* Princeton: Princeton University Press.

Dockner, E. J. (1985). Local stability analysis in optimal control problems with two state variables. In Feichtinger, G. (Ed.), *Optimal control theory and economic analysis 2* (pp. 89–103). Amsterdam: North-Holland.

Dockner, E. J. & Feichtinger, G. (1991). On the optimality of limit cycles in dynamic economic systems. *Journal of Economics, 53*(1), 31–50.

Dockner, E. J. & Feichtinger, G. (1993). Cyclical consumption patterns and rational addiction. *The American Economic Review, 83*(1), 256–263.

Dockner, E. J., Feichtinger, G., & Jørgensen, S. (1985). Tractable classes of nonzero-sum open-loop Nash differential games: Theory and examples. *Journal of Optimization Theory and Applications, 45*(2), 179–197.

Dockner, E. J., Jørgensen, S., Long, N. V., & Sorger, G. (2000). *Differential games in economics and management science.* Cambridge: Cambridge University Press.

Dockner, E. J. & Long, N. V. (1993). International pollution control: Cooperative versus non-cooperative strategies. *Journal of Environmental Economics and Management, 25*(1), 13–29.

Dolcetta, I. C. (1983). On a discrete approximation of the Hamilton-Jacobi equation of dynamic programming. *Applied Mathematics and Optimization, 10*(1), 367–377.

Dorfman, R. (1969). An economic interpretation of optimal control theory. *American Economic Review, 59*(5), 817–831.

Dreyfus, S. E. (1965). *Dynamic programming and the calculus of variations.* New York: Academic.

Dubovickii, A. J. & Miljutin, Y. A. (1965). Extremum problems in the presence of restrictions. *Computational Mathematics and Mathematical Physics, 5*(3), 1–80.

Easterlin, R. A. (1961). The american baby boom in historical perspective. *The American Economic Review, 51*(5), 869–911.

Ehrlich, I. (2000). Uncertain lifetime, life protection, and the value of life saving. *Journal of Health Economics, 19*(3), 341–367.

Ehtamo, H. & Hämäläinen, R. P. (1986). On affine incentives for dynamic decision problems. In Başar, T. (Ed.), *Dynamic games and applications in economics* (pp. 46–63). Berlin: Springer.

Ehtamo, H. & Hämäläinen, R. P. (1993). A cooperative incentive equilibrium for a resource management problem. *Journal of Economic Dynamics and Control, 17*(4), 659–678.

El Ouardighi, F. (2002). The dynamics of cooperation. *International Game Theory Review, 4*(1), 1–16.

Engwerda, J. C. (2005). *LQ Dynamic optimization and differential games.* New York: Wiley.

Evans, G. C. (1924). The dynamics of monopoly. *American Mathematical Monthly, 31*(2), 75–83.

Everingham, S. S. & Rydell, C. P. (1994). *Modeling the demand for cocaine.* RAND Monograph Report.

Everingham, S. S., Rydell, C. P., & Caulkins, J. P. (1995). Cocaine consumption in the U. S.: Estimating past trends and future scenarios. *Socio-Economic Planning Sciences, 29*(4), 305–314.

Falcone, M. (1987). A numerical approach to the infinite horizon problem of deterministic control theory. *Applied Mathematics and Optimization, 15*(1), 1–13.

Farkas, J. (1902). Theorie der einfachen Ungleichungen. *Journal für die reine und angewandte Mathematik, 124*, 1–27.

Feichtinger, G. (1982a). The Nash solution of a maintenance-production differential game. *European Journal of Operations Research, 10*(2), 165–172.

Feichtinger, G. (1982b). Optimal policies for two firms in a noncooperative research project. In Feichtinger, G. (Ed.), *Optimal control theory and economic analysis* (pp. 373–397). Amsterdam: North-Holland.

Feichtinger, G. (1983). A differential games solution to a model of competition between a thief and the police. *Management Science, 29*(6), 686–699.

Feichtinger, G. (1987). Intertemporal optimization of wine consumption at a party: An unusual optimal control model. In Gandolfo, G. & Monzano, F. (Eds.), *Keynesian Theory Planning Models and Quantitive Economics. Essays in Memory of Vittorio Marrama*, volume II (pp. 777–797). Universita Degli Studi di Roma “La Sapienza”.

Feichtinger, G. (1992). Hopf bifurcation in an advertising diffusion model. *Journal of Economic Behavior & Organization, 17*(3), 401–411.

Feichtinger, G. (2001). Environmental policy design and the economics of crime: Some analogies in intertemporal optimization. In P. Kischka, U. Leopold-Wildburger, R. H. Möring, & F. J. Radermacher (Eds.), *Models, Methods and Decision Support for Management* (pp. 23–48). Heidelberg: Physica.

Feichtinger, G., Grienauer, W., & Tragler, G. (2002). Optimal dynamic law enforcement. *European Journal of Operational Research, 141*(1), 58–69.

Feichtinger, G. & Hartl, R. F. (1986). *Optimale Kontrolle ökonomischer Prozesse: Anwendungen des Maximumprinzips in den Wirtschaftswissenschaften.* Berlin: Walter de Gruyter.

Feichtinger, G., Hartl, R. F., Kort, P. M., & Novak, A. J. (2001). Terrorism control in the tourism industry. *Journal of Optimization Theory and Applications, 108*(2), 283–296.

Feichtinger, G., Hartl, R. F., Kort, P. M., & Veliov, V. M. (2005). Environmental policy, the Porter hypothesis and the composition of capital: Effects of learning and technological progress. *Journal of Environmental Economics and Management, 50*(2), 434–446.

Feichtinger, G., Hartl, R. F., Kort, P. M., & Veliov, V. M. (2006a). Anticipation effects of technological progress on capital accumulation: A vintage capital approach. *Journal of Economic Theory, 126*(1), 143–164.

Feichtinger, G., Hartl, R. F., Kort, P. M., & Veliov, V. M. (2006b). Capital accumulation under technological progress and learning: A vintage capital approach. *European Journal of Operations Research, 172*(1), 293–310.

Feichtinger, G., Hartl, R. F., Kort, P. M., & Wirl, F. (2001). The dynamics of a simple relative adjustment cost framework. *German Economic Review, 2*(3), 255–268.

Feichtinger, G., Hartl, R. F., & Sethi, S. P. (1994). Dynamic optimal control models in advertising: Recent developments. *Management Science, 40*(2), 195–226.

Feichtinger, G., Kistner, K. P., & Luhmer, A. (1988). A dynamic model of intensity splitting. *Zeitschrift für Betriebswirtschaft, 11*, 1242–1258. in German.

Feichtinger, G. & Mehlmann, A. (1986). Planning the unusual: Applications of control theory to nonstandard problems. *Acta Applicandae Mathematicae, 7*(1), 79–102.

Feichtinger, G. & Novak, A. J. (2008). Terror and counter-terror operations: A differential game with a cyclical Nash solution. Forthcoming in *Journal of Optimization Theory and Applications.*

Feichtinger, G., Prskawetz, A., & Veliov, V. M. (2004). Age-structured optimal control in population economics. *Theoretical Population Biology, 65*(4), 373–387.

Feichtinger, G. & Sorger, G. (1986). Optimal oscillations in control models: How can constant demand lead to cyclical production? *Operations Research Letters, 5*(6), 277–281.

Feichtinger, G. & Steindl, A. (2006). DNS curves in a production/inventory model. *Journal of Optimization Theory and Applications, 128*(2), 295–308.

Feichtinger, G., Tragler, G., & Veliov, V. M. (2003). Optimality conditions for age-structured control systems. *Journal of Mathematical Analysis and Applications, 288*(1), 47–68.

Feichtinger, G., Tsachev, T., & Veliov, V. M. (2004). Maximum principle for age and duration structured systems: A tool for optimal prevention and treatment of HIV. *Mathematical Population Studies, 11*(1), 3–28.

Feichtinger, G. & Veliov, V. M. (2007). On a distributed control problem arising in dynamic optimization of a fixed-size population. *SIAM Journal of Optimization, 18*(3), 980–1003.

Feichtinger, G. & Wirl, F. (1991). Politico-economic cycles of regulation and deregulation. *European Journal of Political Economy, 7*(4), 469–485.

Feichtinger, G. & Wirl, F. (1994). On the stability and potential cyclicity of corruption in governments subject to popularity constraints. *Mathematical Social Sciences, 28*(2), 113–131.

Feichtinger, G. & Wirl, F. (2000). Instabilities in concave, dynamic, economic optimization. *Journal of Optimization Theory and Applications, 107*(2), 275–286.

Feldbaum, A. A. (1965). *Optimal control systems.* New York: Academic.

Fent, T., Feichtinger, G., & Tragler, G. (2002). A dynamic game of offending and law enforcement. *International Game Theory Review, 4*(1), 71–89.

Fent, T., Feichtinger, G., & Zalesak, M. (1999). Optimal offending in view of the offender's criminal record. *Central European Journal of Operations Research, 7*(2), 111–177.

Fernández, C. E. & Zuazua, E. (2003). Control theory: History, mathematical achievements and perspectives. *Boletin SEMA, 26*, 79–140.

Filar, J. A. & Vrieze, K. (1997). *Competitive markov decision processes.* New York: Springer.

Fisher, R. A. (1930). *The genetical theory of natural selection.* Oxford: Clarendon.

Fisher, W. H. & Hof, F. X. (2005). Status seeking in the small open economy. *Journal of Macroeconomics, 27*(2), 209–232.

Fleming, W. H. (1988). *Future directions in control theory: A mathematical perspective.* Society for Industrial and Applied Mathematics.

Fleming, W. H. & Rishel, R. W. (1975). *Deterministic and stochastic optimal control.* New York: Springer.

Fletcher, R. (1987). *Practical methods of optimization* (2nd ed.). Chichester: Wiley.

Forman, P. & Sánchez-Rón, J. M. (Eds.). (1996). *National military establishments and the advancement of science: Studies in twentieth century history.* Dordrecht: Kluwer.

Forster, B. A. (1977). On a state variable optimal control problem: Consumption-pollution trade-offs. In J. D. Pitchford & S. J. Turnovsky (Eds.), *Applications of Control Theory to Economic Analysis* (pp. 35–56). Amsterdam: North-Holland.

Fraser-Andrews, G. (1999). A multiple-shooting technique for optimal control. *Journal of Optimization Theory and Applications, 102*(2), 299–313.

Friedlander, G. & Joshi, M. (1998). *Introduction to the theory of distributions* (2nd ed.). Cambridge: Cambridge Universtiy Press.

Friedrich, C. J. (1972). *The pathology of politics, violence, betrayal, corruption, secrecy, and propaganda.* New York: Harper & Row.

Frueh, D. P., Ito, T., Li, J. S., Wagner, G., Glaser, S. J., & Khaneja, N. (2005). Sensitivity enhancement in NMR of macromolecules by application of optimal control theory. *Journal of Biomolecular NMR, 32*(1), 23–30.

Fudenberg, D. & Tirole, J. (1991). *Game theory.* Cambridge, MA: MIT.

Gaimon, C. & Thompson, G. L. (1984). A distributed parameter cohort personnel planning model that uses cross-sectional data. *Management Science, 30*(6), 750–764.

Gamkrelidze, R. V. (1978). *Principles of optimal control theory.* New York: Plenum.

Gardiner, K. L. & Schreckengost, R. C. (1987). A system dynamics model for estimating heroin imports into the United States. *System Dynamics Review, 3*(1), 8–27.

Gavrila, C., Feichtinger, G., Tragler, G., Hartl, R. F., & Kort, P. M. (2005). History-dependence in a rational addiction model. *Mathematical Social Sciences, 49*(3), 273–293.

Girsanov, I. V. (1972). *Lectures on mathematical theory of extremum problems.* New York: Springer.

Goetz, R. U. & Zilberman, D. (2000). The dynamics of spatial pollution. *Journal of Economic Dynamics and Control, 24*(1), 143–163.

Goetz, R. U. & Zilberman, D. (2007). The economics of land-zoning: the dynamic approach. *Optimal Control Applications and Methods, 28*(1), 21–43.

Goffe, W. L. (1993). A user's guide to the numerical solution of two-point boundary value problems arising in continuous time dynamic economic models. *Computational Economics, 6*(3-4), 249–255.

Goldstine, H. H. (1980). *A history of the calculus of variations from the 17th through the 19th century.* New York: Springer.

Golub, G. & van Loan, C. (1996). *Matrix computations* (3rd ed.). Baltimore: The Johns Hopkins University Press.

Gordon, H. S. (1954). The economic theory of a common-property resource: The fishery. *The Journal of Political Economy, 62*(2), 124–142.

Gould, J. P. (1970). Diffusion process and optimal advertising policy. In Phelps, E. S. (Ed.), *Microeconomic foundations of employment and inflation theory* (pp. 338–368). London: Macmillan.

Grass, D., Hartl, R. F., & Kort, P. M. (2007). Capital accumulation and embodied technological progress. Working paper.

Großlicht, F. (2003). Optimal dynamic allocation of prevention and treatment in a model of the australian heroin epidemic. Master's thesis, Vienna University of Technology.

Grossman, M. (1972). On the concept of health capital and the demand for health. *Journal of Political Economy, 80*(2), 223–255.

Grüne, L. (1997). An adaptive grid scheme for the discrete Hamilton-Jacobi-Bellman equation. *Numerische Mathematik, 75*(3), 319–337.

Guckenheimer, J. & Holmes, P. (1983). *Nonlinear oscillations, dynamical systems, and bifurcation of vector fields.* New York: Springer.

Hadeler, K. P. (Ed.). (1984). *Perspectives in mathematics*, chapter spread and age structure in epidemic models (pp. 295–320). Basel: Birkhäuser.

Hadley, G. & Kemp, M. C. (1971). *Variational methods in economics.* London: North-Holland.

Hager, M., Neck, R., & Behrens, D. A. (2001). Solving dynamic macroeconomic policy games using the algorithm OPTGAME 1.0. *Optimal Control Applications and Methods, 22*(5–6), 301–332.

Halkin, H. (1974). Necessary conditions for optimal control problems with infinite horizons. *Econometrica, 42*(2), 267–272.

Halkin, H. & Neustadt, L. W. (1966). General necessary conditions for optimization problems. *Proceedings of the National Academy of Sciences of the United States of America, 56*(4), 1066–1071.

Hall, R. E. & Jones, C. I. (2007). The value of life and the rise in health spending. *Quarterly Journal of Economics, 122*(1), 39–72.

Hartl, R. F. (1984). Optimal dynamic advertising policies for hereditary processes. *Journal of Optimization Theory and Applications, 43*(1), 51–72.

Hartl, R. F. (1987). A simple proof of the monotonicity of the state trajectories in autonomous control problems. *Journal of Economic Theory, 40*(1), 211–215.

Hartl, R. F., Kort, P. M., & Feichtinger, G. (2003). Offense control taking into account heterogeneity of age. *Journal of Optimization Theory and Applications, 116*(3), 591–620.

Hartl, R. F., Kort, P. M., Feichtinger, G., & Wirl, F. (2004). Multiple equilibria and thresholds due to relative investment costs. *Journal of Optimization Theory and Applications, 123*(1), 49–82.

Hartl, R. F. & Sethi, S. P. (1983). A note on the free terminal time transversality condition. *Mathematical Methods of Operations Research, 27*(1), 203–208.

Hartl, R. F. & Sethi, S. P. (1984). Optimal control of a class of systems with continuous lags: Dynamic programming approach and economic interpretations. *Journal of Optimization Theory and Applications, 43*(1), 73–88.

Hartl, R. F., Sethi, S. P., & Vickson, R. G. (1995). A survey of the maximum principles for optimal control problems with state constraints. *SIAM Review, 37*(2), 181–218.

Hartman, P. (1982). *Ordinary differential equations* (2nd ed.). Basel: Birkhäuser.

Harwood, H. J. & Myers, T. G. (Eds.). (2003). *Behavioral, ethical, legal, and social implications of immunotherapies and depot medications for treating drug addiction.* Washington, DC: National Academy.

Hassard, B. D., Kazarinoff, N. D., & Wan, Y. H. (1981). *Theory and application of Hopf bifurcation.* Number 41 in London Mathematical Society Lecture Note Series. London: Cambridge University Press.

Haunschmied, J. L., Feichtinger, G., Kort, P. M., & Hartl, R. F. (2005). Keeping up with the techonlogy pace: A DNS-curve and a limit cycle in a technology investment decision problem. *Journal of Economic Behavior and Organization, 57*(4), 509–529.

Haunschmied, J. L., Kort, P. M., Hartl, R. F., & Feichtinger, G. (2003). A DNS-curve in a two-state capital accumulation model: A numerical analysis. *Journal of Economic Dynamics and Control, 27*(4), 701–716.

Haurie, A. (2001). A historical perspective on cooperative differential games. In Altman, E. & Pourtallier, O. (Eds.), *Advances in dynamic games and applications*, volume 6 of *Annals of the international society of dynamic games* (pp. 19–30). Boston: Birkhäuser.

Haurie, A., Sethi, S. P., & Hartl, R. F. (1984). Optimal control of an age-structured population model with applications to social services planning. *Large Scale Systems, 6*, 133–158.

Hestenes, M. R. (1950). A general problem in the calculus of variations with applications to paths of least time. *RAND Research Memorandum, 100*. RM-100.

Hestenes, M. R. (1965). On variational theory and optimal control theory. *SIAM Journal on Control and Optimization, A3*, 23–48.

Hillman, A. L. & Katz, E. (1987). Hierarchical structure and the social costs of bribes and transfers. *Journal of Public Economics, 34*(2), 129–142.

Hirsch, M. W. & Smale, S. (1974). *Differential equations, dynamical systems, and linear algebra*. New York: Academic.

Hirsch, M. W., Smale, S., & Devaney, R. (2002). *Differential equations, dynamical systems and an introduction to chaos* (2nd ed.). Oxford: Elsevier.

Ho, Y. C. (1970). Differential games, dynamic optimization, and generalized control theory. *Journal of Optimization Theory and Applications, 6*(3), 1573–2878.

Hof, F. X. & Wirl, F. (2008). Wealth induced multiple equilibria in small open economy versions of the Ramsey model. Forthcoming in *Homo Oeconomicus*.

Hofbauer, J. & Sigmund, K. (1988). *The theory of evolution and dynamical systems*. Cambridge, U.K.: Cambridge University Press.

Holling, C. S. (1959). The components of predation as revealed by a study of small mammal predation of the European pine sawfly. *Canadian Entomologist, 91*, 293–320.

Homer, J. B. (1993a). Projecting the impact of law enforcement on cocaine prevalence: A system dynamics approach. *Journal of Drug Issues, 23*(2), 281–295.

Homer, J. B. (1993b). A system dynamics model for cocaine prevalence estimation and trend projection. *Journal of Drug Issues, 23*(2), 251–279.

Hommes, C. H. (1991). *Chaotic Dynamics in Economic Models: Some Simple Case-Studies*. Groningen: Wolters-Noordhoff.

Hopf, E. (1943). Abzweigung einer periodischen Lösung von einer stationären Lösung eines Differentialsystems. *Berichte der Sächsischen Akademie der Wissenschaften, Leipzig, 95*, 3–22.

Hotelling, H. (1931). The economics of exhaustible resources. *Journal of Political Economy, 39*(2), 137–175.

Høyrup, J. (1994). *In measure, number, and weight. Studies in mathematics and culture*. New York: State University of New York Press.

Huisman, K. J. (2001). *Technology investment: A game theoretic real options approach*. Dordrecht: Kluwer Academic.

Intriligator, M. D. (1971). *Mathematical optimization and economic theory*. Englewood-Cliffs: Prentice-Hall.

Ioffe, A. D. & Tichomirov, V. M. (1979). *Theory of extremal problems*, volume 6 of *Studies in mathematics and its applications*. Amsterdam: North-Holland.

Isaacs, R. (1965). *Differential games: A mathematical theory with applications to warfare and pursuit, control and optimization*. New York: Wiley.

John, F. (1948). Extremum problems with inequalities as subsidiary conditions. In Friedrichs, K. O., Neugebauer, O. E., & Stoker, J. J. (Eds.), *Studies and Essays presented to Richard Courant on his 60th Birthday* (pp. 187–204). New York: Interscience.

Jørgensen, S. & Zaccour, G. (2004). *Differential games in marketing*. Boston: Kluwer Academic.

Jørgensen, S. & Zaccour, G. (2007). Developments in differential game theory and numerical methods: economic and management applications. *Computational Management Science*, *4*(2), 159–181.

Jorgenson, D. W. (1963). Capital theory and investment behaviour. *The American Economic Review*, *52*(2), 247–259.

Jorgenson, D. W. (1967). The theory of investment behaviour. In Ferber, R. (Ed.), *Determinants of investment behavior* (pp. 129–155). New York: Columbia University Press.

Jost, J. (2005). *Postmodern analysis* (3rd ed.). Berlin: Springer.

Kalish, S. (1983). Monopolist pricing with dynamic demand and production cost. *Marketing Science*, *2*(2), 135–159.

Kamien, M. I. & Schwartz, N. L. (1971). Optimal maintenance and sale age for a machine subject to failure. *Management Science*, *17*(8), B498–B504.

Kamien, M. I. & Schwartz, N. L. (1991). *Dynamic optimization: The calculus of variations and optimal control in economics and management* (2nd ed.). Amsterdam: North-Holland.

Kandel, D. B. (2002). *Stages and pathways of drug involvement: Examining the gateway hypothesis*. New York: Cambridge University Press.

Kaplan, E. H., Mintz, A., Mishal, S., & Samban, C. (2005). What happened to suicide bombings in Israel? Insights from a terror stock model. *Studies in Conflict and Terrorism*, *28*(3), 225–235.

Karatzas, I. & Shreve, S. E. (1998). *Methods of mathematical finance*. New York: Springer.

Kaskosz, B. & Lojasiewicz, S. (1985). A maximum principle for generalized control systems. *Nonlinear analysis: Theory, methods and applications*, *9*(2), 109–130.

Kaya, C. Y., Lucas, S. K., & Simakov, S. T. (2004). Computations for bang–bang constrained optimal control using a mathematical programming formulation. *Optimal Control Applications and Methods*, *25*(6), 295–308.

Kaya, C. Y. & Noakes, J. L. (1996). Computations and time-optimal controls. *Optimal Control Applications and Methods, 1*, *17*(3), 171–185.

Kaya, C. Y. & Noakes, J. L. (2003). Computational algorithm for time-optimal switching control. *Journal of Optimization Theory and Applications, 117*(1), 69–92.

Kelley, A. (1967). The stable, center-stable, center, center-unstable, unstable manifolds. *Journal of Differential Equations, 3*(4), 546–570.

Kelley, H. J., Kopp, R. E., & Moyer, H. G. (1967). Singular extremals. In Leitmann, G. (Ed.), *Topics of optimization* (pp. 63–101). New York: Academic.

Keohane, N. O. & Zeckhauser, R. J. (2003). The ecology of terror defense. *Journal of Risk and Uncertainty, 26*(2–3), 201–29.

Keyfitz, B. L. & Keyfitz, N. (1997). The McKendrick partial differential equation and its uses in epidemiology and population study. *Mathematical and Computer Modelling, 26*(6), 1–9.

Keyfitz, N. (1977). *Applied mathematical demography.* New York: Wiley.

Kierzenka, J. & Shampine, L. F. (2001). A BVP solver based on residual control and the maltab pse. *ACM Transactions on Mathematical Software (TOMS), 27*(3), 299–316.

Kiseleva, T. & Wagener, F. O. O. (2008). The dependence of indifference regions on the discount rate. Preprint.

Kleiman, M. A. R. (1988). Crackdowns: The effects of intensive enforcement on retail heroin dealing. In Chaiken, M. (Ed.), *Street Level Drug Enforcement: Examining the Issues* (pp. 3–34). Washington, DC: National Institute of Justice.

Kleiman, M. A. R. (1993). Enforcement swamping: A positive-feedback mechanism in rates of illicit activity. *Mathematical and Computer Modelling, 17*(2), 65–75.

Kolmanovskii, V. B. & Shaikhet, L. E. (1996). *Control of systems with aftereffect.* Rhode Island: American Mathematical Society.

Koopmans, T. C. (1965). On the concept of optimal economic growth. *Pontificiae Academiae Scientiarum Scripta Varia, 28*(1), 225–300.

Kraft, D. (1994). TOMP–Fortran modules for optimal control calculations. *ACM Transactions on Mathematical Software, 20*(3), 262–281.

Krauskopf, B., Osinga, H. M., & Galán-Vioque, J. (Eds.). (2007). *Numerical continuation methods for dynamical systems: path following and boundary value problems.* Dordrecht: Springer.

Krugman, P. (1991). History versus expectations. *The Quarterly Journal of Economics, 106*(2), 651–67.

Kuhn, M., Prskawetz, A., Wrzaczek, S., & Feichtinger, G. (2007). Health, survival, and consumption over the life cycle: An optimal control approach. Working paper.

Kunkel, P. & von dem Hagen, O. (2000). Numerical solution of infinite-horizon optimal-control problems. *Computational Economics, 16*(3), 189–205.

Kurz, M. (1968). The general instability of a class of competitive growth processes. *Review of Economic Studies, 35*(2), 155–174.

Kurzhanski, A. B. (2007). 50 years of coexistence in control: The contributions of the Russian community. *European Journal of Control, 13*(1), 49–60.

Kuznetsov, Y. A. (1998). *Elements of applied bifurcation theory* (2nd ed.). New York: Springer.

Lawden, D. F. (1964). Optimal trajectories for space navigation. *The Mathematical Gazette, 48*(366), 478–479.

Lehner, M., Meran, G., & Möller, J. (1980). *De Statu Corruptionis. Entscheidungslogische Einübungen in die höhere Amoralität.* Konstanz: Faude.

Leitmann, G. (1974). *Cooperative and non-cooperative many players differential Games.* New York: Springer.

Lempio, F. & Veliov, V. M. (1998). Discrete approximations of differential inclusions. *GAMM Mitteilungen der Gesellschaft für Angewandte Mathematik und Mechanik, 21*(2), 103–135.

Léonard, D. (1981). The signs of the costate variables and the sufficiency conditions in a class of optimal control problems. *Economics Letters, 8*(4), 321–325.

Léonard, D. & Long, N. V. (1992). *Optimal control theory and static optimization in economics.* Cambridge: Cambridge University Press.

Levin, G., Roberts, E. B., & Hirsch, G. B. (1975). *The persistent poppy: a computer-aided search for heroin Policy.* Cambridge, MA: Ballinger Publishing Company.

Levy, D. T., Chaloupka, F., Gitchell, J., Mendez, D., & Warner, K. E. (2002). The use of simulation models for the surveillance, justification and understanding of tobacco control policies. *Health Care Management Science, 5*(2), 113–120.

Lewis, R. M. (1980). Definitions of order and junction conditions in singular optimal control problems. *SIAM Journal on Control and Optimization, 18*(1), 21–32.

Liski, M. (2001). Thin versus thick CO_2 market. *Journal of Environmental Economics and Management, 41*(3), 295–311.

Liviatan, N. & Samuelson, P. A. (1969). Notes on turnpikes: Stable and unstable. *Journal of Economic Theory, 1*, 454–475.

Loewen, P. D. (1993). *Optimal control via nonsmooth analysis*, volume 2 of *CRM Proceedings & Lecture Notes.* Providence, RI: American Mathematical Society.

Long, N. V. & Shimomura, K. (2003). A new proof of the maximum principle. *Economic Theory, 22*(3), 671–674.

Lorenz, E. N. (1963). Deterministic nonperiodic flow. *Journal of the Atmospheric Sciences, 20*(2), 130–141.

Lorenz, H. W. (1993). *Nonlinear dynamical economics and chaotic motion* (2nd ed.). Berlin: Springer.

Lucas, R. E. (1988). On the mechanics of economic development. *Journal of Monetary Economics, 22*(1), 3–42.

Ludwig, T. (1978). *Optimale Expansionspfade der Unternehmung.* Wiesbaden: Gabler.

Luenberger, D. G. (1997). *Investment science.* New York: Oxford University Press.

MacCoun, R. (1998). Toward a psychology of harm reduction. *American Psychologist, 53*(11), 1199–1208.

MacCoun, R., Reuter, P., & Schelling, T. (1996). Assessing alternative drug control regimes. *Journal of Policy Analysis and Management, 15*(3), 330–352.

MacDonald, N. (1989). *Biological delay systems: Linear stability theory.* Cambridge: Cambridge University Press.

Magill, M. J. (1970). *On a general economic theory of motion.* New York: Springer.

Majumdar, M., Mitra, T., & Nishimura, K. (2000). *Optimization and chaos.* Berlin: Springer.

Makris, M. (2001). Necessary conditions for infinite-horizon discounted two-stage optimal control problems. *Journal of Economic Dynamics and Control, 25*(12), 1935–1950.

Malanowski, K., Maurer, H., & Pickenhain, S. (2004). Second order sufficient optimality conditions for state constrained optimal control problems. *Journal of Optimization Theory and Applications, 123*(3), 594–617.

Mäler, K. G., Xepapadeas, A., & de Zeeuw, A. (2003). The economics of shallow lakes. *Environmental and Resource Economics, 26*(4), 603–624.

Mangasarian, O. L. & Fromovitz, S. (1967). The Fritz John necessary conditions in the presence of equality and inequality constraints. *Journal of Mathematical Analysis and Applications, 17*, 37–47.

Marsden, J. & McCracken, M. (1976). *Hopf bifurcation and its applications.* New York: Springer.

Maurer, H., Büskens, C., Kim, J. H., & Kaya, C. Y. (2005). Optimization methods for the verification of second-order sufficient conditions for bang-bang controls. *Optimal Control Methods and Applications, 26*(3), 129–156.

Maurer, H. & Oberle, H. J. (2002). Second order sufficient conditions for optimal control problems with free final time: The Riccati approach. *SIAM Journal for Control and Optimization, 41*(2), 380–403.

Maurer, H. & Pickenhain, S. (1995). Second-order sufficient conditions for control problems with mixed control-state constraints. *Journal of Optimization Theory and Applications, 86*(3), 649–667.

Mautner, K. (2002). A dynamic one-state two-control optimization model of the current australian heroin problem. Master's thesis, Vienna University of Technology.

Mayne, D. Q. (2007). Personal impressions of the dawn of modern control. *European Journal of Control, 13*(1), 61–70.

McIntyre, J. & Paiewonsky, B. (1967). On optimal control with bounded state variables. In C. T. Leondes (Ed.), *Advances in Control Systems*, volume 5 (pp. 389–419). New York: Academic.

McKendrick, A. G. (1926). Applications of mathematics to medical problems. *Proceedings of the Edinburgh Mathematical Society, 44*, 98–130.

McKenzie, L. W. (1986). Optimal economic growth, turnpike theorems and comparative dynamics. In *Handbook of Mathematical Economics*, volume III (pp. 1281–1355). Amsterdam: North-Holland.

McShane, E. J. (1939). On multipliers for Lagrange problems. *American Journal of Mathematics, 61*(4), 809–819.

Mehlmann, A. (1988). *Applied differential games.* New York: Plenum.

Mendez, D. & Warner, K. E. (2000). Smoking prevalence in 2010: Why the healthy people goal is unattainable. *American Journal of Public Health, 90*(3), 401–403.

Mendez, D., Warner, K. E., & Courant, P. N. (1998). Has smoking cessation ceased? Expected trends in the prevalence of smoking in the United States. *American Journal of Epidemiology, 148*(3), 249–258.

Mercenier, J. & Philippe, M. (2001). Temporal aggregation in a multi-sector economy with endogenous growth. *Journal of Economic Dynamics and Control, 25*(8), 1179–1191.

Michel, P. (1982). On the transversality condition in infinite horizon optimal problems. *Econometrica, 50*(4), 975–985.

Michel, V. (1996). Singular optimal control – the state of the art. AGTM-Report 169, Laboratory of Technomathematics, Geomathematics Group, Department of Mathematics, University of Kaiserslautern.

Miele, A. (1962). Extremization of linear integrals by Green's theorem. In Leitmann, G. (Ed.), *Optimization technics with applications to aerospace systems* (pp. 68–98). New York: Academic.

Miller, B. & Rubinovich, E. (2003). *Impulsive control in continuous and discrete-continuous systems.* New York: Kluwer Academic.

Moore, M. H. (1973). Policies to achieve discrimination on the effective price of heroin. *The American Economic Review, 63*(2), 270–277.

Morawetz, J. (2003). Sensitivity analysis in an optimal control model of the australian heroin epidemic. Master's thesis, Vienna University of Technology.

Moyzisch, F. (2003). Sensitivity analysis in a one-state three-control model of the u.s. cocaine epidemic. Master's thesis, Vienna University of Technology.

Müller, J. (1999). Optimal vaccination patterns in age-structured populations. *SIAM Journal on Applied Mathematics, 59*(1), 222–241.

Musto, D. F. (1987). *The American disease: Origins of narcotic control.* New York: Oxford University Press.

Muzicant, J. (1980). *Systeme mit verteilten Parametern in der Bioökonomie: Ein Maximumprinzip zur Kontrolle altersstrukturierter Modelle.* PhD thesis, Vienna University of Technology.

Näslund, B. (1966). A model of capital budgeting under risk. *Journal of Business, 39*(2), 257–271.

Näslund, B. (1969). Optimal rotation and thinning. *Forest Science, 15*(4), 446–451.

Nerlove, M. & Arrow, K. J. (1962). Optimal advertising policy under dynamic conditions. *Economica, 29*(114), 129–142.

Neustadt, L. W. (1976). *Optimization: A theory of necessary conditions*. Princeton University Press.

Nishimura, K. & Sorger, G. (1996). Optimal cycles and chaos: a survey. *Studies in Nonlinear Dynamics and Econometrics*, *1*(1), 11–28.

Oberle, H. J. (1986). Numerical solution of minimax optimal control problems by multiple shooting technique. *Journal of Optimization Theory and Applications*, *50*(2), 331–357.

Oberle, H. J. (2006). Variationsrechnung und Optimale Steuerung. Lecture Notes, University of Hamburg, Department of Mathematics. http://www.math.uni-hamburg.de/home/oberle/skripte/varopt.html.

Office of National Drug Control Policy (1996). *The National Drug Control Strategy: 1996*. The White House.

Orphanides, A. & Zervos, V. (1998). Myopia and addictive behaviour. *The Economic Journal*, *108*(446), 75–91.

Ozdenoren, E., Salant, S., & Silverman, D. (2006). Willpower and the optimal control of visceral urges. NBER Working Paper 12278, National Bureau of Economic Research.

Pampel, T. (2000). *Numerical approximation of generalized connecting orbits*. PhD thesis, University of Bielefeld.

Penot, J.-P. (1997). Multipliers and generalized derivatives of performance functions. *Journal of Optimization Theory and Applications*, *93*(3), 609–618.

Penot, J.-P. (2004). Differentiability properties of optimal value functions. *Canadian Journal of Mathematics*, *56*(4), 825–842.

Pesch, H. J. & Bulirsch, R. (1994). The maximum principle, Bellman's equation, and Carathéodory's work. *Journal of Optimization Theory and Applications*, *80*(2), 199–225.

Pollack, H. A. (2001). Cost-effectiveness of harm reduction in preventing hepatitis C among injection drug users. *Medical Decision Making*, *21*(5), 357–365.

Pontryagin, L. S., Boltyanski, V. G., Gamkrelidze, R. V., & Mishchenko, E. F. (1962). *The mathematical theory of optimal processes*. New York: Wiley.

Pytlak, R. (1999). *Numerical methods for optimal control problems with state constraints*, volume 1707 of *Lecture Notes in Mathematics*. Berlin: Springer.

Ramsey, F. P. (1928). A mathematical theory of saving. *Economic Journal*, *38*(152), 543–559.

Ravn, H. F. (1999). *Discrete time optimal control*. PhD thesis, Technical University of Denmark.

Rinaldi, S., Feichtinger, G., & Wirl, F. (1998). Corruption dynamics in democratic systems. *Complexity*, *3*(5), 53–64.

Robbins, H. (1967). A generalized Legendre-Clebsch condition for the singular cases of optimal control. *IBM Journal of Research and Development*, *11*(2), 361–372.

Rockafellar, R. (1970). *Convex analysis*. Princeton, NJ: Princeton University Press.

Romer, P. (1990). Endogenous technological change. *Journal of Political Economy, 98*(5), 71–102.

Rose-Ackerman, S. (1978). *Corruption: A study in political economy*. New York: Academic.

Rosen, S. (1988). The value of changes in live expectancy. *Journal of Risk and Uncertainty, 1*(3), 285–304.

Rosenzweig, M. L. & MacArthur, R. H. (1963). Graphical representation and stability conditions of predator-prey interactions. *The American Naturalist, 162*(895), 209–223.

Rossi, C. (1999). Estimating the prevalence of injecting drug users on the basis of Markov models of the HIV/AIDS epidemic: Applications to Italian data. *Health Care Management Science, 2*(3), 173–179.

Rossi, C. (2001). A mover-stayer type model for epidemics of problematic drug use. *Bulletin on Narcotics, 53*(1–2), 39–64.

Rudel, S. (2006). Optimal dynamic harm reduction in models of illicit drug consumption. Master's thesis, Vienna University of Technology.

Rydell, C. P., Caulkins, J. P., & Everingham, S. S. (1996). Enforcement or treatment? Modeling the relative efficacy of alternatives for controlling cocaine. *Operations Research, 44*(5), 687–695.

Rydell, C. P. & Everingham, S. S. (1994). *Controlling cocaine: Supply versus demand programs.* MR-331-ONDCP/A/DPRC. Santa Monica, CA: RAND.

Ryder, H. E. & Heal, G. M. (1973). Optimal growth with intertemporally dependent preferences. *Review of Economic Studies, 40*, 1–33.

Sagan, H. (1969). *Introduction to the calculus of variations.* New-York: McGraw-Hill Book Company.

Saglam, H. C. (2002). Optimal pattern of technology adoption under embodiment with a finite planning horizon: A multi-stage optimal control approach. Discussion Paper 2002031, Université Catholique de Louvain, Institut de Recherches Economiques et Sociales (IRES).

Schelling, T. (1967). Economic analysis of organized crime. In *President's Comission on Law Enforcement and the Administration of Justice Task Force.* Washington, DC: Government Printing Office.

Schelling, T. (1971). Dynamic models of segregation. *Journal of Mathematical Sociology, 1*(2), 143–186.

Schelling, T. (1973). Hockey helmets, concealed weapons, and daylight saving: A study of binary choices with externalities. *Journal of Conflict Resolution, 17*(3), 381–428.

Schwartz, L. (1950). *Théorie des distributions.* Paris: Hermann and Cie.

Seidl, A. (2008). *Optimal control of a two-state diffusion model.* PhD thesis, Vienna University of Technology.

Seierstad, A. & Sydsaeter, K. (1977). Sufficient conditions in optimal control theory. *International Economic Review, 18*(2), 367–391.

Seierstad, A. & Sydsaeter, K. (1986). *Optimal control theory with economic applications.* Amsterdam: North-Holland.

Sethi, S. P. (1974). Sufficient conditions for the optimal control of a class of systems with continuous lags. *Journal of Optimization Theory and Applications, 13*(5), 545–552.

Sethi, S. P. (1977). Nearest feasible paths in optimal control problems: Theory, examples, and counterexamples. *Journal of Optimization Theory and Applications, 23*(4), 563–579.

Sethi, S. P. (1978). A survey of management science applications of the deterministic maximum principle. *TIMS Studies in the Management Science, 9*, 33–68.

Sethi, S. P. (1979a). Optimal advertising policy with the contagion model. *Journal of Optimization Theory and Applications, 29*(4), 615–627.

Sethi, S. P. (1979b). Optimal pilfering policies for dynamic continuous thieves. *Management Science, 25*(6), 535–542.

Sethi, S. P. (1983). Deterministic and stochastic optimization of a dynamic advertising model. *Optimal Control Applications and Methods, 4*(2), 179–184.

Sethi, S. P. (1997). *Optimal consumption and investment with bankruptcy.* Norwell, MA: Kluwer Academic.

Sethi, S. P. & Thompson, G. L. (2000). *Optimal control theory applications to management science and economics* (2nd ed.). Boston: Kluwer Academic.

Sethi, S. P. & Zhang, Q. (1994). *Hierarchical decision making in stochastic manufacturing systems.* Systems and Control: Foundations and Applications. Boston, Cambridge, MA: Birkhäuser.

Seydel, R. (1994). *Practical bifurcation and stability analysis: From equilibrium to chaos* (2nd ed.). New York: Springer.

Shell, K. (1967). Optimal program of capital accumulation for an economy in which there is exogenous technical change. In K. Shell (Ed.), *Essays on the Theory of Optimal Economic Growth* (pp. 1–30). Cambridge: MIT.

Shell, K. (1969). Application of Pontryagin's maximum principle to economics. In H. W. Kuhn & G. P. Szegö (Eds.), *Mathematical Systems Theory and Economics*, volume 1. Berlin: Springer.

Shleifer, A. & Vishny, R. W. (1993). Corruption. *Quarterly Journal of Economics, 108*(3), 599–617.

Shub, M. (1987). *Global stability of dynamical systems.* New York: Springer.

Shvartsman, I. A. (2007). New approximation method in the proof of the maximum principle for nonsmooth optimal control problems with state constraints. *Journal of Mathematical Analysis and Applications, 326*(2), 974–1000.

Skiba, A. K. (1978). Optimal growth with a convex-concave production function. *Econometrica, 46*(3), 527–539.

Smith, D. R. (1974). *Variational methods in optimization.* Englewood Cliffs, NJ: Prentice-Hall.

Solow, R. (1956). Technical change and the aggregate production function. *Review of Economics and Statistics, 33*(3), 127–159.

Sparrow, C. (1982). *The Lorenz equations: Bifurcations, chaos, and strange attractors.* New York: Springer.

Stern, L. E. (1984). Criteria of optimality in the infinite-time optimal control problem. *Journal of Optimization Theory and Applications, 44*(3), 497–508.

Strogatz, S. H. (1994). *Nonlinear dynamics and chaos.* Massachusetts: Addison-Wesley.

Sussmann, H. J. & Willems, J. C. (1997). 300 years of optimal control: From the brachystochrone to the maximum principle. *Control Systems Magazine, IEEE, 17*(3), 32–44.

Sussmann, H. J. & Willems, J. C. (2002). The brachistochrone problem and modern control theory. In A. Anzaldo-Meneses, B. Bonnard, J. P. Gauthier, & F. Monroy-Perez (Eds.), *Contemporary Trends in Non-Linear Geometric Control Theory and its Applications* (pp. 113–165). Singapore: World Scientific.

Swan, G. W. (1988). General applications of optimal control theory in cancer chemotherapy. *Mathematical Medicine and Biology, 5*(4), 303–316.

Swaton, N. (2005). Optimal dynamic allocation of prevention, treatment and law enforcement in a one-state model of the u.s. cocaine epidemic. Master's thesis, Vienna University of Technology.

Tengs, T. O., Ahmad, S., Moore, R., & Gage, E. (2004). Federal policy mandating safer cigarettes: A hypothetical simulation of the anticipated population health gains or losses. *Journal of Policy Analysis and Management, 23*(4), 857–872.

Tengs, T. O., Osgood, N. D., & Chen, L. L. (2001). The cost-effectiveness of intensive national school-based anti-tobacco education: Results from the tobacco policy model. *Preventive Medicine, 33*(6), 558–570.

Thompson, G. L. (1968). Optimal maintenance policy and sale date of a machine. *Management Science, 14*(9), 543–550.

Tomiyama, K. (1985). Two-stage optimal control problems and optimality conditions. *Journal of Economic Dynamics and Control, 9*(3), 317–337.

Tomiyama, K. & Rossana, R. J. (1989). Two-stage optimal control problems with an explicit switch point dependence: Optimality criteria and an example of delivery lags and investment. *Journal of Economic Dynamics and Control, 13*(3), 319–337.

Tonelli, L. (1915). Sur une méthode directe du calcul des variations. *Rendiconti del Circolo Matematico di Palermo, 39*, 233–264.

Tragler, G. (1998). *Optimal control of illicit drug consumption: Treatment versus enforcement.* PhD thesis, Vienna University of Technology.

Tragler, G., Caulkins, J. P., & Feichtinger, G. (2001). Optimal dynamic allocation of treatment and enforcement in illicit drug control. *Operations Research, 49*(3), 352–362.

Troger, H. & Steindl, A. (1991). *Nonlinear stability and bifurcation theory.* Vienna: Springer.

Tsutsui, S. & Mino, K. (1990). Non-linear strategies in dynamic competition with sticky prices. *Journal of Economic Theory, 52*(1), 136–161.

Tu, P. N. V. (1991). *Introductory optimization dynamics* (2nd ed.). Berlin: Springer.

Udwadia, F., Leitmann, G., & Lambertini, L. (2006). A dynamical model of terrorism. *Discrete Dynamics in Nature and Society, 2006*, 1–32.

Ushiki, S. (1980). Analytic expressions of unstable manifolds. *Proceedings of the Japan Academy (Series A), 56*(6), 239–244.

Valentine, F. A. (1937). The problem of Lagrange with differential inequalities as added side conditions. In *Contributions of the Theory of the Calculus of Variations.* Chicago: University of Chicago Press.

van Hilten, O., Kort, P. M., & van Loon, P. J. (1993). *Dynamic policies of the firm – An optimal control approach.* Berlin: Springer.

van Loon, P. J. (1985). Investment grants and alternatives to stimulate industry and employment. In Feichtinger, G. (Ed.), *Optimal control theory and economic analysis* (pp. 331–340). Amsterdam: North-Holland.

Verheyen, P. A. (1992). The jump in models with irreversible investments. In Feichtinger, G. (Ed.), *Dynamic Economic Models and Optimal Control*, volume 4 (pp. 75–89). Amsterdam: Elsevier Science.

Verhulst, P. F. (1838). Notice sur la loi que la population suit dans son accroissement. *Correspondance mathématique et physique, 10*, 113–121.

Vinter, R. B. (2000). *Optimal control.* Boston: Birkhäuser.

von Stryk, O. & Bulirsch, R. (1992). Direct and indirect methods for trajectory optimization. *Annals of Operations Research, 37*(1), 357–373.

Wagener, F. O. O. (2003). Skiba points and heteroclinic bifurcations, with applications to the shallow lake system. *Journal of Economic Dynamics and Control, 27*(9), 1533–1561.

Wagener, F. O. O. (2006). Skiba points for small discount rates. *Journal of Optimization Theory and Applications, 128*(2), 261–277.

Wallner, D. (2005). Optimal control of the U. S. cocaine epidemic: Traditional approach vs. harm reduction. Master's thesis, Vienna University of Technology.

Webb, G. F. (1985). *Theory of nonlinear age-dependent population dynamics.* New York: Dekker.

Weiser, M. & Deuflhard, P. (2007). Inexact central path following algorithms for optimal control problems. *SIAM Journal on Control and Optimization, 46*(3), 792–815.

Wiggins, S. (1990). *Introduction to applied nonlinear dynamical systems and chaos.* New York: Springer.

Willems, J. C. (2007). In control, almost from the beginning until the day after tomorrow. *European Journal of Control, 13*(1), 71–81.

Wirl, F. (1992). Cyclical strategies in two-dimensional optimal control models: Necessary conditions and existence. *Annals of Operations Research, 37*(1), 345–356.

Wirl, F. (1999). Complex dynamic environmental policies. *Resource and Energy Economics*, *21*(1), 19–41.

Wirl, F. & Feichtinger, G. (2005). History dependence in concave economies. *Journal of Economic Behavior and Organization*, *57*(4), 390–407.

Wirl, F., Novak, A. J., Feichtinger, G., & Dawid, H. (1997). Indeterminacy of open-loop Nash equilibria: The ruling class versus the tabloid press. In H. G. Natke & Y. Ben-Haim (Eds.), *Uncertainty: Models and Measures* (pp. 124–136). Berlin: Akademie.

Wrzaczek, S., Kuhn, M., & Oeppen, J. (2007). Reproductive value as a factor in the value of life and the shadow price of of a member of the population. In submission.

Xue, A., Teo, K., Lu, Q., & Mei, S. (2006). Polynomial approximations for the stable and unstable manifolds of the hyperbolic equilibrium points using semi-tensor product. *International Journal of Innovative Computing, Information and Control*, *2*(3), 593–608.

Yaari, M. E. (1965). Uncertain lifetime, life insurance, and the theory of the consumer. *The Review of Economic Studies*, *32*(2), 137–150.

Yeung, D. W. K. & Petrosyan, L. A. (2006). *Cooperative stochastic differential games*. New York: Springer.

Yong, J. & Zhou, X. Y. (1999). *Stochastic controls: Hamiltonian systems and HJB equations*. New York: Springer.

Zeidan, V. (1984). First and second order sufficient conditions for optimal control and the calculus of variations. *Applied Mathematics and Optimization*, *11*(1), 209–226.

Zeidan, V. & Zezza, P. (1988). Necessary conditions for optimal control problems: Conjugate points. *SIAM Journal on Control and Optimization*, *26*(3), 592–608.

Zeiler, I. (2004). Prevention, treatment and law enforcement in an optimal control model of cocaine use in the USA. Master's thesis, Vienna University of Technology.

Zeiler, I. (2008). *Epidemics with multiple equilibria and DNS Curves: Optimal control in dynamic models of HIV/AIDS and of illicit drug use*. PhD thesis, Vienna University of Technology.

Glossary

$\mathcal{S}^\infty(x_0)$	Asymptotic solution set, 242
Σ	Asymptotic boundary condition, 329
$\lvert\cdot\rvert$	Absolute value function, 444
$BV([a,\, b])$	Functions of bounded variation, 478
$W(\xi, t)$	Bellman function, 127
∂S	Boundary of set S, 462
$A \times B$	Cartesian product of matrices A and B, 442
$\mathbb{C}$	Complex numbers, 442
$C^0(D, \mathbb{R}^m)$, C^0	Continuous functions, 463
$C^1(D, \mathbb{R}^m)$, C^1	Continuously differentiable functions, 465
$\Omega(x(t), t)$, Ω	Control region, 105
χ_A	Characteristic polynomial of matrix A, 457
$\overline{S}$	Closure of set S, 461
$\bar{x}$	Complex conjugate of x, 457
$f \equiv y_0$	Constant function f, 443
$g \circ f$	Composition function of f and g, 443
$u(\cdot)$	Control (function), 105
$\mathrm{d}f(\hat{x})/\mathrm{d}x$, $f_x(\hat{x})$	Derivative of function f at $\hat{x}$, 465
$\det A$	Determinant of matrix A, 454
$\dim \mathbb{V}$	Dimension of vector space $\mathbb{V}$, 447
δ	Dirac delta function, 480
$\mathcal{D}(\mathbb{R}^n)$	C^∞ functions with compact support, 479
$\mathbb{V}^*$	Dual space of vector space $\mathbb{V}$, 455
$\mathrm{d}f(\hat{x}^\pm)/\mathrm{d}x$, $f_x^\pm(\hat{x})$	Right/left side derivative of function f at $\hat{x}$, 466
$\partial f(x)/\partial v$	Directional derivative of function f in direction v, 467

$\|\cdot\|_s$	Euclidean norm, 459
E	Eigenspace, 457
ξ	Variable for eigenvalue, 456
ν	Variable for eigenvector, 457
$\emptyset$	Empty set, 442
$\underline{t}$	Entry time, 143
$\text{epi}(f)$	Epigraph of function f, 444
$\bar{t}$	Exit time, 143
$\varphi^t(\cdot)$	Flow of a dynamical system, 20
GL_n	General linear group, 451
$H(\cdot)$	Heaviside function, 480
$\mathcal{H}$	Hamiltonian, 109
$\mathcal{H}^*$	Maximized Hamiltonian, 110
A^{-1}	Inverse matrix of A, 451
$f^{-1}(\cdot)$	Inverse function of $f(\cdot)$, 443
Id_X	Identity function on set X, 442
$\inf A$	Infimum of set A, 442
S°	Interior of set S, 461
iff	If and only if, 441
$\tilde{t}$	Junction time, 143
$\text{kern}\, A$	Kernel of matrix A, 450
$\mathbb{L}$	Overall Lagrangian, 210
$\mathcal{L}$	Lagrangian, 201
$O(\|x\|^\alpha)$, $o(\|x\|^\alpha)$	Landau symbols, 444
N_f	Level set of function f, 444
$\lim_{i\to\infty} x_i$	Limes of x_i, 462
$\lim_{x\to a^+} f(x)$	Right-hand limit of function $f(x)$, 464
$\lim_{x\to b^-} f(x)$	Left-hand limit of function $f(x)$, 464
Γ	Limit cycle, 22
$\omega(x_0)$	Positive limit set for x_0, 23
$\alpha(x_0)$	Negative limit set for x_0, 23
$A \cdot B$, AB	Matrix product of A and B, 449
$\mathbb{R}^{m\times n}$	Real $m \times n$-matrices, 448
$\text{argmax}\, f$	Set of maximizers of function f, 469
W^s	Global stable manifold, 43
W^u	Global unstable manifold, 44

W^c_{loc}	Local center manifold, 43
W^s_{loc}	Local stable manifold, 43
W^u_{loc}	Local unstable manifold, 43
$\max A$	Maximum of set A, 442
$\min A$	Minimum of A, 442
$c(x,u,t) \geq 0$	Mixed path (inequality) constraint, 142
$x \mapsto f(x)$	f maps x to $f(x)$, 442
$N(x,\varepsilon)$	ε-Neighborhood of x, 461
$\mathbb{N}$	Natural numbers, 442
$\Vert\cdot\Vert$	Norm, 459
∇	Nabla operator, 467
$S^\perp$	Orthogonal complement of S, 460
$V(u(\cdot))$	Objective functional, 106
$\mathrm{P}(x)$	Optimal costate rule, 241
$\mathrm{Or}(x_0)$	Orbit at x_0, 19
$\perp$	Orthogonal, 460
$C^{0,1}_p(D,\mathbb{R}^k)$	Continuous and piecewise continuously differentiable functions, 466
$C^0_p(D,\mathbb{R}^k)$	Piecewise continuous functions, 464
$C^1_p(D,\mathbb{R}^k)$	Piecewise continuously differentiable functions, 466
$f^{-1}(B)$	Preimage of set B for function f, 442
$\Gamma(\cdot)$	Periodic solution, 22
$\partial f(\hat{x})/\partial x_j$, $f_{x_j}(\hat{x})$	jth partial derivative of f at $\hat{x}$, 466
Θ	Period of a limit cycle, 21
$h(x,t) \geq 0$	Pure state (inequality) constraint, 142
$A \setminus B$	Relative complement of set B in A, 441
$\mathbb{R}$	Real numbers, 442
$\mathbb{R}_+$	Nonnegative real numbers, 442
$\bar{\mathbb{R}}$	Extended real numbers, 442
$\operatorname{range} f$	Range of function f, 442
$\operatorname{rk} A$	Rank of matrix A, 450
$B \not\subset A$	B is not a subset of A, 441
$B \subset A$	B is a subset of A, 441
$B \subsetneq A$	B is a proper subset of A, 441
$\Vert f\Vert_\infty$	Supremum norm of function f, 463
$\Vert f\Vert_{C^1}$	C^1 norm of function f, 465
$\langle x,y\rangle$	Scalar product of vectors x and y, 456
$\sup A$	Supremum of set A, 442

$\operatorname{supp} f$	Support of function f, 479
$\{\}$	Set braces, 441
$\mathrm{d}^2 f(\hat{x})/\mathrm{d}x^2$, $f_{xx}(\hat{x})$	Second derivative of function f at $\hat{x}$, 468
s.t.	Subject to, 10
A'	Transposed matrix of A, 451
$d(x, u, t)$	Total time derivative of the pure state constraint, 147
$\operatorname{tr} A$	Trace of set A, 449
$\mathbb{I}^{(n)}$	$n \times n$ unit matrix, 450
$V^*(x_0)$	Value function for initial state x_0, 108
δG	First variation of G, 215
$\mathbb{Z}$	Integers, 442

Index

abnormal problem, *112*, 163–164, 308
absolute continuity, *465*
absolute value function, *444*
active constraint, *143*
addiction, 270, 322
  model, 183, 314
    multi-stage, 424
adjoint
  equation, *see* costate, equation
  linear ODE, *81*, 350
  variable, *see* costate
adjustment dynamics, 93
admissible
  control, *106*, 391
  direction, *196*
  pair, *105*
  point, *196*
advertising model, 93, 94, 178, 186, 267, 421
age-structured model, 272, 415–420, 436
AIDS, 98, 315, 323, 436
alcohol consumption, 183, 425
anticipation effect, *388*, 427
arc, *108*
Arrow sufficiency conditions, *121*, *154*, *159*
assimilation, 269
asymptotic
  boundary condition
    equilibrium, 286, *350*
    limit cycle, *353*
    proof of, 500
  solution set, *242*, 253

attracting set, *24*
attractor, 13, *25*
Australian heroin drought, 386
autonomous ODE, 13, *19*, 111
  linear, 31–42
  nonlinear, 42–50
autonomous optimal control problem, *111*
  infinite time, 159–168, 241–242

bang-bang control, *133*
basin of attraction, *24*, 235
Bellman function, *127*
Beltrami identity, *230*
bifurcation, *56*
  analysis, 68–70, 74–77, 172, 258–264
  blue sky, *64*, 173
  diagram, 176, 259, 264
  fold, 57, *64*, 258
  global, 56, 260
  heteroclinic, *56*, 260, 262, 366
  indifference, *262*
  local, 56, 260
  pitchfork, *66*
    subcritical, *67*
    supercritical, *66*
  Poincaré–Andronov–Hopf (PAH), 39, *71*, 301
    subcritical, *73*
    supercritical, *73*
  saddle-node, *64*, 258, 263
  theory, 55–77
  transcritical, *65*, 175, 258, 263

big-O, *see* Landau symbols
bijective function, *443*
Bolza problem, *182*
Bolzano–Weierstrass theorem, *462*, 482, 487
boundary
  condition, *85*
  value problem, *see* BVP
boundary arc, *144*, 146, 282, 359, 369, 385
boundary corrector method, 355
boundary of a set, *462*
bounded function, *444*
brachistochrone problem, 230
bribery, 98, 295, 322
bridge building model, 378
Brownian motion, 423
Brusselator, 95
BVP, *18*, 85–89, 110, 328–330, 336–339

C^1 norm, *465*
calculus of variations, 102, 212–228
canonical
  basis, *447*
  system, *110*, 126, 147, 171, 358, 369, 398
capital accumulation
  game, 435
  model, 93, 102, 124, 145, 180, 181, 268, 319, 434
    multi-stage, 427
Carathéodory solution, 97
Cartesian product, *442*
catching up optimality, *156*
cattle-ranching model, 432
Cauchy-Schwarz inequality, *456*
center, 24, *39*
center manifold, *43*, 74
  approximation, 48, 268
  non-uniqueness, 46
  role of, 57
  two-dimensional, 71
chain rule, *466*
chaos, 23, 98
characteristic polynomial, 342, *457*
  recursive formula of, 459
closed set, *461*
closed-loop
  solution, 428
  strategy, *392*, 393, 394
closure of a set, *462*
Cobb–Douglas function, 94, 307
cobweb model, 93, 98
cocaine epidemic, *51–55*, *168–177*, *264–267*, 314
codimension, *97*
codomain of a function, *442*
cold turkey, 424
column vector, *449*
commutative group, *444*
compact set, 51, 192, *462*, 481
complementary slackness condition, *144*, 146, *150*, 177, *201*, *210*
concave function, *471*
cone, *472*
  convex, *472*
  positive, *472*
conjugate point, 250
constraint qualification, 148, *198*
  failing of, 204
  Karush–Kuhn–Tucker, *198*
  of optimal control problem, *144*, 146, *148*, *151*, 153, 228, 359, 369
consumption vs. investment model, *124–127*, *145–147*, *153–154*, *165–167*
consumption–pollution model, 93, 180, 186
  multistage, 425
contact point/time, *143*
continuation method, 330–339
continuity, *463*
continuously differentiable function, *465*
contour line, *444*
control
  singular, *132*
control region, *105*
convergence, *462*
convex
  analysis, 471–472
  cone, *472*
  function, *471*
  hull, *472*
  set, *471*
cooperative game, 434, 435
corner condition, *150*, 225, 289, 357, 361, 385
corrupt government, 298, 379, 395, 430

corruption, 10, 98, 271, 322
  game, *395–402*, 428
  model, *14–16*, 91, *294–306*, 379, 430
    multi-stage, 426
costate, *109*, 118, 211, 384
  discontinuous, 150
  equation, *109*, 147
  sign, *145*, 281
counter-terror measure, 27, 90, 140, 428
  in multi-stage scenario, 386
crackdowns, 137
cream skimming, 169
current-value notation, *111*, 125
cusp point, *204*, 250
cycle, *see* periodic solution
cycle of violence, 323

decreasing function, *444*
delayed system, 420–422
demographic model, 434, 436
depreciation rate, 94, 124, 315, 425
derivative, *465*
determinant, *454*
diagonal matrix, *449*
diagonalizable matrix, *457*
diffeomorphism, *474*
difference
  equation, *18*
  game, *389*
differentiable
  function, *465*
  manifold, *475*
differential
  equation, *see* ODE
  game, 389–415, 434
    cooperative, 434, 435
    linear–quadratic, *395*
    non-zero-sum, 390, 429
    noncooperative, 390, 405, *434*
  inclusion, 97, *242*
diffusion model, 93, 178, 267
Dirac delta function, 424, *480*
direct numerical method, *380*
directional derivative, 215, *467*
discount rate, *106*, 403
distributed parameter control, 383, *417*, 437
distribution (generalized function), *479*
  derivative, *479*
disutility, 183
DNSS
  curve, 236, 310, 366, 375
  point, 236, 247, *253*, 267, 270, 364, 366
Dockner's formula, *343*
domain of a function, *442*
drug, 10, 323
  chemical foundation, 322
  consumption, 270
  control, 278
  enforcement, 137
  epidemic, 54
  law enforcement, 68, 271
  model, 137, *278–294*, 316, 317, *368–377*, 379, 426
    age-structured, *418–420*
    cocaine epidemic, 51–55, 68–70, *74–77*, *168–177*, *264–267*, 314
    constant treatment, 91
    multi-stage, 385–386
  prevention, 278, 280, 291, 292, 294, 386, 418, 421
  price-raising enforcement, 185
  substitution program, 379
  treatment, 54, 68, 75, 169, 185, 279, 284, 291, 292, 294, 316, 317, 386
  use, 322, 323
  user (heavy, light), 52
dual space, *455*, 479
Dubois–Reymond lemma, 214, 220, *477*
duration-specific model, *436*
dynamic game, *see* differential game
dynamic optimization, *see* optimal control problem
dynamic programming, 127–130
dynamical system, *20*

Easterlin cycle, 95
economic equilibrium, 110
economics of crime, 271, 424
  game, 435
eigenspace, 286, *457*
  center, *41*
  stable, *41*
  unstable, *41*
eigenvalue, 32, *457*
eigenvector, 345, 350, 353, *457*
  adjoint, 354

empty set, *441*
end
  constraint, *see* terminal, constraint
  time, *see* terminal, time
enforcement swamping, 14, 271
entry point/time, *143*, 362
envelope theorem, *207*
  proof of, 496
environmental
  game, 430
  model, 93, 180, 186, 238, 322
    age-structured, 436
    multi-stage, 425
epigraph of a function, *444*, 484
equality constraint, 189, *195*
equilibrium, 12, *21*, *110*
  economic, *110*
  solution, *21*
Euclidean vector space, *460*
Euler equation, *217*, 220, 230
exit point/time, *143*, 287, 362
extortion game, 435
extremal, 122, 152, 184
  point, *200*, 212, 221
  solution, *110*
    multiple, 254, 264
  state trajectory, *110*

Farkas lemma, 201, 228, *453*
  proof of the, 483
fashion cycle, 272
feedback strategy, *see* closed-loop, strategy
finite partition, *475*
fire strategy, 27, 139, 387, 388
fire-and-water model, *see* terror model, fire-and-water
first variation, *see* variation
fishery model, 92
fixed point, *see* equilibrium
Floquet
  multiplier, *85*
  theory, 80–85
focus, *38*, 247, 254, 264
Fredholm alternative theorem, *452*
Fritz John
  multiplier, *202*
full rank, *450*
function, *442*
  of bounded variation, 224, 478
functional, 107, *443*
fundamental matrix solution, *79*
fundamental theorem of calculus, *476*
fundamental theorem of the calculus of variations, 478

game theory, *see* differential game
general linear group, *451*
global manifold, *44*
  stable, *44*
  unstable, *45*
global Maximum Principle, *see* Maximum Principle
Gordon–Schäfer model, 92
Gould's model, 178, 267
gradient, 182, 198, 202, *467*
Gram-Schmidt Process, *460*
growth model, 94, *124–127*, *145–147*, *153–154*, *165–167*, 268, 270

half-space, 196, 453, *456*
Hamilton–Jacobi–Bellman equation (HJB), *128*, 427
  proof of the, 129
  stochastic, *423*
Hamiltonian, *109*
  current-value, *111*, 125
  discontinuous, 150
  distributed, *417*
  linear in the control, 132
  maximized, *110*
  maximizing condition, *109*, 212
  objective value by the, 161
  present-value, *111*, 161, 419
  regular, *113*
harm reduction, 323, 384, 385
  model, 315, 386, 434
    multi-stage, 426
Hartman–Grobman theorem, *43*, 348
health and consumption model, 432
health investment, 432, 436
Heaviside function, *480*
Heine–Borel theorem, *462*
heroin dynamics, 51
Hessian matrix, 113, 205, *469*
heteroclinic
  connection, *46*, 262
    computation, 366–367

cycle, *50, 51*
heterogeneity, 27, 51, 52, 98, 270, 383
heterogeneous drug use, 316
higher order derivative, *468*
history-dependence, 236, *253*, 263
HIV, 98, 315, 323, 436
Holling-type function, 91
homeomorphism, 25, 60, *474*
homoclinic
connection, *47*
Hopf bifurcation, *see* bifurcation, Poincaré–Andronov–Hopf (PAH)
de l'Hospital rule, 169, *466*
housing policy, 269
hyperbolic
equilibrium, 30, *42*, 284
limit cycle, *82*
hyperplane, 83, 345, *447*

identity function, *443*
illicit drug, *see* drug
implicit function theorem, 332, *473*
impulse control, *423–424*
inactive constraint, *143*
Inada-conditions, *125*, 269
increasing function, *444*
indifference point, 185, 247, *252*, 270, 273
indirect numerical method, *380*
inequality constraint, *142*, 185, 189, *195*
infimum, *442*, 470
inflow, 69, 169, 307, 387, 407
initial condition, *17*, *107*, 400, *417*
initial value problem (IVP), *17*, 85, 357
initiation
of drug users, 53, 76, 98, 278, 316, 386, 418, 426, 437
of terrorists, 28
term, 75, 169
injection drug use, 51, 317
injective function, *443*
innovator/imitator, 53
integral equation, *18*, 97
integration
by parts, 219, *477*
by substitution, *477*, 485
theory, *475–478*
integro-differential equation, *421*
intensity-splitting model, 272
interior
of a set, *462*
interior arc, *144*, 287, 359, 369, 385
invariant set, *23*
inverse
function, *443*
function theorem, *474*
of a matrix, *450*
invertible matrix, *450*
isocline, *21*, 166, 236, 260
isomorphism, *448*
Itô integral, 423

Jacobian matrix, 27, 42, *467*
Jordan normal form, 32, *458*
Jorgenson's investment model, 182
jump, *464*
of the costate, *150*, 228
of the state, 423
junction point/time, *143*, 225, 360

Karush–Kuhn–Tucker
conditions, *201*
constraint qualification, *198*
kernel, *448*, *450*
kink, *466*

Lagrange
multiplier, 146, *201*, 208, 283, 358, 359, 369
problem, *182*
Lagrange–Karush–Kuhn–Tucker theorem, *201*, 211
weak, *202*, 210
Lagrangian, *201*, 207
approach, 202–204
general, *202*
of optimal control problem, 144, *150*, 210, 282
overall, 211
Landau symbols, *444*
law enforcement, 68, 271, 429, 430, 435
Lawden's spiral, 185
leader–follower game, *402*, *405–415*
Lebesgue integral, 97, 475
left continuity, *464*
left-hand side derivative, *466*
Legendre–Clebsch condition, *113*, 131
generalized, *134*, 138, 185
strict, *113*, 281, 308

Leslie matrix, 415
level set, *444*
LH-model, 51–55, *278–294*, 323, 379
LHE-model, 98
LHY-model, 98
limit, *462*
  right/left-hand, *464*
  set, *23*
limit cycle, *23*, 51, 76, 301
  numerical computation, 302
  numerical computation of a, 344–346
  of saddle-type, 82
  of the canonical system, 347
  stability, 303
linear
  (in)dependent, *447*
  combination, *445*
  equation, *452*
  form, *455*
  transformation, *448*
linear ODE, *see* autonomous, linear ODE
linear–quadratic
  game, *395*
  optimal control problem, *132*
linearization, *13*, 26, 473
Liouville Formula, *80*, 83
Lipschitz continuity, *463*
little-o, *see* Landau symbols
local manifold, *43*
  existence, 43
  stable, *44*
  unstable, *44*
local Maximum Principle, *221*
logistic growth, *91*, 269
Lorenz attractor, 95
Lotka integral equation, 415
Lotka–Volterra model, 98
Lyapunov coefficient, 72, 73

maintenance model, 179
Mangasarian sufficiency conditions, *120*, *154*, *159*, 297
manifold
  center, *43*, 47
  differentiable, *475*
  global, *44*
  local, *43*, *44*
manifold theorem for flows, *43*, 48, 62, 348
Markov
  property, 107
  strategy, *392*, 393, 394
Markov perfect equilibrium, *405*
MatCont, 97
mathematical epidemiology, 415
MATLAB, *97*
matrix, *449*
  ODE, *33*
  product, *450*
  transposition, *451*
maximizer, *469*
  existence, 470
maximum, *442*
  local/global, *189*, *469*
  strict, *469*
Maximum Principle
  economic interpretation, 117–119
  for autonomous system over infinite horizon, *160*
  for constrained variable time, *116*
  for distributed parameter models, *417*
  for general inequality constraints, *149*
  for infinite time horizon, *156*
  for mixed path constraints, *144*
  for pure state constraints, *149*
  for variable terminal time, *116*
  proof of, 130, 222
  with terminal constraints, *111*
  without terminal constraints, *109*
Maxwell set, 272, *273*
Mayer problem, *182*
McKendrick equation, 415, 418, 432, 436
mean value theorem, *473*
methadone maintenance treatment (MMT), 317, *368–377*
Michel's theorem, *160*
  proof of, 484
Minimum Principle, *see* Maximum Principle
mixed path constraint, *142*, 145, 227, 281, 357
monodromy matrix, *82*, 85, 303, 346
monopolist, 102, 178, 180
monotone function, *444*

most rapid approach path (MRAP), 134, 138, 141, 270
multilinear, *454*
multiple drug use model, 316, 323
multiple equilibria, 185, 236, 261, 270, 309, 401
multiple optimal solutions, *see* indifference point or DNSS point
multi-stage optimal control problem, 384–389
multivalued function, 97, 242, 249, *442*
Musto hypothesis, 53, 316

Nabla operator, 417, *467*
Nash equilibrium, 392
  Markovian (MNE), *393*, 394, 405, 411
  open-loop (OLNE), 393, 395, 400, 403, 408
necessary optimality condition
  of optimal control problem, *see* Maximum Principle
  of real-valued problem, *470*
    general, *199*
  of the calculus of variations, 216
  second order, *470*
needle variation, 184, 225
negative (semi)definite matrix, *451*
neighborhood (topological), *461*
neoclassical optimal growth model, 124, 268, 270
Nerlove–Arrow model, 421
Nerlove-Arrow model, 178
node, *38*, 254
  degenerate, *39*
  star, *39*
nonadmissible direction, *197*
noncooperative game, *see* differential game, noncooperative
nondegeneracy condition (bifurcation), 59, 61, 72
nondifferentiable
  function, *465*
  value function, 164–165
nonhyperbolic equilibrium, 47
nonlinear ODE, *see* autonomous, nonlinear ODE
nonsingular matrix, *450*
nonsmooth
  optimization, 128, 189, 437
  systems, 424
noopolitik, *307*
norm, *459*
  topology, *461*
normal
  form, 57–62
  problem, *112*, 125
null matrix, *449*

objective function(al), *106*, *188*
OCMat toolbox, VIII, 325, 381
ODE, 10, *17*, 96, 105
  autonomous, 13, *19*, 111
  nonautonomous, *19*, 33
open set, *461*
open-loop
  Nash solution, 393, 400
open-loop Stackelberg equilibrium (OLSE), *see* Stackelberg equilibrium
open-loop strategy, *392*
optimal
  arc, *108*
  control, *108*
  costate rule, 240, *241*
  dynamics, 239, 260, 264, 492
  solution, *108*, *188*, 485
  state trajectory, *108*
  vector field, 249, 256, 371, 375
    bifurcation, 260, 262
optimal control history, 101–104
optimal control problem, 127, 182, 188, 216
  autonomous, *111*
  discrete, *195*, 209
  finite time horizon, *105*
  infinite time horizon, *105*, 155
  lagged, *see* delayed system
  linear–quadratic, *132*
  singular, *131*
  standard, *107*, 148
  stochastic, 422–423
  with inequality constraint, 142
  with variable terminal time, 116, 117
optimal costate rule, 245
optimal vector field, *242*
optimum, *470*
orbit, *20*, 25, 45, 60, 73, 349

order
of arc, *133*
of indifference point, *252*
of problem, *133*
of pure state constraint, *148*, 149, 359
ordinary differential equation, *see* ODE
orthogonal, 81, *460*
complement, *460*
orthonormal, *460*
outflow, 28, 69, 75, 139, 169, 279, 307, 388, 406
overtaking optimality, *156*

partial derivative, *467*
partial differential equation (PDE), *18*, 383, 415
path, *see* trajectory
path-dependence, *see* history-dependence
periodic solution, *22*, 76, 317, 345, 353
persistent oscillation, 95, 322, 400
phase condition, *345*, 346
phase portrait, 11
analysis, 166, 243–245
Picard–Lindelöf theorem, *18*
piecewise continuity, *464*
piecewise continuous derivative, *466*
pilfering rate, 429
planning horizon, 101, *see* terminal, time
planning the unusual, 186
Poincaré map, *83*
Poincaré–Bendixson theorem, *50*, 95, 399
pollution game, 430
Pontryagin's Maximum Principle, *see* Maximum Principle
positive (semi)definite matrix, *451*
poverty trap, 270
predator–prey model, 91
preimage for a function, *442*
present-value notation, *111*
price dynamics, 93
principal agent game, 430
principal matrix solution, *33*, *79*
principle of optimality, *128*, 252
production–inventory model, 179, 186, 271, 424
profit of optimal control problem, 106, 118
public opinion, 306
pure state constraint, *142*, 148, 153, 158, 178, 180, 183, 185, 225, 269, 357, 361

quasi-admissible direction, *198*
quasiconcave function, *472*

Ramsey model, 268, 272
finite time, *124–127*
general constraints, *153–154*
infinite time, *165–167*, 181
mixed path constraints, *145–147*
rank
linear transformation, *448*
matrix, 331, *450*
rational addiction, 322
reaction function, 402, 412
real vector space, *see* vector space
real-valued function, *443*
recruitment, 436
of drug users, 53
of honest people, 14
of terrorists, 27, 28, 89, 307, 387, 407
reducible matrix, *458*
repeller, 13, *25*, 30, 256, 262
repelling set, *24*, 73, 347
reproductive value, *434*
reputation
for counter-terror, 306
of a drug, 53, 55, 98, 285, 292, 317, 418
of a politician, 299, 428
resale value, 179
resonant term, *72*
Riccati differential equation, 184
Riemann–Stieltjes integral, *476*
right continuity, *464*
right-hand side derivative, *466*
Rosenzweig & MacArthur predator–prey model, 91
row vector, *449*

saddle path, *see* stable, path
saddle point, 38, *42*, 45, 166, 264
stability, *45*, 236, 299
salvage value, *106*, 119, 160, 391, 425

scalar product, 214, *456*, 482
Schelling diagram, 271
scrap value, *see* salvage value
second derivative, *468*
semistable
  equilibrium, *25*, 30, 64, 256, 262
  limit cycle, *25*, 321
separation theorems, 472, 481
set, *441*
shadow price, *117*, 145, 170, 208, 281, 298, 308, 394, 409
shallow lake model, 270
similar matrix, *457*
single-valued function, *442*
singleton, 113, *441*
singular arc, *132*, 138, 185
singular matrix, *450*
sink, *see* attractor
SIR-model, 323
skew-symmetric matrix, *451*
Skiba point, *see* DNSS point
social value of life (SVOL), *433*
Solow growth model, 94
solution of
  IVP, *17*, *18*
  optimal control problem, *108*
source, *see* repeller
span, *446*
spiral, *see* focus
sporadically catching up optimality, *156*
square matrix, *449*
stability of an invariant set, *23*
stable manifold, 38, *44*, *82*
  computation, 347
    BVP approach, 350, 353
    IVP approach, 304, 346, 348, 352
  dimension, 343, 497
  global, 246, 264, 304
stable path, *45*, 166, 168, 250, 262, 351, 371
Stackelberg
  dominance, *405*
  equilibrium, *402*, 403, 405, 412–415, 427
  game, *402*, 411
state
  dynamics, 15, *17*, 30, 105, 109, 138, 161, 209, 395, 421
  trajectory, *106*, 116, 164, 168, 241, 242, 410
state-separable differential game, 395, 402, 404, 435
static optimization, 195–212, 323
steady state, *see* equilibrium
stochastic
  differential equation, 423
  differential game, 437
  Hamilton–Jacobi–Bellman equation, *423*
  optimal control problem, 422–423, 437
  process, 422
strictly in/decreasing function, *444*
structural stability, *26*
subgame perfectness, *405*
subset, *441*
subspace, 41, 57, *446*
sufficiency condition
  of real-valued problem, 470
sufficiency conditions, 393, 404
  Arrow type
    finite time, *121*
    infinite time, *159*
    with constraints, *154*
  Mangasarian type
    finite time, *120*
    infinite time, *159*, 297
    with constraints, *154*
  of static optimization, 205–206
supergradient, 121, *472*, 484
superposition principle, *33*, 78, 92
supremum, 128, *442*, 470
supremum norm, *463*
surjective function, *443*
susceptibles, 52, 89, 315
switching
  function, *132*, 135
  point, 179
  time, 384, 385, 387, 425, 427
symmetric matrix, *451*
system dynamics, *see* state, dynamics

tabloid press, 395, 402, 430
tangent space, *475*
Taylor theorem, 27, 48, *473*
technological progress, 179
technology model, 320, 427

terminal
  constraint, *105*, 107, *142*, 149, 177, 185
  state, *106*, 136
  time, *105*, 116, 119, 127, 179, 195
terror, 10, 324
  collateral damage, 27, 307, 407
  game, *405–415*, 427, 428, 435
  law enforcement, 406
  model, 89, *306–314*, 379
    fire-and-water, *27–30*, 90, *139–141*, 378, 387
    multi-stage, *386–389*, 426
thief–police game, 429, 435
threshold point, *253*
time consistency, *405*
tipping point, *266*, 271
tobacco dynamics, 51
Tonelli's direct optimization method, *122*
topological equivalence, *25*, 60
  local, *26*
  orbital, *25*
trace of a matrix, *449*
trajectory, *19*, 23, 50, 106
transposed matrix, *451*
transversality condition, *109*, 112, 144, 150, 210, 490
  calculus of variation, 220
  differential game, *394*
  economic interpretation of the, 119
  infinite time, 161
    differential game, *394*
  limiting, *159*, 297
  proof of the, 489–490
  violation of the, 162–163
transversality condition (bifurcation), *62*, 76
triangular matrix, *458*
turnpike property, 178, 185

uniform continuity, *464*
unit matrix, *450*
unstable manifold, 38, *82*, 304
unstable path, *45*
unstable set, *24*
unusual optimal control problems, 186
upper bound, 133, *442*
upper triangular matrix, *458*
US cocaine epidemic, *see* drug model, cocaine epidemic
utility, 14, 106, 118, 180, 183, 296, 397, 425, 437
  marginal, 119, 298

vaccination (optimal), 436
value function, 207, 232, 423, *470*
  of optimal control, 118
  of optimal control problem, *108*, 162, 164
    nondifferentiable, 249
  sensitivity, *see* envelope theorem
variation, *215*, 230, 492
  admissible, 213, *215*, 227, 491
variation of constants method, 96
variational equation, *27*, 87, 303, 346, 501
vector field, *20*, 57
  optimal, 249, 256, 371, 375
vector space, 194, 213, *445*
  basis, *447*
  normed, 188, 330, *459*
vector-valued function, *443*
vintage model, *see* age-structured model
viscosity solution, 97, 184

water strategy, 27, 139, 387
weak DNSS
  point, *253*
Weierstrass method, 417
Weierstrass–Erdmann condition, 150, *217*, 225
welfare, 180, 430, 433, 437
Wiener process, 423
Wirl's paradigm, 322
Wronski determinant, *35*, 80

Author Index

Abraham, R. H. 64, 505
Ahmad, S. 51, 527
Alemdar, N. M. 382, 505
Almeder, C. 420, 421, 438, 439, 505
Andronov, A. A. 97, 505
Andvig, J. C. 15, 98, 273, 505
Annemans, L. 51, 505
Apostol, T. M. 204, 505
Arnold, L. 425, 505
Arnold, V. I. 26, 97, 275, 505
Arquilla, J. 309, 506
Arrow, K. J. 103, 127, 155, 166, 168, 178, 184, 186, 506, 523
Arrowsmith, D. K. 20, 26, 51, 97, 506
Arutyunov, A. V. 184, 506
Ascher, U. M. 87, 97, 506
Aubin, J. P. 439, 506
Avriel, M. 234, 506

Başar, T. 392, 393, 397, 436, 506
Barclay, A. 382, 506
Barron, E. N. 184, 506
Barucci, E. 438, 506
Batta, R. 325, 506
Baveja, A. 137, 325, 506
Becker, G. S. 272, 316, 317, 324, 506
Behrens, D. A. 51–53, 55, 75, 77, 98, 171, 269, 280–282, 286, 296, 325, 437, 438, 507, 510, 516
Bell, D. J. 185, 507
Bellman, R. 108, 128, 184, 382, 507
Bensoussan, A. 103, 104, 426, 438, 439, 507
Bertsekas, D. P. 234, 382, 474, 507, 508
Beyn, W. J. 353, 357, 368, 382, 383, 508
Blaquière, A. 426, 508
Bliss, G. A. 214, 235, 508
Boltyanski, V. G. 103, 108, 184, 185, 227, 235, 508, 524
Booß-Bavnbek, B. 326, 508
Boucekkine, R. 387, 429, 436, 508
Breakwell, J. V. 132, 508
Breitner, M. 103, 436, 508
Brito, P. M. B. 326, 508
Brock, W. A. 272, 318, 325, 508
Brokate, M. 418, 438, 508
Bryson, A. E. 185, 509
Bulirsch, R. 101, 103, 382, 524, 528
Bultmann, R. 70, 185, 388, 439, 509
Bushaw, D. W. 103, 509
Büskens, C. 330, 382, 383, 509, 522
Byrd, W. 6, 509

Canon, M. D. 235, 509
Caputo, M. R. 184, 209, 509
Carathéodory, C. 103, 509
Carlson, D. A. 155, 167, 329, 509
Caroff, N. 184, 509

Carpentier, C. 51, 505
Carr, J. 43, 509
Cass, D. 103, 272, 509
Castillo-Chavez, C. 28, 509
Caulkins, J. P. 28, 51–53, 55, 68–70, 75, 77, 98, 137, 138, 169, 171, 185, 186, 269, 271, 273, 274, 280–282, 286, 296, 308, 309, 317, 319, 325, 370, 372, 380, 388, 420, 421, 428, 436, 437, 439, 505–507, 509–511, 513, 525, 527
Cellina, A. 97, 506
Cesari, L. 184, 234, 511
Chaloupka, F. 51, 521
Chander, P. 324, 511
Chen, L. L. 51, 527
Chiang, A. C. 184, 511
Chiarella, C. 98, 511
Chillingworth, D. R. J. 476, 511
Clarke, F. H. 128, 184, 209, 426, 439, 511
Courant, P. N. 51, 523
Crandall, M. G. 97, 184, 511
Cullum, C. D. 235, 509
Cullum, J. 195, 511

Dawid, H. 397, 401, 402, 437, 511, 529
de Hoog, F. R. 382, 511
de Zeeuw, A. 272, 522
Dechert, W. D. 238, 272, 318, 325, 508, 511
Deissenberg, C. 273, 511
Derzko, N. A. 421, 434, 512
Deuflhard, P. 383, 528
Devaney, R. 97, 518
Dietz, K. 417, 512
Dietze, P. 51, 185, 510
Dixit, A. K. 425, 512
Dockner, E. J. 316, 324, 345, 392, 397, 406, 407, 429, 432, 436, 437, 512
Dolcetta, I. C. 382, 512
Dorfman, R. 184, 512
Dreyfus, S. E. 101, 235, 512
Dubovickii, A. J. 235, 512
Dworak, M. 186, 273, 510

Easterlin, R. A. 95, 512
Ehrlich, I. 438, 512
Ehtamo, H. 437, 512
El Ouardighi, F. 436, 513
Engwerda, J. C. 392, 394, 397, 513
Evans, G. C. 102, 513
Everingham, S. S. 51, 52, 169, 280, 281, 286, 292, 294, 295, 325, 511, 513, 525

Falcone, M. 382, 513
Farkas, J. 455, 513
Feichtinger, G. 51–53, 55, 68–70, 75, 77, 93, 94, 98, 114, 136–138, 150, 152, 169, 171, 183–186, 258, 259, 269, 271–275, 280–282, 286, 296, 308, 309, 316, 317, 319, 321, 322, 324, 325, 345, 370, 372, 380, 388, 397, 401, 402, 404, 418–421, 423, 428, 431, 434–439, 505–507, 509–517, 520, 524, 527, 529
Feldbaum, A. A. 103, 515
Fent, T. 437, 515
Fernández, C. E. 101, 102, 515
Filar, J. A. 439, 515
Fisher, R. A. 436, 515
Fisher, W. H. 187, 515
Fleming, W. H. 101, 104, 425, 515
Fletcher, R. 204, 234, 515
Forman, P. 326, 515
Forster, B. A. 180, 515
Frankowska, H. 184, 439, 506, 509
Fraser-Andrews, G. 382, 515
Friedlander, G. 481, 515
Friedrich, C. J. 324, 515
Fromovitz, S. 204, 234, 522
Frueh, D. P. 8, 515
Fudenberg, D. 392, 515

Gage, E. 51, 527
Gaimon, C. 438, 515
Galán-Vioque, J. 332, 334, 520

Gamkrelidze, R. V. 103, 108, 184, 185, 227, 235, 508, 516, 524
Gardiner, K. L. 325, 516
Gavrila, C. 51, 138, 272, 273, 319, 370, 372, 510, 516
Gill, P. 382, 506
Girsanov, I. V. 235, 516
Gitchell, J. 51, 521
Glaser, S. J. 8, 515
Goetz, R. U. 439, 516
Goffe, W. L. 382, 516
Goldstine, H. H. 102, 516
Golub, G. 461, 516
Gordon, H. S. 92, 516
Goryunov, V. V. 275, 505
Gould, J. P. 93, 178, 269, 516
Gozzi, F. 438, 506
Gragnani, A. 98, 510
Grass, D. 308, 309, 380, 429, 436, 510, 516
Greiner, A. 51, 138, 273, 319, 370, 372, 510
Grienauer, W. 273, 513
Großlicht, F. 186, 516
Grossman, M. 438, 516
Grüne, L. 382, 516
Guckenheimer, J. 47, 55–57, 61, 73, 97, 516

Hadeler, K. P. 417, 516
Hadley, G. 103, 516
Hager, M. 438, 516
Halkin, H. 156, 162, 163, 234, 486, 492, 517
Hall, R. E. 438, 517
Hämäläinen, R. P. 437, 512
Hariga, F. 51, 505
Hartl, R. F. 93, 94, 114, 136, 137, 147, 149, 150, 152, 168, 184–186, 271–275, 321, 322, 325, 423, 429, 434, 436, 438, 506, 510, 513, 514, 516–518
Hartman, P. 18, 42, 43, 45, 50, 78, 80, 83, 84, 97, 490, 517
Hartnoll, R. 51, 505
Harwood, H. J. 324, 517
Hassard, B. D. 77, 517
Haunschmied, J. L. 51–53, 55, 75, 137, 138, 273, 280, 286, 319, 321, 322, 325, 370, 372, 506, 507, 510, 517
Haurie, A. 155, 167, 329, 436, 438, 509, 517, 518
Heal, G. M. 187, 324, 525
Hestenes, M. R. 103, 518
Hillman, A. L. 324, 518
Hirsch, G. B. 51, 325, 521
Hirsch, M. W. 32, 50, 97, 518
Ho, Y. C. 185, 436, 509, 518
Hof, F. X. 187, 274, 515, 518
Hofbauer, J. 96, 98, 518
Holling, C. S. 91, 518
Holmes, P. 47, 55–57, 61, 73, 97, 516
Homer, J. B. 51, 325, 518
Hommes, C. H. 96, 518
Hopf, E. 97, 518
Hotelling, H. 102, 518
Høyrup, J. 326, 508, 518
Huisman, K. J.M. 425, 518
Hurst Jr., E. G. 103, 104, 507
Hüsseinov, F. 382, 505

Intriligator, M. D. 103, 127, 518
Ioffe, A. D. 234, 519
Isaacs, R. 103, 436, 519
Ito, T. 8, 515

Jacobson, D. H. 185, 507
James, C. 280, 511
Jensen, R. 184, 506
John, F. 204, 519
Johnson, M. 271, 510
Jones, C. I. 438, 517
Jørgensen, S. 392, 397, 406, 407, 429, 432, 436, 437, 512, 519
Jorgenson, D. W. 182, 519
Joshi, M. 481, 515
Jost, J. 471, 519

Kalish, S. 180, 519
Kamien, M. I. 136, 183, 437, 519
Kandel, D. B. 51, 519
Kaplan, E. H. 326, 519
Karatzas, I. 425, 519
Karlin, S. 186, 506
Karwan, M. H. 325, 506
Kaskosz, B. 439, 519
Katz, E. 324, 518
Kaya, C. Y. 382, 383, 519, 520, 522
Kazarinoff, N. D. 77, 517
Kelley, A. 43, 520
Kelley, H. J. 185, 520
Kemp, M. C. 103, 516
Keohane, N. O. 27, 28, 326, 409, 520
Keyfitz, B. L. 417, 434, 520
Keyfitz, N. 417, 434, 436, 520
Khaneja, N. 8, 515
Kierzenka, J. 334, 520
Kim, J. H.R. 382, 383, 522
Kiseleva, T. 264, 269, 520
Kistner, K. P. 274, 514
Kleiman, M. A. R. 14, 137, 273, 520
Knoll, C. 51, 510
Kolmanovskii, V. B. 422, 520
Koopmans, T. C. 272, 520
Kopp, R. E. 185, 520
Kort, P. M. 51, 137, 138, 182, 272–275, 319, 321, 322, 325, 370, 372, 429, 436, 438, 506, 510, 513, 514, 516, 517, 528
Kraft, D. 382, 520
Krauskopf, B. 332, 334, 520
Krugman, P. 272, 520
Kuhn, M. 435, 436, 439, 520, 529
Kunkel, P. 382, 520
Kurz, M. 103, 127, 155, 166, 168, 184, 238, 273, 506, 520
Kurzhanski, A. B. 104, 521
Kuznetsov, Y. A. 47, 55–57, 62, 63, 72, 73, 97, 264, 270, 332, 334, 344, 347, 382, 521

Lambertini, L. 89, 90, 528
Lawden, D. F. 185, 521
Ledyaev, Yu.S. 209, 426, 511
Lehner, M. 428, 521
Leitmann, G. 89, 90, 436, 521, 528
Leizarowitz, A. 155, 167, 329, 509
Lempio, F. 439, 521
Léonard, D. 96, 97, 145, 184, 196, 234, 521
Lesourne, J. 391
Levin, G. 51, 325, 521
Levy, D. T. 51, 521
Lewis, R. M. 133, 521
Li, J. S. 8, 515
Lions, J. L. 426, 439, 507
Lions, P. L. 97, 184, 511
Liski, M. 272, 521
Liviatan, N. 273, 521
Loewen, P. D. 426, 521
Lojasiewicz, S. 439, 519
Long, N. V. 96, 97, 184, 196, 234, 392, 397, 406, 407, 429, 432, 436, 437, 512, 521
Long, N. Van 184, 521
Lorenz, E. N. 96, 521
Lorenz, H. W. 96, 521
Lu, Q. 351, 529
Lucas, R. E. 272, 521
Lucas, S. K. 382, 519
Ludwig, T. 182, 521
Luenberger, D. G. 382, 522
Luhmer, A. 274, 514
Lyashko, O. V. 275, 505

MacArthur, R. H. 91, 525
MacCoun, R. 325, 522
MacDonald, N. 422, 522
Magill, M. J.P. 102, 522
Majumdar, M. 187, 522
Makris, M. 387, 436, 522
Malanowski, K. 184, 522
Mäler, K. G. 272, 522
Malliaris, A. G. 272, 508
Mangasarian, O. L. 204, 234, 522
Marsden, J. 43, 522
Mattheij, R. M. M. 87, 97, 506

Maurer, H. 184, 330, 382, 383, 509, 522
Mautner, K. 186, 522
Mayne, D. Q. 104, 522
McCracken, M. 43, 522
McIntyre, J. 229, 522
McKendrick, A. G. 417, 522
McKenzie, L. W. 185, 523
McShane, E. J. 103, 523
Mehlmann, A. 186, 428, 436, 514, 523
Mei, S. 351, 529
Mendez, D. 51, 521, 523
Meran, G. 428, 521
Mercenier, J. 382, 523
Michel, P. 486, 523
Michel, V. 134, 523
Miele, A. 134, 185, 523
Miljutin, Y. A. 235, 512
Miller, B. 426, 523
Mino, K. 437, 528
Mintz, A. 326, 519
Mishal, S. 326, 519
Mishchenko, E. F. 103, 108, 184, 185, 227, 235, 524
Mitra, T. 187, 522
Möller, J. 428, 521
Moore, M. H. 137, 523
Moore, R. 51, 527
Morawetz, J. 186, 523
Moyer, H. G. 185, 520
Moyzisch, F. 185, 523
Müller, J. 438, 523
Murphy, K. M. 272, 316, 324, 506
Musto, D. F. 53, 68, 318, 523
Muzicant, J. 421, 523
Myers, T. G. 324, 517

Näslund, B. 103, 104, 507, 523
Neck, R. 438, 507, 516
Nedic, A. 474, 507
Nerlove, M. 178, 523
Neustadt, L. W. 101, 234, 517, 524
Nishimura, K. 187, 238, 272, 511, 522, 524
Nissen, G. 438, 507
Noakes, J. L. 382, 519, 520
Novak, A. J. 325, 397, 401, 402, 404, 437, 438, 511, 513, 514, 529

Oberle, H. J. 223, 235, 382, 522, 524
Oeppen, J. 436, 529
Office of National Drug Control Policy 286, 524
Olsder, G. J. 392, 393, 397, 436, 506
Orphanides, A. 272, 524
Osgood, N. D. 51, 527
Osinga, H. M. 332, 334, 520
Ozdaglar, A. E. 234, 474, 507, 508
Ozdenoren, E. 8, 524

Paiewonsky, B. 229, 522
Pampel, T. 274, 353, 357, 368, 382, 383, 508, 524
Penot, J.-P. 234, 524
Pesch, H. J. 101, 103, 524
Peter, C. 280, 511
Petrosyan, L. A. 436, 529
Philippe, M. 382, 523
Pickenhain, S. 184, 522
Pindyck, R. S. 425, 512
Place, C. M. 20, 26, 51, 97, 506
Polak, E. 235, 509
Pollack, H. A. 319, 524
Pontryagin, L. S. 103, 108, 184, 185, 227, 235, 508, 524
Prskawetz, A. 435, 438, 439, 514, 520
Pytlak, R. 382, 524

Ramsey, F. P. 102, 124, 524
Ravn, H. F. 212, 524
Reuter, P. 325, 522
Rinaldi, S. 98, 524
Rishel, R. W. 425, 515
Ritter, A. 51, 185, 510
Robbins, H. 133, 524
Roberts, E. B. 51, 325, 521
Rockafellar, R. 474, 525
Romer, P. 272, 525
Ronfeldt, D. 309, 506

Rose-Ackerman, S. 324, 525
Rosen, J. 382, 506
Rosen, S. 435, 525
Rosenzweig, M. L. 91, 525
Rossana, R. J. 387, 436, 527
Rossi, C. 51, 325, 525
Rubinovich, E. 426, 523
Rudel, S. 185, 525
Russell, R. D. 87, 97, 506
Rydell, C. P. 51, 52, 169, 280, 281, 286, 292, 294, 295, 325, 511, 513, 525
Ryder, H. E. 187, 324, 525

Sagan, H. 214, 235, 525
Saglam, H. C. 387, 429, 436, 508, 525
Salant, S. 8, 524
Samban, C. 326, 519
Samuelson, P. A. 273, 521
Sánchez-Rón, J. M. 326, 515
Sanderson, W. C. 438, 505
Scarf, H. E. 186, 506
Schelling, T. 271, 272, 325, 522, 525
Schreckengost, R. C. 325, 516
Schwartz, L. 481, 525
Schwartz, N. L. 136, 183, 437, 519
Seidl, A. 318, 525
Seierstad, A. 120, 124, 145, 149, 159, 184, 230, 525, 526
Semmler, W. 273, 353, 357, 368, 382, 383, 508, 511
Sethi, S. P. 104, 147, 149, 150, 152, 183, 185, 186, 238, 272, 421, 423, 425, 426, 431, 434, 438, 512, 514, 517, 518, 526
Seydel, R. 97, 526
Shaikhet, L. E. 422, 520
Shampine, L. F. 334, 520
Shaw, C. D. 64, 505
Shawn, B. 280, 511
Shell, K. 103, 526
Shimomura, K. 184, 521
Shleifer, A. 324, 526
Shreve, S. E. 425, 519
Shub, M. 38, 526
Shvartsman, I. A. 184, 526
Sigmund, K. 96, 98, 518
Silverman, D. 8, 524
Simakov, S. T. 382, 519
Sirakaya, S. 382, 505
Skiba, A. K. 238, 270–272, 526
Smale, S. 32, 50, 97, 518
Smith, D. R. 214, 526
Solow, R. 94, 438, 527
Song, B. 28, 509
Sorger, G. 187, 274, 392, 397, 406, 407, 429, 432, 436, 437, 512, 514, 524
Sparrow, C. 96, 527
Starrett, D. 272, 508
Steindl, A. 97, 273, 514, 527
Stern, L. E. 155, 527
Stern, R. J. 209, 426, 511
Strogatz, S. H. 77, 96, 97, 527
Sussmann, H. J. 102, 235, 527
Swan, G. W. 8, 527
Swaton, N. 185, 527
Sydsaeter, K. 120, 124, 145, 149, 159, 184, 230, 525, 526

Tapiero, C. S. 438, 507
Tecco, J. 51, 505
Tengs, T. O. 51, 527
Teo, K. 351, 529
Thompson, G. L. 104, 183, 185, 186, 421, 425, 426, 434, 438, 512, 515, 526, 527
Tichomirov, V. M. 234, 519
Tirole, J. 392, 515
Tomiyama, K. 387, 436, 527
Tonelli, L. 122, 527
Tragler, G. 51–53, 55, 68–70, 75, 77, 98, 138, 169, 171, 185, 186, 269, 271–274, 280–282, 286, 296, 308, 309, 317, 319, 325, 370, 372, 380, 388, 418–421, 428, 436–439, 505, 507, 509, 510, 513–516, 527
Troger, H. 97, 527
Tsachev, T. 438, 514
Tseng, P. 234, 508

Tsutsui, S. 437, 528
Tu, P. N. V. 184, 528

Udwadia, F. 89, 90, 528
Ushiki, S. 351, 528

Valentine, F. A. 103, 528
Vallée, T. 387, 429, 436, 508
van Hilten, O. 182, 528
van Loan, C. 461, 516
van Loon, P. J.J.M. 182, 528
Vanoverbeke, N. 51, 505
Vasiliev, V. A. 275, 505
Veliov, V. M. 325, 418, 419, 438, 439, 505, 510, 513, 514, 521
Verheyen, P. A. 152, 185, 528
Verhulst, P. F. 98, 528
Vickson, R. G. 147, 149, 150, 152, 185, 517
Vinter, R. B. 108, 122, 124, 184, 506, 528
Vishny, R. W. 324, 526
von dem Hagen, O. 382, 520
von Stryk, O. 382, 528
Vrieze, K. 439, 515

Wagener, F. O. O. 168, 239, 264, 269, 274, 275, 520, 528
Wagner, G. 8, 515
Wallner, D. 171, 185, 317, 325, 388, 428, 436, 510, 528
Wan, Y. H. 77, 517
Ward, C. 6, 509
Warner, K. E. 51, 521, 523
Webb, G. F. 417, 528
Weiser, M. 383, 528
Weiss, R. 382, 511
Wiggins, S. 97, 528
Wilde, L. 324, 511
Willems, J. C. 102, 104, 235, 527, 528
Wirl, F. 98, 258, 259, 273–275, 296, 324, 397, 401, 402, 511, 514, 515, 517, 518, 524, 528, 529
Wolenski, P. R. 209, 426, 511
Wrzaczek, S. 435, 436, 439, 520, 529

Xepapadeas, A. 272, 522
Xue, A. 351, 529

Yaari, M. E. 438, 529
Yegorov, Y. 271, 510
Yeung, D. W. K. 436, 529
Yong, J. 439, 529

Zaccour, G. 392, 397, 436, 519
Zalesak, M. 437, 515
Zeckhauser, R. J. 27, 28, 326, 409, 520
Zeidan, V. 184, 529
Zeiler, I. 171, 185, 325, 529
Zervos, V. 272, 524
Zezza, P. 184, 529
Zhang, Q. 425, 526
Zhou, X. Y. 439, 529
Zilberman, D. 439, 516
Zuazua, E. 101, 102, 515
Zuba, D. 51, 510

MIX
Papier aus verantwortungsvollen Quellen
Paper from responsible sources
FSC® C105338
FSC
www.fsc.org

If you have any concerns about our products,
you can contact us on
ProductSafety@springernature.com

In case Publisher is established outside the EU,
the EU authorized representative is:
Springer Nature Customer Service Center GmbH
Europaplatz 3, 69115 Heidelberg, Germany

Printed by Libri Plureos GmbH
in Hamburg, Germany